QUICK LOOK DRUG BOOK

2005

Leonard L. Lance, RPh, Pharm
Senior Editor
Pharmacist
Lexi-Comp, Inc.
Hudson, Ohio

Charles F. Lacy, Pharm FCSHP
Editor
Vice President, Information Te ologies
Director, Drug Information vices
Professor, Pharmacy Pra ce
Nevada College of Phar cy
Las Vegas, Nevad

Morton P. Goldman, Pha nD, BCPS
Associate Edito
Assistant Director, Pharmacot apy Services
Department of Phar acy
Cleveland Clinic Fou dation
Cleveland, Oh

Lora L. Armstrong, RPh, PharmD, BCPS
Associate Ed or
Director, Pharmacy & erapeutics
Formulary Pro ess
Caremark, Ic.
Northbrook, Ilinois

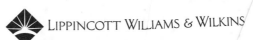

LIPPINCOTT WILLIAMS & WILKINS

Philadelphia • Baltimore • New York • London
Buenos Aires • Hong Kong • Sydney • Tokyo

QICK LOOK
DUG BOOK

2005

Leonard L. Lance, RPh, BSPharm
Senior Editor
Pharmacist
Lexi-Comp, Inc.
Hudson, Ohio

Charles F. Lacy, PharmD, FCSHP
Editor
Vice President, Information Technologies
Director, Drug Information Services
Professor, Pharmacy Practice
Nevada College of Pharmacy
Las Vegas, Nevada

Morton P. Goldman, PharmD, BCPS
Associate Editor
Assistant Director, Pharmacotherapy Services
Department of Pharmacy
Cleveland Clinic Foundation
Cleveland, Ohio

Lora L. Armstrong, RPh, PharmD, BCPS
Associate Editor
Director, Pharmacy & Therapeutics
Formulary Process
Caremark, Inc.
Northbrook, Illinois

NOTICE

This handbook is intended to serve the user as a handy quick reference and not as a complete drug information resource. It does not include information on every therapeutic agent available. The publication covers 1566 commonly used drugs and is specifically designed to present certain important aspects of drug data in a more concise format than is generally found in medical literature or product material supplied by manufacturers.

Although great care was taken to ensure the accuracy of the handbook's content when it went to press, the editors, contributors, and publisher cannot be responsible for the continued accuracy of the supplied information due to ongoing research and new developments in the field. Further, the *Quick Look Drug Book* is not offered as a guide to dosing. The reader, herewith, is advised that information shown under the heading **Usual Dosage** is provided only as an indication of the amount of the drug typically given or taken during therapy. Actual dosing amount for any specific drug should be based on an in-depth evaluation of the individual patient's therapy requirement and strong consideration given to such issues as contraindications, warnings, precautions, adverse reactions, along with the interaction of other drugs. The manufacturers' most current product information or other standard recognized references should always be consulted for such detailed information prior to drug use.

The editors and contributors have written this book in their private capacities. No official support or endorsement by any federal agency or pharmaceutical company is intended or inferred.

This manual was produced using the FormuLex™ Program —
a complete publishing service of Lexi-Comp Inc.

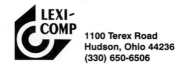

1100 Terex Road
Hudson, Ohio 44236
(330) 650-6506

TABLE OF CONTENTS

ABOUT THE AUTHORS

Leonard L. Lance, RPh, BSPharm

Leonard L. (Bud) Lance has been directly involved in the pharmaceutical industry since receiving his bachelor's degree in pharmacy from Ohio Northern University in 1970. Upon graduation from ONU, Mr Lance spent four years as a navy pharmacist in various military assignments and was instrumental in the development and operation of the first whole hospital I.V. admixture program in a military (Portsmouth Naval Hospital) facility.

After completing his military service, he entered the retail pharmacy field and has managed both an independent and a home I.V. franchise pharmacy operation. Since the late 1970s, Mr Lance has focused much of his interest on using computers to improve pharmacy service. The independent pharmacy he worked for was one of the first retail pharmacy in the State of Ohio to computerize (1977).

His love for computers and pharmacy led him to Lexi-Comp, Inc. in 1988. He developed Lexi-Comp's first drug database in 1989 and was involved in the editing and publishing of Lexi-Comp's first *Drug Information Handbook* in 1990.

As a result of his strong publishing interest, he presently serves in the capacity of pharmacy editor and technical advisor as well as pharmacy (information) database coordinator for Lexi-Comp. Along with the *Quick Look Drug Book*, he provides technical support to Lexi-Comp's *Drug Information Handbook for the Allied Health Professional* and Lexi-Comp's reference publications. Mr Lance also assists approximately 200 major hospitals in producing their own formulary (pharmacy) publications through Lexi-Comp's custom publishing service.

Mr Lance is a member and past president (1984) of the Summit Pharmaceutical Association (SPA). He is also a member of the Ohio Pharmacists Association (OPA), the American Pharmaceutical Association (APhA), and the American Society of Health-System Pharmacists (ASHP).

Charles F. Lacy, PharmD, FCSHP

Dr Lacy is the Vice President for Information Technologies and Professor of Pharmacy Practice at the Nevada College of Pharmacy. In his capacity at the college, Dr Lacy oversees the Library and Learning Resources Center, the Computer Information Systems, and the Drug Information Service. This college-based service provides drug use policy services in addition to traditional drug information resources to the college's affiliated institutions. Prior to his promotion, Dr Lacy was the Facilitative Officer for Clinical Programs where he managed the clinical curriculum, clinical faculty activities, student experiential programs, pharmacy residency programs, and the college's continuing education programs. Currently, Dr Lacy is also the Chairman of the Eureka Development Foundation, a philanthropic group supporting the students at the college and plans and develops new programs for the college.

Prior to coming to the Nevada College of Pharmacy, Dr Lacy was the Clinical Coordinator for the Department of Pharmacy at Cedars-Sinai Medical Center. With over 19 years of clinical experience at one of the nation's largest teaching hospitals, he has developed a reputation as an acknowledged expert in drug information and critical care drug therapy.

Dr Lacy received his doctorate from the University of Southern California School of Pharmacy. Presently, Dr Lacy holds teaching affiliations with the Nevada College of Pharmacy, the University of Southern California School of Pharmacy, the University of California at San Francisco [illegible]chool of Pharmacy, the University of the Pacific School of Pharmacy, Western University of [illegible]alth Sciences School of Pharmacy, and the University of Alberta at Edmonton, School of [illegible]rmacy and Health Sciences.

[illegible]cy is an active member of numerous professional associations including the American [illegible] of Health-System Pharmacists (ASHP), the American College of Clinical Pharmacy [illegible] the American Society of Consultant Pharmacists (ASCP), the American Association of [illegible] of Pharmacy (AACP), American Pharmacists Association (APhA), the Nevada Phar[illegible]nce (NPA), and the California Society of Hospital Pharmacists (CSHP), through which [illegible]red many committees and subcommittees.

Morton P. Goldman, PharmD, BCPS

Dr Goldman received his bachelor's degree in pharmacy from the University of Pittsburgh, College of Pharmacy and his Doctor of Pharmacy degree from the University of Cincinnati, Division of Graduate Studies and Research. He completed his concurrent 2-year hospital pharmacy residency at the V.A. Medical Center in Cincinnati. Dr Goldman is presently the Assistant Director of Pharmacotherapy Services for the Department of Pharmacy at the Cleveland Clinic Foundation (CCF) after having spent over 4 years at CCF as an Infectious Disease pharmacist and 4 years as Clinical Manager. He holds faculty appointments from The University of Toledo, College of Pharmacy and Case Western Reserve University, College of Medicine and is the Pharmacology Curriculum Coordinator for the new Cleveland Clinic Lerner College of Medicine. Dr Goldman is a Board-Certified Pharmacotherapy Specialist (BCPS) with added qualifications in infectious diseases.

In his capacity as Assistant Director of Pharmacotherapy Services at CCF, Dr Goldman remains actively involved in patient care and clinical research with the Department of Infectious Disease, as well as the continuing education of the medical and pharmacy staff. He is an editor of CCF's *Guidelines for Antibiotic Use* and participates in their annual Antimicrobial Review retreat. He is a member of the Pharmacy and Therapeutics Committee and many of its subcommittees. Dr Goldman has authored numerous journal articles and lectures locally and nationally on infectious diseases topics and current drug therapies. He is currently a reviewer for the *Annals of Pharmacotherapy* and the *Journal of the American Medical Association*, an editorial board member of the *Journal of Infectious Disease Pharmacotherapy*, and coauthor of the *Infectious Diseases Handbook*, the *Drug Information Handbook*, and the *Drug Information Handbook for the Allied Health Professional* produced by Lexi-Comp, Inc. He also provides technical support to Lexi-Comp's Clinical Reference Library™ publications.

Dr Goldman is an active member of the Ohio College of Clinical Pharmacy, the Society of Infectious Disease Pharmacists, the American College of Clinical Pharmacy (and is a Fellow of the College), and the American Society of Health-Systems Pharmacists.

Lora L. Armstrong, PharmD, BCPS

Dr Armstrong received her bachelor's degree in pharmacy from Ferris State University and her Doctor of Pharmacy degree from Midwestern University. Dr Armstrong is a Board-Certified Pharmacotherapy Specialist (BCPS).

In her current position, Dr Armstrong serves as the Director of the Pharmacy & Therapeutics Committee process at Caremark, Inc, Prescription Services Division. Caremark is a prescription benefit management company (PBM). Dr Armstrong is responsible for coordination of the Caremark National Pharmacy & Therapeutics Committee and the Caremark Pharmacy & Therapeutics Subcommittee. Dr Armstrong is also responsible for monitoring the pharmaceutical product pipeline, monitoring drug surveillance, and communicating Pharmacy & Therapeutics Committee Formulary information to Caremark's internal and external customers.

Prior to joining Caremark, Inc, Dr Armstrong served as the Director of Drug Information Services at the University of Chicago Hospitals. She obtained 17 years of experience in a variety of clinical settings including critical care, hematology, oncology, infectious diseases, and clinical pharmacokinetics. Dr Armstrong played an active role in the education and training of medical, pharmacy, and nursing staff. She coordinated the Drug Information Center, the medical cente[illegible] Adverse Drug Reaction Monitoring Program, and the continuing Education Program for ph[illegible] cists. She also maintained the hospital's strict formulary program and was the edit[illegible] University of Chicago Hospitals' *Formulary of Accepted Drugs* and the drug informati[illegible] monthly newsletter *Topics in Drug Therapy*.

Dr Armstrong is an active member of the Academy of Managed Care Phar[illegible] American Society of Health-Systems Pharmacists (ASHP), the American Ph[illegible] ation (APhA), the American College of Clinical Pharmacy (ACCP), and th[illegible] peutics Society (P & T Society). Dr Armstrong wrote the chapter entitled [illegible] Used in Endocrinology" in the 4th edition of the textbook *Endocrinol*[illegible] Clinical Instructor of Pharmacy Practice at Midwestern University. Dr Ar[illegible] on the Drug Information Advisory Board for pharmacist.com and on the [illegible] Association Scientific Review Panel for Evaluations of Drug Interactio[illegible]

EDITORIAL ADVISORY PANEL

PREFACE

Working with clinical pharmacists, hospital pharmacy and therapeutics committees, and hospital drug information centers, the editors of this handbook have directly assisted in the development and production of hospital-specific formulary documentation for several hundred major medical institutions in the United States and Canada. The resultant documentation provides pertinent detail concerning use of medications within the hospital and other clinical settings. The most current information on medications has been extracted, reviewed, coalesced, and cross-referenced by the editors to create this *Quick Look Drug Book*.

Thus, this handbook gives the user quick access to data on 1566 medications with cross-referencing to 4902 U.S. and Canadian brand or trade names. Selection of the included medications was based on the analysis of those medications offered in a wide range of hospital formularies. The concise standardized format for data used in this handbook was developed to ensure a consistent presentation of information for all medications.

All generic drug names and synonyms appear in lower case, whereas brand or trade names appear in upper/lower case with the proper trademark information. These three items appear as individual entries in the alphabetical listing of drugs and, thus, there is no requirement for an alphabetical index of drugs.

Mailing and WEB site addresses for Pharmaceutical Manufacturers' and Drug Distributors are provided in the appendix section of this book.

The Indication/Therapeutic Category Index is an expedient mechanism for locating the medication of choice along with its classification. This index will help the user, with knowledge of the disease state, to identify medications which are most commonly used in treatment. All disease states are cross-referenced to a varying number of medications with the most frequently used medication(s) noted.

— L.L. Lance

ACKNOWLEDGMENTS

The *Quick Look Drug Book* exists in its present form as the result of the concerted efforts of the following individuals: Robert D. Kerscher, publisher and president of Lexi-Comp, Inc; Mark Bonfiglio, PharmD, director of pharmacotherapy resources; Stacy S. Robinson, editorial manager; Barbara F. Kerscher, production manager; Cynthia Forney, drug identification database manager; Daniel L. Krinsky, director, pharmacotherapy sales and marketing; Ginger S. Stein, project manager; and David C. Marcus, director of information systems.

Special acknowledgment goes to all Lexi-Comp staff for their contributions to this handbook.

USE OF THE HANDBOOK

The *Quick Look Drug Book* is organized into a drug information section, an appendix, and an indication/therapeutic category index.

The drug information section of the handbook, wherein all drugs are listed alphabetically, details information pertinent to each drug. Extensive cross-referencing is provided by brand name and synonyms.

Drug information is presented in a consistent format and for quick reference will provide the following:

Generic Name	U.S. Adopted Name (USAN) or International Nonproprietary Name (INN) If a drug product is only available in Canada, a ***(Canada only)*** will be attached to that product and will appear with every occurrence of that drug throughout the book
Pronunciation Guide	Subjective aid for pronouncing drug names
Sound-Alike/Look-Alike Issues	Lists drugs with similar sounding names or names that look alike
Synonyms	Official names and some slang
Tall-Man	"Tall-Man" lettering revisions recommended by the FDA
U.S./Canadian Brand Names	Common trade names used in the United States and Canada
Therapeutic Category	Lexi-Comp's own system of logical medication classification
Controlled Substance	Drug Enforcement Agency (DEA) classification for federally scheduled controlled substances
Use	Information pertaining to appropriate use of the drug
Usual Dosage	The amount of the drug to be typically given or taken during therapy
Dosage Forms	Information with regard to form, strength and availability of the drug

Appendix

The appendix offers a compilation of tables, guidelines, and conversion information that can often be helpful when considering patient care.

Indication/Therapeutic Category Index

This index provides a listing of accepted drugs for various disease states thus focus-ng attention on selection of medications most frequently prescribed in relation to a nical diagnosis. Diseases may have other nonofficial drugs for their treatment and indication/therapeutic category index should not be used by itself to determine the opriateness of a particular therapy. The listed indications may encompass vary-egrees of severity and, since certain medications may not be appropriate for a degree of severity, it should not be assumed that the agents listed for specific ons are interchangeable. Also included as a valuable reference is each medi-therapeutic category.

TALL-MAN LETTERS

Confusion between similar drug names is an important cause of medication errors. For years, The Institute for Safe Medication Practices (ISMP), has urged generic manufacturers use a combination of large and small letters as well as bolding (ie, chlorpro**MAZINE** and chlorpro**PAMIDE**) to help distinguish drugs with look-alike names, especially when they share similar strengths. Recently the FDA's Division of Generic Drugs began to issue recommendation letters to manufacturers suggesting this novel way to label their products to help reduce this drug name confusion. Although this project has had marginal success, the method has successfully eliminated problems with products such as diphenhydr**AMINE** and dimenhy**DRINATE**. Hospitals should also follow suit by making similar changes in their own labels, preprinted order forms, computer screens and printouts, and drug storage location labels.

In order for all involved to become more familiar with the FDA's recent suggestion, in this edition of the *Quick Look Drug Book* the "Tall-Man" lettering revisions will be listed in a field called **Tall-Man**.

The following is a list of product names and recommended FDA revisions.

Drug Product	Recommended Revision
acetazolamide	aceta**ZOLAMIDE**
acetohexamide	aceto**HEXAMIDE**
bupropion	bu**PROP**ion
buspirone	bus**PIR**one
chlorpromazine	chlorpro**MAZINE**
chlorpropamide	chlorpro**PAMIDE**
clomiphene	clomi**PHENE**
clomipramine	clomi**PRAMINE**
cycloserine	cyclo**SERINE**
cyclosporine	cyclo**SPORINE**
daunorubicin	**DAUNO**rubicin
dimenhydrinate	dimenhy**DRINATE**
diphenhydramine	diphenhydr**AMINE**
dobutamine	**DOBUT**amine
dopamine	**DOP**amine
doxorubicin	**DOXO**rubicin
glipizide	glipi**ZIDE**
glyburide	gly**BURIDE**
hydralazine	hydr**ALAZINE**
hydroxyzine	hydr**OXY**zine
medroxyprogesterone	medroxy**PROGESTER**one
methylprednisolone	methyl**PREDNIS**olone
methyltestosterone	methyl**TESTOSTER**one

nicardipine	ni**CAR**dipine
nifedipine	**NIFE**dipine
prednisolone	predniso**LONE**
prednisone	predni**SONE**
sulfadiazine	sulfa**DIAZINE**
sulfisoxazole	sulfi**SOXAZOLE**
tolazamide	**TOLAZ**amide
tolbutamide	**TOLBUT**amide
vinblastine	vin**BLAS**tine
vincristine	vin**CRIS**tine

Institute for Safe Medication Practices. "New Tall-Man Lettering Will Reduce Mix-Ups Due to Generic Drug Name Confusion," *ISMP Medication Safety Alert*, September 19, 2001. Available at: http://www.ismp.org.

Institute for Safe Medication Practices. "Prescription Mapping, Can Improve Efficiency While Minimizing Errors With Look-Alike Products," *ISMP Medication Safety Alert*, October 6, 1999. Available at: http://www.ismp.org.

U.S. Pharmacopeia, "USP Quality Review: Use Caution-Avoid Confusion," March 2001, No. 76. Available at: http://www.usp.org.

SAFE WRITING

Health professionals and their support personnel frequently produce handwritten copies of information they see in print; therefore, such information is subjected to even greater possibilities for error or misinterpretation on the part of others. Thus, particular care must be given to how drug names and strengths are expressed when creating written health care documents.

The following are a few examples of safe writing rules suggested by the Institute for Safe Medication Practices, Inc.*

1. There should be a space between a number and its units as it is easier to read. There should be no periods after the abbreviations mg or mL.

Correct	Incorrect
10 mg	10mg
100 mg	100mg

2. Never place a decimal and a zero after a whole number (2 mg is correct and 2.0 mg is incorrect). If the decimal point is not seen because it falls on a line or because individuals are working from copies where the decimal point is not seen, this causes a tenfold overdose.
3. Just the opposite is true for numbers less than one. Always place a zero before a naked decimal (0.5 mL is correct, .5 mL is **in**correct).
4. Never abbreviate the word "unit." The handwritten U or u, looks like a 0 (zero), and may cause a tenfold overdose error to be made.
5. IU is not a safe abbreviation for international units. The handwritten IU looks like IV. Write out international units or use int. units.
6. Q.D. is not a safe abbreviation for once daily, as when the Q is followed by a sloppy dot, it looks like QID which means four times daily.
7. O.D. is not a safe abbreviation for once daily, as it is properly interpreted as meaning "right eye" and has caused liquid medications such as saturated solution of potassium iodide and Lugol's solution to be administered incorrectly. There is no safe abbreviation for once daily. It must be written out in full.
8. Do not use chemical names such as 6-mercaptopurine or 6-thioguanine, as 6-fold overdoses have been given when these were not recognized as chemical names. The proper names of these drugs are mercaptopurine or thioguanine.
9. Do not abbreviate drug names (5FC, 6MP, 5-ASA, MTX, HCTZ CPZ, PF etc) as they are misinterpreted and cause error.
10. Do not use the apothecary system or symbols.
11. Do not abbreviate microgram as μg; instead use mcg as likelihood of misinterpretation.

*From "Safe Writing" by Davis NM, PharmD and Cohen MR, MS tants for Safe Medication Practices, 1143 Wright Drive, Hunti Phone: (215) 947-7566.

12. When writing an outpatient prescription, write a complete prescription. A complete prescription can prevent the prescriber, the pharmacist, and/or the patient from making a mistake and can eliminate the need for further clarification. The legible prescriptions should contain:
    a. patient's full name
    b. for pediatric or geriatric patients: their age (or weight where applicable)
    c. drug name, dosage form and strength; if a drug is new or rarely prescribed, print this information
    d. number or amount to be dispensed
    e. complete instructions for the patient, including the purpose of the medication
    f. when there are recognized contraindications for a prescribed drug, indicate to the pharmacist that you are aware of this fact (ie, when prescribing a potassium salt for a patient receiving an ACE inhibitor, write "K serum leveling being monitored")

ALPHABETICAL LISTING OF DRUGS

1370-999-397 *see* anagrelide *on page 58*

A_1-PI *see* alpha$_1$-proteinase inhibitor *on page 34*

A200® Lice [US-OTC] *see* permethrin *on page 683*

A-200® Maximum Strength [US-OTC] *see* pyrethrins and piperonyl butoxide *on page 751*

A and D® Ointment [US-OTC] *see* vitamin A and vitamin D *on page 915*

abacavir (a BAK a veer)

Synonyms abacavir sulfate; ABC

U.S./Canadian Brand Names Ziagen® [US/Can]

Therapeutic Category Nucleoside Reverse Transcriptase Inhibitor (NRTI)

Use Treatment of HIV infections in combination with other antiretroviral agents

Usual Dosage Oral:

Children: 3 months to 16 years: 8 mg/kg body weight twice daily (maximum 300 mg twice daily) in combination with other antiretroviral agents

Adults: 300 mg twice daily or 600 mg once daily in combination with other antiretroviral agents

Dosage Forms

Solution, oral: 20 mg/mL (240 mL) [strawberry-banana flavor]

Tablet: 300 mg

abacavir and lamivudine (a BAK a veer & la MI vyoo deen)

Synonyms abacavir sulfate and lamivudine; lamivudine and abacavir

U.S./Canadian Brand Names Epzicom™ [US]

Therapeutic Category Antiretroviral Agent, Reverse Transcriptase Inhibitor (Nucleoside)

Use Treatment of HIV infections in combination with other antiretroviral agents

Usual Dosage Oral: Adults: HIV: One tablet (abacavir 600 mg and lamivudine 300 mg) once daily

Dosage Forms Tablet, film-coated: Abacavir 600 mg and lamivudine 300 mg

abacavir, lamivudine, and zidovudine

(a BAK a veer, la MI vyoo deen, & zye DOE vyoo deen)

Synonyms azidothymidine, abacavir, and lamivudine; AZT, abacavir, and lamivudine; compound S, abacavir, and lamivudine; lamivudine, abacavir, and zidovudine; 3TC, abacavir, and zidovudine; ZDV, abacavir, and lamivudine; zidovudine, abacavir, and lamivudine

U.S./Canadian Brand Names Trizivir® [US]

Therapeutic Category Antiretroviral Agent, Nucleoside Reverse Transcriptase Inhibitor (NRTI)

Use Treatment of HIV infection (either alone or in combination with other antiretroviral agents) in patients whose regimen would otherwise contain the components of Trizivir®

Usual Dosage Oral: Adolescents and Adults: 1 tablet twice daily; **Note:** Not recommended for patients <40 kg

Dosage Forms Tablet [film coated]: Abacavir 300 mg, lamivudine 150 mg, and zidovudine 300 mg

bacavir sulfate *see* abacavir *on this page*

acavir sulfate and lamivudine *see* abacavir and lamivudine *on this page*

relix (a ba REL iks)

nyms PPI-149; R-3827

Canadian Brand Names Plenaxis™ [US]

eutic Category Gonadotropin Releasing Hormone Antagonist

liative treatment of advanced symptomatic prostate cancer; treatment is limited to o are not candidates for LHRH therapy, refuse surgical castration, and have one or more of the following complications due to metastases or local encroachment: 1) risk of neurological compromise, 2) ureteral or bladder outlet obstruction, or 3) severe bone pain (persisting despite narcotic analgesia)

Usual Dosage I.M.: Male prostate cancer: 100 mg administered on days 1, 15, 29 (week 4), then every 4 weeks

Dosage Forms Injection, powder for reconstitution [preservative free]: 113 mg [provides 100 mg/2 mL depot suspension when reconstituted; packaged with diluent and syringe]

Abbokinase® [US] *see* urokinase *on page 899*

abbott-43818 *see* leuprolide acetate *on page 509*

ABC *see* abacavir *on previous page*

ABCD *see* amphotericin B cholesteryl sulfate complex *on page 54*

abciximab (ab SIK si mab)

Synonyms C7E3; 7E3

U.S./Canadian Brand Names ReoPro® [US/Can]

Therapeutic Category Platelet Aggregation Inhibitor

Use Prevention of acute cardiac ischemic complications in patients at high risk for abrupt closure of the treated coronary vessel and patients at risk of restenosis; an adjunct with heparin to prevent cardiac ischemic complications in patients with unstable angina not responding to conventional therapy when a percutaneous coronary intervention is scheduled within 24 hours

Usual Dosage I.V.: 0.25 mg/kg bolus administered 10-60 minutes before the start of intervention followed by an infusion of 0.125 mcg/kg/minute (to a maximum of 10 mcg/minute) for 12 hours

Patients with unstable angina not responding to conventional medical therapy and who are planning to undergo percutaneous coronary intervention within 24 hours may be treated with abciximab 0.25 mg/kg intravenous bolus followed by an 18- to 24-hour intravenous infusion of 10 mcg/minute, concluding 1 hour after the percutaneous coronary intervention.

Dosage Forms Injection, solution: 2 mg/mL (5 mL)

Abelcet® [US/Can] *see* amphotericin B lipid complex *on page 55*

Abenol® [Can] *see* acetaminophen *on page 5*

Abilify™ [US] *see* aripiprazole *on page 77*

ABLC *see* amphotericin B lipid complex *on page 55*

A/B® Otic [US] *see* antipyrine and benzocaine *on page 65*

Abreva® [US-OTC] *see* docosanol *on page 285*

absorbable cotton *see* cellulose, oxidized regenerated *on page 174*

absorbable gelatin sponge *see* gelatin (absorbable) *on page 398*

Absorbine® Antifungal *(Discontinued)* *see page 1042*

Absorbine® Jock Itch *(Discontinued)* *see page 1042*

Absorbine Jr.® Antifungal [US-OTC] *see* tolnaftate *on page 870*

acamprosate (a kam PROE sate)

Synonyms acamprosate calcium; calcium acetylhomotaurinate

U.S./Canadian Brand Names Campral® [US]

Therapeutic Category GABA Agonist/Glutamate Antagonist

Use Maintenance of alcohol abstinence

Usual Dosage Oral: Adults: Alcohol abstinence: 666 mg 3 tir be effective in some patients)

Dosage Forms Tablet, enteric coated, as calcium: 333 mg [c sulfites]

acamprosate calcium *see* acamprosate *on previous page*

acarbose (AY car bose)

Sound-Alike/Look-Alike Issues
Precose® may be confused with PreCare®

U.S./Canadian Brand Names Prandase® [Can]; Precose® [US]

Therapeutic Category Antidiabetic Agent, Oral

Use

Monotherapy, as indicated as an adjunct to diet to lower blood glucose in patients with type 2 diabetes mellitus (noninsulin dependent, NIDDM) whose hyperglycemia cannot be managed on diet alone

Combination with a sulfonylurea, metformin, or insulin in patients with type 2 diabetes mellitus (noninsulin dependent, NIDDM) when diet plus acarbose do not result in adequate glycemic control. The effect of acarbose to enhance glycemic control is additive to that of other hypoglycemic agents when used in combination.

Usual Dosage Oral:

Adults: Dosage must be individualized on the basis of effectiveness and tolerance while not exceeding the maximum recommended dose

Initial dose: 25 mg 3 times/day with the first bite of each main meal

Maintenance dose: Should be adjusted at 4- to 8-week intervals based on 1-hour postprandial glucose levels and tolerance. Dosage may be increased from 25 mg 3 times/day to 50 mg 3 times/day. Some patients may benefit from increasing the dose to 100 mg 3 times/day.

Maintenance dose ranges: 50-100 mg 3 times/day.

Maximum dose:

≤60 kg: 50 mg 3 times/day

>60 kg: 100 mg 3 times/day

Patients receiving sulfonylureas: Acarbose given in combination with a sulfonylurea will cause a further lowering of blood glucose and may increase the hypoglycemic potential of the sulfonylurea. If hypoglycemia occurs, appropriate adjustments in the dosage of these agents should be made.

Dosage Forms Tablet: 25 mg, 50 mg, 100 mg

A-Caro-25® [US] *see* beta-carotene *on page 113*

Accolate® [US/Can] *see* zafirlukast *on page 936*

AccuHist® Pediatric *(Discontinued)* *see page 1042*

AccuNeb™ [US] *see* albuterol *on page 25*

Accupril® [US/Can] *see* quinapril *on page 756*

Accuretic™ [US/Can] *see* quinapril and hydrochlorothiazide *on page 756*

Accutane® [US/Can] *see* isotretinoin *on page 489*

ACE *see* captopril *on page 153*

acebutolol (a se BYOO toe lole)

Sound-Alike/Look-Alike Issues
Sectral® may be confused with Factrel®, Seconal®, Septra®

Synonyms acebutolol hydrochloride

U.S./Canadian Brand Names Apo-Acebutolol® [Can]; Gen-Acebutolol [Can]; Monitan® [Can]; Novo-Acebutolol [Can]; Nu-Acebutolol [Can]; Rhotral [Can]; Sectral® [US/Can]

herapeutic Category Antiarrhythmic Agent, Class II; Beta-Adrenergic Blocker

e Treatment of hypertension, ventricular arrhythmias, angina

ual Dosage Oral:

ults:

pertension: 400-800 mg/day (larger doses may be divided); maximum: 1200 mg/ ; usual dose range (JNC 7): 200-800 mg/day in 2 divided doses

icular arrhythmias: Initial: 400 mg/day; maintenance: 600-1200 mg/day in divided

orms Capsule, as hydrochloride: 200 mg, 400 mg

acebutolol hydrochloride *see* acebutolol *on previous page*

Aceon® [US] *see* perindopril erbumine *on page 683*

Acephen® [US-OTC] *see* acetaminophen *on this page*

Acetadote® [US] *see* acetylcysteine *on page 16*

acetaminophen (a seet a MIN oh fen)

Sound-Alike/Look-Alike Issues

Acephen® may be confused with Aciphex™
FeverALL® may be confused with Fiberall®
Tylenol® may be confused with atenolol, timolol, Tuinal®, Tylox®

Synonyms APAP; n-acetyl-p-aminophenol; paracetamol

U.S./Canadian Brand Names Abenol® [Can]; Acephen® [US-OTC]; Apo-Acetaminophen® [Can]; Aspirin Free Anacin® Maximum Strength [US-OTC]; Atasol® [Can]; Cetafen Extra® [US-OTC]; Cetafen® [US-OTC]; Comtrex® Sore Throat Maximum Strength [US-OTC]; ElixSure™ Fever/Pain [US-OTC]; FeverALL® [US-OTC]; Genapap® Children [US-OTC]; Genapap® Extra Strength [US-OTC]; Genapap® Infant [US-OTC]; Genapap® [US-OTC]; Genebs® Extra Strength [US-OTC]; Genebs® [US-OTC]; Mapap® Arthritis [US-OTC]; Mapap® Children's [US-OTC]; Mapap® Extra Strength [US-OTC]; Mapap® Infants [US-OTC]; Mapap® [US-OTC]; Pediatrix [Can]; Redutemp® [US-OTC]; Silapap® Children's [US-OTC]; Silapap® Infants [US-OTC]; Tempra® [Can]; Tylenol® 8 Hour [US-OTC]; Tylenol® Arthritis Pain [US-OTC]; Tylenol® Children's [US-OTC]; Tylenol® Extra Strength [US-OTC]; Tylenol® Infants [US-OTC]; Tylenol® Junior Strength [US-OTC]; Tylenol® Sore Throat [US-OTC]; Tylenol® [US-OTC/Can]; Valorin Extra [US-OTC]; Valorin [US-OTC]

Therapeutic Category Analgesic, Nonnarcotic; Antipyretic

Use Treatment of mild to moderate pain and fever (antipyretic/analgesic); does not have antirheumatic or antiinflammatory effects

Usual Dosage Oral, rectal:

Children <12 years: 10-15 mg/kg/dose every 4-6 hours as needed; do **not** exceed 5 doses (2.6 g) in 24 hours

Note: Higher rectal doses have been studied for use in preoperative pain control in children. However, specific guidelines are not available and dosing may be product dependent. The safety and efficacy of alternating acetaminophen and ibuprofen dosing has not been established.

Adults: 325-650 mg every 4-6 hours or 1000 mg 3-4 times/day; do **not** exceed 4 g/day

Dosage Forms

Caplet (Cefaten® Extra Strength, Genapap® Extra Strength, Genebs® Extra Strength, Mapap® Extra Strength, Tylenol® Extra Strength): 500 mg
Caplet, extended release (Mapap® Arthritis, Tylenol® Arthritis Pain): 650 mg
Capsule (Mapap® Extra Strength): 500 mg
Elixir: 160 mg/5 mL (120 mL, 480 mL, 3780 mL)
Mapap® Children's: 160 mg/5 mL (120 mL) [alcohol free; contains benzoic acid and sodium benzoate; cherry flavor]
Gelcap (Mapap® Extra Strength, Tylenol® Extra Strength): 500 mg
Geltab (Mapap® Extra Strength, Tylenol® Extra Strength): 500 mg
Geltab, extended release (Tylenol® 8 Hour): 650 mg
Liquid, oral: 500 mg/15 mL (240 mL)
Comtrex® Sore Throat Maximum Strength: 500 mg/15 mL (240 mL) [
benzoate; honey lemon flavor]
Genapap® Children: 160 mg/5 mL (120 mL) [contains sodium
grape flavors]
Silapap®: 160 mg/5 mL (120 mL, 240 mL, 480 mL) [su
benzoate; cherry flavor]
Tylenol® Extra Strength: 500 mg/15 mL (240 mL) [contain
flavor]
(Continued)

acetaminophen *(Continued)*

Tylenol® Sore Throat: 500 mg/15 mL (240 mL) [contains sodium benzoate; cherry and honey-lemon flavors]

Solution, oral drops: 80 mg/0.8 mL (15 mL) [droppers are marked at 0.4 mL (40 mg) and at 0.8 mL (80 mg)]

Genapap® Infant: 80 mg/0.8 mL (15 mL) [fruit flavor]

Silapap® Infant's: 80 mg/0.8 mL (15 mL, 30 mL) [contains sodium benzoate; cherry flavor]

Solution, oral: 160 mg/5 mL (120 mL, 480 mL)

Suppository, rectal: 120 mg, 325 mg, 650 mg

Acephen®: 120 mg, 325 mg, 650 mg

FeverALL®: 80 mg, 120 mg, 325 mg, 650 mg

Mapap®: 125 mg, 650 mg

Suspension, oral:

Mapap® Children's: 160 mg/5 mL (120 mL) [contains sodium benzoate; cherry flavor]

Tylenol® Children's: 160 mg/5 mL (120 mL, 240 mL) [contains sodium benzoate; bubblegum, cherry, and grape flavors]

Suspension, oral drops:

Mapap® Infants 80 mg/0.8 mL (15 mL, 30 mL) [contains sodium benzoate; cherry flavor]

Tylenol® Infants: 80 mg/0.8 mL (15 mL, 30 mL) [contains sodium benzoate; cherry and grape flavors]

Syrup, oral (ElixSure™ Fever/Pain): 160 mg/5 mL (120 mL) [bubblegum, cherry, and grape flavors]

Tablet: 325 mg, 500 mg

Aspirin Free Anacin® Extra Strength, Genapap® Extra Strength, Genebs® Extra Strength, Mapap® Extra Strength, Redutemp®, Tylenol® Extra Strength, Valorin Extra: 500 mg

Cetafen®, Genapap®, Genebs®, Mapap®, Tylenol®, Valorin: 325 mg

Tablet, chewable: 80 mg

Genapap® Children: 80 mg [contains phenylalanine 6 mg/tablet; fruit and grape flavors]

Mapap® Children's: 80 mg [contains phenylalanine 3 mg/tablet; bubblegum, fruit, and grape flavors]

Mapap® Junior Strength: 160 mg [contains phenylalanine 12 mg/tablet; grape flavor]

Tylenol® Children's: 80 mg [fruit and grape flavors contain phenylalanine 3 mg/tablet; bubblegum flavor contains phenylalanine 6 mg/tablet]

Tylenol® Junior Strength: 160 mg [contains phenylalanine 6 mg/tablet; fruit and grape flavors]

acetaminophen and chlorpheniramine *see* chlorpheniramine and acetaminophen *on page 188*

acetaminophen and codeine (a seet a MIN oh fen & KOE deen)

Sound-Alike/Look-Alike Issues

Capital® may be confused with Capitrol®

Synonyms codeine and acetaminophen

U.S./Canadian Brand Names Capital® and Codeine [US]; ratio-Emtec [Can]; ratio-Lenoltec [Can]; Triatec-8 [Can]; Triatec-8-Strong [Can]; Triatec-30 [Can]; Tylenol® Elixir with Codeine [Can]; Tylenol® No. 1 [Can]; Tylenol® No. 1 Forte [Can]; Tylenol® No. 2 with Codeine [Can]; Tylenol® No. 3 with Codeine [Can]; Tylenol® No. 4 with Codeine [Can]; Tylenol® with Codeine [US/Can]

herapeutic Category Analgesic, Narcotic

ntrolled Substance C-III; C-V

Relief of mild to moderate pain

l Dosage Doses should be adjusted according to severity of pain and response of atient. Adult doses ≥60 mg codeine fail to give commensurate relief of pain but prolong analgesia and are associated with an appreciably increased incidence effects.

Oral:
Children: Analgesic:
Codeine: 0.5-1 mg codeine/kg/dose every 4-6 hours
Acetaminophen: 10-15 mg/kg/dose every 4 hours up to a maximum of 2.6 g/24 hours for children <12 years; **alternatively, the following can be used:**
3-6 years: 5 mL 3-4 times/day as needed of elixir
7-12 years: 10 mL 3-4 times/day as needed of elixir
>12 years: 15 mL every 4 hours as needed of elixir
Adults:
Antitussive: Based on codeine (15-30 mg/dose) every 4-6 hours (maximum: 360 mg/24 hours based on codeine component)
Analgesic: Based on codeine (30-60 mg/dose) every 4-6 hours (maximum: 4000 mg/24 hours based on acetaminophen component)

Dosage Forms [DSC] = Discontinued product; [Can] = Canadian brand name
Caplet:
ratio-Lenoltec No. 1 [Can], Tylenol® No. 1 [Can]: Acetaminophen 300 mg, codeine phosphate, 8 mg and caffeine 15 mg [not available in the U.S.]
Tylenol® No. 1 Forte [Can]: Acetaminophen 500 mg, codeine phosphate 8 mg, and caffeine 15 mg [not available in the U.S.]
Elixir, oral [C-V]: Acetaminophen 120 mg and codeine phosphate 12 mg per 5 mL (5 mL, 10 mL, 12.5 mL, 15 mL, 120 mL, 480 mL) [contains alcohol 7%]
Tylenol® with Codeine [DSC]: Acetaminophen 120 mg and codeine phosphate 12 mg per 5 mL (480 mL) [contains alcohol 7%; cherry flavor]
Tylenol® Elixir with Codeine [Can]: Acetaminophen 160 mg and codeine phosphate 8 mg per 5 mL (500 mL) [contains alcohol 7%, sucrose 31%; cherry flavor; not available in the U.S.]
Suspension, oral [C-V] (Capital® and Codeine): Acetaminophen 120 mg and codeine phosphate 12 mg per 5 mL (480 mL) [alcohol free; fruit punch flavor]
Tablet [C-III]: Acetaminophen 300 mg and codeine phosphate 15 mg; acetaminophen 300 mg and codeine phosphate 30 mg; acetaminophen 300 mg and codeine phosphate 60 mg
ratio-Emtec [Can], Triatec-30 [Can]: Acetaminophen 300 mg and codeine phosphate 30 mg [not available in the U.S.]
ratio-Lenoltec No. 1 [Can]: Acetaminophen 300 mg, codeine phosphate 8 mg, and caffeine 15 mg [Not available in the U. S.]
ratio-Lenoltec No. 2 [Can], Tylenol® No. 2 with Codeine [Can]: Acetaminophen 300 mg, codeine phosphate 15 mg, and caffeine 15 mg [not available in the U.S.]
ratio-Lenoltec No. 3 [Can], Tylenol® No. 3 with Codeine [Can]: Acetaminophen 300 mg, codeine phosphate 30 mg, and caffeine 15 mg [not available in the U.S.]
ratio-Lenoltec No. 4 [Can], Tylenol® No. 4 with Codeine [Can]: Acetaminophen 300 mg and codeine phosphate 60 mg [not available in the U.S.]
Triatec-8 [Can]: Acetaminophen 325 mg, codeine phosphate 8 mg, and caffeine 30 mg [not available in the U.S.]
Triatec-8 Strong [Can]: Acetaminophen 500 mg, codeine phosphate 8 mg, and caffeine 30 mg [not available in the U.S.]
Tylenol® with Codeine No. 3: Acetaminophen 300 mg and codeine phosphate 30 m[illegible] [contains sodium metabisulfite]
Tylenol® with Codeine No. 4: Acetaminophen 300 mg and codeine phosphate [illegible] [contains sodium metabisulfite]

acetaminophen and diphenhydramine

(a seet a MIN oh fen & dye fen HYE dra meen)

Synonyms diphenhydramine and acetaminophen

U.S./Canadian Brand Names Excedrin® P.M. [US-OTC]; Good[illegible] Legatrin PM® [US-OTC]; Percogesic® Extra Strength [US-O[illegible] Strength [US-OTC]; Tylenol® Severe Allergy [US-OTC]

Therapeutic Category Analgesic, Nonnarcotic

Use Aid in the relief of insomnia accompanied by minor pain

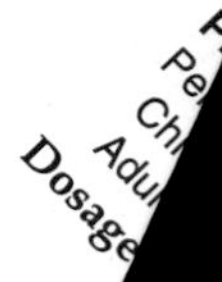

(Continued)

acetaminophen and diphenhydramine *(Continued)*

Usual Dosage Oral: Adults: 50 mg of diphenhydramine HCl (76 mg diphenhydramine citrate) at bedtime or as directed by physician; do not exceed recommended dosage; not for use in children <12 years of age

Dosage Forms [DSC] = Discontinued product

Caplet: Acetaminophen 500 mg and diphenhydramine hydrochloride 25 mg

Excedrin® P.M.: Acetaminophen 500 mg and diphenhydramine citrate 38 mg [contains benzoic acid]

Legatrin PM®: Acetaminophen 500 mg and diphenhydramine hydrochloride 50 mg

Percogesic® Extra Strength: Acetaminophen 500 mg and diphenhydramine hydrochloride 25 mg

Tylenol® PM Extra Strength: Acetaminophen 500 mg and diphenhydramine hydrochloride 25 mg

Tylenol® Severe Allergy: Acetaminophen 500 mg and diphenhydramine hydrochloride 12.5 mg

Gelcap (Tylenol® PM Extra Strength): Acetaminophen 500 mg and diphenhydramine hydrochloride 25 mg [contains benzyl alcohol]

Geltab: Acetaminophen 500 mg and diphenhydramine hydrochloride 25 mg

Excedrin® P.M.: Acetaminophen 500 mg and diphenhydramine citrate 38 mg [contains benzoic acid]

Tylenol® PM Extra Strength: Acetaminophen 500 mg and diphenhydramine hydrochloride 25 mg [contains benzyl alcohol]

Powder for oral solution (Goody's PM® Powder): Acetaminophen 500 mg and diphenhydramine citrate 38 mg

Tablet: Acetaminophen 500 mg and diphenhydramine hydrochloride 25 mg

Anacin® PM Aspirin-Free [DSC], Tylenol® PM Extra Strength: Acetaminophen 500 mg and diphenhydramine hydrochloride 25 mg

Excedrin® P.M.: Acetaminophen 500 mg and diphenhydramine citrate 38 mg [contains benzoic acid]

acetaminophen and hydrocodone *see* hydrocodone and acetaminophen *on page 443*

acetaminophen and oxycodone *see* oxycodone and acetaminophen *on page 656*

acetaminophen and phenyltoloxamine

(a seet a MIN oh fen & fen il to LOKS a meen)

Sound-Alike/Look-Alike Issues

Percogesic® may be confused with paregoric, Percodan®

Synonyms phenyltoloxamine and acetaminophen

U.S./Canadian Brand Names Genesec® [US-OTC]; Percogesic® [US-OTC]; Phenylgesic® [US-OTC]

Therapeutic Category Analgesic, Nonnarcotic

Use Relief of mild to moderate pain

Usual Dosage Oral:

Analgesic: Based on acetaminophen component:

Children: 10-15 mg/kg/dose every 4-6 hours as needed; do **not** exceed 5 doses/24 hours

Adults: 325-650 every 4-6 hours as needed; do **not** exceed 4 g/day

oduct labeling:

cogesic®:

ldren 6-12 years: 1 tablet every 4 hours; do **not** exceed 4 tablets/24 hours

ts: 1-2 tablets every 4 hours; do **not** exceed 8 tablets/24 hours

Forms Tablet: Acetaminophen 325 mg and phenyltoloxamine citrate 30 mg

acetaminophen and pseudoephedrine

(a seet a MIN oh fen & soo doe e FED rin)

Sound-Alike/Look-Alike Issues

Ornex® may be confused with Orexin®, Orinase®

Synonyms pseudoephedrine and acetaminophen

U.S./Canadian Brand Names Alka-Seltzer® Plus Cold and Sinus Liqui-Gels® [US-OTC]; Cetafen Cold® [US-OTC]; Dristan® N.D. [Can]; Dristan® N.D., Extra Strength [Can]; Genapap™ Sinus Maximum Strength [US-OTC]; Infants' Tylenol® Cold [US-OTC]; Mapap® Sinus Maximum Strength [US-OTC]; Medi-Synal [US-OTC]; Ornex® Maximum Strength [US-OTC]; Ornex® [US-OTC]; Sinus-Relief® [US-OTC]; Sinutab® Non Drowsy [Can]; Sinutab® Sinus [US-OTC]; Sudafed® Head Cold and Sinus Extra Strength [Can]; Sudafed® Sinus and Cold [US-OTC]; Sudafed® Sinus Headache [US-OTC]; SudoGest Sinus [US-OTC]; Tylenol® Cold, Infants [US-OTC]; Tylenol® Decongestant [Can]; Tylenol® Sinus [Can]; Tylenol® Sinus, Children's [US-OTC]; Tylenol® Sinus Day Non-Drowsy [US-OTC]

Therapeutic Category Decongestant/Analgesic

Use Relief of mild to moderate pain; relief of congestion

Usual Dosage Oral:

Analgesic: Based on acetaminophen component:

Children: 10-15 mg/kg/dose every 4-6 hours as needed; do **not** exceed 5 doses in 24 hours

Adults: 325-650 mg every 4-6 hours as needed; do **not** exceed 4 g/day

Decongestant: Based on pseudoephedrine component:

Children:

2-6 years: 15 mg every 4 hours; do **not** exceed 90 mg/day

6-12 years: 30 mg every 4 hours; do **not** exceed 180 mg/day

Children >12 years and Adults: 60 mg every 4 hours; do **not** exceed 360 mg/day

Product labeling:

Alka-Seltzer® Plus Cold and Sinus:

Children 6-12 years: 1 dose with water every 4 hours (maximum: 4 doses/24 hours)

Adults: 2 doses with water every 4 hours (maximum: 4 doses/24 hours)

Children's Tylenol® Sinus: Children:

Liquid:

2-5 years (24-47 lb): 1 teaspoonful every 4-6 hours (maximum: 4 doses/24 hours)

6-11 years (48-95 lb): 2 teaspoonfuls every 4-6 hours (maximum: 4 doses/24 hours)

Tablet, chewable:

2-5 years (24-47 lb): 2 tablets every 4-6 hours (maximum: 4 doses/24 hours)

6-11 years (48-95 lb): 4 tablets every 4-6 hours (maximum: 4 doses/24 hours)

Sinutab® Sinus: Children >12 years and Adults: 2 doses every 6 hours (maximum: 8 doses/24 hours)

Dosage Forms

Caplet:

Ornex®: Acetaminophen 325 mg and pseudoephedrine hydrochloride 30 mg

Genapap™ Sinus Maximum Strength, Mapap® Sinus Maximum Strength, Orne
Maximum Strength, Sudafed® Sinus Headache, Tylenol® Sinus Day Non-Dro
Acetaminophen 500 mg and pseudoephedrine hydrochloride 30 mg

Capsule, liquid (Alka-Seltzer® Plus Cold and Sinus, Sudafed® Sinus and Col
minophen 325 mg and pseudoephedrine hydrochloride 30 mg

Gelcap (Tylenol® Sinus Day Non-Drowsy): Acetaminophen 500 mg and
rine hydrochloride 30 mg

Geltab (Mapap® Sinus Maximum Strength, Tylenol® Sinus Day Non-
ophen 500 mg and pseudoephedrine hydrochloride 30 mg

Liquid, oral drops (Infants' Tylenol® Cold): Acetaminophen 80
phedrine 7.5 mg/0.8 mL [contains sodium benzoate; bubble

Suspension (Children's Tylenol® Sinus): Acetaminophen 160
hydrochloride 15 mg/5 mL [contains sodium benzoate; fruit

(Continued)

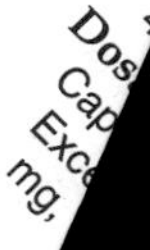

acetaminophen and pseudoephedrine *(Continued)*

Tablet:

Cetafen Cold®, Medi-Synal, Sinus-Relief: Acetaminophen 325 mg and pseudoephedrine hydrochloride 30 mg

Sinutab® Sinus, Sudafed® Sinus Headache, SudoGest Sinus: Acetaminophen 500 mg and pseudoephedrine hydrochloride 30 mg

acetaminophen and tramadol (a seet a MIN oh fen & TRA ma dole)

Synonyms APAP and tramadol; tramadol hydrochloride and acetaminophen

U.S./Canadian Brand Names Ultracet™ [US]

Therapeutic Category Analgesic, Nonnarcotic; Analgesic, Miscellaneous

Use Short-term (≤5 days) management of acute pain

Usual Dosage Oral: Adults: Acute pain: Two tablets every 4-6 hours as needed for pain relief (maximum: 8 tablets/day); treatment should not exceed 5 days

Dosage Forms Tablet: Acetaminophen 325 mg and tramadol hydrochloride 37.5 mg

acetaminophen, aspirin, and caffeine

(a seet a MIN oh fen, AS pir in, & KAF een)

Sound-Alike/Look-Alike Issues

Excedrin® may be confused with Dexatrim®, Dexedrine®

Synonyms aspirin, acetaminophen, and caffeine; aspirin, caffeine and acetaminophen; caffeine, acetaminophen, and aspirin; caffeine, aspirin, and acetaminophen

U.S./Canadian Brand Names Excedrin® Extra Strength [US-OTC]; Excedrin® Migraine [US-OTC]; Fem-Prin® [US-OTC]; Genaced™ [US-OTC]; Goody's® Extra Strength Headache Powder [US-OTC]; Goody's® Extra Strength Pain Relief [US-OTC]; Pain-Off [US-OTC]; Vanquish® Extra Strength Pain Reliever [US-OTC]

Therapeutic Category Analgesic, Nonnarcotic

Use Relief of mild to moderate pain; mild to moderate pain associated with migraine headache

Usual Dosage Oral: Adults:

Analgesic:

Based on **acetaminophen** component:

Mild to moderate pain: 325-650 mg every 4-6 hours as needed; do **not** exceed 4 g/day

Mild to moderate pain associated with migraine headache: 500 mg/dose (in combination with 500 mg aspirin and 130 mg caffeine) every 6 hours while symptoms persist; do not use for longer than 48 hours

Based on **aspirin** component:

Mild to moderate pain: 325-650 mg every 4-6 hours as needed; do **not** exceed 4 g/day

Mild to moderate pain associated with migraine headache: 500 mg/dose (in combination with 500 mg acetaminophen and 130 mg caffeine) every 6 hours; do not use for longer than 48 hours

Product labeling:

Excedrin® Extra Strength, Excedrin® Migraine: Children >12 years and Adults: 2 doses every 6 hours (maximum: 8 doses/24 hours)

Note: When used for migraine, do not use for longer than 48 hours

Goody's® Extra Strength Headache Powder: Children >12 years and Adults: 1 powder, placed on tongue or dissolved in water, every 4-6 hours (maximum: 4 powders/24 hours)

Goody's® Extra Strength Pain Relief Tablets: Children >12 years and Adults: 2 tablets every 4-6 hours (maximum: 8 tablets/24 hours)

/anquish® Extra Strength Pain Reliever: Children >12 years and Adults: 2 tablets every hours (maximum: 12 tablets/24 hours)

age Forms

let:

drin® Extra Strength, Excedrin® Migraine: Acetaminophen 250 mg, aspirin 250 and caffeine 65 mg

Vanquish® Extra Strength Pain Reliever: Acetaminophen 194 mg, aspirin 227 mg, and caffeine 33 mg
Geltab (Excedrin® Extra Strength, Excedrin® Migraine): Acetaminophen 250 mg, aspirin 250 mg, and caffeine 65 mg
Powder (Goody's® Extra Strength Headache Powder): Acetaminophen 260 mg, aspirin 520 mg, and caffeine 32.5 mg [contains lactose]
Tablet:
Excedrin® Extra Strength, Excedrin® Migraine, Genaced™, Pain-Off: Acetaminophen 250 mg, aspirin 250 mg, and caffeine 65 mg
Fem-Prin®: Acetaminophen 194.4 mg, aspirin 226.8 mg, and caffeine 32.4 mg
Goody's® Extra Strength Pain Relief: Acetaminophen 130 mg, aspirin 260 mg, and caffeine 16.25 mg

acetaminophen, butalbital, and caffeine *see* butalbital, acetaminophen, and caffeine *on page 138*

acetaminophen, caffeine, hydrocodone, chlorpheniramine, and phenylephrine *see* hydrocodone, chlorpheniramine, phenylephrine, acetaminophen, and caffeine *on page 446*

acetaminophen, chlorpheniramine, and pseudoephedrine

(a seet a MIN oh fen, klor fen IR a meen, & soo doe e FED rin)

Sound-Alike/Look-Alike Issues
Thera-Flu® may be confused with Tamiflu™, Thera-Flur-N®

Synonyms acetaminophen, pseudoephedrine, and chlorpheniramine; chlorpheniramine, acetaminophen, and pseudoephedrine; chlorpheniramine, pseudoephedrine, and acetaminophen; pseudoephedrine, acetaminophen, and chlorpheniramine; pseudoephedrine, chlorpheniramine, and acetaminophen

U.S./Canadian Brand Names Actifed® Cold and Sinus [US-OTC]; Alka-Seltzer® Plus Cold Liqui-Gels® [US-OTC]; Children's Tylenol® Plus Cold [US-OTC]; Comtrex® Maximum Strength Sinus and Nasal Decongestant [US-OTC]; Sinutab® Sinus & Allergy [Can]; Sinutab® Sinus Allergy Maximum Strength [US-OTC]; Thera-Flu® Cold and Sore Throat Night Time [US-OTC]; Tylenol® Allergy Sinus [US-OTC/Can]

Therapeutic Category Antihistamine/Decongestant/Analgesic

Use Temporary relief of sinus symptoms

Usual Dosage Oral:
Analgesic: Based on **acetaminophen** component:
Children: 10-15 mg/kg/dose every 4-6 hours as needed; do **not** exceed 5 doses in 24 hours
Adults: 325-650 mg every 4-6 hours as needed; do **not** exceed 4 g/day
Antihistamine: Based on **chlorpheniramine maleate** component:
Children:
2-6 years: 1 mg every 4-6 hours (maximum: 6 mg/24 hours)
6-12 years: 2 mg every 4-6 hours (maximum: 12 mg/24 hours)
Children >12 years and Adults: 4 mg every 4-6 hours (maximum: 24 mg/24 hours)
Decongestant: Based on **pseudoephedrine** component:
Children:
2-6 years: 15 mg every 4 hours (maximum: 90 mg/24 hours)
6-12 years: 30 mg every 4 hours (maximum: 180 mg/24 hours)
Children >12 years and Adults: 60 mg every 4 hours (maximum: 360 mg/24

Product labeling:
Alka-Seltzer® Plus Cold Medicine Liqui-Gels®:
Children 6-12 years: 1 softgel every 4 hours with water (maximum: 4
Children >12 years and Adults: 2 softgels every 4 hours with w
doses/24 hours)
Sinutab® Sinus Allergy Maximum Strength: Children >12 year
caplets every 6 hours (maximum: 8 doses/24 hours)
Thera-Flu® Cold and Sore Throat Night Time: Children >12 y
dissolved in hot water every 6 hours (maximum: 4 packets/2

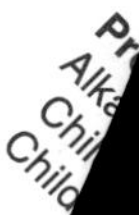

(Continued)

acetaminophen, chlorpheniramine, and pseudoephedrine *(Continued)*

Dosage Forms

Caplet (Actifed® Cold and Sinus, Comtrex® Maximum Strength Sinus and Nasal Decongestant, Sinutab® Sinus Allergy Maximum Strength, Tylenol® Allergy Sinus): Acetaminophen 500 mg, chlorpheniramine maleate 2 mg, and pseudoephedrine hydrochloride 30 mg

Capsule, softgel (Alka-Seltzer® Plus Cold Liqui-Gels®): Acetaminophen 325 mg, chlorpheniramine maleate 2 mg, and pseudoephedrine hydrochloride 30 mg

Gelcap (Tylenol® Allergy Sinus): Acetaminophen 500 mg, chlorpheniramine maleate 2 mg, and pseudoephedrine hydrochloride 30 mg

Geltab (Tylenol® Allergy Sinus): Acetaminophen 500 mg, chlorpheniramine maleate 2 mg, and pseudoephedrine hydrochloride 30 mg

Powder for oral solution [packet] (Thera-Flu® Cold and Sore Throat Night Time): Acetaminophen 650 mg, chlorpheniramine maleate 4 mg, and pseudoephedrine hydrochloride 60 mg [contains phenylalanine 11 mg/packet; lemon flavor]

Suspension (Children's Tylenol® Plus Cold): Acetaminophen 160 mg, chlorpheniramine maleate 1 mg, and pseudoephedrine hydrochloride 15 mg per 5 mL (120 mL) [contains sodium benzoate; grape flavor]

Tablet, chewable (Children's Tylenol® Plus Cold): Acetaminophen 80 mg, chlorpheniramine maleate 0.5 mg, and pseudoephedrine hydrochloride 7.5 mg [contains phenylalanine 6 mg/tablet; grape flavor]

acetaminophen, dextromethorphan, and pseudoephedrine

(a seet a MIN oh fen, deks troe meth OR fan, & soo doe e FED rin)

Synonyms dextromethorphan, acetaminophen, and pseudoephedrine; pseudoephedrine, acetaminophen, and dextromethorphan; pseudoephedrine, dextromethorphan, and acetaminophen

U.S./Canadian Brand Names Alka-Seltzer® Plus Flu Liqui-Gels® [US-OTC]; Comtrex® Non-Drowsy Cold and Cough Relief [US-OTC]; Contac® Cough, Cold and Flu Day & Night™ [Can]; Contac® Severe Cold and Flu/Non-Drowsy [US-OTC]; Infants' Tylenol® Cold Plus Cough Concentrated Drops [US-OTC]; Sudafed® Cold & Cough Extra Strength [Can]; Sudafed® Severe Cold [US-OTC]; Triaminic® Cough and Sore Throat [US-OTC]; Tylenol® Cold Day Non-Drowsy [US-OTC]; Tylenol® Cold Daytime [Can]; Tylenol® Flu Non-Drowsy Maximum Strength [US-OTC]; Vicks® DayQuil® Multi-Symptom Cold and Flu [US-OTC]

Therapeutic Category Cold Preparation

Use Treatment of mild to moderate pain and fever; symptomatic relief of cough and congestion

Usual Dosage Oral:

Analgesic: Based on acetaminophen component:

Children: 10-15 mg/kg/dose every 4-6 hours as needed; do **not** exceed 5 doses/24 hours

Adults: 325-650 mg every 4-7 hours as needed; do **not** exceed 4 g/day

Cough suppressant: Based on dextromethorphan component:

Children 6-12 years: 15 mg every 6-8 hours; do **not** exceed 60 mg/24 hours

Children >12 years and Adults: 10-20 mg every 4-8 hours **or** 30 mg every 8 hours; do **not** exceed 120 mg/24 hours

Decongestant: Based on pseudoephedrine component:

Children:

2-6 years: 15 mg every 4 hours (maximum: 90 mg/24 hours)

6-12 years: 30 mg every 4 hours (maximum: 180 mg/24 hours)

Children >12 years and Adults: 60 mg every 4 hours (maximum: 360 mg/24 hours)

oduct labeling:

-Seltzer® Plus Cold and Flu Liqui-Gels®:

dren 6-12 years: 1 dose every 4 hours (maximum: 4 doses/24 hours)

ren >12 years and Adults: 2 dose every 4 hours (maximum: 4 doses/24 hours)

Infants' Tylenol® Cold Plus Cough Concentrated Drops: Children 2-3 years (24-55 lb): 2 dropperfuls every 4-6 hours (maximum: 4 doses/24 hours)

Sudafed® Severe Cold, Thera-Flu® Non-Drowsy Maximum Strength (gelcap), Tylenol® Flu Non-Drowsy Maximum Strength: Children >12 years and Adults: 2 doses every 6 hours (maximum: 8 doses/24 hours)

Tylenol® Cold Non-Drowsy:

Children 6-11 years: 1 dose every 6 hours (maximum: 4 doses/24 hours)

Children ≥12 years and Adults: 2 doses every 6 hours (maximum: 8 doses/24 hours)

Thera-Flu® Non-Drowsy Maximum Strength: Children >12 years and Adults: 1 packet dissolved in hot water every 6 hours (maximum: 4 packets/24 hours)

Dosage Forms [DSC] = Discontinued product

Caplet:

Contac® Severe Cold and Flu/Non-Drowsy, Sudafed® Severe Cold, Tylenol® Cold Non-Drowsy: Acetaminophen 325 mg, dextromethorphan hydrobromide 15 mg, and pseudoephedrine hydrochloride 30 mg

Comtrex® Non-Drowsy Cold and Cough Relief: Acetaminophen 500 mg, dextromethorphan hydrobromide 15 mg, and pseudoephedrine hydrochloride 30 mg [contains benzoic acid]

Thera-Flu® Severe Cold Non-Drowsy: Acetaminophen 500 mg, dextromethorphan hydrobromide 15 mg, and pseudoephedrine hydrochloride 30 mg [contains lactose] [DSC]

Tylenol® Cold Day Non-Drowsy: Acetaminophen 325 mg dextromethorphan hydrobromide 15 mg, and pseudoephedrine hydrochloride 30 mg

Capsule, liquid:

Alka-Seltzer® Plus Flu Liqui-Gels®: Acetaminophen 325 mg, dextromethorphan hydrobromide 10 mg, and pseudoephedrine hydrochloride 30 mg

Vicks® DayQuil® Multi-Symptom Cold and Flu: Acetaminophen 250 mg, dextromethorphan hydrobromide 10 mg, and pseudoephedrine hydrochloride 30 mg

Gelcap:

Tylenol® Cold Day Non-Drowsy: Acetaminophen 325 mg dextromethorphan hydrobromide 15 mg, and pseudoephedrine hydrochloride 30 mg [contains benzyl alcohol]

Tylenol® Flu Non-Drowsy Maximum Strength: Acetaminophen 500 mg, dextromethorphan hydrobromide 15 mg, and pseudoephedrine hydrochloride 30 mg

Liquid:

Triaminic® Cough and Sore Throat Formula: Acetaminophen 160 mg, dextromethorphan hydrobromide 7.5 mg, and pseudoephedrine hydrochloride 15 mg per 5 mL (120 mL, 240 mL) [contains benzoic acid; grape flavor]

Vicks® DayQuil® Multi-Symptom Cold and Flu: Acetaminophen 325 mg, dextromethorphan hydrobromide 10 mg, and pseudoephedrine hydrochloride 30 mg per 15 mL (175 mL)

Powder for oral solution [packet] (Thera-Flu® Severe Cold Non-Drowsy): Acetaminophen 1000 mg, dextromethorphan hydrobromide 30 mg, and pseudoephedrine hydrochloride 60 mg [contains phenylalanine 17 mg/packet; lemon flavor] [DSC]

Suspension, oral drops (Infants' Tylenol® Cold Plus Cough Concentrated Drops): Acetaminophen 160 mg, dextromethorphan hydrobromide 5 mg, and pseudoephedrine hydrochloride 15 mg per 1.6 mL (15 mL) [1.6 mL = 2 dropperfuls] [cherry flavor]

acetaminophen, dichloralphenazone, and isometheptene *see* acetaminophen, isometheptene, and dichloralphenazone *on this page*

acetaminophen, isometheptene, and dichloralphenazone

(a seet a MIN oh fen, eye soe me THEP teen, & dye KLOR al FEN a zo

Sound-Alike/Look-Alike Issues

Midrin® may be confused with Mydfrin®

Synonyms acetaminophen, dichloralphenazone, and isomethept zone, acetaminophen, and isometheptene; dichloralphenazon acetaminophen; isometheptene, acetaminophen, and dichlor tene, dichloralphenazone, and acetaminophen

U.S./Canadian Brand Names I.D.A. [US]; Midrin® [US]; Mig

(Continued)

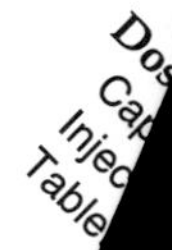

acetaminophen, isometheptene, and dichloralphenazone *(Continued)*

Therapeutic Category Analgesic, Nonnarcotic

Use Relief of migraine and tension headache

Usual Dosage Oral: Adults:

Migraine headache: 2 capsules to start, followed by 1 capsule every hour until relief is obtained (maximum: 5 capsules/12 hours)

Tension headache: 1-2 capsules every 4 hours (maximum: 8 capsules/24 hours)

Dosage Forms Capsule: Acetaminophen 325 mg, isometheptene mucate 65 mg, dichloralphenazone 100 mg

acetaminophen, pseudoephedrine, and chlorpheniramine *see* acetaminophen, chlorpheniramine, and pseudoephedrine *on page 11*

Acetasol® HC [US] *see* acetic acid, propylene glycol diacetate, and hydrocortisone *on next page*

acetazolamide (a set a ZOLE a mide)

Sound-Alike/Look-Alike Issues

acetazolamide may be confused with acetohexamide

Diamox® Sequels® may be confused with Dobutrex®, Trimox®

Tall-Man aceta**ZOLAMIDE**

U.S./Canadian Brand Names Apo-Acetazolamide® [Can]; Diamox® [Can]; Diamox® Sequels® [US]

Therapeutic Category Anticonvulsant; Carbonic Anhydrase Inhibitor

Use Treatment of glaucoma (chronic simple open-angle, secondary glaucoma, preoperatively in acute angle-closure); drug-induced edema or edema due to congestive heart failure (adjunctive therapy); centrencephalic epilepsies (immediate release dosage form); prevention or amelioration of symptoms associated with acute mountain sickness

Usual Dosage Note: I.M. administration is not recommended because of pain secondary to the alkaline pH

Children:

Glaucoma:

Oral: 8-30 mg/kg/day or 300-900 mg/m^2/day divided every 8 hours

I.V.: 20-40 mg/kg/24 hours divided every 6 hours, not to exceed 1 g/day

Edema: Oral, I.V.: 5 mg/kg or 150 mg/m^2 once every day

Epilepsy: Oral: 8-30 mg/kg/day in 1-4 divided doses, not to exceed 1 g/day; sustained release capsule is not recommended for treatment of epilepsy

Adults:

Glaucoma:

Chronic simple (open-angle): Oral: 250 mg 1-4 times/day or 500 mg sustained release capsule twice daily

Secondary, acute (closed-angle): I.V.: 250-500 mg, may repeat in 2-4 hours to a maximum of 1 g/day

Edema: Oral, I.V.: 250-375 mg once daily

Epilepsy: Oral: 8-30 mg/kg/day in 1-4 divided doses; **sustained release capsule is not recommended for treatment of epilepsy**

Mountain sickness: Oral: 250 mg every 8-12 hours (or 500 mg extended release capsules every 12-24 hours)

Therapy should begin 24-48 hours before and continue during ascent and for at least 48 hours after arrival at the high altitude

age Forms

sule, sustained release (Diamox® Sequels®): 500 mg

tion, powder for reconstitution: 500 mg

: 125 mg, 250 mg

acetic acid (a SEE tik AS id)

Sound-Alike/Look-Alike Issues
VōSol® may be confused with Vexol®

Synonyms ethanoic acid

U.S./Canadian Brand Names VōSol® [US]

Therapeutic Category Antibacterial, Otic; Antibacterial, Topical

Use Irrigation of the bladder; treatment of superficial bacterial infections of the external auditory canal

Usual Dosage
Irrigation (note dosage of an irrigating solution depends on the capacity or surface area of the structure being irrigated):
For continuous irrigation of the urinary bladder with 0.25% acetic acid irrigation, the rate of administration will approximate the rate of urine flow; usually 500-1500 mL/24 hours
For periodic irrigation of an indwelling urinary catheter to maintain patency, about 50 mL of 0.25% acetic acid irrigation is required
Otic: Insert saturated wick; keep moist 24 hours; remove wick and instill 5 drops 3-4 times/day

Dosage Forms
Solution for irrigation: 0.25% (250 mL, 500 mL, 1000 mL)
Solution, otic (VōSol®): 2% [in propylene glycol] (15 mL)

acetic acid, hydrocortisone, and propylene glycol diacetate *see* acetic acid, propylene glycol diacetate, and hydrocortisone *on this page*

acetic acid, propylene glycol diacetate, and hydrocortisone
(a SEE tik AS id, PRO pa leen GLY kole dye AS e tate, & hye droe KOR ti sone)

Synonyms acetic acid, hydrocortisone, and propylene glycol diacetate; hydrocortisone, acetic acid, and propylene glycol diacetate; hydrocortisone, propylene glycol diacetate, and acetic acid; propylene glycol diacetate, acetic acid, and hydrocortisone; propylene glycol diacetate, hydrocortisone, and acetic acid

U.S./Canadian Brand Names Acetasol® HC [US]; VōSol® HC [US/Can]

Therapeutic Category Antibiotic/Corticosteroid, Otic

Use Treatment of superficial infections of the external auditory canal caused by organisms susceptible to the action of the antimicrobial, complicated by swelling

Usual Dosage Adults: Otic: Instill 4 drops in ear(s) 3-4 times/day

Dosage Forms Solution, otic drops: Acetic acid 2%, propylene glycol diacetate 3%, and hydrocortisone 1% (10 mL)

acetohexamide (a set oh HEKS a mide)

Sound-Alike/Look-Alike Issues
acetohexamide may be confused with acetazolamide

Tall-Man aceto**HEXAMIDE**

Therapeutic Category Antidiabetic Agent, Oral

Use Adjunct to diet for the management of mild to moderately severe, stable, type 2 diabetes mellitus (noninsulin dependent, NIDDM)

Usual Dosage Oral: Adults:
Initial: 250 mg/day; increase in increments of 250-500 mg daily at intervals of 5 up to 1.5 g/day. Patients on ≤1 g/day can be controlled with once daily adm Patients receiving 1.5 g/day usually benefit from twice daily administratic morning and evening meals. Doses >1.5 g daily are not recommende

Dosage Forms Tablet: 250 mg, 500 mg

acetohydroxamic acid (a SEE toe hye droks am ik AS id)

Sound-Alike/Look-Alike Issues
Lithostat® may be confused with Lithobid®

Synonyms AHA
(Continued)

acetohydroxamic acid *(Continued)*

U.S./Canadian Brand Names Lithostat® [US/Can]

Therapeutic Category Urinary Tract Product

Use Adjunctive therapy in chronic urea-splitting urinary infection

Usual Dosage Oral:

Children: Initial: 10 mg/kg/day

Adults: 250 mg 3-4 times/day for a total daily dose of 10-15 mg/kg/day

Dosage Forms Tablet: 250 mg

Acetoxyl® [Can] *see* benzoyl peroxide *on page 109*

acetoxymethylprogesterone *see* medroxyprogesterone acetate *on page 548*

acetylcholine (a se teel KOE leen)

Sound-Alike/Look-Alike Issues

acetylcholine may be confused with acetylcysteine

Synonyms acetylcholine chloride

U.S./Canadian Brand Names Miochol-E® [US/Can]

Therapeutic Category Cholinergic Agent

Use Produces complete miosis in cataract surgery, keratoplasty, iridectomy and other anterior segment surgery where rapid miosis is required

Usual Dosage Adults: Intraocular: 0.5-2 mL of 1% injection (5-20 mg) instilled into anterior chamber before or after securing one or more sutures

Dosage Forms Powder for intraocular solution, as chloride: 1:100 [10 mg/mL] (2 mL)

acetylcholine chloride *see* acetylcholine *on this page*

acetylcysteine (a se teel SIS teen)

Sound-Alike/Look-Alike Issues

acetylcysteine may be confused with acetylcholine

Mucomyst® may be confused with Mucinex®

Synonyms acetylcysteine sodium; mercapturic acid; NAC; *n*-acetylcysteine; *n*-acetyl-L-cysteine

U.S./Canadian Brand Names Acetadote® [US]; Mucomyst® [US/Can]; Parvolex® [Can]

Therapeutic Category Mucolytic Agent

Use Adjunctive mucolytic therapy in patients with abnormal or viscid mucous secretions in acute and chronic bronchopulmonary diseases; pulmonary complications of surgery and cystic fibrosis; diagnostic bronchial studies; antidote for acute acetaminophen toxicity

Usual Dosage

Acetaminophen poisoning: Children and Adults:

Oral: 140 mg/kg; followed by 17 doses of 70 mg/kg every 4 hours; repeat dose if emesis occurs within 1 hour of administration; therapy should continue until all doses are administered even though the acetaminophen plasma level has dropped below the toxic range

I.V. (Acetadote®): Loading dose: 150 mg/kg over 15 minutes. Maintenance dose: 50 mg/kg infused over 4 hours followed by 100 mg/kg infused over 16 hours. **Note:** To avoid fluid overload in patients <40 kg and those requiring fluid restriction, decrease volume of D_5W proportionally.

Adjuvant therapy in respiratory conditions: **Note:** Patients should receive an aerosolized bronchodilator 10-15 minutes prior to acetylcysteine.

nhalation, nebulization (face mask, mouth piece, tracheostomy): Acetylcysteine 10% nd 20% solution (Mucomyst®) (dilute 20% solution with sodium chloride or sterile ater for inhalation); 10% solution may be used undiluted

nts: 1-2 mL of 20% solution or 2-4 mL of 10% solution until nebulized given 3-4 es/day

Children and Adults: 3-5 mL of 20% solution or 6-10 mL of 10% solution until nebulized given 3-4 times/day; dosing range: 1-10 mL of 20% solution or 2-20 mL of 10% solution every 2-6 hours

Inhalation, nebulization (tent, croupette): Children and Adults: Dose must be individualized; may require up to 300 mL solution/treatment

Direct instillation: Adults:

Into tracheostomy: 1-2 mL of 10% to 20% solution every 1-4 hours

Through percutaneous intrathecal catheter: 1-2 mL of 20% or 2-4 mL of 10% solution every 1-4 hours via syringe attached to catheter

Diagnostic bronchogram: Nebulization or intrathecal: Adults: 1-2 mL of 20% solution or 2-4 mL of 10% solution administered 2-3 times prior to procedure

Dosage Forms

Injection, solution (Acetadote®): 20% [200 mg/mL] (30 mL) [contains disodium edetate]

Solution, as sodium (Mucomyst®): 10% [100 mg/mL] (4 mL, 10 mL, 30 mL); 20% [200 mg/mL] (4 mL, 10 mL, 30 mL)

acetylcysteine sodium *see* acetylcysteine *on previous page*

acetylsalicylic acid *see* aspirin *on page 80*

Aches-N-Pain® *(Discontinued)* *see page 1042*

achromycin *see* tetracycline *on page 851*

Achromycin® Parenteral *(Discontinued)* *see page 1042*

Achromycin® V Capsule *(Discontinued)* *see page 1042*

Achromycin® V Oral Suspension *(Discontinued)* *see page 1042*

aciclovir *see* acyclovir *on page 19*

acidulated phosphate fluoride *see* fluoride *on page 376*

Aci-jel® *(Discontinued)* *see page 1042*

Acilac [Can] *see* lactulose *on page 502*

Aciphex® [US/Can] *see* rabeprazole *on page 758*

acitretin (a si TRE tin)

Sound-Alike/Look-Alike Issues

Soriatane® may be confused with Loxitane®

U.S./Canadian Brand Names Soriatane® [US/Can]

Therapeutic Category Retinoid-like Compound

Use Treatment of severe psoriasis

Usual Dosage Oral: Adults: Individualization of dosage is required to achieve maximum therapeutic response while minimizing side effects

Initial therapy: Therapy should be initiated at 25-50 mg/day, given as a single dose with the main meal

Maintenance doses of 25-50 mg/day may be given after initial response to treatment; the maintenance dose should be based on clinical efficacy and tolerability

Dosage Forms Capsule: 10 mg, 25 mg

Aclovate® [US] *see* alclometasone *on page 27*

acrivastine and pseudoephedrine (AK ri vas teen & soo doe e FE[illegible]

Synonyms pseudoephedrine and acrivastine

U.S./Canadian Brand Names Semprex®-D [US]

Therapeutic Category Antihistamine/Decongestant Combination

Use Temporary relief of nasal congestion, decongest sinus open[illegible] itching of nose or throat, and itchy, watery eyes due to hay [illegible] respiratory allergies

Usual Dosage Oral: Adults: 1 capsule 3-4 times/day

Dosage Forms Capsule: Acrivastine 8 mg and pseudoephedri[illegible]

ACT® *(Discontinued)* *see page 1042*
Actagen-C® *(Discontinued)* *see page 1042*
Actagen® Syrup *(Discontinued)* *see page 1042*
Actagen® Tablet *(Discontinued)* *see page 1042*
Act-A-Med® *(Discontinued)* *see page 1042*
act-D *see* dactinomycin *on page 241*
ACTH *see* corticotropin *on page 228*
ACTH-40® *(Discontinued)* *see page 1042*
ActHIB® [US/Can] *see* *Haemophilus* B conjugate vaccine *on page 426*
Acticin® [US] *see* permethrin *on page 683*
Actidil® *(Discontinued)* *see page 1042*
Actidose-Aqua® [US-OTC] *see* charcoal *on page 180*
Actidose® with Sorbitol [US-OTC] *see* charcoal *on page 180*
Actifed® [Can] *see* triprolidine and pseudoephedrine *on page 889*
Actifed® Allergy Tablet (Night) *(Discontinued)* *see page 1042*
Actifed® Cold and Allergy [US-OTC] *see* triprolidine and pseudoephedrine *on page 889*
Actifed® Cold and Sinus [US-OTC] *see* acetaminophen, chlorpheniramine, and pseudoephedrine *on page 11*
Actifed® Syrup *(Discontinued)* *see page 1042*
Actifed® With Codeine *(Discontinued)* *see page 1042*
Actigall® [US] *see* ursodiol *on page 899*
Actimmune® [US/Can] *see* interferon gamma-1b *on page 480*
Actinex® *(Discontinued)* *see page 1042*
actinomycin *see* dactinomycin *on page 241*
actinomycin Cl *see* dactinomycin *on page 241*
actinomycin D *see* dactinomycin *on page 241*
Actiq® [US/Can] *see* fentanyl *on page 361*
Activase® [US] *see* alteplase *on page 36*
Activase® rt-PA [Can] *see* alteplase *on page 36*
activated carbon *see* charcoal *on page 180*
activated charcoal *see* charcoal *on page 180*
activated dimethicone *see* simethicone *on page 804*
activated ergosterol *see* ergocalciferol *on page 317*
activated methylpolysiloxane *see* simethicone *on page 804*
activated protein C, human, recombinant *see* drotrecogin alfa *on page 297*
Activella™ [US] *see* estradiol and norethindrone *on page 327*
Actonel® [US/Can] *see* risedronate *on page 778*
Actos® [US/Can] *see* pioglitazone *on page 696*
CU-dyne® [US-OTC] *see* povidone-iodine *on page 718*
ular® [US/Can] *see* ketorolac *on page 496*
lar LS™ [US] *see* ketorolac *on page 496*
r® P.F. [US] *see* ketorolac *on page 496*
m® 16 Hours *(Discontinued)* *see page 1042*

Acutrim® II, Maximum Strength ***(Discontinued)*** *see page 1042*

Acutrim® Late Day ***(Discontinued)*** *see page 1042*

ACV *see* acyclovir *on this page*

acycloguanosine *see* acyclovir *on this page*

acyclovir (ay SYE kloe veer)

Sound-Alike/Look-Alike Issues
Zovirax® may be confused with Zostrix®

Synonyms aciclovir; ACV; acycloguanosine

U.S./Canadian Brand Names Alti-Acyclovir [Can]; Apo-Acyclovir® [Can]; Gen-Acyclovir [Can]; Nu-Acyclovir [Can]; ratio-Acyclovir [Can]; Zovirax® [US/Can]

Therapeutic Category Antiviral Agent

Use Treatment of genital herpes simplex virus (HSV), herpes labialis (cold sores), herpes zoster (shingles), HSV encephalitis, neonatal HSV, mucocutaneous HSV, varicella-zoster (chickenpox)

Usual Dosage Note: Obese patients should be dosed using ideal body weight

Genital HSV:
I.V.: Children ≥12 years and Adults (immunocompetent): Initial episode, severe: 5 mg/kg every 8 hours for 5-7 days
Oral:
Adults:
Initial episode: 200 mg every 4 hours while awake (5 times/day) for 10 days (per manufacturer's labeling); 400 mg 3 times/day for 5-10 days has also been reported
Recurrence: 200 mg every 4 hours while awake (5 times/day) for 5 days (per manufacturer's labeling; begin at earliest signs of disease); 400 mg 3 times/day for 5 days has also been reported
Chronic suppression: 400 mg twice daily or 200 mg 3-5 times/day, for up to 12 months followed by re-evaluation (per manufacturer's labeling); 400-1200 mg/day in 2-3 divided doses has also been reported
Topical: Adults (immunocompromised): Ointment: Initial episode: 1/2” ribbon of ointment for a 4” square surface area every 3 hours (6 times/day) for 7 days

Herpes labialis (cold sores): Topical: Children ≥12 years and Adults: Cream: Apply 5 times/day for 4 days

Herpes zoster (shingles):
Oral: Adults (immunocompetent): 800 mg every 4 hours (5 times/day) for 7-10 days
I.V.:
Children <12 years (immunocompromised): 20 mg/kg/dose every 8 hours for 7 days
Children ≥12 years and Adults (immunocompromised): 10 mg/kg/dose or 500 mg/m^2/dose every 8 hours for 7 days

HSV encephalitis: I.V.:
Children 3 months to 12 years: 20 mg/kg/dose every 8 hours for 10 days (per manufacturer's labeling); dosing for 14-21 days also reported
Children ≥12 years and Adults: 10 mg/kg/dose every 8 hours for 10 days (per manufacturer's labeling); 10-15 mg/kg/dose every 8 hours for 14-21 days also reported

Mucocutaneous HSV:
I.V.:
Children <12 years (immunocompromised): 10 mg/kg/dose every 8 hours f
Children ≥12 years and Adults (immunocompromised): 5 mg/kg/dose eve
7 days (per manufacturer's labeling); dosing for up to 14 days also r
Topical: Ointment: Adults (nonlife-threatening, immunocompromis
ointment for a 4” square surface area every 3 hours (6 times/day

Neonatal HSV: I.V.: Neonate: Birth to 3 months: 10 mg/kg/do
days (manufacturer's labeling); 15 mg/kg/dose or 20 mg/kg/do
21 days has also been reported
(Continued)

acyclovir *(Continued)*

Varicella-zoster (chickenpox): Begin treatment within the first 24 hours of rash onset:
Oral:
Children ≥2 years and ≤40 kg (immunocompetent): 20 mg/kg/dose (up to 800 mg/dose) 4 times/day for 5 days
Children >40 kg and Adults (immunocompetent): 800 mg/dose 4 times a day for 5 days
Oral: Adults: 200 mg 3 times/day
I.V.:
Children: 250 mg/m^2/dose every 8 hours or 125 mg/m^2/dose every 6 hours
Adults: 250 mg/m^2/dose every 12 hours and Adults: Allogeneic patients who are HSV and CMV seropositive: 500 mg/m^2/dose (10 mg/kg) every 8 hours; for clinically-symptomatic CMV infection, consider replacing acyclovir with ganciclovir

Dosage Forms
Capsule: 200 mg
Cream, topical: 5% (2 g)
Injection, powder for reconstitution, as sodium: 500 mg, 1000 mg
Injection, solution, as sodium [preservative free]: 25 mg/mL (20 mL, 40 mL); 50 mg/mL (10 mL, 20 mL)
Ointment, topical: 5% (3 g, 15 g)
Suspension, oral: 200 mg/5 mL (480 mL) [banana flavor]
Tablet: 400 mg, 800 mg

AD3L *see* valrubicin *on page 902*

Adacel® [Can] *see* diphtheria, tetanus toxoids, and acellular pertussis vaccine *on page 280*

Adagen™ [US/Can] *see* pegademase (bovine) *on page 670*

Adalat® ***(Discontinued)*** *see page 1042*

Adalat® CC [US] *see* nifedipine *on page 619*

Adalat® XL® [Can] *see* nifedipine *on page 619*

adalimumab (a da LIM yoo mab)

Synonyms antitumor necrosis factor apha (human); D2E7; human antitumor necrosis factor-alpha

U.S./Canadian Brand Names Humira™ [US]

Therapeutic Category Antirheumatic, Disease Modifying; Monoclonal Antibody

Use Treatment of active rheumatoid arthritis (moderate to severe) in patients with inadequate response to one or more disease-modifying antirheumatic drugs (DMARDs)

Usual Dosage SubQ: Adults: Rheumatoid arthritis: 40 mg every other week; may be administered with other DMARDs; patients not taking methotrexate may increase dose to 40 mg/weekly

Dosage Forms Injection, solution [preservative free]: 40 mg/0.8 mL (1 mL) [prefilled glass syringe; packaged with alcohol preps]

adamantanamine hydrochloride *see* amantadine *on page 41*

adapalene (a DAP a leen)

U.S./Canadian Brand Names Differin® [US/Can]

Therapeutic Category Acne Products

Use Treatment of acne vulgaris

Jsual Dosage Topical: Children >12 years and Adults: Apply once daily at bedtime; therapeutic results should be noticed after 8-12 weeks of treatment

sage Forms
eam, topical: 0.1% (15 g, 45 g)
, topical: 0.1% (15 g, 45 g) [alcohol free]
lget, topical: 0.1% (60s)
ion, topical: 0.1% (30 mL)

Adderall® [US] *see* dextroamphetamine and amphetamine *on page 259*

Adderall XR™ [US] *see* dextroamphetamine and amphetamine *on page 259*

adefovir (a DEF o veer)

Synonyms adefovir dipivoxil

U.S./Canadian Brand Names Hepsera™ [US]

Therapeutic Category Antiretroviral Agent, Non-nucleoside Reverse Transcriptase Inhibitor (NNRTI)

Use Treatment of chronic hepatitis B with evidence of active viral replication (based on persistent elevation of ALT/AST or histologic evidence), including patients with lamivudine-resistant hepatitis B

Usual Dosage Oral: Adults: 10 mg once daily

Dosage Forms Tablet, as dipivoxil: 10 mg

adefovir dipivoxil *see* adefovir *on this page*

ADEKs [US-OTC] *see* vitamins (multiple/pediatric) *on page 927*

Adenocard® [US/Can] *see* adenosine *on this page*

Adenoscan® [US] *see* adenosine *on this page*

adenosine (a DEN oh seen)

Synonyms 9-beta-d-ribofuranosyladenine

U.S./Canadian Brand Names Adenocard® [US/Can]; Adenoscan® [US]

Therapeutic Category Antiarrhythmic Agent, Miscellaneous

Use

Adenocard®: Treatment of paroxysmal supraventricular tachycardia (PSVT) including that associated with accessory bypass tracts (Wolff-Parkinson-White syndrome); when clinically advisable, appropriate vagal maneuvers should be attempted prior to adenosine administration; **not effective in atrial flutter, atrial fibrillation, or ventricular tachycardia**

Adenoscan®: Pharmacologic stress agent used in myocardial perfusion thallium-201 scintigraphy

Usual Dosage

Adenocard®: **Rapid I.V. push (over 1-2 seconds) via peripheral line:**

Infants and Children:

Manufacturer's recommendation: <50 kg: 0.05 to 0.1 mg/kg. If conversion of PSVT does not occur within 1-2 minutes, may increase dose by 0.05 to 0.1 mg/kg. May repeat until sinus rhythm is established or to a maximum single dose of 0.3 mg/kg or 12 mg. Follow each dose with normal saline flush. ≥50 kg: Refer to Adults dosing

Pediatric advanced life support (PALS): Treatment of SVT: I.V., I.O.: 0.1 mg/kg; if not effective, administer 0.2 mg/kg of PSVT; medium dose required: 0.15 mg/kg; maximum single dose: 12 mg. Follow each dose with normal saline flush.

Adults: 6 mg; if not effective within 1-2 minutes, 12 mg may be given; may repeat 12 mg bolus if needed

Maximum single dose: 12 mg

Follow each I.V. bolus of adenosine with normal saline flush

Note: Preliminary results in adults suggest adenosine may be administered via a cen*line at lower doses (ie, initial adult dose: 3 mg).*

Adenoscan®: Continuous I.V. infusion via peripheral line: 140 mcg/kg/min minutes using syringe or columetric infusion pump; total dose: 0.84 mg/kg 201 is injected at midpoint (3 minutes) of infusion.

Hemodialysis: Significant drug removal is unlikely based on physiochem tics.

Peritoneal dialysis: Significant drug removal is unlikely based on r acteristics.

Note: Higher doses may be needed for administration via p vein.

(Continued)

adenosine *(Continued)*

Dosage Forms Injection, solution [preservative free]: 3 mg/mL (2 mL)
Adenocard®: 3 mg/mL (2 mL, 4 mL)
Adenoscan®: 3 mg/mL (20 mL, 30 mL)

ADH *see* vasopressin *on page 906*

Adipex-P® [US] *see* phentermine *on page 688*

Adipost® ***(Discontinued)*** *see page 1042*

Adlone® Injection ***(Discontinued)*** *see page 1042*

Adoxa™ [US] *see* doxycycline *on page 294*

Adphen® ***(Discontinued)*** *see page 1042*

ADR *see* doxorubicin *on page 293*

Adrenalin® [US/Can] *see* epinephrine *on page 311*

adrenaline *see* epinephrine *on page 311*

adrenocorticotropic hormone *see* corticotropin *on page 228*

adria *see* doxorubicin *on page 293*

Adriamycin® [Can] *see* doxorubicin *on page 293*

Adriamycin PFS® [US] *see* doxorubicin *on page 293*

Adriamycin RDF® [US] *see* doxorubicin *on page 293*

Adrin® ***(Discontinued)*** *see page 1042*

Adrucil® [US/Can] *see* fluorouracil *on page 378*

adsorbent charcoal *see* charcoal *on page 180*

Adsorbocarpine® Ophthalmic ***(Discontinued)*** *see page 1042*

Adsorbonac® ***(Discontinued)*** *see page 1042*

Adsorbotear® Ophthalmic Solution ***(Discontinued)*** *see page 1042*

Advair® Diskus® [US/Can] *see* fluticasone and salmeterol *on page 382*

Advanced Formula Oxy® Sensitive Gel ***(Discontinued)*** *see page 1042*

Advanced NatalCare® [US] *see* vitamins (multiple/prenatal) *on page 927*

Advantage 24™ [Can] *see* nonoxynol 9 *on page 626*

Advantage-S™ [US-OTC] *see* nonoxynol 9 *on page 626*

Advate [US] *see* antihemophilic factor (recombinant) *on page 63*

Advicor™ [US] *see* niacin and lovastatin *on page 617*

Advil® Children's [US-OTC] *see* ibuprofen *on page 462*

Advil® Cold, Children's [US-OTC] *see* pseudoephedrine and ibuprofen *on page 747*

Advil® Cold & Sinus [US-OTC/Can] *see* pseudoephedrine and ibuprofen *on page 747*

Advil® Infants' [US-OTC] *see* ibuprofen *on page 462*

Advil® Junior [US-OTC] *see* ibuprofen *on page 462*

Advil® Migraine [US-OTC] *see* ibuprofen *on page 462*

dvil® [US-OTC/Can] *see* ibuprofen *on page 462*

rius® [Can] *see* desloratadine *on page 251*

paid® ***(Discontinued)*** *see page 1042*

Bid® [US] *see* flunisolide *on page 373*

Bid®-M [US] *see* flunisolide *on page 373*

ne® ***(Discontinued)*** *see page 1042*

Aerolate® Oral Solution ***(Discontinued)*** *see page 1042*

Aerosporin® Injection ***(Discontinued)*** *see page 1042*

A-Free Prenatal [US] *see* vitamins (multiple/prenatal) *on page 927*

Afrin® Children's Nose Drops ***(Discontinued)*** *see page 1042*

Afrin® Extra Moisturizing [US-OTC] *see* oxymetazoline *on page 658*

Afrinol® ***(Discontinued)*** *see page 1042*

Afrin® Original [US-OTC] *see* oxymetazoline *on page 658*

Afrin® Saline Mist ***(Discontinued)*** *see page 1042*

Afrin® Severe Congestion [US-OTC] *see* oxymetazoline *on page 658*

Afrin® Sinus [US-OTC] *see* oxymetazoline *on page 658*

Afrin® [US-OTC] *see* oxymetazoline *on page 658*

Aftate® Antifungal [US-OTC] *see* tolnaftate *on page 870*

AG *see* aminoglutethimide *on page 45*

agalsidase beta (aye GAL si days BAY ta)

Synonyms alpha-galactosidase-A (human, recombinant); r-h α-GAL

U.S./Canadian Brand Names Fabrazyme® [US]

Therapeutic Category Enzyme

Use Replacement therapy for Fabry disease

Usual Dosage I.V.: Adults: 1 mg/kg every 2 weeks

Dosage Forms Injection, powder for reconstitution: 35 mg [contains mannitol 222 mg/vial; derived from Chinese hamster cells]

Agenerase® [US/Can] *see* amprenavir *on page 57*

Aggrastat® [US/Can] *see* tirofiban *on page 866*

Aggrenox® [US/Can] *see* aspirin and dipyridamole *on page 83*

$AgNO_3$ *see* silver nitrate *on page 804*

Agoral® Maximum Strength Laxative [US-OTC] *see* senna *on page 799*

Agoral® Plain ***(Discontinued)*** *see page 1042*

Agrylin® [US/Can] *see* anagrelide *on page 58*

AGT *see* aminoglutethimide *on page 45*

AHA *see* acetohydroxamic acid *on page 15*

AH-Chew® [US] *see* chlorpheniramine, phenylephrine, and methscopolamine *on page 192*

AH-Chew® II [US] *see* chlorpheniramine, phenylephrine, and methscopolamine *on page 192*

AHF (human) *see* antihemophilic factor (human) *on page 62*

AHF (porcine) *see* antihemophilic factor (porcine) *on page 63*

AHF (recombinant) *see* antihemophilic factor (recombinant) *on page 63*

A-HydroCort® [US] *see* hydrocortisone (systemic) *on page 449*

Airet® ***(Discontinued)*** *see page 1042*

Airomir [Can] *see* albuterol *on page 25*

AKBeta® ***(Discontinued)*** *see page 1042*

Ak-Chlor® Ophthalmic ***(Discontinued)*** *see page 1042*

AK-Con™ [US] *see* naphazoline *on page 604*

AK-Dilate® [US] *see* phenylephrine *on page 689*

AK-Fluor [US] *see* fluorescein sodium *on page 375*

Ak-Homatropine® Ophthalmic ***(Discontinued)*** *see page 104*

Akineton® [US/Can] *see* biperiden *on page 119*

AK-Mycin® ***(Discontinued)*** *see page 1042*

AK-Nefrin® [US] *see* phenylephrine *on page 689*

Akne-Mycin® [US] *see* erythromycin *on page 320*

Akoline® C.B. Tablet ***(Discontinued)*** *see page 1042*

AK-Pentolate® ***(Discontinued)*** *see page 1042*

AK-Poly-Bac® [US] *see* bacitracin and polymyxin B *on page 97*

AK-Pred® [US] *see* prednisolone (ophthalmic) *on page 723*

AK-Spore® H.C. Ophthalmic ***(Discontinued)*** *see page 1042*

AK-Spore® H.C. Otic ***(Discontinued)*** *see page 1042*

AK-Spore® Ophthalmic Ointment ***(Discontinued)*** *see page 1042*

AK-Sulf® [US] *see* sulfacetamide *on page 829*

AK-Taine® ***(Discontinued)*** *see page 1042*

AK-T-Caine™ [US] *see* tetracaine *on page 851*

AKTob® [US] *see* tobramycin *on page 866*

AK-Tracin® ***(Discontinued)*** *see page 1042*

AK-Trol® [US] *see* neomycin, polymyxin B, and dexamethasone *on page 611*

Akwa Tears® [US-OTC] *see* artificial tears *on page 78*

AK-Zol® ***(Discontinued)*** *see page 1042*

Ala-Cort® ***(Discontinued)*** *see page 1042*

Alamag Plus [US-OTC] *see* aluminum hydroxide, magnesium hydroxide, and simethicone *on page 40*

Alamag [US-OTC] *see* aluminum hydroxide and magnesium hydroxide *on page 40*

Alamast™ [US/Can] *see* pemirolast *on page 673*

Ala-Scalp® ***(Discontinued)*** *see page 1042*

Ala-Tet® ***(Discontinued)*** *see page 1042*

Alavert™ Allergy and Sinus [US-OTC] *see* loratadine and pseudoephedrine *on page 530*

Alavert™ [US-OTC] *see* loratadine *on page 530*

Alazide® ***(Discontinued)*** *see page 1042*

Albalon® [US] *see* naphazoline *on page 604*

Albalon®-A Liquifilm [Can] *see* naphazoline and antazoline *on page 604*

Albalon-A® Ophthalmic ***(Discontinued)*** *see page 1042*

albendazole (al BEN da zole)

U.S./Canadian Brand Names Albenza® [US]

Therapeutic Category Anthelmintic

Use Treatment of parenchymal neurocysticercosis caused by *Taenia solium* and cystic hydatid disease of the liver, lung, and peritoneum caused by *Echinococcus granulosus*

Usual Dosage Oral:

Children and Adults:

Neurocysticercosis:

<60 kg: 15 mg/kg/day in 2 divided doses (maximum: 800 mg/day) for 8-30 days

≥60 kg: 400 mg twice daily for 8-30 days

Note: Give concurrent anticonvulsant and steroid therapy during first week.

[illegible]ydatid:

[illegible]60 kg: 15 mg/kg/day in 2 divided doses (maximum: 800 mg/day)

[illegible]0 kg: 400 mg twice daily

Note: Administer dose for three 28-day cycles with a 14-day drug-free interval in between.

Dosage Forms Tablet: 200 mg

Albenza® [US] *see* albendazole *on previous page*

Albert® Docusate [Can] *see* docusate *on page 285*

Albert® Glyburide [Can] *see* glyburide *on page 409*

Albert® Pentoxifylline [Can] *see* pentoxifylline *on page 680*

Albert® Tiafen [Can] *see* tiaprofenic acid *(Canada only) on page 861*

Albumarc® [US] *see* albumin *on this page*

albumin (al BYOO min)

Sound-Alike/Look-Alike Issues

Albutein® may be confused with albuterol

Buminate® may be confused with bumetanide

Synonyms albumin (human); normal human serum albumin; normal serum albumin (human); salt poor albumin; SPA

U.S./Canadian Brand Names Albumarc® [US]; Albuminar® [US]; Albutein® [US]; Buminate® [US]; Plasbumin® [US]; Plasbumin®-5 [Can]; Plasbumin®-25 [Can]

Therapeutic Category Blood Product Derivative

Use Plasma volume expansion and maintenance of cardiac output in the treatment of certain types of shock or impending shock; may be useful for burn patients, ARDS, and cardiopulmonary bypass; other uses considered by some investigators (but not proven) are retroperitoneal surgery, peritonitis, and ascites; unless the condition responsible for hypoproteinemia can be corrected, albumin can provide only symptomatic relief or supportive treatment

Usual Dosage I.V.:

5% should be used in hypovolemic patients or intravascularly-depleted patients

25% should be used in patients in whom fluid and sodium intake must be minimized

Dose depends on condition of patient:

Children: Hypovolemia: 0.5-1 g/kg/dose (10-20 mL/kg/dose of albumin 5%); maximum dose: 6 g/kg/day

Adults: Usual dose: 25 g; initial dose may be repeated in 15-30 minutes if response is inadequate; no more than 250 g should be administered within 48 hours

Hypoproteinemia: 0.5-1 g/kg/dose; repeat every 1-2 days as calculated to replace ongoing losses

Hypovolemia: 0.5-1 g/kg/dose; repeat as needed; maximum dose: 6 g/kg/day

Dosage Forms Injection, solution, human: 5% [50 mg/mL] (50 mL, 250 mL, 500 mL); 25% [250 mg/mL] (50 mL, 100 mL)

Albumarc®: 5% [50 mg/mL] (250 mL, 500 mL); 25% [250 mg/mL] (50 mL, 100 mL)

Albuminar®: 5% [50 mg/mL] (50 mL, 250 mL, 500 mL, 1000 mL); 25% [250 mg/mL] (20 mL, 50 mL, 100 mL)

Albutein®, Buminate®: 5% [50 mg/mL]: (250 mL, 500 mL); 25% [250 mg/mL] (20 mL, 50 mL, 100 mL)

Plasbumin®: 5% [50 mg/mL] (50 mL, 250 mL, 500 mL); 25% [250 mg/mL] (20 mL, 50 mL, 100 mL)

Albuminar® [US] *see* albumin *on this page*

albumin (human) *see* albumin *on this page*

Albumisol® ***(Discontinued)*** *see page 1042*

Albunex® ***(Discontinued)*** *see page 1042*

Albutein® [US] *see* albumin *on this page*

albuterol (al BYOO ter ole)

Sound-Alike/Look-Alike Issues

Albuterol may be confused with Albutein®, atenolol

(Continued)

albuterol *(Continued)*

Proventil® may be confused with Bentyl®, Prilosec® Prinivil®
Salbutamol may be confused with salmeterol
Ventolin® may be confused with phentolamine, Benylin®, Vantin®
Volmax® may be confused with Flomax®

Synonyms albuterol sulfate; salbutamol

U.S./Canadian Brand Names AccuNeb™ [US]; Airomir [Can]; Alti-Salbutamol [Can]; Apo-Salvent® [Can]; Gen-Salbutamol [Can]; PMS-Salbutamol [Can]; Proventil® [US]; Proventil® HFA [US]; Proventil® Repetabs® [US]; ratio-Inspra-Sal [Can]; ratio-Salbutamol [Can]; Rhoxal-salbutamol [Can]; Salbu-2 [Can]; Salbu-4 [Can]; Ventolin® [Can]; Ventolin® Diskus [Can]; Ventolin® HFA [US]; Ventrodisk [Can]; Volmax® [US]; VoSpire ER™ [US]

Therapeutic Category Adrenergic Agonist Agent

Use Bronchodilator in reversible airway obstruction due to asthma or COPD; prevention of exercise-induced bronchospasm

Usual Dosage

Oral:

Children: Bronchospasm (treatment):

2-6 years: 0.1-0.2 mg/kg/dose 3 times/day; maximum dose not to exceed 12 mg/day (divided doses)

6-12 years: 2 mg/dose 3-4 times/day; maximum dose not to exceed 24 mg/day (divided doses) Extended release: 4 mg every 12 hours; maximum dose not to exceed 24 mg/day (divided doses)

Children >12 years and Adults: Bronchospasm (treatment): 2-4 mg/dose 3-4 times/day; maximum dose not to exceed 32 mg/day (divided doses)

Extended release: 8 mg every 12 hours; maximum dose not to exceed 32 mg/day (divided doses). A 4 mg dose every 12 hours may be sufficient in some patients, such as adults of low body weight.

Inhalation: MDI 90 mcg/puff:

Children ≤12 years:

Bronchospasm (acute): 4-8 puffs every 20 minutes for 3 doses, then every 1-4 hours; spacer/holding-chamber device should be used

Exercise-induced bronchospasm (prophylaxis): 1-2 puffs 5 minutes prior to exercise

Children >12 years and Adults:

Bronchospasm (acute): 4-8 puffs every 20 minutes for up to 4 hours, then every 1-4 hours as needed

Exercise-induced bronchospasm (prophylaxis): 2 puffs 5-30 minutes prior to exercise

Children ≥4 years and Adults: Bronchospasm (chronic treatment): 1-2 inhalations every 4-6 hours; maximum: 12 inhalations/day

NIH guidelines: 2 puffs 3-4 times a day as needed; may double dose for mild exacerbations

Nebulization:

Children ≤12 years:

Bronchospasm (treatment): 0.05 mg/kg every 4-6 hours; minimum dose: 1.25 mg, maximum dose: 2.5 mg 2-12 years: AccuNeb™: 0.63 mg or 1.25 mg 3-4 times/day, as needed, delivered over 5-15 minutes Children >40 kg, patients with more severe asthma, or children 11-12 years: May respond better with a 1.25 mg dose

Bronchospasm (acute): Solution 0.5%: 0.15 mg/kg (minimum dose: 2.5 mg) every 20 minutes for 3 doses, then 0.15-0.3 mg/kg (up to 10 mg) every 1-4 hours as needed; may also use 0.5 mg/kg/hour by continuous infusion. Continuous nebulized albuterol at 0.3 mg/kg/hour has been used safely in the treatment of severe status asthmaticus in children; continuous nebulized doses of 3 mg/kg/hour ± 2.2 mg/kg/hour in children whose mean age was 20.7 months resulted in no cardiac toxicity; the optimal dosage for continuous nebulization remains to be determined.

Note: Use of the 0.5% solution should be used for bronchospasm (acute or treatment) in children <15 kg. AccuNeb™ has not been studied for the treatment of acute bronchospasm; use of the 0.5% concentrated solution may be more appropriate.

Children >12 years and Adults:
Bronchospasm (treatment): 2.5 mg, diluted to a total of 3 mL, 3-4 times/day over 5-15 minutes NIH guidelines: 1.25-5 mg every 4-8 hours
Bronchospasm (acute) in intensive care patients: 2.5-5 mg every 20 minutes for 3 doses, then 2.5-10 mg every 1-4 hours as needed, **or** 10-15 mg/hour continuously

Dosage Forms [DSC] = Discontinued product
Aerosol, oral: 90 mcg/dose (17 g) [200 doses]
Proventil®: 90 mcg/dose (17 g) [200 doses]
Ventolin® [DSC]: 90 mcg/dose (6.8 g) [80 doses]; (17 g) [200 doses]
Aerosol, oral, as sulfate [chlorofluorocarbon free]:
Proventil® HFA: 90 mcg/dose (6.7 g) [200 doses]
Ventolin® HFA: 90 mcg/dose (18 g) [200 doses]
Solution for oral inhalation, as sulfate: 0.083% (3 mL); 0.5% (20 mL)
AccuNeb™: 0.63 mg/3 mL (3 mL); 1.25 mg/3 mL (3 mL)
Proventil®: 0.083% (3 mL); 0.5% (20 mL)
Syrup, as sulfate: 2 mg/5 mL (480 mL)
Tablet, as sulfate: 2 mg, 4 mg
Tablet, extended release, as sulfate:
Proventil® Repetabs®: 4 mg
Volmax®, VoSpire ER™: 4 mg, 8 mg

albuterol and ipratropium *see* ipratropium and albuterol *on page 483*

albuterol sulfate *see* albuterol *on page 25*

Alcaine® [US/Can] *see* proparacaine *on page 738*

Alcalak [US-OTC] *see* calcium carbonate *on page 144*

alclometasone (al kloe MET a sone)

Sound-Alike/Look-Alike Issues
Aclovate® may be confused with Accolate®

Synonyms alclometasone dipropionate

U.S./Canadian Brand Names Aclovate® [US]

Therapeutic Category Corticosteroid, Topical

Use Treatment of inflammation of corticosteroid-responsive dermatosis (low potency topical corticosteroid)

Usual Dosage Topical: Apply a thin film to the affected area 2-3 times/day. Therapy should be discontinued when control is achieved; if no improvement is seen, reassessment of diagnosis may be necessary.

Dosage Forms
Cream, as dipropionate: 0.05% (15 g, 45 g, 60 g)
Ointment, as dipropionate: 0.05% (15 g, 45 g, 60 g)

alclometasone dipropionate *see* alclometasone *on this page*

alcohol, absolute *see* alcohol (ethyl) *on this page*

alcohol, dehydrated *see* alcohol (ethyl) *on this page*

alcohol (ethyl) (AL koe hol ETH il)

Sound-Alike/Look-Alike Issues
ethanol may be confused with Ethyol®, Ethamolin®

Synonyms alcohol, absolute; alcohol, dehydrated; ethanol; ethyl alcohol; EtOH

U.S./Canadian Brand Names Biobase™ [Can]; Biobase-G™ [Can]; Diluso[illegible] Duonalc® [Can]; Duonalc-E® Mild [Can]; Lavacol® [US-OTC]

Therapeutic Category Intravenous Nutritional Therapy; Pharmaceutica[illegible]

Use Topical antiinfective; pharmaceutical aid; therapeutic neurolysis (ne[illegible] block); replenishment of fluid and carbohydrate calories

Usual Dosage
Oral: **Note:** Oral dosing is not recommended outside of a hospit[illegible]
600 mg/kg [equivalent to 1.8 mL/kg using a 43% solution]

(Continued)

alcohol (ethyl) *(Continued)*

Maintenance dose: Nondrinker: 66 mg/kg/hour [equivalent to 0.2 mL/kg/hour using a 43% solution] Chronic drinker: 154 mg/kg/hour [equivalent to 0.46 mL/kg/hour using a 43% solution]

Dosage adjustment for hemodialysis: Maintenance dose: Nondrinker: 169 mg/kg/hour [equivalent to 0.5 mL/kg/hour using a 43% solution] Chronic drinker: 257 mg/kg/hour [equivalent to 0.77 mL/kg/hour using a 43% solution]

I.V.: Initial dose: 600 mg/kg [equivalent to 7.6 mL/kg using a 10% solution]

Maintenance dose: Nondrinker: 66 mg/kg/hour [equivalent to 0.83 mL/kg/hour using a 10% solution] Chronic drinker: 154 mg/kg/hour [equivalent to 1.96 mL/kg/hour using a 10% solution]

Antiseptic: Children and Adults: Liquid denatured alcohol: Topical: Apply 1-3 times/day as needed

Therapeutic neurolysis (nerve or ganglion block): Adults: Dehydrated alcohol injection: Intraneural: Dosage variable depending upon the site of injection (eg, trigeminal neuralgia: 0.05-0.5 mL as a single injection per interspace vs subarachnoid injection: 0.5-1 mL as a single injection per interspace); single doses >1.5 mL are seldom required

Replenishment of fluid and carbohydrate calories: Adults: Dehydrated alcohol infusion: Alcohol 5% and dextrose 5%: 1-2 L/day by slow infusion

Dosage Forms

Infusion [in D_5W, dehydrated]: Alcohol 5% (1000 mL); alcohol 10% (1000 mL)

Injection, solution [dehydrated]: 98% (1 mL, 5 mL)

Liquid, topical [denatured] (Lavacol®): 70% (473 mL)

Alcomicin® [Can] *see* gentamicin *on page 403*

Alconefrin® Nasal Solution *(Discontinued)* *see page 1042*

Aldactazide® [US] *see* hydrochlorothiazide and spironolactone *on page 443*

Aldactazide 25® [Can] *see* hydrochlorothiazide and spironolactone *on page 443*

Aldactazide 50® [Can] *see* hydrochlorothiazide and spironolactone *on page 443*

Aldactone® [US/Can] *see* spironolactone *on page 821*

Aldara™ [US/Can] *see* imiquimod *on page 467*

aldesleukin (al des LOO kin)

Sound-Alike/Look-Alike Issues

aldesleukin may be confused with oprelvekin

Proleukin® may be confused with oprelvekin

Synonyms epidermal thymocyte activating factor; ETAF; IL-2; interleukin-2; lymphocyte mitogenic factor; NSC-373364; T-cell growth factor; TCGF; thymocyte stimulating factor

U.S./Canadian Brand Names Proleukin® [US/Can]

Therapeutic Category Biological Response Modulator

Use Treatment of metastatic renal cell cancer, melanoma

Usual Dosage Refer to individual protocols.

I.V.:

Renal cell carcinoma: 600,000 int. units/kg every 8 hours for a maximum of 14 doses; repeat after 9 days of rest for a total of 28 doses per course. Re-evaluate at 4 weeks. Retreat if needed 7 weeks after hospital discharge from previous course.

Melanoma:

Single-agent use: 600,000 int. units/kg every 8 hours for a maximum of 14 doses; repeat after 9 days of rest for a total of 28 doses per course. Re-evaluate at 4 weeks. Retreat if needed 7 weeks after hospital discharge from previous course.

In combination with cytotoxic agents: 24 million int. units/m^2 days 12-16 and 19-23

ubQ:

ingle-agent doses: 3-18 million int. units/day for 5 days weekly and repeated weekly to 6 weeks

In combination with interferon:

5 million int. units/m^2 3 times/week

1.8 million int. units/m^2 twice daily 5 days/week for 6 weeks

Investigational regimen: SubQ: 11 million int. units (flat dose) daily x 4 days per week for 4 consecutive weeks; repeat every 6 weeks

Dosage Forms Injection, powder for reconstitution: 22 x 10^6 int. units [18 million int. units/mL = 1.1 mg/mL when reconstituted]

Aldex™ [US] *see* guaifenesin and phenylephrine *on page 418*

Aldoclor® *(Discontinued)* *see page 1042*

Aldomet® *(Discontinued)* *see page 1042*

Aldoril® [US] *see* methyldopa and hydrochlorothiazide *on page 569*

Aldoril® D [US] *see* methyldopa and hydrochlorothiazide *on page 569*

Aldoril® D50 *(Discontinued)* *see page 1042*

Aldroxicon II [US-OTC] *see* aluminum hydroxide, magnesium hydroxide, and simethicone *on page 40*

Aldroxicon I [US-OTC] *see* aluminum hydroxide, magnesium hydroxide, and simethicone *on page 40*

Aldurazyme® [US] *see* laronidase *on page 507*

alefacept (a LE fa sept)

Synonyms B 9273; BG 9273; human LFA-3/IgG(1) fusion protein; LFA-3/IgG(1) fusion protein, human

U.S./Canadian Brand Names Amevive® [US]

Therapeutic Category Monoclonal Antibody

Controlled Substance Alefacept will be distributed directly to physician offices or to a specialty pharmacy; injections are intended to be administered in the physician's office

Use Treatment of moderate to severe plaque psoriasis in adults who are candidates for systemic therapy or phototherapy

Usual Dosage Adults:

I.M.: 15 mg once weekly; usual duration of treatment: 12 weeks

I.V.: 7.5 mg once weekly; usual duration of treatment: 12 weeks

A second course of treatment may be initiated at least 12 weeks after completion of the initial course of treatment, provided CD4$^+$ T-lymphocyte counts are within the normal range.

Note: CD4$^+$ T-lymphocyte counts should be monitored before initiation of treatment and weekly during therapy. Dosing should be withheld if CD4$^+$ counts are <250 cells/μL, and dosing should be permanently discontinued if CD4$^+$ lymphocyte counts remain at <250 cell/μL for longer than 1 month.

Dosage Forms [DSC] = Discontinued product

Injection, powder for reconstitution: 7.5 mg [for I.V. administration; supplied with SWFI] [DSC]

Injection, powder for reconstitution: 15 mg [for I.M. administration; supplied with SWFI'

alemtuzumab (ay lem TU zoo mab)

Synonyms campath-1H; DNA-derived humanized monoclonal antibody; hu IgG1 anti-CD52 monoclonal antibody

U.S./Canadian Brand Names Campath® [US]

Therapeutic Category Antineoplastic Agent, Monoclonal Antibody

Use Treatment of B-cell chronic lymphocytic leukemia (B-CLL)

Usual Dosage Note: **Dose escalation is required;** usually accomr Do not exceed single doses >30 mg or cumulative doses >90 m with diphenhydramine and acetaminophen 30 minutes before initi (Continued)

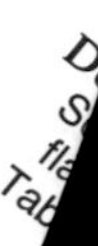

alemtuzumab *(Continued)*

antiinfective prophylaxis. Discontinue therapy during serious infection, serious hematologic or other serious toxicity until the event resolves. Permanently discontinue if evidence of autoimmune anemia or autoimmune thrombocytopenia occurs.

I.V. infusion: Adults: B-CLL: **Note:** A similar dosing regimen has been successfully administered subcutaneously (Lundin, 2002):

Initial: 3 mg/day as a 2-hour infusion; increase to 10 mg/day, then to 30 mg/day as tolerated

Maintenance: 30 mg/day 3 times/week on alternate days for up to 12 weeks

Dosage adjustment for hematologic toxicity (severe neutropenia or thrombocytopenia, not autoimmune):

First occurrence: ANC <250/µL and/or platelet count ≤25,000/µL: Hold therapy; resume at same dose when ANC ≥500/µL and platelet count ≥50,000/µL. If delay between dosing is ≥7 days, restart at 3 mg/day and escalate as tolerated.

Second occurrence: ANC <250/µL and/or platelet count ≤25,000/µL: Hold therapy; resume at 10 mg/day when ANC ≥500/µL and platelet count ≥50,000/µL. If delay between dosing is ≥7 days, restart at 3 mg/day and escalate as tolerated.

Third occurrence: ANC <250/µL and/or platelet count ≤25,000/µL: Permanently discontinue therapy

Patients with a baseline ANC ≤500/µL and/or a baseline platelet count ≤25,000/µL at initiation of therapy: If ANC and/or platelet counts decreased to ≤50% of the baseline value, hold therapy. When ANC and/or platelet count return to baseline, resume therapy. If delay between dosing is ≥7 days, restart at 3 mg/day and escalate as tolerated.

Dosage Forms Injection, solution: 10 mg/mL (3 mL)

alendronate (a LEN droe nate)

Sound-Alike/Look-Alike Issues

Fosamax® may be confused with Flomax®

Synonyms alendronate sodium

U.S./Canadian Brand Names Fosamax® [US/Can]; Novo-Alendronate [Can]

Therapeutic Category Bisphosphonate Derivative

Use Treatment and prevention of osteoporosis in postmenopausal females; treatment of osteoporosis in males; Paget disease of the bone in patients who are symptomatic, at risk for future complications, or with alkaline phosphatase ≥2 times the upper limit of normal; treatment of glucocorticoid-induced osteoporosis in males and females with low bone mineral density who are receiving a daily dosage ≥7.5 mg of prednisone (or equivalent)

Usual Dosage Oral: Adults: **Note:** Patients treated with glucocorticoids and those with Paget disease should receive adequate amounts of calcium and vitamin D.

Osteoporosis in postmenopausal females:

Prophylaxis: 5 mg once daily **or** 35 mg once weekly

Treatment: 10 mg once daily **or** 70 mg once weekly

Osteoporosis in males: 10 mg once daily **or** 70 mg once weekly

Osteoporosis secondary to glucocorticoids in males and females: Treatment: 5 mg once daily; a dose of 10 mg once daily should be used in postmenopausal females who are not receiving estrogen.

Paget disease of bone in males and females: 40 mg once daily for 6 months

Retreatment: Relapses during the 12 months following therapy occurred in 9% of patients who responded to treatment. Specific retreatment data are not available. Retreatment with alendronate may be considered, following a 6-month post-treatment evaluation period, in patients who have relapsed based on increases in serum alkaline phosphatase, which should be measured periodically. Retreatment may also be considered in those who failed to normalize their serum alkaline phosphatase.

sage Forms

lution, oral, as monosodium trihydrate: 70 mg/75 mL [contains parabens; raspberry vor]

let, as sodium: 5 mg, 10 mg, 35 mg, 40 mg, 70 mg

alendronate sodium *see* alendronate *on previous page*

Aler-Dryl [US-OTC] *see* diphenhydramine *on page 277*

Alertec® [Can] *see* modafinil *on page 587*

Alesse® [US/Can] *see* ethinyl estradiol and levonorgestrel *on page 339*

Aleve® [US-OTC] *see* naproxen *on page 605*

Alfenta® [US/Can] *see* alfentanil *on this page*

alfentanil (al FEN ta nil)

Sound-Alike/Look-Alike Issues

alfentanil may be confused with Anafranil®, fentanyl, remifentanil, sufentanil

Alfenta® may be confused with Sufenta®

Synonyms alfentanil hydrochloride

U.S./Canadian Brand Names Alfenta® [US/Can]

Therapeutic Category Analgesic, Narcotic; General Anesthetic

Controlled Substance C-II

Use Analgesic adjunct given by continuous infusion or in incremental doses in maintenance of anesthesia with barbiturate or N_2O or a primary anesthetic agent for the induction of anesthesia in patients undergoing general surgery in which endotracheal intubation and mechanical ventilation are required

Usual Dosage Doses should be titrated to appropriate effects; wide range of doses is dependent upon desired degree of analgesia/anesthesia

Children <12 years: Dose not established

Adults: Anesthesia of ≤30 minutes: Initial (induction): 8-20 mcg/kg, then 3-5 mcg/kg/dose or 0.5-1 mcg/kg/minute for maintenance; total dose: 8-40 mcg/kg; higher doses used for longer anesthesia required procedures

Dosage Forms Injection, solution, as hydrochloride [preservative free]: 500 mcg/mL (2 mL, 5 mL, 10 mL, 20 mL)

alfentanil hydrochloride *see* alfentanil *on this page*

Alferon® N [US/Can] *see* interferon alfa-n3 *on page 479*

alfuzosin (al FYOO zoe sin)

Synonyms alfuzosin hydrochloride

U.S./Canadian Brand Names Uroxatral™ [US]

Therapeutic Category Alpha-Adrenergic Blocking Agent

Use Treatment of the functional symptoms of benign prostatic hyperplasia (BPH)

Usual Dosage Oral: Adults: 10 mg once daily

Dosage Forms Tablet, extended release, as hydrochloride: 10 mg

alfuzosin hydrochloride *see* alfuzosin *on this page*

alglucerase (al GLOO ser ase)

Sound-Alike/Look-Alike Issues

Ceredase® may be confused with Cerezyme®

Synonyms glucocerebrosidase

U.S./Canadian Brand Names Ceredase® [US]

Therapeutic Category Enzyme

Use Replacement therapy for Gaucher disease (type 1)

Usual Dosage I.V.: Children and Adults: Initial: 30-60 units/kg every 2 weeks individualized based on disease severity; average dose: 60 units/kg eve Range: 2.5 units/kg 3 times/week to 60 units/kg 1-4 times/week. Once pa is well established, dose may be reduced every 3-6 months to determ therapy.

Dosage Forms Injection, solution [preservative free]: 10 units/mL (5 mL) [contains human albumin 1%]

Alimta® [US] *see* pemetrexed *on page 673*

Alinia® [US] *see* nitazoxanide *on page 621*

alitretinoin (a li TRET i noyn)

Sound-Alike/Look-Alike Issues
Panretin® may be confused with pancreatin

U.S./Canadian Brand Names Panretin® [US/Can]

Therapeutic Category Antineoplastic Agent, Miscellaneous; Retinoic Acid Derivative

Use **Orphan drug:** Topical treatment of cutaneous lesions in AIDS-related Kaposi sarcoma

Usual Dosage Topical: Apply gel twice daily to cutaneous Kaposi sarcoma lesions

Dosage Forms Gel: 0.1% (60 g tube)

Alka-Mints® [US-OTC] *see* calcium carbonate *on page 144*

Alka-Seltzer® Gas Relief [US-OTC] *see* simethicone *on page 804*

Alka-Seltzer® Plus Cold and Cough [US-OTC] *see* chlorpheniramine, phenylephrine, and dextromethorphan *on page 191*

Alka-Seltzer® Plus Cold and Sinus Liqui-Gels® [US-OTC] *see* acetaminophen and pseudoephedrine *on page 9*

Alka-Seltzer® Plus Cold Liqui-Gels® [US-OTC] *see* acetaminophen, chlorpheniramine, and pseudoephedrine *on page 11*

Alka-Seltzer® Plus Flu Liqui-Gels® [US-OTC] *see* acetaminophen, dextromethorphan, and pseudoephedrine *on page 12*

Alkeran® [US/Can] *see* melphalan *on page 550*

Allbee® C-800 + Iron [US-OTC] *see* vitamin B complex combinations *on page 915*

Allbee® C-800 [US-OTC] *see* vitamin B complex combinations *on page 915*

Allbee® with C [US-OTC] *see* vitamin B complex combinations *on page 915*

Allegra® [US/Can] *see* fexofenadine *on page 366*

Allegra® 60 mg Capsule *(Discontinued)* *see page 1042*

Allegra-D® [US/Can] *see* fexofenadine and pseudoephedrine *on page 366*

Aller-Chlor® [US-OTC] *see* chlorpheniramine *on page 187*

Allercon® Tablet *(Discontinued)* *see page 1042*

Allerdryl® [Can] *see* diphenhydramine *on page 277*

Allerest® 12 Hour Capsule *(Discontinued)* *see page 1042*

Allerest® 12 Hour Nasal Solution *(Discontinued)* *see page 1042*

Allerest® Eye Drops *(Discontinued)* *see page 1042*

Allerest® Maximum Strength Allergy and Hay Fever [US-OTC] *see* chlorpheniramine and pseudoephedrine *on page 189*

Allerfrim® [US-OTC] *see* triprolidine and pseudoephedrine *on page 889*

Allerfrin® Syrup *(Discontinued)* *see page 1042*

Allerfrin® Tablet *(Discontinued)* *see page 1042*

Allerfrin® With Codeine *(Discontinued)* *see page 1042*

llergan® [US] *see* antipyrine and benzocaine *on page 65*

lerMax® [US-OTC] *see* diphenhydramine *on page 277*

rnix [Can] *see* diphenhydramine *on page 277*

rphed® [US-OTC] *see* triprolidine and pseudoephedrine *on page 889*

sol® [US] *see* naphazoline *on page 604*

Jr [US] *see* guaifenesin *on page 415*

allopurinol (al oh PURE i nole)

Sound-Alike/Look-Alike Issues

allopurinol may be confused with Apresoline®

Zyloprim® may be confused with Xylo-Pfan®, ZORprin®

Synonyms allopurinol sodium

U.S./Canadian Brand Names Aloprim™ [US]; Apo-Allopurinol® [Can]; Zyloprim® [US/Can]

Therapeutic Category Xanthine Oxidase Inhibitor

Use

Oral: Prevention of attack of gouty arthritis and nephropathy; treatment of secondary hyperuricemia which may occur during treatment of tumors or leukemia; prevention of recurrent calcium oxalate calculi

I.V.: Treatment of elevated serum and urinary uric acid levels when oral therapy is not tolerated in patients with leukemia, lymphoma, and solid tumor malignancies who are receiving cancer chemotherapy

Usual Dosage

Oral: Doses >300 mg should be given in divided doses.

Children ≤10 years: Secondary hyperuricemia associated with chemotherapy: 10 mg/kg/day in 2-3 divided doses **or** 200-300 $mg/m^2/day$ in 2-4 divided doses, maximum: 800 mg/24 hours

Alternative (manufacturer labeling): <6 years: 150 mg/day in 3 divided doses; 6-10 years: 300 mg/day in 2-3 divided doses

Children >10 years and Adults:

Secondary hyperuricemia associated with chemotherapy: 600-800 mg/day in 2-3 divided doses for prevention of acute uric acid nephropathy for 2-3 days starting 1-2 days before chemotherapy

Gout: Mild: 200-300 mg/day; Severe: 400-600 mg/day; to reduce the possibility of acute gouty attacks, initiate dose at 100 mg/day and increase weekly to recommended dosage.

Recurrent calcium oxalate stones: 200-300 mg/day in single or divided doses

I.V.: Hyperuricemia secondary to chemotherapy: Intravenous daily dose can be given as a single infusion or in equally divided doses at 6-, 8-, or 12-hour intervals. A fluid intake sufficient to yield a daily urinary output of at least 2 L in adults and the maintenance of a neutral or, preferably, slightly alkaline urine are desirable.

Children ≤10 years: Starting dose: 200 $mg/m^2/day$

Children >10 years and Adults: 200-400 $mg/m^2/day$ (max: 600 mg/day)

Dosage Forms

Injection, powder for reconstitution, as sodium (Aloprim™): 500 mg

Tablet (Zyloprim®): 100 mg, 300 mg

allopurinol sodium *see* allopurinol *on this page*

Almacone Double Strength® [US-OTC] *see* aluminum hydroxide, magnesium hydroxide, and simethicone *on page 40*

Almacone® [US-OTC] *see* aluminum hydroxide, magnesium hydroxide, and simethicone *on page 40*

Almora® [US-OTC] *see* magnesium gluconate *on page 537*

almotriptan (al moh TRIP tan)

Synonyms almotriptan malate

U.S./Canadian Brand Names Axert™ [US/Can]

Therapeutic Category Serotonin $5\text{-}HT_{1D}$ Receptor Agonist

Use Acute treatment of migraine with or without aura

Usual Dosage Oral: Adults: Migraine: Initial: 6.25-12.5 mg in a single d headache returns, repeat the dose after 2 hours; no more than 2 dose period

Note: If the first dose is ineffective, diagnosis needs to be re-eval treating more than 4 migraines/month has not been established.

Dosage Forms Tablet, as malate: 6.25 mg, 12.5 mg

almotriptan malate *see* almotriptan *on previous page*

Alocril™ [US/Can] *see* nedocromil (ophthalmic) *on page 608*

Aloe Vesta® 2-n-1 Antifungal [US-OTC] *see* miconazole *on page 578*

Alomide® [US/Can] *see* lodoxamide tromethamine *on page 526*

Alophen® [US-OTC] *see* bisacodyl *on page 120*

Aloprim™ [US] *see* allopurinol *on previous page*

Alor® 5/500 ***(Discontinued)*** *see page 1042*

Alora® [US] *see* estradiol *on page 324*

alosetron (a LOE se tron)

Sound-Alike/Look-Alike Issues

Lotronex® may be confused with Lovenox®, Protonix®

U.S./Canadian Brand Names Lotronex® [US]

Therapeutic Category 5-HT$_3$ Receptor Antagonist

Use Treatment of irritable bowel syndrome (IBS) in women with severe diarrhea-predominant IBS who have failed to respond to conventional therapy

Usual Dosage Oral: Adults: Female: Initial: 1 mg once daily for 4 weeks, with or without food; if tolerated, but response is inadequate, may be increased after 4 weeks to 1 mg twice daily. If response is inadequate after 4 weeks of twice daily dosing, discontinue treatment.

Note: Discontinue immediately if constipation or signs/symptoms of ischemic colitis occur. Do not reinitiate in patients who develop ischemic colitis.

Dosage Forms Tablet: 0.5 mg, 1 mg

Aloxi™ [US] *see* palonosetron *on page 661*

alpha$_1$-antitrypsin *see* alpha$_1$-proteinase inhibitor *on this page*

alpha$_1$-PI *see* alpha$_1$-proteinase inhibitor *on this page*

alpha$_1$-proteinase inhibitor (al fa won-PRO tee in ase in HI bi tor)

Synonyms A$_1$-PI; alpha$_1$-antitrypsin; alpha$_1$-PI; alpha$_1$-proteinase inhibitor, human; α_1-PI

U.S./Canadian Brand Names Aralast™ [US]; Prolastin® [US/Can]; Zemaira™ [US]

Therapeutic Category Antitrypsin Deficiency Agent

Use Replacement therapy in congenital alpha$_1$-antitrypsin deficiency with clinical emphysema

Usual Dosage I.V.: Adults: 60 mg/kg once weekly

Dosage Forms

Injection, powder for reconstitution [single-dose vial]:

Aralast™, Prolastin®: 500 mg, 1000 mg [packaged with diluent]

Zemaira™: 1000 mg [packaged with diluent]

alpha$_1$-proteinase inhibitor, human *see* alpha$_1$-proteinase inhibitor *on this page*

alpha-galactosidase-A (human, recombinant) *see* agalsidase beta *on page 23*

Alphagan® ***(Discontinued)*** *see page 1042*

Alphagan® P [US/Can] *see* brimonidine *on page 127*

lphamul® ***(Discontinued)*** *see page 1042*

hanate® [US] *see* antihemophilic factor (human) *on page 62*

haNine® SD [US] *see* factor IX *on page 354*

aquin HP [US] *see* hydroquinone *on page 454*

alprazolam (al PRAY zoe lam)

Sound-Alike/Look-Alike Issues

alprazolam may be confused with alprostadil, lorazepam, triazolam

Xanax® may be confused with Lanoxin®, Tenex®, Tylox®, Xopenex®, Zantac®, Zyrtec®

U.S./Canadian Brand Names Alprazolam Intensol® [US]; Alti-Alprazolam [Can]; Apo-Alpraz® [Can]; Gen-Alprazolam [Can]; Novo-Alprazol [Can]; Nu-Alprax [Can]; Xanax® [US/Can]; Xanax TS™ [Can]; Xanax XR® [US]

Therapeutic Category Benzodiazepine

Controlled Substance C-IV

Use Treatment of anxiety disorder (GAD); panic disorder, with or without agoraphobia; anxiety associated with depression

Usual Dosage Oral: **Note:** Treatment >4 months should be re-evaluated to determine the patient's continued need for the drug

Adults:

Anxiety: Immediate release: Effective doses are 0.5-4 mg/day in divided doses; the manufacturer recommends starting at 0.25-0.5 mg 3 times/day; titrate dose upward; maximum: 4 mg/day

Anxiety associated with depression: Immediate release: Average dose required: 2.5-3 mg/day in divided doses

Panic disorder:

Immediate release: Initial: 0.5 mg 3 times/day; dose may be increased every 3-4 days in increments ≤1 mg/day; many patients obtain relief at 2 mg/day, as much as 10 mg/day may be required

Extended release: 0.5-1 mg once daily; may increase dose every 3-4 days in increments ≤1 mg/day (range: 3-6 mg/day)

Switching from immediate release to extended release: Patients may be switched to extended release tablets by taking the total daily dose of the immediate release tablets and giving it once daily using the extended release preparation.

Dose reduction: Abrupt discontinuation should be avoided. Daily dose may be decreased by 0.5 mg every 3 days, however, some patients may require a slower reduction. If withdrawal symptoms occur, resume previous dose and discontinue on a less rapid schedule.

Dosage Forms

Solution, oral (Alprazolam Intensol®): 1 mg/mL (30 mL)

Tablet (Xanax®): 0.25 mg, 0.5 mg, 1 mg, 2 mg

Tablet, extended release (Xanax XR®): 0.5 mg, 1 mg, 2 mg, 3 mg

Alprazolam Intensol® [US] *see* alprazolam *on this page*

alprostadil (al PROS ta dill)

Sound-Alike/Look-Alike Issues

alprostadil may be confused with alprazolam

Synonyms PGE_1; prostaglandin E_1

U.S./Canadian Brand Names Caverject® [US/Can]; Caverject® Impulse™ [Can]; Edex® [US]; Muse® [Can]; Muse® Pellet [US]; Prostin® VR [Can]; Prostin VR Pediatric® [US]

Therapeutic Category Prostaglandin

Use

Prostin VR Pediatric®: Temporary maintenance of patency of ductus arteriosu[illegible] neonates with ductal-dependent congenital heart disease until surgery ca[illegible] performed. These defects include cyanotic (eg, pulmonary atresia, pulmonary s[illegible] tricuspid atresia, Fallot's tetralogy, transposition of the great vessels) and [illegible] (eg, interruption of aortic arch, coarctation of aorta, hypoplastic left ven[illegible] disease

Caverject®: Treatment of erectile dysfunction of vasculogenic, psychog[illegible] genic etiology; adjunct in the diagnosis of erectile dysfunction

Edex®, Muse®: Treatment of erectile dysfunction of vasculogeni[illegible] neurogenic etiology

(Continued)

alprostadil *(Continued)*

Usual Dosage

Patent ductus arteriosus (Prostin VR Pediatric®):

I.V. continuous infusion into a large vein, or alternatively through an umbilical artery catheter placed at the ductal opening: 0.05-0.1 mcg/kg/minute with therapeutic response, rate is reduced to lowest effective dosage; with unsatisfactory response, rate is increased gradually; maintenance: 0.01-0.4 mcg/kg/minute

PGE$_1$ is usually given at an infusion rate of 0.1 mcg/kg/minute, but it is often possible to reduce the dosage to 1/2 or even 1/10 without losing the therapeutic effect. The mixing schedule is as follows. Infusion rates deliver 0.1 mcg/kg/minute:

Therapeutic response is indicated by increased pH in those with acidosis or by an increase in oxygenation (PO$_2$) usually evident within 30 minutes

Erectile dysfunction:

Caverject®, Edex®: Intracavernous: Individualize dose by careful titration; doses >40 mcg (Edex®) or >60 mcg (Caverject®) are not recommended: Initial dose must be titrated in physicians office. Patient must stay in the physician's office until complete detumescence occurs; if there is no response, then the next higher dose may be given within 1 hour; if there is still no response, a 1-day interval before giving the next dose is recommended; increasing the dose or concentration in the treatment of impotence results in increasing pain and discomfort

Vasculogenic, psychogenic, or mixed etiology: Initiate dosage titration at 2.5 mcg, increasing by 2.5 mcg to a dose of 5 mcg and then in increments of 5-10 mcg depending on the erectile response until the dose produces an erection suitable for intercourse, not lasting >1 hour; if there is absolutely no response to initial 2.5 mcg dose, the second dose may be increased to 7.5 mcg, followed by increments of 5-10 mcg

Neurogenic etiology (eg, spinal cord injury): Initiate dosage titration at 1.25 mcg, increasing to a dose of 2.5 mcg and then 5 mcg; increase further in increments 5 mcg until the dose is reached that produces an erection suitable for intercourse, not lasting >1 hour

Maintenance: Once appropriate dose has been determined, patient may self-administer injections at a frequency of no more than 3 times/week with at least 24 hours between doses

Muse® Pellet: Intraurethral:

Initial: 125-250 mcg

Maintenance: Administer as needed to achieve an erection; duration of action is about 30-60 minutes; use only two systems per 24-hour period

Dosage Forms [DSC] = Discontinued product

Injection, powder for reconstitution:

Caverject®: 10 mcg, 20 mcg, 40 mcg [contains lactose; diluent contains benzyl alcohol]

Caverject® Impulse™: 10 mcg, 20 mcg [prefilled injection system; contains lactose; diluent contains benzyl alcohol]

Edex®: 10 mcg, 20 mcg, 40 mcg [contains lactose; diluent contains benzyl alcohol; also packaged in kits containing diluent, syringe, and alcohol swab]

Injection, solution: 500 mcg/mL (1 mL)

Caverject® [DSC]: 20 mcg/mL (2 mL)

Prostin VR Pediatric®: 500 mcg/mL (1 mL) [contains dehydrated alcohol]

Pellet, urethral (Muse®): 125 mcg, 250 mcg, 500 mcg, 1000 mcg

Alrex® [US/Can] *see* loteprednol *on page 532*

AL-Rr® Oral *(Discontinued)* *see page 1042*

ltace® [US/Can] *see* ramipril *on page 762*

amist [US-OTC] *see* sodium chloride *on page 810*

plase (AL te plase)

nd-Alike/Look-Alike Issues

plase may be confused with Altace™

Synonyms alteplase, recombinant; alteplase, tissue plasminogen activator, recombinant; tPA

U.S./Canadian Brand Names Activase® [US]; Activase® rt-PA [Can]; Cathflo™ Activase® [US/Can]

Therapeutic Category Fibrinolytic Agent

Use Management of acute myocardial infarction for the lysis of thrombi in coronary arteries; management of acute massive pulmonary embolism (PE) in adults

Acute myocardial infarction (AMI): Chest pain ≥20 minutes, ≤12-24 hours; S-T elevation ≥0.1 mV in at least two ECG leads

Acute pulmonary embolism (APE): Age ≤75 years: Documented massive pulmonary embolism by pulmonary angiography or echocardiography or high probability lung scan with clinical shock

Cathflo™ Activase®: Restoration of central venous catheter function

Usual Dosage

I.V.:

Coronary artery thrombi: Front loading dose (weight-based):

Patients >67 kg: Total dose: 100 mg over 1.5 hours; infuse 15 mg over 1-2 minutes. Infuse 50 mg over 30 minutes. See "Note."

Patients ≤67 kg: Total dose: 1.25 mg/kg; infuse 15 mg I.V. bolus over 1-2 minutes, then infuse 0.75 mg/kg (not to exceed 50 mg) over next 30 minutes, followed by 0.5 mg/kg over next 60 minutes (not to exceed 35 mg). See "Note."

Note: Concurrently, begin heparin 60 units/kg bolus (maximum: 4000 units) followed by continuous infusion of 12 units/kg/hour (maximum: 1000 units/hour) and adjust to aPTT target of 1.5-2 times the upper limit of control. Infuse remaining 35 mg of alteplase over the next hour.

Acute pulmonary embolism: 100 mg over 2 hours.

Acute ischemic stroke: Doses should be given within the first 3 hours of the onset of symptoms; recommended total dose: 0.9 mg/kg (maximum dose should not exceed 90 mg) infused over 60 minutes.

Load with 0.09 mg/kg (10% of the 0.9 mg/kg dose) as an I.V. bolus over 1 minute, followed by 0.81 mg/kg (90% of the 0.9 mg/kg dose) as a continuous infusion over 60 minutes. Heparin should not be started for 24 hours or more after starting alteplase for stroke.

Intracatheter: Central venous catheter clearance: Cathflo™ Activase®:

Patients ≥10 to <30 kg: 110% of the internal lumen volume of the catheter (≤2 mg [1 mg/mL]); retain in catheter for ≤2 hours; may instill a second dose if catheter remains occluded

Patients ≥30 kg: 2 mg (1 mg/mL); retain in catheter for ≤2 hours; may instill a second dose if catheter remains occluded

Advisory Panel to the Society for Cardiovascular and Interventional Radiology on Thrombolytic Therapy recommendation: ≤2 mg/hour and subtherapeutic heparin (aPTT <1.5 times baseline)

Dosage Forms Injection, powder for reconstitution, recombinant:

Activase®: 50 mg [29 million int. units]; 100 mg [58 million int. units]

Cathflo™ Activase®: 2 mg

alteplase, recombinant *see* alteplase *on previous page*

alteplase, tissue plasminogen activator, recombinant *see* alteplase *on previous page*

ALternaGel® [US-OTC] *see* aluminum hydroxide *on page 39*

Alti-Acyclovir [Can] *see* acyclovir *on page 19*

Alti-Alprazolam [Can] *see* alprazolam *on page 35*

Alti-Amiodarone [Can] *see* amiodarone *on page 47*

Alti-Amoxi-Clav® [Can] *see* amoxicillin and clavulanate potassium *on*

Alti-Azathioprine [Can] *see* azathioprine *on page 93*

Alti-Captopril [Can] *see* captopril *on page 153*

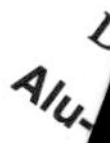

Alti-Clindamycin [Can] *see* clindamycin *on page 210*

Alti-Clobazam [Can] *see* clobazam *(Canada only) on page 212*

Alti-Clonazepam [Can] *see* clonazepam *on page 215*

Alti-CPA [Can] *see* cyproterone *(Canada only) on page 238*

Alti-Desipramine [Can] *see* desipramine *on page 251*

Alti-Diltiazem CD [Can] *see* diltiazem *on page 273*

Alti-Divalproex [Can] *see* valproic acid and derivatives *on page 901*

Alti-Domperidone [Can] *see* domperidone *(Canada only) on page 288*

Alti-Doxazosin [Can] *see* doxazosin *on page 291*

Alti-Flunisolide [Can] *see* flunisolide *on page 373*

Alti-Fluoxetine [Can] *see* fluoxetine *on page 379*

Alti-Flurbiprofen [Can] *see* flurbiprofen *on page 381*

Alti-Fluvoxamine [Can] *see* fluvoxamine *on page 385*

Alti-Ipratropium [Can] *see* ipratropium *on page 482*

Alti-Metformin [Can] *see* metformin *on page 560*

Alti-Minocycline [Can] *see* minocycline *on page 583*

Alti-Moclobemide [Can] *see* moclobemide *(Canada only) on page 587*

Alti-MPA [Can] *see* medroxyprogesterone acetate *on page 548*

Altinac™ [US] *see* tretinoin (topical) *on page 879*

Alti-Nadolol [Can] *see* nadolol *on page 599*

Alti-Nortriptyline [Can] *see* nortriptyline *on page 629*

Alti-Ranitidine [Can] *see* ranitidine hydrochloride *on page 763*

Alti-Salbutamol [Can] *see* albuterol *on page 25*

Alti-Sotalol [Can] *see* sotalol *on page 819*

Alti-Sulfasalazine [Can] *see* sulfasalazine *on page 833*

Alti-Terazosin [Can] *see* terazosin *on page 845*

Alti-Ticlopidine [Can] *see* ticlopidine *on page 862*

Alti-Timolol [Can] *see* timolol *on page 863*

Alti-Trazodone [Can] *see* trazodone *on page 877*

Alti-Verapamil [Can] *see* verapamil *on page 908*

Alti-Zopiclone [Can] *see* zopiclone *(Canada only) on page 944*

Altocor™ ***(Discontinued)*** *see page 1042*

Altoprev™ [US] *see* lovastatin *on page 533*

altretamine (al TRET a meen)

Synonyms hexamethylmelamine; HEXM; HMM; HXM; NSC-13875

U.S./Canadian Brand Names Hexalen® [US/Can]

Therapeutic Category Antineoplastic Agent

Use Palliative treatment of persistent or recurrent ovarian cancer

Usual Dosage Refer to individual protocols. Oral:

Adults: 4-12 mg/kg/day in 3-4 divided doses for 21-90 days

Alternatively: 240-320 mg/m^2/day in 3-4 divided doses for 21 days, repeated every 6 weeks

Alternatively: 260 mg/m^2/day for 14-21 days of a 28-day cycle in 4 divided doses

Alternatively: 150 mg/m^2/day in 3-4 divided doses for 14 days of a 28-day cycle

osage Forms Gelcap: 50 mg [contains lactose]

Cap® [US-OTC] *see* aluminum hydroxide *on next page*

Aludrox® *(Discontinued)* *see page 1042*

aluminum chloride hexahydrate

(a LOO mi num KLOR ide heks a HYE drate)

Sound-Alike/Look-Alike Issues

Drysol™ may be confused with Drisdol®

U.S./Canadian Brand Names Certain Dri® [US-OTC]; Drysol™ [US]; Xerac AC™ [US]

Therapeutic Category Topical Skin Product

Use Astringent in the management of hyperhidrosis

Usual Dosage Topical: Adults: Apply once daily at bedtime; once excessive sweating has stopped, may decrease to once or twice weekly, or as needed. Wash treated area in the morning.

Dosage Forms

Solution, topical: 20% in SD alcohol 40 (35 mL, 37.5 mL, 60 mL) [contains ethyl alcohol]
- Certain Dri®: 12% (36 mL)
- Drysol™: 20% (35 mL, 37.5 mL, 60 mL) [contains ethyl alcohol 93%]
- Xerac AC™: 6.25% (35 mL, 60 mL) [contains ethyl alcohol 95%]

aluminum hydroxide (a LOO mi num hye DROKS ide)

U.S./Canadian Brand Names ALternaGel® [US-OTC]; Alu-Cap® [US-OTC]; Amphojel® [Can]; Basaljel® [Can]

Therapeutic Category Antacid

Use Treatment of hyperacidity; hyperphosphatemia

Usual Dosage Oral:

Hyperphosphatemia:
- Children: 50-150 mg/kg/24 hours in divided doses every 4-6 hours, titrate dosage to maintain serum phosphorus within normal range
- Adults: Initial: 300-600 mg 3 times/day with meals

Antacid: Adults: 600-1200 mg between meals and at bedtime

Dosage Forms

Capsule (Alu-Cap®): 400 mg

Suspension, oral: 320 mg/5 mL (473 mL)
- ALternaGel®: 600 mg/5 mL (360 mL)

aluminum hydroxide and magnesium carbonate

(a LOO mi num hye DROKS ide & mag NEE zhum KAR bun nate)

Synonyms magnesium carbonate and aluminum hydroxide

U.S./Canadian Brand Names Gaviscon® Extra Strength [US-OTC]; Gaviscon® Liquid [US-OTC]

Therapeutic Category Antacid

Use Temporary relief of symptoms associated with gastric acidity

Usual Dosage Oral: Adults:

Liquid:
- Gaviscon® Regular Strength: 15-30 mL 4 times/day after meals and at bedtime
- Gaviscon® Extra Strength Relief: 15-30 mL 4 times/day after meals

Tablet (Gaviscon® Extra Strength Relief): Chew 2-4 tablets 4 times/day

Dosage Forms

Liquid:
- Gaviscon®: Aluminum hydroxide 31.7 mg and magnesium carbonate 119.3 mL (355 mL) [contains sodium 0.57 mEq/5 mL]
- Gaviscon® Extra Strength: Aluminum hydroxide 84.6 mg and magnesi 79.1 mg per 5 mL (355 mL) [contains sodium 0.9 mEq/5 mL]

Tablet, chewable (Gaviscon® Extra Strength): Aluminum hydroxide 16 sium carbonate 105 mg [contains sodium 1.3 mEq/tablet]

aluminum hydroxide and magnesium hydroxide

(a LOO mi num hye DROKS ide & mag NEE zhum hye DROK side)

Synonyms magnesium hydroxide and aluminum hydroxide

U.S./Canadian Brand Names Alamag [US-OTC]; Diovol® [Can]; Diovol® Ex [Can]; Gelusil® [Can]; Gelusil® Extra Strength [Can]; Mylanta® [Can]; Rulox [US]; Rulox No. 1 [US]; Univol® [Can]

Therapeutic Category Antacid

Use Antacid, hyperphosphatemia in renal failure

Usual Dosage Oral: 5-10 mL 4-6 times/day, between meals and at bedtime; may be used every hour for severe symptoms

Dosage Forms [DSC] = Discontinued product

Suspension: Aluminum hydroxide 225 mg and magnesium hydroxide 200 mg per 5 mL (360 mL)

Alamag, Rulox: Aluminum hydroxide 225 mg and magnesium hydroxide 200 mg per 5 mL (360 mL)

Suspension, high potency (Maalox® TC) [DSC]: Aluminum hydroxide 600 mg and magnesium hydroxide 300 mg per 5 mL (360 mL)

Tablet, chewable:

Alamag: Aluminum hydroxide 300 mg and magnesium hydroxide 150 mg

Rulox No. 1: Aluminum hydroxide 200 mg and magnesium hydroxide 200 mg

aluminum hydroxide, magnesium hydroxide, and simethicone

(a LOO mi num hye DROKS ide, mag NEE zhum hye DROKS ide, & sye METH i kone)

Sound-Alike/Look-Alike Issues

Maalox® may be confused with Maox®, Monodox®

Mylanta® may be confused with Mynatal®

Synonyms magnesium hydroxide, aluminum hydroxide, and simethicone; simethicone, aluminum hydroxide, and magnesium hydroxide

U.S./Canadian Brand Names Alamag Plus [US-OTC]; Aldroxicon II [US-OTC]; Aldroxicon I [US-OTC]; Almacone Double Strength® [US-OTC]; Almacone® [US-OTC]; Diovol Plus® [Can]; Maalox® Max [US-OTC]; Maalox® [US-OTC]; Mylanta® Double Strength [Can]; Mylanta® Extra Strength [Can]; Mylanta® Liquid [US-OTC]; Mylanta® Maximum Strength Liquid [US-OTC]; Mylanta® Regular Strength [Can]

Therapeutic Category Antacid; Antiflatulent

Use Temporary relief of hyperacidity associated with gas; may also be used for indications associated with other antacids

Usual Dosage Oral: Adults: 10-20 mL or 2-4 tablets 4-6 times/day between meals and at bedtime; may be used every hour for severe symptoms

Dosage Forms

Liquid: Aluminum hydroxide 200 mg, magnesium hydroxide 200 mg, and simethicone 20 mg per 5 mL (360 mL); aluminum hydroxide 400 mg, magnesium hydroxide 400 mg, and simethicone 40 mg per 5 mL (360 mL)

Aldroxicon I: Aluminum hydroxide 200 mg, magnesium hydroxide 200 mg, and simethicone 20 mg per 5 mL (30 mL)

Aldroxicon II: Aluminum hydroxide 400 mg, magnesium hydroxide 400 mg, and simethicone 40 mg per 5 mL (30 mL)

Almacone®: Aluminum hydroxide 200 mg, magnesium hydroxide 200 mg, and simethicone 20 mg per 5 mL (360 mL)

Almacone Double Strength: Aluminum hydroxide 400 mg, magnesium hydroxide 400 mg, and simethicone 40 mg per 5 mL (360 mL)

Maalox®: Aluminum hydroxide 200 mg, magnesium hydroxide 200 mg, and simethicone 20 mg per 5 mL (360 mL, 770 mL) [lemon and mint flavors]

Maalox® Max: Aluminum hydroxide 400 mg, magnesium hydroxide 400 mg, and simethicone 40 mg per 5 mL (360 mL, 770 mL) [cherry, vanilla creme, and wild berry flavors]

Mylanta®: Aluminum hydroxide 200 mg, magnesium hydroxide 200 mg, and simethicone 20 mg per 5 mL (180 mL, 360 mL, 720 mL) [original, cherry, and mint flavors]

Mylanta® Maximum Strength: Aluminum hydroxide 400 mg, magnesium hydroxide 400 mg, and simethicone 40 mg per 5 mL (180 mL, 360 mL, 720 mL) [original, cherry, and mint flavors]
Suspension (Alamag Plus): Aluminum hydroxide 225 mg, magnesium hydroxide 200 mg, and simethicone 25 mg per 5 mL (360 mL)
Tablet, chewable: Aluminum hydroxide 200 mg, magnesium hydroxide 200 mg, and simethicone 25 mg
Alamag Plus: Aluminum hydroxide 200 mg, magnesium hydroxide 200 mg, and simethicone 25 mg [cherry flavor]
Almacone®: Aluminum hydroxide 200 mg, magnesium hydroxide 200 mg, and simethicone 20 mg [peppermint flavor]

aluminum sucrose sulfate, basic *see* sucralfate *on page 827*

aluminum sulfate and calcium acetate

(a LOO mi num SUL fate & KAL see um AS e tate)

Synonyms calcium acetate and aluminum sulfate

U.S./Canadian Brand Names Domeboro® [US-OTC]; Pedi-Boro® [US-OTC]

Therapeutic Category Topical Skin Product

Use Astringent wet dressing for relief of inflammatory conditions of the skin and to reduce weeping that may occur in dermatitis

Usual Dosage Topical: Soak affected area in the solution 2-4 times/day for 15-30 minutes or apply wet dressing soaked in the solution for more extended periods; rewet dressing with solution 2-4 times/day every 15-30 minutes

Dosage Forms

Powder, for topical solution:
Domeboro®: Aluminum sulfate 1191 mg and calcium acetate 938 mg per packet (12s, 100s)
Pedi-Boro®: Aluminum sulfate 49% and calcium acetate 51% per packet (12s, 100s)
Tablet, effervescent, for topical solution (Domeboro®): Aluminum sulfate 878 mg and calcium acetate 604 mg

Alupent® [US] *see* metaproterenol *on page 559*

Alupent® Inhalation Solution *(Discontinued)* *see page 1042*

Alustra™ [US] *see* hydroquinone *on page 454*

Alu-Tab® *(Discontinued)* *see page 1042*

amantadine (a MAN ta deen)

Sound-Alike/Look-Alike Issues

amantadine may be confused with ranitidine, rimantadine
Symmetrel® may be confused with Synthroid®

Synonyms adamantanamine hydrochloride; amantadine hydrochloride

U.S./Canadian Brand Names Endantadine® [Can]; PMS-Amantadine [Can]; Symmetrel® [US/Can]

Therapeutic Category Anti-Parkinson Agent; Antiviral Agent

Use Prophylaxis and treatment of influenza A viral infection; treatment of parkinsonism; treatment of drug-induced extrapyramidal symptoms

Usual Dosage Oral:

Children:
Influenza A treatment:
1-9 years: 5 mg/kg/day in 2 divided doses (manufacturers range: 4.4-8.8 mg/ maximum dose: 150 mg/day
≥10 years and <40 kg: 5 mg/kg/day; maximum dose: 150 mg/day
10-12 years and ≥40 kg: 100 mg twice daily.
≥13 years: Refer to Adults dosing

(Continued)

amantadine *(Continued)*

Note: Initiate within 24-48 hours after onset of symptoms; discontinue as soon as possible based on clinical response (generally within 3-5 days or within 24-48 hours after symptoms disappear)

Influenza A prophylaxis: Refer to "Influenza A treatment" dosing

Note: Continue treatment throughout the peak influenza activity in the community or throughout the entire influenza season in patients who cannot be vaccinated. Development of immunity following vaccination takes ~2 weeks; amantadine therapy should be considered for high-risk patients from the time of vaccination until immunity has developed. For children <9 years receiving influenza vaccine for the first time, amantadine prophylaxis should continue for 6 weeks (4 weeks after the first dose and 2 weeks after the second dose)

Adults:

Drug-induced extrapyramidal symptoms: 100 mg twice daily; may increase to 300-400 mg/day, if needed

Influenza A viral infection: 100 mg twice daily; initiate within 24-48 hours after onset of symptoms; discontinue as soon as possible based on clinical response (generally within 3-5 days or within 24-48 hours after symptoms disappear)

Influenza A prophylaxis: 100 mg twice daily

Note: Continue treatment throughout the peak influenza activity in the community or throughout the entire influenza season in patients who cannot be vaccinated. Development of immunity following vaccination takes ~2 weeks; amantadine therapy should be considered for high-risk patients from the time of vaccination until immunity has developed

Dosage Forms

Capsule, as hydrochloride: 100 mg

Syrup, as hydrochloride (Symmetrel®): 50 mg/5 mL (480 mL) [raspberry flavor]

Tablet, as hydrochloride (Symmetrel®): 100 mg

amantadine hydrochloride *see* amantadine *on previous page*

Amaphen® *(Discontinued)* *see page 1042*

Amaryl® [US/Can] *see* glimepiride *on page 405*

Amatine® [Can] *see* midodrine *on page 581*

ambenonium (am be NOE nee um)

Synonyms ambenonium chloride

U.S./Canadian Brand Names Mytelase® [US/Can]

Therapeutic Category Cholinergic Agent

Use Treatment of myasthenia gravis

Usual Dosage Oral: Adults: 5-25 mg 3-4 times/day

Dosage Forms Caplet, as chloride [scored]: 10 mg [contains lactose and sucrose]

ambenonium chloride *see* ambenonium *on this page*

Ambi 10® *(Discontinued)* *see page 1042*

Ambien® [US/Can] *see* zolpidem *on page 943*

Ambifed-G [US] *see* guaifenesin and pseudoephedrine *on page 419*

Ambifed-G DM [US] *see* guaifenesin, pseudoephedrine, and dextromethorphan *on page 422*

Ambi® Skin Tone *(Discontinued)* *see page 1042*

AmBisome® [US/Can] *see* amphotericin B liposomal *on page 55*

mcinonide (am SIN oh nide)

.S./Canadian Brand Names Amcort® [Can]; Cyclocort® [US/Can]

herapeutic Category Corticosteroid, Topical

Use Relief of the inflammatory and pruritic manifestations of corticosteroid-responsive dermatoses (high potency corticosteroid)

Usual Dosage Topical: Adults: Apply in a thin film 2-3 times/day. Therapy should be discontinued when control is achieved; if no improvement is seen, reassessment of diagnosis may be necessary.

Dosage Forms

Cream: 0.1% (15 g, 30 g, 60 g) [contains benzyl alcohol]

Lotion: 0.1% (60 mL)

Cyclocort®: 0.1% (20 mL, 60 mL) [contains benzyl alcohol]

Ointment: 0.1% (30 g, 60 g) [contains benzyl alcohol]

Cyclocort®: 0.1% (15 g, 30 g, 60 g) [contains benzyl alcohol]

Amcort® [Can] *see* amcinonide *on previous page*

Amcort® Injection *(Discontinued)* *see page 1042*

Amen® *(Discontinued)* *see page 1042*

Amerge® [US/Can] *see* naratriptan *on page 606*

Americaine® Anesthetic Lubricant [US] *see* benzocaine *on page 107*

Americaine® [US-OTC] *see* benzocaine *on page 107*

A-methapred® [US] *see* methylprednisolone *on page 572*

amethocaine hydrochloride *see* tetracaine *on page 851*

amethopterin *see* methotrexate *on page 565*

Ametop™ [Can] *see* tetracaine *on page 851*

Amevive® [US] *see* alefacept *on page 29*

amfepramone *see* diethylpropion *on page 269*

AMG 073 *see* cinacalcet *on page 200*

Amibid LA *(Discontinued)* *see page 1042*

Amicar® [US/Can] *see* aminocaproic acid *on page 45*

Amidal [US] *see* guaifenesin and phenylephrine *on page 418*

Amidate® [US/Can] *see* etomidate *on page 351*

amifostine (am i FOS teen)

Sound-Alike/Look-Alike Issues

Ethyol® may be confused with ethanol

Synonyms ethiofos; gammaphos; WR2721; YM-08310

U.S./Canadian Brand Names Ethyol® [US/Can]

Therapeutic Category Antidote

Use Reduce the incidence of moderate to severe xerostomia in patients undergoing postoperative radiation treatment for head and neck cancer, where the radiation port includes a substantial portion of the parotid glands. Reduce the cumulative renal toxicity associated with repeated administration of cisplatin in patients with advanced ovarian cancer or nonsmall-cell lung cancer.

Usual Dosage Adults:

Cisplatin-induced renal toxicity, reduction: I.V.: 740-910 mg/m^2 once daily 30 minutes prior to cytotoxic therapy

Note: Doses >740 mg/m^2 are associated with a higher incidence of hypotension a[illegible] may require interruption of therapy or dose modification for subsequent cycles [illegible] 910 mg/m^2 doses, the manufacturer suggests the following blood pressure[illegible] adjustment schedule:

The infusion of amifostine should be interrupted if the systolic bloo[illegible] decreases significantly from baseline, as defined below:

Decrease of 20 mm Hg if baseline systolic blood pressure <100

Decrease of 25 mm Hg if baseline systolic blood pressure 100-119

Decrease of 30 mm Hg if baseline systolic blood pressure 120-13[illegible]

(Continued)

amifostine *(Continued)*

Decrease of 40 mm Hg if baseline systolic blood pressure 140-179
Decrease of 50 mm Hg if baseline systolic blood pressure ≥180

If the blood pressure returns to normal within 5 minutes (assisted by fluid administration and postural management) and the patient is asymptomatic, the infusion may be restarted so that the full dose of amifostine may be administered. If the full dose of amifostine cannot be administered, the dose of amifostine for subsequent cycles should be 740 mg/m^2.

Xerostomia from head and neck cancer, reduction:
I.V.: 200mg/m^2/day during radiation therapy **or**
SubQ: 500 mg/day during radiation therapy

Dosage Forms Injection, powder for reconstitution: 500 mg

Amigesic® [US/Can] *see* salsalate *on page 793*

amikacin (am i KAY sin)

Sound-Alike/Look-Alike Issues
amikacin may be confused with Amicar®
Amikin® may be confused with Amicar®

Synonyms amikacin sulfate

U.S./Canadian Brand Names Amikin® [US/Can]

Therapeutic Category Aminoglycoside (Antibiotic)

Use Treatment of serious infections due to organisms resistant to gentamicin and tobramycin including *Pseudomonas*, *Proteus*, *Serratia*, and other gram-positive bacilli (bone infections, respiratory tract infections, endocarditis, and septicemia); documented infection of mycobacterial organisms susceptible to amikacin

Usual Dosage Individualization is critical because of the low therapeutic index

Use of ideal body weight (IBW) for determining the mg/kg/dose appears to be more accurate than dosing on the basis of total body weight (TBW)

In morbid obesity, dosage requirement may best be estimated using a dosing weight of IBW + 0.4 (TBW - IBW)

Initial and periodic peak and trough plasma drug levels should be determined, particularly in critically-ill patients with serious infections or in disease states known to significantly alter aminoglycoside pharmacokinetics (eg, cystic fibrosis, burns, or major surgery)

Infants, Children, and Adults: I.M., I.V.: 5-7.5 mg/kg/dose every 8 hours

Some clinicians suggest a daily dose of 15-20 mg/kg for all patients with normal renal function. This dose is at least as efficacious with similar, if not less, toxicity than conventional dosing.

Dosage Forms Injection, solution, as sulfate: 50 mg/mL (2 mL, 4 mL); 62.5 mg/mL (8 mL); 250 mg/mL (2 mL, 4 mL) [contains metabisulfite]

amikacin sulfate *see* amikacin *on this page*

Amikin® [US/Can] *see* amikacin *on this page*

amiloride (a MIL oh ride)

Sound-Alike/Look-Alike Issues
amiloride may be confused with amiodarone, amlodipine

Synonyms amiloride hydrochloride

U.S./Canadian Brand Names Midamor® [Can]

Therapeutic Category Diuretic, Potassium Sparing

Use Counteracts potassium loss induced by other diuretics in the treatment of hypertension or edematous conditions including CHF, hepatic cirrhosis, and hypoaldosteronism; usually used in conjunction with more potent diuretics such as thiazides or loop diuretics

sual Dosage Oral:
hildren: Although safety and efficacy in children have not been established by the DA, a dosage of 0.625 mg/kg/day has been used in children weighing 6-20 kg.

Adults: 5-10 mg/day (up to 20 mg)
Hypertension (JNC 7): 5-10 mg/day in 1-2 divided doses
Dosage Forms Tablet, as hydrochloride: 5 mg

amiloride and hydrochlorothiazide
(a MIL oh ride & hye droe klor oh THYE a zide)

Synonyms hydrochlorothiazide and amiloride
U.S./Canadian Brand Names Apo-Amilzide® [Can]; Moduret® [Can]; Moduretic® [Can]; Novamilor [Can]; Nu-Amilzide [Can]
Therapeutic Category Diuretic, Combination
Use Potassium-sparing diuretic; antihypertensive
Usual Dosage Adults: Oral: Start with 1 tablet/day, then may be increased to 2 tablets/day if needed; usually given in a single dose
Dosage Forms Tablet: Amiloride hydrochloride 5 mg and hydrochlorothiazide 50 mg

amiloride hydrochloride *see* amiloride *on previous page*

Amin-Aid® *(Discontinued)* *see page 1042*

Aminate Fe-90 [US] *see* vitamins (multiple/prenatal) *on page 927*

2-amino-6-mercaptopurine *see* thioguanine *on page 857*

2-amino-6-trifluoromethoxy-benzothiazole *see* riluzole *on page 777*

aminobenzylpenicillin *see* ampicillin *on page 56*

aminocaproic acid (a mee noe ka PROE ik AS id)

Sound-Alike/Look-Alike Issues
Amicar® may be confused with amikacin, Amikin®
Synonyms epsilon aminocaproic acid
U.S./Canadian Brand Names Amicar® [US/Can]
Therapeutic Category Hemostatic Agent
Use Treatment of excessive bleeding from fibrinolysis
Usual Dosage Acute bleeding syndrome:
Adults: Oral, I.V.: 4-5 g during the first hour, followed by 1 g/hour for 8 hours or until bleeding controlled (maximum daily dose: 30 g)
Initial: I.V.: 0.1 g/kg over 30-60 minutes
Maintenance: Oral: 1-3 g every 6 hours
Dosage Forms
Injection, solution: 250 mg/mL (20 mL) [contains benzyl alcohol]
Syrup: 1.25 g/5 mL (240 mL, 480 mL)
Amicar®: 1.25 g/5 mL (480 mL) [raspberry flavor]
Tablet [scored]: 500 mg, 1000 mg

Amino-Cerv™ [US] *see* urea *on page 897*

aminoglutethimide (a mee noe gloo TETH i mide)

Sound-Alike/Look-Alike Issues
Cytadren® may be confused with cytarabine
Synonyms AG; AGT; BA-16038; elipten
U.S./Canadian Brand Names Cytadren® [US]
Therapeutic Category Antineoplastic Agent
Use Suppression of adrenal function in selected patients with Cushing syndrome
Usual Dosage Oral: Adults: Adrenal suppression: 250 mg every 6 hours may increased at 1- to 2-week intervals to a total of 2 g/day
Dosage Forms Tablet [scored]: 250 mg

aminolevulinic acid (a MEE noh lev yoo lin ik AS id)

Synonyms aminolevulinic acid hydrochloride
U.S./Canadian Brand Names Levulan® [Can]; Levulan® Kerastick™ [US]
(Continued)

aminolevulinic acid *(Continued)*

Therapeutic Category Photosensitizing Agent, Topical; Porphyrin Agent, Topical

Use Treatment of minimally to moderately thick actinic keratoses (grade 1 or 2) of the face or scalp; to be used in conjunction with blue light illumination

Usual Dosage Adults: Topical: Apply to actinic keratoses (**not** perilesional skin) followed 14-18 hours later by blue light illumination. Application/treatment may be repeated at a treatment site after 8 weeks.

Dosage Forms Powder for topical solution: 20% (1s, 6s) [2-component system containing aminolevulinic acid hydrochloride 354 mg (powder) and diluent containing ethanol 48% (1.5 mL) packaged together in an applicator tube]

aminolevulinic acid hydrochloride *see* aminolevulinic acid *on previous page*

aminophylline (am in OFF i lin)

Sound-Alike/Look-Alike Issues

aminophylline may be confused with amitriptyline, ampicillin

Synonyms theophylline ethylenediamine

U.S./Canadian Brand Names Phyllocontin®-350 [Can]; Phyllocontin® [Can]

Therapeutic Category Theophylline Derivative

Use Bronchodilator in reversible airway obstruction due to asthma or COPD; increase diaphragmatic contractility

Usual Dosage

Treatment of acute bronchospasm: I.V.:

Loading dose (in patients not currently receiving aminophylline or theophylline): 6 mg/kg (based on aminophylline) administered I.V. over 20-30 minutes; administration rate should not exceed 25 mg/minute (aminophylline)

Approximate I.V. maintenance dosages are based upon **continuous infusions**; bolus dosing (often used in children <6 months of age) may be determined by multiplying the hourly infusion rate by 24 hours and dividing by the desired number of doses/day

6 weeks to 6 months: 0.5 mg/kg/hour

6 months to 1 year: 0.6-0.7 mg/kg/hour

1-9 years: 1 mg/kg/hour

9-16 years and smokers: 0.8 mg/kg/hour

Adults, nonsmoking: 0.5 mg/kg/hour

Older patients and patients with cor pulmonale: 0.3 mg/kg/hour

Patients with congestive heart failure: 0.1-0.2 mg/kg/hour

Dosage should be adjusted according to serum level measurements during the first 12- to 24-hour period.

Bronchodilator: Oral: Children ≥45 kg and Adults: Initial: 380 mg/day (equivalent to theophylline 300 mg/day) in divided doses every 6-8 hours; may increase dose after 3 days; maximum dose: 928 mg/day (equivalent to theophylline 800 mg/day)

Dosage Forms [DSC] = Discontinued product

Injection, solution: 25 mg/mL (10 mL, 20 mL)

Liquid, oral [DSC]: 105 mg/5 mL (500 mL) [apricot flavor]

Tablet: 100 mg, 200 mg

aminosalicylate sodium (a MEE noe sa LIS i late SOW dee um)

Synonyms PAS

Therapeutic Category Nonsteroidal Antiinflammatory Drug (NSAID)

Use Treatment of tuberculosis with combination drugs

Usual Dosage Oral:

Children: 150-300 mg/kg/day in 3-4 equally divided doses

Adults: 150 mg/kg/day in 2-3 equally divided doses (usually 12-14 g/day)

Dosage Forms Tablet: 500 mg

aminosalicylic acid *see* mesalamine *on page 556*

ιinoxin® [US-OTC] *see* pyridoxine *on page 752*

amiodarone (a MEE oh da rone)

Sound-Alike/Look-Alike Issues

amiodarone may be confused with amiloride, amrinone

Cordarone® may be confused with Cardura®, Cordran®

Synonyms amiodarone hydrochloride

U.S./Canadian Brand Names Alti-Amiodarone [Can]; Cordarone® [US/Can]; Gen-Amiodarone [Can]; Novo-Amiodarone [Can]; Pacerone® [US]; Rhoxal-amiodarone [Can]

Therapeutic Category Antiarrhythmic Agent, Class III

Use

Oral: Management of life-threatening recurrent ventricular fibrillation (VF) or hemodynamically unstable ventricular tachycardia (VT)

I.V.: Initiation of treatment and prophylaxis of frequency recurring VF and unstable VT in patients refractory to other therapy. Also, used for patients when oral amiodarone is indicated, but who are unable to take oral medication.

Usual Dosage Note: Lower loading and maintenance doses are preferable in women and all patients with low body weight.

Oral:

Adults:

Ventricular arrhythmias: 800-1600 mg/day in 1-2 doses for 1-3 weeks, then when adequate arrhythmia control is achieved, decrease to 600-800 mg/day in 1-2 doses for 1 month; maintenance: 400 mg/day. Lower doses are recommended for supraventricular arrhythmias.

I.V.:

Adults:

Breakthrough VF or VT: 150 mg supplemental doses in 100 mL D_5W over 10 minutes

Pulseless VF or VT: I.V. push: Initial: 300 mg in 20-30 mL NS or D_5W; if VF or VT recurs, supplemental dose of 150 mg followed by infusion of 1 mg/minute for 6 hours, then 0.5 mg/minute (maximum daily dose: 2.2 g)

Recommendations for conversion to intravenous amiodarone after oral administration: During long-term amiodarone therapy (ie, ≥4 months), the mean plasma-elimination half-life of the active metabolite of amiodarone is 61 days. Replacement therapy may not be necessary in such patients if oral therapy is discontinued for a period <2 weeks, since any changes in serum amiodarone concentrations during this period may **not** be clinically significant.

Dosage Forms

Injection, solution, as hydrochloride: 50 mg/mL (3 mL, 18 mL) [contains benzyl alcohol and polysorbate (Tween®) 80]

Cordarone®: 50 mg/mL (30 mL) [contains benzyl alcohol and polysorbate (Tween®) 80]

Tablet, as hydrochloride [scored]: 200 mg

Cordarone®: 200 mg

Pacerone®: 100 mg [not scored], 200 mg, 400 mg

amiodarone hydrochloride *see* amiodarone *on this page*

Amipaque® *(Discontinued)* *see page 1042*

Ami-Tex LA [US] *see* guaifenesin and phenylephrine *on page 418*

Ami-Tex PSE [US] *see* guaifenesin and pseudoephedrine *on page 419*

Amitone® [US-OTC] *see* calcium carbonate *on page 144*

amitriptyline (a mee TRIP ti leen)

Sound-Alike/Look-Alike Issues

amitriptyline may be confused with aminophylline, imipramine, nortriptyline

Elavil® may be confused with Aldoril®, Eldepryl®, enalapril, Equanil®, Mellaril®, O Plavix®

Synonyms amitriptyline hydrochloride

U.S./Canadian Brand Names Apo-Amitriptyline® [Can]; Levate® [Can]; PM line [Can]

(Continued)

amitriptyline *(Continued)*

Therapeutic Category Antidepressant, Tricyclic (Tertiary Amine)

Use Relief of symptoms of depression

Usual Dosage

Adolescents: Depressive disorders: Oral: Initial: 25-50 mg/day; may administer in divided doses; increase gradually to 100 mg/day in divided doses

Adults:

Depression:

Oral: 50-150 mg/day single dose at bedtime or in divided doses; dose may be gradually increased up to 300 mg/day

I.M.: 20-30 mg 4 times/day

Dosage Forms [DSC] = Discontinued product

Injection, as hydrochloride: 10 mg/mL (10 mL) [DSC]

Tablet, as hydrochloride: 10 mg, 25 mg, 50 mg, 75 mg, 100 mg, 150 mg

amitriptyline and chlordiazepoxide

(a mee TRIP ti leen & klor dye az e POKS ide)

Synonyms chlordiazepoxide and amitriptyline

U.S./Canadian Brand Names Limbitrol® DS [US]; Limbitrol® [US/Can]

Therapeutic Category Antidepressant, Tricyclic (Tertiary Amine)

Controlled Substance C-IV

Use Treatment of moderate to severe anxiety and/or agitation and depression

Usual Dosage Initial: 3-4 tablets in divided doses; this may be increased to 6 tablets/day as required; some patients respond to smaller doses and can be maintained on 2 tablets

Dosage Forms Tablet:

5-12.5 (Limbitrol®): Amitriptyline hydrochloride 12.5 mg and chlordiazepoxide 5 mg [contains lactose]

10-25 (Limbitrol® DS): Amitriptyline hydrochloride 25 mg and chlordiazepoxide 10 mg [contains lactose]

amitriptyline and perphenazine (a mee TRIP ti leen & per FEN a zeen)

Synonyms perphenazine and amitriptyline

U.S./Canadian Brand Names Etrafon® [Can]; Triavil® [US/Can]

Therapeutic Category Antidepressant/Phenothiazine

Use Treatment of patients with moderate to severe anxiety and depression

Usual Dosage Oral: 1 tablet 2-4 times/day

Dosage Forms Tablet:

2-10 (Triavil®): Amitriptyline hydrochloride 10 mg and perphenazine 2 mg

2-25 (Triavil®): Amitriptyline hydrochloride 25 mg and perphenazine 2 mg

4-10: Amitriptyline hydrochloride 10 mg and perphenazine 4 mg

4-25 (Triavil®): Amitriptyline hydrochloride 25 mg and perphenazine 4 mg

4-50: Amitriptyline hydrochloride 50 mg and perphenazine 4 mg

amitriptyline hydrochloride *see* amitriptyline *on previous page*

AmLactin® [US-OTC] *see* lactic acid with ammonium hydroxide *on page 501*

amlexanox (am LEKS an oks)

U.S./Canadian Brand Names Aphthasol® [US]

Therapeutic Category Antiinflammatory Agent, Locally Applied

Use Treatment of aphthous ulcers (ie, canker sores)

Usual Dosage Administer (0.5 cm - ¼") directly on ulcers 4 times/day following oral hygiene, after meals, and at bedtime

Dosage Forms Paste: 5% (5 g) [contains benzyl alcohol]

amlodipine (am LOE di peen)

Sound-Alike/Look-Alike Issues

amlodipine may be confused with amiloride

Norvasc® may be confused with Navane®, Norvir®, Vascor®

Synonyms amlodipine besylate

U.S./Canadian Brand Names Norvasc® [US/Can]

Therapeutic Category Calcium Channel Blocker

Use Treatment of hypertension and angina

Usual Dosage Oral:

Children 6-17 years: Hypertension: 2.5-5 mg once daily

Adults:

Hypertension: Initial dose: 5 mg once daily; maximum dose: 10 mg once daily. In general, titrate in 2.5 mg increments over 7-14 days. Usual dosage range (JNC 7): 2.5-10 mg once daily.

Angina: Usual dose: 5-10 mg

Dosage Forms Tablet, as besylate [equivalent to amlodipine base]: 2.5 mg, 5 mg, 10 mg

amlodipine and atorvastatin (am LOW di peen & a TORE va sta tin)

Synonyms atorvastatin calcium and amlodipine besylate

U.S./Canadian Brand Names Caduet® [US]

Therapeutic Category Antilipemic Agent, HMG-CoA Reductase Inhibitor; Calcium Channel Blocker

Use For use when treatment with both agents is appropriate:

Amlodipine is used for the treatment of hypertension and angina.

Atorvastatin is used with dietary therapy for the following:

Hyperlipidemias: To reduce elevations in total cholesterol, LDL-C, apolipoprotein B, and triglycerides in patients with primary hypercholesterolemia (elevations of 1 or more components are present in Fredrickson type IIa, IIb, III, and IV hyperlipidemias); treatment of homozygous familial hypercholesterolemia

Heterozygous familial hypercholesterolemia (HeFH): In adolescent patients (10-17 years of age, females >1 year postmenarche) with HeFH having LDL-C ≥190 mg/dL **or** LDL ≥160 mg/dL with positive family history of premature cardiovascular disease (CVD) or with 2 or more CVD risk factors in the adolescent patient

Usual Dosage Oral: Children 10-17 years (females >1 year postmenarche) and Adults: Treatment of hypertension/angina and hyperlipidemias: Dose is individualized, given once daily and substituted for each individual component. See individual agents. Maximum dose: Amlodipine 10 mg/day, atorvastatin 80 mg/day.

Dosage Forms

Tablet:

5/10: Amlodipine 5 mg and atorvastatin 10 mg

5/20: Amlodipine 5 mg and atorvastatin 20 mg

5/40: Amlodipine 5 mg and atorvastatin 40 mg

5/80: Amlodipine 5 mg and atorvastatin 80 mg

10/10: Amlodipine 10 mg and atorvastatin 10 mg

10/20: Amlodipine 10 mg and atorvastatin 20 mg

10/40: Amlodipine 10 mg and atorvastatin 40 mg

10/80: Amlodipine 10 mg and atorvastatin 80 mg

amlodipine and benazepril (am LOE di peen & ben AY ze pril)

Synonyms benazepril and amlodipine

U.S./Canadian Brand Names Lotrel® [US]

Therapeutic Category Antihypertensive Agent, Combination

Use Treatment of hypertension

Usual Dosage Oral: Adults: Dose is individualized, given once daily

Dosage Forms

Capsule:

Amlodipine 2.5 mg and benazepril hydrochloride 10 mg

(Continued)

amlodipine and benazepril *(Continued)*

Amlodipine 5 mg and benazepril hydrochloride 10 mg
Amlodipine 5 mg and benazepril hydrochloride 20 mg
Amlodipine 10 mg and benazepril hydrochloride 20 mg

amlodipine besylate *see* amlodipine *on previous page*

Ammens® Medicated Deodorant [US-OTC] *see* zinc oxide *on page 940*

ammonapse *see* sodium phenylbutyrate *on page 814*

ammonia spirit (aromatic) (a MOE nee ah SPEAR it air oh MAT ik)

Synonyms smelling salts
Therapeutic Category Respiratory Stimulant
Use Respiratory and circulatory stimulant, treatment of fainting
Usual Dosage Used as "smelling salts" to treat or prevent fainting
Dosage Forms Solution for inhalation [ampul]: 1.7% to 2.1% (0.33 mL)

ammonium chloride (a MOE nee um KLOR ide)

Therapeutic Category Electrolyte Supplement, Oral
Use Treatment of hypochloremic states or metabolic alkalosis
Usual Dosage Metabolic alkalosis: The following equations represent different methods of correction utilizing either the serum HCO_3^-, the serum chloride, or the base excess

Dosing of mEq NH_4Cl via the chloride-deficit method (hypochloremia):

Dose of mEq NH_4Cl = [0.2 L/kg x body weight (kg)] x [103 - observed serum chloride]; administer 50% of dose over 12 hours, then re-evaluate

Note: 0.2 L/kg is the estimated chloride volume of distribution and 103 is the average normal serum chloride concentration (mEq/L)

Dosing of mEq NH_4Cl via the bicarbonate-excess method (refractory hypochloremic metabolic alkalosis):

Dose of NH_4Cl = [0.5 L/kg x body weight (kg)] x (observed serum HCO_3^- - 24); administer 50% of dose over 12 hours, then re-evaluate

Note: 0.5 L/kg is the estimated bicarbonate volume of distribution and 24 is the average normal serum bicarbonate concentration (mEq/L)

These equations will yield different requirements of ammonium chloride

Dosage Forms Injection, solution: Ammonium 5 mEq/mL and chloride 5 mEq/mL (20 mL) [equivalent to ammonium chloride 267.5 mg/mL]

ammonium lactate *see* lactic acid with ammonium hydroxide *on page 501*

Amnesteem™ [US] *see* isotretinoin *on page 489*

amobarbital (am oh BAR bi tal)

Synonyms amylobarbitone
U.S./Canadian Brand Names Amytal® [US/Can]
Therapeutic Category Barbiturate
Controlled Substance C-II
Use Hypnotic in short-term treatment of insomnia; reduce anxiety and provide sedation preoperatively
Usual Dosage

Children:
- Sedative: I.M., I.V. : 6-12 years: Manufacturer's dosing range: 65- 500 mg
- Hypnotic: I.M.: 2-3 mg/kg (maximum: 500 mg)

Adults:
- Hypnotic: I.M., I.V.: 65-200 mg at bedtime (maximum I.M. dose: 500 mg)
- Sedative: I.M., I.V.: 30-50 mg 2-3 times/day

Dosage Forms Injection, powder for reconstitution, as sodium: 500 mg

amobarbital and secobarbital (am oh BAR bi tal & see koe BAR bi tal)

Synonyms secobarbital and amobarbital

Therapeutic Category Barbiturate

Controlled Substance C-II

Use Short-term treatment of insomnia

Usual Dosage Adults: Oral: 1-2 capsules at bedtime

Dosage Forms Capsule: Amobarbital 50 mg and secobarbital 50 mg

Amonidrin® Tablet *(Discontinued)* *see page 1042*

AMO Vitrax® *(Discontinued)* *see page 1042*

amoxapine (a MOKS a peen)

Sound-Alike/Look-Alike Issues

amoxapine may be confused with amoxicillin, Amoxil®

Therapeutic Category Antidepressant, Tricyclic (Secondary Amine)

Use Treatment of depression, psychotic depression, depression accompanied by anxiety or agitation

Usual Dosage Oral:

Children: Not established in children <16 years of age.

Adolescents: Initial: 25-50 mg/day; increase gradually to 100 mg/day; may administer as divided doses or as a single dose at bedtime

Adults: Initial: 25 mg 2-3 times/day, if tolerated, dosage may be increased to 100 mg 2-3 times/day; may be given in a single bedtime dose when dosage <300 mg/day

Elderly: Initial: 25 mg at bedtime increased by 25 mg weekly for outpatients and every 3 days for inpatients if tolerated; usual dose: 50-150 mg/day, but doses up to 300 mg may be necessary

Maximum daily dose:

Inpatient: 600 mg

Outpatient: 400 mg

Dosage Forms Tablet: 25 mg, 50 mg, 100 mg, 150 mg

amoxicillin (a moks i SIL in)

Sound-Alike/Look-Alike Issues

amoxicillin may be confused with amoxapine, Amoxil®, Atarax®

Amoxil® may be confused with amoxapine, amoxicillin

Trimox® may be confused with Diamox®, Tylox®

Synonyms amoxicillin trihydrate; amoxycillin; *p*-hydroxyampicillin

U.S./Canadian Brand Names Amoxil® [US/Can]; Apo-Amoxi® [Can]; DisperMox™ [US]; Gen-Amoxicillin [Can]; Lin-Amox [Can]; Moxilin® [US]; Novamoxin® [Can]; Nu-Amoxi [Can]; PMS-Amoxicillin [Can]; Trimox® [US]

Therapeutic Category Penicillin

Use Treatment of otitis media, sinusitis, and infections caused by susceptible organisms involving the respiratory tract, skin, and urinary tract; prophylaxis of bacterial endocarditis in patients undergoing surgical or dental procedures; as part of a multidrug regimen for *H. pylori* eradication

Usual Dosage Oral:

Children ≤3 months: 20-30 mg/kg/day divided every 12 hours

Children: >3 months and <40 kg: Dosing range: 20-50 mg/kg/day in divided doses every 8-12 hours

Ear, nose, throat, genitourinary tract, or skin/skin structure infections:

Mild to moderate: 25 mg/kg/day in divided doses every 12 hours **or** 20 mg/kg/day in divided doses every 8 hours

Severe: 45 mg/kg/day in divided doses every 12 hours **or** 40 mg/kg/day in divided doses every 8 hours

Acute otitis media due to highly-resistant strains of *S. pneumoniae:* Doses as high as 80-90 mg/kg/day divided every 12 hours have been used

(Continued)

amoxicillin *(Continued)*

Lower respiratory tract infections: 45 mg/kg/day in divided doses every 12 hours **or** 40 mg/kg/day in divided doses every 8 hours
Subacute bacterial endocarditis prophylaxis: 50 mg/kg 1 hour before procedure only with documented susceptible organisms:
<40 kg: 15 mg/kg every 8 hours
≥40 kg: 500 mg every 8 hours

Adults: Dosing range: 250-500 mg every 8 hours or 500-875 mg twice daily; maximum dose: 2-3 g/day
Ear, nose, throat, genitourinary tract or skin/skin structure infections:
Mild to moderate: 500 mg every 12 hours **or** 250 mg every 8 hours
Severe: 875 mg every 12 hours **or** 500 mg every 8 hours
Lower respiratory tract infections: 875 mg every 12 hours **or** 500 mg every 8 hours
Endocarditis prophylaxis: 2 g 1 hour before procedure
Helicobacter pylori eradication: 1000 mg twice daily; requires combination therapy with at least one other antibiotic and an acid-suppressing agent (proton pump inhibitor or H_2 blocker)

Dosage Forms [DSC] = Discontinued product
Capsule, as trihydrate: 250 mg, 500 mg
Amoxil®, Moxilin®, Trimox®: 250 mg, 500 mg
Powder for oral suspension, as trihydrate: 125 mg/5 mL (80 mL, 100 mL, 150 mL); 200 mg/5 mL (50 mL, 75 mL, 100 mL); 250 mg/5 mL (80 mL, 100 mL, 150 mL); 400 mg/5 mL (50 mL, 75 mL, 100 mL)
Amoxil®: 125 mg/5 mL (150 mL) [contains sodium benzoate; strawberry flavor] [DSC]; 200 mg/5 mL (5 mL, 50 mL, 75 mL, 100 mL) [contains sodium benzoate; bubblegum flavor]; 250 mg/5 mL (100 mL, 150 mL) [contains sodium benzoate; bubblegum flavor]; 400 mg/5 mL (5 mL, 50 mL, 75 mL, 100 mL) [contains sodium benzoate; bubblegum flavor]
Moxilin®: 250 mg/5 mL (100 mL, 150 mL)
Trimox®: 125 mg/5 mL (80 mL, 100 mL, 150 mL); 250 mg/5 mL (80 mL, 100 mL, 150 mL) [contains sodium benzoate; raspberry-strawberry flavor]
Powder for oral suspension, as trihydrate [drops] (Amoxil®): 50 mg/mL (15 mL [DSC], 30 mL) [bubblegum flavor]
Tablet, as trihydrate [film coated] (Amoxil®): 500 mg, 875 mg
Tablet, chewable, as trihydrate: 125 mg, 200 mg, 250 mg, 400 mg
Amoxil®: 200 mg [contains phenylalanine 1.82 mg/tablet; cherry banana peppermint flavor]; 400 mg [contains phenylalanine 3.64 mg/tablet; cherry banana peppermint flavor]
Tablet, for oral suspension, as trihydrate (DisperMox™): 200 mg [contains phenylalanine 5.6 mg; strawberry flavor]; 400 mg [contains phenylalanine 5.6 mg; strawberry flavor]; 600 mg [contains phenylalanine 11.23 mg; strawberry flavor]

amoxicillin and clavulanate potassium

(a moks i SIL in & klav yoo LAN ate poe TASS ee um)

Sound-Alike/Look-Alike Issues
Augmentin® may be confused with Azulfidine®

Synonyms amoxicillin and clavulanic acid

U.S./Canadian Brand Names Alti-Amoxi-Clav® [Can]; Apo-Amoxi-Clav [Can]; Augmentin® [US/Can]; Augmentin ES-600® [US]; Augmentin XR™ [US]; Clavulin® [Can]; ratio-AmoxiClav

Therapeutic Category Penicillin

Use Treatment of otitis media, sinusitis, and infections caused by susceptible organisms involving the lower respiratory tract, skin and skin structure, and urinary tract; spectrum same as amoxicillin with additional coverage of beta-lactamase producing *B. catarrhalis*, *H. influenzae*, *N. gonorrhoeae*, and *S. aureus* (not MRSA). The expanded coverage of this combination makes it a useful alternative when amoxicillin resistance is present and patients cannot tolerate alternative treatments.

Usual Dosage

Infants <3 months: 30 mg/kg/day divided every 12 hours using the 125 mg/5 mL suspension

Children ≥3 months and <40 kg:

Otitis media: 90 mg/kg/day divided every 12 hours for 10 days

Lower respiratory tract infections, severe infections, sinusitis: 45 mg/kg/day divided every 12 hours **or** 40 mg/kg/day divided every 8 hours

Less severe infections: 25 mg/kg/day divided every 12 hours or 20 mg/kg/day divided every 8 hours

Children >40 kg and Adults: 250-500 mg every 8 hours or 875 mg every 12 hours

Children ≥16 years and Adults:

Acute bacterial sinusitis: Extended release tablet: Two 1000 mg tablets every 12 hours for 10 days

Community-acquired pneumonia: Extended release tablet: Two 1000 mg tablets every 12 hours for 7-10 days

Dosage Forms

Powder for oral suspension: 200: Amoxicillin 200 mg and clavulanate potassium 28.5 mg per 5 mL (100 mL) [contains phenylalanine]; 400: Amoxicillin 400 mg and clavulanate potassium 57 mg per 5 mL (100 mL) [contains phenylalanine]

Augmentin®:

125: Amoxicillin 125 mg and clavulanate potassium 31.25 mg per 5 mL (75 mL, 100 mL, 150 mL) [banana flavor]

200: Amoxicillin 200 mg and clavulanate potassium 28.5 mg per 5 mL (50 mL, 75 mL, 100 mL) [contains phenylalanine 7 mg/5 mL; orange-raspberry flavor]

250: Amoxicillin 250 mg and clavulanate potassium 62.5 mg per 5 mL (75 mL, 100 mL, 150 mL) [orange flavor]

400: Amoxicillin 400 mg and clavulanate potassium 57 mg per 5 mL (50 mL, 75 mL, 100 mL) [contains phenylalanine 7 mg/5 mL; orange-raspberry flavor]

Augmentin ES-600®: Amoxicillin 600 mg and clavulanic potassium 42.9 mg per 5 mL (75 mL, 125 mL, 200 mL) [contains phenylalanine 7 mg/5 mL; orange flavor]

Tablet: 500: Amoxicillin trihydrate 500 mg and clavulanate potassium 125 mg; 875: Amoxicillin trihydrate 875 mg and clavulanate potassium 125 mg

Augmentin®:

250: Amoxicillin trihydrate 250 mg and clavulanate potassium 125 mg

500: Amoxicillin trihydrate 500 mg and clavulanate potassium 125 mg

875: Amoxicillin trihydrate 875 mg and clavulanate potassium 125 mg

Tablet, chewable: 200: Amoxicillin trihydrate 200 mg and clavulanate potassium 28.5 mg [contains phenylalanine]; 400: Amoxicillin trihydrate 400 mg and clavulanate potassium 57 mg [contains phenylalanine]

Augmentin®:

125: Amoxicillin trihydrate 125 mg and clavulanate potassium 31.25 mg [lemon-lime flavor]

200: Amoxicillin trihydrate 200 mg and clavulanate potassium 28.5 mg [contains phenylalanine 2.1 mg/tablet; cherry-banana flavor]

250: Amoxicillin trihydrate 250 mg and clavulanate potassium 62.5 mg [lemon-lime flavor]

400: Amoxicillin trihydrate 400 mg and clavulanate potassium 57 mg [contains phenylalanine 4.2 mg/tablet; cherry-banana flavor]

Tablet, extended release (Augmentin XR™): Amoxicillin 1000 mg and clavulanic acid 62.5 mg

amoxicillin and clavulanic acid *see* amoxicillin and clavulanate potassium *on previous page*

amoxicillin, lansoprazole, and clarithromycin *see* lansoprazole, amoxicillin, and clarithromycin *on page 506*

amoxicillin trihydrate *see* amoxicillin *on page 51*

Amoxil® [US/Can] *see* amoxicillin *on page 51*

amoxycillin *see* amoxicillin *on page 51*

amphetamine and dextroamphetamine *see* dextroamphetamine and amphetamine *on page 259*

Amphocin® [US] *see* amphotericin B (conventional) *on this page*

Amphojel® *(Discontinued)* *see page 1042*

Amphojel® [Can] *see* aluminum hydroxide *on page 39*

Amphotec® [US/Can] *see* amphotericin B cholesteryl sulfate complex *on this page*

amphotericin B cholesteryl sulfate complex

(am foe TER i sin bee kole LES te ril SUL fate KOM plecks)

Sound-Alike/Look-Alike Issues

Amphotec® may be confused with Abelcet®, AmBisome®

Synonyms ABCD; amphotericin B colloidal dispersion

U.S./Canadian Brand Names Amphotec® [US/Can]

Therapeutic Category Antifungal Agent

Use Treatment of invasive aspergillosis in patients who have failed amphotericin B deoxycholate treatment, or who have renal impairment or experience unacceptable toxicity which precludes treatment with amphotericin B deoxycholate in effective doses.

Usual Dosage Children and Adults: I.V.:

Premedication: For patients who experience chills, fever, hypotension, nausea, or other nonanaphylactic infusion-related immediate reactions, premedicate with the following drugs, 30-60 minutes prior to drug administration: a nonsteroidal (eg, ibuprofen, choline magnesium trisalicylate) with or without diphenhydramine; or acetaminophen with diphenhydramine; or hydrocortisone 50-100 mg. If the patient experiences rigors during the infusion, meperidine may be administered.

Range: 3-4 mg/kg/day (infusion of 1 mg/kg/hour); maximum: 7.5 mg/kg/day

Dosage Forms Injection, powder for reconstitution: 50 mg, 100 mg

amphotericin B colloidal dispersion *see* amphotericin B cholesteryl sulfate complex *on this page*

amphotericin B (conventional) (am foe TER i sin bee con VEN sha nal)

Sound-Alike/Look-Alike Issues

Amphocin® may be confused with Abelcet®, AmBisome®, Amphotec®

Fungizone® may be confused with Abelcet®, AmBisome®, Amphotec®

Synonyms amphotericin B desoxycholate

U.S./Canadian Brand Names Amphocin® [US]; Fungizone® [US/Can]

Therapeutic Category Antifungal Agent

Use Treatment of severe systemic and central nervous system infections caused by susceptible fungi such as *Candida* species, *Histoplasma capsulatum, Cryptococcus neoformans, Aspergillus* species, *Blastomyces dermatitidis, Torulopsis glabrata*, and *Coccidioides immitis*; fungal peritonitis; irrigant for bladder fungal infections; and topically for cutaneous and mucocutaneous candidal infections; used in fungal infection in patients with bone marrow transplantation, amebic meningoencephalitis, ocular aspergillosis (intraocular injection), candidal cystitis (bladder irrigation), chemoprophylaxis (low-dose I.V.), immunocompromised patients at risk of aspergillosis (intranasal/nebulized), refractory meningitis (intrathecal), coccidioidal arthritis (intraarticular/I.M.).

Low-dose amphotericin B 0.1-0.25 mg/kg/day has been administered after bone marrow transplantation to reduce the risk of invasive fungal disease. Alternative routes of administration and extemporaneous preparations have been used when standard antifungal therapy is not available (eg, inhalation, intraocular injection, subconjunctival application, intracavitary administration into various joints and the pleural space).

Usual Dosage

I.V.: Premedication: For patients who experience chills, fever, hypotension, nausea, or other nonanaphylactic infusion-related immediate reactions, premedicate with the following drugs, 30-60 minutes prior to drug administration: a nonsteroidal (eg, ibuprofen, choline magnesium trisalicylate) with or without diphenhydramine; or acetaminophen with diphenhydramine; or hydrocortisone 50-100 mg. If the patient experiences rigors during the infusion, meperidine may be administered.

Infants and Children:

Test dose: I.V.: 0.1 mg/kg/dose to a maximum of 1 mg; infuse over 30-60 minutes. Many clinicians believe a test dose is unnecessary.

Maintenance dose: 0.25-1 mg/kg/day given once daily; infuse over 2-6 hours. Once therapy has been established, amphotericin B can be administered on an every-other-day basis at 1-1.5 mg/kg/dose; cumulative dose: 1.5-2 g over 6-10 week.

Adults:

Test dose: 1 mg infused over 20-30 minutes. Many clinicians believe a test dose is unnecessary.

Maintenance dose: Usual: 0.25-1.5 mg/kg/day; 1-1.5 mg/kg over 4-6 hours every other day may be given once therapy is established; aspergillosis, mucormycosis, rhinocerebral phycomycosis often require 1-1.5 mg/kg/day; do not exceed 1.5 mg/kg/day

Duration of therapy varies with nature of infection: Usual duration is 4-12 weeks or cumulative dose of 1-4 g

I.T.: Meningitis, coccidioidal or cryptococcal:

Children.: 25-100 mcg every 48-72 hours; increase to 500 mcg as tolerated

Adults: Initial: 25-300 mcg every 48-72 hours; increase to 500 mcg to 1 mg as tolerated; maximum total dose: 15 mg has been suggested

Oral: 1 mL (100 mg) 4 times/day

Topical: Apply to affected areas 2-4 times/day for 1-4 weeks of therapy depending on nature and severity of infection

Bladder irrigation: Candidal cystitis: Irrigate with 50 mcg/mL solution instilled periodically or continuously for 5-10 days or until cultures are clear

Dosage Forms

Cream (Fungizone®): 3% (20 g)

Injection, powder for reconstitution, as desoxycholate (Amphocin®; Fungizone®): 50 mg

Lotion (Fungizone®): 3% (30 mL)

amphotericin B desoxycholate *see* amphotericin B (conventional) *on previous page*

amphotericin B lipid complex (am foe TER i sin bee LIP id KOM pleks)

Sound-Alike/Look-Alike Issues

Abelcet® may be confused with Amphocin®, Fungizone®

Synonyms ABLC

U.S./Canadian Brand Names Abelcet® [US/Can]

Therapeutic Category Antifungal Agent

Use Treatment of aspergillosis or any type of progressive fungal infection in patients who are refractory to or intolerant of conventional amphotericin B therapy

Usual Dosage Children and Adults: I.V.:

Premedication: For patients who experience chills, fever, hypotension, nausea, or other nonanaphylactic infusion-related immediate reactions, premedicate with the following drugs, 30-60 minutes prior to drug administration: a nonsteroidal (eg, ibuprofen, choline magnesium trisalicylate) with or without diphenhydramine; or acetaminophen with diphenhydramine; or hydrocortisone 50-100 mg. If the patient experiences rigors during the infusion, meperidine may be administered.

Range: 2.5-5 mg/kg/day as a single infusion

Dosage Forms Injection, suspension: 5 mg/mL (20 mL)

amphotericin B liposomal (am foe TER i sin bee lye po SO mal)

Sound-Alike/Look-Alike Issues

AmBisome® may be confused with Abelcet®, Amphocin®, Amphotec®, Fungizone®

Synonyms L-AmB

U.S./Canadian Brand Names AmBisome® [US/Can]

Therapeutic Category Antifungal Agent, Systemic

(Continued)

amphotericin B liposomal *(Continued)*

Use Empirical therapy for presumed fungal infection in febrile, neutropenic patients. Treatment of patients with *Aspergillus* species, *Candida* species and/or *Cryptococcus* species infections refractory to amphotericin B desoxycholate, or in patients where renal impairment or unacceptable toxicity precludes the use of amphotericin B desoxycholate. Treatment of cryptococcal meningitis in HIV-infected patients. Treatment of visceral leishmaniasis.

Usual Dosage Children and Adults: I.V.:

Note: Premedication: For patients who experience chills, fever, hypotension, nausea, or other nonanaphylactic infusion-related immediate reactions, premedicate with the following drugs, 30-60 minutes prior to drug administration: a nonsteroidal (eg, ibuprofen, choline magnesium trisalicylate) with or without diphenhydramine; or acetaminophen with diphenhydramine; or hydrocortisone 50-100 mg. If the patient experiences rigors during the infusion, meperidine may be administered.

Empiric therapy: Recommended initial dose: 3 mg/kg/day

Systemic fungal infections (*Aspergillus, Candida, Cryptococcus*): Recommended initial dose of 3-5 mg/kg/day

Cryptococcal meningitis in HIV-infected patients: 6 mg/kg/day

Treatment of visceral leishmaniasis:

Immunocompetent patients: 3 mg/kg/day on days 1-5, and 3 mg/kg/day on days 14 and 21; a repeat course may be given in patients who do not achieve parasitic clearance

Immunocompromised patients: 4 mg/kg/day on days 1-5, and 4 mg/kg/day on days 10, 17, 24, 31, and 38

Dosage Forms Injection, powder for reconstitution: 50 mg

ampicillin (am pi SIL in)

Sound-Alike/Look-Alike Issues

ampicillin may be confused with aminophylline

Synonyms aminobenzylpenicillin; ampicillin sodium; ampicillin trihydrate

U.S./Canadian Brand Names Apo-Ampi® [Can]; Novo-Ampicillin [Can]; Nu-Ampi [Can]; Principen® [US]

Therapeutic Category Penicillin

Use Treatment of susceptible bacterial infections (nonbeta-lactamase-producing organisms); susceptible bacterial infections caused by streptococci, pneumococci, nonpenicillinase-producing staphylococci, *Listeria*, meningococci; some strains of *H. influenzae*, *Salmonella*, *Shigella*, *E. coli*, *Enterobacter*, and *Klebsiella*

Usual Dosage

Infants and Children:

Mild-to-moderate infections:

I.M., I.V.: 100-150 mg/kg/day in divided doses every 6 hours (maximum: 2-4 g/day)

Oral: 50-100 mg/kg/day in doses divided every 6 hours (maximum: 2-4 g/day)

Severe infections/meningitis: I.M., I.V.: 200-400 mg/kg/day in divided doses every 6 hours (maximum: 6-12 g/day)

Endocarditis prophylaxis: I.M., I.V.:

Dental, oral, respiratory tract, or esophageal procedures: 50 mg/kg within 30 minutes prior to procedure in patients unable to take oral amoxicillin

Genitourinary and gastrointestinal tract (except esophageal) procedures: High-risk patients: 50 mg/kg (maximum: 2 g) within 30 minutes prior to procedure, followed by ampicillin 25 mg/kg (or amoxicillin 25 mg/kg orally) 6 hours later; must be used in combination with gentamicin. Moderate-risk patients: 50 mg/kg within 30 minutes prior to procedure

Adults:

Susceptible infections:

Oral: 250-500 mg every 6 hours

I.M., I.V.: 250-500 mg every 6 hours

Sepsis/meningitis: I.M., I.V.: 150-250 mg/kg/24 hours divided every 3-4 hours (range: 6-12 g/day)

Endocarditis prophylaxis: I.M., I.V.:

Dental, oral, respiratory tract, or esophageal procedures: 2 g within 30 minutes prior to procedure in patients unable to take oral amoxicillin

Genitourinary and gastrointestinal tract (except esophageal) procedures: High-risk patients: 2 g within 30 minutes prior to procedure, followed by ampicillin 1 g (or amoxicillin 1 g orally) 6 hours later; must be used in combination with gentamicin Moderate-risk patients: 2 g within 30 minutes prior to procedure

Dosage Forms

Capsule (Principen®): 250 mg, 500 mg

Injection, powder for reconstitution, as sodium: 125 mg, 250 mg, 500 mg, 1 g, 2 g, 10 g

Powder for oral suspension (Principen®): 125 mg/5 mL (100 mL, 200 mL); 250 mg/5 mL (100 mL, 200 mL)

ampicillin and sulbactam (am pi SIL in & SUL bak tam)

Synonyms sulbactam and ampicillin

U.S./Canadian Brand Names Unasyn® [US/Can]

Therapeutic Category Penicillin

Use Treatment of susceptible bacterial infections involved with skin and skin structure, intra-abdominal infections, gynecological infections; spectrum is that of ampicillin plus organisms producing beta-lactamases such as *S. aureus*, *H. influenzae*, *E. coli*, *Klebsiella*, *Acinetobacter*, *Enterobacter*, and anaerobes

Usual Dosage Unasyn® (ampicillin/sulbactam) is a combination product. Dosage recommendations for Unasyn® are based on the ampicillin component.

Children ≥1 year: I.V.:

Mild-to-moderate infections: 100-150 mg ampicillin/kg/day (150-300 mg Unasyn®) divided every 6 hours; maximum: 8 g ampicillin/day (12 g Unasyn®)

Severe infections: 200-400 mg ampicillin/kg/day divided every 6 hours; maximum: 8 g ampicillin/day (12 g Unasyn®)

Adults: I.M., I.V.: 1-2 g ampicillin (1.5-3 g Unasyn®) every 6 hours; maximum: 8 g ampicillin/day (12 g Unasyn®)

Dosage Forms Injection, powder for reconstitution: 3 g [ampicillin sodium 2 g and sulbactam sodium 1 g]; 15 g [ampicillin sodium 10 g and sulbactam sodium 5 g] [bulk package]

Unasyn®: 1.5 g [ampicillin sodium 1 g and sulbactam sodium 0.5 g]; 3 g [ampicillin sodium 2 g and sulbactam sodium 1 g]; 15 g [ampicillin sodium 10 g and sulbactam sodium 5 g] [bulk package]

ampicillin sodium *see* ampicillin *on previous page*

ampicillin trihydrate *see* ampicillin *on previous page*

amprenavir (am PRE na veer)

U.S./Canadian Brand Names Agenerase® [US/Can]

Therapeutic Category Protease Inhibitor

Use Treatment of HIV infections in combination with at least two other antiretroviral agents; oral solution should only be used when capsules or other protease inhibitors are not therapeutic options

Usual Dosage Oral: **Note:** Capsule and oral solution are **not** interchangeable on a mg-per-mg basis.

Capsule:

Children 4-12 years and older (<50 kg): 20 mg/kg twice daily or 15 mg/kg 3 times daily; maximum: 2400 mg/day

Children >13 years (>50 kg) and Adults: 1200 mg twice daily

Note: Dosage adjustments for amprenavir when administered in combination therapy: Efavirenz: Adjustments necessary for both agents: Amprenavir 1200 mg 3 times/day (single protease inhibitor) **or** Amprenavir 1200 mg twice daily plus ritonavir 200 mg twice daily. Ritonavir: Adjustments necessary for both agents: Amprenavir 1200 mg plus ritonavir 200 mg once daily **or** Amprenavir 600 mg plus ritonavir 100 mg twice daily

(Continued)

amprenavir *(Continued)*

Solution:

Children 4-12 years or older (up to 16 years weighing <50 kg): 22.5 mg/kg twice daily or 17 mg/kg 3 times daily; maximum: 2800 mg/day

Children 13-16 years (weighing at least 50 kg) or >16 years and Adults: 1400 mg twice daily

Dosage Forms

Capsule: 50 mg, 150 mg

Solution, oral [use only when there are no other options]: 15 mg/mL (240 mL) [contains propylene glycol 550 mg/mL and vitamin E 46 int. units/mL; grape-bubblegum-peppermint flavor]

AMPT *see* metyrosine *on page 577*

amrinone lactate *see* inamrinone *on page 469*

Amvisc® *(Discontinued)* *see page 1042*

Amvisc® Plus *(Discontinued)* *see page 1042*

amyl nitrite (AM il NYE trite)

Synonyms isoamyl nitrite

Therapeutic Category Vasodilator

Use Coronary vasodilator in angina pectoris; adjunct in treatment of cyanide poisoning; produce changes in the intensity of heart murmurs

Usual Dosage Nasal inhalation:

Cyanide poisoning: Children and Adults: Inhale the vapor from a 0.3 mL crushed ampul every minute for 15-30 seconds until I.V. sodium nitrite infusion is available

Angina: Adults: 1-6 inhalations from 1 crushed ampul; may repeat in 3-5 minutes

Dosage Forms Vapor for inhalation [crushable glass perles]: 0.3 mL

amyl nitrite, sodium thiosulfate, and sodium nitrite *see* sodium nitrite, sodium thiosulfate, and amyl nitrite *on page 813*

amylobarbitone *see* amobarbital *on page 50*

Amytal® [US/Can] *see* amobarbital *on page 50*

Anabolin® *(Discontinued)* *see page 1042*

Anacin-3® (all products) *(Discontinued)* *see page 1042*

Anacin® PM Aspirin Free *(Discontinued)* *see page 1042*

Anadrol® [US] *see* oxymetholone *on page 659*

Anafranil® [US/Can] *see* clomipramine *on page 214*

anagrelide (an AG gre lide)

Synonyms 1370-999-397; anagrelide hydrochloride; BL4162A; 6,7-dichloro-1,5-dihydroimidazo [2,1b] quinazolin-2(3H)-one monohydrochloride

U.S./Canadian Brand Names Agrylin® [US/Can]

Therapeutic Category Platelet Reducing Agent

Use Treatment of essential thrombocythemia (ET) and thrombocythemia associated with chronic myelogenous leukemia (CML), polycythemia vera, and other myeloproliferative disorders

Usual Dosage Adults: Oral: 0.5 mg 4 times/day or 1 mg twice daily

Maintain for ≥1 week, then adjust to the lowest effective dose to reduce and maintain platelet count <600,000/µL ideally to the normal range; the dose must not be increased by >0.5 mg/day in any 1 week; maximum dose: 10 mg/day or 2.5 mg/dose

Dosage Forms Capsule: 0.5 mg, 1 mg

anagrelide hydrochloride *see* anagrelide *on this page*

Anaids® Tablet *(Discontinued)* *see page 1042*

anakinra (an a KIN ra)

Synonyms IL-1Ra; interleukin-1 receptor antagonist

U.S./Canadian Brand Names Kineret™ [US/Can]

Therapeutic Category Antirheumatic, Disease Modifying

Use Reduction of signs and symptoms of moderately- to severely-active rheumatoid arthritis in adult patients who have failed one or more disease-modifying antirheumatic drugs (DMARDs); may be used alone or in combination with DMARDs (other than tumor necrosis factor-blocking agents)

Usual Dosage Adults: SubQ: Rheumatoid arthritis: 100 mg once daily (administer at approximately the same time each day)

Dosage Forms Injection, solution [preservative free]: 100 mg/0.67 mL (1 mL) [prefilled syringe]

Ana-Kit® [US] *see* epinephrine and chlorpheniramine *on page 313*

Analpram-HC® [US] *see* pramoxine and hydrocortisone *on page 720*

AnaMantle® HC [US] *see* lidocaine and hydrocortisone *on page 520*

Anamine® Syrup *(Discontinued)* *see page 1042*

Anandron® [Can] *see* nilutamide *on page 620*

Anaplex® Liquid *(Discontinued)* *see page 1042*

Anaprox® [US/Can] *see* naproxen *on page 605*

Anaprox® DS [US/Can] *see* naproxen *on page 605*

Anaspaz® [US] *see* hyoscyamine *on page 459*

anastrozole (an AS troe zole)

Synonyms ICI-D1033; ZD1033

U.S./Canadian Brand Names Arimidex® [US/Can]

Therapeutic Category Antineoplastic Agent

Use Treatment of locally-advanced or metastatic breast cancer (ER-positive or hormone receptor unknown) in postmenopausal women; treatment of advanced breast cancer in postmenopausal women with disease progression following tamoxifen therapy; adjuvant treatment of early ER-positive breast cancer in postmenopausal women

Usual Dosage Refer to individual protocols. Breast cancer: Adults: Oral: 1 mg once daily

Dosage Forms Tablet: 1 mg

Anatrast® [US] *see* radiological/contrast media (ionic) *on page 759*

Anatuss® *(Discontinued)* *see page 1042*

Anbesol® Baby [US-OTC/Can] *see* benzocaine *on page 107*

Anbesol® Maximum Strength [US-OTC] *see* benzocaine *on page 107*

Anbesol® [US-OTC] *see* benzocaine *on page 107*

Ancef® [US] *see* cefazolin *on page 166*

Ancobon® [US/Can] *see* flucytosine *on page 372*

Andehist DM NR Drops [US] *see* carbinoxamine, pseudoephedrine, and dextromethorphan *on page 159*

Andehist NR Drops [US] *see* carbinoxamine and pseudoephedrine *on page 157*

Andehist NR Syrup [US] *see* brompheniramine and pseudoephedrine *on page 129*

Andriol® [Can] *see* testosterone *on page 848*

Androcur® [Can] *see* cyproterone *(Canada only) on page 238*

Androcur® Depot [Can] *see* cyproterone *(Canada only) on page 238*

Androderm® [US/Can] *see* testosterone *on page 848*

Andro/Fem® *(Discontinued)* *see page 1042*

AndroGel® [US/Can] *see* testosterone *on page 848*

Android® [US] *see* methyltestosterone *on page 573*

Andro-L.A.® Injection *(Discontinued)* *see page 1042*

Androlone® *(Discontinued)* *see page 1042*

Androlone®-D *(Discontinued)* *see page 1042*

Andropository [Can] *see* testosterone *on page 848*

Andropository® Injection *(Discontinued)* *see page 1042*

Anectine® *(Discontinued)* *see page 1042*

Anemagen™ OB [US] *see* vitamins (multiple/prenatal) *on page 927*

Anergan® 25 Injection *(Discontinued)* *see page 1042*

Anestacon® [US] *see* lidocaine *on page 518*

aneurine hydrochloride *see* thiamine *on page 856*

Anexate® [Can] *see* flumazenil *on page 373*

Anexsia® [US] *see* hydrocodone and acetaminophen *on page 443*

Angio Conray® [US] *see* radiological/contrast media (ionic) *on page 759*

Angiomax® [US/Can] *see* bivalirudin *on page 122*

Angiovist® [US] *see* radiological/contrast media (ionic) *on page 759*

Angiscein® [US] *see* fluorescein sodium *on page 375*

anisindione (an is in DY one)

Therapeutic Category Anticoagulant (Other)

Use Prophylaxis and treatment of venous thrombosis, pulmonary embolism, and thromboembolic disorders; atrial fibrillation with risk of embolism; adjunct in the prophylaxis of systemic embolism following myocardial infarction

Usual Dosage Oral: Adults:

Initial: 300 mg on first day, 200 mg on second day, 100 mg on third day

Maintenance dosage: Established by daily PT/INR determinations; range: 25-250 mg/day

Note: When discontinuing therapy, manufacturer recommends tapering dose over 3-4 weeks.

Dosage Forms Tablet: 50 mg

Anodynos-DHC® *(Discontinued)* *see page 1042*

Anolor 300 [US] *see* butalbital, acetaminophen, and caffeine *on page 138*

Anoquan® *(Discontinued)* *see page 1042*

Ansaid® [US/Can] *see* flurbiprofen *on page 381*

ansamycin *see* rifabutin *on page 775*

Antabuse® [US] *see* disulfiram *on page 283*

Antagon® [US/Can] *see* ganirelix *on page 397*

antazoline and naphazoline *see* naphazoline and antazoline *on page 604*

Antazoline-V® Ophthalmic *(Discontinued)* *see page 1042*

Anthra-Derm® *(Discontinued)* *see page 1042*

Anthraforte® [Can] *see* anthralin *on this page*

anthralin (AN thra lin)

Synonyms dithranol

U.S./Canadian Brand Names Anthraforte® [Can]; Anthranol® [Can]; Anthrascalp® [Can]; Drithocreme® [US]; Dritho-Scalp® [US]; Micanol® [Can]; Psoriatec™ [US]

Therapeutic Category Keratolytic Agent

Use Treatment of psoriasis (quiescent or chronic psoriasis)

Usual Dosage Adults: Topical: Generally, apply once a day or as directed. The irritant potential of anthralin is directly related to the strength being used and each patient's individual tolerance. Always commence treatment using a short, daily contact time (5-10 minutes) for at least 1 week using the lowest strength possible. Contact time may be gradually increased (to 20-30 minutes) as tolerated.

Skin application: Apply sparingly only to psoriatic lesions and rub gently and carefully into the skin until absorbed. Avoid applying an excessive quantity which may cause unnecessary soiling and staining of the clothing or bed linen.

Scalp application: Comb hair to remove scalar debris, wet hair and, after suitably parting, rub cream well into the lesions, taking care to prevent the cream from spreading onto the forehead,

Remove by washing or showering; optimal period of contact will vary according to the strength used and the patient's response to treatment. Continue treatment until the skin is entirely clear (ie, when there is nothing to feel with the fingers and the texture is normal).

Dosage Forms

Cream:

Dritho-Cream®, Psoriatec™: 1% (50 g)

Dritho-Scalp®: 0.5% (50 g)

Anthranol® [Can] *see* anthralin *on previous page*

Anthrascalp® [Can] *see* anthralin *on previous page*

anthrax vaccine, adsorbed (AN thraks vak SEEN, ad SORBED)

Synonyms AVA

U.S./Canadian Brand Names BioThrax™ [US]

Therapeutic Category Vaccine

Use Immunization against *Bacillus anthracis.* Recommended for individuals who may come in contact with animal products which come from anthrax endemic areas and may be contaminated with *Bacillus anthracis* spores; recommended for high-risk persons such as veterinarians and other handling potentially infected animals. Routine immunization for the general population is not recommended.

The Department of Defense is implementing an anthrax vaccination program against the biological warfare agent anthrax, which will be administered to all active duty and reserve personnel.

Usual Dosage SubQ:

Children <18 years: Safety and efficacy have not been established

Children ≥18 years and Adults:

Primary immunization: Three injections of 0.5 mL each given 2 weeks apart, followed by three additional injections given at 6-, 12-, and 18 months; it is not necessary to restart the series if a dose is not given on time; resume as soon as practical

Subsequent booster injections: 0.5 mL at 1-year intervals are recommended for immunity to be maintained

Dosage Forms Injection, suspension: 5 mL [vial stopper contains dry natural rubber]

Antiben® ***(Discontinued)*** *see page 1042*

AntibiOtic® Ear [US] *see* neomycin, polymyxin B, and hydrocortisone *on page 611*

anti-CD11a *see* efalizumab *on page 304*

anti-CD20 monoclonal antibody *see* rituximab *on page 780*

anti-CD20-murine monoclonal antibody I-131 *see* tositumomab and iodine I 131 tositumomab *on page 873*

antidigoxin fab fragments, ovine *see* digoxin immune Fab *on page 271*

antidiuretic hormone *see* vasopressin *on page 906*

antihemophilic factor (human) (an tee hee moe FIL ik FAK tor HYU man)

Synonyms AHF (human); factor VIII (human)

U.S./Canadian Brand Names Alphanate® [US]; Hemofil® M [US/Can]; Humate-P® [US/Can]; Koāte®-DVI [US]; Monarc® M [US]; Monoclate-P® [US]

Therapeutic Category Blood Product Derivative

Use Management of hemophilia A for patients in whom a deficiency in factor VIII has been demonstrated; can be of significant therapeutic value in patients with acquired factor VIII inhibitors not exceeding 10 Bethesda units/mL

Humate-P®: In addition, indicated as treatment of spontaneous bleeding in patients with severe von Willebrand disease and in mild and moderate von Willebrand disease where desmopressin is known or suspected to be inadequate

Orphan status: Alphanate®: Management of von Willebrand disease

Usual Dosage Children and Adults: I.V.: Individualize dosage based on coagulation studies performed prior to treatment and at regular intervals during treatment; 1 AHF unit is the activity present in 1 mL of normal pooled human plasma; dosage should be adjusted to actual vial size currently stocked in the pharmacy. (General guidelines presented; consult individual product labeling for specific dosing recommendations.)

Dosage based on desired factor VIII increase (%):

To calculate dosage needed based on desired factor VIII increase (%):

Body weight (kg) x 0.5 int. units/kg x desired factor VIII increase (%) = int. units factor VIII required

For example:

50 kg x 0.5 int. units/kg x 30 (% increase) = 750 int. units factor VIII

Dosage based on expected factor VIII increase (%):

It is also possible to calculate the **expected** % factor VIII increase:

(# int. units administered x 2%/int. units/kg) divided by body weight (kg) = expected % factor VIII increase

For example:

(1400 int. units x 2%/int. units/kg) divided by 70 kg = 40%

General guidelines:

Minor Hemorrhage: Required peak postinfusion AHF level: 20% to 40% (10-20 int. units/kg), repeat dose every 12-24 hours for 1-3 days until bleeding is resolved or healing achieved; mild superficial or early hemorrhages may respond to a single dose

Moderate hemorrhage: Required peak postinfusion AHF level: 30% to 60% (15-30 int. units/kg): Infuse every 12-24 hours for ≥3 days until pain and disability are resolved

Alternatively, a loading dose to achieve 50% (25 int. units/kg) may be given, followed by 10-15 int. units/kg dose given every 8-12 hours; may be needed for >7 days

Severe/life-threatening hemorrhage: Required peak postinfusion AHF level: 60% to 100% (30-50 int. units/kg): Infuse every 8-24 hours until threat is resolved

Alternatively, a loading dose to achieve 80% to 100% (40-50 int. units/kg) may be given, followed by 20-25 int. units/kg dose given every 8-12 hours for ≥14 days

Minor surgery: Required peak postinfusion AHF level: 30% to 80% (15-40 int. units/kg): Highly dependent upon procedure and specific product recommendations; for some procedures, may be administered as a single infusion plus oral antifibrinolytic therapy within 1 hour; in other procedures, may repeat dose every 12-24 hours as needed

Major surgery: Required peak pre- and postsurgery AHF level: 80% to 100% (40-50 int. units/kg): Administer every 6-24 hours until healing is complete (10-14 days)

Prophylaxis: May also be given on a regular schedule to prevent bleeding

If bleeding is not controlled with adequate dose, test for presence of inhibitor. It may not be possible or practical to control bleeding if inhibitor titers >10 Bethesda units/mL; antihemophilic factor (porcine) may be considered as an alternative

von Willebrand disease:

Treatment of hemorrhage in von Willebrand disease (Humate-P®): 1 int. units of factor VIII per kg of body weight would be expected to raise circulating vWF:RC of approximately 3.5-4 int. units/dL

Type 1, mild (if desmopressin is not appropriate): Major hemorrhage:

Loading dose: 40-60 int. units/kg

Maintenance dose: 40-50 int. units/kg every 8-12 hours for 3 days, keeping vWF:RC of nadir >50%; follow with 40-50 int. units/kg daily for up to 7 days

Type 1, moderate or severe:

Minor hemorrhage: 40-50 int. units/kg for 1-2 doses

Major hemorrhage: Loading dose: 50-75 int. units/kg Maintenance dose: 40-60 int. units/kg daily for up to 7 days

Types 2 and 3:

Minor hemorrhage: 40-50 int. units/kg for 1-2 doses

Major hemorrhage: Loading dose: 60-80 int. units/kg Maintenance dose: 40-60 int. units/kg every 8-12 hours for 3 days, keeping vWF:RC of nadir >50%; follow with 40-60 int. units/kg daily for up to 7 days

Dosage Forms Injection, human [single-dose vial]: Labeling on cartons and vials indicates number of int. units

antihemophilic factor (porcine) (an tee hee moe FIL ik FAK ter POR seen)

Synonyms AHF (porcine); factor VIII (porcine)

U.S./Canadian Brand Names Hyate:C® [US]

Therapeutic Category Antihemophilic Agent

Use Management of hemophilia A in patients with antibodies to human factor VIII (consider use of human factor VIII in patients with antibody titer of <5 Bethesda units/mL); management of previously nonhemophilic patients with spontaneously-acquired inhibitors to human factor VIII, regardless of initial antihuman inhibitor titer

Usual Dosage Clinical response should be used to assess efficacy

Initial dose:

Antibody level to human factor VIII <50 Bethesda units/mL: 100-150 porcine units/kg (body weight) is recommended

Antibody level to human factor VIII >50 Bethesda units/mL: Activity of the antibody to antihemophilic (porcine) should be determined; **an antiporcine antibody level** >20 Bethesda units/mL indicates that the patient is unlikely to benefit from treatment; for lower titers, a dose of 100-150 porcine units/kg is recommended

The initial dose may also be calculated using the following method:

1. Determine patient's antibody titer against porcine factor VIII
2. Calculate average plasma volume: (body weight kg) (average blood volume) (1 - hematocrit) = plasma volume (body weight kg) (80 mL/kg) (1 - hematocrit) = plasma volume **Note:** A hematocrit of 50% = 0.5 for the equation
3. Neutralizing dose: (plasma volume mL) (antibody titer Bethesda units/mL) = neutralizing dose units This is the predicted dose required to neutralize the circulating antibodies. An incremental dose must be added to the neutralizing dose in order to increase the plasma factor VIII to the desired level.
4. Incremental dose: (desired plasma factor VIII level) (body weight) divided by 1.5 = incremental dose units
5. Total dose = neutralizing dose + incremental dose = total dose units

If a patient has previously been treated with Hyate:C®, this may provide a guide to his likely response and, therefore, assist in estimation of the preliminary dose

Subsequent doses: Following administration of the initial dose, if the recovery of factor VIII in the patient's plasma is not sufficient, another larger dose should be administered; if recovery after the second dose is still insufficient, a third and larger dose may prove effective. Once appropriate factor VIII levels are achieved, dosing can be repeated every 6-8 hours.

Dosage Forms Injection, powder for reconstitution: 400-700 porcine units [to be reconstituted with 20 mL SWFI]

antihemophilic factor (recombinant)

(an tee hee moe FIL ik FAK tor ree KOM be nant)

Synonyms AHF (recombinant); factor VIII (recombinant); rAHF

U.S./Canadian Brand Names Advate [US]; Helixate® FS [US/Can]; Kogenate® [Can]; Kogenate® FS [US/Can]; Recombinate™ [US/Can]; ReFacto® [US/Can]

Therapeutic Category Blood Product Derivative

(Continued)

antihemophilic factor (recombinant) *(Continued)*

Use Management of hemophilia A (classic hemophilia) for patients in whom a deficiency in factor VIII has been demonstrated; prevention and control of bleeding episodes; perioperative management of hemophilia A; can be of significant therapeutic value in patients with acquired factor VIII inhibitors not exceeding 10 Bethesda units/mL

Usual Dosage Children and Adults: I.V.: Individualize dosage based on coagulation studies performed prior to treatment and at regular intervals during treatment; 1 AHF unit is the activity present in 1 mL of normal pooled human plasma; dosage should be adjusted to actual vial size currently stocked in the pharmacy. (General guidelines presented; consult individual product labeling for specific dosing recommendations.)

Dosage based on desired factor VIII increase (%):

To calculate dosage needed based on desired factor VIII increase (%):

Body weight (kg) x 0.5 int. units/kg x desired factor VIII increase (%) = int. units factor VIII required

For example:

50 kg x 0.5 int. units/kg x 30 (% increase) = 750 int. units factor VIII

Dosage based on expected factor VIII increase (%):

It is also possible to calculate the **expected** % factor VIII increase:

(# int. units administered x 2%/int. units/kg) divided by body weight (kg) = expected % factor VIII increase

For example:

(1400 int. units x 2%/int. units/kg) divided by 70 kg = 40%

General guidelines:

Minor hemorrhage: Required peak postinfusion AHF level: 20% to 40% (10-20 int. units/kg); mild superficial or early hemorrhages may respond to a single dose; may repeat dose every 12-24 hours for 1-3 days until bleeding is resolved or healing achieved

Moderate hemorrhage/minor surgery: Required peak postinfusion AHF level: 30% to 60% (15-30 int. units/kg); repeat dose at 12-24 hours if needed; some products suggest continuing for ≥3 days until pain and disability are resolved

Severe/life-threatening hemorrhage: Required peak postinfusion AHF level: Initial dose: 80% to 100% (40-50 int. units/kg); maintenance dose: 40% to 50% (20-25 int. units/kg) every 8-12 hours until threat is resolved

Major surgery: Required peak pre- and postsurgery AHF level: ~100% (50 int. units/kg) give first dose prior to surgery and repeat every 6-12 hours until healing complete (10-14 days)

Prophylaxis: May also be given on a regular schedule to prevent bleeding

If bleeding is not controlled with adequate dose, test for presence of inhibitor. It may not be possible or practical to control bleeding if inhibitor titers >10 Bethesda units/mL; antihemophilic factor (porcine) may be considered as an alternative

Dosage Forms

Injection, powder for reconstitution, recombinant [preservative free]:

Advate: 250 int. units, 500 int. units, 1000 int. units, 1500 int. units [plasma/albumin free]

Helixate® FS, Kogenate® FS: 250 int. units, 500 int. units, 1000 int. units [contains sucrose 28 mg/vial]

Recombinate™: 250 int. units, 500 units, 1000 int. units [contains human albumin 12.5 mg/mL; packaging contains natural rubber latex]

ReFacto®: 250 int. units, 500 units, 1000 int. units, 2000 int. units [contains sucrose]

Antihist-1® ***(Discontinued)*** *see page 1042*

Antihist-D® ***(Discontinued)*** *see page 1042*

anti-inhibitor coagulant complex

(an tee-in HI bi tor coe AG yoo lant KOM pleks)

Synonyms coagulant complex inhibitor

U.S./Canadian Brand Names Autoplex® T [US]; Feiba VH® [US]; Feiba VH Immuno® [Can]

Therapeutic Category Hemophilic Agent

Use Patients with factor VIII inhibitors who are to undergo surgery or those who are bleeding

Usual Dosage Dosage range: 25-100 factor VIII correctional units per kg depending on the severity of hemorrhage

Dosage Forms

Injection, powder for reconstitution:

Autoplex® T: Each bottle is labeled with correctional units of factor VIII [with heparin 2 units/mL; packaging contains natural rubber latex]

Feiba VH®: Each bottle is labeled with correctional units of factor VIII [heparin free; packaging contains natural rubber latex]

Antilirium® *(Discontinued)* *see page 1042*

Antiminth® *(Discontinued)* *see page 1042*

Antinea® Cream *(Discontinued)* *see page 1042*

Antiphlogistine Rub A-535 Capsaicin [Can] *see* capsaicin *on page 153*

Antiphlogistine Rub A-535 No Odour [Can] *see* triethanolamine salicylate *on page 884*

antipyrine and benzocaine (an tee PYE reen & BEN zoe kane)

Sound-Alike/Look-Alike Issues

Auralgan® may be confused with Ophthalgan®

Synonyms benzocaine and antipyrine

U.S./Canadian Brand Names A/B® Otic [US]; Allergan® [US]; Auralgan® [Can]; Aurodex® [US]; Auroto® [US]

Therapeutic Category Otic Agent, Analgesic; Otic Agent, Ceruminolytic

Use Temporary relief of pain and reduction of swelling associated with acute congestive and serous otitis media, swimmer's ear, otitis externa; facilitates ear wax removal

Usual Dosage Otic: Fill ear canal; moisten cotton pledget, place in external ear, repeat every 1-2 hours until pain and congestion are relieved; for ear wax removal instill drops 3-4 times/day for 2-3 days

Dosage Forms

Solution, otic: Antipyrine 5.4% and benzocaine 1.4% (15 mL)

A/B Otic, Allergen®, Aurodex, Auroto: Antipyrine 5.4% and benzocaine 1.4% (15 mL)

Antispas® Injection *(Discontinued)* *see page 1042*

antithrombin III (an tee THROM bin three)

Synonyms AT III; heparin cofactor I

U.S./Canadian Brand Names Thrombate III® [US/Can]

Therapeutic Category Blood Product Derivative

Use Treatment of hereditary antithrombin III deficiency in connection with surgical or obstetrical procedures; thromboembolism

Usual Dosage Adults:

Initial dose: Dosing is individualized based on pretherapy AT-III levels. The initial dose should raise antithrombin III levels (AT-III) to 120% and may be calculated based on the following formula:

Initial dosage (int. units) = [desired AT-III level % - baseline AT-III level %] x body weight (kg) divided by 1.4%/int. units/kg (eg, if a 70 kg adult patient had a baseline AT-III level of 57%, the initial dose would be (120% - 57%) x 70/1.4%/int. units/kg = 3150 int. units).

(Continued)

antithrombin III *(Continued)*

Maintenance dose: Subsequent dosing should be targeted to keep levels between 80% to 120% which may be achieved by administering 60% of the initial dose every 24 hours. Adjustments may be made by adjusting dose or interval. Maintain level within normal range for 2-8 days depending on type of surgery or procedure.

Dosage Forms Injection, powder for reconstitution [preservative free]: 500 int. units, 1000 int. units [contains heparin; packaged with diluent]

antithymocyte globulin (equine) (an te THY moe site GLOB yu lin, E kwine)

Sound-Alike/Look-Alike Issues

Atgam® may be confused with Ativan®

Synonyms horse antihuman thymocyte gamma globulin

U.S./Canadian Brand Names Atgam® [US/Can]

Therapeutic Category Immunosuppressant Agent

Use Prevention and treatment of acute renal allograft rejection; treatment of moderate to severe aplastic anemia in patients not considered suitable candidates for bone marrow transplantation

Usual Dosage An intradermal skin test is recommended prior to administration of the initial dose of ATG; use 0.1 mL of a 1:1000 dilution of ATG in normal saline. A positive skin reaction consists of a wheal ≥10 mm in diameter. If a positive skin test occurs, the first infusion should be administered in a controlled environment with intensive life support immediately available. A systemic reaction precludes further administration of the drug. The absence of a reaction does **not** preclude the possibility of an immediate sensitivity reaction.

Premedication with diphenhydramine, hydrocortisone, and acetaminophen is recommended prior to first dose.

Children: I.V.:

Aplastic anemia protocol: 10-20 mg/kg/day for 8-14 days; then administer every other day for 7 more doses; addition doses may be given every other day for 21 total doses in 28 days

Renal allograft: 5-25 mg/kg/day

Adults: I.V.:

Aplastic anemia protocol: 10-20 mg/kg/day for 8-14 days, then administer every other day for 7 more doses, for a total of 21 doses in 28 days

Renal allograft:

Rejection prophylaxis: 15 mg/kg/day for 14 days followed by 14 days of alternative day therapy at the same dose; the first dose should be administered within 24 hours before or after transplantation

Rejection treatment: 10-15 mg/kg/day for 14 days, then administer every other day for 10-14 days up to 21 doses in 28 days

Dosage Forms Injection, solution: 50 mg/mL (5 mL)

antithymocyte globulin (rabbit) (an te THY moe site GLOB yu lin RAB bit)

Synonyms antithymocyte immunoglobulin; ATG

U.S./Canadian Brand Names Thymoglobulin® [US]

Therapeutic Category Immunosuppressant Agent

Use Treatment of renal transplant acute rejection in conjunction with concomitant immunosuppression

Usual Dosage I.V.: 1.5 mg/kg/day for 7-14 days

Dosage Forms Injection, powder for reconstitution: 25 mg vial [packaged with diluent]

antithymocyte immunoglobulin *see* antithymocyte globulin (rabbit) *on this page*

antitumor necrosis factor apha (human) *see* adalimumab *on page 20*

Anti-Tuss® Expectorant *(Discontinued)* *see page 1042*

anti-VEGF monoclonal antibody *see* bevacizumab *on page 117*

antivenin *(Crotalidae)* polyvalent

(an tee VEN in (kroe TAL ih die) pol i VAY lent)

Synonyms crotaline antivenin, polyvalent; North and South American antisnake-bite serum; pit viper antivenin; snake (pit viper) antivenin

U.S./Canadian Brand Names Antivenin Polyvalent [Equine] [US]; CroFab™ [Ovine] [US]

Therapeutic Category Antivenin

Use Neutralization of venoms of North and South American crotalids: Rattlesnake, copperhead, cottonmouth, tropical moccasins, fer-de-lance, bushmaster

Usual Dosage Children and Adults: Crotalid envenomation:

Antivenin polyvalent (equine): I.M., I.V.: Initial sensitivity test: 0.02-0.03 mL of a 1:10 dilution of normal horse serum or antivenin given intracutaneously; also give a control test using normal saline in the opposite extremity. A positive reaction occurs within 5-30 minutes. A negative reaction does not rule out the possibility of an immediate or delayed reaction with treatment.

Minimal envenomation: 20-40 mL (2-4 vials)

Moderate envenomation: 50-90 mL (5-9 vials)

Severe envenomation: 100-150 mL (10-15 vials) or more

Note: The entire initial dose of antivenin should be administered as soon as possible to be most effective (within 4 hours after the bite). I.V. is the preferred route of administration. When administered I.V., infuse the initial 5-10 mL dilution over 3-5 minutes while carefully observing the patient for signs and symptoms of sensitivity reactions. If no reaction occurs, continue infusion at a safe I.V. fluid delivery rate. Additional doses of antivenin are based on clinical response to the initial dose. If swelling continues to progress, symptoms increase in severity, hypotension occurs, or decrease in hematocrit appears, an additional 10-50 mL (1-5 vials) should be administered.

Antivenin polyvalent (ovine): I.V.: Minimal or moderate envenomation:

Initial dose: 4-6 vials, dependent upon patient response. Treatment should begin within 6 hours of snakebite; monitor for 1 hour following infusion. Repeat with an additional 4-6 vials if control is not achieved with initial dose. Continue to treat with 4- to 6-vial doses until complete arrest of local manifestations, coagulation tests, and systemic signs are normal. Administer I.V. over 60 minutes at a rate of 25-50 mL/hour for the first 10 minutes. If no allergic reaction is observed, increase rate to 250 mL/hour. Monitor closely

Maintenance dose: Once control is achieved, administer 2 vials every 6 hours for up to 18 hours; optimal dosing past 18 hours has not been established; however, treatment may be continued if deemed necessary based on the patients condition

Dosage Forms Injection, powder for reconstitution:

Antivenin polyvalent [equine]: Derived from *Croatus adamanteus, C. atrox, C. durissus terrificous,* and *Bothrops atrox* snake venoms [equine origin; contains phenol and thimerosal; packaged with diluent]

CroFab™ [ovine]: Derived from *Croatus adamanteus, C. atrox, C. scutulatus,* and *Agkistrodon piscivorus* snake venoms [ovine origin; contains thimerosal; manufactured with papain]

antivenin *(Latrodectus mactans)* (an tee VEN in lak tro DUK tus MAK tans)

Synonyms black widow spider species antivenin (*Latrodectus mactans*)

Therapeutic Category Antivenin

Use Treatment of patients with symptoms of black widow spider bites

Usual Dosage

Children <12 years (severe or shock): I.V.: 2.5 mL in 10-50 mL over 15 minutes

Children and Adults: I.M.: 2.5 mL

Dosage Forms Injection, powder for reconstitution: 6000 antivenin units [equine origin; contains thimerosal; packaged with diluent]

antivenin *(Micrurus fulvius)* (an tee VEN in mye KRU rus FUL vee us)

Synonyms North American coral snake antivenin

Therapeutic Category Antivenin

(Continued)

antivenin *(Micrurus fulvius)* *(Continued)*

Use Neutralization of venoms of Eastern coral snake and Texas coral snake, but does **not** neutralize venom of Arizona or Sonoran coral snake

Usual Dosage I.V.: Children and Adults: 3-5 vials by slow injection (dependent on severity of signs/symptoms; some patients may need more than 10 vials)

Dosage Forms Injection, powder for reconstitution: Derived from *Micrurus fulvius* venom [equine origin; contains phenol and thimerosal; packaged with diluent]

Antivenin Polyvalent [Equine] [US] *see* antivenin *(Crotalidae)* polyvalent *on previous page*

Antivert® [US/Can] *see* meclizine *on page 546*

Antivert® Chewable Tablet *(Discontinued)* *see page 1042*

Antizol® [US] *see* fomepizole *on page 387*

Antrizine® *(Discontinued)* *see page 1042*

Antrocol® Capsule & Tablet *(Discontinued)* *see page 1042*

Anturane® *(Discontinued)* *see page 1042*

Anucort™ HC [US] *see* hydrocortisone (rectal) *on page 448*

Anusol-HC® Suppository [US] *see* hydrocortisone (rectal) *on page 448*

Anusol® Ointment [US-OTC] *see* pramoxine *on page 720*

Anuzinc [Can] *see* zinc sulfate *on page 941*

Anxanil® Oral *(Discontinued)* *see page 1042*

Anzemet® [US/Can] *see* dolasetron *on page 287*

Apacet® *(Discontinued)* *see page 1042*

APAP *see* acetaminophen *on page 5*

APAP and tramadol *see* acetaminophen and tramadol *on page 10*

Apaphen® *(Discontinued)* *see page 1042*

Apatate® [US-OTC] *see* vitamin B complex combinations *on page 915*

ApexiCon™ [US] *see* diflorasone *on page 269*

ApexiCon™ E [US] *see* diflorasone *on page 269*

Aphedrid™ [US-OTC] *see* triprolidine and pseudoephedrine *on page 889*

Aphrodyne® [US] *see* yohimbine *on page 936*

Aphthasol® [US] *see* amlexanox *on page 48*

Apidra™ [US] *see* insulin preparations *on page 474*

A.P.L.® *(Discontinued)* *see page 1042*

Aplisol® [US] *see* tuberculin tests *on page 893*

Aplitest® *(Discontinued)* *see page 1042*

aplonidine *see* apraclonidine *on page 74*

Apo-Acebutolol® [Can] *see* acebutolol *on page 4*

Apo-Acetaminophen® [Can] *see* acetaminophen *on page 5*

Apo-Acetazolamide® [Can] *see* acetazolamide *on page 14*

Apo-Acyclovir® [Can] *see* acyclovir *on page 19*

Apo-Allopurinol® [Can] *see* allopurinol *on page 33*

Apo-Alpraz® [Can] *see* alprazolam *on page 35*

Apo-Amilzide® [Can] *see* amiloride and hydrochlorothiazide *on page 45*

Apo-Amitriptyline® [Can] *see* amitriptyline *on page 47*

Apo-Amoxi® [Can] *see* amoxicillin *on page 51*

Apo-Diltiaz® [Can] *see* diltiazem *on page 273*
Apo-Diltiaz CD® [Can] *see* diltiazem *on page 273*
Apo-Diltiaz SR® [Can] *see* diltiazem *on page 273*
Apo-Dimenhydrinate® [Can] *see* dimenhydrinate *on page 274*
Apo-Dipivefrin® [Can] *see* dipivefrin *on page 281*
Apo-Dipyridamole FC® [Can] *see* dipyridamole *on page 282*
Apo-Divalproex® [Can] *see* valproic acid and derivatives *on page 901*
Apo-Docusate-Calcium® [Can] *see* docusate *on page 285*
Apo-Docusate-Sodium® [Can] *see* docusate *on page 285*
Apo-Domperidone® [Can] *see* domperidone *(Canada only) on page 288*
Apo-Doxazosin® [Can] *see* doxazosin *on page 291*
Apo-Doxepin® [Can] *see* doxepin *on page 292*
Apo-Doxy® [Can] *see* doxycycline *on page 294*
Apo-Doxy Tabs® [Can] *see* doxycycline *on page 294*
Apo-Erythro Base® [Can] *see* erythromycin *on page 320*
Apo-Erythro E-C® [Can] *see* erythromycin *on page 320*
Apo-Erythro-ES® [Can] *see* erythromycin *on page 320*
Apo-Erythro-S® [Can] *see* erythromycin *on page 320*
Apo-Etodolac® [Can] *see* etodolac *on page 350*
Apo-Famotidine® [Can] *see* famotidine *on page 356*
Apo-Fenofibrate® [Can] *see* fenofibrate *on page 360*
Apo-Feno-Micro® [Can] *see* fenofibrate *on page 360*
Apo-Ferrous Gluconate® [Can] *see* ferrous gluconate *on page 364*
Apo-Ferrous Sulfate® [Can] *see* ferrous sulfate *on page 364*
Apo-Flavoxate® [Can] *see* flavoxate *on page 369*
Apo-Fluconazole® [Can] *see* fluconazole *on page 371*
Apo-Flunisolide® [Can] *see* flunisolide *on page 373*
Apo-Fluoxetine® [Can] *see* fluoxetine *on page 379*
Apo-Fluphenazine® [Can] *see* fluphenazine *on page 380*
Apo-Fluphenzaine Decanoate® [Can] *see* fluphenazine *on page 380*
Apo-Flurazepam® [Can] *see* flurazepam *on page 381*
Apo-Flurbiprofen® [Can] *see* flurbiprofen *on page 381*
Apo-Flutamide® [Can] *see* flutamide *on page 382*
Apo-Fluvoxamine® [Can] *see* fluvoxamine *on page 385*
Apo-Folic® [Can] *see* folic acid *on page 385*
Apo-Furosemide® [Can] *see* furosemide *on page 393*
Apo-Gabapentin® [Can] *see* gabapentin *on page 395*
Apo-Gain® [Can] *see* minoxidil *on page 584*
Apo-Gemfibrozil® [Can] *see* gemfibrozil *on page 400*
Apo-Gliclazide® [Can] *see* gliclazide *(Canada only) on page 405*
Apo-Glyburide® [Can] *see* glyburide *on page 409*
Apo-Haloperidol® [Can] *see* haloperidol *on page 428*
Apo-Haloperidol LA® [Can] *see* haloperidol *on page 428*
Apo-Hydralazine® [Can] *see* hydralazine *on page 440*

Apo-Minocycline® [Can] *see* minocycline *on page 583*

Apo-Misoprostil® [Can] *see* misoprostol *on page 585*

Apo-Moclobemide® [Can] *see* moclobemide *(Canada only) on page 587*

apomorphine (a poe MOR feen)

Synonyms apomorphine hydrochloride; apomorphine hydrochloride hemihydrate

U.S./Canadian Brand Names Apokyn™ [US]

Therapeutic Category Anti-Parkinson Agent (Dopamine Agonist)

Use Treatment of hypomobility, "off" episodes with Parkinson disease

Usual Dosage SubQ: Adults: Begin antiemetic therapy 3 days prior to initiation and continue for 2 months before reassessing need.

Parkinson disease, "off" episode: Initial test dose 2 mg, **medical supervision required; see "Note"**. Subsequent dosing is based on both tolerance and response to initial test dose.

If patient tolerates test dose and responds: Starting dose: 2 mg as needed; may increase dose in 1 mg increments every few days; maximum dose: 6 mg

If patient tolerates but does not respond to 2 mg test dose: Second test dose: 4 mg

If patient tolerates and responds to 4 mg test dose: Starting dose: 3 mg, as needed for "off" episodes; may increase dose in 1 mg increments every few days; maximum dose 6 mg

If patient does not tolerate 4 mg test dose: Third test dose: 3 mg

If patient tolerates 3 mg test dose: Starting dose: 2 mg as needed for "off" episodes; may increase dose in 1 mg increments to a maximum of 3 mg

If therapy is interrupted for >1 week, restart at 2 mg and gradually titrate dose.

Note: Medical supervision is required for all test doses with standing and supine blood pressure monitoring predose and 20-, 40-, and 60 minutes postdose. If subsequent test doses are required, wait >2 hours before another test dose is given; next test dose should be timed with another "off" episode. If a single dose is ineffective for a particular "off" episode, then a second dose should not be given. The average dosing frequency was 3 times/day in the development program with limited experience in dosing >5 times/day and with total daily doses >20 mg. Apomorphine is intended to treat the "off" episodes associated with levodopa therapy of Parkinson disease and has not been studied in levodopa-naive Parkinson patients.

Dosage Forms Injection, solution, as hydrochloride: 10 mg/mL (2 mL) [contains sodium metabisulfite]; (3 mL) [multidose cartridge; contains sodium metabisulfite and benzyl alcohol]

apomorphine hydrochloride *see* apomorphine *on this page*

apomorphine hydrochloride hemihydrate *see* apomorphine *on this page*

Apo-Nabumetone® [Can] *see* nabumetone *on page 598*

Apo-Nadol® [Can] *see* nadolol *on page 599*

Apo-Napro-Na® [Can] *see* naproxen *on page 605*

Apo-Napro-Na DS® [Can] *see* naproxen *on page 605*

Apo-Naproxen® [Can] *see* naproxen *on page 605*

Apo-Naproxen SR® [Can] *see* naproxen *on page 605*

Apo-Nefazodone® [Can] *see* nefazodone *on page 608*

Apo-Nifed® [Can] *see* nifedipine *on page 619*

Apo-Nifed PA® [Can] *see* nifedipine *on page 619*

Apo-Nitrofurantoin® [Can] *see* nitrofurantoin *on page 622*

Apo-Nizatidine® [Can] *see* nizatidine *on page 625*

Apo-Norflox® [Can] *see* norfloxacin *on page 628*

Apo-Nortriptyline® [Can] *see* nortriptyline *on page 629*

Apo-Oflox® [Can] *see* ofloxacin *on page 640*

Apo-Trimebutine® [Can] *see* trimebutine *(Canada only) on page 886*

Apo-Trimethoprim® [Can] *see* trimethoprim *on page 887*

Apo-Trimip® [Can] *see* trimipramine *on page 888*

Apo-Verap® [Can] *see* verapamil *on page 908*

Apo-Warfarin® [Can] *see* warfarin *on page 933*

Apo-Zidovudine® [Can] *see* zidovudine *on page 939*

Apo-Zopiclone® [Can] *see* zopiclone *(Canada only) on page 944*

APPG *see* penicillin G procaine *on page 676*

apraclonidine (a pra KLOE ni deen)

Sound-Alike/Look-Alike Issues

Iopidine® may be confused with indapamide, iodine, Lodine®

Synonyms aplonidine; apraclonidine hydrochloride; p-aminoclonidine

U.S./Canadian Brand Names Iopidine® [US/Can]

Therapeutic Category Alpha$_2$-Adrenergic Agonist Agent, Ophthalmic

Use Prevention and treatment of postsurgical intraocular pressure (IOP) elevation; short-term, adjunctive therapy in patients who require additional reduction of IOP

Usual Dosage Adults: Ophthalmic:

0.5%: Instill 1-2 drops in the affected eye(s) 3 times/day

1%: Instill 1 drop in operative eye 1 hour prior to anterior segment laser surgery, second drop in eye immediately upon completion of procedure

Dosage Forms Solution, ophthalmic, as hydrochloride: 0.5% (5 mL, 10 mL); 1% (0.1 mL) [contains benzalkonium chloride]

apraclonidine hydrochloride *see* apraclonidine *on this page*

aprepitant (ap RE pi tant)

Synonyms L 754030; MK 869

U.S./Canadian Brand Names Emend® [US]

Therapeutic Category Antiemetic

Use Prevention of acute and delayed nausea and vomiting associated with highly-emetogenic chemotherapy in combination with a corticosteroid and 5-HT$_3$ receptor antagonist

Usual Dosage Oral: Adults: 125 mg on day 1, followed by 80 mg on days 2 and 3; should be used in combination with a corticosteroid and 5-HT$_3$ receptor antagonist

In clinical trials, the following regimen was used:

Aprepitant: Oral: 125 mg day 1, followed by 80 mg on days 2 and 3

Dexamethasone: Oral: 12 mg on day 1, followed 8 mg on days 2, 3, and 4

Ondansetron: I.V.: 32 mg on day 1

Dosage Forms

Capsule: 80 mg, 125 mg

Combination package: 80 mg (2 capsules) and 125 mg (1 capsule)

Apresazide® *(Discontinued)* *see page 1042*

Apresoline® *(Discontinued)* *see page 1042*

Apresoline® [Can] *see* hydralazine *on page 440*

Apri® [US] *see* ethinyl estradiol and desogestrel *on page 335*

Aprodine® [US-OTC] *see* triprolidine and pseudoephedrine *on page 889*

aprotinin (a proe TYE nin)

U.S./Canadian Brand Names Trasylol® [US/Can]

Therapeutic Category Hemostatic Agent

Use Reduction or prevention of blood loss in patients undergoing coronary artery bypass surgery when a high risk of excessive bleeding exists, including open heart reoperation, pre-existing coagulopathies, operations on the great vessels, and when a patient's beliefs prohibit blood transfusions

Usual Dosage

Test dose: **All** patients should receive a 1 mL I.V. test dose at least 10 minutes prior to the loading dose to assess the potential for allergic reactions. **Note:** To avoid physical incompatibility with heparin when adding to pump-prime solution, each agent should be added during recirculation to assure adequate dilution.

Regimen A (standard dose):

2 million units (280 mg) loading dose I.V. over 20-30 minutes
2 million units (280 mg) into pump prime volume
500,000 units/hour (70 mg/hour) I.V. during operation

Regimen B (low dose):

1 million units (140 mg) loading dose I.V. over 20-30 minutes
1 million units (140 mg) into pump prime volume
250,000 units/hour (35 mg/hour) I.V. during operation

Dosage Forms Injection, solution: 1.4 mg/mL [10,000 KIU/mL] (100 mL, 200 mL)

Aquacare® [US-OTC] *see* urea *on page 897*

Aquachloral® Supprettes® [US] *see* chloral hydrate *on page 181*

Aquacort® [Can] *see* hydrocortisone (topical) *on page 451*

Aqua Gem E® [US-OTC] *see* vitamin E *on page 918*

AquaLase™ [US] *see* balanced salt solution *on page 99*

Aqua Lube Plus [US-OTC] *see* nonoxynol 9 *on page 626*

AquaMEPHYTON® *(Discontinued)* *see page 1042*

AquaMEPHYTON® [Can] *see* phytonadione *on page 693*

Aquanil™ HC [US] *see* hydrocortisone (topical) *on page 451*

Aquaphilic® With Carbamide [US-OTC] *see* urea *on page 897*

Aquaphyllin® *(Discontinued)* *see page 1042*

AquaSite® [US-OTC] *see* artificial tears *on page 78*

Aquasol A® [US] *see* vitamin A *on page 914*

Aquasol E® [US-OTC] *see* vitamin E *on page 918*

Aquatab® C [US] *see* guaifenesin, pseudoephedrine, and dextromethorphan *on page 422*

Aquatab® D [US] *see* guaifenesin and pseudoephedrine *on page 419*

Aquatab® DM [US] *see* guaifenesin and dextromethorphan *on page 416*

AquaTar® *(Discontinued)* *see page 1042*

Aquatensen® [US/Can] *see* methyclothiazide *on page 568*

Aquazide® H [US] *see* hydrochlorothiazide *on page 441*

aqueous procaine penicillin G *see* penicillin G procaine *on page 676*

Aquest® *(Discontinued)* *see page 1042*

arabinosylcytosine *see* cytarabine *on page 239*

ara-C *see* cytarabine *on page 239*

Aralast™ [US] *see* alpha$_1$-proteinase inhibitor *on page 34*

Aralen® [US/Can] *see* chloroquine phosphate *on page 186*

Aralen® Phosphate With Primaquine Phosphate *(Discontinued)* *see page 1042*

Aramine® *(Discontinued)* *see page 1042*

Aramine® [Can] *see* metaraminol *on page 559*

Aranesp® [US/Can] *see* darbepoetin alfa *on page 245*

Arava® [US/Can] *see* leflunomide *on page 508*

Arcotinic® Tablet *(Discontinued)* *see page 1042*

Arduan® *(Discontinued)* *see page 1042*

Aredia® [US/Can] *see* pamidronate *on page 662*

argatroban (ar GA troh ban)

Therapeutic Category Anticoagulant, Thrombin Inhibitor

Use Prophylaxis or treatment of thrombosis in adults with heparin-induced thrombocytopenia; adjunct to percutaneous coronary intervention (PCI) in patients who have or are at risk of thrombosis associated with heparin-induced thrombocytopenia

Usual Dosage I.V.: Adults:

Heparin-induced thrombocytopenia:

Initial dose: 2 mcg/kg/minute

Maintenance dose: Measure aPTT after 2 hours, adjust dose until the steady-state aPTT is 1.5-3.0 times the initial baseline value, not exceeding 100 seconds; dosage should not exceed 10 mcg/kg/minute

Conversion to oral anticoagulant: Because there may be a combined effect on the INR when argatroban is combined with warfarin, loading doses of warfarin should not be used. Warfarin therapy should be started at the expected daily dose.

Patients receiving ≤2 mcg/kg/minute of argatroban: Argatroban therapy can be stopped when the combined INR on warfarin and argatroban is >4; repeat INR measurement in 4-6 hours; if INR is below therapeutic level, argatroban therapy may be restarted. Repeat procedure daily until desired INR on warfarin alone is obtained.

Patients receiving >2 mcg/kg/minute of argatroban: Reduce dose of argatroban to 2 mcg/kg/minute; measure INR for argatroban and warfarin 4-6 hours after dose reduction; argatroban therapy can be stopped when the combined INR on warfarin and argatroban is >4. Repeat INR measurement in 4-6 hours; if INR is below therapeutic level, argatroban therapy may be restarted. Repeat procedure daily until desired INR on warfarin alone is obtained.

Note: Critically-ill patients with normal hepatic function became excessively anticoagulated with FDA-approved or lower starting doses of argatroban (Reichert MG, 2003). Doses between 0.15-1.3 mcg/kg/minute were required to maintain aPTTs in the target range. Another report of a cardiac patient with anasarca secondary to acute renal failure had a reduction in argatroban clearance similar to patient with hepatic dysfunction (de Denus S, 2003). Reduced clearance may have been attributed to reduced perfusion to the liver. Consider reducing starting dose to 0.5-1 mcg/kg/minute in critically-ill patients who may have impaired hepatic perfusion (eg, patients requiring vasopressors, having decreased cardiac output, having fluid overload).

Percutaneous coronary intervention (PCI):

Initial: Begin infusion of 25 mcg/kg/minute and administer bolus dose of 350 mcg/kg (over 3-5 minutes). ACT should be checked 5-10 minutes after bolus infusion; proceed with procedure if ACT >300 seconds. Following initial bolus:

ACT <300 seconds: Give an additional 150 mcg/kg bolus, and increase infusion rate to 30 mcg/kg/minute (recheck ACT in 5-10 minutes)

ACT >450 seconds: Decrease infusion rate to 15 mcg/kg/minute (recheck ACT in 5-10 minutes)

Once a therapeutic ACT (300-450 seconds) is achieved, infusion should be continued at this dose for the duration of the procedure.

Impending abrupt closure, thrombus formation during PCI, or inability to achieve ACT >300 sec: An additional bolus of 150 mcg/kg, followed by an increase in infusion rate to 40 mcg/kg/minute may be administered.

Dosage Forms Injection, solution: 100 mg/mL (2.5 mL) [contains dehydrated alcohol 1000 mg/mL]

arginine (AR ji neen)

Synonyms arginine hydrochloride

U.S./Canadian Brand Names R-Gene® [US]

Therapeutic Category Diagnostic Agent

Use Pituitary function test (growth hormone)

Usual Dosage I.V.: Pituitary function test:

Children: 500 mg kg/dose administered over 30 minutes

Adults: 30 g (300 mL) administered over 30 minutes

Dosage Forms Injection, solution, as hydrochloride: 10% [100 mg/mL = 950 mOsm/L] (300 mL) [contains chloride 0.475 mEq/mL]

arginine hydrochloride *see* arginine *on previous page*

8-arginine vasopressin *see* vasopressin *on page 906*

Argyrol® S.S. *(Discontinued)* *see page 1042*

Aricept® [US/Can] *see* donepezil *on page 288*

Arimidex® [US/Can] *see* anastrozole *on page 59*

aripiprazole (ay ri PIP ray zole)

Synonyms BMS 337039; OPC-14597

U.S./Canadian Brand Names Abilify™ [US]

Therapeutic Category Antipsychotic Agent, Quinolone

Use Treatment of schizophrenia, bipolar mania (acute mania and mixed episodes)

Usual Dosage Oral:

Adults:

Schizophrenia: 10-15 mg once daily; may be increased to a maximum of 30 mg once daily (efficacy at dosages above 10-15 mg has not been shown to be increased). Dosage titration should not be more frequent than every 2 weeks.

Bipolar mania, acute mania and mixed episodes: 30 mg once daily; may require a decrease to 15 mg based on tolerability (15% of patients had dose decreased); safety of doses >30 mg/day has not been evaluated

Dosage Forms Tablet: 5 mg, 10 mg, 15 mg, 20 mg, 30 mg [contains lactose]

Aristocort® A Topical [US] *see* triamcinolone (topical) *on page 882*

Aristocort® Forte Injection [US] *see* triamcinolone (systemic) *on page 881*

Aristocort® Intralesional Injection [US] *see* triamcinolone (systemic) *on page 881*

Aristocort® Tablet [US/Can] *see* triamcinolone (systemic) *on page 881*

Aristocort® Topical [US] *see* triamcinolone (topical) *on page 882*

Aristospan® Intraarticular Injection [US/Can] *see* triamcinolone (systemic) *on page 881*

Aristospan® Intralesional Injection [US/Can] *see* triamcinolone (systemic) *on page 881*

Arixtra® [US/Can] *see* fondaparinux *on page 388*

Arlidin® *(Discontinued)* *see page 1042*

Arm-a-Med® Isoetharine *(Discontinued)* *see page 1042*

Arm-a-Med® Isoproterenol *(Discontinued)* *see page 1042*

Arm-a-Med® Metaproterenol *(Discontinued)* *see page 1042*

A.R.M.® Caplet *(Discontinued)* *see page 1042*

Armour® Thyroid [US] *see* thyroid *on page 860*

A.R.M® [US-OTC] *see* chlorpheniramine and pseudoephedrine *on page 189*

Aromasin® [US/Can] *see* exemestane *on page 353*

Arrestin® *(Discontinued)* *see page 1042*

arsenic trioxide (AR se nik tri OKS id)

Synonyms NSC-706363

U.S./Canadian Brand Names Trisenox™ [US]

Therapeutic Category Antineoplastic Agent, Miscellaneous

Use Induction of remission and consolidation in patients with acute promyelocytic leukemia (APL) which is specifically characterized by t(15;17) translocation or PML/RAR-alpha gene expression. Should be used only in those patients who have relapsed or are refractory to retinoid and anthracycline chemotherapy.

Orphan drug: Treatment of myelodysplastic syndrome; multiple myeloma; chronic myeloid leukemia (CML); acute myelocytic leukemia (AML)

Usual Dosage I.V.: Children >5 years and Adults:

Induction: 0.15 mg/kg/day; administer daily until bone marrow remission; maximum induction: 60 doses

Consolidation: 0.15 mg/kg/day starting 3-6 weeks after completion of induction therapy; maximum consolidation: 25 doses over 5 weeks

Dosage Forms Injection, solution [preservative free]: 1 mg/mL (10 mL)

Artane® *(Discontinued)* *see page 1042*

Artha-G® *(Discontinued)* *see page 1042*

ArthriCare® for Women Extra Moisturizing [US-OTC] *see* capsaicin *on page 153*

ArthriCare® for Women Multi-Action [US-OTC] *see* capsaicin *on page 153*

ArthriCare® for Women Silky Dry [US-OTC] *see* capsaicin *on page 153*

ArthriCare® for Women Ultra Strength [US-OTC] *see* capsaicin *on page 153*

Arthritis Foundation® Ibuprofen *(Discontinued)* *see page 1042*

Arthritis Foundation® Nighttime *(Discontinued)* *see page 1042*

Arthritis Foundation® Pain Reliever, Aspirin Free *(Discontinued)* *see page 1042*

Arthropan® *(Discontinued)* *see page 1042*

Arthrotec® [US/Can] *see* diclofenac and misoprostol *on page 267*

Articulose-50® Injection *(Discontinued)* *see page 1042*

artificial tears (ar ti FISH il tears)

Sound-Alike/Look-Alike Issues

Isopto® Tears may be confused with Isoptin®

Murocel® may be confused with Murocoll-2®

Synonyms hydroxyethylcellulose; polyvinyl alcohol

U.S./Canadian Brand Names Akwa Tears® [US-OTC]; AquaSite® [US-OTC]; Bion® Tears [US-OTC]; HypoTears PF [US-OTC]; HypoTears [US-OTC]; Isopto® Tears [US]; Liquifilm® Tears [US-OTC]; Moisture® Eyes PM [US-OTC]; Moisture® Eyes [US-OTC]; Murine® Tears [US-OTC]; Murocel® [US-OTC]; Nature's Tears® [US-OTC]; Nu-Tears® II [US-OTC]; Nu-Tears® [US-OTC]; OcuCoat® PF [US-OTC]; OcuCoat® [US-OTC]; Puralube® Tears [US-OTC]; Refresh® Tears [US-OTC]; Refresh® [US-OTC]; Teardrops® [Can]; Teargen® II [US-OTC]; Teargen® [US-OTC]; Tearisol® [US-OTC]; Tears Again® [US-OTC]; Tears Naturale® Free [US-OTC]; Tears Naturale® II [US-OTC]; Tears Naturale® [US-OTC]; Tears Plus® [US-OTC]; Tears Renewed® [US-OTC]; Ultra Tears® [US-OTC]; Viva-Drops® [US-OTC]

Therapeutic Category Ophthalmic Agent, Miscellaneous

Use Ophthalmic lubricant; for relief of dry eyes and eye irritation

Usual Dosage Ophthalmic: Use as needed to relieve symptoms, 1-2 drops into eye(s) 3-4 times/day

Dosage Forms Solution, ophthalmic: 15 mL and 30 mL dropper bottles

asa *see* aspirin *on page 80*

A.S.A.® *(Discontinued)* *see page 1042*

5-ASA *see* mesalamine *on page 556*

Asacol® [US/Can] *see* mesalamine *on page 556*

Asaphen [Can] *see* aspirin *on next page*

Asaphen E.C. [Can] *see* aspirin *on next page*

Asbron-G® Elixir *(Discontinued)* *see page 1042*

Asbron-G® Tablet *(Discontinued)* *see page 1042*

ascorbic acid (a SKOR bik AS id)

Synonyms vitamin C

U.S./Canadian Brand Names C-500-GR™ [US-OTC]; Cecon® [US-OTC]; Cevi-Bid® [US-OTC]; C-Gram [US-OTC]; Dull-C® [US-OTC]; Proflavanol C™ [Can]; Revitalose C-1000® [Can]; Vita-C® [US-OTC]

Therapeutic Category Vitamin, Water Soluble

Use Prevention and treatment of scurvy and to acidify the urine

Usual Dosage Oral, I.M., I.V., SubQ:

Recommended daily allowance (RDA):
- <6 months: 30 mg
- 6 months to 1 year: 35 mg
- 1-3 years: 15 mg; upper limit of intake should not exceed 400 mg/day
- 4-8 years: 25 mg; upper limit of intake should not exceed 650 mg/day
- 9-13 years: 45 mg; upper limit of intake should not exceed 1200 mg/day
- 14-18 years: Upper limit of intake should not exceed 1800 mg/day
  - Male: 75 mg
  - Female: 65 mg
- Adults: Upper limit of intake should not exceed 2000 mg/day
  - Male: 90 mg
  - Female: 75 mg;
- Pregnant female:
  - ≤18 years: 80 mg; upper limit of intake should not exceed 1800 mg/day
  - 19-50 years: 85 mg; upper limit of intake should not exceed 2000 mg/day
- Lactating female:
  - ≤18 years: 15 mg; upper limit of intake should not exceed 1800 mg/day
  - 19-50 years: 20 mg; upper limit of intake should not exceed 2000 mg/day
- Adult smoker: Add an additional 35 mg/day

Children:
- Scurvy: 100-300 mg/day in divided doses for at least 2 weeks
- Urinary acidification: 500 mg every 6-8 hours
- Dietary supplement: 35-100 mg/day

Adults:
- Scurvy: 100-250 mg 1-2 times/day for at least 2 weeks
- Urinary acidification: 4-12 g/day in 3-4 divided doses
- Prevention and treatment of colds: 1-3 g/day
- Dietary supplement: 50-200 mg/day

Dosage Forms

Capsule: 500 mg, 1000 mg
- C-500-GR™: 500 mg

Capsule, timed release: 500 mg

Crystal (Vita-C®): 4 g/teaspoonful (100 g)

Injection, solution: 250 mg/mL (2 mL, 30 mL); 500 mg/mL (50 mL)
- Cenolate®: 500 mg/mL (1 mL, 2 mL) [contains sodium hydrosulfite]

Powder, solution (Dull-C®): 4 g/teaspoonful (100 g, 500 g)

Solution, oral (Cecon®): 90 mg/mL (50 mL)

Tablet: 100 mg, 250 mg, 500 mg, 1000 mg
- C-Gram: 1000 mg

Tablet, chewable: 100 mg, 250 mg, 500 mg [some products may contain aspartame]

Tablet, timed release: 500 mg, 1000 mg, 1500 mg
- Cevi-Bid®: 500 mg

ascorbic acid and ferrous sulfate *see* ferrous sulfate and ascorbic acid *on page 365*

Ascorbicap® *(Discontinued)* *see page 1042*

Ascriptin® Extra Strength [US-OTC] *see* aspirin *on this page*

Ascriptin® [US-OTC] *see* aspirin *on this page*

Asendin® *(Discontinued)* *see page 1042*

Asmalix® *(Discontinued)* *see page 1042*

asparaginase (a SPIR a ji nase)

Sound-Alike/Look-Alike Issues
asparaginase may be confused with pegaspargase

Synonyms *E. coli* asparaginase; *Erwinia* asparaginase; L-asparaginase; NSC-106977 (*Erwinia*); NSC-109229 (*E. coli*)

U.S./Canadian Brand Names Elspar® [US/Can]; Kidrolase® [Can]

Therapeutic Category Antineoplastic Agent

Use Treatment of acute lymphocytic leukemia, lymphoma

Usual Dosage Refer to individual protocols.

Children:
- I.V.:
  - Infusion for induction: 1000 units/kg/day for 10 days
  - Consolidation: 6000-10,000 units/m^2/day for 14 days
- I.M.: 6000 units/m^2 on days 4, 7, 10, 13, 16, 19, 22, 25, 28

Adults:
- I.V. infusion single agent for induction:
  - 200 units/kg/day for 28 days **or**
  - 5000-10,000 units/m^2/day for 7 days every 3 weeks **or**
  - 10,000-40,000 units every 2-3 weeks
- I.M. as single agent: 6000-12,000 units/m^2; reconstitution to 10,000 units/mL may be necessary

Some institutions recommended the following precautions for asparaginase administration: Have parenteral epinephrine, diphenhydramine, and hydrocortisone available at the bedside. Have a freely running I.V. in place. Have a physician readily accessible. Monitor the patient closely for 30-60 minutes. Avoid administering the drug at night.

Some practitioners recommend a desensitization regimen for patients who react to a test dose, or are being retreated following a break in therapy. Doses are doubled and given every 10 minutes until the total daily dose for that day has been administered. For example, if a patient was to receive a total dose of 4000 units, he/she would receive injections 1 through 12 during the desensitization

Dosage Forms Injection, powder for reconstitution: 10,000 units

aspart, insulin *see* insulin preparations *on page 474*

A-Spas® *(Discontinued)* *see page 1042*

Aspercin Extra [US-OTC] *see* aspirin *on this page*

Aspercin [US-OTC] *see* aspirin *on this page*

Aspergum® [US-OTC] *see* aspirin *on this page*

aspirin (AS pir in)

Sound-Alike/Look-Alike Issues
aspirin may be confused with Afrin®, Asendin®
Ascriptin® may be confused with Aricept®
Ecotrin® may be confused with Akineton®, Edecrin®, Epogen®
Halfprin® may be confused with Halfan®, Haltran®
ZORprin® may be confused with Zyloprim®

Synonyms acetylsalicylic acid; asa

U.S./Canadian Brand Names Asaphen [Can]; Asaphen E.C. [Can]; Ascriptin® Extra Strength [US-OTC]; Ascriptin® [US-OTC]; Aspercin Extra [US-OTC]; Aspercin [US-OTC]; Aspergum® [US-OTC]; Bayer® Aspirin Extra Strength [US-OTC]; Bayer® Aspirin Regimen Adult Low Strength [US-OTC]; Bayer® Aspirin Regimen Children's [US-OTC]; Bayer® Aspirin Regimen Regular Strength [US-OTC]; Bayer® Aspirin [US-OTC]; Bayer® Extra Strength Arthritis Pain Regimen [US-OTC]; Bayer® Plus Extra Strength [US-OTC]; Bayer® Women's Aspirin Plus Calcium [US-OTC]; Bufferin® Extra Strength [US-OTC]; Bufferin® [US-OTC]; Buffinol Extra [US-OTC]; Buffinol [US-OTC]; Easprin® [US]; Ecotrin® Low Strength [US-OTC]; Ecotrin® Maximum Strength [US-OTC]; Ecotrin® [US-OTC]; Entrophen® [Can]; Halfprin® [US-OTC]; Novasen [Can]; St Joseph® Adult Aspirin [US-OTC]; Sureprin 81™ [US-OTC]; ZORprin® [US]

Therapeutic Category Analgesic, Nonnarcotic; Antiplatelet Agent; Antipyretic; Nonsteroidal Antiinflammatory Drug (NSAID)

Use Treatment of mild-to-moderate pain, inflammation, and fever; may be used as prophylaxis of myocardial infarction; prophylaxis of stroke and/or transient ischemic episodes; management of rheumatoid arthritis, rheumatic fever, osteoarthritis, and gout (high dose); adjunctive therapy in revascularization procedures (coronary artery bypass graft [CABG], percutaneous transluminal coronary angioplasty [PTCA], carotid endarterectomy), stent implantation

Usual Dosage

Children:

Analgesic and antipyretic: Oral, rectal: 10-15 mg/kg/dose every 4-6 hours, up to a total of 4 g/day

Antiinflammatory: Oral: Initial: 60-90 mg/kg/day in divided doses; usual maintenance: 80-100 mg/kg/day divided every 6-8 hours; monitor serum concentrations

Antiplatelet effects: Adequate pediatric studies have not been performed; pediatric dosage is derived from adult studies and clinical experience and is not well established; suggested doses have ranged from 3-5 mg/kg/day to 5-10 mg/kg/day given as a single daily dose. Doses are rounded to a convenient amount (eg, 1/2 of 80 mg tablet).

Mechanical prosthetic heart valves: 6-20 mg/kg/day given as a single daily dose (used in combination with an oral anticoagulant in children who have systemic embolism despite adequate oral anticoagulation therapy (INR 2.5-3.5) and used in combination with low-dose anticoagulation (INR 2-3) and dipyridamole when full-dose oral anticoagulation is contraindicated)

Blalock-Taussig shunts: 3-5 mg/kg/day given as a single daily dose

Kawasaki disease: Oral: 80-100 mg/kg/day divided every 6 hours; monitor serum concentrations; after fever resolves: 3-5 mg/kg/day once daily; in patients without coronary artery abnormalities, give lower dose for at least 6-8 weeks or until ESR and platelet count are normal; in patients with coronary artery abnormalities, low-dose aspirin should be continued indefinitely

Antirheumatic: Oral: 60-100 mg/kg/day in divided doses every 4 hours

Adults:

Analgesic and antipyretic: Oral, rectal: 325-650 mg every 4-6 hours up to 4 g/day

Antiinflammatory: Oral: Initial: 2.4-3.6 g/day in divided doses; usual maintenance: 3.6-5.4 g/day; monitor serum concentrations

Myocardial infarction prophylaxis: 75-325 mg/day; use of a lower aspirin dosage has been recommended in patients receiving ACE inhibitors

Acute myocardial infarction: 160-325 mg/day (have patient chew tablet if not taking aspirin before presentation)

CABG: 325 mg/day starting 6 hours following procedure

PTCA: Initial: 80-325 mg/day starting 2 hours before procedure; longer pretreatment durations (up to 24 hours) should be considered if lower dosages (80-100 mg) are used

Stent implantation: Oral: 325 mg 2 hours prior to implantation and 160-325 mg daily thereafter

Carotid endarterectomy: 81-325 mg/day preoperatively and daily thereafter

Acute stroke : 160-325 mg/day, initiated within 48 hours (in patients who are not candidates for thrombolytics and are not receiving systemic anticoagulation)

(Continued)

aspirin *(Continued)*

Stroke prevention/TIA: 30-325 mg/day (dosages up to 1300 mg/day in 2-4 divided doses have been used in clinical trials)

Dosage Forms

Caplet:
- Bayer® Aspirin: 325 mg [film coated]
- Bayer® Aspirin Extra Strength: 500 mg [film coated]
- Bayer® Extra Strength Arthritis Pain Regimen: 500 mg [enteric coated]
- Bayer® Women's Aspirin Plus Calcium: 81 mg [contains elemental calcium 300 mg]

Caplet, buffered (Ascriptin® Extra Strength): 500 mg [contains aluminum hydroxide, calcium carbonate, and magnesium hydroxide]

Gelcap (Bayer® Aspirin Extra Strength): 500 mg

Gum (Aspergum®): 227 mg [cherry or orange flavor]

Suppository, rectal: 300 mg, 600 mg

Tablet: 325 mg
- Aspercin: 325 mg
- Aspercin Extra: 500 mg
- Bayer® Aspirin: 325 mg [film coated]

Tablet, buffered: 325 mg
- Ascriptin®: 325 mg [contains aluminum hydroxide, calcium carbonate, and magnesium hydroxide]
- Bayer® Plus Extra Strength: 500 mg [contains calcium carbonate]
- Bufferin®: 325 mg [contains citric acid]
- Bufferin® Extra Strength: 500 mg [contains citric acid]
- Buffinol: 325 mg [contains magnesium oxide]
- Buffinol Extra: 500 mg [contains magnesium oxide]

Tablet, chewable: 81 mg
- Bayer® Aspirin Regimen Children's Chewable: 81 mg [cherry, mint or orange flavor]
- St. Joseph® Adult Aspirin: 81 mg [orange flavor]

Tablet, controlled release (ZORprin®): 800 mg

Tablet, enteric coated: 81 mg, 325 mg, 500 mg, 650 mg
- Bayer® Aspirin Regimen Adult Low Strength, Ecotrin® Low Strength, St. Joseph Adult Aspirin: 81 mg
- Bayer® Aspirin Regimen Regular Strength, Ecotrin®: 325 mg
- Easprin®: 975 mg
- Ecotrin® Maximum Strength: 500 mg
- Halfprin: 81 mg, 162 mg
- Sureprin 81™: 81 mg

aspirin, acetaminophen, and caffeine *see* acetaminophen, aspirin, and caffeine *on page 10*

aspirin and carisoprodol *see* carisoprodol and aspirin *on page 162*

aspirin and codeine (AS pir in & KOE deen)

Synonyms codeine and aspirin

U.S./Canadian Brand Names Coryphen® Codeine [Can]

Therapeutic Category Analgesic, Narcotic

Controlled Substance C-III

Use Relief of mild to moderate pain

Usual Dosage Oral:

Children:
- Aspirin: 10 mg/kg/dose every 4 hours
- Codeine: 0.5-1 mg/kg/dose every 4 hours

Adults: 1-2 tablets every 4-6 hours as needed for pain

Dosage Forms Tablet:
- #3: Aspirin 325 mg and codeine phosphate 30 mg
- #4: Aspirin 325 mg and codeine phosphate 60 mg

aspirin and dipyridamole (AS pir in & dye peer ID a mole)

Sound-Alike/Look-Alike Issues

Aggrenox® may be confused with Aggrastat®

Synonyms aspirin and extended-release dipyridamole

U.S./Canadian Brand Names Aggrenox® [US/Can]

Therapeutic Category Antiplatelet Agent

Use Reduction in the risk of stroke in patients who have had transient ischemia of the brain or completed ischemic stroke due to thrombosis

Usual Dosage Adults: Oral: 1 capsule (dipyridamole 200 mg, aspirin 25 mg) twice daily.

Dosage Forms Capsule: Dipyridamole (extended release) 200 mg and aspirin 25 mg [contains lactose]

aspirin and extended-release dipyridamole *see* aspirin and dipyridamole *on this page*

aspirin and hydrocodone *see* hydrocodone and aspirin *on page 445*

aspirin and meprobamate (AS pir in & me proe BA mate)

Synonyms meprobamate and aspirin

U.S./Canadian Brand Names Equagesic® [US]; 292 MEP® [Can]

Therapeutic Category Skeletal Muscle Relaxant

Controlled Substance C-IV

Use Adjunct to treatment of skeletal muscular disease in patients exhibiting tension and/or anxiety

Usual Dosage Oral: 1 tablet 3-4 times/day

Dosage Forms Tablet: Aspirin 325 mg and meprobamate 200 mg

aspirin and methocarbamol *see* methocarbamol and aspirin *on page 565*

aspirin and oxycodone *see* oxycodone and aspirin *on page 657*

aspirin and pravastatin (AS pir in & PRA va stat in)

Synonyms buffered aspirin and pravastatin sodium; pravastatin and aspirin

U.S./Canadian Brand Names Pravigard™ PAC [US]

Therapeutic Category Antilipemic Agent, HMG-CoA Reductase Inhibitor; Salicylate

Use Combination therapy in patients who need treatment with aspirin and pravastatin to reduce the incidence of cardiovascular events, including myocardial infarction, stroke, and death.

Usual Dosage Oral: Adults: Initial: Pravastatin 40 mg with aspirin (either 81 mg or 325 mg); both medications taken once daily. If pravastatin 40 mg does not achieve the desired cholesterol result, dosage may be increased to 80 mg once daily with aspirin (either 81 mg or 325 mg) once daily. Some patients may achieve/maintain goal cholesterol levels at a pravastatin dosage of 20 mg.

Dosage Forms Combination package (Pravigard™ PAC) [each administration card contains]:

81/20:

Tablet: Aspirin, buffered 81 mg (5/card) [contains calcium carbonate, and magnesium oxide, and magnesium carbonate]

Tablet (Pravachol®): Pravastatin sodium 20 mg (5/card) [contains lactose]

81/40:

Tablet: Aspirin, buffered 81 mg (5/card) [contains calcium carbonate, and magnesium oxide, and magnesium carbonate]

Tablet (Pravachol®): Pravastatin sodium 40 mg (5/card) [contains lactose]

81/80:

Tablet: Aspirin, buffered 81 mg (5/card) [contains calcium carbonate, and magnesium oxide, and magnesium carbonate]

Tablet (Pravachol®): Pravastatin sodium 80 mg (5/card) [contains lactose]

(Continued)

aspirin and pravastatin *(Continued)*

325/20:

Tablet: Aspirin, buffered 325 mg (5/card) [contains calcium carbonate, and magnesium oxide, and magnesium carbonate]

Tablet (Pravachol®): Pravastatin sodium 20 mg (5/card) [contains lactose]

325/40:

Tablet: Aspirin, buffered 325 mg (5/card) [contains calcium carbonate, and magnesium oxide, and magnesium carbonate]

Tablet (Pravachol®): Pravastatin sodium 40 mg (5/card) [contains lactose]

325/80:

Tablet: Aspirin, buffered 325 mg (5/card) [contains calcium carbonate, and magnesium oxide, and magnesium carbonate]

Tablet (Pravachol®): Pravastatin sodium 80 mg (5/card) [contains lactose]

aspirin and propoxyphene *see* propoxyphene and aspirin *on page 740*

aspirin, caffeine and acetaminophen *see* acetaminophen, aspirin, and caffeine *on page 10*

aspirin, caffeine, and butalbital *see* butalbital, aspirin, and caffeine *on page 138*

aspirin, carisoprodol, and codeine *see* carisoprodol, aspirin, and codeine *on page 162*

Aspirin Free Anacin® *(Discontinued)* *see page 1042*

Aspirin Free Anacin® Maximum Strength [US-OTC] *see* acetaminophen *on page 5*

aspirin, orphenadrine, and caffeine *see* orphenadrine, aspirin, and caffeine *on page 649*

Asproject® *(Discontinued)* *see page 1042*

Astelin® [US/Can] *see* azelastine *on page 93*

AsthmaHaler® Mist *(Discontinued)* *see page 1042*

AsthmaNefrin® *(Discontinued)* *see page 1042*

Astramorph/PF™ [US] *see* morphine sulfate *on page 591*

Atabrine® Tablet *(Discontinued)* *see page 1042*

Atacand® [US/Can] *see* candesartan *on page 151*

Atacand HCT™ [US] *see* candesartan and hydrochlorothiazide *on page 151*

Atacand® Plus [Can] *see* candesartan and hydrochlorothiazide *on page 151*

Atapryl® *(Discontinued)* *see page 1042*

Atarax® [US/Can] *see* hydroxyzine *on page 458*

Atasol® [Can] *see* acetaminophen *on page 5*

atazanavir (at a za NA veer)

Synonyms atazanavir sulfate; BMS-232632

U.S./Canadian Brand Names Reyataz® [US]

Therapeutic Category Antiretroviral Agent, Protease Inhibitor

Use Treatment of HIV-1 infections in combination with at least two other antiretroviral agents

Note: In patients with prior virologic failure, coadministration with ritonavir is recommended.

Usual Dosage Oral: Adults:

Antiretroviral-naive patients: 400 mg once daily; administer with food

Antiretroviral-experienced patients: 300 mg once daily **plus** ritonavir 100 mg once daily; administer with food

Coadministration with efavirenz:

Antiretroviral-naive patients: It is recommended that atazanavir 300 mg plus ritonavir 100 mg be given with efavirenz 600 mg (all as a single daily dose); administer with food

Antiretroviral-experienced patients: Recommendations have not been established.

Coadministration with didanosine buffered formulations: Administer atazanavir 2 hours before or 1 hour after didanosine buffered formulations

Coadministration with tenofovir: The manufacturer recommends that atazanavir 300 mg plus ritonavir 100 mg be given with tenofovir 300 mg (all as a single daily dose); administer with food

Dosage Forms Capsules, as sulfate: 100 mg, 150 mg, 200 mg

atazanavir sulfate *see* atazanavir *on previous page*

atenolol (a TEN oh lole)

Sound-Alike/Look-Alike Issues

atenolol may be confused with albuterol, Altenol®, timolol, Tylenol®

Tenormin® may be confused with Imuran®, Norpramin®, thiamine, Trovan®

U.S./Canadian Brand Names Apo-Atenol® [Can]; Gen-Atenolol [Can]; Novo-Atenol [Can]; Nu-Atenol [Can]; PMS-Atenolol [Can]; Rhoxal-atenolol [Can]; Tenolin [Can]; Tenormin® [US/Can]

Therapeutic Category Beta-Adrenergic Blocker

Use Treatment of hypertension, alone or in combination with other agents; management of angina pectoris, postmyocardial infarction patients

Usual Dosage

Oral:

Children: 0.8-1 mg/kg/dose given daily; range of 0.8-1.5 mg/kg/day; maximum dose: 2 mg/kg/day

Adults:

Hypertension: 25-50 mg once daily, may increase to 100 mg/day. Doses >100 mg are unlikely to produce any further benefit.

Angina pectoris: 50 mg once daily, may increase to 100 mg/day. Some patients may require 200 mg/day.

Postmyocardial infarction: Follow I.V. dose with 100 mg/day or 50 mg twice daily for 6-9 days postmyocardial infarction.

I.V.:

Hypertension: Dosages of 1.25-5 mg every 6-12 hours have been used in short-term management of patients unable to take oral enteral beta-blockers

Postmyocardial infarction: Early treatment: 5 mg slow I.V. over 5 minutes; may repeat in 10 minutes. If both doses are tolerated, may start oral atenolol 50 mg every 12 hours or 100 mg/day for 6-9 days postmyocardial infarction.

Dosage Forms

Injection, solution: 0.5 mg/mL (10 mL)

Tablet: 25 mg, 50 mg, 100 mg

atenolol and chlorthalidone (a TEN oh lole & klor THAL i done)

Synonyms chlorthalidone and atenolol

U.S./Canadian Brand Names Tenoretic® [US/Can]

Therapeutic Category Antihypertensive Agent, Combination

Use Treatment of hypertension with a cardioselective beta-blocker and a diuretic

Usual Dosage Adults: Oral: Initial (based on atenolol component): 50 mg once daily, then individualize dose until optimal dose is achieved

Dosage Forms Tablet:

50: Atenolol 50 mg and chlorthalidone 25 mg

100: Atenolol 100 mg and chlorthalidone 25 mg

ATG *see* antithymocyte globulin (rabbit) *on page 66*

Atgam® [US/Can] *see* antithymocyte globulin (equine) *on page 66*

AT III *see* antithrombin III *on page 65*

Ativan® [US/Can] *see* lorazepam *on page 530*

Atolone® Oral *(Discontinued)* *see page 1042*

atomoxetine (AT oh mox e teen)

Synonyms atomoxetine hydrochloride; LY139603; methylphenoxy-benzene propanamine; tomoxetine

U.S./Canadian Brand Names Strattera™ [US]

Therapeutic Category Norepinephrine Reuptake Inhibitor, Selective

Use Treatment of attention deficit/hyperactivity disorder (ADHD)

Usual Dosage Oral:

Children and Adolescents ≤70 kg: ADHD: Initial: 0.5 mg/kg/day, increase after minimum of 3 days to ~1.2 mg/kg/day; may administer as either a single daily dose or two evenly divided doses in morning and late afternoon/early evening. Maximum daily dose: 1.4 mg/kg or 100 mg, whichever is less. In patients receiving effective CYP2D6 inhibitors (eg, paroxetine, fluoxetine, quinidine), do not exceed 1.2 mg/kg.

Children and Adolescents >70 kg: Refer to Adults dosing

Adults:

ADHD: Initial: 40 mg/day, increased after minimum of 3 days to ~80 mg/day; may administer as either a single daily dose or two evenly divided doses in morning and late afternoon/early evening. May increase to 100 mg in 2-4 additional weeks to achieve optimal response. In patients receiving effective CYP2D6 inhibitors (eg, paroxetine, fluoxetine, quinidine), do not exceed 80 mg/day.

Dosage Forms Capsule: 10 mg, 18 mg, 25 mg, 40 mg, 60 mg

atomoxetine hydrochloride *see* atomoxetine *on this page*

atorvastatin (a TORE va sta tin)

Sound-Alike/Look-Alike Issues

Lipitor® may be confused with Levatol®

U.S./Canadian Brand Names Lipitor® [US/Can]

Therapeutic Category HMG-CoA Reductase Inhibitor

Use

Primary prevention of CVD in high-risk patients

Used with dietary therapy for the following:

Hyperlipidemias: To reduce elevations in total cholesterol, LDL-C, apolipoprotein B, and triglycerides in patients with primary hypercholesterolemia (elevations of 1 or more components are present in Fredrickson type IIa, IIb, III, and IV hyperlipidemias)

Treatment of homozygous familial hypercholesterolemia

Heterozygous familial hypercholesterolemia (HeFH): In adolescent patients (10-17 years of age, females >1 year postmenarche) with HeFH having LDL-C ≥190 mg/dL **or** LDL ≥160 mg/dL with positive family history of premature cardiovascular disease (CVD) or with 2 or more CVD risk factors in the adolescent patient

Usual Dosage Oral: **Note:** Doses should be individualized according to the baseline LDL-cholesterol levels, the recommended goal of therapy, and patient response; adjustments should be made at intervals of 2-4 weeks

Children 10-17 years (females >1 year postmenarche): HeFH: 10 mg once daily (maximum: 20 mg/day)

Adults:

Hyperlipidemias: Initial: 10-20 mg once daily; patients requiring >45% reduction in LDL-C may be started at 40 mg once daily; range: 10-80 mg once daily

Primary prevention of CVD: 10 mg once daily

Dosage Forms Tablet: 10 mg, 20 mg, 40 mg, 80 mg

atorvastatin calcium and amlodipine besylate *see* amlodipine and atorvastatin *on page 49*

atovaquone (a TOE va kwone)

U.S./Canadian Brand Names Mepron® [US/Can]

Therapeutic Category Antiprotozoal

Use Acute oral treatment of mild to moderate *Pneumocystis carinii* pneumonia (PCP) in patients who are intolerant to co-trimoxazole; prophylaxis of PCP in patients intolerant to co-trimoxazole; treatment/suppression of *Toxoplasma gondii* encephalitis, primary prophylaxis of HIV-infected persons at high risk for developing *Toxoplasma gondii* encephalitis

Usual Dosage Oral: Adolescents 13-16 years and Adults:

Prevention of PCP: 1500 mg once daily with food

Treatment of mild to moderate PCP: 750 mg twice daily with food for 21 days

Dosage Forms Suspension, oral: 750 mg/5 mL (5 mL, 210 mL) [contains benzyl alcohol; citrus flavor]

atovaquone and proguanil (a TOE va kwone & pro GWA nil)

Synonyms proguanil and atovaquone

U.S./Canadian Brand Names Malarone™ [US/Can]

Therapeutic Category Antimalarial Agent

Use Prevention or treatment of acute, uncomplicated *P. falciparum* malaria

Usual Dosage Oral:

Children (dosage based on body weight):

Prevention of malaria: Start 1-2 days prior to entering a malaria-endemic area, continue throughout the stay and for 7 days after returning. Take as a single dose, once daily.

11-20 kg: Atovaquone/proguanil 62.5 mg/25 mg
21-30 kg: Atovaquone/proguanil 125 mg/50 mg
31-40 kg: Atovaquone/proguanil 187.5 mg/75 mg
>40 kg: Atovaquone/proguanil 250 mg/100 mg

Treatment of acute malaria: Take as a single dose, once daily for 3 consecutive days.

5-8 kg: Atovaquone/proguanil 125 mg/50 mg
9-10 kg: Atovaquone/proguanil 187.5 mg/75 mg
11-20 kg: Atovaquone/proguanil 250 mg/100 mg
21-30 kg: Atovaquone/proguanil 500 mg/200 mg
31-40 kg: Atovaquone/proguanil 750 mg/300 mg
>40 kg: Atovaquone/proguanil 1 g/400 mg

Adults:

Prevention of malaria: Atovaquone/proguanil 250 mg/100 mg once daily; start 1-2 days prior to entering a malaria-endemic area, continue throughout the stay and for 7 days after returning

Treatment of acute malaria: Atovaquone/proguanil 1 g/400 mg as a single dose, once daily for 3 consecutive days

Dosage Forms

Tablet: Atovaquone 250 mg and proguanil hydrochloride 100 mg

Tablet, pediatric: Atovaquone 62.5 mg and proguanil hydrochloride 25 mg

Atozine® Oral *(Discontinued)* *see page 1042*

atracurium (a tra KYOO ree um)

Synonyms atracurium besylate

U.S./Canadian Brand Names Tracrium® [US]

Therapeutic Category Skeletal Muscle Relaxant

Use Adjunct to general anesthesia to facilitate endotracheal intubation and to relax skeletal muscles during surgery; to facilitate mechanical ventilation in ICU patients; does not relieve pain or produce sedation

Usual Dosage I.V. (not to be used I.M.): Dose to effect; doses must be individualized due to interpatient variability; use ideal body weight for obese patients

Children 1 month to 2 years: Initial: 0.3-0.4 mg/kg followed by maintenance doses as needed to maintain neuromuscular blockade

(Continued)

atracurium *(Continued)*

Children >2 years to Adults: 0.4-0.5 mg/kg, then 0.08-0.1 mg/kg 20-45 minutes after initial dose to maintain neuromuscular block, followed by repeat doses of 0.08-0.1 mg/kg at 15- to 25-minute intervals

Initial dose after succinylcholine for intubation (balanced anesthesia): Adults: 0.2-0.4 mg/kg

Pretreatment/priming: 10% of intubating dose given 3-5 minutes before initial dose

Continuous infusion:

Surgery: Initial: 9-10 mcg/kg/minute at initial signs of recovery from bolus dose; block usually maintained by a rate of 5-9 mcg/kg/minute under balanced anesthesia

ICU: Block usually maintained by rate of 11-13 mcg/kg/minute (rates for pediatric patients may be higher)

Dosage Forms

Injection, as besylate: 10 mg/mL (10 mL) [contains benzyl alcohol]

Injection, as besylate [preservative free]: 10 mg/mL (5 mL)

atracurium besylate *see* atracurium *on previous page*

Atrohist® Plus *(Discontinued)* *see page 1042*

Atromid-S® *(Discontinued)* *see page 1042*

Atropair® *(Discontinued)* *see page 1042*

AtroPen® [US] *see* atropine *on this page*

atropine (A troe peen)

Synonyms atropine sulfate

U.S./Canadian Brand Names AtroPen® [US]; Atropine-Care® [US]; Dioptic's Atropine Solution [Can]; Isopto® Atropine [US/Can]; Minim's Atropine Solution [Can]; Sal-Tropine™ [US]

Therapeutic Category Anticholinergic Agent

Use

Injection: Preoperative medication to inhibit salivation and secretions; treatment of symptomatic sinus bradycardia; AV block (nodal level); ventricular asystole; antidote for organophosphate pesticide poisoning

Ophthalmic: Produce mydriasis and cycloplegia for examination of the retina and optic disc and accurate measurement of refractive errors; uveitis

Oral: Inhibit salivation and secretions

Usual Dosage

Neonates, Infants, and Children: Doses <0.1 mg have been associated with paradoxical bradycardia.

Inhibit salivation and secretions (preanesthesia): Oral, I.M., I.V., SubQ:

<5 kg: 0.02 mg/kg/dose 30-60 minutes preop then every 4-6 hours as needed. Use of a minimum dosage of 0.1 mg in neonates <5 kg will result in dosages >0.02 mg/kg. There is no documented minimum dosage in this age group.

>5 kg: 0.01-0.02 mg/kg/dose to a maximum 0.4 mg/dose 30-60 minutes preop; minimum dose: 0.1 mg

Alternate dosing:

3-7 kg (7-16 lb): 0.1 mg

8-11 kg (17-24 lb): 0.15 mg

11-18 kg (24-40 lb): 0.2 mg

18-29 kg (40-65 lb): 0.3 mg

>30 kg (>65 lb): 0.4 mg

Bradycardia: I.V., intratracheal: 0.02 mg/kg, minimum dose 0.1 mg, maximum single dose: 0.5 mg in children and 1 mg in adolescents; may repeat in 5-minute intervals to a maximum total dose of 1 mg in children or 2 mg in adolescents. (**Note:** For intratracheal administration, the dosage must be diluted with normal saline to a total volume of 1-5 mL). When treating bradycardia in neonates, reserve use for those patients unresponsive to improved oxygenation and epinephrine.

Prehospital ("in the field"): I.M.:

Birth to <2 years: Mild-to-moderate symptoms: 0.05 mg/kg; severe symptoms: 0.1 mg/kg

2-10 years: Mild-to-moderate symptoms: 1 mg; severe symptoms: 2 mg

>10 years: Mild-to-moderate symptoms: 2 mg; severe symptoms: 4 mg

Hospital/emergency department: I.M.:

Birth to <2 years: Mild-to-moderate symptoms: 0.05 mg/kg I.M. **or** 0.02 mg/kg I.V.; severe symptoms: 0.1 mg/kg I.M. **or** 0.02 mg/kg I.V.

2-10 years: Mild-to-moderate symptoms: 1 mg; severe symptoms: 2 mg

>10 years: Mild-to-moderate symptoms: 2 mg; severe symptoms: 4 mg

Children: Organophosphate or carbamate poisoning:

I.V.: 0.03-0.05 mg/kg every 10-20 minutes until atropine effect, then every 1-4 hours for at least 24 hours

I.M. (AtroPen®): Mild symptoms: Administer dose listed below as soon as exposure is known or suspected. If severe symptoms develop after first dose, 2 additional doses should be repeated in 10 minutes; do not administer more than 3 doses. Severe symptoms: Immediately administer 3 doses as follows:

<6.8 kg (15 lbs): Use of **AtroPen® formulation not recommended;** administer atropine 0.05 mg/kg

6.8-18 kg (15-40 lbs): 0.5 mg/dose

18-41 kg (40-90 lbs): 1 mg/dose

>41 kg (>90 lbs): 2 mg/dose

Adults (doses <0.5 mg have been associated with paradoxical bradycardia):

Asystole or pulseless electrical activity: I.V.: 1 mg; repeat in 3-5 minutes if asystole persists; total dose of 0.04 mg/kg; may give intratracheally in 10 mL NS (intratracheal dose should be 2-2.5 times the I.V. dose)

Inhibit salivation and secretions (preanesthesia):

I.M., I.V., SubQ: 0.4-0.6 mg 30-60 minutes preop and repeat every 4-6 hours as needed

Bradycardia: I.V.: 0.5-1 mg every 5 minutes, not to exceed a total of 3 mg or 0.04 mg/kg; may give intratracheally in 10 mL NS (intratracheal dose should be 2-2.5 times the I.V. dose)

Neuromuscular blockade reversal: I.V.: 25-30 mcg/kg 60 seconds before neostigmine or 7-10 mcg/kg in combination with edrophonium

Organophosphate or carbamate poisoning:

I.V.: 2 mg, followed by 2 mg every 5-60 minutes until adequate atropinization has occurred; initial doses of up to 6 mg may be used in life-threatening cases

I.M. (AtroPen®): Mild symptoms: Administer 2 mg as soon as exposure is known or suspected. If severe symptoms develop after first dose, 2 additional doses should be repeated in 10 minutes; do not administer more than 3 doses. Severe symptoms: Immediately administer three 2 mg doses.

Note: Pralidoxime is a component of the management of nerve agent toxicity; consult pralidoxime monograph for specific route and dose. For prehospital ("in the field") management, repeat atropine I.M. (children: 0.05-0.1 mg/kg; adults: 2 mg) at 5-10 minute intervals until secretions have diminished and breathing is comfortable or airway resistance has returned to near normal. For hospital management, repeat atropine I.M. (infants 1 mg; all others: 2 mg) at 5-10 minute intervals until secretions have diminished and breathing is comfortable or airway resistance has returned to near normal.

Mydriasis, cycloplegia (preprocedure): Ophthalmic (1% solution): Instill 1-2 drops 1 hour before procedure.

Uveitis: Ophthalmic:

1% solution: Instill 1-2 drops 4 times/day

Ointment: Apply a small amount in the conjunctival sac up to 3 times/day; compress the lacrimal sac by digital pressure for 1-3 minutes after instillation

Dosage Forms

Injection, solution, as sulfate: 0.05 mg/mL (5 mL); 0.1 mg/mL (5 mL, 10 mL); 0.4 mg/mL (0.5 mL, 1 mL, 20 mL); 0.5 mg/mL (1 mL); 1 mg/mL (1 mL)

AtroPen® [prefilled auto-injector]: 2 mg/0.7 mL (0.7 mL)

(Continued)

atropine *(Continued)*

Ointment, ophthalmic, as sulfate: 1% (3.5 g)
Solution, ophthalmic, as sulfate: 1% (5 mL, 15 mL)
Atropine-Care®: 1% (2 mL)
Isopto® Atropine: 1% (5 mL, 15 mL)
Tablet, as sulfate (Sal-Tropine™): 0.4 mg

atropine and difenoxin *see* difenoxin and atropine *on page 269*

atropine and diphenoxylate *see* diphenoxylate and atropine *on page 279*

Atropine-Care® [US] *see* atropine *on page 88*

atropine, hyoscyamine, scopolamine, and phenobarbital *see* hyoscyamine, atropine, scopolamine, and phenobarbital *on page 460*

atropine soluble tablet ***(Discontinued)*** *see page 1042*

atropine sulfate *see* atropine *on page 88*

Atropisol® ***(Discontinued)*** *see page 1042*

Atrovent® [US/Can] *see* ipratropium *on page 482*

A/T/S® [US] *see* erythromycin *on page 320*

attapulgite (at a PULL gite)

Sound-Alike/Look-Alike Issues
Kaopectate® may be confused with Kayexalate®

U.S./Canadian Brand Names Kaopectate® [Can]

Therapeutic Category Antidiarrheal

Use Symptomatic treatment of diarrhea

Usual Dosage Adequate controlled clinical studies documenting the efficacy of attapulgite are lacking; its usage and dosage has been primarily empiric; the following are manufacturer's recommended dosages
Oral: Give after each bowel movement
Children:
3-6 years: 300-750 mg/dose; maximum dose: 7 doses/day or 2250 mg/day
6-12 years: 600-1500 mg/dose; maximum dose: 7 doses/day or 4500 mg/day
Children >12 years and Adults: 1200-3000 mg/dose; maximum dose: 8 doses/day or 9000 mg/day

Dosage Forms [DSC] = Discontinued product
Caplet (Kaopectate® Maximum Strength [DSC]): 750 mg
Liquid, oral concentrate: Activated attapulgite 600 mg/15 mL (120 mL, 180 mL, 240 mL); activated attapulgite 750 mg/15 mL (120 mL, 360 mL)
Children's Kaopectate® [DSC]: Activated attapulgite 300 mg/7.5 mL (180 mL) [cherry flavor]
Diasorb®: Activated attapulgite 750 mg/5 mL (120 mL) [cola flavor; sugar free]
Kaopectate® Advanced Formula [DSC]: Activated attapulgite 750 mg/15 mL (90 mL, 240 mL, 360 mL) [peppermint flavor]

Attenuvax® [US] *see* measles virus vaccine (live) *on page 545*

Augmentin® [US/Can] *see* amoxicillin and clavulanate potassium *on page 52*

Augmentin ES-600® [US] *see* amoxicillin and clavulanate potassium *on page 52*

Augmentin XR™ [US] *see* amoxicillin and clavulanate potassium *on page 52*

Auralgan® [Can] *see* antipyrine and benzocaine *on page 65*

auranofin (au RANE oh fin)

Sound-Alike/Look-Alike Issues
Ridaura® may be confused with Cardura®

U.S./Canadian Brand Names Ridaura® [US/Can]

Therapeutic Category Gold Compound

Use Management of active stage of classic or definite rheumatoid arthritis in patients that do not respond to or tolerate other agents; psoriatic arthritis; adjunctive or alternative therapy for pemphigus

Usual Dosage Oral:

Children: Initial: 0.1 mg/kg/day divided daily; usual maintenance: 0.15 mg/kg/day in 1-2 divided doses; maximum: 0.2 mg/kg/day in 1-2 divided doses

Adults: 6 mg/day in 1-2 divided doses; after 3 months may be increased to 9 mg/day in 3 divided doses; if still no response after 3 months at 9 mg/day, discontinue drug

Dosage Forms Capsule: 3 mg [29% gold]

Aureomycin® *(Discontinued)* *see page 1042*

Aurodex® [US] *see* antipyrine and benzocaine *on page 65*

Aurolate® [US] *see* gold sodium thiomalate *on page 412*

aurothioglucose (aur oh thye oh GLOO kose)

Therapeutic Category Gold Compound

Use Management of active stage of classic or definite rheumatoid or psoriatic arthritis in patients that do not respond to or tolerate other agents

Usual Dosage I.M. (doses should initially be administered at weekly intervals):

Children 6-12 years: Initial: 0.25 mg/kg/dose first week; increment at 0.25 mg/kg/dose increasing with each weekly dose; maintenance: 0.75-1 mg/kg/dose weekly not to exceed 25 mg/dose to a total of 20 doses, then every 2-4 weeks

Adults: 10 mg first week; 25 mg second and third week; then 50 mg/week until 800 mg to 1 g cumulative dose has been administered - if improvement occurs without adverse reactions, administer 25-50 mg every 2-3 weeks, then every 3-4 weeks

Dosage Forms Injection, suspension: 50 mg/mL [gold 50%] (10 mL)

Auroto® [US] *see* antipyrine and benzocaine *on page 65*

Autoplex® T [US] *see* anti-inhibitor coagulant complex *on page 65*

AVA *see* anthrax vaccine, adsorbed *on page 61*

Avagard™ [US-OTC] *see* chlorhexidine gluconate *on page 183*

Avage™ [US] *see* tazarotene *on page 840*

Avalide® [US/Can] *see* irbesartan and hydrochlorothiazide *on page 484*

Avandamet™ [US/Can] *see* rosiglitazone and metformin *on page 786*

Avandia® [US/Can] *see* rosiglitazone *on page 785*

Avapro® [US/Can] *see* irbesartan *on page 483*

Avapro® HCT *see* irbesartan and hydrochlorothiazide *on page 484*

AVAR™ [US] *see* sulfur and sulfacetamide *on page 834*

AVAR™ Cleanser [US] *see* sulfur and sulfacetamide *on page 834*

AVAR™ Green [US] *see* sulfur and sulfacetamide *on page 834*

Avastin™ [US] *see* bevacizumab *on page 117*

Avaxim® [Can] *see* hepatitis A vaccine *on page 432*

Avaxim®-Pediatric [Can] *see* hepatitis A vaccine *on page 432*

AVC™ *(Discontinued)* *see page 1042*

Avelox® [US/Can] *see* moxifloxacin *on page 593*

Avelox® I.V. [US] *see* moxifloxacin *on page 593*

Aventyl® [Can] *see* nortriptyline *on page 629*

Aventyl® HCl [US] *see* nortriptyline *on page 629*

Aviane™ [US] *see* ethinyl estradiol and levonorgestrel *on page 339*

Avinza™ [US] *see* morphine sulfate *on page 591*

Avita® [US] *see* tretinoin (topical) *on page 879*

Avitene® [US] *see* collagen hemostat *on page 225*

Avitene® Flour [US] *see* collagen hemostat *on page 225*

Avitene® Ultrafoam [US] *see* collagen hemostat *on page 225*

Avitene® UltraWrap™ [US] *see* collagen hemostat *on page 225*

Avlosulfon® *(Discontinued)* *see page 1042*

Avodart™ [US] *see* dutasteride *on page 299*

Avonex® [US/Can] *see* interferon beta-1a *on page 479*

Axert™ [US/Can] *see* almotriptan *on page 33*

Axid® [US/Can] *see* nizatidine *on page 625*

Axid® AR [US-OTC] *see* nizatidine *on page 625*

Axotal® *(Discontinued)* *see page 1042*

AY-25650 *see* triptorelin *on page 890*

Aygestin® [US] *see* norethindrone *on page 627*

Ayr® Baby Saline [US-OTC] *see* sodium chloride *on page 810*

Ayr® Saline Mist [US-OTC] *see* sodium chloride *on page 810*

Ayr® Saline [US-OTC] *see* sodium chloride *on page 810*

azacitidine (ay za SYE ti deen)

Synonyms AZA-CR; 5-azacytidine; 5-AZC; ladakamycin; NSC-102816

U.S./Canadian Brand Names Vidaza™ [US]

Therapeutic Category Antineoplastic Agent, Antimetabolite (Pyrimidine)

Use Treatment of myelodysplastic syndrome (MDS)

Usual Dosage

I.V.:

Children:

Pediatric AML and ANLL: 250 mg/m^2 days 4 and 5 every 4 weeks

Pediatric AML induction: 300 mg/m^2 days 5 and 6

Adults:

Acute leukemia: 50-150 mg/m^2 days 1 through 5 of induction 200 mg/m^2 CIVI days 7 through 9 of induction

CML (accelerated phase and blast crisis): 50-150 mg/m^2 days 1 through 5 of induction

AML induction: 150 mg/m^2 days 3 through 5 and 8 through 10, **then** 150 mg/m^2 days 1 through 5 and 8 through 10 (cycle 2 consolidation)

AML consolidation: 150 mg/m^2 CIVI days 1 through 7 for 3 cycles

AML maintenance: 150 mg/m^2 days 1 through 3 every 6 weeks

MDS: 75-150 mg/m^2 CIVI days 1 through 7 every 4 weeks

SubQ: MDS: 75 mg/m^2/day for 7 days repeated every 4 weeks. Dose may be increased to 100 mg/m^2/day if no benefit is observed after 2 cycles and no toxicity other than nausea and vomiting have occurred. Treatment is recommended for at least 4 cycles.

Dosage Forms Injection, powder for suspension: 100 mg [contains mannitol 100 mg]

AZA-CR *see* azacitidine *on this page*

Azactam® [US/Can] *see* aztreonam *on page 95*

5-azacytidine *see* azacitidine *on this page*

Azasan® [US] *see* azathioprine *on next page*

azatadine (a ZA ta deen)

Therapeutic Category Antihistamine

Use Treatment of perennial and seasonal allergic rhinitis and chronic urticaria

Usual Dosage Children >12 years and Adults: Oral: 1-2 mg twice daily

Dosage Forms Tablet, as maleate: 1 mg

azatadine and pseudoephedrine (a ZA ta deen & soo doe e FED rin)

Synonyms pseudoephedrine and azatadine

Therapeutic Category Antihistamine/Decongestant Combination

Use Perennial and seasonal allergic rhinitis and other allergic symptoms including urticaria

Usual Dosage Adults: 1 tablet twice daily

Dosage Forms Tablet: Azatadine maleate 1 mg and pseudoephedrine sulfate 120 mg

azathioprine (ay za THYE oh preen)

Sound-Alike/Look-Alike Issues

azathioprine may be confused with azatadine, azidothymidine, Azulfidine®

Imuran® may be confused with Elmiron®, Enduron®, Imdur®, Inderal®, Tenormin®

Synonyms azathioprine sodium

U.S./Canadian Brand Names Alti-Azathioprine [Can]; Apo-Azathioprine® [Can]; Azasan® [US]; Gen-Azathioprine [Can]; Imuran® [US/Can]

Therapeutic Category Immunosuppressant Agent

Use Adjunct with other agents in prevention of rejection of kidney transplants; also used in severe active rheumatoid arthritis unresponsive to other agents; other autoimmune diseases (ITP, SLE, MS, Crohn disease)

Usual Dosage **I.V. dose is equivalent to oral dose** (dosing should be based on ideal body weight):

Children and Adults: Renal transplantation: Oral, I.V.: 2-5 mg/kg/day to start, then 1-3 mg/kg/day maintenance

Adults: Rheumatoid arthritis: Oral: 1 mg/kg/day for 6-8 weeks; increase by 0.5 mg/kg every 4 weeks until response or up to 2.5 mg/kg/day

Dosage Forms

Injection, powder for reconstitution, as sodium: 100 mg

Tablet [scored]: 50 mg

Azasan®: 25 mg, 50 mg, 75 mg, 100 mg

Imuran®: 50 mg

azathioprine sodium *see* azathioprine *on this page*

5-AZC *see* azacitidine *on previous page*

Azdone® ***(Discontinued)*** *see page 1042*

azelaic acid (a zeh LAY ik AS id)

U.S./Canadian Brand Names Azelex® [US]; Finacea™ [US]

Therapeutic Category Topical Skin Product

Use Topical treatment of mild to moderate inflammatory acne vulgaris; treatment of mild to moderate rosacea

Finacea™: Not FDA-approved for the treatment of acne

Usual Dosage Topical:

Adolescents ≥12 years and Adults: Acne vulgaris: Cream 20%: After skin is thoroughly washed and patted dry, gently but thoroughly massage a thin film of azelaic acid cream into the affected areas twice daily, in the morning and evening. The duration of use can vary and depends on the severity of the acne. In the majority of patients with inflammatory lesions, improvement of the condition occurs within 4 weeks.

Adults: Rosacea: Gel 15%: Massage gently into affected areas of the face twice daily

Dosage Forms

Cream (Azelex®): 20% (30 g, 50 g) [contains benzoic acid and propylene glycol]

Gel (Finacea™): 15% (30 g) [contains benzoic acid and propylene glycol]

azelastine (a ZEL as teen)

Sound-Alike/Look-Alike Issues

Optivar® may be confused with Optiray®

(Continued)

azelastine *(Continued)*

Synonyms azelastine hydrochloride

U.S./Canadian Brand Names Astelin® [US/Can]; Optivar® [US]

Therapeutic Category Antihistamine; Antihistamine, Ophthalmic

Use

Nasal spray: Treatment of the symptoms of seasonal allergic rhinitis such as rhinorrhea, sneezing, and nasal pruritus in children ≥5 years of age and adults; treatment of the symptoms of vasomotor rhinitis in children ≥12 years of age and adults

Ophthalmic: Treatment of itching of the eye associated with seasonal allergic conjunctivitis in children ≥3 years of age and adults

Usual Dosage

Children 5-11 years: Seasonal allergic rhinitis: Intranasal: 1 spray each nostril twice daily

Children ≥12 years and Adults: Seasonal allergic rhinitis or vasomotor rhinitis: Intranasal: 2 sprays (137 mcg/spray) each nostril twice daily

Children ≥3 years and Adults: Itching eyes due to seasonal allergic conjunctivitis: Ophthalmic: Instill 1 drop into affected eye(s) twice daily

Dosage Forms

Solution, intranasal spray, as hydrochloride (Astelin®): 1 mg/mL [137 mcg/spray] (17 mL, 30 mL) [contains benzalkonium chloride]

Solution, ophthalmic, as hydrochloride (Optivar®): 0.05% (6 mL) [contains benzalkonium chloride]

azelastine hydrochloride *see* azelastine *on previous page*

Azelex® [US] *see* azelaic acid *on previous page*

azidothymidine *see* zidovudine *on page 939*

azidothymidine, abacavir, and lamivudine *see* abacavir, lamivudine, and zidovudine *on page 2*

azithromycin (az ith roe MYE sin)

Sound-Alike/Look-Alike Issues

azithromycin may be confused with erythromycin

Zithromax® may be confused with Zinacef®

Synonyms azithromycin dihydrate; Zithromax® TRI-PAK™; Zithromax® Z-PAK®

U.S./Canadian Brand Names Zithromax® [US/Can]

Therapeutic Category Macrolide (Antibiotic)

Use Treatment of acute otitis media due to *H. influenzae, M. catarrhalis*, or *S. pneumoniae*; pharyngitis/tonsillitis due to *S. pyogenes*; treatment of mild-to-moderate upper and lower respiratory tract infections, infections of the skin and skin structure, community-acquired pneumonia, pelvic inflammatory disease (PID), sexually-transmitted diseases (urethritis/cervicitis), pharyngitis/tonsillitis (alternative to first-line therapy), and genital ulcer disease (chancroid) due to susceptible strains of *C. trachomatis, M. catarrhalis, H. influenzae, S. aureus, S. pneumoniae, Mycoplasma pneumoniae*, and *C. psittaci*; acute bacterial exacerbations of chronic obstructive pulmonary disease (COPD) due to *H. influenzae, M. catarrhalis*, or *S. pneumoniae*; acute bacterial sinusitis

Usual Dosage

Oral:

Children ≥6 months:

Community-acquired pneumonia: 10 mg/kg on day 1 (maximum: 500 mg/day) followed by 5 mg/kg/day once daily on days 2-5 (maximum: 250 mg/day)

Bacterial sinusitis: 10 mg/kg once daily for 3 days (maximum: 500 mg/day)

Otitis media: 1-day regimen: 30 mg/kg as a single dose (maximum dose: 1500 mg) 3-day regimen: 10 mg/kg once daily for 3 days (maximum: 500 mg/day) 5-day regimen: 10 mg/kg on day 1 (maximum: 500 mg/day) followed by 5 mg/kg/day once daily on days 2-5 (maximum: 250 mg/day)

Children ≥2 years: Pharyngitis, tonsillitis: 12 mg/kg/day once daily for 5 days (maximum: 500 mg/day)

Children: 5 mg/kg/day once daily (maximum dose: 250 mg/day) or 20 mg/kg (maximum dose: 1200 mg) once weekly given alone or in combination with rifabutin

Adolescents ≥16 years and Adults:

Respiratory tract, skin and soft tissue infections: 500 mg on day 1 followed by 250 mg/day on days 2-5 (maximum: 500 mg/day) Alternative regimen: Bacterial exacerbation of COPD: 500 mg/day for a total of 3 days

Bacterial sinusitis: 500 mg/day for a total of 3 days

Urethritis/cervicitis: Due to *C. trachomatis*: 1 g as a single dose Due to *N. gonorrhoeae*: 2 g as a single dose

Chancroid due to *H. ducreyi*: 1 g as a single dose

I.V.: Adults:

Community-acquired pneumonia: 500 mg as a single dose for at least 2 days, follow I.V. therapy by the oral route with a single daily dose of 500 mg to complete a 7-10 day course of therapy

Pelvic inflammatory disease (PID): 500 mg as a single dose for 1-2 days, follow I.V. therapy by the oral route with a single daily dose of 250 mg to complete a 7-day course of therapy

Dosage Forms

Injection, powder for reconstitution, as dihydrate: 500 mg

Powder for oral suspension, as dihydrate: 100 mg/5 mL (15 mL); 200 mg/5 mL (15 mL, 22.5 mL, 30 mL) [cherry creme de vanilla and banana flavor]; 1 g [single-dose packet; cherry creme de vanilla and banana flavor]

Tablet, as dihydrate: 250 mg, 500 mg, 600 mg

Zithromax® TRI-PAK™ [unit-dose pack]: 500 mg (3s)

Zithromax® Z-PAK® [unit-dose pack]: 250 mg (6s)

azithromycin dihydrate *see* azithromycin *on previous page*

Azlin® Injection *(Discontinued)* *see page 1042*

Azmacort® [US] *see* triamcinolone (inhalation, oral) *on page 880*

Azo Gantanol® *(Discontinued)* *see page 1042*

Azo Gantrisin® *(Discontinued)* *see page 1042*

Azo-Gesic® [US-OTC] *see* phenazopyridine *on page 685*

Azopt® [US/Can] *see* brinzolamide *on page 127*

Azo-Standard® [US-OTC] *see* phenazopyridine *on page 685*

AZT *see* zidovudine *on page 939*

AZT™ [Can] *see* zidovudine *on page 939*

AZT + 3TC *see* zidovudine and lamivudine *on page 939*

AZT, abacavir, and lamivudine *see* abacavir, lamivudine, and zidovudine *on page 2*

azthreonam *see* aztreonam *on this page*

aztreonam (AZ tree oh nam)

Synonyms azthreonam

U.S./Canadian Brand Names Azactam® [US/Can]

Therapeutic Category Antibiotic, Miscellaneous

Use Treatment of patients with urinary tract infections, lower respiratory tract infections, septicemia, skin/skin structure infections, intraabdominal infections, and gynecological infections caused by susceptible gram-negative bacilli

Usual Dosage

Children >1 month: I.M., I.V.:

Mild-to-moderate infections: 30 mg/kg every 8 hours

Moderate-to-severe infections: 30 mg/kg every 6-8 hours; maximum: 120 mg/kg/day (8 g/day)

Cystic fibrosis: 50 mg/kg/dose every 6-8 hours (ie, up to 200 mg/kg/day); maximum: 8 g/day

(Continued)

aztreonam *(Continued)*

Adults:
Urinary tract infection: I.M., I.V.: 500 mg to 1 g every 8-12 hours
Moderately-severe systemic infections: 1 g I.V. or I.M. or 2 g I.V. every 8-12 hours
Severe systemic or life-threatening infections (especially caused by *Pseudomonas aeruginosa*): I.V.: 2 g every 6-8 hours; maximum: 8 g/day

Dosage Forms
Infusion [premixed]: 1 g (50 mL); 2 g (50 mL)
Injection, powder for reconstitution: 500 mg, 1 g, 2 g

Azulfidine® [US] *see* sulfasalazine *on page 833*

Azulfidine® EN-tabs® [US] *see* sulfasalazine *on page 833*

Azulfidine® Suspension *(Discontinued)* *see page 1042*

B1 *see* tositumomab and iodine I 131 tositumomab *on page 873*

B1 antibody *see* tositumomab and iodine I 131 tositumomab *on page 873*

B2036-PEG *see* pegvisomant *on page 672*

B 9273 *see* alefacept *on page 29*

BA-16038 *see* aminoglutethimide *on page 45*

Babee® Cof Syrup [US-OTC] *see* dextromethorphan *on page 261*

Babee® Teething® [US-OTC] *see* benzocaine *on page 107*

BabyBIG® [US] *see* botulism immune globulin (intravenous-human) *on page 125*

Baby Gasz [US-OTC] *see* simethicone *on page 804*

BAC *see* benzalkonium chloride *on page 107*

B-A-C® *(Discontinued)* *see page 1042*

Bacid® [US-OTC/Can] *see* Lactobacillus *on page 501*

Baciguent® [US/Can] *see* bacitracin *on this page*

BaciiM® [US] *see* bacitracin *on this page*

bacillus calmette-Guérin (BCG) live *see* BCG vaccine *on page 101*

bacitracin (bas i TRAY sin)

Sound-Alike/Look-Alike Issues
bacitracin may be confused with Bactrim®, Bactroban®

U.S./Canadian Brand Names Baciguent® [US/Can]; BaciiM® [US]

Therapeutic Category Antibiotic, Ophthalmic; Antibiotic, Topical; Antibiotic, Miscellaneous

Use Treatment of susceptible bacterial infections mainly; has activity against gram-positive bacilli; due to toxicity risks, systemic and irrigant uses of bacitracin should be limited to situations where less toxic alternatives would not be effective

Usual Dosage **Do not administer I.V.:**
Infants: I.M.:
≤2.5 kg: 900 units/kg/day in 2-3 divided doses
>2.5 kg: 1000 units/kg/day in 2-3 divided doses
Children: I.M.: 800-1200 units/kg/day divided every 8 hours
Adults: Oral:
Antibiotic-associated colitis: 25,000 units 4 times/day for 7-10 days
Children and Adults:
Topical: Apply 1-5 times/day
Ophthalmic, ointment: Instill 1/4" to 1/2" ribbon every 3-4 hours into conjunctival sac for acute infections, or 2-3 times/day for mild to moderate infections for 7-10 days
Irrigation, solution: 50-100 units/mL in normal saline, lactated Ringer's, or sterile water for irrigation; soak sponges in solution for topical compresses 1-5 times/day or as needed during surgical procedures

Dosage Forms [DSC] = Discontinued product

Injection, powder for reconstitution (BaciiM®): 50,000 units

Ointment, ophthalmic (AK-Tracin® [DSC]): 500 units/g (3.5 g)

Ointment, topical: 500 units/g (0.9 g, 15 g, 30 g, 120 g, 454 g)

Baciguent®: 500 units/g (15 g, 30 g)

bacitracin and polymyxin B (bas i TRAY sin & pol i MIKS in bee)

Sound-Alike/Look-Alike Issues

Betadine® may be confused with Betagan®, betaine

Synonyms polymyxin B and bacitracin

U.S./Canadian Brand Names AK-Poly-Bac® [US]; Betadine® First Aid Antibiotics + Moisturizer [US-OTC]; LID-Pack® [Can]; Optimyxin® [Can]; Polycidin® Ophthalmic Ointment [Can]; Polysporin® Ophthalmic [US]; Polysporin® Topical [US-OTC]

Therapeutic Category Antibiotic, Ophthalmic; Antibiotic, Topical

Use Treatment of superficial infections caused by susceptible organisms

Usual Dosage Children and Adults:

Ophthalmic ointment: Instill 1/2" ribbon in the affected eye(s) every 3-4 hours for acute infections or 2-3 times/day for mild to moderate infections for 7-10 days

Topical ointment/powder: Apply to affected area 1-4 times/day; may cover with sterile bandage if needed

Dosage Forms

Ointment, ophthalmic (AK-Poly-Bac®, Polysporin®): Bacitracin 500 units and polymyxin B sulfate 10,000 units per g (3.5 g)

Ointment, topical [OTC]: Bacitracin 500 units and polymyxin B sulfate 10,000 units per g in white petrolatum (15 g, 30 g)

Betadine® First Aid Antibiotics + Moisturizer: Bacitracin 500 units and polymyxin B sulfate 10,000 units per g (14 g)

Polysporin®: Bacitracin 500 units and polymyxin B sulfate 10,000 units per g (15 g, 30 g)

Powder, topical (Polysporin®): Bacitracin 500 units and polymyxin B sulfate 10,000 units per g (10 g)

bacitracin, neomycin, and polymyxin B

(bas i TRAY sin, nee oh MYE sin, & pol i MIKS in bee)

Synonyms neomycin, bacitracin, and polymyxin B; polymyxin B, bacitracin, and neomycin; triple antibiotic

U.S./Canadian Brand Names Neosporin® Neo To Go® [US-OTC]; Neosporin® Ophthalmic Ointment [US/Can]; Neosporin® Topical [US-OTC]; Neotopic® [Can]

Therapeutic Category Antibiotic, Ophthalmic; Antibiotic, Topical

Use Helps prevent infection in minor cuts, scrapes and burns; short-term treatment of superficial external ocular infections caused by susceptible organisms

Usual Dosage Children and Adults:

Ophthalmic: Ointment: Instill 1/2" into the conjunctival sac every 3-4 hours for 7-10 days for acute infections

Topical: Apply 1-3 times/day to infected area; may cover with sterile bandage as needed

Dosage Forms

Ointment, ophthalmic (Neosporin®): Bacitracin 400 units, neomycin 3.5 mg, and polymyxin B 10,000 units per g (3.5 g)

Ointment, topical: Bacitracin 400 units, neomycin 3.5 mg, and polymyxin B 5000 units per g (0.9 g, 15 g, 30 g, 454 g)

Neosporin®: Bacitracin 400 units, neomycin 3.5 mg, and polymyxin B 5000 units per g (15 g, 30 g)

Neosporin® Neo To Go®: Bacitracin 400 units, neomycin 3.5 mg, and polymyxin B 5000 units per g (0.9 g)

bacitracin, neomycin, polymyxin B, and hydrocortisone

(bas i TRAY sin, nee oh MYE sin, pol i MIKS in bee, & hye droe KOR ti sone)

Synonyms hydrocortisone, bacitracin, neomycin, and polymyxin B; neomycin, bacitracin, polymyxin B, and hydrocortisone; polymyxin B, bacitracin, neomycin, and hydrocortisone

U.S./Canadian Brand Names Cortisporin® Ointment [US/Can]

Therapeutic Category Antibiotic/Corticosteroid, Ophthalmic; Antibiotic/Corticosteroid, Topical

Use Prevention and treatment of susceptible inflammatory conditions where bacterial infection (or risk of infection) is present

Usual Dosage Children and Adults:

Ophthalmic: Ointment: Instill ½" ribbon to inside of lower lid every 3-4 hours until improvement occurs

Topical: Apply sparingly 2-4 times/day. Therapy should be discontinued when control is achieved; if no improvement is seen, reassessment of diagnosis may be necessary.

Dosage Forms [DSC] = Discontinued product

Ointment, ophthalmic (AK-Spore® H.C. [DSC], Cortisporin®): Bacitracin 400 units, neomycin sulfate 3.5 mg, polymyxin B 10,000 units, and hydrocortisone 10 mg per g (3.5 g)

Ointment, topical (Cortisporin®): Bacitracin 400 units, neomycin 3.5 mg, polymyxin B 5000 units, and hydrocortisone 10 mg per g (15 g)

bacitracin, neomycin, polymyxin B, and lidocaine

(bas i TRAY sin, nee oh MYE sin, pol i MIKS in bee, & LYE doe kane)

Therapeutic Category Antibiotic, Topical

Use Prevention and treatment of susceptible superficial topical infections

Usual Dosage Adults: Topical: Apply 1-4 times/day to infected areas; cover with sterile bandage if needed

Dosage Forms Ointment, topical: Bacitracin 500 units, neomycin base 3.5 g, polymyxin B sulfate 5000 units, and lidocaine 40 mg per g (15 g, 30 g)

baclofen (BAK loe fen)

Sound-Alike/Look-Alike Issues

baclofen may be confused with Bactroban®

Lioresal® may be confused with lisinopril, Loniten®, Lotensin®

U.S./Canadian Brand Names Apo-Baclofen® [Can]; Gen-Baclofen [Can]; Lioresal® [US/Can]; Liotec [Can]; Nu-Baclo [Can]; PMS-Baclofen [Can]

Therapeutic Category Skeletal Muscle Relaxant

Use Treatment of reversible spasticity associated with multiple sclerosis or spinal cord lesions

Orphan drug: Intrathecal: Treatment of intractable spasticity caused by spinal cord injury, multiple sclerosis, and other spinal disease (spinal ischemia or tumor, transverse myelitis, cervical spondylosis, degenerative myelopathy)

Usual Dosage

Oral (avoid abrupt withdrawal of drug):

Children:

2-7 years: Initial: 10-15 mg/24 hours divided every 8 hours; titrate dose every 3 days in increments of 5-15 mg/day to a maximum of 40 mg/day

≥8 years: Maximum: 60 mg/day in 3 divided doses

Adults: 5 mg 3 times/day, may increase 5 mg/dose every 3 days to a maximum of 80 mg/day

Hiccups: Adults: Usual effective dose: 10-20 mg 2-3 times/day

Intrathecal:

Test dose: 50-100 mcg, doses >50 mcg should be given in 25 mcg increments, separated by 24 hours. A screening dose of 25 mcg may be considered in very small patients. Patients not responding to screening dose of 100 mcg should not be considered for chronic infusion/implanted pump.

Maintenance: After positive response to test dose, a maintenance intrathecal infusion can be administered via an implanted intrathecal pump. Initial dose via pump: Infusion at a 24-hour rate dosed at twice the test dose. Avoid abrupt discontinuation.

Dosage Forms

Injection, solution, intrathecal [preservative free] (Lioresal®): 50 mcg/mL (1 mL); 500 mcg/mL (20 mL); 2000 mcg/mL (5 mL)

Tablet: 10 mg, 20 mg

Bactocill® ***(Discontinued)*** *see page 1042*

BactoShield® ***(Discontinued)*** *see page 1042*

BactoShield® CHG [US-OTC] *see* chlorhexidine gluconate *on page 183*

Bactrim™ [US] *see* sulfamethoxazole and trimethoprim *on page 831*

Bactrim™ DS [US] *see* sulfamethoxazole and trimethoprim *on page 831*

Bactrim™ I.V. Infusion ***(Discontinued)*** *see page 1042*

Bactroban® [US/Can] *see* mupirocin *on page 595*

Bactroban® Nasal [US] *see* mupirocin *on page 595*

baking soda *see* sodium bicarbonate *on page 809*

BAL *see* dimercaprol *on page 275*

balanced salt solution (BAL anced salt soe LOO shun)

U.S./Canadian Brand Names AquaLase™ [US]; BSS® [US/Can]; BSS® Plus [US/Can]; Eye-Stream® [Can]

Therapeutic Category Ophthalmic Agent, Miscellaneous

Use Intraocular or extraocular irrigating solution

Usual Dosage Adults: Ophthalmic irrigation: Based on standard for each surgical procedure

Dosage Forms

Solution, ophthalmic [irrigation; preservative free]: Sodium chloride 0.64%, potassium chloride 0.075%, calcium chloride 0.048%, magnesium chloride 0.03%, sodium acetate 0.39%, sodium citrate 0.17% (18 mL, 200 mL, 250 mL, 500 mL)

AquaLase™: Sodium chloride 0.64%, potassium chloride 0.075%, calcium chloride 0.048%, magnesium chloride 0.03%, sodium acetate 0.39%, sodium citrate 0.17% (90 mL)

BSS®: Sodium chloride 0.64%, potassium chloride 0.075%, calcium chloride 0.048%, magnesium chloride 0.03%, sodium acetate 0.39%, sodium citrate 0.17% (15 mL, 30 mL, 250 mL, 500 mL)

BSS Plus®: Sodium chloride 0.71%, potassium chloride 0.038%, calcium chloride 0.154%, magnesium chloride 0.02%, sodium phosphate 0.42%, sodium bicarbonate 0.21%, dextrose 0.92%, glutathione 0.018% (500 mL)

Baldex® ***(Discontinued)*** *see page 1042*

BAL in Oil® [US] *see* dimercaprol *on page 275*

Balmex® [US-OTC] *see* zinc oxide *on page 940*

Balminil® [Can] *see* xylometazoline *on page 935*

Balminil® Decongestant [Can] *see* pseudoephedrine *on page 745*

Balminil® DM D [Can] *see* pseudoephedrine and dextromethorphan *on page 746*

Balminil® DM + Decongestant + Expectorant [Can] *see* guaifenesin, pseudoephedrine, and dextromethorphan *on page 422*

Balminil® DM E [Can] *see* guaifenesin and dextromethorphan *on page 416*

Balminil® Expectorant [Can] *see* guaifenesin *on page 415*

Balnetar® [US-OTC/Can] *see* coal tar *on page 219*

balsalazide (bal SAL a zide)

Sound-Alike/Look-Alike Issues

Colazal® may be confused with Clozaril®

Synonyms balsalazide disodium

U.S./Canadian Brand Names Colazal® [US]

Therapeutic Category 5-Aminosalicylic Acid Derivative; Antiinflammatory Agent

Use Treatment of mild to moderate active ulcerative colitis

Usual Dosage Oral: Adults: 2.25 g (three 750 mg capsules) 3 times/day for 8-12 weeks

Dosage Forms Capsule: 750 mg

balsalazide disodium *see* balsalazide *on this page*

balsam peru, trypsin, and castor oil *see* trypsin, balsam peru, and castor oil *on page 892*

Bancap® *(Discontinued)* *see page 1042*

Bancap HC® [US] *see* hydrocodone and acetaminophen *on page 443*

Band-Aid® Hurt-Free™ Antiseptic Wash [US-OTC] *see* lidocaine *on page 518*

Banesin® *(Discontinued)* *see page 1042*

Banophen® Decongestant Capsule *(Discontinued)* *see page 1042*

Banophen® [US-OTC] *see* diphenhydramine *on page 277*

Banthine® *(Discontinued)* *see page 1042*

Bantron® *(Discontinued)* *see page 1042*

Barbidonna® *(Discontinued)* *see page 1042*

Barbita® *(Discontinued)* *see page 1042*

Barc™ Liquid *(Discontinued)* *see page 1042*

Baricon® [US] *see* radiological/contrast media (ionic) *on page 759*

barium sulfate *see* radiological/contrast media (ionic) *on page 759*

Barobag® [US] *see* radiological/contrast media (ionic) *on page 759*

Baro-CAT® [US] *see* radiological/contrast media (ionic) *on page 759*

Baroflave® [US] *see* radiological/contrast media (ionic) *on page 759*

Barosperse® [US] *see* radiological/contrast media (ionic) *on page 759*

Bar-Test® [US] *see* radiological/contrast media (ionic) *on page 759*

Basaljel® *(Discontinued)* *see page 1042*

Basaljel® [Can] *see* aluminum hydroxide *on page 39*

base ointment *see* zinc oxide *on page 940*

basiliximab (ba si LIKS i mab)

U.S./Canadian Brand Names Simulect® [US/Can]

Therapeutic Category Immunosuppressant Agent

Use Prophylaxis of acute organ rejection in renal transplantation

Usual Dosage **Note:** Patients previously administered basiliximab should only be re-exposed to a subsequent course of therapy with extreme caution.

I.V.:

Children <35 kg: Renal transplantation: 10 mg within 2 hours prior to transplant surgery, followed by a second 10 mg dose 4 days after transplantation; the second dose should be withheld if complications occur (including severe hypersensitivity reactions or graft loss)

Children ≥35 kg and Adults: Renal transplantation: 20 mg within 2 hours prior to transplant surgery, followed by a second 20 mg dose 4 days after transplantation; the second dose should be withheld if complications occur (including severe hypersensitivity reactions or graft loss)

Dosage Forms Injection, powder for reconstitution: 10 mg, 20 mg

Bausch & Lomb® Computer Eye Drops [US-OTC] *see* glycerin *on page 410*

Bausch & Lomb® Earwax Removal [US-OTC] *see* carbamide peroxide *on page 155*

Baycol® ***(Discontinued)*** *see page 1042*

Bayer® Aspirin Extra Strength [US-OTC] *see* aspirin *on page 80*

Bayer® Aspirin Regimen Adult Low Strength [US-OTC] *see* aspirin *on page 80*

Bayer® Aspirin Regimen Children's [US-OTC] *see* aspirin *on page 80*

Bayer® Aspirin Regimen Regular Strength [US-OTC] *see* aspirin *on page 80*

Bayer® Aspirin [US-OTC] *see* aspirin *on page 80*

Bayer® Extra Strength Arthritis Pain Regimen [US-OTC] *see* aspirin *on page 80*

Bayer® Plus Extra Strength [US-OTC] *see* aspirin *on page 80*

Bayer® Women's Aspirin Plus Calcium [US-OTC] *see* aspirin *on page 80*

BayGam® [US/Can] *see* immune globulin (intramuscular) *on page 468*

BayHep B® [US/Can] *see* hepatitis B immune globulin *on page 433*

Baypress® ***(Discontinued)*** *see page 1042*

BayRab® [US/Can] *see* rabies immune globulin (human) *on page 759*

BayRho-D® Full-Dose [US/Can] *see* Rh_o(D) immune globulin *on page 771*

BayRho-D® Mini-Dose [US] *see* Rh_o(D) immune globulin *on page 771*

BayTet™ [US/Can] *see* tetanus immune globulin (human) *on page 849*

Baza® Antifungal [US-OTC] *see* miconazole *on page 578*

Baza® Clear [US-OTC] *see* vitamin A and vitamin D *on page 915*

B-Caro-T™ [US] *see* beta-carotene *on page 113*

BCG, live *see* BCG vaccine *on this page*

BCG vaccine (bee see jee vak SEEN)

Synonyms bacillus calmette-Guérin (BCG) live; BCG, live

U.S./Canadian Brand Names ImmuCyst® [Can]; Oncotice™ [Can]; Pacis™ [Can]; TherаCys® [US]; TICE® BCG [US]

Therapeutic Category Biological Response Modulator

Use Immunization against tuberculosis and immunotherapy for cancer; treatment of bladder cancer

BCG vaccine is not routinely recommended for use in the U.S. for prevention of tuberculosis

BCG vaccine is strongly recommended for infants and children with negative tuberculin skin tests who:

- are at high risk of intimate and prolonged exposure to persistently untreated or ineffectively treated patients with infectious pulmonary tuberculosis, and
- cannot be removed from the source of exposure, and
- cannot be placed on long-term preventive therapy
- are continuously exposed with tuberculosis who have bacilli resistant to isoniazid and rifampin

BCG is also recommended for tuberculin-negative infants and children in groups in which the rate of new infections exceeds 1% per year and for whom the usual surveillance and treatment programs have been attempted but are not operationally feasible

(Continued)

BCG vaccine *(Continued)*

Usual Dosage Children >1 month and Adults:

Immunization against tuberculosis (TICE® BCG): 0.2-0.3 mL percutaneous; initial lesion usually appears after 10-14 days consisting of small red papule at injection site and reaches maximum diameter of 3 mm in 4-6 weeks; conduct postvaccinal tuberculin test (ie, 5 TU of PPD) in 2-3 months; if test is negative, repeat vaccination

Immunotherapy for bladder cancer:

Intravesical treatment: Instill into bladder for 2 hours

TheraCys®: One dose instilled into bladder once weekly for 6 weeks followed by one treatment at 3, 6, 12, 18, and 24 months after initial treatment

TICE® BCG: One dose instilled into the bladder once weekly for 6 weeks followed by once monthly for 6-12 months

Dosage Forms Injection, powder for reconstitution, intravesical:

TheraCys®: 81 mg [with diluent]

TICE® BCG: 50 mg

BCNU *see* carmustine *on page 162*

B complex combinations *see* vitamin B complex combinations *on page 915*

B-D™ Glucose [US-OTC] *see* glucose (instant) *on page 408*

Bebulin® VH [US] *see* factor IX complex (human) *on page 355*

becaplermin (be KAP ler min)

Sound-Alike/Look-Alike Issues

Regranex® may be confused with Granulex®, Repronex®

Synonyms recombinant human platelet-derived growth factor B; rPDGF-BB

U.S./Canadian Brand Names Regranex® [US/Can]

Therapeutic Category Topical Skin Product

Use Debridement adjunct for the treatment of diabetic ulcers that occur on the lower limbs and feet

Usual Dosage Topical: Adults:

Diabetic ulcers: Apply appropriate amount of gel once daily with a cotton swab or similar tool, as a coating over the ulcer

The amount of becaplermin to be applied will vary depending on the size of the ulcer area. To calculate the length of gel applied to the ulcer, measure the greatest length of the ulcer by the greatest width of the ulcer in inches. Tube size will determine the formula used in the calculation. For a 15 or 7.5 g tube, multiply length x width x 0.6. For a 2 g tube, multiply length x width x 1.3.

Note: If the ulcer does not decrease in size by ~30% after 10 weeks of treatment or complete healing has not occurred in 20 weeks, continued treatment with becaplermin gel should be reassessed.

Dosage Forms Gel, topical: 0.01% (15 g)

beclomethasone (be kloe METH a sone)

Sound-Alike/Look-Alike Issues

Vanceril® may be confused with Vancenase®

Synonyms beclomethasone dipropionate

U.S./Canadian Brand Names Apo-Beclomethasone® [Can]; Beconase® AQ [US]; Gen-Beclo [Can]; Nu-Beclomethasone [Can]; Propaderm® [Can]; QVAR® [US/Can]; Rivanase AQ [Can]; Vanceril® AEM [Can]

Therapeutic Category Adrenal Corticosteroid

Use

Oral inhalation: Maintenance and prophylactic treatment of asthma; includes those who require corticosteroids and those who may benefit from a dose reduction/elimination of systemically administered corticosteroids. Not for relief of acute bronchospasm

Nasal aerosol: Symptomatic treatment of seasonal or perennial rhinitis and to prevent recurrence of nasal polyps following surgery

Usual Dosage Nasal inhalation and oral inhalation dosage forms are not to be used interchangeably

Aqueous inhalation, nasal (Beconase® AQ): Children ≥6 years and Adults: 1-2 inhalations each nostril twice daily; total dose 168-336 mcg/day

Intranasal (Beconase®):

Children 6-12 years: 1 inhalation in each nostril 3 times/day; total dose 252 mcg/day

Children ≥12 years and Adults: 1 inhalation in each nostril 2-4 times/day or 2 inhalations each nostril twice daily (total dose 168-336 mcg/day); usual maximum maintenance: 1 inhalation in each nostril 3 times/day (252 mcg/day)

Oral inhalation (doses should be titrated to the lowest effective dose once asthma is controlled) (QVAR®):

Children 5-11 years: Initial: 40 mcg twice daily; maximum dose: 80 mcg twice daily

Children ≥12 years and Adults:

Patients previously on bronchodilators only: Initial dose 40-80 mcg twice daily; maximum dose: 320 mcg twice day

Patients previously on inhaled corticosteroids: Initial dose 40-160 mcg twice daily; maximum dose: 320 mcg twice daily

Dosage Forms [DSC] = Discontinued product

Aerosol for oral inhalation, as dipropionate (QVAR®): 40 mcg/inhalation [100 metered doses] (7.3 g); 80 mcg/inhalation [100 metered doses] (7.3 g)

Aerosol, intranasal, as dipropionate (Beconase® [DSC]): 42 mcg/inhalation: [80 metered doses] (6.7 g); [200 metered doses] (16.8 g)

Suspension, intranasal, aqueous, as dipropionate [spray] (Beconase® AQ): 42 mcg/inhalation [180 metered doses] (25 g)

beclomethasone dipropionate *see* beclomethasone *on previous page*

Beclovent® *(Discontinued)* *see page 1042*

Becomject-100® *(Discontinued)* *see page 1042*

Beconase® *(Discontinued)* *see page 1042*

Beconase® AQ [US] *see* beclomethasone *on previous page*

Becotin® Pulvules® *(Discontinued)* *see page 1042*

Beepen-VK® *(Discontinued)* *see page 1042*

Beesix® *(Discontinued)* *see page 1042*

behenyl alcohol *see* docosanol *on page 285*

Belix® Oral *(Discontinued)* *see page 1042*

belladonna (bel a DON a)

Therapeutic Category Anticholinergic Agent

Use Decrease gastrointestinal activity in functional bowel disorders and to delay gastric emptying as well as decrease gastric secretion

Usual Dosage Tincture: Oral:

Children: 0.03 mL/kg 3 times/day

Adults: 0.6-1 mL 3-4 times/day

Dosage Forms Tincture: Belladonna alkaloids (principally hyoscyamine and atropine) 0.3 mg/mL with alcohol 65% to 70% (120 mL, 480 mL, 3780 mL)

belladonna and opium (bel a DON a & OH pee um)

Synonyms opium and belladonna

U.S./Canadian Brand Names B&O Supprettes® [US]

Therapeutic Category Analgesic, Narcotic

Controlled Substance C-II

Use Relief of moderate to severe pain associated with rectal or bladder tenesmus that may occur in postoperative states and neoplastic situations; pain associated with ureteral spasms not responsive to non-narcotic analgesics and to space intervals between injections of opiates

(Continued)

belladonna and opium *(Continued)*

Usual Dosage Rectal: Adults: 1 suppository 1-2 times/day, up to 4 doses/day

Dosage Forms Suppository:

#15 A: Belladonna extract 16.2 mg and opium 30 mg

#16 A: Belladonna extract 16.2 mg and opium 60 mg

belladonna, phenobarbital, and ergotamine tartrate

(bel a DON a, fee noe BAR bi tal, & er GOT a meen TAR trate)

Synonyms ergotamine tartrate, belladonna, and phenobarbital; phenobarbital, belladonna, and ergotamine tartrate

U.S./Canadian Brand Names Bellamine S [US]; Bellergal® Spacetabs® [Can]; Bel-Tabs [US]

Therapeutic Category Ergot Alkaloid and Derivative

Use Management and treatment of menopausal disorders, GI disorders, and recurrent throbbing headache

Usual Dosage Oral: 1 tablet each morning and evening

Dosage Forms Tablet: Belladonna alkaloids 0.2 mg, phenobarbital 40 mg, and ergotamine tartrate 0.6 mg

Bellafoline® *(Discontinued)* *see page 1042*

Bellamine S [US] *see* belladonna, phenobarbital, and ergotamine tartrate *on this page*

Bellatal® *(Discontinued)* *see page 1042*

Bellergal-S® *(Discontinued)* *see page 1042*

Bellergal® Spacetabs® [Can] *see* belladonna, phenobarbital, and ergotamine tartrate *on this page*

Bel-Tabs [US] *see* belladonna, phenobarbital, and ergotamine tartrate *on this page*

Bemote® *(Discontinued)* *see page 1042*

Bena-D® *(Discontinued)* *see page 1042*

Benadryl® 50 mg Capsule *(Discontinued)* *see page 1042*

Benadryl® Allergy and Sinus Fastmelt™ [US-OTC] *see* diphenhydramine and pseudoephedrine *on page 279*

Benadryl® Allergy/Sinus [US-OTC] *see* diphenhydramine and pseudoephedrine *on page 279*

Benadryl® Allergy [US-OTC/Can] *see* diphenhydramine *on page 277*

Benadryl® Children's Allergy and Cold Fastmelt™ [US-OTC] *see* diphenhydramine and pseudoephedrine *on page 279*

Benadryl® Children's Allergy and Sinus [US-OTC] *see* diphenhydramine and pseudoephedrine *on page 279*

Benadryl® Cold/Flu *(Discontinued)* *see page 1042*

Benadryl® Dye-Free Allergy [US-OTC] *see* diphenhydramine *on page 277*

Benadryl® Gel Extra Strength [US-OTC] *see* diphenhydramine *on page 277*

Benadryl® Gel [US-OTC] *see* diphenhydramine *on page 277*

Benadryl® Injection [US] *see* diphenhydramine *on page 277*

Benahist® Injection *(Discontinued)* *see page 1042*

Ben-Allergin-50® Injection *(Discontinued)* *see page 1042*

Ben-Aqua® *(Discontinued)* *see page 1042*

benazepril (ben AY ze pril)

Sound-Alike/Look-Alike Issues

benazepril may be confused with Benadryl®

Lotensin® may be confused with Lioresal®, Loniten®, lovastatin

Synonyms benazepril hydrochloride

U.S./Canadian Brand Names Lotensin® [US/Can]

Therapeutic Category Angiotensin-Converting Enzyme (ACE) Inhibitor

Use Treatment of hypertension, either alone or in combination with other antihypertensive agents

Usual Dosage Oral: Hypertension:

Children ≥6 years: Initial: 0.2 mg/kg/day as monotherapy; dosing range: 0.1-0.6 mg/kg/day (maximum dose: 40 mg/day)

Adults: Initial: 10 mg/day in patients not receiving a diuretic; 20-40 mg/day as a single dose or 2 divided doses; the need for twice-daily dosing should be assessed by monitoring peak (2-6 hours after dosing) and trough responses.

Note: Patients taking diuretics should have them discontinued 2-3 days prior to starting benazepril. If they cannot be discontinued, then initial dose should be 5 mg; restart after blood pressure is stabilized if needed.

Dosage Forms Tablet, as hydrochloride: 5 mg, 10 mg, 20 mg, 40 mg

benazepril and amlodipine *see* amlodipine and benazepril *on page 49*

benazepril and hydrochlorothiazide

(ben AY ze pril & hye droe klor oh THYE a zide)

Synonyms hydrochlorothiazide and benazepril

U.S./Canadian Brand Names Lotensin® HCT [US]

Therapeutic Category Antihypertensive Agent, Combination

Use Treatment of hypertension

Usual Dosage Dose is individualized

Dosage Forms Tablet:

5/6.25: Benazepril 5 mg and hydrochlorothiazide 6.25 mg

10/12.5: Benazepril 10 mg and hydrochlorothiazide 12.5 mg

20/12.5: Benazepril 20 mg and hydrochlorothiazide 12.5 mg

20/25: Benazepril 20 mg and hydrochlorothiazide 25 mg

benazepril hydrochloride *see* benazepril *on this page*

bendroflumethiazide (ben droe floo meth EYE a zide)

Therapeutic Category Diuretic, Thiazide

Use Management of mild to moderate hypertension, edema associated with congestive heart failure, pregnancy, or nephrotic syndrome; reportedly does not alter serum electrolyte concentrations appreciably at recommended doses

Usual Dosage Oral:

Children: Initial: 0.1-0.4 mg/kg/day in 1-2 doses; maintenance dose: 0.05-0.1 mg/kg/day in 1-2 doses; maximum dose: 20 mg/day

Adults: 2.5-20 mg/day or twice daily in divided doses

Dosage Forms Tablet: 5 mg

BeneFix® [US/Can] *see* factor IX *on page 354*

Benemid® *(Discontinued)* *see page 1042*

Benicar™ [US] *see* olmesartan *on page 642*

Benicar HCT™ [US] *see* olmesartan and hydrochlorothiazide *on page 643*

Benoject® *(Discontinued)* *see page 1042*

Benoquin® [US] *see* monobenzone *on page 590*

Benoxyl® [Can] *see* benzoyl peroxide *on page 109*

benserazide and levodopa *(Canada only)*

(ben SER a zide & lee voe DOE pa)

Synonyms levodopa and benserazide

U.S./Canadian Brand Names Prolopa® [Can]

Therapeutic Category Anti-Parkinson Agent

Use Treatment of Parkinson disease (except drug-induced Parkinsonism)

Usual Dosage Oral: Adults: **Note:** Dosage expressed as levodopa/benserazide:

Initial: 100/25 mg 1-2 times/day, increase every 3-4 days until therapeutic effect; optimal dosage: 400/100 mg to 800/200 mg/day divided into 4-6 doses

Note: 200/50 mg used only when maintenance therapy is reached and not to exceed levodopa 1000-1200 mg/benserazide 250-300 mg per day

Patients previously on levodopa: Allow 12 hours or more to lapse between last dose of levodopa; start at 15% of previous levodopa dosage

Note: Dosages should be introduced gradually, individualized, and continued for 3-6 weeks before assessing benefit. Decrease dosage in patients with dystonia.

Dosage Forms Capsule:

50-12.5: Levodopa 50 mg and benserazide 12.5 mg

100-25: Levodopa 100 mg and benserazide 25 mg

200-50: Levodopa 200 mg and benserazide 50 mg

bentoquatam (ben to KWA tam)

Synonyms quaternium-18 bentonite

U.S./Canadian Brand Names IvyBlock® [US-OTC]

Therapeutic Category Protectant, Topical

Use Skin protectant for the prevention of allergic contact dermatitis to poison oak, ivy, and sumac

Usual Dosage Children >6 years and Adults: Topical: Apply to skin 15 minutes prior to potential exposure to poison ivy, poison oak, or poison sumac, and reapply every 4 hours

Dosage Forms Lotion: 5% (120 mL) [contains benzyl alcohol]

Bentyl® [US] *see* dicyclomine *on page 267*

Bentyl® Injection *(Discontinued)* *see page 1042*

Bentylol® [Can] *see* dicyclomine *on page 267*

Benuryl™ [Can] *see* probenecid *on page 729*

Benylin® 3.3 mg-D-E [Can] *see* guaifenesin, pseudoephedrine, and codeine *on page 422*

Benylin® Adult [US-OTC] *see* dextromethorphan *on page 261*

Benylin® Cough Syrup *(Discontinued)* *see page 1042*

Benylin DM® *(Discontinued)* *see page 1042*

Benylin® DM-D [Can] *see* pseudoephedrine and dextromethorphan *on page 746*

Benylin® DM-D-E [Can] *see* guaifenesin, pseudoephedrine, and dextromethorphan *on page 422*

Benylin® DM-E [Can] *see* guaifenesin and dextromethorphan *on page 416*

Benylin® E Extra Strength [Can] *see* guaifenesin *on page 415*

Benylin® Expectorant [US-OTC] *see* guaifenesin and dextromethorphan *on page 416*

Benylin® Pediatric [US-OTC] *see* dextromethorphan *on page 261*

Benzac® [US] *see* benzoyl peroxide *on page 109*

Benzac® AC [US/Can] *see* benzoyl peroxide *on page 109*

Benzac® AC Gel *(Discontinued)* *see page 1042*

Benzac® AC Wash [US] *see* benzoyl peroxide *on page 109*

BenzaClin® [US] *see* clindamycin and benzoyl peroxide *on page 211*

Benzac® W [US] *see* benzoyl peroxide *on page 109*

Benzac® W Gel *(Discontinued)* *see page 1042*

Benzac® W Gel [Can] *see* benzoyl peroxide *on page 109*

Benzac® W Wash [US/Can] *see* benzoyl peroxide *on page 109*

Benzagel® [US] *see* benzoyl peroxide *on page 109*

Benzagel® Wash [US] *see* benzoyl peroxide *on page 109*

benzalkonium chloride (benz al KOE nee um KLOR ide)

Sound-Alike/Look-Alike Issues
Benza® may be confused with Benzac®

Synonyms BAC

U.S./Canadian Brand Names Benza® [US-OTC]; HandClens® [US-OTC]; 3M™ Cavilon™ Skin Cleanser [US-OTC]; Zephiran® [US-OTC]

Therapeutic Category Antibacterial, Topical

Use Surface antiseptic and germicidal preservative

Usual Dosage Thoroughly rinse anionic detergents and soaps from the skin or other areas prior to use of solutions because they reduce the antibacterial activity of BAC. To protect metal instruments stored in BAC solution, add crushed Anti-Rust Tablets, 4 tablets/quart, to antiseptic solution, change solution at least once weekly. Not to be used for storage of aluminum or zinc instruments, instruments with lenses fastened by cement, lacquered catheters, or some synthetic rubber goods.

Dosage Forms [DSC] = Discontinued product
Solution, topical:
Benza®: 1:750 (60 mL, 240 mL, 480 mL, 3840 mL)
HandClens®: 0.13% (120 mL, 480 mL, 800 mL)
Ony-Clear [DSC]: 1% (30 mL)
Zephiran®: 1:750 (240 mL, 3840 mL) [aqueous]
Solution, topical spray (3M™ Cavilon™ Skin Cleanser): 0.11% (240 mL)

Benzamycin® [US] *see* erythromycin and benzoyl peroxide *on page 321*

Benzamycin® Pak [US] *see* erythromycin and benzoyl peroxide *on page 321*

Benzashave® [US] *see* benzoyl peroxide *on page 109*

benzathine benzylpenicillin *see* penicillin G benzathine *on page 675*

benzathine penicillin G *see* penicillin G benzathine *on page 675*

Benza® [US-OTC] *see* benzalkonium chloride *on this page*

Benzedrex® [US-OTC] *see* propylhexedrine *on page 742*

benzene hexachloride *see* lindane *on page 522*

benzhexol hydrochloride *see* trihexyphenidyl *on page 886*

benzmethyzin *see* procarbazine *on page 731*

benzocaine (BEN zoe kane)

Sound-Alike/Look-Alike Issues
Orabase®-B may be confused with Orinase®

Synonyms ethyl aminobenzoate

U.S./Canadian Brand Names Americaine® Anesthetic Lubricant [US]; Americaine® [US-OTC]; Anbesol® Baby [US-OTC/Can]; Anbesol® Maximum Strength [US-OTC]; Anbesol® [US-OTC]; Babee® Teething® [US-OTC]; Benzodent® [US-OTC]; Chiggerex® [US-OTC]; Chiggertox® [US-OTC]; Cylex® [US-OTC]; Detane® [US-OTC]; Foille® Medicated First Aid [US-OTC]; Foille® Plus [US-OTC]; Foille® [US-OTC]; HDA® Toothache [US-OTC]; Hurricaine® [US]; Lanacane® [US-OTC]; Mycinettes® [US-OTC]; Orabase®-B [US-OTC]; Orajel® Baby Nighttime [US-OTC]; Orajel® Baby [US-OTC]; Orajel®
(Continued)

benzocaine *(Continued)*

Maximum Strength [US-OTC]; Orajel® [US-OTC]; Orasol® [US-OTC]; Solarcaine® [US-OTC]; Trocaine® [US-OTC]; Zilactin® Baby [US-OTC/Can]; Zilactin®-B [US-OTC/Can]

Therapeutic Category Local Anesthetic

Use Temporary relief of pain associated with local anesthetic for pruritic dermatosis, pruritus, minor burns, acute congestive and serous otitis media, swimmer's ear, otitis externa, toothache, minor sore throat pain, canker sores, hemorrhoids, rectal fissures, anesthetic lubricant for passage of catheters and endoscopic tubes; nonprescription diet aid

Usual Dosage Children and Adults:

Mucous membranes: Dosage varies depending on area to be anesthetized and vascularity of tissues

Oral mouth/throat preparations: Refer to specific package labeling or as directed by physician. **Note:** Do not administer for >2 days or use in children <2 years of age, unless directed by physician.

Topical: Apply to affected area as needed

Dosage Forms

Aerosol, oral spray (Hurricaine®): 20% (60 mL) [cherry flavor]

Aerosol, topical spray:

- Americaine®: 20% (20 mL, 120 mL)
- Foille®: 5% (97.5 mL) [contains chloroxylenol 0.63%]
- Foille® Plus: 5% (105 mL) [contains chloroxylenol 0.63% and alcohol 57.33%]
- Solarcaine®: 20% (90 mL, 120 mL, 135 mL) [contains triclosan, alcohol 0.13%]

Cream, topical: 5% (30 g, 454 g)

- Lanacane®: 20% (30g)

Gel, oral:

- Anbesol® 6.3% (7.5 g)
- Anbesol® Baby, Detane®, Orajel® Baby: 7.5% (7.5 g, 10 g, 15 g)
- Anbesol® Maximum Strength, Orajel® Maximum Strength: 20% (6 g, 7.5 g, 10 g)
- HDA® Toothache: 6.5% (15 mL) [contains benzyl alcohol]
- Hurricaine®: 20% (5 g, 30 g) [mint, pina colada, watermelon, and wild cherry flavors]
- Orabase-B®: 20% (7 g)
- Orajel®, Orajel® Baby Nighttime, Zilactin®-B, Zilactin® Baby: 10% (6 g, 7.5 g, 10 g)

Gel, topical (Americaine® Anesthetic Lubricant): 20% (2.5 g, 28 g) [contains 0.1% benzethonium chloride

Liquid, oral:

- Anbesol®, Orasol®: 6.3% (9 mL, 15 mL, 30 mL)
- Anbesol® Maximum Strength: 20% (9 mL, 14 mL)
- Hurricaine®: 20% (30 mL) [pina colada and wild cherry flavors]
- Orajel®: 10% (13 mL) [contains tartrazine]
- Orajel® Baby: 7.5% (13 mL)

Liquid, topical (Chiggertox®): 2% (30 mL)

Lotion, oral (Babee® Teething): 2.5% (15 mL)

Lozenge:

- Cylex®, Mycinettes®: 15 mg [Cylex® contains cetylpyridinium chloride 5 mg]
- Trocaine®: 10 mg

Ointment, oral (Benzodent®): 20% (30 g)

Ointment, topical:

- Chiggerex®: 2% (52 g)
- Foille® Medicated First Aid: 5% (3.5 g, 28 g) [contains chloroxylenol 0.1%, benzyl alcohol; corn oil base]

Paste, oral (Orabase®-B): 20% (7 g)

benzocaine and antipyrine *see* antipyrine and benzocaine *on page 65*

benzocaine and cetylpyridinium chloride *see* cetylpyridinium and benzocaine *on page 179*

benzocaine, butyl aminobenzoate, tetracaine, and benzalkonium chloride

(BEN zoe kane, BYOO til a meen oh BENZ oh ate, TET ra kane, & benz al KOE nee um KLOR ide)

Synonyms tetracaine hydrochloride, benzocaine butyl aminobenzoate, and benzalkonium chloride

U.S./Canadian Brand Names Cetacaine® [US]

Therapeutic Category Local Anesthetic

Use Topical anesthetic to control pain or gagging

Usual Dosage Apply to affected area for approximately 1 second or less

Dosage Forms

Aerosol, topical: Benzocaine 14%, butyl aminobenzoate 2%, tetracaine hydrochloride 2%, and benzalkonium chloride 0.5% (56 g) [also packaged in a kit with various sized cannulas]

Gel, topical: Benzocaine 14%, butyl aminobenzoate 2%, tetracaine hydrochloride 2%, and benzalkonium chloride 0.5% (29 g)

Liquid, topical: Benzocaine 14%, butyl aminobenzoate 2%, tetracaine hydrochloride 2%, and benzalkonium chloride 0.5% (56 mL)

benzocaine, gelatin, pectin, and sodium carboxymethylcellulose

(BEN zoe kane, JEL a tin, PEK tin, & SOW dee um kar box ee meth il SEL yoo lose)

Therapeutic Category Local Anesthetic

Use Topical anesthetic and emollient for oral lesions

Usual Dosage Topical: Apply 2-4 times/day

Dosage Forms Paste: Benzocaine 20%, gelatin, pectin, and sodium carboxymethylcellulose (5 g, 15 g)

Benzocol® *(Discontinued)* *see page 1042*

Benzodent® [US-OTC] *see* benzocaine *on page 107*

benzoin (BEN zoyn)

Synonyms gum benjamin

Therapeutic Category Pharmaceutical Aid; Protectant, Topical

Use Protective application for irritations of the skin; sometimes used in boiling water as steam inhalants for their expectorant and soothing action

Usual Dosage Apply 1-2 times/day

Dosage Forms [DSC] = Discontinued product

Tincture, USP: (15 mL, 60 mL, 120 mL, 480 mL, 4000 mL)

TinBen®: 120 mL [DSC]

Tincture, USP [spray]: 120 mL

benzonatate (ben ZOE na tate)

U.S./Canadian Brand Names Tessalon® [US/Can]

Therapeutic Category Antitussive

Use Symptomatic relief of nonproductive cough

Usual Dosage Children >10 years and Adults: Oral: 100 mg 3 times/day or every 4 hours up to 600 mg/day

Dosage Forms

Capsule: 100 mg

Tessalon®: 100 mg, 200 mg

benzoyl peroxide (BEN zoe il peer OKS ide)

Sound-Alike/Look-Alike Issues

Benoxyl® may be confused with Brevoxyl®, Peroxyl®

Benzac® may be confused with Benza®

(Continued)

benzoyl peroxide *(Continued)*

Brevoxyl® may be confused with Benoxyl®
Fostex® may be confused with pHisoHex®

U.S./Canadian Brand Names Acetoxyl® [Can]; Benoxyl® [Can]; Benzac® [US]; Benzac® AC [US/Can]; Benzac® AC Wash [US]; Benzac® W [US]; Benzac® W Gel [Can]; Benzac® W Wash [US/Can]; Benzagel® [US]; Benzagel® Wash [US]; Benzashave® [US]; Brevoxyl® [US]; Brevoxyl® Cleansing [US]; Brevoxyl® Wash [US]; Clearplex [US-OTC]; Clinac™ BPO [US]; Del Aqua® [US]; Desquam-E™ [US]; Desquam-X® [US/Can]; Exact® Acne Medication [US-OTC]; Fostex® 10% BPO [US-OTC]; Loroxide® [US-OTC]; Neutrogena® Acne Mask [US-OTC]; Neutrogena® On The Spot® Acne Treatment [US-OTC]; Oxy 10® Balanced Medicated Face Wash [US-OTC]; Oxy 10® Balance Spot Treatment [US-OTC]; Oxyderm™ [Can]; Palmer's® Skin Success Acne [US-OTC]; PanOxyl® [US/Can]; PanOxyl®-AQ [US/Can]; PanOxyl® Aqua Gel [US]; PanOxyl® Bar [US-OTC]; Seba-Gel™ [US]; Solugel® [Can]; Triaz® [US]; Triaz® Cleanser [US]; Zapzyt® [US-OTC]

Therapeutic Category Acne Products

Use Adjunctive treatment of mild to moderate acne vulgaris and acne rosacea

Usual Dosage Children and Adults:

Cleansers: Wash once or twice daily; control amount of drying or peeling by modifying dose frequency or concentration

Topical: Apply sparingly once daily; gradually increase to 2-3 times/day if needed. If excessive dryness or peeling occurs, reduce dose frequency or concentration; if excessive stinging or burning occurs, remove with mild soap and water; resume use the next day.

Dosage Forms [DSC] = Discontinued product

Cream, topical:
- Benzashave®: 5% (120 g); 10% (120 g)
- Exact® Acne Medication: 5% (18 g)
- Neutrogena® Acne Mask: 5% (60 g)
- Neutrogena® On The Spot® Acne Treatment: 2.5% (22.5 g)

Gel, topical: 2.5% (60 g); 5% (45 g, 60 g, 90 g); 10% (45 g, 60 g, 90 g)
- Benzac® [alcohol based]: 5% (60 g); 10% (60 g) [contains alcohol 12%]
- Benzac® AC [water based]: 2.5% (60 g); 5% (60 g); 10% (60 g)
- Benzac® W [water based]: 2.5% (60 g); 5% (60 g); 10% (60 g)
- Benzagel®: 5% (45 g); 10% (45 g)
- Benzagel® Wash [water based]: 10% (60 g)
- Brevoxyl®: 4% (43 g, 90 g); 8% (43 g, 90 g)
- Clearplex: 5% (45 g); 10% (45 g)
- Clinac™ BPO: 7% (45 g, 90 g) [90 g DSC]
- Desquam-E™ [water based]: 2.5% (42.5 g); 5% (42.5 g); 10% (42.5 g) [emollient gel]
- Desquam-X®: 5% (42.5 g, 90 g); 10% (42.5 g, 90 g)
- Fostex® 10% BPO: 10% (45 g)
- Oxy 10® Balance Spot Treatment: 5% (30 g); 10% (30 g)
- PanOxyl® [alcohol based]: 5% (57 g, 113 g); 10% (57 g, 113 g)
- PanOxyl® AQ [water based]: 2.5% (57 g, 113 g); 5% (57 g, 113 g); 10% (57 g, 113 g)
- PanOxyl® Aqua Gel [water based]: 10% (42.5 g)
- Seba-Gel™: 5% (60 g, 90 g); 10% (60 g, 90 g)
- Triaz®: 3% (42.5 g); 6% (42.5 g); 10% (42.5 g)
- Triaz® Cleanser: 3% (170 g, 340 g); 6% (170 g, 340 g); 10% (170 g, 340 g)
- Zapzyt®: 10% (30 g)

Liquid, topical: 2.5% (240 mL); 5% (120 mL, 150 mL, 240 mL); 10% (150 mL, 240 mL)
- Benzac® AC Wash [water based]: 2.5% (240 mL); 5% (240 mL); 10% (240 mL)
- Benzac® W Wash [water based]: 5% (240 mL); 10% (240 mL)
- Del-Aqua®: 5% (45 mL); 10% (45 mL)
- Desquam-X®: 5% (150 mL)
- Oxy-10® Balance Medicated Face Wash: 10% (240 mL)

Lotion, topical: 5% (30 mL); 10% (30 mL)
- Brevoxyl® Cleansing: 4% (297 g); 8% (297 g) [in a lathering vehicle]

Brevoxyl® Wash: 4% (170 g); 8% (170 g) [in a lathering vehicle]
Fostex® 10% BPO: 10% (150 mL)
Loroxide®: 5.5% (26 mL)
Palmer's® Skin Success Acne: 10% (30 mL) [contains vitamin E and aloe]
Soap, topical [bar]:
Desquam-X®: 10% (113 g)
Fostex® 10% BPO: 10% (113 g)
PanOxyl® Bar: 5% (113 g); 10% (113 g)

benzoyl peroxide and clindamycin *see* clindamycin and benzoyl peroxide *on page 211*

benzoyl peroxide and erythromycin *see* erythromycin and benzoyl peroxide *on page 321*

benzoyl peroxide and hydrocortisone

(BEN zoe il peer OKS ide & hye droe KOR ti sone)

Synonyms hydrocortisone and benzoyl peroxide

U.S./Canadian Brand Names Vanoxide-HC® [US/Can]

Therapeutic Category Acne Products

Use Treatment of acne vulgaris and oily skin

Usual Dosage Topical: Shake well; apply thin film 1-3 times/day, gently massage into skin

Dosage Forms Lotion: Benzoyl peroxide 5% and hydrocortisone acetate 0.5% (25 mL)

benzphetamine (benz FET a meen)

Synonyms benzphetamine hydrochloride

U.S./Canadian Brand Names Didrex® [US/Can]

Therapeutic Category Anorexiant

Controlled Substance C-III

Use Short-term adjunct in exogenous obesity

Usual Dosage Adults: Oral: Dose should be individualized based on patient response: Initial: 25-50 mg once daily; titrate to 25-50 mg 1-3 times/day; once-daily dosing should be administered midmorning or midafternoon; maximum dose: 50 mg 3 times/day

Dosage Forms Tablet, as hydrochloride: 50 mg

benzphetamine hydrochloride *see* benzphetamine *on this page*

benztropine (BENZ troe peen)

Sound-Alike/Look-Alike Issues

benztropine may be confused with bromocriptine

Synonyms benztropine mesylate

U.S./Canadian Brand Names Apo-Benztropine® [Can]; Cogentin® [US/Can]

Therapeutic Category Anticholinergic Agent; Anti-Parkinson Agent

Use Adjunctive treatment of Parkinson disease; treatment of drug-induced extrapyramidal symptoms (except tardive dyskinesia)

Usual Dosage Use in children ≤3 years of age should be reserved for life-threatening emergencies

Drug-induced extrapyramidal symptom: Oral, I.M., I.V.:
Children >3 years: 0.02-0.05 mg/kg/dose 1-2 times/day
Adults: 1-4 mg/dose 1-2 times/day
Acute dystonia: Adults: I.M., I.V.: 1-2 mg
Parkinsonism: Oral: Adults: 0.5-6 mg/day in 1-2 divided doses; if one dose is greater, administer at bedtime; titrate dose in 0.5 mg increments at 5- to 6-day intervals

Dosage Forms

Injection, solution, as mesylate (Cogentin®): 1 mg/mL (2 mL)
Tablet, as mesylate: 0.5 mg, 1 mg, 2 mg

benztropine mesylate *see* benztropine *on this page*

benzydamine *(Canada only)* (ben ZID a meen)

Synonyms benzydamine hydrochloride

U.S./Canadian Brand Names Apo-Benzydamine® [Can]; Dom-Benzydamine [Can]; Novo-Benzydamine [Can]; PMS-Benzydamine [Can]; ratio-Benzydamine [Can]; Sun-Benz® [Can]; Tantum® [Can]

Therapeutic Category Analgesic, Topical

Use Symptomatic treatment of pain associated with acute pharyngitis; treatment of pain associated with radiation-induced oropharyngeal mucositis

Usual Dosage Oral rinse: Adults:

Radiation-associated mucositis: 15 mL as a gargle or rinse 3-4 times/day; contact between the liquid and the oral mucosa should be maintained for at least 30 seconds, followed by expulsion from the mouth. Clinical studies maintained contact for ~2 minutes, up to 8 times/day. Patient should not swallow the liquid. Begin treatment 1day prior to initiation of radiation therapy and continue daily during treatment. Continue oral rinse treatments after the completion of radiation therapy until desired result/healing is achieved.

Acute pharyngitis: Gargle with 15 mL every 1½-3 hours until symptoms resolve. Patient should expel solution from mouth following use; solution should not be swallowed.

Dosage Forms Oral rinse, as hydrochloride: 0.15% (100 mL, 250 mL)

benzydamine hydrochloride *see* benzydamine *(Canada only)* *on this page*

benzylpenicillin benzathine *see* penicillin G benzathine *on page 675*

benzylpenicillin potassium *see* penicillin G (parenteral/aqueous) *on page 676*

benzylpenicillin sodium *see* penicillin G (parenteral/aqueous) *on page 676*

benzylpenicilloyl-polylysine (BEN zil pen i SIL oyl-pol i LIE seen)

Synonyms penicilloyl-polylysine; PPL

U.S./Canadian Brand Names Pre-Pen® [US]

Therapeutic Category Diagnostic Agent

Use Adjunct in assessing the risk of administering penicillin (penicillin or benzylpenicillin) in adults with a history of clinical penicillin hypersensitivity

Usual Dosage PPL is administered by a scratch technique or by intradermal injection. For initial testing, PPL should always be applied via the scratch technique. **Do not administer intradermally to patients who have positive reactions to a scratch test.** PPL test alone does not identify those patients who react to a minor antigenic determinant and does not appear to predict reliably the occurrence of late reactions.

Scratch test: Use scratch technique with a 20-gauge needle to make 3-5 mm nonbleeding scratch on epidermis, apply a small drop of solution to scratch, rub in gently with applicator or toothpick. A positive reaction consists of a pale wheal surrounding the scratch site which develops within 10 minutes and ranges from 5-15 mm or more in diameter.

Intradermal test: Use intradermal test with a tuberculin syringe with a 26- to 30-gauge short bevel needle; a dose of 0.01-0.02 mL is injected intradermally. A control of 0.9% sodium chloride should be injected at least 1.5" from the PPL test site. Most skin responses to the intradermal test will develop within 5-15 minutes.

Interpretation:

(-) Negative: No reaction

(±) Ambiguous: Wheal only slightly larger than original bleb with or without erythematous flare and larger than control site

(+) Positive: Itching and marked increase in size of original bleb

Control site should be reactionless

Dosage Forms Injection, solution: 6 x 10^{-5} M (0.25 mL)

bepridil (BE pri dil)

Sound-Alike/Look-Alike Issues

bepridil may be confused with Prepidil®

Vascor® may be confused with Norvasc®

Synonyms bepridil hydrochloride
U.S./Canadian Brand Names Vascor® [Can]
Therapeutic Category Calcium Channel Blocker
Use Treatment of chronic stable angina; due to side effect profile, reserve for patients who have been intolerant of other antianginal therapy; bepridil may be used alone or in combination with nitrates or beta-blockers
Usual Dosage Adults: Oral: Initial: 200 mg/day, then adjust dose at 10-day intervals until optimal response is achieved; usual dose: 300 mg/day; maximum daily dose: 400 mg
Dosage Forms Tablet, as hydrochloride: 200 mg, 300 mg

bepridil hydrochloride *see* bepridil *on previous page*

beractant (ber AKT ant)

Sound-Alike/Look-Alike Issues
Survanta® may be confused with Sufenta®
Synonyms bovine lung surfactant; natural lung surfactant
U.S./Canadian Brand Names Survanta® [US/Can]
Therapeutic Category Lung Surfactant
Use Prevention and treatment of respiratory distress syndrome (RDS) in premature infants

Prophylactic therapy: Body weight <1250 g in infants at risk for developing or with evidence of surfactant deficiency (administer within 15 minutes of birth)
Rescue therapy: Treatment of infants with RDS confirmed by x-ray and requiring mechanical ventilation (administer as soon as possible - within 8 hours of age)

Usual Dosage
Prophylactic treatment: Administer 100 mg phospholipids (4 mL/kg) intratracheal as soon as possible; as many as 4 doses may be administered during the first 48 hours of life, no more frequently than 6 hours apart. The need for additional doses is determined by evidence of continuing respiratory distress; if the infant is still intubated and requiring at least 30% inspired oxygen to maintain a PaO_2 ≤80 torr.
Rescue treatment: Administer 100 mg phospholipids (4 mL/kg) as soon as the diagnosis of RDS is made; may repeat if needed, no more frequently than every 6 hours to a maximum of 4 doses
Dosage Forms Suspension for inhalation: 25 mg/mL (4 mL, 8 mL)

Berocca® *(Discontinued)* *see page 1042*

Berocca® Plus *(Discontinued)* *see page 1042*

Berotec® [Can] *see* fenoterol *(Canada only) on page 361*

Berubigen® *(Discontinued)* *see page 1042*

Beta-2® *(Discontinued)* *see page 1042*

Betacaine® [Can] *see* lidocaine *on page 518*

beta-carotene (BAY tah-KARE oh teen)

U.S./Canadian Brand Names A-Caro-25® [US]; B-Caro-T™ [US]; Lumitene™ [US]
Therapeutic Category Vitamin, Fat Soluble
Use Reduce the severity of photosensitivity reactions in patients with erythropoietic protoporphyria (EPP)
Usual Dosage Oral:
Children <14 years: 30-150 mg/day
Adults: 30-300 mg/day
Dosage Forms
Capsule: 10,000 int. units (6 mg); 25,000 int. units (15 mg)
A-Caro-25®, B-Caro-T™: 25,000 int. units (15 mg)
Lumitene™: 50,000 int. units (30 mg)
Tablet: 10,000 int. units

Betachron® *(Discontinued)* *see page 1042*

Betaderm® [Can] *see* betamethasone (topical) *on page 116*

Betadine® First Aid Antibiotics + Moisturizer [US-OTC] *see* bacitracin and polymyxin B *on page 97*

Betadine® Ophthalmic [US] *see* povidone-iodine *on page 718*

Betadine® [US-OTC/Can] *see* povidone-iodine *on page 718*

9-beta-d-ribofuranosyladenine *see* adenosine *on page 21*

Betagan® [US/Can] *see* levobunolol *on page 511*

betahistine *(Canada only)* (bay ta HISS teen)

Synonyms betahistine dihydrochloride

U.S./Canadian Brand Names Serc® [Can]

Therapeutic Category Antihistamine

Use Treatment of Ménière disease (to decrease episodes of vertigo)

Usual Dosage Oral: Adults: 8-16 mg 3 times/day; administration with meals is recommended

Dosage Forms Tablet, as dihydrochloride: 8 mg, 16 mg

betahistine dihydrochloride *see* betahistine *(Canada only) on this page*

betaine anhydrous (BAY tayne an HY drus)

Sound-Alike/Look-Alike Issues

betaine may be confused with Betadine®

U.S./Canadian Brand Names Cystadane® [US/Can]

Therapeutic Category Homocystinuria Agent

Use **Orphan drug:** Treatment of homocystinuria to decrease elevated homocysteine blood levels; included within the category of homocystinuria are deficiencies or defects in cystathionine beta-synthase (CBS), 5,10-methylenetetrahydrofolate reductase (MTHFR), and cobalamin cofactor metabolism (CBL).

Usual Dosage

Children <3 years: Dosage may be started at 100 mg/kg/day and then increased weekly by 100 mg/kg increments

Children ≥3 years and Adults: Oral: 6 g/day administered in divided doses of 3 g twice daily. Dosages of up to 20 g/day have been necessary to control homocysteine levels in some patients.

Dosage in all patients can be gradually increased until plasma homocysteine is undetectable or present only in small amounts

Dosage Forms Powder for oral solution: 1 g/scoop (180 g) [1 scoop = 1.7 mL]

Betaject™ [Can] *see* betamethasone (topical) *on page 116*

Betalene® Topical *(Discontinued)* *see page 1042*

Betalin® S *(Discontinued)* *see page 1042*

Betaloc® [Can] *see* metoprolol *on page 575*

Betaloc® Durules® *see* metoprolol *on page 575*

betamethasone and calcipotriol *(Canada only)*

(bay ta METH a sone & kal si POE try ole)

Synonyms calcipotriol and betamethasone dipropionate

U.S./Canadian Brand Names Dovobet® [Can]

Therapeutic Category Corticosteroid, Topical; Vitamin D Analog

Use Treatment of psoriasis vulgaris

Usual Dosage Topical: Adults: Psoriasis vulgaris: Apply to affected area once daily (maximum recommended dose: 100 g/week); treatment may be discontinued when response is noted. Treatment should generally be limited to 4 weeks.

Dosage Forms Cream: Calcipotriol 50 mcg and betamethasone 0.5 mg per gram (3 g, 30 g, 60 g, 100 g, 120 g)

betamethasone and clotrimazole

(bay ta METH a sone & kloe TRIM a zole)

Sound-Alike/Look-Alike Issues

Lotrisone® may be confused with Lotrimin®

Synonyms clotrimazole and betamethasone

U.S./Canadian Brand Names Lotriderm® [Can]; Lotrisone® [US]

Therapeutic Category Antifungal/Corticosteroid

Use Topical treatment of various dermal fungal infections (including tinea pedis, cruris, and corpora in patients ≥17 years of age)

Usual Dosage

Children <17 years: Do not use

Children ≥17 years and Adults:

Tinea corporis, tinea cruris: Topical: Massage into affected area twice daily, morning and evening; do not use for longer than 2 weeks; reevaluate after 1 week if no clinical improvement; do not exceed 45 g cream/week or 45 mL lotion/week

Tinea pedis: Topical: Massage into affected area twice daily, morning and evening; do not use for longer than 4 weeks; reevaluate after 2 weeks if no clinical improvement; do not exceed 45 g cream/week or 45 mL lotion/week

Dosage Forms

Cream: Betamethasone dipropionate 0.05% and clotrimazole 1% (15 g, 45 g) [contains benzyl alcohol]

Lotion: Betamethasone dipropionate 0.05% and clotrimazole 1% (30 mL) [contains benzyl alcohol]

betamethasone dipropionate *see* betamethasone (topical) *on next page*

betamethasone dipropionate, augmented *see* betamethasone (topical) *on next page*

betamethasone sodium phosphate *see* betamethasone (systemic) *on this page*

betamethasone (systemic) (bay ta METH a sone sis TEM ik)

Synonyms betamethasone sodium phosphate; flubenisolone

U.S./Canadian Brand Names Celestone® [US]; Celestone® Soluspan® [US/Can]

Therapeutic Category Adrenal Corticosteroid

Use Inflammatory dermatoses such as seborrheic or atopic dermatitis, neurodermatitis, anogenital pruritus, psoriasis, inflammatory phase of xerosis

Usual Dosage Base dosage on severity of disease and patient response

Children: Use lowest dose listed as initial dose for adrenocortical insufficiency (physiologic replacement)

I.M.: 0.0175-0.125 mg base/kg/day divided every 6-12 hours **or** 0.5-7.5 mg base/m^2/day divided every 6-12 hours

Oral: 0.0175-0.25 mg/kg/day divided every 6-8 hours **or** 0.5-7.5 mg/m^2/day divided every 6-8 hours

Adolescents and Adults:

Oral: 2.4-4.8 mg/day in 2-4 doses; range: 0.6-7.2 mg/day

I.M.: Betamethasone sodium phosphate and betamethasone acetate: 0.6-9 mg/day (generally, $^1/_3$ to $^1/_2$ of oral dose) divided every 12-24 hours

Adults:

Intrabursal, intra-articular, intradermal: 0.25-2 mL

Intralesional: Rheumatoid arthritis/osteoarthritis:

Very large joints: 1-2 mL

Large joints: 1 mL

Medium joints: 0.5-1 mL

Small joints: 0.25-0.5 mL

(Continued)

betamethasone (systemic) *(Continued)*

Dosage Forms

Injection, suspension (Celestone® Soluspan®): Betamethasone sodium phosphate 3 mg/mL and betamethasone acetate 3 mg/mL [6 mg/mL] (5 mL)

Syrup, as base (Celestone®): 0.6 mg/5 mL (118 mL)

betamethasone (topical) (bay ta METH a sone TOP i kal)

Sound-Alike/Look-Alike Issues

Luxiq® may be confused with Lasix®

Synonyms betamethasone dipropionate; betamethasone dipropionate, augmented; betamethasone valerate

U.S./Canadian Brand Names Betaderm® [Can]; Betaject™ [Can]; Beta-Val® [US]; Betnesol® [Can]; Betnovate® [Can]; Celestoderm®-EV/2 [Can]; Celestoderm®-V [Can]; Diprolene® [US]; Diprolene® AF [US]; Diprolene® Glycol [Can]; Diprosone® [Can]; Ectosone [Can]; Luxiq® [US]; Maxivate® [US]; Prevex® B [Can]; Taro-Sone® [Can]; Topisone® [Can]; Valisone® Scalp Lotion [Can]

Therapeutic Category Corticosteroid, Topical

Use Inflammatory dermatoses such as seborrheic or atopic dermatitis, neurodermatitis, anogenital pruritus, psoriasis, inflammatory phase of xerosis

Usual Dosage Topical: Apply thin film 2-4 times/day. Therapy should be discontinued when control is achieved; if no improvement is seen, reassessment of diagnosis may be necessary.

Dosage Forms [DSC] = Discontinued product

Note: Potency expressed as betamethasone base.

Cream, topical, as dipropionate: 0.05% (15 g, 45 g)
 Maxivate®: 0.05% (45 g)
Cream, topical, as dipropionate augmented (Diprolene® AF): 0.05% (15 g, 50 g)
Cream, topical, as valerate: 0.1% (15 g, 45 g)
 Beta-Val®: 0.1% (15 g, 45 g)
Foam, topical, as valerate (Luxiq®): 0.12% (50 g, 100 g) [contains alcohol 60.4%]
Gel, topical, as dipropionate augmented: 0.05% (15 g, 50 g)
 Diprolene® [DSC]: 0.05% (15 g, 50 g)
Lotion, topical, as dipropionate: 0.05% (60 mL)
 Maxivate®: 0.05% (60 mL)
Lotion, topical, as dipropionate augmented (Diprolene®): 0.05% (30 mL, 60 mL)
Lotion, topical, as valerate (Beta-Val®): 0.1% (60 mL)
Ointment, topical, as dipropionate: 0.05% (15 g, 45 g)
 Maxivate®: 0.05% (45 g)
Ointment, topical, as dipropionate augmented: 0.05% (15 g, 50 g)
 Diprolene®: 0.05% (15 g, 50 g)
Ointment, topical, as valerate: 0.1% (15 g, 45 g)

betamethasone valerate *see* betamethasone (topical) *on this page*

Betapace® [US] *see* sotalol *on page 819*

Betapace AF® [US/Can] *see* sotalol *on page 819*

Betapen®-VK *(Discontinued)* *see page 1042*

Betasept® [US-OTC] *see* chlorhexidine gluconate *on page 183*

Betaseron® [US/Can] *see* interferon beta-1b *on page 480*

Betatar® [US-OTC] *see* coal tar *on page 219*

Beta-Val® [US] *see* betamethasone (topical) *on this page*

Beta-Val® Ointment (only) *(Discontinued)* *see page 1042*

Betaxin® [Can] *see* thiamine *on page 856*

betaxolol (be TAKS oh lol)

Sound-Alike/Look-Alike Issues

betaxolol may be confused with bethanechol, labetalol

Synonyms betaxolol hydrochloride

U.S./Canadian Brand Names Betoptic® S [US/Can]; Kerlone® [US]

Therapeutic Category Beta-Adrenergic Blocker

Use Treatment of chronic open-angle glaucoma and ocular hypertension; management of hypertension

Usual Dosage Adults:

Ophthalmic: Instill 1 drop twice daily.

Oral: 5-10 mg/day; may increase dose to 20 mg/day after 7-14 days if desired response is not achieved. Initial dose in elderly: 5 mg/day.

Dosage Forms

Solution, ophthalmic, as hydrochloride: 0.5% (5 mL, 10 mL, 15 mL) [contains benzalkonium chloride]

Suspension, ophthalmic, as hydrochloride (Betoptic® S): 0.25% (2.5 mL, 5 mL, 10 mL, 15 mL) [contains benzalkonium chloride]

Tablet, as hydrochloride (Kerlone®): 10 mg, 20 mg

betaxolol hydrochloride *see* betaxolol *on this page*

Betaxon® *(Discontinued)* *see page 1042*

bethanechol (be THAN e kole)

Sound-Alike/Look-Alike Issues

bethanechol may be confused with betaxolol

Synonyms bethanechol chloride

U.S./Canadian Brand Names Duvoid® [Can]; Myotonachol® [Can]; PMS-Bethanechol [Can]; Urecholine® [US]

Therapeutic Category Cholinergic Agent

Use Nonobstructive urinary retention and retention due to neurogenic bladder

Usual Dosage Oral:

Adults:

Urinary retention, neurogenic bladder, and/or bladder atony:

Oral: Initial: 10-50 mg 2-4 times/day (some patients may require dosages of 50-100 mg 4 times/day). To determine effective dose, may initiate at a dose of 5-10 mg, with additional doses of 5-10 mg hourly until an effective cumulative dose is reached. Cholinergic effects at higher oral dosages may be cumulative.

SubQ: Initial: 2.575 mg, may repeat in 15-30 minutes (maximum cumulative initial dose: 10.3 mg); subsequent doses may be given 3-4 times daily as needed (some patients may require more frequent dosing at 2.5- to 3-hour intervals). Chronic neurogenic atony may require doses of 7.5-10 every 4 hours.

Dosage Forms Tablet, as chloride: 5 mg, 10 mg, 25 mg, 50 mg

bethanechol chloride *see* bethanechol *on this page*

Betimol® [US] *see* timolol *on page 863*

Betnesol® [Can] *see* betamethasone (topical) *on previous page*

Betnovate® [Can] *see* betamethasone (topical) *on previous page*

Betoptic® *(Discontinued)* *see page 1042*

Betoptic® S [US/Can] *see* betaxolol *on this page*

bevacizumab (be vuh SIZ uh mab)

Synonyms anti-VEGF monoclonal antibody; rhuMAb-VEGF

U.S./Canadian Brand Names Avastin™ [US]

Therapeutic Category Antineoplastic Agent, Monoclonal Antibody; Vaccine, Recombinant

Use Treatment of metastatic colorectal cancer as a component of multidrug therapy

(Continued)

bevacizumab *(Continued)*

Usual Dosage I.V.: Adults: Colorectal cancer: 5-10 mg/kg every 2 weeks

Dosage Forms Injection, solution [preservative free]: 25 mg/mL (4 mL, 16 mL)

bexarotene (beks AIR oh teen)

U.S./Canadian Brand Names Targretin® [US/Can]

Therapeutic Category Retinoic Acid Derivative; Vitamin A Derivative; Vitamin, Fat Soluble

Use

Oral: Treatment of cutaneous manifestations of cutaneous T-cell lymphoma in patients who are refractory to at least one prior systemic therapy

Topical: Treatment of cutaneous lesions in patients with refractory cutaneous T-cell lymphoma (stage 1A and 1B) or who have not tolerated other therapies

Usual Dosage

Oral: 300 mg/m^2/day taken as a single daily dose. If there is no tumor response after 8 weeks and the initial dose was well tolerated, then an increase to 400 mg/m^2/day can be made with careful monitoring. Maintain as long as the patient is deriving benefit.

If the initial dose is not tolerated, then it may be adjusted to 200 mg/m^2/day, then to 100 mg/m^2/day or temporarily suspended if necessary to manage toxicity

Topical: Apply once every other day for first week, then increase on a weekly basis to once daily, 2 times/day, 3 times/day, and finally 4 times/day, according to tolerance

Dosage Forms

Capsule: 75 mg

Gel: 1% (60 g)

Bexophene® *(Discontinued)* *see page 1042*

Bextra® [US/Can] *see* valdecoxib *on page 900*

Bexxar® [US] *see* tositumomab and iodine I 131 tositumomab *on page 873*

bezafibrate *(Canada only)* (be za FYE brate)

U.S./Canadian Brand Names Bezalip® [Can]; PMS-Bezafibrate [Can]

Therapeutic Category Antihyperlipidemic Agent, Miscellaneous

Use Adjunct to diet and other therapeutic measures for treatment of type IIa and IIb mixed hyperlipidemia, to regulate lipid and apoprotein levels (reduce serum TG, LDL-cholesterol, and apolipoprotein B, increase HDL-cholesterol and apolipoprotein A); treatment of adult patients with high to very high triglyceride levels (Fredrickson classification type IV and V hyperlipidemias), who are at high risk of sequelae and complications from their dyslipidemia.

Usual Dosage Oral: Adults:

Immediate release: 200 mg 2-3 times/day; may reduce to 200 mg twice daily in patients with good response

Sustained release: 400 mg once daily

Dosage Forms

Tablet, immediate release: 200 mg

Tablet, sustained release: 400 mg

Bezalip® [Can] *see* bezafibrate *(Canada only) on this page*

BG 9273 *see* alefacept *on page 29*

Biamine® Injection *(Discontinued)* *see page 1042*

Biavax® II *(Discontinued)* *see page 1042*

Biaxin® [US/Can] *see* clarithromycin *on page 207*

Biaxin® XL [US/Can] *see* clarithromycin *on page 207*

bicalutamide (bye ka LOO ta mide)

Synonyms CDX; ICI-176334

U.S./Canadian Brand Names Casodex® [US/Can]

Therapeutic Category Androgen

Use In combination therapy with LHRH agonist analogues in treatment of advanced prostatic carcinoma

Usual Dosage Adults: Oral: 50-150 mg/day

Dosage Forms Tablet: 50 mg

Bicillin® C-R [US] *see* penicillin G benzathine and penicillin G procaine *on page 675*

Bicillin® C-R 900/300 [US] *see* penicillin G benzathine and penicillin G procaine *on page 675*

Bicillin® L-A [US] *see* penicillin G benzathine *on page 675*

BiCNU® [US/Can] *see* carmustine *on page 162*

BIG-IV *see* botulism immune globulin (intravenous-human) *on page 125*

Bilezyme® Tablet *(Discontinued)* *see page 1042*

Bilopaque® *(Discontinued)* *see page 1042*

Biltricide® [US/Can] *see* praziquantel *on page 722*

bimatoprost (bi MAT oh prost)

U.S./Canadian Brand Names Lumigan® [US/Can]

Therapeutic Category Ophthalmic Agent, Miscellaneous

Use Reduction of intraocular pressure (IOP) in patients with open-angle glaucoma or ocular hypertension; should be used in patients who are intolerant of other IOP-lowering medications or failed treatment with another IOP-lowering medication

Usual Dosage Ophthalmic: Adult: Open-angle glaucoma or ocular hypertension: Instill 1 drop into affected eye(s) once daily in the evening; do not exceed once-daily dosing (may decrease IOP-lowering effect). If used with other topical ophthalmic agents, separate administration by at least 5 minutes.

Dosage Forms Solution, ophthalmic: 0.03% (2.5 mL, 5 mL, 7.5 mL) [contains benzalkonium chloride]

Biobase™ [Can] *see* alcohol (ethyl) *on page 27*

Biobase-G™ [Can] *see* alcohol (ethyl) *on page 27*

Biocef® [US] *see* cephalexin *on page 176*

Bioclate® *(Discontinued)* *see page 1042*

BioCox® *(Discontinued)* *see page 1042*

Biodine® *(Discontinued)* *see page 1042*

Biofed [US-OTC] *see* pseudoephedrine *on page 745*

Biomox® *(Discontinued)* *see page 1042*

Bion® Tears [US-OTC] *see* artificial tears *on page 78*

Biopatch® *(Discontinued)* *see page 1042*

BioQuin® Durules™ [Can] *see* quinidine *on page 756*

Bio-Statin® [US] *see* nystatin *on page 637*

BioThrax™ [US] *see* anthrax vaccine, adsorbed *on page 61*

Biozyme-C® *(Discontinued)* *see page 1042*

biperiden (bye PER i den)

Synonyms biperiden hydrochloride; biperiden lactate

U.S./Canadian Brand Names Akineton® [US/Can]

Therapeutic Category Anticholinergic Agent; Anti-Parkinson Agent

(Continued)

biperiden *(Continued)*

Use Adjunct in the therapy of all forms of Parkinsonism; control of extrapyramidal symptoms secondary to antipsychotics

Usual Dosage Oral: Adults:

Parkinsonism: 2 mg 3-4 times/day

Extrapyramidal: 2 mg 1-3 times/day

Dosage Forms Tablet, as hydrochloride: 2 mg

biperiden hydrochloride *see* biperiden *on previous page*

biperiden lactate *see* biperiden *on previous page*

Biphetamine® *(Discontinued)* *see page 1042*

Bisac-Evac™ [US-OTC] *see* bisacodyl *on this page*

bisacodyl (bis a KOE dil)

Sound-Alike/Look-Alike Issues

Doxidan® may be confused with doxepin

Modane® may be confused with Matulane®, Moban®

U.S./Canadian Brand Names Alophen® [US-OTC]; Apo-Bisacodyl® [Can]; Bisac-Evac™ [US-OTC]; Bisacodyl Unisert® [US-OTC]; Carter's Little Pills® [Can]; Correctol® Tablets [US-OTC]; Doxidan® *(reformulation)* [US-OTC]; Dulcolax® [US-OTC/Can]; Femilax™ [US-OTC]; Fleet® Bisacodyl Enema [US-OTC]; Fleet® Stimulant Laxative [US-OTC]; Gentlax® [US-OTC]; Modane Tablets® [US-OTC]; Veracolate [US-OTC]

Therapeutic Category Laxative

Use Treatment of constipation; colonic evacuation prior to procedures or examination

Usual Dosage

Children:

Oral: >6 years: 5-10 mg (0.3 mg/kg) at bedtime or before breakfast

Rectal suppository:

<2 years: 5 mg as a single dose

>2 years: 10 mg

Adults:

Oral: 5-15 mg as single dose (up to 30 mg when complete evacuation of bowel is required)

Rectal suppository: 10 mg as single dose

Dosage Forms

Enema (Fleet® Bisacodyl Enema): 10 mg/30 mL (37 mL)

Suppository, rectal (Bisac-Evac™, Bisacodyl Uniserts®; Dulcolax®): 10 mg

Tablet, delayed release (Doxidan®): 5 mg

Tablet, enteric coated (Alophen®; Bisac-Evac™, Correctol®, Dulcolax®, Femilax™, Fleet® Stimulant Laxative, Gentlax®, Modane®, Veracolate): 5 mg

Bisacodyl Unisert® [US-OTC] *see* bisacodyl *on this page*

bis-chloronitrosourea *see* carmustine *on page 162*

bismatrol *see* bismuth *on this page*

bismuth (BIZ muth)

Sound-Alike/Look-Alike Issues

Kaopectate® may be confused with Kayexalate®

Synonyms bismatrol; bismuth subgallate; bismuth subsalicylate; pink bismuth

U.S./Canadian Brand Names Children's Kaopectate® (reformulation) [US-OTC]; Diotame® [US-OTC]; Kaopectate® Extra Strength [US-OTC]; Kaopectate® [US-OTC]; Pepto-Bismol® Maximum Strength [US-OTC]; Pepto-Bismol® [US-OTC]

Therapeutic Category Antidiarrheal

Use

Subsalicylate formulation: Symptomatic treatment of mild, nonspecific diarrhea; control of traveler's diarrhea (enterotoxigenic *Escherichia coli*); as part of a multidrug regimen for *H. pylori* eradication to reduce the risk of duodenal ulcer recurrence

Subgallate formulation: An aid to reduce fecal odors from a colostomy or ileostomy

Usual Dosage Oral:

Treatment of nonspecific diarrhea, control/relieve traveler's diarrhea: Subsalicylate (doses based on 262 mg/15 mL liquid or 262 mg tablets):

Children: Up to 8 doses/24 hours:

3-6 years: $^{1}/_{3}$ tablet or 5 mL every 30 minutes to 1 hour as needed

6-9 years: $^{2}/_{3}$ tablet or 10 mL every 30 minutes to 1 hour as needed

9-12 years: 1 tablet or 15 mL every 30 minutes to 1 hour as needed

Children >12 years and Adults: 2 tablets or 30 mL every 30 minutes to 1 hour as needed up to 8 doses/24 hours

Helicobacter pylori eradication: Adults: 524 mg 4 times/day with meals and at bedtime; requires combination therapy

Control of fecal odor in ileostomy or colostomy: Children ≥12 years and Adults: Subgallate: 200-400 mg up to 4 times/day

Dosage Forms

Caplet, as subsalicylate (Pepto-Bismol®): 262 mg [sugar free; contains sodium 2 mg]

Liquid, as subsalicylate: 262 mg/15 mL (240 mL, 360 mL, 480 mL); 525 mg/15 mL (240 mL, 360 mL)

Children's Kaopectate®: 87 mg/5 mL (180 mL) [contains sodium 3.3 mg/5 mL; cherry flavor]

Diotame®: 262 mg/15 mL (30 mL)

Kaopectate®: 262 mg/15 mL (240 mL) [contains sodium 10 mg/15 mL; regular and peppermint flavor]

Kaopectate® Extra Strength: 525 mg/15 mL (240 mL) [contains sodium 11 mg/15 mL; peppermint flavor]

Pepto-Bismol®: 262 mg/15 mL (120 mL, 240 mL, 360 mL, 480 mL) [sugar free; contains sodium 6 mg/15 mL and benzoic acid; wintergreen flavor]

Pepto-Bismol® Maximum Strength: 525 mg/15 mL (120 mL, 240 mL, 360 mL) [sugar free; contains sodium 6 mg/15 mL and benzoic acid; wintergreen flavor]

Tablet, as subgallate: 200 mg

Tablet, chewable, as subsalicylate: 262 mg

Diotame®: 262 mg

Pepto-Bismol®: 262 mg [sugar free; contains sodium <1 mg; cherry flavor]

bismuth subgallate *see* bismuth *on previous page*

bismuth subsalicylate *see* bismuth *on previous page*

bismuth subsalicylate, metronidazole, and tetracycline

(BIZ muth sub sa LIS i late, me troe NI da zole, & tet ra SYE kleen)

Synonyms bismuth subsalicylate, tetracycline, and metronidazole; metronidazole, bismuth subsalicylate, and tetracycline; metronidazole, tetracycline, and bismuth subsalicylate; tetracycline, bismuth subsalicylate, and metronidazole; tetracycline, metronidazole, and bismuth subsalicylate

U.S./Canadian Brand Names Helidac® [US]

Therapeutic Category Antidiarrheal

Use In combination with an H_2 antagonist, as part of a multidrug regimen for *H. pylori* eradication to reduce the risk of duodenal ulcer recurrence

Usual Dosage Adults: Chew 2 bismuth subsalicylate 262.4 mg tablets, swallow 1 metronidazole 250 mg tablet, and swallow 1 tetracycline 500 mg capsule 4 times/day at meals and bedtime, plus an H_2 antagonist (at the appropriate dose) for 14 days; follow with 8 oz of water; the H_2 antagonist should be continued for a total of 28 days

Dosage Forms Combination package [each package contains 14 blister cards (2-week supply); each card contains the following]:

Capsule: Tetracycline hydrochloride: 500 mg (4)

(Continued)

bismuth subsalicylate, metronidazole, and tetracycline *(Continued)*

Tablet: Bismuth subsalicylate [chewable]: 262.4 mg (8)
Tablet: Metronidazole: 250 mg (4)

bismuth subsalicylate, tetracycline, and metronidazole *see* bismuth subsalicylate, metronidazole, and tetracycline *on previous page*

bisoprolol (bis OH proe lol)

Sound-Alike/Look-Alike Issues
Zebeta® may be confused with DiaBeta®
Synonyms bisoprolol fumarate
U.S./Canadian Brand Names Monocor® [Can]; Zebeta® [US/Can]
Therapeutic Category Beta-Adrenergic Blocker
Use Treatment of hypertension, alone or in combination with other agents
Usual Dosage Oral:
Adults: 2.5-5 mg once daily, may be increased to 10 mg, and then up to 20 mg once daily, if necessary
Hypertension (JNC 7): 2.5-10 mg once daily
Dosage Forms Tablet, as fumarate: 5 mg, 10 mg

bisoprolol and hydrochlorothiazide

(bis OH proe lol & hye droe klor oh THYE a zide)
Sound-Alike/Look-Alike Issues
Ziac® may be confused with Tiazac®, Zerit®
Synonyms hydrochlorothiazide and bisoprolol
U.S./Canadian Brand Names Ziac® [US/Can]
Therapeutic Category Antihypertensive Agent, Combination
Use Treatment of hypertension
Usual Dosage Oral: Adults: Dose is individualized, given once daily
Dosage Forms
Tablet:
2.5/6.25: Bisoprolol fumarate 2.5 mg and hydrochlorothiazide 6.25 mg
5/6.25: Bisoprolol fumarate 5 mg and hydrochlorothiazide 6.25 mg
10/6.25: Bisoprolol fumarate 10 mg and hydrochlorothiazide 6.25 mg

bisoprolol fumarate *see* bisoprolol *on this page*

bistropamide *see* tropicamide *on page 892*

bivalirudin (bye VAL i roo din)

Synonyms hirulog
U.S./Canadian Brand Names Angiomax® [US/Can]
Therapeutic Category Anticoagulant (Other)
Use Anticoagulant used in conjunction with aspirin for patients with unstable angina undergoing percutaneous transluminal coronary angioplasty (PTCA)
Usual Dosage Adults: Anticoagulant in patients with unstable angina undergoing PTCA (treatment should be started just prior to PTCA): I.V.: Initial: Bolus: 1 mg/kg, followed by continuous infusion: 2.5 mg/kg/hour over 4 hours; if needed, infusion may be continued at 0.2 mg/kg/hour for up to 20 hours; patients should also receive aspirin 300-325 mg/day
Dosage Forms Injection, powder for reconstitution: 250 mg

BL4162A *see* anagrelide *on page 58*

black widow spider species antivenin (*Latrodectus mactans*) *see* antivenin (*Latrodectus mactans*) *on page 67*

Blanex® Capsule *(Discontinued)* *see page 1042*

BlemErase® Lotion *(Discontinued)* *see page 1042*

Blenoxane® [US/Can] *see* bleomycin *on this page*

bleo *see* bleomycin *on this page*

bleomycin (blee oh MYE sin)

Sound-Alike/Look-Alike Issues
bleomycin may be confused with Cleocin®

Synonyms bleo; bleomycin sulfate; BLM; NSC-125066

U.S./Canadian Brand Names Blenoxane® [US/Can]

Therapeutic Category Antineoplastic Agent

Use Treatment of squamous cell carcinomas, melanomas, sarcomas, testicular carcinoma, Hodgkin lymphoma, and non-Hodgkin lymphoma

Orphan drug: Sclerosing agent for malignant pleural effusion

Usual Dosage Refer to individual protocols; 1 unit = 1 mg

May be administered I.M., I.V., SubQ, or intracavitary

Children and Adults:

Test dose for lymphoma patients: I.M., I.V., SubQ: Because of the possibility of an anaphylactoid reaction, ≤2 units of bleomycin for the first 2 doses; monitor vital signs every 15 minutes; wait a minimum of 1 hour before administering remainder of dose; if no acute reaction occurs, then the regular dosage schedule may be followed

Single-agent therapy:

I.M./I.V./SubQ: Squamous cell carcinoma, lymphoma, testicular carcinoma: 0.25-0.5 units/kg (10-20 units/m^2) 1-2 times/week

CIV: 15 units/m^2 over 24 hours daily for 4 days

Combination-agent therapy:

I.M./I.V.: 3-4 units/m^2

I.V.: ABVD: 10 units/m^2 on days 1 and 15

Maximum cumulative lifetime dose: 400 units

Pleural sclerosing: 60-240 units as a single infusion. Dose may be repeated at intervals of several days if fluid continues to accumulate (mix in 50-100 mL of D_5W, NS, or SWFI); may add lidocaine 100-200 mg to reduce local discomfort.

Dosage Forms Injection, powder for reconstitution, as sulfate: 15 units, 30 units

bleomycin sulfate *see* bleomycin *on this page*

Bleph®-10 [US] *see* sulfacetamide *on page 829*

Blephamide® [US/Can] *see* sulfacetamide and prednisolone *on page 829*

Blis-To-Sol® [US-OTC] *see* tolnaftate *on page 870*

BLM *see* bleomycin *on this page*

Blocadren® [US] *see* timolol *on page 863*

BMS-232632 *see* atazanavir *on page 84*

BMS 337039 *see* aripiprazole *on page 77*

Bonamine™ [Can] *see* meclizine *on page 546*

Bonefos® [Can] *see* clodronate disodium *(Canada only)* *on page 213*

Bonine® [US-OTC/Can] *see* meclizine *on page 546*

Bontril® [Can] *see* phendimetrazine *on page 685*

Bontril PDM® [US] *see* phendimetrazine *on page 685*

Bontril® Slow-Release [US] *see* phendimetrazine *on page 685*

boric acid (BOR ik AS id)

Therapeutic Category Pharmaceutical Aid

Use

Ophthalmic: Mild antiseptic used for inflamed eyelids

Otic: Prophylaxis of swimmer's ear

(Continued)

boric acid *(Continued)*

Topical ointment: Temporary relief of chapped, chafed, or dry skin, diaper rash, abrasions, minor burns, sunburn, insect bites, and other skin irritations

Usual Dosage

Ophthalmic: Apply to lower eyelid 1-2 times/day

Otic: Place 2-4 drops in ears

Topical: Apply as needed

Dosage Forms

Ointment:

Ophthalmic: 5% (3.5 g); 10% (3.5 g)

Topical: 5% (52.5 g); 10% (28 g)

Topical (Borofax®): 5% boric acid and lanolin (1¾ oz)

Solution, otic: 2.75% with isopropyl alcohol (30 mL)

bortezomib (bore TEZ oh mib)

Synonyms LDP-341; MLN341; PS-341

U.S./Canadian Brand Names Velcade™ [US]

Therapeutic Category Proteasome Inhibitor

Use Treatment of multiple myeloma in patients who have had two prior therapies and had disease progression during the previous therapy

Usual Dosage I.V.: Adults: Multiple myeloma: 1.3 mg/m^2 twice weekly for 2 weeks on days 1, 4, 8, 11, followed by a 10-day rest period on days 12-21. Consecutive doses should be separated by at least 72 hours. One treatment cycle is equal to 21 days.

Dosage Forms Injection, powder for reconstitution [preservative free]: 3.5 mg [contains mannitol 35 mg]

bosentan (boe SEN tan)

U.S./Canadian Brand Names Tracleer® [US/Can]

Therapeutic Category Endothelin Antagonist

Controlled Substance Bosentan (Tracleer™) is available only through a limited distribution program directly from the manufacturer (Actelion Pharmaceuticals 1-866-228-3546). It will not be available through wholesalers or individual pharmacies.

Use Treatment of pulmonary artery hypertension (PAH) in patients with World Health Organization (WHO) Class III or IV symptoms to improve exercise capacity and decrease the rate of clinical deterioration

Usual Dosage Oral: Adults: Initial: 62.5 mg twice daily for 4 weeks; increase to maintenance dose of 125 mg twice daily; adults <40 kg should be maintained at 62.5 mg twice daily

Note: When discontinuing treatment, consider a reduction in dosage to 62.5 mg twice daily for 3-7 days (to avoid clinical deterioration).

Dosage Forms Tablet: 62.5 mg, 125 mg

B&O Supprettes® [US] *see* belladonna and opium *on page 103*

Botox® [US] *see* botulinum toxin type A *on this page*

Botox® Cosmetic [US/Can] *see* botulinum toxin type A *on this page*

botulinum toxin type A (BOT yoo lin num TOKS in type aye)

Synonyms BTX-A

U.S./Canadian Brand Names Botox® [US]; Botox® Cosmetic [US/Can]

Therapeutic Category Ophthalmic Agent, Toxin

Use Treatment of strabismus and blepharospasm associated with dystonia (including benign essential blepharospasm or VII nerve disorders in patients ≥12 years of age); cervical dystonia (spasmodic torticollis) in patients ≥16 years of age; temporary improvement in the appearance of lines/wrinkles of the face (moderate to severe glabellar lines associated with corrugator and/or procerus muscle activity) in adult patients ≤65 years of age; treatment of severe primary axillary hyperhidrosis in adults not adequately controlled with topical treatments

Orphan drug: Treatment of dynamic muscle contracture in pediatric cerebral palsy patients

Usual Dosage

Cervical dystonia: Children ≥16 years and Adults: I.M.: For dosing guidance, the mean dose is 236 units (25th to 75th percentile range 198-300 units) divided among the affected muscles in patients previously treated with botulinum toxin. Initial dose in previously untreated patients should be lower. Sequential dosing should be based on the patient's head and neck position, localization of pain, muscle hypertrophy, patient response, and previous adverse reactions. The total dose injected into the sternocleidomastoid muscles should be ≤100 units to decrease the occurrence of dysphagia.

Blepharospasm: Children ≥12 years and Adults: I.M.: Initial dose: 1.25-2.5 units injected into the medial and lateral pretarsal orbicularis oculi of the upper and lower lid; dose may be increased up to twice the previous dose if the response from the initial dose lasted ≤2 months; maximum dose per site: 5 units; cumulative dose in a 30-day period: ≤200 units. Tolerance may occur if treatments are given more often than every 3 months, but the effect is not usually permanent.

Strabismus: Children ≥12 years and Adults: I.M.:

Initial dose: Vertical muscles and for horizontal strabismus <20 prism diopters: 1.25-2.5 units in any one muscle Horizontal strabismus of 20-50 prism diopters: 2.5-5 units in any one muscle Persistent VI nerve palsy >1 month: 1.5-2.5 units in the medial rectus muscle

Re-examine patients 7-14 days after each injection to assess the effect of that dose. Subsequent doses for patients experiencing incomplete paralysis of the target may be increased up to twice the previous administered dose. The maximum recommended dose as a single injection for any one muscle is 25 units. Do not administer subsequent injections until the effects of the previous dose are gone.

Primary axillary hyperhidrosis: Adults ≥18 years: Intradermal: 50 units/axilla. Injection area should be defined by standard staining techniques. Injections should be evenly distributed into multiple sites (10-15), administered in 0.1-0.2 mL aliquots, ~1-2 cm apart.

Reduction of glabellar lines: Adults ≤65 years: I.M.: An effective dose is determined by gross observation of the patient's ability to activate the superficial muscles injected. The location, size and use of muscles may vary markedly among individuals. Inject 0.1 mL dose into each of five sites, two in each corrugator muscle and one in the procerus muscle (total dose 0.5 mL).

Dosage Forms Injection, powder for reconstitution [preservative free] (Botox®, Botox® Cosmetic): *Clostridium botulinum* toxin type A 100 units [contains human albumin]

botulinum toxin type B (BOT yoo lin num TOKS in type bee)

U.S./Canadian Brand Names Myobloc® [US]

Therapeutic Category Neuromuscular Blocker Agent, Toxin

Use Treatment of cervical dystonia (spasmodic torticollis)

Usual Dosage

Children: Not established in pediatric patients

Adults: Cervical dystonia: I.M.: Initial: 2500-5000 units divided among the affected muscles in patients **previously treated** with botulinum toxin; initial dose in **previously untreated** patients should be lower. Subsequent dosing should be optimized according to patient's response.

Dosage Forms Injection, solution [single-dose vial]: 5000 units/mL (0.5 mL, 1 mL, 2 mL) [contains albumin 0.05%]

botulism immune globulin (intravenous-human)

(BOT yoo lism i MYUN GLOB you lin, in tra VEE nus-HYU man)

Synonyms BIG-IV

U.S./Canadian Brand Names BabyBIG® [US]

Therapeutic Category Immune Globulin

Controlled Substance Available from the California Department of Health

Use Treatment of infant botulism caused by toxin type A or B

(Continued)

botulism immune globulin (intravenous-human) *(Continued)*

Usual Dosage I.V.: Children <1 year: Infant botulism: 1 mL/kg (50 mg/kg) as a single dose; infuse at 0.5 mL/kg/hour (25 mg/kg/hour) for the first 15 minutes; if well tolerated, may increase to 1 mL/kg/hour (50 mg/kg/hour)

Dosage Forms Injection, powder for reconstitution [preservative free]: ~100 mg [contains albumin 1% and sucrose 5%; packaged with SWFI]

Boudreaux's® Butt Paste [US-OTC] *see* zinc oxide *on page 940*

bovine lung surfactant *see* beractant *on page 113*

Breathe Right® Saline [US-OTC] *see* sodium chloride *on page 810*

Breezee® Mist Antifungal *(Discontinued)* *see page 1042*

Breonesin® *(Discontinued)* *see page 1042*

Brethaire® *(Discontinued)* *see page 1042*

Brethine® [US] *see* terbutaline *on page 846*

bretylium (bre TIL ee um)

Sound-Alike/Look-Alike Issues
bretylium may be confused with Brevibloc®

Synonyms bretylium tosylate

Therapeutic Category Antiarrhythmic Agent, Class III

Use Treatment of ventricular tachycardia and fibrillation; treatment of other serious ventricular arrhythmias resistant to lidocaine

Usual Dosage **Note:** Patients should undergo defibrillation/cardioversion before and after bretylium doses as necessary.

Children (**Note:** Not well established, although the following dosing has been suggested):

I.M.: 2-5 mg/kg as a single dose

I.V.: Acute ventricular fibrillation: Initial: 5 mg/kg, then attempt electrical defibrillation; repeat with 10 mg/kg if ventricular fibrillation persists at 15- to 30-minute intervals to maximum total of 30 mg/kg.

Maintenance dose: I.M., I.V.: 5 mg/kg every 6 hours

Adults:

Immediate life-threatening ventricular arrhythmias (ventricular fibrillation, unstable ventricular tachycardia): Initial dose: I.V.: 5 mg/kg (undiluted) over 1 minute; if arrhythmia persists, administer 10 mg/kg (undiluted) over 1 minute and repeat as necessary (usually at 15- to 30-minute intervals) up to a total dose of 30-35 mg/kg.

Other life-threatening ventricular arrhythmias:

Initial dose: I.M., I.V.: 5-10 mg/kg, may repeat every 1-2 hours if arrhythmia persists; administer I.V. dose (diluted) over 8-10 minutes.

Maintenance dose: I.M.: 5-10 mg/kg every 6-8 hours; I.V. (diluted): 5-10 mg/kg every 6 hours; I.V. infusion (diluted): 1-2 mg/minute (little experience with doses >40 mg/kg/day)

Example dilution: 2 g/250 mL D_5W (infusion pump should be used for I.V. infusion administration)

Rate of I.V. infusion: 1-4 mg/minute 1 mg/minute = 7 mL/hour 2 mg/minute = 15 mL/hour 3 mg/minute = 22 mL/hour 4 mg/minute = 30 mL/hour

Dosage Forms
Injection, solution, as tosylate: 50 mg/mL (10 mL)
Injection, solution, as tosylate [premixed in D_5W]: 2 mg/mL (250 mL); 4 mg/mL (250 mL)

bretylium tosylate *see* bretylium *on this page*

Bretylol® *(Discontinued)* *see page 1042*

Brevibloc® [US/Can] *see* esmolol *on page 322*

Brevicon® [US] *see* ethinyl estradiol and norethindrone *on page 342*

Brevicon® 0.5/35 [Can] *see* ethinyl estradiol and norethindrone *on page 342*

Brevicon® 1/35 [Can] *see* ethinyl estradiol and norethindrone *on page 342*

Brevital® Sodium [US/Can] *see* methohexital *on page 565*

Brevoxyl® [US] *see* benzoyl peroxide *on page 109*

Brevoxyl® Cleansing [US] *see* benzoyl peroxide *on page 109*

Brevoxyl® Wash [US] *see* benzoyl peroxide *on page 109*

Bricanyl® *(Discontinued)* *see page 1042*

brimonidine (bri MOE ni deen)

Sound-Alike/Look-Alike Issues
brimonidine may be confused with bromocriptine

Synonyms brimonidine tartrate

U.S./Canadian Brand Names Alphagan® P [US/Can]; PMS-Brimonidine Tartrate [Can]; ratio-Brimonidine [Can]

Therapeutic Category Alpha$_2$-Adrenergic Agonist Agent, Ophthalmic

Use Lowering of intraocular pressure (IOP) in patients with open-angle glaucoma or ocular hypertension

Usual Dosage Ophthalmic: Children ≥2 years of age and Adults: Glaucoma (Alphagan®, Alphagan® P): Instill 1 drop in affected eye(s) 3 times/day (approximately every 8 hours)

Dosage Forms
Solution, ophthalmic, as tartrate: 0.15% (5 mL, 10 mL, 15 mL)

brimonidine tartrate *see* brimonidine *on this page*

brinzolamide (brin ZOH la mide)

U.S./Canadian Brand Names Azopt® [US/Can]

Therapeutic Category Carbonic Anhydrase Inhibitor

Use Lowers intraocular pressure in patients with ocular hypertension or open-angle glaucoma

Usual Dosage Ophthalmic: Adults: Instill 1 drop in affected eye(s) 3 times/day

Dosage Forms Suspension, ophthalmic: 1% (5 mL, 10 mL, 15 mL) [contains benzalkonium chloride]

Brioschi® [US-OTC] *see* sodium bicarbonate *on page 809*

British anti-lewisite *see* dimercaprol *on page 275*

BRL 43694 *see* granisetron *on page 413*

Brofed® [US] *see* brompheniramine and pseudoephedrine *on page 129*

Bromaline® Elixir *(Discontinued)* *see page 1042*

Bromaline® [US-OTC] *see* brompheniramine and pseudoephedrine *on page 129*

Bromanate® DC *(Discontinued)* *see page 1042*

Bromarest® *(Discontinued)* *see page 1042*

Bromatapp® *(Discontinued)* *see page 1042*

Bromaxefed RF [US] *see* brompheniramine and pseudoephedrine *on page 129*

bromazepam *(Canada only)* (broe MA ze pam)

U.S./Canadian Brand Names Apo-Bromazepam® [Can]; Gen-Bromazepam [Can]; Lectopam® [Can]; Novo-Bromazepam [Can]; Nu-Bromazepam [Can]

Therapeutic Category Benzodiazepine; Sedative

Use Short-term, symptomatic treatment of anxiety

Usual Dosage Oral: Adults: Initial: 6-18 mg/day in equally divided doses; initial course of treatment should not last longer than 1 week; optimal dosage range: 6-30 mg/day

Dosage Forms Tablet: 1.5 mg, 3 mg, 6 mg

Brombay® *(Discontinued)* *see page 1042*

Bromfed® *(Discontinued)* *see page 1042*

Bromfed-PD® *(Discontinued)* *see page 1042*

Bromfenex® [US] *see* brompheniramine and pseudoephedrine *on next page*

Bromfenex® PD [US] *see* brompheniramine and pseudoephedrine *on next page*

Bromhist Pediatric [US] *see* brompheniramine and pseudoephedrine *on next page*

bromocriptine (broe moe KRIP teen)

Sound-Alike/Look-Alike Issues

bromocriptine may be confused with benztropine, brimonidine

Parlodel® may be confused with pindolol, Provera®

Synonyms bromocriptine mesylate

U.S./Canadian Brand Names Apo-Bromocriptine® [Can]; Parlodel® [US/Can]; PMS-Bromocriptine [Can]

Therapeutic Category Anti-Parkinson Agent; Ergot Alkaloid and Derivative

Use

Amenorrhea with or without galactorrhea; infertility or hypogonadism; prolactin-secreting adenomas; acromegaly; Parkinson disease

A previous indication for prevention of postpartum lactation was withdrawn voluntarily by Sandoz Pharmaceuticals Corporation.

Usual Dosage Oral:

Children: Prolactin-secreting adenoma:

11-15 years (based on limited information): Initial: 1.25-2.5 mg daily; dosage may be increased as tolerated to achieve a therapeutic response (range 2.5-10 mg daily).

≥16 years: Refer to Adults dosing

Adults:

Parkinsonism: 1.25 mg 2 times/day, increased by 2.5 mg/day in 2- to 4-week intervals (usual dose range is 30-90 mg/day in 3 divided doses), though elderly patients can usually be managed on lower doses

Neuroleptic malignant syndrome: 2.5-5 mg 3 times/day

Hyperprolactinemia: 2.5 mg 2-3 times/day

Acromegaly: Initial: 1.25-2.5 mg increasing as necessary every 3-7 days; usual dose: 20-30 mg/day

Prolactin-secreting adenomas: Initial: 1.25-2.5 mg/day; may be increased as tolerated every 2-7 days until optimal response (range: 2.5-15 mg/day)

Dosage Forms

Capsule, as mesylate: 5 mg

Tablet, as mesylate: 2.5 mg

bromocriptine mesylate *see* bromocriptine *on this page*

Bromphen® *(Discontinued)* *see page 1042*

Bromphen® DC With Codeine *(Discontinued)* *see page 1042*

brompheniramine (brome fen IR a meen)

Synonyms parabromdylamine

Therapeutic Category Antihistamine

Use Perennial and seasonal allergic rhinitis and other allergic symptoms including urticaria

Usual Dosage

Oral:

Children:

<6 years: 0.125 mg/kg/dose administered every 6 hours; maximum: 6-8 mg/day

6-12 years: 2-4 mg every 6-8 hours; maximum: 12-16 mg/day

Adults: 4 mg every 4-6 hours or 8 mg of sustained release form every 8-12 hours or 12 mg of sustained release every 12 hours; maximum: 24 mg/day

I.M., I.V., S.C.:
Children <12 years: 0.5 mg/kg/24 hours divided every 6-8 hours
Adults: 5-50 mg every 4-12 hours, maximum: 40 mg/24 hours

Dosage Forms
Capsule, as maleate: 4 mg
Elixir, as maleate: 2 mg/5 mL with 3% alcohol (120 mL)
Liquid, as maleate: 2 mg/5 mL (60 mL, 120 mL, 240 mL)
Solution, as maleate: 2 mg/5 mL (10 mL)
Tablet, as maleate: 4 mg
Tablet, sustained release, as maleate: 6 mg, 12 mg

brompheniramine and pseudoephedrine

(brome fen IR a meen & soo doe e FED rin)

Synonyms brompheniramine maleate and pseudoephedrine hydrochloride; brompheniramine maleate and pseudoephedrine sulfate; pseudoephedrine and brompheniramine

U.S./Canadian Brand Names Andehist NR Syrup [US]; Brofed® [US]; Bromaline® [US-OTC]; Bromaxefed RF [US]; Bromfenex® [US]; Bromfenex® PD [US]; Bromhist Pediatric [US]; Children's Dimetapp® Elixir Cold & Allergy [US-OTC]; Histex™ SR [US]; Lodrane® [US]; Lodrane® 12D [US]; Lodrane® LD [US]; Rondec® Syrup [US]; Touro™ Allergy [US]

Therapeutic Category Antihistamine/Decongestant Combination

Use Temporary relief of symptoms of seasonal and perennial allergic rhinitis, and vasomotor rhinitis, including nasal obstruction

Usual Dosage Oral:
Capsule, long acting:
Based on 60 mg pseudoephedrine:
Children 6-12 years: 1 capsule every 12 hours
Children ≥12 years and Adults: 1-2 capsules every 12 hours
Based on 120 mg pseudoephedrine: Children ≥12 years and Adults: 1 capsule every 12 hours
Liquid:
Based on brompheniramine 1 mg/pseudoephedrine 15 mg per 1 mL: Children:
1-3 months: 0.25 mL 4 times/day
3-6 months: 0.5 mL 4 times/day
6-12 months: 0.75 mL 4 times/day
12-24 months: 1 mL 4 times/day
Based on brompheniramine 1 mg/pseudoephedrine 15 mg per 5 mL: Children:
6-11 months (6-8 kg): 2.5 mL every 6-8 hours (maximum: 4 doses/24 hours)
12-23 months (8-10 kg): 3.75 mL every 6-8 hours (maximum: 4 doses/24 hours)
2-6 years: 5 mL every 6-8 hours (maximum: 4 doses/24 hours)
6-12 years: 10 mL every 6-8 hours (maximum: 4 doses/24 hours)
>12 years and Adults: 20 mg every 4 hours (maximum: 4 doses/24 hours)
Based on brompheniramine 4 mg/pseudoephedrine 30 mg:
Children 2-6 years: 2.5 mL 3 times/day
Children >6 years and Adults: 5 mL 3 times/day
Brompheniramine 4 mg/pseudoephedrine 45 mg per 5 mL:
Children 2-6 years: 2.5 mL 4 times/day
Children >6 years and Adults: 5 mL 4 times/day
Tablet, extended release: Based on pseudoephedrine 45 mg:
Children 6-12 years: 1 tablet every 12 hours
Children ≥12 years and Adults: 1-2 tablets every 12 hours

Dosage Forms [DSC] = Discontinued product
Capsule, extended release: Brompheniramine maleate 6 mg and pseudoephedrine hydrochloride 60 mg; Brompheniramine maleate 12 mg and pseudoephedrine hydrochloride 120 mg
Bromfed® [DSC], Bromfenex®: Brompheniramine maleate 12 mg and pseudoephedrine hydrochloride 120 mg
Bromfed-PD® [DSC], Bromfenex® PD, Lodrane® LD: Brompheniramine maleate 6 mg and pseudoephedrine hydrochloride 60 mg
(Continued)

brompheniramine and pseudoephedrine *(Continued)*

Histex™ SR: Brompheniramine maleate 10 mg and pseudoephedrine hydrochloride 120 mg

Capsule, sustained release (Touro™ Allergy): Brompheniramine maleate 5.75 mg and pseudoephedrine hydrochloride 60 mg

Elixir: Brompheniramine maleate 1 mg and pseudoephedrine hydrochloride 15 mg per 5 mL (120 mL, 480 mL)

Children's Dimetapp® Elixir Cold & Allergy: Brompheniramine maleate 1 mg and pseudoephedrine hydrochloride 15 mg per 5 mL (240 mL) [alcohol free; contains sodium benzoate; grape flavor]

Liquid (Lodrane®): Brompheniramine maleate 4 mg and pseudoephedrine hydrochloride 60 mg per 5 mL (480 mL) [alcohol free, dye free, sugar free; cherry flavor]

Liquid, oral drops (AccuHist® Pediatric [DSC], Bromhist Pediatric): Brompheniramine maleate 1 mg and pseudoephedrine hydrochloride 15 mg per 1 mL (30 mL) [contains sodium benzoate; cherry flavor]

Solution (Bromaline®): Brompheniramine maleate 1 mg and pseudoephedrine hydrochloride 15 mg per 5 mL (120 mL, 480 mL) [alcohol free; contains sodium benzoate; grape flavor]

Syrup: Brompheniramine maleate 4 mg and pseudoephedrine sulfate 45 mg per 5 mL (120 mL, 480 mL)

Andehist NR: Brompheniramine maleate 4 mg and pseudoephedrine sulfate 45 mg per 5 mL (473 mL) [raspberry flavor]

Brofed®: Brompheniramine maleate 4 mg and pseudoephedrine hydrochloride 30 mg per 5 mL(480 mL) [mint flavor]

Bromaxefed RF: Brompheniramine maleate 4 mg and pseudoephedrine hydrochloride 45 mg per 5 mL (120 mL, 480 mL) [alcohol free; cherry flavor]

Rondec®: Brompheniramine maleate 4 mg and pseudoephedrine hydrochloride 45 mg per 5 mL (120 mL, 480 mL) [cherry flavor]

Tablet, extended release (Lodrane® 12D): Brompheniramine maleate 6 mg and pseudoephedrine hydrochloride 45 mg

brompheniramine maleate and pseudoephedrine hydrochloride *see* brompheniramine and pseudoephedrine *on previous page*

brompheniramine maleate and pseudoephedrine sulfate *see* brompheniramine and pseudoephedrine *on previous page*

Brompheril® ***(Discontinued)*** *see page 1042*

Bronchial® ***(Discontinued)*** *see page 1042*

Bronchial Mist® ***(Discontinued)*** *see page 1042*

Broncho Saline® [US-OTC] *see* sodium chloride *on page 810*

Bronitin® Mist ***(Discontinued)*** *see page 1042*

Bronkephrine® ***(Discontinued)*** *see page 1042*

Bronkometer® ***(Discontinued)*** *see page 1042*

Bronkosol® ***(Discontinued)*** *see page 1042*

Brontex® [US] *see* guaifenesin and codeine *on page 416*

Brotane® ***(Discontinued)*** *see page 1042*

BSS® [US/Can] *see* balanced salt solution *on page 99*

BSS® Plus [US/Can] *see* balanced salt solution *on page 99*

BTX-A *see* botulinum toxin type A *on page 124*

B-type natriuretic peptide (human) *see* nesiritide *on page 614*

Bucladin®-S Softab® ***(Discontinued)*** *see page 1042*

budesonide (byoo DES oh nide)

U.S./Canadian Brand Names Entocort® [Can]; Entocort™ EC [US]; Gen-Budesonide AQ [Can]; Pulmicort® [Can]; Pulmicort Respules® [US]; Pulmicort Turbuhaler® [US]; Rhinocort® Aqua® [US]; Rhinocort® Turbuhaler® [Can]

Therapeutic Category Adrenal Corticosteroid

Use

Intranasal: Children ≥6 years of age and Adults: Management of symptoms of seasonal or perennial rhinitis

Nebulization: Children 12 months to 8 years: Maintenance and prophylactic treatment of asthma

Oral capsule: Treatment of active Crohn disease (mild to moderate) involving the ileum and/or ascending colon

Oral inhalation: Maintenance and prophylactic treatment of asthma; includes patients who require corticosteroids and those who may benefit from systemic dose reduction/elimination

Usual Dosage

Nasal inhalation: (Rhinocort® Aqua®): Children ≥6 years and Adults: 64 mcg/day as a single 32 mcg spray in each nostril. Some patients who do not achieve adequate control may benefit from increased dosage. A reduced dosage may be effective after initial control is achieved.

Maximum dose: Children <12 years: 128 mcg/day; Adults: 256 mcg/day

Nebulization: Children 12 months to 8 years: Pulmicort Respules®: Titrate to lowest effective dose once patient is stable; start at 0.25 mg/day or use as follows:

Previous therapy of bronchodilators alone: 0.5 mg/day administered as a single dose or divided twice daily (maximum daily dose: 0.5 mg)

Previous therapy of inhaled corticosteroids: 0.5 mg/day administered as a single dose or divided twice daily (maximum daily dose: 1 mg)

Previous therapy of oral corticosteroids: 1 mg/day administered as a single dose or divided twice daily (maximum daily dose: 1 mg)

Oral inhalation:

Children ≥6 years:

Previous therapy of bronchodilators alone: 200 mcg twice initially which may be increased up to 400 mcg twice daily

Previous therapy of inhaled corticosteroids: 200 mcg twice initially which may be increased up to 400 mcg twice daily

Previous therapy of oral corticosteroids: The highest recommended dose in children is 400 mcg twice daily

Adults:

Previous therapy of bronchodilators alone: 200-400 mcg twice initially which may be increased up to 400 mcg twice daily

Previous therapy of inhaled corticosteroids: 200-400 mcg twice initially which may be increased up to 800 mcg twice daily

Previous therapy of oral corticosteroids: 400-800 mcg twice daily which may be increased up to 800 mcg twice daily

NIH Guidelines (NIH, 1997) (give in divided doses twice daily):

Children:

"Low" dose: 100-200 mcg/day

"Medium" dose: 200-400 mcg/day (1-2 inhalations/day)

"High" dose: >400 mcg/day (>2 inhalation/day)

Adults:

"Low" dose: 200-400 mcg/day (1-2 inhalations/day)

"Medium" dose: 400-600 mcg/day (2-3 inhalations/day)

"High" dose: >600 mcg/day (>3 inhalation/day)

Oral: Adults: Crohn disease: 9 mg once daily in the morning; safety and efficacy have not been established for therapy duration >8 weeks; recurring episodes may be treated with a repeat 8-week course of treatment

(Continued)

budesonide *(Continued)*

Note: Treatment may be tapered to 6 mg once daily for 2 weeks prior to complete cessation. Patients receiving CYP3A4 inhibitors should be monitored closely for signs and symptoms of hypercorticism; dosage reduction may be required.

Dosage Forms

Capsule, enteric coated (Entocort™ EC): 3 mg

Powder for oral inhalation (Pulmicort Turbuhaler®): 200 mcg/inhalation (104 g) [delivers ~160 mcg/inhalation; 200 metered doses]

Additional dosage strengths available in Canada: 100 mcg/inhalation, 400 mcg/inhalation

Suspension for oral inhalation (Pulmicort Respules®): 0.25 mg/2 mL (30s), 0.5 mg/2 mL (30s)

Suspension, nasal spray (Rhinocort® Aqua®): 32 mcg/inhalation (8.6 g) [120 metered doses]

budesonide and eformoterol *see* budesonide and formoterol *(Canada only) on this page*

budesonide and formoterol *(Canada only)*

(byoo DES oh nide & for MOH te rol)

Synonyms budesonide and eformoterol; eformoterol and budesonide; formoterol fumarate dehydrate and budesonide

U.S./Canadian Brand Names Symbicort® [Can]

Therapeutic Category $Beta_2$-Adrenergic Agonist Agent; Corticosteroid, Inhalant (Oral)

Use Treatment of asthma in patients ≥12 years of age where combination therapy is indicated

Usual Dosage Oral inhalation: Children ≥12 years and Adults: 1-2 inhalations once or twice daily

Maximum long-term maintenance dose: 4 inhalations/day; in periods of worsening asthma, this may be temporarily increased to 4 inhalations twice daily

Manufacturer's recommendation: Initial: Symbicort® 200 once or twice daily to establish symptom control. Following the establishment of response/symptom control: Titrate to the lowest dosage possible to maintain control (may substitute Symbicort® 100).

Dosage Forms

Powder for oral inhalation:

Symbicort® 100 Turbuhaler®: Budesonide 100 mcg and formoterol dehydrate 6 mcg per inhalation (available in 60 or 120 metered doses) [delivers ~80 mcg budesonide and 4.5 mcg formoterol per inhalation; contains lactose]

Symbicort® 200 Turbuhaler®: Budesonide 200 mcg and formoterol dehydrate 6 mcg per inhalation (available in 60 or 120 metered doses) [delivers ~160 mcg budesonide and 4.5 mcg formoterol per inhalation; contains lactose]

buffered aspirin and pravastatin sodium *see* aspirin and pravastatin *on page 83*

Buffered®, Tri-buffered *(Discontinued)* *see page 1042*

Bufferin® Extra Strength [US-OTC] *see* aspirin *on page 80*

Bufferin® [US-OTC] *see* aspirin *on page 80*

Buffinol Extra [US-OTC] *see* aspirin *on page 80*

Buffinol [US-OTC] *see* aspirin *on page 80*

Buf-Puf® Acne Cleansing Bar *(Discontinued)* *see page 1042*

bumetanide (byoo MET a nide)

Sound-Alike/Look-Alike Issues

bumetanide may be confused with Buminate®

Bumex® may be confused with Brevibloc®, Buprenex®, bupropion, Permax®

U.S./Canadian Brand Names Bumex® [US/Can]; Burinex® [Can]

Therapeutic Category Diuretic, Loop

Use Management of edema secondary to congestive heart failure or hepatic or renal disease including nephrotic syndrome; may be used alone or in combination with antihypertensives in the treatment of hypertension; can be used in furosemide-allergic patients

Usual Dosage

Oral, I.M., I.V.:

Neonates: 0.01-0.05 mg/kg/dose every 24-48 hours

Infants and Children: 0.015-0.1 mg/kg/dose every 6-24 hours (maximum dose: 10 mg/day)

Adults:

Edema:

Oral: 0.5-2 mg/dose (maximum dose: 10 mg/day) 1-2 times/day

I.M., I.V.: 0.5-1 mg/dose; may repeat in 2-3 hours for up to 2 doses if needed (maximum dose: 10 mg/day)

Continuous I.V. infusion: 0.9-1 mg/hour

Hypertension: Oral: 0.5 mg daily (maximum dose: 5 mg/day); usual dosage range (JNC 7): 0.5-2 mg/day in 2 divided doses

Dosage Forms

Injection, solution: 0.25 mg/mL (2 mL, 4 mL, 10 mL) [contains benzyl alcohol]

Tablet (Bumex®): 0.5 mg, 1 mg, 2 mg

Bumex® [US/Can] *see* bumetanide *on previous page*

Bumex® Injection *(Discontinued)* *see page 1042*

Buminate® [US] *see* albumin *on page 25*

Buphenyl® [US] *see* sodium phenylbutyrate *on page 814*

bupivacaine (byoo PIV a kane)

Sound-Alike/Look-Alike Issues

bupivacaine may be confused with mepivacaine, ropivacaine

Marcaine® may be confused with Narcan®

Synonyms bupivacaine hydrochloride

U.S./Canadian Brand Names Marcaine® Spinal [US]; Marcaine® [US/Can]; Sensorcaine®-MPF [US]; Sensorcaine® [US/Can]

Therapeutic Category Local Anesthetic

Use Local anesthetic (injectable) for peripheral nerve block, infiltration, sympathetic block, caudal or epidural block, retrobulbar block

Usual Dosage Dose varies with procedure, depth of anesthesia, vascularity of tissues, duration of anesthesia and condition of patient. Some formulations contain metabisulfites (in epinephrine-containing injection); do not use solutions containing preservatives for caudal or epidural block.

Local anesthesia: Infiltration: 0.25% infiltrated locally; maximum: 175 mg

Caudal block (with or without epinephrine, preservative free):

Children: 1-3.7 mg/kg

Adults: 15-30 mL of 0.25% or 0.5%

Epidural block (other than caudal block - with or without epinephrine, preservative free):

Administer in 3-5 mL increments, allowing sufficient time to detect toxic manifestations of inadvertent I.V. or I.T. administration:

Children: 1.25 mg/kg/dose

Adults: 10-20 mL of 0.25% or 0.5%

Surgical procedures requiring a high degree of muscle relaxation and prolonged effects **only**: 10-20 mL of 0.75% (**Note:** Not to be used in obstetrical cases)

Maxillary and mandibular infiltration and nerve block: 9 mg (1.8 mL) of 0.5% (with epinephrine) per injection site; a second dose may be administered if necessary to produce adequate anesthesia after allowing up to 10 minutes for onset, up to a maximum of 90 mg per dental appointment

(Continued)

bupivacaine *(Continued)*

Obstetrical anesthesia: Incremental dose: 3-5 mL of 0.5% (not exceeding 50-100 mg in any dosing interval); allow sufficient time to detect toxic manifestations or inadvertent I.V. or I.T. injection

Peripheral nerve block: 5 mL of 0.25 or 0.5%; maximum: 400 mg/day

Sympathetic nerve block: 20-50 mL of 0.25%

Retrobulbar anesthesia: 2-4 mL of 0.75%

Spinal anesthesia: Solution of 0.75% bupivacaine in 8.25% dextrose is used:

Lower extremity and perineal procedures: 1 mL

Lower abdominal procedures: 1.6 mL

Obstetrical:

Normal vaginal delivery: 0.8 mL (higher doses may be required in some patients)

Cesarean section: 1-1.4 mL

Dosage Forms

Injection, solution, as hydrochloride [preservative free]: 0.25% [2.5 mg/mL] (10 mL, 20 mL, 30 mL, 50 mL); 0.5% [5 mg/mL] (10 mL, 20 mL, 30 mL); 0.75% [7.5 mg/mL] (10 mL, 20 mL, 30 mL)

Marcaine®: 0.25% [2.5 mg/mL] (10 mL, 30 mL, 50 mL); 0.5% [5 mg/mL] (10 mL, 30 mL); 0.75% [7.5 mg/mL] (10 mL, 30 mL)

Marcaine® Spinal: 0.75% [7.5 mg/mL] (2 mL) [in dextrose 8.25%]

Sensorcaine®-MPF: 0.25% [2.5 mg/mL] (10 mL, 30 mL); 0.5% [5 mg/mL] (10 mL, 30 mL); 0.75% [7.5 mg/mL] (10 mL, 30 mL)

Injection, solution, as hydrochloride (Marcaine®, Sensorcaine®): 0.25% [2.5 mg/mL] (50 mL); 0.5% [5 mg/mL] (50 mL) [contains methylparaben]

Injection, solution, with epinephrine 1:200,000, as hydrochloride [preservative free]: 0.25% [2.5 mg/mL] (10 mL, 30 mL); 0.5 % [5 mg/mL] (30 mL)

Marcaine®: 0.25% [2.5 mg/mL] (10 mL, 30 mL); 0.5% [5 mg/mL] (3 mL, 10 mL, 30 mL); 0.75% [7.5 mg/mL] (30 mL) [contains sodium metabisulfite]

Sensorcaine®-MPF: 0.25% [2.5 mg/mL] (10 mL, 30 mL); 0.5% [5 mg/mL] (10 mL, 30 mL); 0.75% [7.5 mg/mL] (30 mL) [contains sodium metabisulfite]

Injection, solution, with epinephrine 1:200,000, as hydrochloride [with preservative] (Marcaine®, Sensorcaine®): 0.25% [2.5 mg/mL] (50 mL); 0.5% [5 mg/mL] (50 mL) [contains methylparaben and sodium metabisulfite]

bupivacaine hydrochloride *see* bupivacaine *on previous page*

Buprenex® [US/Can] *see* buprenorphine *on this page*

buprenorphine (byoo pre NOR feen)

Sound-Alike/Look-Alike Issues

Buprenex® may be confused with Brevibloc®, Bumex®

Synonyms buprenorphine hydrochloride

U.S./Canadian Brand Names Buprenex® [US/Can]; Subutex® [US]

Therapeutic Category Analgesic, Narcotic

Controlled Substance C-V

Use

Injection: Management of moderate to severe pain

Tablet: Treatment of opioid dependence

Usual Dosage **Long-term use is not recommended**

Note: These are guidelines and do not represent the maximum doses that may be required in all patients. Doses should be titrated to pain relief/prevention. In high-risk patients (eg, elderly, debilitated, presence of respiratory disease) and/or concurrent CNS depressant use, reduce dose by one-half. Buprenorphine has an analgesic ceiling.

Acute pain (moderate to severe):

Children 2-12 years: I.M., slow I.V.: 2-6 mcg/kg every 4-6 hours

Children ≥13 years and Adults:

I.M.: Initial: Opiate-naive: 0.3 mg every 6-8 hours as needed; initial dose (up to 0.3 mg) may be repeated once in 30-60 minutes after the initial dose if needed; usual dosage range: 0.15-0.6 mg every 4-8 hours as needed

Slow I.V.: Initial: Opiate-naive: 0.3 mg every 6-8 hours as needed; initial dose (up to 0.3 mg) may be repeated once in 30-60 minutes after the initial dose if needed

Sublingual: Children ≥16 years and Adults: Opioid dependence:

Induction: Range: 12-16 mg/day (doses during an induction study used 8 mg on day 1, followed by 16 mg on day 2; induction continued over 3-4 days). Treatment should begin at least 4 hours after last use of heroin or short-acting opioid, preferably when first signs of withdrawal appear. Titrating dose to clinical effectiveness should be done as rapidly as possible to prevent undue withdrawal symptoms and patient drop-out during the induction period.

Maintenance: Target dose: 16 mg/day; range: 4-24 mg/day; patients should be switched to the buprenorphine/naloxone combination product for maintenance and unsupervised therapy

Dosage Forms

Injection, solution (Buprenex®): 0.3 mg/mL (1 mL)

Tablet, sublingual (Subutex®): 2 mg, 8 mg

buprenorphine and naloxone (byoo pre NOR feen & nal OKS one)

Synonyms buprenorphine hydrochloride and naloxone hydrochloride dihydrate; naloxone and buprenorphine; naloxone hydrochloride dihydrate and buprenorphine hydrochloride

U.S./Canadian Brand Names Suboxone® [US]

Therapeutic Category Analgesic, Narcotic

Controlled Substance C-III; Prescribing of tablets for opioid dependence is limited to physicians who have met the qualification criteria and have received a DEA number specific to prescribing this product. Tablets will be available through pharmacies and wholesalers which normally provide controlled substances.

Use Treatment of opioid dependence

Usual Dosage Sublingual: Children ≥16 years and Adults: Opioid dependence: **Note:** This combination product is not recommended for use during the induction period; initial treatment should begin using buprenorphine oral tablets. Patients should be switched to the combination product for maintenance and unsupervised therapy.

Maintenance: Target dose (based on buprenorphine content): 16 mg/day; range: 4-24 mg/day

Dosage Forms Tablet, sublingual: Buprenorphine 2 mg and naloxone 0.5 mg; buprenorphine 8 mg and naloxone 2 mg [lemon-lime flavor]

buprenorphine hydrochloride *see* buprenorphine *on previous page*

buprenorphine hydrochloride and naloxone hydrochloride dihydrate *see* buprenorphine and naloxone *on this page*

bupropion (byoo PROE pee on)

Sound-Alike/Look-Alike Issues

bupropion may be confused with Bumex®, BuSpar®, buspirone

Wellbutrin® may be confused with Wellcovorin®

Wellbutrin SR® may be confused with Wellbutrin XL™

Zyban® may be confused with Zagam®

Tall-Man bu**PROP**ion

U.S./Canadian Brand Names Wellbutrin® [US/Can]; Wellbutrin SR® [US]; Wellbutrin XL™ [US]; Zyban® [US/Can]

Therapeutic Category Antidepressant, Aminoketone

Use Treatment of depression; adjunct in smoking cessation

(Continued)

bupropion *(Continued)*

Usual Dosage Oral:

Adults:

Depression:

Immediate release: 100 mg 3 times/day; begin at 100 mg twice daily; may increase to a maximum dose of 450 mg/day

Sustained release: Initial: 150 mg/day in the morning; may increase to 150 mg twice daily by day 4 if tolerated; target dose: 300 mg/day given as 150 mg twice daily; maximum dose: 400 mg/day given as 200 mg twice daily

Extended release: Initial: 150 mg/day in the morning; may increase as early as day 4 of dosing to 300 mg/day; maximum dose: 450 mg/day

Smoking cessation (Zyban®): Initiate with 150 mg once daily for 3 days; increase to 150 mg twice daily; treatment should continue for 7-12 weeks

Dosage Forms

Tablet, as hydrochloride (Wellbutrin®): 75 mg, 100 mg

Tablet, extended release, as hydrochloride (Wellbutrin XL™): 150 mg, 300 mg

Tablet, sustained release, as hydrochloride: 100 mg, 150 mg [equivalent to Wellbutrin® SR], 150 mg [equivalent to Zyban®]

Wellbutrin® SR: 100 mg, 150 mg, 200 mg

Zyban®: 150 mg

Burinex® [Can] *see* bumetanide *on page 132*

Burnamycin [US-OTC] *see* lidocaine *on page 518*

Burn Jel [US-OTC] *see* lidocaine *on page 518*

Burn-O-Jel [US-OTC] *see* lidocaine *on page 518*

Buscopan® [Can] *see* scopolamine *on page 796*

buserelin acetate *(Canada only)* (BYOO se rel in AS e tate)

Therapeutic Category Luteinizing Hormone-Releasing Hormone Analog

Use For the palliative treatment of patients with hormone-dependent advanced carcinoma of the prostate gland (Stage D). Buserelin is also indicated for the treatment of endometriosis in patients who do not require surgery as primary therapy. The duration of treatment is usually 6 months and should not exceed 9 months. Experience with buserelin for the management of endometriosis has been limited to women 18 years of age and older.

Usual Dosage Buserelin should be administered at approximately equal time intervals to ensure that the desired therapeutic effect is maintained.

Prostatic Cancer: Initial Treatment: For the first 7 days of treatment give buserelin 500 mcg (0.5 mL) every 8 hours by S.C. injection. For patient comfort, vary the injection site.

Maintenance Treatment: Depending upon patient preference, or physician recommendation, maintenance treatment may be by daily S.C. injection or by intranasal administration 3 times daily. During maintenance dosing by the S.C. route, the buserelin dose is 200 mcg (0.2 mL) daily. For patient comfort, vary the site of injection.

During maintenance dosing by the intranasal administration route, the buserelin dose is 400 mcg (200 mcg into each nostril) 3 times daily using the metered-dose pump (nebulizer) provided. Each pump action delivers 100 mcg buserelin acetate or 0.1mL solution.

Endometriosis: The dose of buserelin in patients with endometriosis is 400 mcg (200 mcg into each nostril) 3 times daily using the metered-dose pump (nebulizer) provided. Each pump action delivers 100 mcg or 0.1 mL solution. The treatment duration is usually 6 months and should not exceed 9 months.

Dosage Forms Injection, depot: 6.6 mg [2 month]; 9.9 mg [3 month]

BuSpar® [US/Can] *see* buspirone *on next page*

Buspirex [Can] *see* buspirone *on next page*

buspirone (byoo SPYE rone)

Sound-Alike/Look-Alike Issues

buspirone may be confused with bupropion, risperidone

BuSpar® may be confused with bupropion

Synonyms buspirone hydrochloride

Tall-Man bus**PIR**one

U.S./Canadian Brand Names Apo-Buspirone® [Can]; BuSpar® [US/Can]; Buspirex [Can]; Gen-Buspirone [Can]; Lin-Buspirone [Can]; Novo-Buspirone [Can]; Nu-Buspirone [Can]; PMS-Buspirone [Can]

Therapeutic Category Antianxiety Agent

Use Management of generalized anxiety disorder (GAD)

Usual Dosage Oral:

Generalized anxiety disorder:

Children and Adolescents: Initial: 5 mg daily; increase in increments of 5 mg/day at weekly intervals as needed, to a maximum dose of 60 mg/day divided into 2-3 doses

Adults: 15 mg/day (7.5 mg twice daily); may increase in increments of 5 mg/day every 2-4 days to a maximum of 60 mg/day; target dose for most people is 30 mg/day (15 mg twice daily)

Dosage Forms Tablet, as hydrochloride: 5 mg, 7.5 mg, 10 mg, 15 mg, 30 mg

BuSpar®: 5 mg, 10 mg, 15 mg, 30 mg

buspirone hydrochloride *see* buspirone *on this page*

busulfan (byoo SUL fan)

Sound-Alike/Look-Alike Issues

busulfan may be confused with Butalan®

Myleran® may be confused with melphalan, Mylicon®

U.S./Canadian Brand Names Busulfex® [US/Can]; Myleran® [US/Can]

Therapeutic Category Antineoplastic Agent

Use

Oral: Chronic myelogenous leukemia; conditioning regimens for bone marrow transplantation

I.V.: Combination therapy with cyclophosphamide as a conditioning regimen prior to allogeneic hematopoietic progenitor cell transplantation for chronic myelogenous leukemia

Usual Dosage Busulfan should be based on adjusted ideal body weight because actual body weight, ideal body weight, or other factors can produce significant differences in busulfan clearance among lean, normal, and obese patients; refer to individual protocols

Children:

For remission induction of CML: Oral: 0.06-0.12 mg/kg/day **OR** 1.8-4.6 mg/m^2/day; titrate dosage to maintain leukocyte count above 40,000/mm^3; reduce dosage by 50% if the leukocyte count reaches 30,000-40,000/mm^3; discontinue drug if counts fall to ≤20,000/mm^3

BMT marrow-ablative conditioning regimen:

Oral: 1 mg/kg/dose (ideal body weight) every 6 hours for 16 doses

I.V.: ≤12 kg: 1.1 mg/kg/dose (ideal body weight) every 6 hours for 16 doses >12 kg: 0.8 mg/kg/dose (ideal body weight) every 6 hours for 16 doses Adjust dose to desired AUC [1125 µmol(min)] using the following formula: Adjusted dose (mg) = Actual dose (mg) x [target AUC µmol(min) / actual AUC µmol(min)]

Adults:

For remission induction of CML: Oral: 4-8 mg/day (may be as high as 12 mg/day); Maintenance doses: Controversial, range from 1-4 mg/day to 2 mg/week; treatment is continued until WBC reaches 10,000-20,000 cells/mm^3 at which time drug is discontinued; when WBC reaches 50,000/mm^3, maintenance dose is resumed

BMT marrow-ablative conditioning regimen:

Oral: 1 mg/kg/dose (ideal body weight) every 6 hours for 16 doses

(Continued)

busulfan *(Continued)*

I.V.: 0.8 mg/kg (ideal body weight or actual body weight, whichever is lower) every 6 hours for 4 days (a total of 16 doses)

I.V. dosing in morbidly obese patients: Dosing should be based on adjusted ideal body weight (AIBW) which should be calculated as ideal body weight (IBW) + 0.25 times (actual weight minus ideal body weight) AIBW = IBW + 0.25 x (AW - IBW)

Dosage Forms

Injection, solution (Busulfex®): 6 mg/mL (10 mL)

Tablet (Myleran®): 2 mg

Busulfex® [US/Can] *see* busulfan *on previous page*

butabarbital sodium (byoo ta BAR bi tal SOW dee um)

Sound-Alike/Look-Alike Issues

butabarbital may be confused with butalbital

U.S./Canadian Brand Names Butisol Sodium® [US]

Therapeutic Category Barbiturate

Controlled Substance C-III

Use Sedative; hypnotic

Usual Dosage Oral:

Children: Preoperative sedation: 2-6 mg/kg/dose (maximum: 100 mg)

Adults:

Sedative: 15-30 mg 3-4 times/day

Hypnotic: 50-100 mg

Preop: 50-100 mg 1-1½ hours before surgery

Dosage Forms

Elixir, as sodium: 30 mg/5 mL (480 mL) [contains alcohol 7% and tartrazine]

Tablet, as sodium: 30 mg, 50 mg [contains tartrazine]

Butace® *(Discontinued)* *see page 1042*

Butalan® *(Discontinued)* *see page 1042*

butalbital, acetaminophen, and caffeine

(byoo TAL bi tal, a seet a MIN oh fen, & KAF een)

Sound-Alike/Look-Alike Issues

Fioricet® may be confused with Fiorinal®, Lorcet®

Repan® may be confused with Riopan®

Synonyms acetaminophen, butalbital, and caffeine

U.S./Canadian Brand Names Anolor 300 [US]; Esgic® [US]; Esgic-Plus™ [US]; Fioricet® [US]; Repan® [US]; Zebutal™ [US]

Therapeutic Category Barbiturate/Analgesic

Use Relief of the symptomatic complex of tension or muscle contraction headache

Usual Dosage Adults: Oral: 1-2 tablets or capsules every 4 hours; not to exceed 6/day

Dosage Forms

Capsule:

Anolor 300, Esgic®: Butalbital 50 mg, caffeine 40 mg, and acetaminophen 325 mg

Esgic-Plus™, Zebutal™: Butalbital 50 mg, caffeine 40 mg, and acetaminophen 500 mg

Tablet: Esgic®, Fioricet®, Repan®: Butalbital 50 mg, caffeine 40 mg, and acetaminophen 325 mg

butalbital, aspirin, and caffeine (byoo TAL bi tal, AS pir in, & KAF een)

Sound-Alike/Look-Alike Issues

Fiorinal® may be confused with Fioricet®, Florical®, Florinef®

Synonyms aspirin, caffeine, and butalbital; butalbital compound

U.S./Canadian Brand Names Fiorinal® [US/Can]

Therapeutic Category Barbiturate/Analgesic

Controlled Substance C-III (Fiorinal®)

Use Relief of the symptomatic complex of tension or muscle contraction headache
Usual Dosage Oral: Adults: 1-2 tablets or capsules every 4 hours; not to exceed 6/day
Dosage Forms Capsule (Fiorinal®): Butalbital 50 mg, caffeine 40 mg, and aspirin 325 mg

butalbital, aspirin, caffeine, and codeine

(byoo TAL bi tal, AS pir in, KAF een, & KOE deen)

Sound-Alike/Look-Alike Issues
Fiorinal® may be confused with Fioricet®, Florical®, Florinef®
Phrenilin® may be confused with Phenergan®, Trinalin®

Synonyms codeine and butalbital compound; codeine, butalbital, aspirin, and caffeine
U.S./Canadian Brand Names Fiorinal®-C 1/2 [Can]; Fiorinal®-C 1/4 [Can]; Fiorinal® With Codeine [US]; Phrenilin® With Caffeine and Codeine [US]; Tecnal C 1/2 [Can]; Tecnal C 1/4 [Can]
Therapeutic Category Analgesic, Narcotic; Barbiturate
Controlled Substance C-III
Use Mild to moderate pain when sedation is needed
Usual Dosage Adults: Oral: 1-2 capsules every 4 hours as needed for pain; up to 6/day
Dosage Forms Capsule: Butalbital 50 mg, caffeine 40 mg, aspirin 325 mg, and codeine phosphate 30 mg
Fioricet® with Codeine: Butalbital 50 mg, caffeine 40 mg, acetaminophen 325 mg, and codeine phosphate 30 mg [may contain benzyl alcohol]
Phrenilin® with Caffeine and Codeine: Butalbital 50 mg, caffeine 40 mg, acetaminophen 325 mg, and codeine phosphate 30 mg [contains benzyl alcohol and lactose]

butalbital compound *see* butalbital, aspirin, and caffeine *on previous page*

butenafine (byoo TEN a fine)

Synonyms butenafine hydrochloride
U.S./Canadian Brand Names Lotrimin® Ultra™ [US-OTC]; Mentax® [US]
Therapeutic Category Antifungal Agent
Use Topical treatment of tinea pedis (athlete's foot), tinea cruris (jock itch), tinea corporis (ringworm), and tinea versicolor
Usual Dosage Children >12 years and Adults: Topical:
Tinea corporis, tinea cruris, or tinea versicolor: Apply once daily for 2 weeks to affected area and surrounding skin
Tinea pedis: Apply once daily for 4 weeks or twice daily for 7 days to affected area and surrounding skin (7-day regimen may have lower efficacy)
Dosage Forms Cream, as hydrochloride:
Lotrimin® Ultra™: 1% (12 g, 24 g) [contains benzyl alcohol and sodium benzoate]
Mentax®: 1% (15 g, 30 g) [contains benzyl alcohol and sodium benzoate]

butenafine hydrochloride *see* butenafine *on this page*

Buticaps® *(Discontinued)* *see page 1042*

Butisol Sodium® [US] *see* butabarbital sodium *on previous page*

butoconazole (byoo toe KOE na zole)

Sound-Alike/Look-Alike Issues
Mycelex® may be confused with Myoflex®

Synonyms butoconazole nitrate
U.S./Canadian Brand Names Femstat® One [Can]; Gynazole-1® [US]; Mycelex®-3 [US-OTC]
Therapeutic Category Antifungal Agent
Use Local treatment of vulvovaginal candidiasis
Usual Dosage Adults: Female:
Femstat®-3 [OTC]: Insert 1 applicatorful (~5 g) intravaginally at bedtime for 3 consecutive days
(Continued)

butoconazole *(Continued)*

Gynazole-1®: Insert 1 applicatorful (~5 g) intravaginally as a single dose; treatment may need to be extended for up to 6 days in pregnant women (use in pregnancy during 2nd or 3rd trimester only)

Dosage Forms

Cream, vaginal, as nitrate:

Mycelex®-3: 2% (5 g) [prefilled applicator], (20 g) [with disposable applicator]

Gynazole-1®: 2% (5 g) [prefilled applicator]

butoconazole nitrate *see* butoconazole *on previous page*

butorphanol (byoo TOR fa nole)

Sound-Alike/Look-Alike Issues

Stadol® may be confused with Haldol®, sotalol

Synonyms butorphanol tartrate

U.S./Canadian Brand Names Apo-Butorphanol® [Can]; PMS-Butorphanol [Can]; Stadol® [US]; Stadol NS™ [Can]

Therapeutic Category Analgesic, Narcotic

Controlled Substance C-IV

Use

Parenteral: Management of moderate to severe pain; preoperative medication; supplement to balanced anesthesia; management of pain during labor

Nasal spray: Management of moderate to severe pain, including migraine headache pain

Usual Dosage Note: These are guidelines and do not represent the maximum doses that may be required in all patients. Doses should be titrated to pain relief/prevention. Butorphanol has an analgesic ceiling.

Adults:

Parenteral:

Acute pain (moderate to severe):

I.M.: Initial: 2 mg, may repeat every 3-4 hours as needed; usual range: 1-4 mg every 3-4 hours as needed

I.V.: Initial: 1 mg, may repeat every 3-4 hours as needed; usual range: 0.5-2 mg every 3-4 hours as needed

Preoperative medication: I.M.: 2 mg 60-90 minutes before surgery

Supplement to balanced anesthesia: I.V.: 2 mg shortly before induction and/or an incremental dose of 0.5-1 mg (up to 0.06 mg/kg), depending on previously administered sedative, analgesic, and hypnotic medications

Pain during labor (fetus >37 weeks gestation and no signs of fetal distress):

I.M., I.V.: 1-2 mg; may repeat in 4 hours

Note: Alternative analgesia should be used for pain associated with delivery or if delivery is anticipated within 4 hours

Nasal spray:

Moderate to severe pain (including migraine headache pain): Initial: 1 spray (~1 mg per spray) in 1 nostril; if adequate pain relief is not achieved within 60-90 minutes, an additional 1 spray in 1 nostril may be given; may repeat initial dose sequence in 3-4 hours after the last dose as needed

Alternatively, an initial dose of 2 mg (1 spray in each nostril) may be used in patients who will be able to remain recumbent (in the event drowsiness or dizziness occurs); additional 2 mg doses should not be given for 3-4 hours

Note: In some clinical trials, an initial dose of 2 mg (as 2 doses 1 hour apart or 2 mg initially - 1 spray in each nostril) has been used, followed by 1 mg in 1 hour; side effects were greater at these dosages

Dosage Forms

Injection, solution, as tartrate [preservative free] (Stadol®): 1 mg/mL (1 mL); 2 mg/mL (1 mL, 2 mL)

Injection, solution, as tartrate [with preservative] (Stadol®): 2 mg/mL (10 mL)

Solution, intranasal spray, as tartrate: 10 mg/mL (2.5 mL) [14-15 doses]

Stadol® NS [DSC]: 10 mg/mL (2.5 mL)

butorphanol tartrate *see* butorphanol *on previous page*

B vitamin combinations *see* vitamin B complex combinations *on page 915*

BW-430C *see* lamotrigine *on page 503*

BW524W91 *see* emtricitabine *on page 307*

Byclomine® Injection *(Discontinued)* *see page 1042*

Bydramine® Cough Syrup *(Discontinued)* *see page 1042*

C2B8 *see* rituximab *on page 780*

C2B8 monoclonal antibody *see* rituximab *on page 780*

C7E3 *see* abciximab *on page 3*

C8-CCK *see* sincalide *on page 806*

311C90 *see* zolmitriptan *on page 943*

C225 *see* cetuximab *on page 179*

C-500-GR™ [US-OTC] *see* ascorbic acid *on page 79*

cabergoline (ca BER go leen)

U.S./Canadian Brand Names Dostinex® [US/Can]

Therapeutic Category Ergot-like Derivative

Use Treatment of hyperprolactinemic disorders, either idiopathic or due to pituitary adenomas

Usual Dosage Initial dose: Oral: 0.25 mg twice weekly; the dose may be increased by 0.25 mg twice weekly up to a maximum of 1 mg twice weekly according to the patient's serum prolactin level. Dosage increases should not occur more rapidly than every 4 weeks. Once a normal serum prolactin level is maintained for 6 months, the dose may be discontinued and prolactin levels monitored to determine if cabergoline is still required. The durability of efficacy beyond 24 months of therapy has not been established.

Dosage Forms Tablet: 0.5 mg

Caduet® [US] *see* amlodipine and atorvastatin *on page 49*

Caelyx® [Can] *see* doxorubicin (liposomal) *on page 294*

Cafatine-PB® *(Discontinued)* *see page 1042*

Cafetrate® *(Discontinued)* *see page 1042*

caffeine, acetaminophen, and aspirin *see* acetaminophen, aspirin, and caffeine *on page 10*

caffeine and sodium benzoate (KAF een & SOW dee um BEN zoe ate)

Synonyms sodium benzoate and caffeine

Therapeutic Category Diuretic, Miscellaneous

Use Emergency stimulant in acute circulatory failure; as a diuretic; and to relieve spinal puncture headache

Usual Dosage

Children: I.M., I.V., S.C.: 8 mg/kg every 4 hours as needed

Adults: I.M., I.V.: 500 mg, maximum single dose: 1 g

Dosage Forms Injection, solution: Caffeine 121 mg and sodium benzoate 129 mg per mL (2 mL); caffeine 125 mg and sodium benzoate 125 mg per mL (2 mL)

caffeine, aspirin, and acetaminophen *see* acetaminophen, aspirin, and caffeine *on page 10*

caffeine (citrated) (KAF een SIT rated)

Therapeutic Category Respiratory Stimulant; Stimulant

Use Central nervous system stimulant; used in the treatment of apnea of prematurity (28 to <33 weeks gestational age). Has several advantages over theophylline in the treatment of neonatal apnea, its half-life is about 3 times as long, allowing once daily dosing, drug levels do not need to be drawn at peak and trough; has a wider therapeutic window, allowing more room between an effective concentration and toxicity.

Usual Dosage Apnea of prematurity: Neonates:

Loading dose (usually administered I.V.): 10-20 mg/kg as caffeine citrate (5-10 mg/kg as caffeine base). If theophylline has been administered to the patient within the previous 3 days, a full or modified loading dose (50% to 75% of a loading dose) may be given (caffeine is a significant metabolite of theophylline in the newborn).

Maintenance dose: Oral, I.V.: 5 mg/kg/day as caffeine citrate (2.5 mg/kg/day as caffeine base) once daily starting 24 hours after the loading dose. Maintenance dose is adjusted based on patient's response (efficacy and adverse effects), and serum caffeine concentrations.

Dosage Forms

Injection: 20 mg/mL as caffeine citrate [equivalent to 10 mg/mL caffeine base] (3 mL)

Solution, oral: 20 mg/mL as caffeine citrate [equivalent to 10 mg/mL caffeine base] (3 mL)

caffeine, hydrocodone, chlorpheniramine, phenylephrine, and acetaminophen *see* hydrocodone, chlorpheniramine, phenylephrine, acetaminophen, and caffeine *on page 446*

caffeine, orphenadrine, and aspirin *see* orphenadrine, aspirin, and caffeine *on page 649*

Caladryl® Spray *(Discontinued)* *see page 1042*

Calan® [US/Can] *see* verapamil *on page 908*

Calan® SR [US] *see* verapamil *on page 908*

Calcarb 600 [US-OTC] *see* calcium carbonate *on page 144*

Calcibind® [US/Can] *see* cellulose sodium phosphate *on page 175*

Calci-Chew® [US-OTC] *see* calcium carbonate *on page 144*

Calciday-667® *(Discontinued)* *see page 1042*

Calciferol™ [US] *see* ergocalciferol *on page 317*

Calcijex® [US] *see* calcitriol *on next page*

Calcimar® *(Discontinued)* *see page 1042*

Calcimar® [Can] *see* calcitonin *on next page*

Calci-Mix® [US-OTC] *see* calcium carbonate *on page 144*

Calciparine® Injection *(Discontinued)* *see page 1042*

calcipotriene (kal si POE try een)

U.S./Canadian Brand Names Dovonex® [US]

Therapeutic Category Antipsoriatic Agent

Use Treatment of moderate plaque psoriasis

Usual Dosage Topical: Adults: Apply in a thin film to the affected skin twice daily and rub in gently and completely

Dosage Forms

Cream: 0.005% (60 g, 120 g)

Ointment: 0.005% (60 g, 120 g)

Solution, topical: 0.005% (60 mL)

calcipotriol and betamethasone dipropionate *see* betamethasone and calcipotriol *(Canada only) on page 114*

Calcite-500 [Can] *see* calcium carbonate *on next page*

calcitonin (kal si TOE nin)

Sound-Alike/Look-Alike Issues
calcitonin may be confused with calcitriol
Miacalcin® may be confused with Micatin®

Synonyms calcitonin (salmon)

U.S./Canadian Brand Names Calcimar® [Can]; Caltine® [Can]; Miacalcin® [US]; Miacalcin® NS [Can]

Therapeutic Category Polypeptide Hormone

Use Calcitonin (salmon): Treatment of Paget disease of bone (osteitis deformans); adjunctive therapy for hypercalcemia; used in postmenopausal osteoporosis and osteogenesis imperfecta

Usual Dosage Salmon calcitonin:
Children: Dosage not established
Adults:
Paget disease: I.M., SubQ: Initial: 100 units/day; maintenance: 50 units/day or 50-100 units every 1-3 days
Hypercalcemia: Initial: I.M., SubQ: 4 units/kg every 12 hours; may increase up to 8 units/kg every 12 hours to a maximum of every 6 hours
Osteogenesis imperfecta: I.M., SubQ: 2 units/kg 3 times/week
Postmenopausal osteoporosis:
I.M., SubQ: 100 units/day
Intranasal: 200 units (1 spray)/day

Dosage Forms
Injection, solution, calcitonin-salmon: 200 int. units/mL (2 mL)
Solution, nasal spray, calcitonin-salmon: 200 int. units/0.09 mL (3.7 mL) [contains benzalkonium chloride]

calcitonin (salmon) *see* calcitonin *on this page*

Cal-Citrate® 250 [US-OTC] *see* calcium citrate *on page 147*

calcitriol (kal si TRYE ole)

Sound-Alike/Look-Alike Issues
calcitriol may be confused with Calciferol®, calcitonin

Synonyms 1,25 dihydroxycholecalciferol

U.S./Canadian Brand Names Calcijex® [US]; Rocaltrol® [US/Can]

Therapeutic Category Vitamin D Analog

Use Management of hypocalcemia in patients on chronic renal dialysis; management of secondary hyperparathyroidism in moderate-to-severe chronic renal failure; management of hypocalcemia in hypoparathyroidism and pseudohypoparathyroidism

Usual Dosage Individualize dosage to maintain calcium levels of 9-10 mg/dL
Renal failure:
Children:
Oral: 0.25-2 mcg/day have been used (with hemodialysis); 0.014-0.041 mcg/kg/day (not receiving hemodialysis); increases should be made at 4- to 8-week intervals
I.V.: 0.01-0.05 mcg/kg 3 times/week if undergoing hemodialysis
Adults:
Oral: 0.25 mcg/day or every other day (may require 0.5-1 mcg/day); increases should be made at 4- to 8-week intervals
I.V.: 0.5 mcg/day 3 times/week (may require from 0.5-3 mcg/day given 3 times/week) if undergoing hemodialysis
Hypoparathyroidism/pseudohypoparathyroidism: Oral (evaluate dosage at 2- to 4-week intervals):
Children:
<1 year: 0.04-0.08 mcg/kg once daily
1-5 years: 0.25-0.75 mcg once daily
Children >6 years and Adults: 0.5-2 mcg once daily
(Continued)

calcitriol *(Continued)*

Vitamin D-dependent rickets: Children and Adults: Oral: 1 mcg once daily
Vitamin D-resistant rickets (familial hypophosphatemia): Children and Adults: Oral: Initial: 0.015-0.02 mcg/kg once daily; maintenance: 0.03-0.06 mcg/kg once daily; maximum dose: 2 mcg once daily
Hypocalcemia in premature infants: Oral: 1 mcg once daily for 5 days
Hypocalcemic tetany in premature infants: I.V.: 0.05 mcg/kg once daily for 5-12 days

Dosage Forms
Capsule (Rocaltrol®): 0.25 mcg, 0.5 mcg [each strength contains coconut oil]
Injection, solution: 1 mcg/mL (1 mL); 2 mcg/mL (2 mL)
Calcijex®: 1 mcg/mL (1 mL)
Solution, oral (Rocaltrol®): 1 mcg/mL (15 mL) [contains palm seed oil]

calcium acetate (KAL see um AS e tate)

Sound-Alike/Look-Alike Issues
PhosLo® may be confused with Phos-Flur®, ProSom™

U.S./Canadian Brand Names PhosLo® [US]

Therapeutic Category Electrolyte Supplement, Oral

Use
Oral: Control of hyperphosphatemia in end-stage renal failure; does not promote aluminum absorption
I.V.: Calcium supplementation in parenteral nutrition therapy

Usual Dosage
Dietary Reference Intake:
0-6 months: 210 mg/day
7-12 months: 270 mg/day
1-3 years: 500 mg/day
4-8 years: 800 mg/day
Adults, Male/Female:
9-18 years: 1300 mg/day
19-50 years: 1000 mg/day
≥51 years: 1200 mg/day
Female: Pregnancy: Same as for Adults, Male/Female
Female: Lactating: Same as for Adults, Male/Female

Oral: Adults, on dialysis: Initial: 1334 mg with each meal, can be increased gradually to bring the serum phosphate value <6 mg/dL as long as hypercalcemia does not develop (usual dose: 2001-2868 mg calcium acetate with each meal); do not give additional calcium supplements
I.V.: Dose is dependent on the requirements of the individual patient; in central venous total parental nutrition (TPN), calcium is administered at a concentration of 5 mEq (10 mL)/L of TPN solution; the additive maintenance dose in neonatal TPN is 0.5 mEq calcium/kg/day (1.0 mL/kg/day)
Neonates: 70-200 mg/kg/day
Infants and Children: 70-150 mg/kg/day
Adolescents: 18-35 mg/kg/day

Dosage Forms Note: Elemental calcium listed in brackets:
Gelcap (PhosLo®): 667 mg [169 mg]
Injection, solution: 0.5 mEq/mL (10 mL, 50 mL, 100 mL)
Tablet (PhosLo®): 667 mg [169 mg]

calcium acetate and aluminum sulfate *see* aluminum sulfate and calcium acetate *on page 41*

calcium acetylhomotaurinate *see* acamprosate *on page 3*

calcium carbonate (KAL see um KAR bun ate)

Sound-Alike/Look-Alike Issues
Florical® may be confused with Fiorinal®

Mylanta® may be confused with Mynatal®
Nephro-Calci® may be confused with Nephrocaps®
Os-Cal® may be confused with Asacol®

U.S./Canadian Brand Names Alcalak [US-OTC]; Alka-Mints® [US-OTC]; Amitone® [US-OTC]; Apo-Cal® [Can]; Calcarb 600 [US-OTC]; Calci-Chew® [US-OTC]; Calci-Mix® [US-OTC]; Calcite-500 [Can]; Cal-Gest [US-OTC]; Cal-Mint [US-OTC]; Caltrate® [Can]; Caltrate® 600 [US-OTC]; Chooz® [US-OTC]; Florical® [US-OTC]; Mylanta® Children's [US-OTC]; Nephro-Calci® [US-OTC]; Os-Cal® [Can]; Os-Cal® 500 [US-OTC]; Oysco 500 [US-OTC]; Oyst-Cal 500 [US-OTC]; Titralac™ Extra Strength [US-OTC]; Titralac™ [US-OTC]; Tums® 500 [US-OTC]; Tums® E-X [US-OTC]; Tums® Smooth Dissolve [US-OTC]; Tums® Ultra [US-OTC]; Tums® [US-OTC]

Therapeutic Category Antacid; Electrolyte Supplement, Oral

Use As an antacid, and treatment and prevention of calcium deficiency or hyperphosphatemia (eg, osteoporosis, osteomalacia, mild/moderate renal insufficiency, hypoparathyroidism, postmenopausal osteoporosis, rickets); has been used to bind phosphate

Usual Dosage Oral (dosage is in terms of elemental calcium):

Dietary Reference Intake:
0-6 months: 210 mg/day
7-12 months: 270 mg/day
1-3 years: 500 mg/day
4-8 years: 800 mg/day
Adults, Male/Female:
9-18 years: 1300 mg/day
19-50 years: 1000 mg/day
≥51 years: 1200 mg/day
Female: Pregnancy: Same as for Adults, Male/Female
Female: Lactating: Same as for Adults, Male/Female

Hypocalcemia (dose depends on clinical condition and serum calcium level): Dose expressed in mg of **elemental calcium**
Neonates: 50-150 mg/kg/day in 4-6 divided doses; not to exceed 1 g/day
Children: 45-65 mg/kg/day in 4 divided doses
Adults: 1-2 g or more/day in 3-4 divided doses

Adults:
Dietary supplementation: 500 mg to 2 g divided 2-4 times/day
Antacid: Dosage based on acid-neutralizing capacity of specific product; generally, 1-2 tablets or 5-10 mL every 2 hours; maximum: 7000 mg calcium carbonate per 24 hours; specific product labeling should be consulted

Adults >51 years: Osteoporosis: 1200 mg/day

Dosage Forms

Capsule:
Calci-Mix®: 1250 mg [equivalent to elemental calcium 500 mg]
Florical®: 364 mg [equivalent to elemental calcium 145.6 mg; contains sodium fluoride 8.3 mg]

Powder: 1600 mg/teaspoonful (960 g)

Suspension, oral: 1250 mg/5 mL (5 mL, 500 mL) [equivalent to elemental calcium 500 mg/5 mL; mint flavor]

Tablet: 1250 mg [equivalent to elemental calcium 500 mg]; 1500 mg [equivalent to elemental calcium 600 mg]
Calcarb 600, Caltrate® 600, Nephro-Calci®: 1500 mg [equivalent to elemental calcium 600 mg]
Florical®: 364 mg [equivalent to elemental calcium 145.6 mg; contains sodium fluoride 8.3 mg]
Os-Cal® 500, Oysco 500, Oyst-Cal 500: 1250 mg [equivalent to elemental calcium 500 mg]

Tablet, chewable: 500 mg [equivalent to elemental calcium 200 mg]; 650 mg [equivalent to elemental calcium 260 mg]; 750 mg [equivalent to elemental calcium 300 mg]
Alcalak: 420 mg [equivalent to elemental calcium 168 mg]

(Continued)

calcium carbonate *(Continued)*

Alka-Mints®: 850 mg [equivalent to elemental calcium 340 mg; assorted and spearmint flavors]
Amitone®: 420 mg [equivalent to elemental calcium 168 mg; spearmint flavor]
Cal-Gest: 500 mg [equivalent to elemental calcium 200 mg]
Calci-Chew®: 1250 mg [equivalent to elemental calcium 500 mg; cherry, lemon, and orange flavors]
Cal-Mint: 650 mg [equivalent to elemental calcium 260 mg; mint flavor]
Chooz®: 500 mg [equivalent to elemental calcium 200 mg; contains phenylalanine]
Mylanta® Children's: 400 mg [equivalent to elemental calcium 160 mg; bubblegum flavor]
Os-Cal® 500: 1250 mg [equivalent to elemental calcium 500 mg; Bavarian cream flavor]
Titralac™: 420 mg [equivalent to elemental calcium 168 mg; sugar free; mint flavor]
Titralac™ Extra Strength: 750 mg [equivalent to elemental calcium 300 mg; sugar free; mint flavor]
Tums®: 500 mg [equivalent to elemental calcium 200 mg; assorted fruit (contains tartrazine) and peppermint flavors]
Tums® E-X: 750 mg [equivalent to elemental calcium 300 mg; assorted fruit (contains tartrazine), fresh blend, tropical assorted fruit, wintergreen (contains tartrazine), and assorted berry flavors]
Tums® Extra Strength Sugar Free: 750 mg [equivalent to elemental calcium 300 mg; sugar free; contains phenylalanine <1 mg/tablet; orange cream flavor]
Tums® Smooth Dissolve: 750 mg [equivalent to elemental calcium 300 mg; assorted fruit (contains tartrazine) and peppermint flavors]
Tums® Ultra®: 1000 mg [equivalent to elemental calcium 400 mg; assorted mint, assorted berry, and tropical assorted berry (contains tartrazine) flavors]

calcium carbonate and magnesium hydroxide

(KAL see um KAR bun ate & mag NEE zhum hye DROKS ide)

Sound-Alike/Look-Alike Issues
Mylanta® may be confused with Mynatal®

Synonyms magnesium hydroxide and calcium carbonate

U.S./Canadian Brand Names Mylanta® Gelcaps® [US-OTC]; Mylanta® Supreme [US-OTC]; Mylanta® Ultra [US-OTC]; Rolaids®, Extra Strength [US-OTC]; Rolaids® [US-OTC]

Therapeutic Category Antacid

Use Hyperacidity

Usual Dosage Adults: Oral: 2-4 tablets between meals, at bedtime, or as directed by healthcare provider

Dosage Forms
Gelcap (Mylanta® Gelcaps®): Calcium carbonate 550 mg and magnesium hydroxide 125 mg
Suspension (Mylanta® Supreme): Calcium carbonate 400 mg and magnesium hydroxide 135 mg per 5 mL (30 mL, 360 mL, 720 mL) [cherry and mint flavors]
Tablet, chewable:
Mylanta® Ultra: Calcium carbonate 700 mg and magnesium hydroxide 300 mg [cherry créme and cool mint flavors]
Rolaids®: Calcium carbonate 550 mg and magnesium hydroxide 110 mg [original, cherry, and spearmint flavors]
Rolaids® Extra Strength: Calcium carbonate 675 mg and magnesium hydroxide 135 mg [cool strawberry, fresh mint, fruit, and tropical fruit punch flavors]

calcium carbonate and simethicone

(KAL see um KAR bun ate & sye METH i kone)

Synonyms simethicone and calcium carbonate

U.S./Canadian Brand Names Titralac™ Plus [US-OTC]

Therapeutic Category Antacid; Antiflatulent

Use Relief of acid indigestion, heartburn

Usual Dosage Oral (OTC labeling): Adults: Two tablets every 2-3 hours as needed (maximum: 19 tablets/24 hours)

Dosage Forms Tablet, chewable: Calcium carbonate 420 mg and simethicone 21 mg [equivalent to elemental calcium 168 mg; sugar free; spearmint flavor]

calcium carbonate, magnesium hydroxide, and famotidine *see* famotidine, calcium carbonate, and magnesium hydroxide *on page 357*

calcium chloride (KAL see um KLOR ide)

Therapeutic Category Electrolyte Supplement, Oral

Use Cardiac resuscitation when epinephrine fails to improve myocardial contractions, cardiac disturbances of hyperkalemia, hypocalcemia, or calcium channel blocking agent toxicity; emergent treatment of hypocalcemic tetany, treatment of hypermagnesemia

Usual Dosage Note: Calcium chloride is 3 times as potent as calcium gluconate

Cardiac arrest in the presence of hyperkalemia or hypocalcemia, magnesium toxicity, or calcium antagonist toxicity: I.V.:

Infants and Children: 20 mg/kg; may repeat in 10 minutes if necessary

Adults: 2-4 mg/kg (10% solution), repeated every 10 minutes if necessary

Hypocalcemia: I.V.:

Children (manufacturer's recommendation): 2.7-5 mg/kg/dose every 4-6 hours

Alternative pediatric dosing: Infants and Children: 10-20 mg/kg/dose (infants <1 mEq; children 1-7 mEq), repeat every 4-6 hours if needed

Adults: 500 mg to 1 g (7-14 mEq)/dose repeated every 4-6 hours if needed

Hypocalcemic tetany: I.V.:

Infants and Children: 10 mg/kg (0.5-0.7 mEq/kg) over 5-10 minutes; may repeat after 6-8 hours or follow with an infusion with a maximum dose of 200 mg/kg/day

Adults: 1 g over 10-30 minutes; may repeat after 6 hours

Hypocalcemia secondary to citrated blood transfusion: I.V.:

Neonates, Infants, and Children: Give 0.45 mEq **elemental** calcium for each 100 mL citrated blood infused

Adults: 1.35 mEq calcium with each 100 mL of citrated blood infused

Dosage Forms Injection, solution [preservative free]: 10% [100 mg/mL] (10 mL) [equivalent to elemental calcium 27.2 mg/mL, calcium 1.36 mEq/mL]

calcium citrate (KAL see um SIT rate)

Sound-Alike/Look-Alike Issues

Citracal® may be confused with Citrucel®

U.S./Canadian Brand Names Cal-Citrate® 250 [US-OTC]; Citracal® [US-OTC]; Osteocit® [Can]

Therapeutic Category Electrolyte Supplement, Oral

Use Antacid; treatment and prevention of calcium deficiency or hyperphosphatemia (eg, osteoporosis, osteomalacia, mild/moderate renal insufficiency, hypoparathyroidism, postmenopausal osteoporosis, rickets)

Usual Dosage Oral: Dosage is in terms of elemental calcium

Dietary Reference Intake:

0-6 months: 210 mg/day

7-12 months: 270 mg/day

1-3 years: 500 mg/day

4-8 years: 800 mg/day

Adults, Male/Female:

9-18 years: 1300 mg/day

19-50 years: 1000 mg/day

≥51 years: 1200 mg/day

Female: Pregnancy: Same as for Adults, Male/Female

Female: Lactating: Same as for Adults, Male/Female

Dietary supplement: Usual dose: 500 mg to 2 g 2-4 times/day

(Continued)

calcium citrate *(Continued)*

Dosage Forms

Granules: 760 mg/teaspoonful (480 g)
Tablet: Elemental calcium 200 mg, 250 mg
Cal-Citrate®: Elemental calcium 250 mg
Citracal®: 950 mg [equivalent to elemental calcium 200 mg]

calcium disodium edetate *see* edetate calcium disodium *on page 302*

Calcium Disodium Versenate® [US] *see* edetate calcium disodium *on page 302*

calcium EDTA *see* edetate calcium disodium *on page 302*

calcium glubionate (KAL see um gloo BYE oh nate)

Sound-Alike/Look-Alike Issues
calcium glubionate may be confused with calcium gluconate

Therapeutic Category Electrolyte Supplement, Oral

Use Adjunct in treatment and prevention of postmenopausal osteoporosis; treatment and prevention of calcium depletion or hyperphosphatemia (eg, osteoporosis, osteomalacia, mild/moderate renal insufficiency, hypoparathyroidism, rickets)

Usual Dosage Dosage is in terms of **elemental** calcium

Dietary Reference Intake:
0-6 months: 210 mg/day
7-12 months: 270 mg/day
1-3 years: 500 mg/day
4-8 years: 800 mg/day
Adults, Male/Female:
9-18 years: 1300 mg/day
19-50 years: 1000 mg/day
≥51 years: 1200 mg/day
Female: Pregnancy: Same as for Adults, Male/Female
Female: Lactating: Same as for Adults, Male/Female

Syrup is a hyperosmolar solution; dosage is in terms of calcium glubionate, elemental calcium is in parentheses
Neonatal hypocalcemia: 1200 mg (77 mg Ca^{++})/kg/day in 4-6 divided doses
Maintenance: Infants and Children: 600-2000 mg (38-128 mg Ca^{++})/kg/day in 4 divided doses up to a maximum of 9 g (575 mg Ca^{++})/day
Adults: 6-18 g (~0.5-1 g Ca^{++})/day in divided doses

Dosage Forms Syrup: 1.8 g/5 mL (480 mL) [equivalent to elemental calcium 115 mg/5 mL]

calcium gluceptate ***(Discontinued)*** *see page 1042*

calcium gluconate (KAL see um GLOO koe nate)

Sound-Alike/Look-Alike Issues
calcium gluconate may be confused with calcium glubionate

Therapeutic Category Electrolyte Supplement, Oral

Use Treatment and prevention of hypocalcemia; treatment of tetany, cardiac disturbances of hyperkalemia, cardiac resuscitation when epinephrine fails to improve myocardial contractions, hypocalcemia, or calcium channel blocker toxicity; calcium supplementation

Usual Dosage Dosage is in terms of **elemental** calcium

Dietary Reference Intake:
0-6 months: 210 mg/day
7-12 months: 270 mg/day
1-3 years: 500 mg/day
4-8 years: 800 mg/day
9-18 years: 1300 mg/day

Adults, Male/Female:
19-50 years: 1000 mg/day
≥51 years: 1200 mg/day
Female: Pregnancy: Same as for Adults, Male/Female
Female: Lactating: Same as for Adults, Male/Female
Hypocalcemia: I.V.:
Neonates: 200-800 mg/kg/day as a continuous infusion or in 4 divided doses
Infants and Children: 200-500 mg/kg/day as a continuous infusion or in 4 divided doses
Adults: 2-15 g/24 hours as a continuous infusion or in divided doses
Hypocalcemia: Oral:
Children: 200-500 mg/kg/day divided every 6 hours
Adults: 500 mg to 2 g 2-4 times/day
Osteoporosis/bone loss: Oral: 1000-1500 mg in divided doses/day
Hypocalcemia secondary to citrated blood infusion: I.V.: Give 0.45 mEq **elemental** calcium for each 100 mL citrated blood infused
Hypocalcemic tetany: I.V.:
Neonates: 100-200 mg/kg/dose, may follow with 500 mg/kg/day in 3-4 divided doses or as an infusion
Infants and Children: 100-200 mg/kg/dose (0.5-0.7 mEq/kg/dose) over 5-10 minutes; may repeat every 6-8 hours **or** follow with an infusion of 500 mg/kg/day
Adults: 1-3 g (4.5-16 mEq) may be administered until therapeutic response occurs
Calcium antagonist toxicity, magnesium intoxication, or cardiac arrest in the presence of hyperkalemia or hypocalcemia: Calcium chloride is recommended calcium salt: I.V.:
Infants and Children: 60-100 mg/kg/dose (maximum: 3 g/dose)
Adults: 500-800 mg; maximum: 3 g/dose
Maintenance electrolyte requirements for total parenteral nutrition: I.V.: Daily requirements: Adults: 8-16 mEq/1000 kcal/24 hours

Dosage Forms
Injection, solution [preservative free]: 10% [100 mg/mL] (10 mL, 50 mL, 100 mL, 200 mL) [equivalent to elemental calcium 9 mg/mL; calcium 0.46 mEq/mL]
Powder: 347 mg/tablespoonful (480 g)
Tablet: 500 mg [equivalent to elemental calcium 45 mg]; 650 mg [equivalent to elemental calcium 58.5 mg]; 975 mg [equivalent to elemental calcium 87.75 mg]

calcium lactate (KAL see um LAK tate)

Therapeutic Category Electrolyte Supplement, Oral
Use Adjunct in prevention of postmenopausal osteoporosis; treatment and prevention of calcium depletion
Usual Dosage Oral (in terms of calcium lactate):
Dietary Reference Intake (in terms of elemental calcium):
0-6 months: 210 mg/day
7-12 months: 270 mg/day
1-3 years: 500 mg/day
4-8 years: 800 mg/day
Adults, Male/Female:
9-18 years: 1300 mg/day
19-50 years: 1000 mg/day
≥51 years: 1200 mg/day
Female: Pregnancy: Same as Adults, Male/Female
Female: Lactating: Same as Adults, Male/Female
Children: 500 mg/kg/day divided every 6-8 hours; maximum daily dose: 9 g
Adults: 1.5-3 g divided every 8 hours
Dosage Forms Tablet: 650 mg [equivalent to elemental calcium 84.5 mg]

calcium leucovorin *see* leucovorin *on page 509*

calcium pantothenate *see* pantothenic acid *on page 666*

calcium phosphate (tribasic) (KAL see um FOS fate tri BAY sik)

Synonyms tricalcium phosphate

U.S./Canadian Brand Names Posture® [US-OTC]

Therapeutic Category Electrolyte Supplement, Oral

Use Adjunct in prevention of postmenopausal osteoporosis; treatment and prevention of calcium depletion

Usual Dosage Oral (dosage is in terms of elemental calcium):

Dietary Reference Intake:

0-6 months: 210 mg/day
7-12 months: 270 mg/day
1-3 years: 500 mg/day
4-8 years: 800 mg/day
Adults, Male/Female:
9-18 years: 1300 mg/day
19-50 years: 1000 mg/day
≥51 years: 1200 mg/day
Female: Pregnancy: Same as for Adults, Male/Female
Female: Lactating: Same as for Adults, Male/Female

Prevention of osteoporosis:
Children: 45-65 mg/kg/day
Adults: 1-2 g/day

Dosage Forms Tablet: 1565.2 mg [equivalent to elemental calcium 600 mg; sugar free]

CaldeCORT® [US] *see* hydrocortisone (topical) *on page 451*

Calderol® *(Discontinued)* *see page 1042*

calfactant (cal FAC tant)

U.S./Canadian Brand Names Infasurf® [US]

Therapeutic Category Lung Surfactant

Use Prevention of respiratory distress syndrome (RDS) in premature infants at high risk for RDS and for the treatment ("rescue") of premature infants who develop RDS

Prophylaxis: Therapy at birth with calfactant is indicated for premature infants <29 weeks of gestational age at significant risk for RDS. Should be administered as soon as possible, preferably within 30 minutes after birth.

Treatment: For infants ≤72 hours of age with RDS (confirmed by clinical and radiologic findings) and requiring endotracheal intubation.

Usual Dosage Intratracheal administration **only**: Each dose is 3 mL/kg body weight at birth; should be administered every 12 hours for a total of up to 3 doses

Dosage Forms Suspension, intratracheal [preservative free]: 35 mg/mL (6 mL)

Cal-Gest [US-OTC] *see* calcium carbonate *on page 144*

Cal-Mint [US-OTC] *see* calcium carbonate *on page 144*

Calm-X® Oral *(Discontinued)* *see page 1042*

Calmylin with Codeine [Can] *see* guaifenesin, pseudoephedrine, and codeine *on page 422*

Cal-Nate™ [US] *see* vitamins (multiple/prenatal) *on page 927*

Calphron® *(Discontinued)* *see page 1042*

Cal-Plus® *(Discontinued)* *see page 1042*

Caltine® [Can] *see* calcitonin *on page 143*

Caltrate® [Can] *see* calcium carbonate *on page 144*

Caltrate® 600 [US-OTC] *see* calcium carbonate *on page 144*

Caltrate Jr.® *(Discontinued)* *see page 1042*

Camalox® Suspension & Tablet *(Discontinued)* *see page 1042*

Camila™ [US] *see* norethindrone *on page 627*

Campath® [US] *see* alemtuzumab *on page 29*

campath-1H *see* alemtuzumab *on page 29*

Campho-Phenique® [US-OTC] *see* camphor and phenol *on this page*

camphor and phenol (KAM for & FEE nole)

Synonyms phenol and camphor

U.S./Canadian Brand Names Campho-Phenique® [US-OTC]

Therapeutic Category Topical Skin Product

Use Relief of pain and itching associated with minor burns, sunburn, minor cuts, insect bites, minor skin irritation; temporary relief of pain from cold sores

Usual Dosage Topical: Adults: Relief of pain/itching: Apply 1-3 times/day

Dosage Forms

Gel, topical (Campho-Phenique®): Camphor 10.8% and phenol 4.7% (7 g, 15 g)

Liquid, topical: Camphor 10.8% and phenol 4.7% (45 mL)

Campho-Phenique®: Camphor 10.8% and phenol 4.7% (22.5 mL, 45 mL)

camphorated tincture of opium *see* paregoric *on page 667*

camphor, menthol, and phenol (KAM for, MEN thol, & FEE nole)

Therapeutic Category Topical Skin Product

Use Relief of dry, itching skin

Usual Dosage Topical: Apply as needed for dry skin

Dosage Forms Lotion, topical: Camphor 0.5%, menthol 0.5%, and phenol 0.5% in emollient base (240 mL)

Campral® [US] *see* acamprosate *on page 3*

Camptosar® [US/Can] *see* irinotecan *on page 484*

camptothecin-11 *see* irinotecan *on page 484*

Canasa™ [US] *see* mesalamine *on page 556*

Cancidas® [US/Can] *see* caspofungin *on page 164*

candesartan (kan de SAR tan)

Sound-Alike/Look-Alike Issues

Atacand® may be confused with antacid

Synonyms candesartan cilexetil

U.S./Canadian Brand Names Atacand® [US/Can]

Therapeutic Category Angiotensin II Receptor Antagonist

Use Alone or in combination with other antihypertensive agents in treating essential hypertension

Usual Dosage Adults: Oral:

Hypertension: Usual dose is 4-32 mg once daily; dosage must be individualized. Blood pressure response is dose-related over the range of 2-32 mg. The usual recommended starting dose of 16 mg once daily when it is used as monotherapy in patients who are not volume depleted. It can be administered once or twice daily with total daily doses ranging from 8-32 mg. Larger doses do not appear to have a greater effect and there is relatively little experience with such doses.

Dosage Forms Tablet, as cilexetil: 4 mg, 8 mg, 16 mg, 32 mg

candesartan and hydrochlorothiazide

(kan de SAR tan & hye droe klor oh THYE a zide)

Synonyms candesartan cilexetil and hydrochlorothiazide

U.S./Canadian Brand Names Atacand HCT™ [US]; Atacand® Plus [Can]

Therapeutic Category Antihypertensive Agent, Combination

Use Treatment of hypertension; combination product should not be used for initial therapy

(Continued)

candesartan and hydrochlorothiazide *(Continued)*

Usual Dosage Oral: Adults: Replacement therapy: Combination product can be substituted for individual agents; maximum therapeutic effect would be expected within 4 weeks

Usual dosage range:

Candesartan: 8-32 mg/day, given once daily or twice daily in divided doses

Hydrochlorothiazide: 12.5-50 mg once daily

Dosage Forms Tablet:

16-12.5: Candesartan 16 mg and hydrochlorothiazide 12.5 mg

32-12.5: Candesartan 32 mg and hydrochlorothiazide 12.5 mg

candesartan cilexetil *see* candesartan *on previous page*

candesartan cilexetil and hydrochlorothiazide *see* candesartan and hydrochlorothiazide *on previous page*

Candida albicans (Monilia) (KAN dee da AL bi kans mo NIL ya)

Synonyms *Monilia* skin test

U.S./Canadian Brand Names Candin® [US]

Therapeutic Category Diagnostic Agent

Use Screen for detection of nonresponsiveness to antigens in immunocompromised individuals

Usual Dosage Intradermal: 0.1 mL, examine reaction site in 24-48 hours; induration of ≥5 mm in diameter is a positive reaction

Dosage Forms Injection, solution: 0.1 mL/dose (1 mL)

Candin® [US] *see Candida albicans (Monilia) on this page*

Candistatin® [Can] *see* nystatin *on page 637*

Canesten® Topical [Can] *see* clotrimazole *on page 218*

Canesten® Vaginal [Can] *see* clotrimazole *on page 218*

Cankaid® [US-OTC] *see* carbamide peroxide *on page 155*

Cantharone® ***(Discontinued)*** *see page 1042*

Cantharone Plus® ***(Discontinued)*** *see page 1042*

Cantil® [US/Can] *see* mepenzolate *on page 552*

Capastat® Sulfate [US] *see* capreomycin *on this page*

capecitabine (kap eh SITE a bean)

U.S./Canadian Brand Names Xeloda® [US/Can]

Therapeutic Category Antineoplastic Agent, Antimetabolite

Use Treatment of metastatic colorectal cancer, metastatic breast cancer

Usual Dosage Oral: Adults: 2500 mg/m²/day in 2 divided doses (~12 hours apart) at the end of a meal for 2 weeks followed by a 1- or 2-week rest period

Dosage Forms Tablet: 150 mg, 500 mg

Capex™ [US/Can] *see* fluocinolone *on page 374*

Capital® and Codeine [US] *see* acetaminophen and codeine *on page 6*

Capitrol® [US/Can] *see* chloroxine *on page 187*

Capoten® [US/Can] *see* captopril *on next page*

Capozide® [US/Can] *see* captopril and hydrochlorothiazide *on page 154*

capreomycin (kap ree oh MYE sin)

Sound-Alike/Look-Alike Issues

Capastat® may be confused with Cepastat®

Synonyms capreomycin sulfate

U.S./Canadian Brand Names Capastat® Sulfate [US]
Therapeutic Category Antibiotic, Miscellaneous
Use Treatment of tuberculosis in conjunction with at least one other antituberculosis agent
Usual Dosage I.M., I.V.:
Infants and Children: 15-30 mg/kg/day, up to 1 g/day maximum
Adults: 1 g/day (not to exceed 20 mg/kg/day) for 60-120 days, followed by 1 g 2-3 times/week
Dosage Forms Injection, powder for reconstitution, as sulfate: 1 g

capreomycin sulfate *see* capreomycin *on previous page*

Capsagel® [US-OTC] *see* capsaicin *on this page*

capsaicin (kap SAY sin)

Sound-Alike/Look-Alike Issues
Zostrix® may be confused with Zestril®, Zovirax®
U.S./Canadian Brand Names Antiphlogistine Rub A-535 Capsaicin [Can]; ArthriCare® for Women Extra Moisturizing [US-OTC]; ArthriCare® for Women Multi-Action [US-OTC]; ArthriCare® for Women Silky Dry [US-OTC]; ArthriCare® for Women Ultra Strength [US-OTC]; Capsagel® [US-OTC]; Capzasin-HP® [US-OTC]; Zostrix®-HP [US-OTC/Can]; Zostrix® [US-OTC/Can]
Therapeutic Category Analgesic, Topical
Use Topical treatment of pain associated with postherpetic neuralgia, rheumatoid arthritis, osteoarthritis, diabetic neuropathy; postsurgical pain
Usual Dosage Children ≥2 years and Adults: Topical: Apply to affected area at least 3-4 times/day; application frequency less than 3-4 times/day prevents the total depletion, inhibition of synthesis, and transport of substance P resulting in decreased clinical efficacy and increased local discomfort
Dosage Forms
Cream, topical: 0.025% (60 g); 0.075% (60 g)
ArthriCare® for Women Multi-Action: 0.025% (42 g) [contains menthol]
ArthriCare® for Women Silky Dry: 0.025% (42 g)
ArthriCare® for Women Ultra Strength: 0.075% (42 g) [contains benzalkonium chloride and menthol]
Capzasin-P®: 0.025% (45 g)
Capzasin-HP®: 0.075% (45 g)
Zostrix®: 0.025% (60 g)
Zostrix®-HP: 0.075% (60 g)
Gel, topical (Capsagel®): 0.025% (60 g); 0.05% (60 g); 0.075% (30 g)
Lotion, topical (ArthriCare® for Women Extra Moisturizing): 0.025% (120 mL, 240 mL)
Patch, topical (TheraPatch® Warm): 0.09% (6s) [DSC]
Stick (Zostrix® HP): 0.075% (21 g) [DSC]

captopril (KAP toe pril)

Sound-Alike/Look-Alike Issues
captopril may be confused with Capitrol®, carvedilol
Synonyms ACE
U.S./Canadian Brand Names Alti-Captopril [Can]; Apo-Capto® [Can]; Capoten® [US/Can]; Gen-Captopril [Can]; Novo-Captopril [Can]; Nu-Capto [Can]; PMS-Captopril [Can]
Therapeutic Category Angiotensin-Converting Enzyme (ACE) Inhibitor
Use Management of hypertension; treatment of congestive heart failure, left ventricular dysfunction after myocardial infarction, diabetic nephropathy
Usual Dosage Note: Dosage must be titrated according to patient's response; use lowest effective dose. Oral:
Infants: Initial: 0.15-0.3 mg/kg/dose; titrate dose upward to maximum of 6 mg/kg/day in 1-4 divided doses; usual required dose: 2.5-6 mg/kg/day
Children: Initial: 0.5 mg/kg/dose; titrate upward to maximum of 6 mg/kg/day in 2-4 divided doses
(Continued)

captopril *(Continued)*

Older Children: Initial: 6.25-12.5 mg/dose every 12-24 hours; titrate upward to maximum of 6 mg/kg/day

Adolescents: Initial: 12.5-25 mg/dose given every 8-12 hours; increase by 25 mg/dose to maximum of 450 mg/day

Adults:

Acute hypertension (urgency/emergency): 12.5-25 mg, may repeat as needed (may be given sublingually, but no therapeutic advantage demonstrated)

Hypertension:

Initial dose: 12.5-25 mg 2-3 times/day; may increase by 12.5-25 mg/dose at 1- to 2-week intervals up to 50 mg 3 times/day; maximum dose: 150 mg 3 times/day; add diuretic before further dosage increases

Usual dose range (JNC 7): 25-100 mg/day in 2 divided doses

Congestive heart failure:

Initial dose: 6.25-12.5 mg 3 times/day in conjunction with cardiac glycoside and diuretic therapy; initial dose depends upon patient's fluid/electrolyte status

Target dose: 50 mg 3 times/day

Maximum dose: 150 mg 3 times/day

LVD after MI: Initial dose: 6.25 mg followed by 12.5 mg 3 times/day; then increase to 25 mg 3 times/day during next several days and then over next several weeks to target dose of 50 mg 3 times/day

Diabetic nephropathy: 25 mg 3 times/day; other antihypertensives often given concurrently

Dosage Forms Tablet: 12.5 mg, 25 mg, 50 mg, 100 mg

captopril and hydrochlorothiazide

(KAP toe pril & hye droe klor oh THYE a zide)

Synonyms hydrochlorothiazide and captopril

U.S./Canadian Brand Names Capozide® [US/Can]

Therapeutic Category Antihypertensive Agent, Combination

Use Management of hypertension and treatment of congestive heart failure

Usual Dosage Oral: Adults: Hypertension, CHF: May be substituted for previously titrated dosages of the individual components; alternatively, may initiate as follows:

Initial: Single tablet (captopril 25 mg/hydrochlorothiazide 15 mg) taken once daily; daily dose of captopril should not exceed 150 mg; daily dose of hydrochlorothiazide should not exceed 50 mg

Dosage Forms Tablet:

25/15: Captopril 25 mg and hydrochlorothiazide 15 mg

25/25: Captopril 25 mg and hydrochlorothiazide 25 mg

50/15: Captopril 50 mg and hydrochlorothiazide 15 mg

50/25: Captopril 50 mg and hydrochlorothiazide 25 mg

Capzasin-HP® [US-OTC] *see* capsaicin *on previous page*

Capzasin-P® *(Discontinued)* *see page 1042*

Carac™ [US] *see* fluorouracil *on page 378*

Carafate® [US] *see* sucralfate *on page 827*

Carapres® [Can] *see* clonidine *on page 215*

carbachol (KAR ba kole)

Sound-Alike/Look-Alike Issues

Isopto® Carbachol may be confused with Isopto® Carpine

Synonyms carbacholine; carbamylcholine chloride

U.S./Canadian Brand Names Carbastat® [Can]; Isopto® Carbachol [US/Can]; Miostat® [US/Can]

Therapeutic Category Cholinergic Agent

Use Lowers intraocular pressure in the treatment of glaucoma; cause miosis during surgery

Usual Dosage Adults:

Ophthalmic: Instill 1-2 drops up to 3 times/day

Intraocular: 0.5 mL instilled into anterior chamber before or after securing sutures

Dosage Forms [DSC] = Discontinued product

Solution, intraocular (Carbastat® [DSC], Miostat®): 0.01% (1.5 mL)

Solution, ophthalmic (Isopto® Carbachol): 1.5% (15 mL); 3% (30 mL) [contains benzalkonium chloride]

carbacholine *see* carbachol *on previous page*

carbamazepine (kar ba MAZ e peen)

Sound-Alike/Look-Alike Issues

Carbatrol® may be confused with Cartrol®

Epitol® may be confused with Epinal®

Tegretol® may be confused with Mebaral®, Tegrin®, Toradol®, Trental®

Synonyms CBZ

U.S./Canadian Brand Names Apo-Carbamazepine® [Can]; Carbatrol® [US]; Epitol® [US]; Gen-Carbamazepine CR [Can]; Novo-Carbamaz [Can]; Nu-Carbamazepine® [Can]; PMS-Carbamazepine [Can]; Taro-Carbamzepine Chewable [Can]; Tegretol® [US/Can]; Tegretol®-XR [US]

Therapeutic Category Anticonvulsant

Use Partial seizures with complex symptomatology (psychomotor, temporal lobe), generalized tonic-clonic seizures (grand mal), mixed seizure patterns

Usual Dosage Oral (dosage must be adjusted according to patient's response and serum concentrations):

Children:

<6 years: Initial: 5 mg/kg/day; dosage may be increased every 5-7 days to 10 mg/kg/day; then up to 20 mg/kg/day if necessary; administer in 2-4 divided doses

6-12 years: Initial: 100 mg twice daily or 10 mg/kg/day in 2 divided doses; increase by 100 mg/day at weekly intervals depending upon response; usual maintenance: 20-30 mg/kg/day in 2-4 divided doses (maximum dose: 1000 mg/day)

Children >12 years and Adults: 200 mg twice daily to start, increase by 200 mg/day at weekly intervals until therapeutic levels achieved; usual dose: 400-1200 mg/day in 2-4 divided doses; maximum dose: 12-15 years: 1000 mg/day, >15 years: 1200 mg/day; some patients have required up to 1.6-2.4 g/day

Trigeminal or glossopharyngeal neuralgia: Initial: 100 mg twice daily with food, gradually increasing in increments of 100 mg twice daily as needed; usual maintenance: 400-800 mg daily in 2 divided doses; maximum dose: 1200 mg/day

Dosage Forms

Capsule, extended release (Carbatrol®): 100 mg, 200 mg, 300 mg

Suspension, oral: 100 mg/5 mL (10 mL, 450 mL)

Tegretol®: 100 mg/5 mL (450 mL) [citrus vanilla flavor]

Tablet (Epitol®, Tegretol®): 200 mg

Tablet, chewable (Tegretol®): 100 mg

Tablet, extended release (Tegretol®-XR): 100 mg, 200 mg, 400 mg

carbamide *see* urea *on page 897*

carbamide peroxide (KAR ba mide per OKS ide)

Synonyms urea peroxide

U.S./Canadian Brand Names Bausch & Lomb® Earwax Removal [US-OTC]; Cankaid® [US-OTC]; Debrox® [US-OTC]; Dent's Ear Wax [US-OTC]; E•R•O [US-OTC]; Gly-Oxide® [US-OTC]; Murine® Ear [US-OTC]; Orajel® Perioseptic® Spot Treatment [US-OTC]

Therapeutic Category Antiinfective Agent, Oral; Otic Agent, Ceruminolytic

(Continued)

carbamide peroxide *(Continued)*

Use Relief of minor inflammation of gums, oral mucosal surfaces and lips including canker sores and dental irritation; emulsify and disperse ear wax

Usual Dosage Children and Adults:

Oral: Solution (should not be used for >7 days): Oral preparation should not be used in children <2 years of age; apply several drops undiluted on affected area 4 times/day after meals and at bedtime; expectorate after 2-3 minutes **or** place 10 drops onto tongue, mix with saliva, swish for several minutes, expectorate

Otic:

Children <12 years: Tilt head sideways and individualize the dose according to patient size; 3 drops (range: 1-5 drops) twice daily for up to 4 days, tip of applicator should not enter ear canal; keep drops in ear for several minutes by keeping head tilted and placing cotton in ear

Children ≥12 years and Adults: Tilt head sideways and instill 5-10 drops twice daily up to 4 days, tip of applicator should not enter ear canal; keep drops in ear for several minutes by keeping head tilted and placing cotton in ear

Dosage Forms

Solution, oral: 10% (60 mL)

Cankaid®: 10% (22 mL) [in anhydrous glycerol]

Gly-Oxide®: 10% (15 mL, 60 mL) [contains glycerin]

Orajel® Perioseptic® Spot Treatment: 15% (13.3 mL) [contains anhydrous glycerin]

Solution, otic: 6.5% (15 mL)

Debrox®: 6.5% (15 mL, 30 mL) [contains propylene glycol]

Bausch & Lomb Earwax Removal, Dent's Ear Wax, E•R•O, Murine® Ear: 6.5% (15 mL)

carbamylcholine chloride *see* carbachol *on page 154*

Carbastat® *(Discontinued)* *see page 1042*

Carbastat® [Can] *see* carbachol *on page 154*

Carbatrol® [US] *see* carbamazepine *on previous page*

Carbaxefed DM RF [US] *see* carbinoxamine, pseudoephedrine, and dextromethorphan *on page 159*

Carbaxefed RF [US] *see* carbinoxamine and pseudoephedrine *on next page*

carbenicillin (kar ben i SIL in)

Synonyms carbenicillin indanyl sodium; carindacillin

U.S./Canadian Brand Names Geocillin® [US]

Therapeutic Category Penicillin

Use Treatment of serious urinary tract infections and prostatitis caused by susceptible gram-negative aerobic bacilli

Usual Dosage Oral:

Children: 30-50 mg/kg/day divided every 6 hours; maximum dose: 2-3 g/day

Adults: 1-2 tablets every 6 hours for urinary tract infections or 2 tablets every 6 hours for prostatitis

Dosage Forms Tablet [film coated]: 382 mg [contains sodium 23 mg/tablet]

carbenicillin indanyl sodium *see* carbenicillin *on this page*

carbetapentane and chlorpheniramine

(kar bay ta PEN tane & klor fen IR a meen)

Synonyms carbetapentane tannate and chlorpheniramine tannate; chlorpheniramine and carbetapentane

U.S./Canadian Brand Names Tannic-12 [US]; Tannic-12 S [US]; Tannihist-12 RF [US]; Tussi-12® [US]; Tussi-12 S™ [US]; Tussizone-12 RF™ [US]

Therapeutic Category Antihistamine/Antitussive

Use Symptomatic relief of cough associated with upper respiratory tract conditions, such as the common cold, bronchitis, bronchial asthma

Usual Dosage Oral:

Children: Based on carbetapentane 30 mg and chlorpheniramine 4 mg per 5 mL suspension:

2-6 years: 2.5-5 mL every 12 hours

>6 years: 5-10 mL every 12 hours

Adults: Based on carbetapentane 60 mg and chlorpheniramine 5 mg per tablet: 1-2 tablets every 12 hours

Dosage Forms

Suspension:

Tannate 12 S: Carbetapentane tannate 30 mg and chlorpheniramine tannate 4 mg per 5 mL (120 mL, 480 mL)

Tannic-12 S: Carbetapentane tannate 30 mg and chlorpheniramine tannate 4 mg per 5 mL (120 mL) [contains benzoic acid; strawberry flavor]

Tannihist-12 RF: Carbetapentane tannate 30 mg and chlorpheniramine tannate 4 mg per 5 mL (120 mL, 480 mL) [strawberry-black currant flavor]

Tussi-12 S™: Carbetapentane tannate 30 mg and chlorpheniramine tannate 4 mg per 5 mL (120 mL) [contains benzoic acid and tartrazine; strawberry-currant flavor]

Tussizone-12 RF™: Carbetapentane tannate 30 mg and chlorpheniramine tannate 4 mg per 5 mL (120 mL, 480 mL) [contains benzoic acid and tartrazine; strawberry-black currant flavor]

Tablet (Tannic-12, Tussi-12®, Tussizone-12 RF™): Carbetapentane tannate 60 mg and chlorpheniramine tannate 5 mg

carbetapentane, ephedrine, phenylephrine, and chlorpheniramine *see* chlorpheniramine, ephedrine, phenylephrine, and carbetapentane *on page 190*

carbetapentane tannate and chlorpheniramine tannate *see* carbetapentane and chlorpheniramine *on previous page*

carbetocin *(Canada only)* (kar BE toe sin)

Therapeutic Category Uteronic Agent

Use For the prevention of uterine atony and postpartum hemorrhage following elective cesarean section under epidural or spinal anesthesia.

Usual Dosage A single I.V. dose of 100 mcg (1 mL) is administered by bolus injection, over 1 minute, only when delivery of the infant has been completed by cesarean section under epidural anesthetic. Carbetocin can be administered either before or after delivery of the placenta

Dosage Forms Injection: 1 mcg/mL (1 mL)

carbidopa (kar bi DOE pa)

U.S./Canadian Brand Names Lodosyn® [US]

Therapeutic Category Anti-Parkinson Agent; Dopaminergic Agent (Anti-Parkinson)

Use Given with levodopa in the treatment of parkinsonism to enable a lower dosage of levodopa to be used and a more rapid response to be obtained and to decrease side-effects

Usual Dosage Oral: Adults: 70-100 mg/day; maximum daily dose: 200 mg

Dosage Forms Tablet: 25 mg

carbidopa and levodopa *see* levodopa and carbidopa *on page 513*

carbidopa, levodopa, and entacapone *see* levodopa, carbidopa, and entacapone *on page 513*

carbinoxamine and pseudoephedrine

(kar bi NOKS a meen & soo doe e FED rin)

Synonyms pseudoephedrine and carbinoxamine

U.S./Canadian Brand Names Andehist NR Drops [US]; Carbaxefed RF [US]; Carboxine-PSE [US]; Hydro-Tussin™-CBX [US]; Palgic®-D [US]; Palgic®-DS [US]; (Continued)

carbinoxamine and pseudoephedrine *(Continued)*

Pediatex™-D [US]; Rondec® Drops [US]; Rondec® Tablets [US]; Rondec-TR® [US]; Sildec [US]

Therapeutic Category Antihistamine/Decongestant Combination

Use Seasonal and perennial allergic rhinitis; vasomotor rhinitis

Usual Dosage Oral:

Children:

Drops (Andehist NR, Carbaxefed RF, Rondec®, Sildec):
- 1-3 months: 0.25 mL 4 times/day
- 3-6 months: 0.5 mL 4 times/day
- 6-12 months: 0.75 mL 4 times/day
- 12-24 months: 1 mL 4 times/day

Liquid (Pediatex™-D):
- 1-3 months: 1.25 mL up to 4 times/day
- 3-6 months: 2.5 mL up to 4 times/day
- 6-9 months: 3.75 mL up to 4 times/day
- 9-18 months: 3.75-5 mL up to 4 times/day
- 18 months to 6 years: 5 mL 3-4 times/day
- >6 years: Refer to Adults dosing

Syrup (Hydro-Tussin™-CBX, Palgic®-DS):
- 1-3 months: 1.25 mL up to 4 times/day
- 3-6 months: 2.5 mL up to 4 times/day
- 6-9 months: 3.75 mL up to 4 times/day
- 9-18 months: 3.75-5 mL up to 4 times/day
- 18 months to 6 years: 5 mL 3-4 times/day
- >6 years: Refer to Adults dosing

Tablet (Rondec®): ≥6 years: Refer to Adults dosing

Tablet, timed release:
- 6-12 years (Palgic®-D): One-half tablet every 12 hours
- ≥12 years (Palgic®-D, Rondec-TR®): Refer to Adults dosing

Adults:
- Liquid (Pediatex™-D): 10 mL 4 times/day
- Syrup (Hydro-Tussin™-CBX, Palgic®-DS): 10 mL 4 times/day
- Tablet (Rondec®): 1 tablet 4 times a day
- Tablet, timed release (Palgic®-D, Rondec-TR®): 1 tablet every 12 hours

Dosage Forms

Liquid (Pediatex™-D): Carbinoxamine maleate 2 mg and pseudoephedrine hydrochloride 20 mg per 5 mL (480 mL) [alcohol free, dye free, sugar free; cotton candy flavor]

Solution, oral drops:
- Andehist NR: Carbinoxamine maleate 1 mg and pseudoephedrine hydrochloride 15 mg per mL (30 mL) [alcohol and sugar free; raspberry flavor]
- Carbaxefed RF, Rondec®: Carbinoxamine maleate 1 mg and pseudoephedrine hydrochloride 15 mg per mL (30 mL) [alcohol free; contains sodium benzoate; cherry flavor]
- Sildec: Carbinoxamine maleate 1 mg and pseudoephedrine hydrochloride 15 mg per mL (30 mL) [raspberry flavor]

Solution: Carbinoxamine maleate 2 mg and pseudoephedrine hydrochloride 25 mg per 5 mL (480 mL)
- Carboxine-PSE: Carbinoxamine maleate 2 mg and pseudoephedrine hydrochloride 20 mg per 5 mL (480 mL) [peach flavor]

Syrup: Carbinoxamine maleate 2 mg and pseudoephedrine hydrochloride 25 mg per 5 mL (480 mL)
- Hydro-Tussin™-CBX, Palgic® DS: Carbinoxamine maleate 2 mg and pseudoephedrine hydrochloride 25 mg per 5 mL (480 mL) [alcohol, dye, and sugar free; strawberry/pineapple flavor]

Tablet (Rondec®): Carbinoxamine maleate 4 mg and pseudoephedrine hydrochloride 60 mg

Tablet, timed release:
Palgic®-D: Carbinoxamine maleate 8 mg and pseudoephedrine hydrochloride 80 mg [dye free]
Rondec-TR®: Carbinoxamine maleate 8 mg and pseudoephedrine hydrochloride 120 mg

carbinoxamine, dextromethorphan, and pseudoephedrine *see* carbinoxamine, pseudoephedrine, and dextromethorphan *on this page*

carbinoxamine, pseudoephedrine, and dextromethorphan

(kar bi NOKS a meen, soo doe e FED rin, & deks troe meth OR fan)

Sound-Alike/Look-Alike Issues
Tussafed® may be confused with Tussafin®

Synonyms carbinoxamine, dextromethorphan, and pseudoephedrine; dextromethorphan, carbinoxamine, and pseudoephedrine; dextromethorphan, pseudoephedrine, and carbinoxamine; pseudoephedrine, carbinoxamine, and dextromethorphan; pseudoephedrine, dextromethorphan, and carbinoxamine

U.S./Canadian Brand Names Andehist DM NR Drops [US]; Carbaxefed DM RF [US]; Decahist-DM [US]; Pediatex™-DM [US]; Rondec®-DM Drops [US]; Slidec-DM [US]; Tussafed® [US]

Therapeutic Category Antihistamine/Decongestant/Antitussive

Use Relief of coughs and upper respiratory symptoms, including nasal congestion, associated with allergy or the common cold

Usual Dosage Oral:
Drops (Rondec®-DM): Infants and Children:
1-3 months: 1/4 mL 4 times/day
3-6 months: 1/2 mL 4 times/day
6-12 months: 3/4 mL 4 times/day
12-24 months: 1 mL 4 times/day
Liquid (Pediatex™-DM):
Children 18 months to 6 years: 2.5 mL 4 times/day
Children 6-12 years: 5 mL 4 times/day
Children ≥12 years and Adults: 10 mL 4 times/day
Syrup (Tussafed®):
Children 18 months to 6 years: 2.5 mL 4 times/day
Children >6 years and Adults: 5 mL 4 times/day

Dosage Forms
Liquid:
Decahist-DM: Carbinoxamine maleate 2 mg, pseudoephedrine hydrochloride 15 mg and dextromethorphan hydrobromide 15 mg per 5 mL (480 mL) [peach flavor]
Pediatex™-DM: Carbinoxamine maleate 2 mg, pseudoephedrine hydrochloride 15 mg and dextromethorphan hydrobromide 15 mg per 5 mL (480 mL) [alcohol free, dye free, sugar free; cotton candy flavor]
Liquid, oral drops: Carbinoxamine maleate 1 mg, pseudoephedrine hydrochloride 15 mg and dextromethorphan hydrobromide 4 mg per mL (30 mL)
Andehist DM NR: Carbinoxamine maleate 1 mg, pseudoephedrine hydrochloride 15 mg and dextromethorphan hydrobromide 4 mg per mL (30 mL) [alcohol and sugar free; grape flavor]
Carbaxefed DM RF: Carbinoxamine maleate 1 mg, pseudoephedrine hydrochloride 15 mg and dextromethorphan hydrobromide 4 mg per mL (30 mL) [alcohol free; grape flavor]
Rondec® DM: Carbinoxamine maleate 1 mg, pseudoephedrine hydrochloride 15 mg and dextromethorphan hydrobromide 4 mg per mL (30 mL) [alcohol free; contains sodium benzoate; grape flavor]
Sildec-DM: Carbinoxamine maleate 1 mg, pseudoephedrine hydrochloride 15 mg and dextromethorphan hydrobromide 4 mg per mL (30 mL)
Syrup, oral (Tussafed®): Carbinoxamine maleate 4 mg, pseudoephedrine hydrochloride 60 mg, and dextromethorphan hydrobromide 15 mg per 5 mL (480 mL) [alcohol and sugar free]

Carbiset® Tablet *(Discontinued)* *see page 1042*

Carbiset-TR® Tablet *(Discontinued)* *see page 1042*

Carbocaine® *(Discontinued)* *see page 1042*

Carbocaine® [Can] *see* mepivacaine *on page 554*

Carbodec® Syrup *(Discontinued)* *see page 1042*

Carbodec® Tablet *(Discontinued)* *see page 1042*

Carbodec® TR Tablet *(Discontinued)* *see page 1042*

carbol-fuchsin solution (kar bol-FOOK sin soe LOO shun)

Synonyms Castellani paint
U.S./Canadian Brand Names Castellani Paint Modified [US]
Therapeutic Category Antifungal Agent
Use Treatment of superficial mycotic infections
Usual Dosage Topical: Apply to affected area 2-4 times/day
Dosage Forms Solution, topical: Phenol 1.5%, alcohol 13%, basic fuchsin, resorcinol, acetone (30 mL, 480 mL)

carbolic acid *see* phenol *on page 687*

Carbolith™ [Can] *see* lithium *on page 525*

carboplatin (KAR boe pla tin)

Sound-Alike/Look-Alike Issues
carboplatin may be confused with cisplatin
Paraplatin® may be confused with Platinol®-AQ
Synonyms CBDCA
U.S./Canadian Brand Names Paraplatin-AQ [Can]; Paraplatin® [US]
Therapeutic Category Antineoplastic Agent
Use Treatment of ovarian cancer
Usual Dosage Refer to individual protocols. IVPB, I.V. infusion, intraperitoneal:
Children:
Solid tumor: 300-600 mg/m^2 once every 4 weeks
Brain tumor: 175 mg/m^2 weekly for 4 weeks every 6 weeks, with a 2-week recovery period between courses
Adults:
Ovarian cancer: 300-360 mg/m^2 I.V. every 3-4 weeks
Autologous BMT: I.V.: 1600 mg/m^2 (total dose) divided over 4 days **requires BMT (ie, FATAL without BMT)**
Dosage Forms
Injection, powder for reconstitution: 50 mg, 150 mg, 450 mg
Injection, solution: 10 mg/mL (5 mL, 15 mL, 45 mL, 60 mL)

carbopol 940 *(Canada only)* (KAR boe pol nine forty)

Therapeutic Category Ophthalmic Agent, Miscellaneous
Use Artificial tear
Usual Dosage Ophthalmic: Use as needed for dry eyes
Dosage Forms Gel, ophthalmic: 20 mg (10 g)

carboprost *see* carboprost tromethamine *on this page*

carboprost tromethamine (KAR boe prost tro METH a meen)

Synonyms carboprost
U.S./Canadian Brand Names Hemabate® [US/Can]
Therapeutic Category Prostaglandin
Use Termination of pregnancy and refractory postpartum uterine bleeding

Usual Dosage I.M.: Adults:

Abortion: Initial: 250 mcg, then 250 mcg at 1½-hour to 3½-hour intervals depending on uterine response; a 500 mcg dose may be given if uterine response is not adequate after several 250 mcg doses; do not exceed 12 mg total dose or continuous administration for >2 days

Refractory postpartum uterine bleeding: Initial: 250 mcg; may repeat at 15- to 90-minute intervals to a total dose of 2 mg

Bladder irrigation for hemorrhagic cystitis (refer to individual protocols): [0.4-1.0 mg/dL as solution] 50 mL instilled into bladder 4 times/day for 1 hour

Dosage Forms Injection, solution: Carboprost 250 mcg and tromethamine 83 mcg per mL (1 mL) [contains benzyl alcohol]

carbose D *see* carboxymethylcellulose *on this page*

Carboxine-PSE [US] *see* carbinoxamine and pseudoephedrine *on page 157*

carboxymethylcellulose (kar boks ee meth il SEL yoo lose)

Synonyms carbose D; carboxymethylcellulose sodium

U.S./Canadian Brand Names Celluvisc™ [Can]; Refresh® Liquigel [US-OTC]; Refresh® Plus [US-OTC/Can]; Tears Again® Gel Drops™ [US-OTC]; Tears Again® Night and Day™ [US-OTC]; Theratears® [US]

Therapeutic Category Ophthalmic Agent, Miscellaneous

Use Artificial tear substitute

Usual Dosage Ophthalmic: Adults: Instill 1-2 drops into eye(s) 3-4 times/day

Dosage Forms

Gel, ophthalmic, as sodium (Tears Again® Night and Day™): 1.5% (3.5 g)

Solution ophthalmic, as sodium:

Refresh Liquigel™: 1% (15 mL) [liquid gel formulation]

Refresh Plus®: 0.5% (0.4 mL) [preservative free; available in packages of 30 or 50]

Refresh Tears®: 0.5% (15 mL)

Tears Again® Gel Drops™: 0.7% (15 mL)

Theratears®: 0.25% (0.6 mL [preservative free], 15 mL)

carboxymethylcellulose sodium *see* carboxymethylcellulose *on this page*

Carcocaps® [US-OTC] *see* charcoal *on page 180*

Cardem® ***(Discontinued)*** *see page 1042*

Cardene® [US] *see* nicardipine *on page 617*

Cardene® I.V. [US] *see* nicardipine *on page 617*

Cardene® SR [US] *see* nicardipine *on page 617*

Cardilate® ***(Discontinued)*** *see page 1042*

Cardio-Green® ***(Discontinued)*** *see page 1042*

Cardioquin® ***(Discontinued)*** *see page 1042*

Cardizem® [US/Can] *see* diltiazem *on page 273*

Cardizem® CD [US/Can] *see* diltiazem *on page 273*

Cardizem® Injection ***(Discontinued)*** *see page 1042*

Cardizem® LA [US] *see* diltiazem *on page 273*

Cardizem® SR ***(Discontinued)*** *see page 1042*

Cardizem® SR [Can] *see* diltiazem *on page 273*

Cardura® [US] *see* doxazosin *on page 291*

Cardura-1™ [Can] *see* doxazosin *on page 291*

Cardura-2™ [Can] *see* doxazosin *on page 291*

Cardura-4™ [Can] *see* doxazosin *on page 291*

CareNate™ 600 [US] *see* vitamins (multiple/prenatal) *on page 927*

Carimune™ [US] *see* immune globulin (intravenous) *on page 468*

carindacillin *see* carbenicillin *on page 156*

carisoprodate *see* carisoprodol *on this page*

carisoprodol (kar i soe PROE dole)

Synonyms carisoprodate; isobamate
U.S./Canadian Brand Names Soma® [US/Can]
Therapeutic Category Skeletal Muscle Relaxant
Use Skeletal muscle relaxant
Usual Dosage Oral: Adults: 350 mg 3-4 times/day; take last dose at bedtime; compound: 1-2 tablets 4 times/day
Dosage Forms Tablet: 350 mg

carisoprodol and aspirin (kar i soe PROE dole & AS pir in)

Synonyms aspirin and carisoprodol
U.S./Canadian Brand Names Soma® Compound [US]
Therapeutic Category Skeletal Muscle Relaxant
Use Skeletal muscle relaxant
Usual Dosage Oral: Adults: 1-2 tablets 4 times/day
Dosage Forms Tablet: Carisoprodol 200 mg and aspirin 325 mg

carisoprodol, aspirin, and codeine

(kar i soe PROE dole, AS pir in, and KOE deen)
Synonyms aspirin, carisoprodol, and codeine; codeine, aspirin, and carisoprodol
U.S./Canadian Brand Names Soma® Compound w/Codeine [US]
Therapeutic Category Skeletal Muscle Relaxant
Controlled Substance C-III
Use Skeletal muscle relaxant
Usual Dosage Oral: Adults: 1 or 2 tablets 4 times/day
Dosage Forms Tablet: Carisoprodol 200 mg, aspirin 325 mg, and codeine phosphate 16 mg

Carmol® 10 [US-OTC] *see* urea *on page 897*

Carmol® 20 [US-OTC] *see* urea *on page 897*

Carmol® 40 [US] *see* urea *on page 897*

Carmol® Deep Cleaning [US] *see* urea *on page 897*

Carmol-HC® [US] *see* urea and hydrocortisone *on page 898*

Carmol® Scalp [US] *see* sulfacetamide *on page 829*

carmustine (kar MUS teen)

Synonyms BCNU; bis-chloronitrosourea; carmustinum; NSC-409962; WR-139021
U.S./Canadian Brand Names BiCNU® [US/Can]; Gliadel® [US]
Therapeutic Category Antineoplastic Agent
Use
Injection: Treatment of brain tumors (glioblastoma, brainstem glioma, medulloblastoma, astrocytoma, ependymoma, and metastatic brain tumors), multiple myeloma, Hodgkin disease, non-Hodgkin lymphomas, melanoma, lung cancer, colon cancer
Wafer (implant): Adjunct to surgery in patients with recurrent glioblastoma multiforme; adjunct to surgery and radiation in patients with high-grade malignant glioma
Usual Dosage
Refer to individual protocols. I.V.:
Children: 200-250 mg/m^2 every 4-6 weeks as a single dose
Adults: Usual dosage (per manufacturer labeling): 150-200 mg/m^2 every 6 weeks as a single dose or divided into daily injections on 2 successive days

Alternative regimens:
75-120 mg/m^2 days 1 and 2 every 6-8 weeks **or**
50-80 mg/m^2 days 1,2,3 every 6-8 weeks
Primary brain cancer:
150-200 mg/m^2 every 6-8 weeks as a single dose **or**
75-120 mg/m^2 days 1 and 2 every 6-8 weeks **or**
20-65 mg/m^2 every 4-6 weeks **or**
0.5-1 mg/kg every 4-6 weeks **or**
40-80 mg/m^2/day for 3 days every 6-8 weeks
Autologous BMT: ALL OF THE FOLLOWING DOSES ARE FATAL WITHOUT BMT
Combination therapy: Up to 300-900 mg/m^2
Single-agent therapy: Up to 200 mg/m^2 (fatal necrosis is associated with doses >2 g/m^2)
Implantation (wafer): Adults: Recurrent glioblastoma multiforme, malignant glioma: Up to 8 wafers may be placed in the resection cavity (total dose 62.6 mg); should the size and shape not accommodate 8 wafers, the maximum number of wafers allowed should be placed

Dosage Forms
Injection, powder for reconstitution (BiCNU®): 100 mg [packaged with 3 mL of absolute alcohol as diluent]
Wafer (Gliadel®): 7.7 mg (8s)

carmustinum *see* carmustine *on previous page*

Carnitor® [US/Can] *see* levocarnitine *on page 512*

Caroid® *(Discontinued)* *see page 1042*

Carrington Antifungal [US-OTC] *see* miconazole *on page 578*

carteolol (KAR tee oh lole)

Sound-Alike/Look-Alike Issues
carteolol may be confused with carvedilol
Cartrol® may be confused with Carbatrol®
Ocupress® may be confused with Ocufen®

Synonyms carteolol hydrochloride

U.S./Canadian Brand Names Cartrol® Oral [Can]; Ocupress® Ophthalmic [Can]

Therapeutic Category Beta-Adrenergic Blocker

Use Management of hypertension; treatment of chronic open-angle glaucoma and intraocular hypertension

Usual Dosage Adults:
Oral: 2.5 mg as a single daily dose, with a maintenance dose normally 2.5-5 mg once daily; doses >10 mg do not increase response and may in fact decrease effect.
Ophthalmic: Instill 1 drop in affected eye(s) twice daily.

Dosage Forms [DSC] = Discontinued product
Solution, ophthalmic, as hydrochloride: 1% (5 mL, 10 mL, 15 mL) [contains benzalkonium chloride]
Ocupress® [DSC]: 1% (5 mL, 10 mL, 15 mL) [contains benzalkonium chloride]
Tablet, as hydrochloride (Cartrol®): 2.5 mg, 5 mg

carteolol hydrochloride *see* carteolol *on this page*

Carter's Little Pills® *(Discontinued)* *see page 1042*

Carter's Little Pills® [Can] *see* bisacodyl *on page 120*

Cartia XT™ [US] *see* diltiazem *on page 273*

Cartrol® *(Discontinued)* *see page 1042*

Cartrol® Oral [Can] *see* carteolol *on this page*

carvedilol (KAR ve dil ole)

Sound-Alike/Look-Alike Issues
carvedilol may be confused with captopril, carteolol

U.S./Canadian Brand Names Coreg® [US/Can]

(Continued)

carvedilol *(Continued)*

Therapeutic Category Beta-Adrenergic Blocker

Use Mild to severe heart failure of ischemic or cardiomyopathic origin (usually in addition to standardized therapy); left ventricular dysfunction following myocardial infarction (MI); management of hypertension

Usual Dosage Oral: Adults: Reduce dosage if heart rate drops to <55 beats/minute.

Hypertension: 6.25 mg twice daily; if tolerated, dose should be maintained for 1-2 weeks, then increased to 12.5 mg twice daily. Dosage may be increased to a maximum of 25 mg twice daily after 1-2 weeks. Maximum dose: 50 mg/day

Congestive heart failure: 3.125 mg twice daily for 2 weeks; if this dose is tolerated, may increase to 6.25 mg twice daily. Double the dose every 2 weeks to the highest dose tolerated by patient. (Prior to initiating therapy, other heart failure medications should be stabilized and fluid retention minimized.)

Maximum recommended dose:

Mild to moderate heart failure: <85 kg: 25 mg twice daily >85 kg: 50 mg twice daily

Severe heart failure: 25 mg twice daily

Left ventricular dysfunction following MI: Initial 3.125-6.25 mg twice daily; increase dosage incrementally (ie, from 6.25 to 12.5 mg twice daily) at intervals of 3-10 days, based on tolerance, to a target dose of 25 mg twice daily. **Note**: Should be initiated only after patient is hemodynamically stable and fluid retention has been minimized.

Dosage Forms Tablet: 3.125 mg, 6.25 mg, 12.5 mg, 25 mg

Casodex® [US/Can] *see* bicalutamide *on page 119*

caspofungin (kas poe FUN jin)

Synonyms caspofungin acetate

U.S./Canadian Brand Names Cancidas® [US/Can]

Therapeutic Category Antifungal Agent, Systemic

Use Treatment of invasive *Aspergillus* infections in patients who are refractory or intolerant of other therapy; treatment of candidemia and other *Candida* infections (intra-abdominal abscesses, esophageal, peritonitis, pleural space); empirical treatment for presumed fungal infections in febrile neutropenic patient

Usual Dosage I.V.:

Children: Safety and efficacy in pediatric patients have not been established

Adults: **Note:** Duration of caspofungin treatment should be determined by patient status and clinical response. Empiric therapy should be given until neutropenia resolves. In patients with positive cultures, treatment should continue until 14 days after last positive culture. In neutropenic patients, treatment should be given at least 7 days after both signs and symptoms of infection **and** neutropenia resolve.

Invasive *Aspergillus*: Initial dose: 70 mg on day 1; subsequent dosing: 50 mg/day

Invasive candidiasis: Initial dose: 70 mg on day 1; subsequent dosing: 50 mg/day

Empiric therapy: Initial dose: 70 mg on day 1; subsequent dosing: 50 mg/day; may increase up to 70 mg/day if tolerated, but clinical response is inadequate

Esophageal candidiasis: 50 mg/day; **Note:** The majority of patients studied for this indication also had oropharyngeal involvement.

Concomitant use of an enzyme inducer:

Patients receiving rifampin: 70 mg caspofungin daily

Patients receiving carbamazepine, dexamethasone, efavirenz, nevirapine, **or** phenytoin (and possibly other enzyme inducers) may require an increased daily dose of caspofungin (70 mg/day).

Dosage Forms Injection, powder for reconstitution, as acetate: 50 mg, 70 mg

caspofungin acetate *see* caspofungin *on this page*

Castellani paint *see* carbol-fuchsin solution *on page 160*

Castellani Paint Modified [US] *see* carbol-fuchsin solution *on page 160*

castor oil (KAS tor oyl)

Synonyms oleum ricini

U.S./Canadian Brand Names Purge® [US-OTC]

Therapeutic Category Laxative

Use Preparation for rectal or bowel examination or surgery; rarely used to relieve constipation; also applied to skin as emollient and protectant

Usual Dosage Oral: Oil:

Children 2-11 years: 5-15 mL as a single dose

Children ≥12 years and Adults: 15-60 mL as a single dose

Dosage Forms [DSC] = Discontinued product

Emulsion, oral (Emulsoil® [DSC]): 95% (60 mL)

Oil, oral: 100% (60 mL, 120 mL, 480 mL, 3840 mL)

Purge®: 95% (30 mL, 60 mL) [lemon flavor]

castor oil, trypsin, and balsam peru *see* trypsin, balsam peru, and castor oil *on page 892*

Cataflam® [US/Can] *see* diclofenac *on page 266*

Catapres® [US] *see* clonidine *on page 215*

Catapres-TTS® [US] *see* clonidine *on page 215*

Catarase® 1:5000 *(Discontinued)* *see page 1042*

Cathflo™ Activase® [US/Can] *see* alteplase *on page 36*

Caverject® [US/Can] *see* alprostadil *on page 35*

Caverject® Impulse™ [Can] *see* alprostadil *on page 35*

CB-1348 *see* chlorambucil *on page 182*

CBDCA *see* carboplatin *on page 160*

CBZ *see* carbamazepine *on page 155*

CCNU *see* lomustine *on page 527*

C-Crystals® *(Discontinued)* *see page 1042*

2-CdA *see* cladribine *on page 207*

CDDP *see* cisplatin *on page 205*

CDX *see* bicalutamide *on page 119*

Cebid® *(Discontinued)* *see page 1042*

Ceclor® [US/Can] *see* cefaclor *on this page*

Ceclor® CD [US] *see* cefaclor *on this page*

Cecon® [US-OTC] *see* ascorbic acid *on page 79*

Cedax® [US] *see* ceftibuten *on page 172*

Cedilanid-D® Injection *(Discontinued)* *see page 1042*

Cedocard®-SR [Can] *see* isosorbide dinitrate *on page 488*

CEE *see* estrogens (conjugated/equine) *on page 329*

CeeNU® [US/Can] *see* lomustine *on page 527*

Ceepryn® *(Discontinued)* *see page 1042*

cefaclor (SEF a klor)

Sound-Alike/Look-Alike Issues

cefaclor may be confused with cephalexin

U.S./Canadian Brand Names Apo-Cefaclor® [Can]; Ceclor® [US/Can]; Ceclor® CD [US]; Novo-Cefaclor [Can]; Nu-Cefaclor [Can]; PMS-Cefaclor [Can]; Raniclor™ [US]

Therapeutic Category Cephalosporin (Second Generation)

(Continued)

cefaclor *(Continued)*

Use Treatment of susceptible bacterial infections including otitis media, lower respiratory tract infections, acute exacerbations of chronic bronchitis, pharyngitis and tonsillitis, urinary tract infections, skin and skin structure infections

Usual Dosage Oral:

Children >1 month: Dosing range: 20-40 mg/kg/day divided every 8-12 hours; maximum dose: 1 g/day

Otitis media: 40 mg/kg/day divided every 12 hours

Pharyngitis: 20 mg/kg/day divided every 12 hours

Adults: Dosing range: 250-500 mg every 8 hours

Extended release tablets:

Acute bacterial exacerbations of or secondary infections with chronic bronchitis: 500 mg every 12 hours for 7 days

Pharyngitis, tonsillitis, uncomplicated skin and skin structure infections: 375 mg every 12 hours for 10 days

Dosage Forms

Capsule (Ceclor®): 250 mg, 500 mg

Powder for oral suspension: 125 mg/5 mL (75 mL, 150 mL); 187 mg/5 mL (50 mL, 100 mL); 250 mg/5 mL (75 mL, 150 mL); 375 mg/5 mL (50 mL, 100 mL)

Ceclor®: 125 mg/5 mL (150 mL); 187 mg/5 mL (100 mL); 250 mg/5 mL (75 mL, 150 mL); 375 mg/5 mL (100 mL)

Tablet, chewable (Raniclor™): 125 mg [contains phenylalanine 2.8 mg; fruity flavor], 187 mg [contains phenylalanine 4.2 mg; fruity flavor], 250 mg [contains phenylalanine 5.6 mg; fruity flavor], 375 mg [contains phenylalanine 8.4 mg; fruity flavor]

Tablet, extended release (Ceclor® CD): 375 mg, 500 mg

cefadroxil (sef a DROKS il)

Synonyms cefadroxil monohydrate

U.S./Canadian Brand Names Apo-Cefadroxil® [Can]; Duricef® [US/Can]; Novo-Cefadroxil [Can]

Therapeutic Category Cephalosporin (First Generation)

Use Treatment of susceptible bacterial infections, including those caused by group A beta-hemolytic *Streptococcus*; prophylaxis against bacterial endocarditis in patients who are allergic to penicillin and undergoing surgical or dental procedures

Usual Dosage Oral:

Children: 30 mg/kg/day divided twice daily up to a maximum of 2 g/day

Adults: 1-2 g/day in 2 divided doses

Prophylaxis against bacterial endocarditis:

Children: 50 mg/kg 1 hour prior to the procedure

Adults: 2 g 1 hour prior to the procedure

Dosage Forms

Capsule, as monohydrate: 500 mg

Powder for oral suspension, as monohydrate: 250 mg/5 mL (50 mL, 100 mL); 500 mg/5 mL (75 mL, 100 mL) [contains sodium benzoate; orange-pineapple flavor]

Tablet, as monohydrate: 1 g

cefadroxil monohydrate *see* cefadroxil *on this page*

Cefadyl® *(Discontinued)* *see page 1042*

Cefanex® *(Discontinued)* *see page 1042*

cefazolin (sef A zoe lin)

Sound-Alike/Look-Alike Issues

cefazolin may be confused with cefprozil, cephalexin, cephalothin

Synonyms cefazolin sodium

U.S./Canadian Brand Names Ancef® [US]

Therapeutic Category Cephalosporin (First Generation)

Use Treatment of respiratory tract, skin and skin structure, genital, urinary tract, biliary tract, bone and joint infections, and septicemia due to susceptible gram-positive cocci (except enterococcus); some gram-negative bacilli including *E. coli*, *Proteus*, and *Klebsiella* may be susceptible; perioperative prophylaxis

Usual Dosage I.M., I.V.:

Children >1 month: 25-100 mg/kg/day divided every 6-8 hours; maximum: 6 g/day

Adults: 250 mg to 2 g every 6-12 (usually 8) hours, depending on severity of infection; maximum dose: 12 g/day

Dosage Forms

Infusion [premixed in D_5W]: 500 mg (50 mL); 1 g (50 mL)

Injection, powder for reconstitution: 500 mg, 1 g, 10 g, 20 g

Ancef®: 1 g, 10 g

cefazolin sodium *see* cefazolin *on previous page*

cefdinir (SEF di ner)

Synonyms CFDN

U.S./Canadian Brand Names Omnicef® [US/Can]

Therapeutic Category Cephalosporin (Third Generation)

Use Treatment of community-acquired pneumonia, acute exacerbations of chronic bronchitis, acute bacterial otitis media, acute maxillary sinusitis, pharyngitis/tonsillitis, and uncomplicated skin and skin structure infections.

Usual Dosage Oral:

Children: 7 mg/kg/dose twice daily for 5-10 days or 14 mg/kg/dose once daily for 10 days (maximum: 600 mg/day)

Adolescents and Adults: 300 mg twice daily or 600 mg once daily for 10 days

Dosage Forms

Capsule: 300 mg

Powder for oral suspension: 125 mg/5 mL (60 mL, 100 mL) [contains sodium benzoate; strawberry flavor]

cefditoren (sef de TOR en)

Synonyms cefditoren pivoxil

U.S./Canadian Brand Names Spectracef™ [US]

Therapeutic Category Antibiotic, Cephalosporin

Use Treatment of acute bacterial exacerbation of chronic bronchitis or community-acquired pneumonia (due to susceptible organisms including *Haemophilus influenzae, Haemophilus parainfluenzae, Streptococcus pneumoniae*-penicillin susceptible only, *Moraxella catarrhalis*); pharyngitis or tonsillitis (*Streptococcus pyogenes*); and uncomplicated skin and skin-structure infections (*Staphylococcus aureus*-not MRSA, *Streptococcus pyogenes*)

Usual Dosage Oral: Children ≥12 years and Adults:

Acute bacterial exacerbation of chronic bronchitis: 400 mg twice daily for 10 days

Community-acquired pneumonia: 400 mg twice daily for 14 days

Pharyngitis, tonsillitis, uncomplicated skin and skin structure infections: 200 mg twice daily for 10 days

Dosage Forms Tablet, as pivoxil: 200 mg [equivalent to cefditoren; contains sodium caseinate]

cefditoren pivoxil *see* cefditoren *on this page*

cefepime (SEF e pim)

Synonyms cefepime hydrochloride

U.S./Canadian Brand Names Maxipime® [US/Can]

Therapeutic Category Cephalosporin (Fourth Generation)

(Continued)

cefepime *(Continued)*

Use Treatment of uncomplicated and complicated urinary tract infections, including pyelonephritis caused by typical urinary tract pathogens; monotherapy for febrile neutropenia; uncomplicated skin and skin structure infections caused by *Streptococcus pyogenes*; moderate to severe pneumonia caused by pneumococcus, *Pseudomonas aeruginosa*, and other gram-negative organisms; complicated intra-abdominal infections (in combination with metronidazole). Also active against methicillin-susceptible staphylococci, *Enterobacter* sp, and many other gram-negative bacilli.

Children 2 months to 16 years: Empiric therapy of febrile neutropenia patients, uncomplicated skin/soft tissue infections, pneumonia, and uncomplicated/complicated urinary tract infections.

Usual Dosage

Children:

Febrile neutropenia: I.V.: 50 mg/kg every 8 hours for 7-10 days

Uncomplicated skin/soft tissue infections, pneumonia, and complicated/uncomplicated UTI: I.V.: 50 mg/kg twice daily

Adults:

Most infections: I.V.: 1-2 g every 12 hours for 7-10 days; higher doses or more frequent administration may be required in pseudomonal infections

Urinary tract infections, mild to moderate: I.M., I.V.: 500-1000 mg every 12 hours

Monotherapy for febrile neutropenic patients: I.V.: 2 g every 8 hours for 7 days or until the neutropenia resolves

Dosage Forms Injection, powder for reconstitution, as hydrochloride: 500 mg, 1 g, 2 g

cefepime hydrochloride *see* cefepime *on previous page*

cefixime (sef IKS eem)

Sound-Alike/Look-Alike Issues

Suprax® may be confused with Sporanox®, Surbex®

U.S./Canadian Brand Names Suprax® [US/Can]

Therapeutic Category Cephalosporin (Third Generation)

Use Treatment of urinary tract infections, otitis media, respiratory infections due to susceptible organisms including *S. pneumoniae* and *S. pyogenes, H. influenzae* and many Enterobacteriaceae; uncomplicated cervical/urethral gonorrhea due to *N. gonorrhoeae*

Usual Dosage Oral:

Children ≥6 months: 8 mg/kg/day divided every 12-24 hours

Children >50 kg or >12 years and Adults: 400 mg/day divided every 12-24 hours

Uncomplicated cervical/urethral gonorrhea due to *N. gonorrhoeae*: 400 mg as a single dose

For *S. pyogenes* infections, treat for 10 days; use suspension for otitis media due to increased peak serum levels as compared to tablet form

Dosage Forms

Powder for oral suspension: 100 mg/5 mL (50 mL, 75 mL, 100 mL) [contains sodium benzoate; strawberry flavor]

Tablet [film coated]: 400 mg

Cefizox® [US/Can] *see* ceftizoxime *on page 172*

Cefobid® *(Discontinued)* *see page 1042*

Cefotan® [US/Can] *see* cefotetan *on next page*

cefotaxime (sef oh TAKS eem)

Sound-Alike/Look-Alike Issues

cefotaxime may be confused with cefoxitin, ceftizoxime, cefuroxime

Synonyms cefotaxime sodium

U.S./Canadian Brand Names Claforan® [US/Can]

Therapeutic Category Cephalosporin (Third Generation)

Use Treatment of susceptible infection in respiratory tract, skin and skin structure, bone and joint, urinary tract, gynecologic as well as septicemia, and documented or suspected meningitis. Active against most gram-negative bacilli (not *Pseudomonas*) and gram-positive cocci (not enterococcus). Active against many penicillin-resistant pneumococci.

Usual Dosage

Infants and Children 1 month to 12 years: I.M., I.V.: <50 kg: 50-180 mg/kg/day in divided doses every 4-6 hours

Meningitis: 200 mg/kg/day in divided doses every 6 hours

Children >12 years and Adults:

Uncomplicated infections: I.M., I.V.: 1 g every 12 hours

Moderate/severe infections: I.M., I.V.: 1-2 g every 8 hours

Infections commonly needing higher doses (eg, septicemia): I.V.: 2 g every 6-8 hours

Life-threatening infections: I.V.: 2 g every 4 hours

Preop: I.M., I.V.: 1 g 30-90 minutes before surgery

C-section: 1 g as soon as the umbilical cord is clamped, then 1 g I.M., I.V. at 6- and 12-hour intervals

Dosage Forms

Infusion, as sodium [premixed in D_5W] (Claforan®): 1 g (50 mL); 2 g (50 mL)

Injection, powder for reconstitution, as sodium: 500 mg, 1 g, 2 g, 10 g, 20 g

Claforan®: 500 mg, 1 g, 2 g, 10 g [contains sodium 50.5 mg (2.2 mEq) per cefotaxime 1 g]

cefotaxime sodium *see* cefotaxime *on previous page*

cefotetan (SEF oh tee tan)

Sound-Alike/Look-Alike Issues

cefotetan may be confused with cefoxitin, Ceftin®

Cefotan® may be confused with Ceftin®

Synonyms cefotetan disodium

U.S./Canadian Brand Names Cefotan® [US/Can]

Therapeutic Category Cephalosporin (Second Generation)

Use Used predominantly for respiratory tract, skin and skin structure, bone and joint, urinary tract and gynecologic as well as septicemia; surgical prophylaxis; intra-abdominal infections and other mixed infections; active against gram-negative enteric bacilli including *E. coli*, *Klebsiella*, and *Proteus*; less active against staphylococci and streptococci than first generation cephalosporins, but active against anaerobes including *Bacteroides fragilis*

Usual Dosage

Adolescents and Adults: I.V.: Pelvic inflammatory disease: 2 g every 12 hours; used in combination with doxycycline

Adults: I.M., I.V.: 1-6 g/day in divided doses every 12 hours; usual dose: 1-2 g every 12 hours for 5-10 days; 1-2 g may be given every 24 hours for urinary tract infection

Preoperative prophylaxis: I.M., I.V.: 1-2 g 30-60 minutes prior to surgery; when used for cesarean section, dose should be given as soon as umbilical cord is clamped

Dosage Forms

Infusion [premixed iso-osmotic solution]: 1 g (50 mL); 2 g (50 mL) [contains sodium 80 mg/g (3.5 mEq/g)]

Injection, powder for reconstitution: 1 g, 2 g, 10 g [contains sodium 80 mg/g (3.5 mEq/g)]

cefotetan disodium *see* cefotetan *on this page*

cefoxitin (se FOKS i tin)

Sound-Alike/Look-Alike Issues

cefoxitin may be confused with cefotaxime, cefotetan, Cytoxan®

Mefoxin® may be confused with Lanoxin®

Synonyms cefoxitin sodium

(Continued)

cefoxitin *(Continued)*

U.S./Canadian Brand Names Mefoxin® [US/Can]

Therapeutic Category Cephalosporin (Second Generation)

Use Less active against staphylococci and streptococci than first generation cephalosporins, but active against anaerobes including *Bacteroides fragilis*; active against gram-negative enteric bacilli including *E. coli*, *Klebsiella*, and *Proteus*; used predominantly for respiratory tract, skin and skin structure, bone and joint, urinary tract and gynecologic as well as septicemia; surgical prophylaxis; intra-abdominal infections and other mixed infections; indicated for bacterial *Eikenella corrodens* infections

Usual Dosage

Infants >3 months and Children: I.M., I.V.:

Mild to moderate infection: 80-100 mg/kg/day in divided doses every 4-6 hours

Severe infection: 100-160 mg/kg/day in divided doses every 4-6 hours; maximum dose: 12 g/day

Perioperative prophylaxis: 30-40 mg/kg 30-60 minutes prior to surgery followed by 30-40 mg/kg/dose every 6 hours for no more than 24 hours after surgery depending on the procedure

Adolescents and Adults: I.M., I.V.: Perioperative prophylaxis: 1-2 g 30-60 minutes prior to surgery followed by 1-2 g every 6-8 hours for no more than 24 hours after surgery depending on the procedure

Adults: I.M., I.V.: 1-2 g every 6-8 hours (I.M. injection is painful); up to 12 g/day

Pelvic inflammatory disease:

Inpatients: I.V.: 2 g every 6 hours **plus** doxycycline 100 mg I.V. or 100 mg orally every 12 hours until improved, followed by doxycycline 100 mg orally twice daily to complete 14 days

Outpatients: I.M.: 2 g **plus** probenecid 1 g orally as a single dose, followed by doxycycline 100 mg orally twice daily for 14 days

Dosage Forms

Infusion, as sodium [premixed iso-osmotic solution]: 1 g (50 mL); 2 g (50 mL) [contains sodium 53.8 mg/g (2.3 mEq/g)]

Injection, powder for reconstitution, as sodium: 1 g, 2 g, 10 g [contains sodium 53.8 mg/g (2.3 mEq/g)]

cefoxitin sodium *see* cefoxitin *on previous page*

cefpodoxime (sef pode OKS eem)

Sound-Alike/Look-Alike Issues

Vantin® may be confused with Ventolin®

Synonyms cefpodoxime proxetil

U.S./Canadian Brand Names Vantin® [US/Can]

Therapeutic Category Cephalosporin (Second Generation)

Use Treatment of susceptible acute, community-acquired pneumonia caused by *S. pneumoniae* or nonbeta-lactamase producing *H. influenzae*; acute uncomplicated gonorrhea caused by *N. gonorrhoeae*; uncomplicated skin and skin structure infections caused by *S. aureus* or *S. pyogenes*; acute otitis media caused by *S. pneumoniae*, *H. influenzae*, or *M. catarrhalis*; pharyngitis or tonsillitis; and uncomplicated urinary tract infections caused by *E. coli*, *Klebsiella*, and *Proteus*

Usual Dosage Oral:

Children 2 months to 12 years:

Acute otitis media: 10 mg/kg/day divided every 12 hours (400 mg/day) for 5 days (maximum: 200 mg/dose)

Acute maxillary sinusitis: 10 mg/kg/day divided every 12 hours for 10 days (maximum: 200 mg/dose)

Pharyngitis/tonsillitis: 10 mg/kg/day in 2 divided doses for 5-10 days (maximum: 100 mg/dose)

Children ≥12 years and Adults:

Acute community-acquired pneumonia and bacterial exacerbations of chronic bronchitis: 200 mg every 12 hours for 14 days and 10 days, respectively

Acute maxillary sinusitis: 200 mg every 12 hours for 10 days
Skin and skin structure: 400 mg every 12 hours for 7-14 days
Uncomplicated gonorrhea (male and female) and rectal gonococcal infections (female): 200 mg as a single dose
Pharyngitis/tonsillitis: 100 mg every 12 hours for 5-10 days
Uncomplicated urinary tract infection: 100 mg every 12 hours for 7 days

Dosage Forms
Granules for oral suspension: 50 mg/5 mL (50 mL, 75 mL, 100 mL); 100 mg/5 mL (50 mL, 75 mL, 100 mL) [contains sodium benzoate; lemon creme flavor]
Tablet [film coated]: 100 mg, 200 mg

cefpodoxime proxetil *see* cefpodoxime *on previous page*

cefprozil (sef PROE zil)

Sound-Alike/Look-Alike Issues
cefprozil may be confused with cefazolin, cefuroxime
Cefzil® may be confused with Cefol®, Ceftin®, Kefzol®

U.S./Canadian Brand Names Cefzil® [US/Can]

Therapeutic Category Cephalosporin (Second Generation)

Use Treatment of otitis media and infections involving the respiratory tract and skin and skin structure; active against methicillin-sensitive staphylococci, many streptococci, and various gram-negative bacilli including *E. coli*, some *Klebsiella*, *P. mirabilis*, *H. influenzae*, and *Moraxella*.

Usual Dosage Oral:
Infants and Children >6 months to 12 years: Otitis media: 15 mg/kg every 12 hours for 10 days
Pharyngitis/tonsillitis:
Children 2-12 years: 7.5 -15 mg/kg/day divided every 12 hours for 10 days (administer for >10 days if due to *S. pyogenes*); maximum: 1 g/day
Children >13 years and Adults: 500 mg every 24 hours for 10 days
Uncomplicated skin and skin structure infections:
Children 2-12 years: 20 mg/kg every 24 hours for 10 days; maximum: 1 g/day
Children >13 years and Adults: 250 mg every 12 hours, or 500 mg every 12-24 hours for 10 days
Secondary bacterial infection of acute bronchitis or acute bacterial exacerbation of chronic bronchitis: 500 mg every 12 hours for 10 days

Dosage Forms
Powder for oral suspension, as anhydrous: 125 mg/5 mL (50 mL, 75 mL, 100 mL); 250 mg/5 mL (50 mL, 75 mL, 100 mL) [contains phenylalanine 28 mg/5 mL and sodium benzoate; bubblegum flavor]
Tablet, as anhydrous: 250 mg, 500 mg

ceftazidime (SEF tay zi deem)

Sound-Alike/Look-Alike Issues
ceftazidime may be confused with ceftizoxime
Tazicef® may be confused with Tazidime®

U.S./Canadian Brand Names Fortaz® [US/Can]; Tazicef® [US]

Therapeutic Category Cephalosporin (Third Generation)

Use Treatment of documented susceptible *Pseudomonas aeruginosa* infection and infections due to other susceptible aerobic gram-negative organisms; empiric therapy of a febrile, granulocytopenic patient

Usual Dosage
Infants and Children 1 month to 12 years: I.V.: 30-50 mg/kg/dose every 8 hours; maximum dose: 6 g/day
Adults: I.M., I.V.: 500 mg to 2 g every 8-12 hours
Urinary tract infections: 250-500 mg every 12 hours

Dosage Forms [DSC] = Discontinued product
Infusion, as sodium [premixed iso-osmotic solution] (Fortaz®): 1 g (50 mL); 2 g (50 mL)
(Continued)

ceftazidime *(Continued)*

Injection, powder for reconstitution:
Ceptaz® [DSC]: 10 g [L-arginine formulation]
Fortaz®: 500 mg, 1 g, 2 g, 6 g [contains sodium carbonate]
Tazicef®: 1 g, 2 g, 6 g [contains sodium carbonate]

ceftibuten (sef TYE byoo ten)

U.S./Canadian Brand Names Cedax® [US]

Therapeutic Category Cephalosporin (Third Generation)

Use Oral cephalosporin for treatment of bronchitis, otitis media, and pharyngitis/tonsillitis due to *H. influenzae* and *M. catarrhalis*, both beta-lactamase-producing and nonproducing strains, as well as *S. pneumoniae* (weak) and *S. pyogenes*

Usual Dosage Oral:
Children <12 years: 9 mg/kg/day for 10 days; maximum daily dose: 400 mg
Children ≥12 years and Adults: 400 mg once daily for 10 days; maximum: 400 mg

Dosage Forms
Capsule: 400 mg
Powder for oral suspension: 90 mg/5 mL (30 mL, 60 mL, 120 mL) [contains sodium benzoate; cherry flavor]

Ceftin® [US/Can] *see* cefuroxime *on next page*

Ceftin® Tablet 125 mg *(Discontinued)* *see page 1042*

ceftizoxime (sef ti ZOKS eem)

Sound-Alike/Look-Alike Issues
ceftizoxime may be confused with cefotaxime, ceftazidime, cefuroxime

Synonyms ceftizoxime sodium

U.S./Canadian Brand Names Cefizox® [US/Can]

Therapeutic Category Cephalosporin (Third Generation)

Use Treatment of susceptible bacterial infection, mainly respiratory tract, skin and skin structure, bone and joint, urinary tract and gynecologic, as well as septicemia; active against many gram-negative bacilli (not *Pseudomonas*), some gram-positive cocci (not *Enterococcus*), and some anaerobes

Usual Dosage I.M., I.V.:
Children ≥6 months: 150-200 mg/kg/day divided every 6-8 hours (maximum of 12 g/24 hours)
Adults: 1-2 g every 8-12 hours, up to 2 g every 4 hours or 4 g every 8 hours for life-threatening infections

Dosage Forms
Infusion [premixed iso-osmotic solution]: 1 g (50 mL); 2 g (50 mL)
Injection, powder for reconstitution: 1 g, 2 g, 10 g

ceftizoxime sodium *see* ceftizoxime *on this page*

ceftriaxone (sef trye AKS one)

Sound-Alike/Look-Alike Issues
Rocephin® may be confused with Roferon®

Synonyms ceftriaxone sodium

U.S./Canadian Brand Names Rocephin® [US/Can]

Therapeutic Category Cephalosporin (Third Generation)

Use Treatment of lower respiratory tract infections, acute bacterial otitis media, skin and skin structure infections, bone and joint infections, intra-abdominal and urinary tract infections, pelvic inflammatory disease (PID), uncomplicated gonorrhea, bacterial septicemia, and meningitis; used in surgical prophylaxis

Usual Dosage
Infants and Children:
Usual dose: I.M., I.V.:
Mild-to-moderate infections: 50-75 mg/kg/day in 1-2 divided doses every 12-24 hours (maximum: 2 g/day); continue until at least 2 days after signs and symptoms of infection have resolved
Serious infections: 80-100 mg/kg/day in 1-2 divided doses (maximum: 4 g/day)
Gonococcal infection, uncomplicated: I.M.: 125 mg in a single dose
Meningitis: I.M., I.V.:
Uncomplicated: Loading dose of 100 mg/kg (maximum: 4 g), followed by 100 mg/kg/day divided every 12-24 hours (maximum: 4 g/day); usual duration of treatment is 7-14 days
Gonococcal, complicated: <45 kg: 50 mg/kg/day given every 12 hours (maximum: 2 g/day); usual duration of treatment is 10-14 days >45 kg: I.V.: 1-2 g every 12 hours; usual duration of treatment is 10-14 days
Otitis media: I.M., I.V.:
Acute: 50 mg/kg in a single dose (maximum: 1 g)
Adults: Usual dose: I.M., I.V.: 1-2 g every 12-24 hours, depending on the type and severity of infection
Gonococcal infection, uncomplicated: I.M.: 125-250 mg in a single dose
PID: I.M.: 250 mg in a single dose
Surgical prophylaxis: I.V.: 1 g 30 minutes to 2 hours before surgery

Dosage Forms Note: Contains sodium 83 mg (3.6 mEq) per ceftriaxone 1 g
Infusion [premixed in dextrose]: 1 g (50 mL); 2 g (50 mL)
Injection, powder for reconstitution: 250 mg, 500 mg, 1 g, 2 g, 10 g

ceftriaxone sodium *see* ceftriaxone *on previous page*

cefuroxime (se fyoor OKS eem)

Sound-Alike/Look-Alike Issues
cefuroxime may be confused with cefotaxime, cefprozil, ceftizoxime, deferoxamine
Ceftin® may be confused with Cefotan®, cefotetan, Cefzil®, Cipro®
Zinacef® may be confused with Zithromax®

Synonyms cefuroxime axetil; cefuroxime sodium

U.S./Canadian Brand Names Apo-Cefuroxime® [Can]; Ceftin® [US/Can]; Kefurox® [Can]; ratio-Cefuroxime [Can]; Zinacef® [US/Can]

Therapeutic Category Cephalosporin (Second Generation)

Use Treatment of infections caused by staphylococci, group B streptococci, *H. influenzae* (type A and B), *E. coli*, *Enterobacter*, *Salmonella*, and *Klebsiella*; treatment of susceptible infections of the lower respiratory tract, otitis media, urinary tract, skin and soft tissue, bone and joint, sepsis and gonorrhea

Usual Dosage Note: Cefuroxime axetil film-coated tablets and oral suspension are not bioequivalent and are not substitutable on a mg/mg basis
Children ≥3 months to 12 years:
Pharyngitis, tonsillitis: Oral:
Suspension: 20 mg/kg/day (maximum: 500 mg/day) in 2 divided doses for 10 days
Tablet: 125 mg every 12 hours for 10 days
Acute otitis media, impetigo: Oral:
Suspension: 30 mg/kg/day (maximum: 1 g/day) in 2 divided doses for 10 days
Tablet: 250 mg twice daily for 10 days
I.M., I.V.: 75-150 mg/kg/day divided every 8 hours; maximum dose: 6 g/day
Meningitis: Not recommended (doses of 200-240 mg/kg/day divided every 6-8 hours have been used); maximum dose: 9 g/day
Acute bacterial maxillary sinusitis:
Suspension: 30 mg/kg/day in 2 divided doses for 10 days; maximum dose: 1 g/day
Tablet: 250 mg twice daily for 10 days
Children ≥13 years and Adults:
Oral: 250-500 mg twice daily for 10 days (5 days in selected patients with acute bronchitis)
(Continued)

cefuroxime *(Continued)*

Uncomplicated urinary tract infection: 125-250 mg every 12 hours for 7-10 days
Uncomplicated gonorrhea: 1 g as a single dose
Early Lyme disease: 500 mg twice daily for 20 days
I.M., I.V.: 750 mg to 1.5 g/dose every 8 hours or 100-150 mg/kg/day in divided doses every 6-8 hours; maximum: 6 g/24 hours

Dosage Forms [DSC] = Discontinued product
Infusion, as sodium [premixed] (Zinacef®): 750 mg (50 mL); 1.5 g (50 mL) [contains sodium 4.8 mEq (111 mg) per 750 mg]
Injection, powder for reconstitution, as sodium (Zinacef®): 750 mg, 1.5 g, 7.5 g [contains sodium 4.8 mEq (111 mg) per 750 mg]
Powder for oral suspension, as axetil (Ceftin®): 125 mg/5 mL (100 mL) [contains phenylalanine 11.8 mg/5 mL; tutti-frutti flavor]; 250 mg/5 mL (50 mL, 100 mL) [contains phenylalanine 25.2 mg/5 mL; tutti-frutti flavor]
Tablet, as axetil: 250 mg, 500 mg
Ceftin®: 250 mg, 500 mg

cefuroxime axetil *see* cefuroxime *on previous page*

cefuroxime sodium *see* cefuroxime *on previous page*

Cefzil® [US/Can] *see* cefprozil *on page 171*

Celebrex® [US/Can] *see* celecoxib *on this page*

celecoxib (ce le COX ib)

Sound-Alike/Look-Alike Issues
Celebrex® may be confused with Celexa®, Cerebra®, Cerebyx®

U.S./Canadian Brand Names Celebrex® [US/Can]

Therapeutic Category Nonsteroidal Antiinflammatory Drug (NSAID), COX-2 Selective

Use Relief of the signs and symptoms of osteoarthritis; relief of the signs and symptoms of rheumatoid arthritis in adults; decreasing intestinal polyps in familial adenomatous polyposis (FAP); management of acute pain; treatment of primary dysmenorrhea

Usual Dosage Adults: Oral:
Acute pain or primary dysmenorrhea: Initial dose: 400 mg, followed by an additional 200 mg if needed on day 1; maintenance dose: 200 mg twice daily as needed
Familial adenomatous polyposis (FAP): 400 mg twice daily
Osteoarthritis: 200 mg/day as a single dose or in divided dose twice daily
Rheumatoid arthritis: 100-200 mg twice daily

Dosage Forms Capsule: 100 mg, 200 mg, 400 mg

Celectol® *(Discontinued)* *see page 1042*

Celestoderm®-EV/2 [Can] *see* betamethasone (topical) *on page 116*

Celestoderm®-V [Can] *see* betamethasone (topical) *on page 116*

Celestone® [US] *see* betamethasone (systemic) *on page 115*

Celestone® Soluspan® [US/Can] *see* betamethasone (systemic) *on page 115*

Celexa™ [US/Can] *see* citalopram *on page 205*

CellCept® [US/Can] *see* mycophenolate *on page 596*

Cellugel® [US] *see* hydroxypropyl methylcellulose *on page 457*

cellulose, oxidized regenerated

(SEL yoo lose, OKS i dyzed re JEN er aye ted)

Sound-Alike/Look-Alike Issues
Surgicel® may be confused with Serentil®

Synonyms absorbable cotton; oxidized regenerated cellulose

U.S./Canadian Brand Names Surgical® Fibrillar [US]; Surgicel® [US]; Surgicel® NuKnit [US]

Therapeutic Category Hemostatic Agent

Use Hemostatic; temporary packing for the control of capillary, venous, or small arterial hemorrhage

Usual Dosage Minimal amounts of the fabric strip are laid on the bleeding site or held firmly against the tissues until hemostasis occurs; remove excess material

Dosage Forms

Fabric, fibrous:
Surgicel® Fibrillar:
1" x 2" (10s)
2" x 4" (10s)
4" x 4" (10s)

Fabric, knitted:
Surgicel® NuKnit:
1" x 1" (24s)
1" x 3½" (10s)
3" x 4" (24s)
6" x 9" (10s)

Fabric, sheer weave:
Surgicel®:
½" x 2" (24s)
2" x 3" (24s)
2" x 14" (24s)
4" x 8" (24s)

cellulose sodium phosphate (sel yoo lose SOW dee um FOS fate)

Synonyms CSP; sodium cellulose phosphate

U.S./Canadian Brand Names Calcibind® [US/Can]

Therapeutic Category Urinary Tract Product

Use Adjunct to dietary restriction to reduce renal calculi formation in absorptive hypercalciuria type I

Usual Dosage Adults: Oral: 5 g 3 times/day with meals; decrease dose to 5 g with main meal and 2.5 g with each of two other meals when urinary calcium declines to <150 mg/day

Dosage Forms Powder: 2.5 g/scoop (45 g)

Celluvisc™ [Can] *see* carboxymethylcellulose *on page 161*

Celontin® [US/Can] *see* methsuximide *on page 568*

Cena-K® *(Discontinued)* *see page 1042*

Cenestin® [US/Can] *see* estrogens (conjugated A/synthetic) *on page 329*

Cenocort® A-40 *(Discontinued)* *see page 1042*

Cenocort® Forte *(Discontinued)* *see page 1042*

Centrax® Capsule & Tablet *(Discontinued)* *see page 1042*

Centrum® Kids Rugrats™ Complete [US-OTC] *see* vitamins (multiple/pediatric) *on page 927*

Centrum® Kids Rugrats™ Extra Calcium [US-OTC] *see* vitamins (multiple/pediatric) *on page 927*

Centrum® Kids Rugrats™ Extra C [US-OTC] *see* vitamins (multiple/pediatric) *on page 927*

Centrum® Performance™ [US-OTC] *see* vitamins (multiple/oral) *on page 927*

Centrum® Silver® [US-OTC] *see* vitamins (multiple/oral) *on page 927*

Centrum® [US-OTC] *see* vitamins (multiple/oral) *on page 927*

Cēpacol® [Can] *see* cetylpyridinium and benzocaine *on page 179*

Cēpacol® Gold [US-OTC] *see* cetylpyridinium *on page 179*

Cēpacol® Maximum Strength [US-OTC] *see* dyclonine *on page 300*

Cēpacol Viractin® [US-OTC] *see* tetracaine *on page 851*

Cēpastat® Extra Strength [US-OTC] *see* phenol *on page 687*

Cēpastat® [US-OTC] *see* phenol *on page 687*

cephalexin (sef a LEKS in)

Sound-Alike/Look-Alike Issues
cephalexin may be confused with cefaclor, cefazolin, cephalothin, ciprofloxacin

Synonyms cephalexin monohydrate

U.S./Canadian Brand Names Apo-Cephalex® [Can]; Biocef® [US]; Keflex® [US]; Keftab® [Can]; Novo-Lexin® [Can]; Nu-Cephalex® [Can]; Panixine DisperDose™ [US]

Therapeutic Category Cephalosporin (First Generation)

Use Treatment of susceptible bacterial infections including respiratory tract infections, otitis media, skin and skin structure infections, bone infections and genitourinary tract infections, including acute prostatitis; alternative therapy for acute bacterial endocarditis prophylaxis

Usual Dosage Oral:

Children >1 year: Dosing range: 25-50 mg/kg/day every 6-8 hours; more severe infections: 50-100 mg/kg/day in divided doses every 6-8 hours; maximum: 4 g/24 hours

Otitis media: 75-100 mg/kg/day in 4 divided doses

Streptococcal pharyngitis, skin and skin structure infections: 25-50 mg/kg/day divided every 12 hours

Uncomplicated cystitis: Children >15 years: Refer to Adults dosing

Prophylaxis of bacterial endocarditis (dental, oral, respiratory tract, or esophageal procedures): 50 mg/kg 1 hour prior to procedure (maximum: 2 g)

Adults: Dosing range: 250-1000 mg every 6 hours; maximum: 4 g/day

Streptococcal pharyngitis, skin and skin structure infections: 500 mg every 12 hours

Uncomplicated cystitis: 500 mg every 12 hours for 7-14 days

Prophylaxis of bacterial endocarditis (dental, oral, respiratory tract, or esophageal procedures): 2 g 1 hour prior to procedure

Dosage Forms

Capsule: 250 mg, 500 mg

Biocef®: 500 mg

Keflex®: 250 mg, 500 mg

Powder for oral suspension: 125 mg/5 mL (100 mL, 200 mL); 250 mg/5 mL (100 mL, 200 mL)

Biocef®: 125 mg/5 mL (100 mL); 250 mg/5 mL (100 mL)

Tablet, for oral suspension (Panixine DisperDose™): 125 mg [contains phenylalanine 2.8 mg; peppermint flavor], 250 mg [contains phenylalanine 5.6 mg; peppermint flavor]

cephalexin monohydrate *see* cephalexin *on this page*

cephalothin (sef A loe thin)

Sound-Alike/Look-Alike Issues
cephalothin may be confused with cefazolin, cephalexin

Synonyms cephalothin sodium

Therapeutic Category Cephalosporin (First Generation)

Use Treatment of infections when caused by susceptible strains in respiratory, genitourinary, gastrointestinal, skin and soft tissue, bone and joint infections; septicemia; treatment of susceptible gram-positive bacilli and cocci (never enterococcus); some gram-negative bacilli including *E. coli*, *Proteus*, and *Klebsiella* may be susceptible

Usual Dosage I.V.:

Neonates:

Postnatal age <7 days:

<2000 g: 20 mg every 12 hours

>2000 g: 20 mg every 8 hours

Postnatal age >7 days:

<2000 g: 20 mg every 8 hours

>2000 g: 20 mg every 6 hours

Children: 75-125 mg/kg/day divided every 4-6 hours; maximum dose: 10 g in a 24-hour period

Adults: 500 mg to 2 g every 4-6 hours

Dosage Forms [DSC] = Discontinued product

Infusion, as sodium [frozen]: 1 g (50 mL); 2 g (50 mL) [DSC]

cephalothin sodium *see* cephalothin *on previous page*

cephradine (SEF ra deen)

Sound-Alike/Look-Alike Issues

cephradine may be confused with cephapirin

Velosef® may be confused with Vasosulf®

U.S./Canadian Brand Names Velosef® [US]

Therapeutic Category Cephalosporin (First Generation)

Use Treatment of infections when caused by susceptible strains in respiratory, genitourinary, gastrointestinal, skin and soft tissue, bone and joint infections; treatment of susceptible gram-positive bacilli and cocci (never enterococcus); some gram-negative bacilli including *E. coli*, *Proteus*, and *Klebsiella* may be susceptible

Usual Dosage Oral:

Children ≥9 months: Usual dose: 25-50 mg/kg/day in divided doses every 6 hours

Otitis media: 75-100 mg/kg/day in divided doses every 6 or 12 hours (maximum: 4 g/day)

Adults: 250-500 mg every 6-12 hours

Dosage Forms [DSC] = Discontinued product

Capsule: 250 mg, 500 mg [DSC]

Powder for oral suspension: 250 mg/5 mL (100 mL) [fruit flavor]

Cephulac® ***(Discontinued)*** *see page 1042*

Ceptaz® ***(Discontinued)*** *see page 1042*

Cerebyx® [US/Can] *see* fosphenytoin *on page 391*

Ceredase® [US] *see* alglucerase *on page 31*

Cerespan® ***(Discontinued)*** *see page 1042*

Cerezyme® [US/Can] *see* imiglucerase *on page 466*

Certain Dri® [US-OTC] *see* aluminum chloride hexahydrate *on page 39*

Cerubidine® [US/Can] *see* daunorubicin hydrochloride *on page 246*

Cerumenex® [US/Can] *see* triethanolamine polypeptide oleate-condensate *on page 884*

Cervidil® [US/Can] *see* dinoprostone *on page 275*

C.E.S.® [Can] *see* estrogens (conjugated/equine) *on page 329*

Cesamet® ***(Discontinued)*** *see page 1042*

Cetacaine® [US] *see* benzocaine, butyl aminobenzoate, tetracaine, and benzalkonium chloride *on page 109*

Cetacort® [US] *see* hydrocortisone (topical) *on page 451*

Cetafen Cold® [US-OTC] *see* acetaminophen and pseudoephedrine *on page 9*

Cetafen Extra® [US-OTC] *see* acetaminophen *on page 5*

Cetafen® [US-OTC] *see* acetaminophen *on page 5*

Cetamide™ [Can] *see* sulfacetamide *on page 829*

Cetane® ***(Discontinued)*** *see page 1042*

Ceta-Plus® [US] *see* hydrocodone and acetaminophen *on page 443*

Cetapred® Ophthalmic ***(Discontinued)*** *see page 1042*

cetirizine (se TI ra zeen)

Sound-Alike/Look-Alike Issues

Zyrtec® may be confused with Serax®, Xanax®, Zantac®, Zyprexa®

Synonyms cetirizine hydrochloride; P-071; UCB-P071

U.S./Canadian Brand Names Apo-Cetirizine® [Can]; Reactine™ [Can]; Zyrtec® [US]

Therapeutic Category Antihistamine

Use Perennial and seasonal allergic rhinitis and other allergic symptoms including urticaria; chronic idiopathic urticaria

Usual Dosage Oral:

Children:

6-12 months: Chronic urticaria, perennial allergic rhinitis: 2.5 mg once daily

12 months to <2 years: Chronic urticaria, perennial allergic rhinitis: 2.5 mg once daily; may increase to 2.5 mg every 12 hours if needed

2-5 years: Chronic urticaria, perennial or seasonal allergic rhinitis: Initial: 2.5 mg once daily; may be increased to 2.5 mg every 12 hours **or** 5 mg once daily

Children ≥6 years and Adults: Chronic urticaria, perennial or seasonal allergic rhinitis: 5-10 mg once daily, depending upon symptom severity

Dosage Forms

Syrup, as hydrochloride: 5 mg/5 mL (120 mL, 480 mL) [banana-grape flavor]

Tablet, as hydrochloride: 5 mg, 10 mg

Tablet, chewable, as hydrochloride: 5 mg, 10 mg [grape flavor]

cetirizine and pseudoephedrine (se TI ra zeen & soo doe e FED rin)

Synonyms cetirizine hydrochloride and pseudoephedrine hydrochloride; pseudoephedrine hydrochloride and cetirizine hydrochloride

U.S./Canadian Brand Names Reactine® Allergy and Sinus [Can]; Zyrtec-D 12 Hour™ [US]

Therapeutic Category Antihistamine/Decongestant Combination

Use Treatment of symptoms of seasonal or perennial allergic rhinitis

Usual Dosage Oral: Children ≥12 years and Adults: Seasonal/perennial allergic rhinitis: 1 tablet twice daily

Dosage Forms Tablet, extended release: Cetirizine hydrochloride 5 mg and pseudoephedrine hydrochloride 120 mg

cetirizine hydrochloride *see* cetirizine *on this page*

cetirizine hydrochloride and pseudoephedrine hydrochloride *see* cetirizine and pseudoephedrine *on this page*

cetrorelix (se troh REE liks)

Synonyms cetrorelix acetate

U.S./Canadian Brand Names Cetrotide™ [US/Can]

Therapeutic Category Antigonadotropic Agent

Use Inhibits premature luteinizing hormone (LH) surges in women undergoing controlled ovarian stimulation

Usual Dosage SubQ: Adults: Female: Used in conjunction with controlled ovarian stimulation therapy using gonadotropins (FSH, HMG):

Single-dose regimen: 3 mg given when serum estradiol levels show appropriate stimulation response, usually stimulation day 7 (range days 5-9). If hCG is not administered within 4 days, continue cetrorelix at 0.25 mg/day until hCG is administered

Multiple-dose regimen: 0.25 mg morning or evening of stimulation day 5, or morning of stimulation day 6; continue until hCG is administered.

Dosage Forms Injection, powder for reconstitution: 0.25 mg, 3 mg [supplied with SWFI in prefilled syringe]

cetrorelix acetate *see* cetrorelix *on this page*

Cetrotide™ [US/Can] *see* cetrorelix *on this page*

cetuximab (se TUK see mab)

Synonyms C225; IMC-C225

U.S./Canadian Brand Names Erbitux™ [US]

Therapeutic Category Antineoplastic Agent, Monoclonal Antibody; Epidermal Growth Factor Receptor (EGFR) Inhibitor

Use Treatment of epidermal growth factor receptor (EGFR) expressing, metastatic colorectal carcinoma; may be used in combination with irinotecan in patients who are refractory to irinotecan-based chemotherapy or as a single agent in patients who are intolerant to irinotecan-based chemotherapy.

Usual Dosage I.V.: Adults:

Colorectal cancer:

Initial loading dose: 400 mg/m^2 infused over 120 minutes

Maintenance dose: 250 mg/m^2 infused over 60 minutes

Dosage Forms Injection, solution [preservative free]: 2 mg/mL (50 mL)

cetylpyridinium (SEE til peer i DI nee um)

Synonyms cetylpyridinium chloride; CPC

U.S./Canadian Brand Names Cēpacol® Gold [US-OTC]

Therapeutic Category Local Anesthetic

Use Antiseptic to aid in the prevention and reduction of plaque and gingivitis, and to freshen breath

Usual Dosage Children ≥6 years and Adults: Oral (OTC labeling): Rinse or gargle to freshen mouth; may be used before or after brushing

Dosage Forms Liquid, as chloride [mouthwash/gargle]: 0.05% (120 mL, 360 mL, 720 mL, 960 mL) [contains alcohol 14% and tartrazine]

cetylpyridinium and benzocaine
(SEE til peer i DI nee um & BEN zoe kane)

Synonyms benzocaine and cetylpyridinium chloride; cetylpyridinium chloride and benzocaine

U.S./Canadian Brand Names Cēpacol® [Can]; Kank-A® [Can]

Therapeutic Category Local Anesthetic

Use Symptomatic relief of sore throat

Usual Dosage Antiseptic/anesthetic: Oral: Dissolve in mouth as needed for sore throat

Dosage Forms Troche: Cetylpyridinium chloride 1:1500 and benzocaine 10 mg (18s)

cetylpyridinium chloride *see* cetylpyridinium *on this page*

cetylpyridinium chloride and benzocaine *see* cetylpyridinium and benzocaine *on this page*

Cevalin® *(Discontinued)* *see page 1042*

Cevi-Bid® [US-OTC] *see* ascorbic acid *on page 79*

cevimeline (se vi ME leen)

Sound-Alike/Look-Alike Issues

Evoxac® may be confused with Eurax®

Synonyms cevimeline hydrochloride

U.S./Canadian Brand Names Evoxac® [US/Can]

Therapeutic Category Cholinergic Agent

Use Treatment of symptoms of dry mouth in patients with Sjögren syndrome

Usual Dosage Adults: Oral: 30 mg 3 times/day

Dosage Forms Capsule, as hydrochloride: 30 mg

cevimeline hydrochloride *see* cevimeline *on this page*

CFDN *see* cefdinir *on page 167*

CG *see* chorionic gonadotropin (human) *on page 197*

CGP-42446 *see* zoledronic acid *on page 942*

CGP 57148B *see* imatinib *on page 465*

C-Gram [US-OTC] *see* ascorbic acid *on page 79*

Charcadole® [Can] *see* charcoal *on this page*

Charcadole® Aqueous [Can] *see* charcoal *on this page*

Charcadole® TFS [Can] *see* charcoal *on this page*

CharcoAid® *(Discontinued)* *see page 1042*

CharcoAid® G [US-OTC] *see* charcoal *on this page*

charcoal (CHAR kole)

Sound-Alike/Look-Alike Issues

Actidose® may be confused with Actos®

Synonyms activated carbon; activated charcoal; adsorbent charcoal; liquid antidote; medicinal carbon; medicinal charcoal

U.S./Canadian Brand Names Actidose-Aqua® [US-OTC]; Actidose® with Sorbitol [US-OTC]; Carcocaps® [US-OTC]; Charcadole® [Can]; Charcadole® Aqueous [Can]; Charcadole® TFS [Can]; CharcoAid® G [US-OTC]; Charcoal Plus® DS [US-OTC]; EZ-Char™ [US-OTC]; Kerr Insta-Char® [US-OTC]

Therapeutic Category Antidote

Use Emergency treatment in poisoning by drugs and chemicals; aids the elimination of certain drugs and improves decontamination of excessive ingestions of sustained - release products or in the presence of bezoars; repetitive doses have proven useful to enhance the elimination of certain drugs (eg, theophylline, phenobarbital, and aspirin); repetitive doses for gastric dialysis in uremia to adsorb various waste products; dietary supplement (digestive aid)

Usual Dosage Oral:

Acute poisoning: **Note:** ~10 g of activated charcoal for each 1 g of toxin is considered adequate; this may require multiple doses. If sorbitol is also used, sorbitol dose should not exceed 1.5 g/kg. When using multiple doses of charcoal, sorbitol should be given with every other dose (not to exceed 2 doses/day).

Children: 1 g/kg as a single dose; if multiple doses are needed, additional doses can be given as 0.25 g/kg every hour or equivalent (ie, 0.5 g/kg every 2 hours) **or**

>1 year-12 years: 25-50 g as a single dose; smaller doses (10-25 g) may be used in children 1-5 years due to smaller gut lumen capacity

Children >12 years and Adults: 25-100 g as a single dose; if multiple doses are needed, additional doses may be given as 12.5 g/hour or equivalent (ie, 25 g every 2 hours)

Dietary supplement: Adult: 500-520 mg after meals; may repeat in 2 hours if needed (maximum 10 g/day)

Dosage Forms [DSC] = Discontinued product

Capsule, activated (Charcocaps®): 260 mg

Granules, activated (CharcoAid® G): 15 g (120 mL)

Liquid, activated:

Actidose-Aqua®: 15 g (72 mL); 25 g (120 mL); 50 g (240 mL)

Kerr Insta-Char®: 25 g (120 mL) [cherry flavor]; 50 g (240 mL) [unflavored or cherry flavor]

Liqui-Char® [DSC]: 15 g (75 mL); 25 g (120 mL)

Liquid, activated [with sorbitol]:

Actidose® with Sorbitol, Liqui-Char® [DSC]: 25 g (120 mL); 50 g (240 mL)

Kerr Insta-Char®: 25 g (120 mL); 50 g (240 mL) [cherry flavor]

Pellets, activated (EZ-Char™): 25 g

Powder for suspension, activated: 30 g, 240 g

Tablets, activated (Charcoal Plus® DS): 250 mg

Charcoal Plus® DS [US-OTC] *see* charcoal *on this page*

Charcocaps® *(Discontinued)* *see page 1042*

Chealamide® ***(Discontinued)*** *see page 1042*

Chemet® [US/Can] *see* succimer *on page 826*

Chenix® Tablet ***(Discontinued)*** *see page 1042*

Cheracol® [US] *see* guaifenesin and codeine *on page 416*

Cheracol® D [US-OTC] *see* guaifenesin and dextromethorphan *on page 416*

Cheracol® Plus [US-OTC] *see* guaifenesin and dextromethorphan *on page 416*

Cheratussin DAC [US] *see* guaifenesin, pseudoephedrine, and codeine *on page 422*

CHG *see* chlorhexidine gluconate *on page 183*

Chibroxin® ***(Discontinued)*** *see page 1042*

chicken pox vaccine *see* varicella virus vaccine *on page 905*

Chiggerex® [US-OTC] *see* benzocaine *on page 107*

Chiggertox® [US-OTC] *see* benzocaine *on page 107*

Children's Dimetapp® Elixir Cold & Allergy [US-OTC] *see* brompheniramine and pseudoephedrine *on page 129*

Children's Hold® ***(Discontinued)*** *see page 1042*

Children's Kaopectate® ***(Discontinued)*** *see page 1042*

Children's Kaopectate® (reformulation) [US-OTC] *see* bismuth *on page 120*

Children's Sudafed® Cough & Cold [US-OTC] *see* pseudoephedrine and dextromethorphan *on page 746*

Children's Tylenol® Plus Cold [US-OTC] *see* acetaminophen, chlorpheniramine, and pseudoephedrine *on page 11*

children's vitamins *see* vitamins (multiple/pediatric) *on page 927*

Chirocaine® ***(Discontinued)*** *see page 1042*

Chirocaine® [Can] *see* levobupivacaine *on page 511*

Chlo-Amine® Oral ***(Discontinued)*** *see page 1042*

Chlorafed® Liquid ***(Discontinued)*** *see page 1042*

chloral *see* chloral hydrate *on this page*

chloral hydrate (KLOR al HYE drate)

Synonyms chloral; hydrated chloral; trichloroacetaldehyde monohydrate

U.S./Canadian Brand Names Aquachloral® Supprettes® [US]; PMS-Chloral Hydrate [Can]; Somnote™ [US]

Therapeutic Category Hypnotic, Nonbarbiturate

Controlled Substance C-IV

Use Short-term sedative and hypnotic (<2 weeks), sedative/hypnotic for diagnostic procedures; sedative prior to EEG evaluations

Usual Dosage

Children:

Sedation or anxiety: Oral, rectal: 5-15 mg/kg/dose every 8 hours (maximum: 500 mg/dose)

Prior to EEG: Oral, rectal: 20-25 mg/kg/dose, 30-60 minutes prior to EEG; may repeat in 30 minutes to maximum of 100 mg/kg or 2 g total

Hypnotic: Oral, rectal: 20-40 mg/kg/dose up to a maximum of 50 mg/kg/24 hours or 1 g/dose or 2 g/24 hours

Conscious sedation: Oral: 50-75 mg/kg/dose 30-60 minutes prior to procedure; may repeat 30 minutes after initial dose if needed, to a total maximum dose of 120 mg/kg or 1 g total

Adults: Oral, rectal:

Sedation, anxiety: 250 mg 3 times/day

(Continued)

chloral hydrate *(Continued)*

Hypnotic: 500-1000 mg at bedtime or 30 minutes prior to procedure, not to exceed 2 g/24 hours

Dosage Forms

Capsule (Somnote™): 500 mg

Suppository, rectal (Aquachloral® Supprettes®): 325 mg [contains tartrazine], 650 mg

Syrup: 500 mg/5 mL (480 mL) [contains sodium benzoate]

chlorambucil (klor AM byoo sil)

Sound-Alike/Look-Alike Issues

chlorambucil may be confused with Chloromycetin®

Leukeran® may be confused with Alkeran®, leucovorin, Leukine®

Synonyms CB-1348; chlorambucilum; chloraminophene; chlorbutinum; NSC-3088; WR-139013

U.S./Canadian Brand Names Leukeran® [US/Can]

Therapeutic Category Antineoplastic Agent

Use Management of chronic lymphocytic leukemia, Hodgkin and non-Hodgkin lymphoma; breast and ovarian carcinoma; Waldenström macroglobulinemia, testicular carcinoma, thrombocythemia, choriocarcinoma

Usual Dosage Refer to individual protocols. Oral:

Children:

General short courses: 0.1-0.2 mg/kg/day **or** 4.5 mg/m^2/day for 3-6 weeks for remission induction (usual: 4-10 mg/day); maintenance therapy: 0.03-0.1 mg/kg/day (usual: 2-4 mg/day)

Nephrotic syndrome: 0.1-0.2 mg/kg/day every day for 5-15 weeks with low-dose prednisone

Chronic lymphocytic leukemia (CLL):

Biweekly regimen: Initial: 0.4 mg/kg/dose every 2 weeks; increase dose by 0.1 mg/kg every 2 weeks until a response occurs and/or myelosuppression occurs

Monthly regimen: Initial: 0.4 mg/kg, increase dose by 0.2 mg/kg every 4 weeks until a response occurs and/or myelosuppression occurs

Malignant lymphomas:

Non-Hodgkin lymphoma: 0.1 mg/kg/day

Hodgkin lymphoma: 0.2 mg/kg/day

Adults: 0.1-0.2 mg/kg/day **or**

3-6 mg/m^2/day for 3-6 weeks, then adjust dose on basis of blood counts **or**

0.4 mg/kg and increased by 0.1 mg/kg biweekly or monthly **or**

14 mg/m^2/day for 5 days, repeated every 21-28 days

Dosage Forms Tablet [film coated]: 2 mg

chlorambucilum *see* chlorambucil *on this page*

chloraminophene *see* chlorambucil *on this page*

chloramphenicol (klor am FEN i kole)

Sound-Alike/Look-Alike Issues

Chloromycetin® may be confused with chlorambucil, Chlor-Trimeton®

U.S./Canadian Brand Names Chloromycetin® [Can]; Chloromycetin® Sodium Succinate [US]; Diochloram® [Can]; Pentamycetin® [Can]

Therapeutic Category Antibiotic, Ophthalmic; Antibiotic, Otic; Antibiotic, Miscellaneous

Use Treatment of serious infections due to organisms resistant to other less toxic antibiotics or when its penetrability into the site of infection is clinically superior to other antibiotics to which the organism is sensitive; useful in infections caused by *Bacteroides, H. influenzae, Neisseria meningitidis, Salmonella*, and *Rickettsia*; active against many vancomycin-resistant enterococci

Usual Dosage

Meningitis: I.V.: Infants >30 days and Children: 50-100 mg/kg/day divided every 6 hours

Other infections: I.V.:
Infants >30 days and Children: 50-75 mg/kg/day divided every 6 hours; maximum daily dose: 4 g/day
Adults: 50-100 mg/kg/day in divided doses every 6 hours; maximum daily dose: 4 g/day

Dosage Forms Injection, powder for reconstitution (Chloromycetin® Sodium Succinate): 1 g [contains sodium ~52 mg/g (2.25 mEq/g)]

ChloraPrep® [US-OTC] *see* chlorhexidine gluconate *on this page*

Chloraseptic® Gargle [US-OTC] *see* phenol *on page 687*

Chloraseptic® Mouth Pain Spray [US-OTC] *see* phenol *on page 687*

Chloraseptic® Rinse [US-OTC] *see* phenol *on page 687*

Chloraseptic® Spray for Kids [US-OTC] *see* phenol *on page 687*

Chloraseptic® Spray [US-OTC] *see* phenol *on page 687*

Chlorate® Oral *(Discontinued)* *see page 1042*

chlorbutinum *see* chlorambucil *on previous page*

chlordiazepoxide (klor dye az e POKS ide)

Sound-Alike/Look-Alike Issues
Librium® may be confused with Librax®

Synonyms methaminodiazepoxide hydrochloride

U.S./Canadian Brand Names Apo-Chlordiazepoxide® [Can]; Librium® [US]

Therapeutic Category Benzodiazepine

Controlled Substance C-IV

Use Management of anxiety disorder or for the short-term relief of symptoms of anxiety; withdrawal symptoms of acute alcoholism; preoperative apprehension and anxiety

Usual Dosage
Children:
<6 years: Not recommended
>6 years: Anxiety: Oral, I.M.: 0.5 mg/kg/24 hours divided every 6-8 hours
Adults:
Anxiety:
Oral: 15-100 mg divided 3-4 times/day
I.M., I.V.: Initial: 50-100 mg followed by 25-50 mg 3-4 times/day as needed
Preoperative anxiety: I.M.: 50-100 mg prior to surgery
Ethanol withdrawal symptoms: Oral, I.V.: 50-100 mg to start, dose may be repeated in 2-4 hours as necessary to a maximum of 300 mg/24 hours
Note: Up to 300 mg may be given I.M. or I.V. during a 6-hour period, but not more than this in any 24-hour period.

Dosage Forms
Capsule, as hydrochloride: 5 mg, 10 mg, 25 mg
Injection, powder for reconstitution, as hydrochloride: 100 mg [diluent contains benzyl alcohol, polysorbate 80, and propylene glycol]

chlordiazepoxide and amitriptyline *see* amitriptyline and chlordiazepoxide *on page 48*

chlordiazepoxide and clidinium *see* clidinium and chlordiazepoxide *on page 210*

chlorethazine *see* mechlorethamine *on page 546*

chlorethazine mustard *see* mechlorethamine *on page 546*

Chlorgest-HD® Elixir *(Discontinued)* *see page 1042*

chlorhexidine gluconate (klor HEKS i deen GLOO koe nate)

Sound-Alike/Look-Alike Issues
Peridex® may be confused with Precedex™

(Continued)

chlorhexidine gluconate *(Continued)*

Synonyms CHG

U.S./Canadian Brand Names Avagard™ [US-OTC]; BactoShield® CHG [US-OTC]; Betasept® [US-OTC]; ChloraPrep® [US-OTC]; Chlorostat® [US-OTC]; Dyna-Hex® [US-OTC]; Hibiclens® [US-OTC]; Hibidil® 1:2000 [Can]; Hibistat® [US-OTC]; Operand® Chlorhexidine Gluconate [US-OTC]; ORO-Clense [Can]; Peridex® [US]; Periochip® [US]; PerioGard® [US]; SpectroGram 2™ [Can]

Therapeutic Category Antibiotic, Oral Rinse; Antibiotic, Topical

Use Skin cleanser for surgical scrub, cleanser for skin wounds, preoperative skin preparation, germicidal hand rinse, and as antibacterial dental rinse. Chlorhexidine is active against gram-positive and gram-negative organisms, facultative anaerobes, aerobes, and yeast.

Orphan drug: Peridex®: Oral mucositis with cytoreductive therapy when used for patients undergoing bone marrow transplant

Usual Dosage Adults:

Oral rinse (Peridex®, PerioGard®):

Floss and brush teeth, completely rinse toothpaste from mouth and swish 15 mL (one capful) undiluted oral rinse around in mouth for 30 seconds, then expectorate. Caution patient not to swallow the medicine and instruct not to eat for 2-3 hours after treatment. (Cap on bottle measures 15 mL.)

Treatment of gingivitis: Oral prophylaxis: Swish for 30 seconds with 15 mL chlorhexidine, then expectorate; repeat twice daily (morning and evening). Patient should have a re-evaluation followed by a dental prophylaxis every 6 months.

Periodontal chip: One chip is inserted into a periodontal pocket with a probing pocket depth ≥5 mm. Up to 8 chips may be inserted in a single visit. Treatment is recommended every 3 months in pockets with a remaining depth ≥5 mm. If dislodgment occurs 7 days or more after placement, the subject is considered to have had the full course of treatment. If dislodgment occurs within 48 hours, a new chip should be inserted. The chip biodegrades completely and does not need to be removed. Patients should avoid dental floss at the site of PerioChip® insertion for 10 days after placement because flossing might dislodge the chip.

Insertion of periodontal chip: Pocket should be isolated and surrounding area dried prior to chip insertion. The chip should be grasped using forceps with the rounded edges away from the forceps. The chip should be inserted into the periodontal pocket to its maximum depth. It may be maneuvered into position using the tips of the forceps or a flat instrument.

Cleanser:

Surgical scrub: Scrub 3 minutes and rinse thoroughly, wash for an additional 3 minutes

Hand sanitizer (Avagard™): Dispense 1 pumpful in palm of one hand; dip fingertips of opposite hand into solution and work it under nails. Spread remainder evenly over hand and just above elbow, covering all surfaces. Repeat on other hand. Dispense another pumpful in each hand and reapply to each hand up to the wrist. Allow to dry before gloving.

Hand wash: Wash for 15 seconds and rinse

Hand rinse: Rub 15 seconds and rinse

Dosage Forms

Chip, for periodontal pocket insertion (PerioChip®): 2.5 mg

Liquid, topical [surgical scrub]:

Avagard™: 1% (500 mL) [contains ethyl alcohol and moisturizers]

BactoShield® CHG: 2% (120 mL, 480 mL, 750 mL, 1000 mL, 3800 mL); 4% (120 mL, 480 mL, 750 mL, 1000 mL, 3800 mL) [contains isopropyl alcohol]

Betasept®: 4% (120 mL, 240 mL, 480 mL, 960 mL, 3840 mL) [contains isopropyl alcohol]

ChloraPrep®: 2% (0.67 mL, 1.5 mL, 3 mL, 10.5 mL) [contains isopropyl alcohol 70%; prefilled applicator]

Chlorostat®: 2% (360 mL, 3840 mL) [contains isopropyl alcohol]

Dyna-Hex: 2% (120 mL, 960 mL, 3840 mL); 4% (120 mL, 960 mL, 3840 mL)

Hibiclens®: 4% (15 mL, 120 mL, 240 mL, 480 mL, 960 mL, 3840 mL) [contains isopropyl alcohol]
Operand® Chlorhexidine Gluconate: 2% (120 mL); 4% (120 mL, 240 mL, 480 mL, 960 mL, 3840 mL) [contains isopropyl alcohol]
Liquid, oral rinse: 0.12% (480 mL)
Peridex®: 0.12% (480 mL) [contains alcohol 11.6%]
PerioGard®: 0.12% (480 mL) [contains alcohol 11.6%; mint flavor]
Liquid, topical: Hibistat®: 0.5% (240 mL, 480 mL) [contains isopropyl alcohol]
Pad [prep pad]: Hibistat®: 0.5% (50s) [contains isopropyl alcohol]
Sponge/Brush (BactoShield® CHG, Hibiclens®): 4% per sponge/brush [contains isopropyl alcohol]

chlormeprazine *see* prochlorperazine *on page 731*

Chlor-Mes-D [US] *see* chlorpheniramine, phenylephrine, and methscopolamine *on page 192*

2-chlorodeoxyadenosine *see* cladribine *on page 207*

chloroethane *see* ethyl chloride *on page 349*

Chlorofon-A® Tablet *(Discontinued)* *see page 1042*

Chloromag® [US] *see* magnesium chloride *on page 536*

Chloromycetin® [Can] *see* chloramphenicol *on page 182*

Chloromycetin® Cream *(Discontinued)* *see page 1042*

Chloromycetin® Kapseals® *(Discontinued)* *see page 1042*

Chloromycetin® Ophthalmic *(Discontinued)* *see page 1042*

Chloromycetin® Otic *(Discontinued)* *see page 1042*

Chloromycetin® Palmitate Oral Suspension *(Discontinued)* *see page 1042*

Chloromycetin® Sodium Succinate [US] *see* chloramphenicol *on page 182*

chlorophyll (KLOR oh fil)

Synonyms chlorophyllin

U.S./Canadian Brand Names Nullo® [US-OTC]

Therapeutic Category Gastrointestinal Agent, Miscellaneous

Use Control fecal odors in colostomy or ileostomy

Usual Dosage

Oral: Children >12 years and Adults: 100-200 mg/day in divided doses; may increase to 300 mg/day if odor is not controlled (maximum: 300 mg/day)

Ostomy: Tablet: May also place 1-2 tablets in empty pouch each time it is reused or changed.

Dosage Forms [DSC] = Discontinued product

Caplet (Nullo®): Chlorophyllin copper complex 100 mg
Tablet (Nullo®): Chlorophyllin copper complex 33.3 mg [DSC]

chlorophyllin *see* chlorophyll *on this page*

chloroprocaine (klor oh PROE kane)

Sound-Alike/Look-Alike Issues

Nesacaine® may be confused with Neptazane®

Synonyms chloroprocaine hydrochloride

U.S./Canadian Brand Names Nesacaine®-CE [Can]; Nesacaine®-MPF [US]; Nesacaine® [US]

Therapeutic Category Local Anesthetic

Use Infiltration anesthesia and peripheral and epidural anesthesia

Usual Dosage Dosage varies with anesthetic procedure, the area to be anesthetized, the vascularity of the tissues, depth of anesthesia required, degree of muscle relaxation required, and duration of anesthesia; range.

(Continued)

chloroprocaine *(Continued)*

Children >3 years (normally developed): Maximum dose (without epinephrine): 11 mg/kg
Infiltration: 0.5% to 1%
Nerve block: 1% to 1.5%
Adults:
Maximum single dose (without epinephrine): 11 mg/kg; maximum dose: 800 mg
Maximum single dose (with epinephrine): 14 mg/kg; maximum dose: 1000 mg
Infiltration and peripheral nerve block: 1% to 2%: 0.5-40 mL
Mandibular: 2%: 2-3 mL; total dose 40-60 mg
Infraorbital: 2%: 0.5-1 mL; total dose 10-20 mg
Brachial plexus: 2%; 30-40 mL; total dose 600-800 mg
Digital (without epinephrine): 1%; 3-4 mL; total dose: 30-40 mg
Pudendal: 2%; 10 mL each side; total dose: 400 mg
Paracervical: 1%; 3 mL per each of four sites
Epidural block: Preservative-free: 2%: 5 mL; 3%: 3 mL
Caudal: 2% or 3%: 15-25 mL; may repeat at 40-60 minute intervals
Lumbar: 2% or 3%: 2-2.5 mL per segment; usual total volume: 15-25 mL; may repeat with doses that are 2-6 mL less than initial dose every 40-50 minutes.

Dosage Forms

Injection, solution, as hydrochloride (Nesacaine®): 1% (30 mL); 2% (30 mL) [contains disodium EDTA and methylparaben]
Injection, solution, as hydrochloride [preservative free]: (Nesacaine®-MPF): 2% (20 mL); 3% (20 mL)

chloroprocaine hydrochloride *see* chloroprocaine *on previous page*

Chloroptic® Ophthalmic Solution *(Discontinued)* *see page 1042*

Chloroptic-P® Ophthalmic *(Discontinued)* *see page 1042*

Chloroptic® SOP *(Discontinued)* *see page 1042*

chloroquine phosphate (KLOR oh kwin FOS fate)

U.S./Canadian Brand Names Aralen® [US/Can]

Therapeutic Category Aminoquinoline (Antimalarial)

Use Suppression or chemoprophylaxis of malaria; treatment of uncomplicated or mild to moderate malaria; extraintestinal amebiasis

Usual Dosage Oral:

Suppression or prophylaxis of malaria:
Children: Administer 5 mg base/kg/week on the same day each week (not to exceed 300 mg base/dose); begin 1-2 weeks prior to exposure; continue for 4-6 weeks after leaving endemic area; if suppressive therapy is not begun prior to exposure, double the initial loading dose to 10 mg base/kg and administer in 2 divided doses 6 hours apart, followed by the usual dosage regimen
Adults: 500 mg/week (300 mg base) on the same day each week; begin 1-2 weeks prior to exposure; continue for 4-6 weeks after leaving endemic area; if suppressive therapy is not begun prior to exposure, double the initial loading dose to 1 g (600 mg base) and administer in 2 divided doses 6 hours apart, followed by the usual dosage regimen
Acute attack:
Children: 10 mg/kg (base) on day 1, followed by 5 mg/kg (base) 6 hours later and 5 mg/kg (base) on days 2 and 3
Adults: 1 g (600 mg base) on day 1, followed by 500 mg (300 mg base) 6 hours later, followed by 500 mg (300 mg base) on days 2 and 3
Extraintestinal amebiasis:
Children: 10 mg/kg (base) once daily for 2-3 weeks (up to 300 mg base/day)
Adults: 1 g/day (600 mg base) for 2 days followed by 500 mg/day (300 mg base) for at least 2-3 weeks
Note: Not considered first-line agent.

Dosage Forms

Tablet, as phosphate: 250 mg [equivalent to 150 mg base]; 500 mg [equivalent to 300 mg base]

Aralen®: 500 mg [equivalent to 300 mg base]

Chloroserpine® ***(Discontinued)*** *see page 1042*

Chlorostat® [US-OTC] *see* chlorhexidine gluconate *on page 183*

chlorothiazide (klor oh THYE a zide)

U.S./Canadian Brand Names Diuril® [US/Can]

Therapeutic Category Diuretic, Thiazide

Use Management of mild to moderate hypertension; adjunctive treatment of edema

Usual Dosage Note: The manufacturer states that I.V. and oral dosing are equivalent. Some clinicians may use lower I.V. doses, however, because of chlorothiazide's poor oral absorption. I.V. dosing in infants and children has not been well established.

Infants <6 months:

Oral: 20-40 mg/kg/day in 2 divided doses (maximum dose: 375 mg/day)

Oral: 10-20 mg/kg/day in 2 divided doses (maximum dose: 375 mg/day in children <2 years or 1 g/day in children 2-12 years)

Adults:

Hypertension: Oral: 500 mg to 2 g/day divided in 1-2 doses (manufacturer labeling); doses of 125-500 mg/day have also been recommended

Edema: Oral, I.V.: 500 mg to 1 g once or twice daily. Intermittent treatment (ie, therapy on alternate days) may be appropriate for some patients.

Dosage Forms

Injection, powder for reconstitution, as sodium: 500 mg

Suspension, oral: 250 mg/5 mL (237 mL) [contains alcohol 0.5% and benzoic acid]

Tablet: 250 mg, 500 mg

chloroxine (klor OKS een)

Sound-Alike/Look-Alike Issues

Capitrol® may be confused with Capital®, captopril

U.S./Canadian Brand Names Capitrol® [US/Can]

Therapeutic Category Antiseborrheic Agent, Topical

Use Treatment of dandruff or seborrheic dermatitis of the scalp

Usual Dosage Use twice weekly, massage into wet scalp, avoid contact with eyes, lather should remain on the scalp for approximately 3 minutes, then rinsed; application should be repeated and the scalp rinsed thoroughly

Dosage Forms Shampoo, topical: 2% (110 g) [contains benzyl alcohol]

Chlorphed® ***(Discontinued)*** *see page 1042*

Chlorphed®-LA Nasal Solution ***(Discontinued)*** *see page 1042*

chlorpheniramine (klor fen IR a meen)

Sound-Alike/Look-Alike Issues

Chlor-Trimeton® may be confused with Chloromycetin®

Synonyms chlorpheniramine maleate; CTM

U.S./Canadian Brand Names Aller-Chlor® [US-OTC]; Chlorphen [US-OTC]; Chlor-Trimeton® [US-OTC]; Chlor-Tripolon® [Can]; Diabetic Tussin® Allergy Relief [US-OTC]; Novo-Pheniram® [Can]

Therapeutic Category Antihistamine

Use Perennial and seasonal allergic rhinitis and other allergic symptoms including urticaria

Usual Dosage

Children: Oral: 0.35 mg/kg/day in divided doses every 4-6 hours

2-6 years: 1 mg every 4-6 hours, not to exceed 6 mg in 24 hours

(Continued)

chlorpheniramine *(Continued)*

6-12 years: 2 mg every 4-6 hours, not to exceed 12 mg/day or sustained release 8 mg at bedtime

Children >12 years and Adults: Oral: 4 mg every 4-6 hours, not to exceed 24 mg/day or sustained release 8-12 mg every 8-12 hours, not to exceed 24 mg/day

Dosage Forms

Syrup, as maleate:

Aller-Chlor®: 2 mg/5 mL (120 mL)

Diabetic Tussin® Allergy Relief: 2 mg/5 mL (120 mL) [alcohol free, dye free, sugar free]

Tablet, as maleate (Aller-Chlor®, Chlor-Trimeton®, Chlorphen): 4 mg

Tablet, extended release, as maleate (Chlor-Trimeton®): 12 mg

chlorpheniramine, acetaminophen, and pseudoephedrine *see* acetaminophen, chlorpheniramine, and pseudoephedrine *on page 11*

chlorpheniramine and acetaminophen

(klor fen IR a meen & a seet a MIN oh fen)

Synonyms acetaminophen and chlorpheniramine

U.S./Canadian Brand Names Coricidin® HBP Cold and Flu [US-OTC]

Therapeutic Category Antihistamine/Analgesic

Use Symptomatic relief of congestion, headache, aches and pains of colds and flu

Usual Dosage Adults: Oral: 2 tablets every 4 hours

Dosage Forms Tablet: Chlorpheniramine maleate 2 mg and acetaminophen 325 mg

chlorpheniramine and carbetapentane *see* carbetapentane and chlorpheniramine *on page 156*

chlorpheniramine and hydrocodone *see* hydrocodone and chlorpheniramine *on page 445*

chlorpheniramine and phenylephrine (klor fen IR a meen & fen il EF rin)

Sound-Alike/Look-Alike Issues

Rynatan® may be confused with Rynatuss®

Synonyms chlorpheniramine maleate and phenylephrine hydrochloride; chlorpheniramine tannate and phenylephrine tannate; phenylephrine and chlorpheniramine

U.S./Canadian Brand Names Dallergy-JR® [US]; Ed A-Hist® [US]; Histatab® Plus [US-OTC]; Rynatan® [US]; Rynatan® Pediatric Suspension [US]

Therapeutic Category Antihistamine/Decongestant Combination

Use Temporary relief of nasal congestion and eustachian tube congestion as well as runny nose, sneezing, itching of nose or throat, itchy and watery eyes

Usual Dosage General dosing guidelines; consult specific product labeling. Antihistamine/decongestant: Oral:

Children:

2-6 years: Chlorpheniramine tannate 4.5 mg and phenylephrine tannate 5 mg per 5 mL: 2.5-5 mL every 12 hours

6-12 years:

Chlorpheniramine maleate 4 mg and phenylephrine hydrochloride 20 mg every 12 hours **or**

Chlorpheniramine tannate 4.5 mg and phenylephrine tannate 5 mg per 5 mL: 5-10 mL every 12 hours

≥12 years: Chlorpheniramine maleate 8 mg and phenylephrine hydrochloride 40 mg every 12 hours

Adults:

Chlorpheniramine maleate 8 mg and phenylephrine hydrochloride 40 mg every 12 hours **or**

Chlorpheniramine tannate 9 mg and phenylephrine tannate 25 mg every 12 hours

Dosage Forms

Capsule, extended release (Dallergy-JR®): Chlorpheniramine maleate 4 mg and phenylephrine hydrochloride 20 mg

Liquid (Ed A-Hist®): Chlorpheniramine maleate 4 mg and phenylephrine hydrochloride 10 mg per 5 mL (480 mL)

Suspension, oral (Rynatan® Pediatric Suspension): Chlorpheniramine tannate 4.5 mg and phenylephrine tannate 5 mg per 5 mL (480 mL) [contains benzoic acid and tartrazine; strawberry flavor]

Tablet:

Histatab® Plus: Chlorpheniramine maleate 2 mg and phenylephrine hydrochloride 5 mg

Rynatan®: Chlorpheniramine tannate 9 mg and phenylephrine tannate 25 mg

chlorpheniramine and pseudoephedrine

(klor fen IR a meen & soo doe e FED rin)

Sound-Alike/Look-Alike Issues

Allerest® may be confused with Sinarest®

Synonyms chlorpheniramine maleate and pseudoephedrine hydrochloride; chlorpheniramine tannate and pseudoephedrine tannate; dexchlorpheniramine tannate and pseudoephedrine tannate; pseudoephedrine and chlorpheniramine

U.S./Canadian Brand Names Allerest® Maximum Strength Allergy and Hay fever [US-OTC]; A.R.M® [US-OTC]; Chlor-Trimeton® Allergy D [US-OTC]; C-Phed Tannate [US]; Deconamine® [US]; Deconamine® SR [US]; Genaphed® Plus [US-OTC]; Hayfebrol® [US-OTC]; Histex™ [US]; Kronofed-A® [US]; Kronofed-A®-Jr [US]; PediaCare® Cold and Allergy [US-OTC]; Rhinosyn-PD® [US-OTC]; Rhinosyn® [US-OTC]; Sudafed® Sinus & Allergy [US-OTC]; Tanafed® [US]; Tanafed DP™ [US]; Triaminic® Cold and Allergy [US-OTC/Can]

Therapeutic Category Antihistamine/Decongestant Combination

Use Relief of nasal congestion associated with the common cold, hay fever, and other allergies, sinusitis, eustachian tube blockage, and vasomotor and allergic rhinitis

Usual Dosage General dosing guidelines; consult specific product labeling. Rhinitis/decongestant: Oral:

Children:

2-6 years:

Chlorpheniramine maleate 1 mg and pseudoephedrine hydrochloride 15 mg every 4-6 hours

Chlorpheniramine tannate 4.5 mg and pseudoephedrine tannate 75 mg (Tanafed®): 2.5-5 mL every 12 hours (maximum: 10 mL/24 hours)

Dexchlorpheniramine tannate 2.5 mg and pseudoephedrine tannate 75 mg (Tanafed DP™): 2.5-5 mL every 12 hours (maximum: 10 mL/24 hours)

6-12 years:

Chlorpheniramine maleate 2 mg and pseudoephedrine hydrochloride 30 mg every 4-6 hours

Chlorpheniramine tannate 4.5 mg and pseudoephedrine tannate 75 mg (Tanafed®): 5-10 mL every 12 hours (maximum: 20 mL/24 hours)

Dexchlorpheniramine tannate 2.5 mg and pseudoephedrine tannate 75 mg (Tanafed DP™): 5-10 mL every 12 hours (maximum: 20 mL/24 hours)

Children ≥12 years and Adults:

Chlorpheniramine maleate 4 mg and pseudoephedrine hydrochloride 60 mg every 4-6 hours (immediate release products) or every 12 hours (extended release products)

Chlorpheniramine tannate 4.5 mg and pseudoephedrine tannate 75 mg (Tanafed®): 10-20 mL every 12 hours (maximum: 40 mL/24 hours)

Dexchlorpheniramine tannate 2.5 mg and pseudoephedrine tannate 75 mg (Tanafed DP™): 5-10 mL every 12 hours: (maximum: 20 mL/24 hours)

Dosage Forms [DSC] = Discontinued product

Caplet (A.R.M.®): Chlorpheniramine maleate 4 mg and pseudoephedrine hydrochloride 60 mg

Capsule, extended release: Chlorpheniramine maleate 8 mg and pseudoephedrine hydrochloride 120 mg

Capsule, sustained release:

Deconamine® SR, Kronofed-A®: Chlorpheniramine maleate 8 mg and pseudoephedrine hydrochloride 120 mg

(Continued)

chlorpheniramine and pseudoephedrine *(Continued)*

Kronofed-A®-Jr: Chlorpheniramine maleate 4 mg and pseudoephedrine hydrochloride 60 mg

Liquid:

Hayfebrol®: Chlorpheniramine maleate 2 mg and pseudoephedrine hydrochloride 30 mg per 5 mL (120 mL)

Histex™: Chlorpheniramine maleate 2 mg and pseudoephedrine sulfate 30 mg per 5 mL (480 mL) [peach flavor]

PediaCare® Cold and Allergy: Chlorpheniramine maleate 1 mg and pseudoephedrine sulfate 15 mg per 5 mL (120 mL) [alcohol free; bubblegum flavor]

Triaminic® Cold and Allergy: Chlorpheniramine maleate 1 mg and pseudoephedrine sulfate 15 mg per 5 mL (120 mL) [orange flavor]

Suspension: Chlorpheniramine tannate 4.5 mg and pseudoephedrine tannate 75 mg per 5 mL (120 mL, 480 mL)

C-Phed Tannate: Chlorpheniramine tannate 4.5 mg and pseudoephedrine tannate 75 mg per 5 mL (120 mL, 480 mL) [strawberry-banana flavor]

Tanafed®: Chlorpheniramine tannate 4.5 mg and pseudoephedrine tannate 75 mg per 5 mL (120 mL, 480 mL) [contains sodium benzoate; strawberry-banana flavor]

Tanafed DP™: Dexchlorpheniramine tannate 2.5 mg and pseudoephedrine tannate 75 mg (120 mL, 480 mL) [contains sodium benzoate; strawberry-banana flavor]

Syrup:

Deconamine®: Chlorpheniramine maleate 2 mg and pseudoephedrine sulfate 30 mg per 5 mL (480 mL) [alcohol free, dye free; contains sodium benzoate; grape flavor]

Rhinosyn PD®, Ryna® [DSC]: Chlorpheniramine maleate 2 mg and pseudoephedrine sulfate 30 mg per 5 mL (120 mL)

Rhinosyn®: Chlorpheniramine maleate 4 mg and pseudoephedrine sulfate 60 mg per 5 mL (120 mL, 480 mL)

Tablet: Chlorpheniramine maleate 4 mg and pseudoephedrine hydrochloride 60 mg

Allerest® Maximum Strength Allergy and Hay Fever: Chlorpheniramine maleate 2 mg and pseudoephedrine hydrochloride 30 mg

Chlor-Trimeton® Allergy D, Genaphed® Plus, Sudafed® Sinus & Allergy: Chlorpheniramine maleate 4 mg and pseudoephedrine hydrochloride 60 mg

Deconamine®: Chlorpheniramine maleate 4 mg and pseudoephedrine hydrochloride 60 mg [dye free]

Tablet, chewable (Triaminic® Cold and Allergy): Chlorpheniramine maleate 1 mg and pseudoephedrine sulfate 15 mg [contains phenylalanine 17.6 mg/tablet; orange flavor]

chlorpheniramine, ephedrine, phenylephrine, and carbetapentane

(klor fen IR a meen, e FED rin, fen il EF rin, & kar bay ta PEN tane)

Sound-Alike/Look-Alike Issues

Rynatuss® may be confused with Rynatan®

Synonyms carbetapentane, ephedrine, phenylephrine, and chlorpheniramine; ephedrine, chlorpheniramine, phenylephrine, and carbetapentane; phenylephrine, ephedrine, chlorpheniramine, and carbetapentane

U.S./Canadian Brand Names Rynatuss® [US]; Rynatuss® Pediatric [US]; Tetra Tannate Pediatric [US]

Therapeutic Category Antihistamine/Decongestant/Antitussive

Use Symptomatic relief of cough with a decongestant and an antihistamine

Usual Dosage Oral:

Children:

<2 years: Titrate dose individually

2-6 years: 2.5-5 mL every 12 hours

>6 years: 5-10 mL every 12 hours

Adults: 1-2 tablets every 12 hours

Dosage Forms

Suspension (Rynatuss® Pediatric, Tetra Tannate Pediatric): Carbetapentane tannate 30 mg, ephedrine tannate 5 mg, phenylephrine tannate 5 mg, and chlorpheniramine tannate 4 mg per 5 mL (240 mL, 480 mL) [contains tartrazine and benzoic acid; strawberry flavor]

Tablet (Rynatuss®): Carbetapentane tannate 60 mg, ephedrine tannate 10 mg, phenylephrine tannate 10 mg, and chlorpheniramine tannate 5 mg

chlorpheniramine, hydrocodone, phenylephrine, acetaminophen, and caffeine *see* hydrocodone, chlorpheniramine, phenylephrine, acetaminophen, and caffeine *on page 446*

chlorpheniramine maleate *see* chlorpheniramine *on page 187*

chlorpheniramine maleate and phenylephrine hydrochloride *see* chlorpheniramine and phenylephrine *on page 188*

chlorpheniramine maleate and pseudoephedrine hydrochloride *see* chlorpheniramine and pseudoephedrine *on page 189*

chlorpheniramine, phenylephrine, and dextromethorphan

(klor fen IR a meen, fen il EF rin, & deks troe meth OR fan)

Synonyms dextromethorphan, chlorpheniramine, and phenylephrine; phenylephrine, chlorpheniramine, and dextromethorphan

U.S./Canadian Brand Names Alka-Seltzer® Plus Cold and Cough [US-OTC]; Coldtuss DR [US]; Corfen DM [US]; De-Chlor DM [US]; De-Chlor DR [US]; Dex PC [US]; Tri-Vent™ DPC [US]

Therapeutic Category Antihistamine/Decongestant/Antitussive

Use Temporary relief of cough and upper respiratory symptoms associated with allergies or the common cold

Usual Dosage Oral: Relief of cough and cold symptoms:

Children:

2-6 years (Tri-Vent™ DPC): 2.5 mL every 6 hours (maximum: 10 mL/24 hours)

6-12 years (Tri-Vent™ DPC): 5 mL every 6 hours (maximum: 20 mL/24 hours)

Children ≥12 years and Adults:

Alka-Seltzer® Plus Cold and Cough: 2 tablets dissolved in water every 4 hours (maximum: 8 tablets/24 hours)

Tri-Vent™ DPC: 10 mL every 6 hours (maximum: 40 mL/24 hours)

Dosage Forms

Liquid: Chlorpheniramine maleate 4 mg, phenylephrine hydrochloride 10 mg, and dextromethorphan hydrobromide 15 mg per 5 mL (480 mL)

Corfen DM: Chlorpheniramine maleate 4 mg, phenylephrine hydrochloride 10 mg, and dextromethorphan hydrobromide 15 mg per 5 mL (480 mL) [grape flavor]

De-Chlor DM: Chlorpheniramine maleate 2 mg, phenylephrine hydrochloride 10 mg, and dextromethorphan hydrobromide 15 mg per 5 mL (480 mL) [strawberry flavor]

De-Chlor DR: Chlorpheniramine maleate 2 mg, phenylephrine hydrochloride 6 mg, and dextromethorphan hydrobromide 15 mg per 5 mL (480 mL) [strawberry flavor]

Syrup: Chlorpheniramine maleate 2 mg, phenylephrine hydrochloride 10 mg, and dextromethorphan hydrobromide 15 mg per 5 mL (480 mL)

Coldtuss DR: Chlorpheniramine maleate 4 mg, phenylephrine hydrochloride 6 mg, and dextromethorphan hydrobromide 15 mg per 5 mL (480 mL) [strawberry flavor]

Dex PC: Chlorpheniramine maleate 2 mg, phenylephrine hydrochloride 6 mg, and dextromethorphan hydrobromide 15 mg per 5 mL (480 mL) [strawberry flavor]

Tri-Ven™ DPC: Chlorpheniramine maleate 2 mg, phenylephrine hydrochloride 6 mg, and dextromethorphan hydrobromide 15 mg per 5 mL (480 mL) [alcohol free; contains sodium benzoate; strawberry flavor]

Tablet, effervescent (Alka-Seltzer® Plus Cold and Cough): Chlorpheniramine maleate 2 mg, phenylephrine hydrochloride 5 mg, and dextromethorphan hydrobromide 10 mg [contains phenylalanine 11 mg/tablet and sodium 504 mg/tablet]

chlorpheniramine, phenylephrine, and methscopolamine

(klor fen IR a meen, fen il EF rin, & meth skoe POL a meen)

Synonyms methscopolamine, chlorpheniramine, and phenylephrine; phenylephrine, chlorpheniramine, and methscopolamine

U.S./Canadian Brand Names AH-Chew® [US]; AH-Chew® II [US]; Chlor-Mes-D [US]; Dallergy® [US]; Dehistine [US]; Drize®-R [US]; Extendryl [US]; Extendryl JR [US]; Extendryl SR [US]; Hista-Vent® DA [US]; PCM [US]; PCM Allergy [US]

Therapeutic Category Antihistamine/Decongestant/Anticholinergic

Use Treatment of upper respiratory symptoms such as respiratory congestion, allergic rhinitis, vasomotor rhinitis, sinusitis, and allergic skin reactions of urticaria and angioedema

Usual Dosage

Children 6-11 years: Relief of respiratory symptoms: Oral:

- Extendryl chewable tablet: One tablet every 4 hours; do not exceed 4 doses in 24 hours
- Dallergy®: One-half caplet every 12 hours
- Extendryl JR: One capsule every 12 hours
- Extendryl syrup: 2.5-5 mL, may repeat up to every 4 hours depending on age and body weight

Children ≥12 years and Adults: Relief of respiratory symptoms: Oral: **Note:** If disturbances in urination occur in patients without renal impairment, medication should be discontinued for 1-2 days and should then be restarted at a lower dose

- Dallergy®, Extendryl SR: One capsule every 12 hours
- Extendryl: 1-2 chewable tablets every 4 hours
- Extendryl syrup: 5-10 mL every 3-4 hours (4 times/day)

Dosage Forms [DSC] = Discontinued product

Caplet, extended release (Dallergy®): Chlorpheniramine maleate 12 mg, phenylephrine hydrochloride 20 mg, and methscopolamine nitrate 2.5 mg

Capsule, extended release:

- Extendryl JR: Chlorpheniramine maleate 4 mg, phenylephrine hydrochloride 10 mg, and methscopolamine nitrate 1.25 mg
- Extendryl SR: Chlorpheniramine maleate 8 mg, phenylephrine hydrochloride 20 mg, and methscopolamine nitrate 2.5 mg

Liquid (Chlor-Mes-D): Chlorpheniramine maleate 2 mg, phenylephrine hydrochloride 10 mg, and methscopolamine nitrate 0.625 mg per 5 mL (480 mL)

Syrup:

- Dallergy®: Chlorpheniramine maleate 2 mg, phenylephrine hydrochloride 10 mg, and methscopolamine nitrate 0.625 mg per 5 mL (480 mL)
- Dehistine: Chlorpheniramine maleate 2 mg, phenylephrine hydrochloride 10 mg, and methscopolamine nitrate 1.25 mg per 5 mL (480 mL) [root beer flavor]
- Extendryl: Chlorpheniramine maleate 2 mg, phenylephrine hydrochloride 10 mg, and methscopolamine nitrate 1.25 mg per 5 mL (480 mL) [contains sodium benzoate; root beer flavor]

Tablet:

- Dallergy®: Chlorpheniramine maleate 4 mg, phenylephrine hydrochloride 10 mg, and methscopolamine nitrate 1.25 mg [scored]
- Vanex Forte™-D [DSC]: Chlorpheniramine maleate 8 mg, phenylephrine hydrochloride 20 mg, and methscopolamine nitrate 2.5 mg [dye free; scored]

Tablet, chewable:

- AH-Chew®: Chlorpheniramine maleate 2 mg, phenylephrine hydrochloride 10 mg, and methscopolamine nitrate 1.25 mg [grape flavor]
- AH-Chew® II: Chlorpheniramine maleate 2 mg, phenylephrine hydrochloride 15 mg, and methscopolamine nitrate 1.25 mg [grape flavor]
- Extendryl: Chlorpheniramine maleate 2 mg, phenylephrine hydrochloride 10 mg, and methscopolamine nitrate 1.25 mg [root beer flavor]
- PCM: Chlorpheniramine maleate 2 mg, phenylephrine hydrochloride 10 mg, and methscopolamine nitrate 1.25 mg

Tablet, extended release: Chlorpheniramine maleate 8 mg, phenylephrine hydrochloride 20 mg, and methscopolamine nitrate 2.5 mg
  Drize®-R: Chlorpheniramine maleate 8 mg, phenylephrine hydrochloride 20 mg, and methscopolamine nitrate 2.5 mg [dye free; scored]
  Hista-Vent® DA: Chlorpheniramine maleate 8 mg, phenylephrine hydrochloride 20 mg, and methscopolamine nitrate 2.5 mg [scored]
  PCM Allergy: Chlorpheniramine maleate 12 mg, phenylephrine hydrochloride 20 mg, and methscopolamine nitrate 2.5 mg

chlorpheniramine, phenylephrine, and phenyltoloxamine

(klor fen IR a meen, fen il EF rin, & fen il tole LOKS a meen)

Synonyms phenylephrine, chlorpheniramine, and phenyltoloxamine; phenyltoloxamine, chlorpheniramine, and phenylephrine

U.S./Canadian Brand Names Comhist® [US]; Nalex®-A [US]

Therapeutic Category Antihistamine/Decongestant Combination

Use Symptomatic relief of rhinitis and nasal congestion due to colds or allergy

Usual Dosage Oral:

Children:
- 2-6 years: Nalex®-A liquid: 1.25-2.5 mL every 4-6 hours
- 6-12 years:
  - Nalex®-A liquid: 5 mL every 4-6 hours
  - Nalex®-A tablet: 1/2 tablet 2-3 times/day

Children >12 years and Adults:
- Nalex®-A liquid: 10 mL every 4-6 hours
- Nalex®-A tablet: 1 tablet 2-3 times/day

Dosage Forms

Liquid (Nalex®-A): Chlorpheniramine maleate 2.5 mg, phenylephrine hydrochloride 5 mg, and phenyltoloxamine citrate 7.5 mg per 5 mL (480 mL) [alcohol free, sugar free; cotton candy flavor]

Tablet: (Comhist®): Chlorpheniramine maleate 2 mg, phenylephrine hydrochloride 10 mg, and phenyltoloxamine citrate 25 mg

Tablet, prolonged release (Nalex®-A): Chlorpheniramine maleate 4 mg, phenylephrine hydrochloride 20 mg, and phenyltoloxamine citrate 40 mg

chlorpheniramine, phenylephrine, codeine, and potassium iodide

(klor fen IR a meen, fen il EF rin, KOE deen, & poe TASS ee um EYE oh dide)

Synonyms codeine, chlorpheniramine, phenylephrine, and potassium iodide; phenylephrine, chlorpheniramine, codeine, and potassium iodide; potassium iodide, chlorpheniramine, phenylephrine, and codeine

U.S./Canadian Brand Names Pediacof® [US]

Therapeutic Category Antihistamine/Decongestant/Antitussive

Controlled Substance C-IV

Use Symptomatic relief of rhinitis, nasal congestion and cough due to colds or allergy

Usual Dosage Children 6 months to 12 years: 1.25-10 mL every 4-6 hours

Dosage Forms Syrup (Pediacof®): Chlorpheniramine maleate 0.75 mg, phenylephrine hydrochloride 2.5 mg, codeine phosphate 5 mg, and potassium iodide 75 mg per 5 mL (480 mL) [contains alcohol 5% and sodium benzoate; raspberry flavor]

chlorpheniramine, pseudoephedrine, and acetaminophen *see* acetaminophen, chlorpheniramine, and pseudoephedrine *on page 11*

chlorpheniramine, pseudoephedrine, and codeine

(klor fen IR a meen, soo doe e FED rin, & KOE deen)

Synonyms codeine, chlorpheniramine, and pseudoephedrine; pseudoephedrine, chlorpheniramine, and codeine

U.S./Canadian Brand Names Dihistine® DH [US]

(Continued)

chlorpheniramine, pseudoephedrine, and codeine *(Continued)*

Therapeutic Category Antihistamine/Decongestant/Antitussive

Controlled Substance C-V

Use Temporary relief of cough associated with minor throat or bronchial irritation or nasal congestion due to common cold, allergic rhinitis, or sinusitis

Usual Dosage Oral:

Children:

25-50 lb: 1.25-2.50 mL every 4-6 hours, up to 4 doses in 24-hour period

50-90 lb: 2.5-5 mL every 4-6 hours, up to 4 doses in 24-hour period

Adults: 10 mL every 4-6 hours, up to 4 doses in 24-hour period

Dosage Forms

Elixir: Chlorpheniramine maleate 2 mg, pseudoephedrine hydrochloride 30 mg, and codeine phosphate 10 mg per 5 mL (120 mL, 480 mL)

Dihistine® DH: Chlorpheniramine maleate 2 mg, pseudoephedrine hydrochloride 30 mg, and codeine phosphate 10 mg per 5 mL (120 mL, 480 mL) [contains alcohol; grape flavor]

chlorpheniramine tannate and phenylephrine tannate *see* chlorpheniramine and phenylephrine *on page 188*

chlorpheniramine tannate and pseudoephedrine tannate *see* chlorpheniramine and pseudoephedrine *on page 189*

Chlorphen [US-OTC] *see* chlorpheniramine *on page 187*

Chlor-Pro® Injection ***(Discontinued)*** *see page 1042*

chlorpromazine (klor PROE ma zeen)

Sound-Alike/Look-Alike Issues

chlorpromazine may be confused with chlorpropamide, clomipramine, Compazine®, prochlorperazine, promethazine

Synonyms chlorpromazine hydrochloride; CPZ

Tall-Man chlorpro**MAZINE**

U.S./Canadian Brand Names Apo-Chlorpromazine® [Can]; Largactil® [Can]; Novo-Chlorpromazine [Can]

Therapeutic Category Phenothiazine Derivative

Use Control of mania; treatment of schizophrenia; control of nausea and vomiting; relief of restlessness and apprehension before surgery; acute intermittent porphyria; adjunct in the treatment of tetanus; intractable hiccups; combativeness and/or explosive hyperexcitable behavior in children 1-12 years of age and in short-term treatment of hyperactive children

Usual Dosage

Children ≥6 months:

Schizophrenia/psychoses:

Oral: 0.5-1 mg/kg/dose every 4-6 hours; older children may require 200 mg/day or higher

I.M., I.V.: 0.5-1 mg/kg/dose every 6-8 hours <5 years (22.7 kg): Maximum: 40 mg/day 5-12 years (22.7-45.5 kg): Maximum: 75 mg/day

Nausea and vomiting:

Oral: 0.5-1 mg/kg/dose every 4-6 hours as needed

I.M., I.V.: 0.5-1 mg/kg/dose every 6-8 hours <5 years (22.7 kg): Maximum: 40 mg/day 5-12 years (22.7-45.5 kg): Maximum: 75 mg/day

Adults:

Schizophrenia/psychoses:

Oral: Range: 30-2000 mg/day in 1-4 divided doses, initiate at lower doses and titrate as needed; usual dose: 400-600 mg/day; some patients may require 1-2 g/day

I.M., I.V.: Initial: 25 mg, may repeat (25-50 mg) in 1-4 hours, gradually increase to a maximum of 400 mg/dose every 4-6 hours until patient is controlled; usual dose: 300-800 mg/day

Intractable hiccups: Oral, I.M.: 25-50 mg 3-4 times/day

Nausea and vomiting:
Oral: 10-25 mg every 4-6 hours
I.M., I.V.: 25-50 mg every 4-6 hours

Dosage Forms [DSC] = Discontinued product
Injection, solution, as hydrochloride (Thorazine® [DSC]): 25 mg/mL (10 mL) [contains benzyl alcohol, sodium bisulfite, and sodium sulfite]
Tablet, as hydrochloride: 10 mg, 25 mg, 50 mg, 100 mg, 200 mg

chlorpromazine hydrochloride *see* chlorpromazine *on previous page*

chlorpropamide (klor PROE pa mide)

Sound-Alike/Look-Alike Issues
chlorpropamide may be confused with chlorpromazine
Diabinese® may be confused with DiaBeta®, Dialume®

Tall-Man chlorpro**PAMIDE**

U.S./Canadian Brand Names Apo-Chlorpropamide® [Can]; Diabinese® [US]; Novo-Propamide [Can]

Therapeutic Category Antidiabetic Agent, Oral

Use Management of blood sugar in type 2 diabetes mellitus (noninsulin dependent, NIDDM)

Usual Dosage Oral: The dosage of chlorpropamide is variable and should be individualized based upon the patient's response
Initial dose:
Adults: 250 mg/day in mild to moderate diabetes in middle-aged, stable diabetic
Elderly: 100-125 mg/day in older patients
Subsequent dosages may be increased or decreased by 50-125 mg/day at 3- to 5-day intervals
Maintenance dose: 100-250 mg/day; severe diabetics may require 500 mg/day; avoid doses >750 mg/day

Dosage Forms Tablet: 100 mg, 250 mg

Chlor-Rest® Tablet *(Discontinued)* *see page 1042*

Chlortab® *(Discontinued)* *see page 1042*

chlorthalidone (klor THAL i done)

U.S./Canadian Brand Names Apo-Chlorthalidone® [Can]; Thalitone® [US]

Therapeutic Category Diuretic, Miscellaneous

Use Management of mild to moderate hypertension when used alone or in combination with other agents; treatment of edema associated with congestive heart failure or nephrotic syndrome. Recent studies have found chlorthalidone effective in the treatment of isolated systolic hypertension in the elderly.

Usual Dosage Oral:
Children (nonapproved): 2 mg/kg/dose 3 times/week or 1-2 mg/kg/day
Adults: 25-100 mg/day or 100 mg 3 times/week; usual dosage range (JNC 7): 12.5-25 mg/day

Dosage Forms
Tablet: 25 mg, 50 mg, 100 mg
Thalitone®: 15 mg

chlorthalidone and atenolol *see* atenolol and chlorthalidone *on page 85*

chlorthalidone and clonidine *see* clonidine and chlorthalidone *on page 216*

Chlor-Trimeton® Allergy D [US-OTC] *see* chlorpheniramine and pseudoephedrine *on page 189*

Chlor-Trimeton® Syrup *(Discontinued)* *see page 1042*

Chlor-Trimeton® [US-OTC] *see* chlorpheniramine *on page 187*

Chlor-Tripolon® [Can] *see* chlorpheniramine *on page 187*

Chlor-Tripolon ND® [Can] *see* loratadine and pseudoephedrine *on page 530*

chlorzoxazone (klor ZOKS a zone)

Sound-Alike/Look-Alike Issues
Parafon Forte® may be confused with Fam-Pren Forte

U.S./Canadian Brand Names Parafon Forte® [Can]; Parafon Forte® DSC [US]; Strifon Forte® [Can]

Therapeutic Category Skeletal Muscle Relaxant

Use Symptomatic treatment of muscle spasm and pain associated with acute musculoskeletal conditions

Usual Dosage Oral:
Children: 20 mg/kg/day or 600 mg/m^2/day in 3-4 divided doses
Adults: 250-500 mg 3-4 times/day up to 750 mg 3-4 times/day

Dosage Forms
Caplet (Parafon Forte® DSC): 500 mg
Tablet: 250 mg, 500 mg

Cholac® [US] *see* lactulose *on page 502*

Cholan-HMB® *(Discontinued)* *see page 1042*

Cholebrine® [US] *see* radiological/contrast media (ionic) *on page 759*

cholecalciferol (kole e kal SI fer ole)

Synonyms D_3

U.S./Canadian Brand Names Delta-D® [US]; D-Vi-Sol® [Can]

Therapeutic Category Vitamin D Analog

Use Dietary supplement, treatment of vitamin D deficiency, or prophylaxis of deficiency

Usual Dosage Adults: Oral: 400-1000 units/day

Dosage Forms
Tablet: 1000 int. units
Delta-D®: 400 int. units

Choledyl® *(Discontinued)* *see page 1042*

Choledyl SA® *(Discontinued)* *see page 1042*

cholera vaccine (all products) *(Discontinued)* *see page 1042*

cholestyramine resin (koe LES tir a meen REZ in)

U.S./Canadian Brand Names Novo-Cholamine [Can]; Novo-Cholamine Light [Can]; PMS-Cholestyramine [Can]; Prevalite® [US]; Questran® [US/Can]; Questran® Light [US]; Questran® Light Sugar Free [Can]

Therapeutic Category Bile Acid Sequestrant

Use Adjunct in the management of primary hypercholesterolemia; pruritus associated with elevated levels of bile acids; diarrhea associated with excess fecal bile acids; binding toxicologic agents; pseudomembraneous colitis

Usual Dosage Oral (dosages are expressed in terms of anhydrous resin):
Children: 240 mg/kg/day in 3 divided doses; need to titrate dose depending on indication
Adults: 4 g 1-2 times/day to a maximum of 24 g/day and 6 doses/day

Dosage Forms
Powder for oral suspension: 4 g of resin/5.7 g of powder (5.7 g packets, 240 g can) [light formulation]; 4 g of resin/9 g of powder (9 g packets, 378 g can)
Prevalite®: 4 g of resin/5.5 g of powder (5.5 g packets, 231 g can) [contains phenylalanine 14.1 mg/5.5 g; orange flavor]
Questran®: 4 g of resin/9 g of powder (9 g packets, 378 g can)
Questran® Light: 4 g of resin/5 g of powder (5 g packets, 210 g can) [contains phenylalanine 16.8 g/5 g]

choline magnesium trisalicylate

(KOE leen mag NEE zhum trye sa LIS i late)

Synonyms tricosal

Therapeutic Category Analgesic, Nonnarcotic; Nonsteroidal Antiinflammatory Drug (NSAID)

Use Management of osteoarthritis, rheumatoid arthritis, and other arthritis; acute painful shoulder

Usual Dosage Oral (based on total salicylate content):

Children <37 kg: 50 mg/kg/day given in 2 divided doses; 2250 mg/day for heavier children

Adults: 500 mg to 1.5 g 2-3 times/day **or** 3 g at bedtime; usual maintenance dose: 1-4.5 g/day

Dosage Forms

Liquid: 500 mg/5 mL (240 mL) [choline salicylate 293 mg and magnesium salicylate 362 mg per 5 mL; cherry cordial flavor]

Tablet: 500 mg [choline salicylate 293 mg and magnesium salicylate 362 mg]; 750 mg [choline salicylate 440 mg and magnesium salicylate 544 mg]; 1000 mg [choline salicylate 587 mg and magnesium salicylate 725 mg]

Cholografin® Meglumine [US] *see* radiological/contrast media (ionic) *on page 759*

Choloxin® ***(Discontinued)*** *see page 1042*

chondroitin sulfate and sodium hyaluronate

(kon DROY tin SUL fate-SOW de um hye a loo ROE nate)

Synonyms sodium hyaluronate-chrondroitin sulfate

U.S./Canadian Brand Names Viscoat® [US]

Therapeutic Category Ophthalmic Agent, Viscoelastic

Use Surgical aid in anterior segment procedures, protects corneal endothelium and coats intraocular lens thus protecting it

Usual Dosage Carefully introduce (using a 27-gauge needle or cannula) into anterior chamber after thoroughly cleaning the chamber with a balanced salt solution

Dosage Forms Solution, ophthalmic: Sodium chondroitin 4% and sodium hyaluronate 3% (0.5 mL)

Chooz® [US-OTC] *see* calcium carbonate *on page 144*

Chorex® ***(Discontinued)*** *see page 1042*

choriogonadotropin alfa *see* chorionic gonadotropin (recombinant) *on this page*

chorionic gonadotropin (human)

(kor ee ON ik goe NAD oh troe pin HYU man)

Synonyms CG; HCG

Therapeutic Category Gonadotropin

Use Treatment of hypogonadotropic hypogonadism, prepubertal cryptorchidism; induce ovulation

Usual Dosage Children: I.M.:

Prepubertal cryptorchidism: 1000-2000 units/m^2/dose 3 times/week for 3 weeks

Hypogonadotropic hypogonadism: 500-1000 USP units 3 times/week for 3 weeks, followed by the same dose twice weekly for 3 weeks

Dosage Forms Powder for injection: 5000 units, 10,000 units

chorionic gonadotropin (recombinant)

(kor ee ON ik goe NAD oh troe pin ree KOM be nant)

Synonyms choriogonadotropin alfa; r-hCG

U.S./Canadian Brand Names Ovidrel® [US]

Therapeutic Category Gonadotropin; Ovulation Stimulator

(Continued)

chorionic gonadotropin (recombinant) *(Continued)*

Use As part of an assisted reproductive technology (ART) program, induces ovulation in infertile females who have been pretreated with follicle stimulating hormones (FSH); induces ovulation and pregnancy in infertile females when the cause of infertility is functional

Usual Dosage SubQ: Adults: Female: Assisted reproductive technologies (ART) and ovulation induction: 250 mcg given 1 day following the last dose of follicle stimulating agent. Use only after adequate follicular development has been determined. Hold treatment when there is an excessive ovarian response.

Dosage Forms

Injection, powder for reconstitution: 285 mcg [packaged with 1 mL SWFI; delivers 250 mcg r-hCG following reconstitution] [DSC]

Injection, solution : 257.5 mcg/0.515 mL (0.515 mL) [prefilled syringe; delivers 250 mcg r-hCG/0.5 mL]

Choron® *(Discontinued)* *see page 1042*

Chromagen® OB [US] *see* vitamins (multiple/prenatal) *on page 927*

chromium *see* trace metals *on page 874*

Chronovera® [Can] *see* verapamil *on page 908*

Chronulac® *(Discontinued)* *see page 1042*

Chymex® *(Discontinued)* *see page 1042*

Cialis® [US] *see* tadalafil *on page 838*

Cibacalcin® *(Discontinued)* *see page 1042*

ciclopirox (sye kloe PEER oks)

Sound-Alike/Look-Alike Issues

Loprox® may be confused with Lonox®

Synonyms ciclopirox olamine

U.S./Canadian Brand Names Loprox® [US/Can]; Penlac™ [US/Can]

Therapeutic Category Antifungal Agent

Use

Cream/suspension: Treatment of tinea pedis (athlete's foot), tinea cruris (jock itch), tinea corporis (ringworm), cutaneous candidiasis, and tinea versicolor (pityriasis)

Gel: Treatment of tinea pedis (athlete's foot), tinea corporis (ringworm); seborrheic dermatitis of the scalp

Lacquer: Topical treatment of mild to moderate onychomycosis of the fingernails and toenails

Shampoo: Treatment of seborrheic dermatitis of the scalp

Usual Dosage Topical:

Children >10 years and Adults: Tinea pedis, tinea cruris, tinea corporis, cutaneous candidiasis, and tinea versicolor: Cream/suspension: Apply twice daily, gently massage into affected areas; if no improvement after 4 weeks of treatment, re-evaluate the diagnosis

Children >16 years and Adults:

Tinea pedis, tinea corporis, seborrheic dermatitis of the scalp: Gel: Apply twice daily, gently massage into affected areas and surrounding skin; if no improvement after 4 weeks of treatment, re-evaluate diagnosis

Seborrheic dermatitis of the scalp: Shampoo: Apply to wet hair, lather, and leave in place ~3 minute; rinse. Repeat twice weekly for 4 weeks; allow a minimum of 3 days between applications.

Onychomycosis of the fingernails and toenails: Children ≥12 years and Adults: Lacquer (solution): Apply to affected nails daily (as a part of a comprehensive management program for onychomycosis)

Dosage Forms

Cream, as olamine (Loprox®): 0.77% (15 g, 30 g, 90 g)

Gel (Loprox®): 0.77% (30 g, 45 g, 100 g)

Shampoo (Loprox®): 1% (120 mL)
Solution, topical [nail lacquer] (Penlac™): 8% (6.6 mL)
Suspension, topical, as olamine (Loprox®): 0.77% (30 mL, 60 mL)

ciclopirox olamine *see* ciclopirox *on previous page*

cidecin *see* daptomycin *on page 245*

cidofovir (si DOF o veer)

U.S./Canadian Brand Names Vistide® [US]

Therapeutic Category Antiviral Agent

Use Treatment of cytomegalovirus (CMV) retinitis in patients with acquired immunodeficiency syndrome (AIDS). **Note:** Should be administered with probenecid.

Usual Dosage

Induction: 5 mg/kg I.V. over 1 hour once weekly for 2 consecutive weeks

Maintenance: 5 mg/kg over 1 hour once every other week

Administer with probenecid - 2 g orally 3 hours prior to each cidofovir dose and 1 g at 2 and 8 hours after completion of the infusion (total: 4 g)

Hydrate with 1 L of 0.9% NS I.V. prior to cidofovir infusion; a second liter may be administered over a 1- to 3-hour period immediately following infusion, if tolerated

Dosage Forms Injection, solution [preservative free]: 75 mg/mL (5 mL)

cilazapril *(Canada only)* (sye LAY za pril)

Synonyms cilazapril monohydrate

U.S./Canadian Brand Names Inhibace® [Can]

Therapeutic Category Angiotensin-Converting Enzyme (ACE) Inhibitor

Use Management of hypertension; treatment of congestive heart failure

Usual Dosage Oral:

Hypertension: 2.5-5 mg once daily (maximum dose: 10 mg/day)

Congestive heart failure: Initial: 0.5 mg once daily; if tolerated, after 5 days increase to 1 mg/day (lowest maintenance dose); may increase to maximum of 2.5 mg once daily

Dosage Forms Tablet: 1 mg, 2.5 mg, 5 mg

cilazapril monohydrate *see* cilazapril *(Canada only)* *on this page*

cilostazol (sil OH sta zol)

Sound-Alike/Look-Alike Issues

Pletal® may be confused with Plendil®

Synonyms OPC-13013

U.S./Canadian Brand Names Pletal® [US/Can]

Therapeutic Category Platelet Aggregation Inhibitor

Use Symptomatic management of peripheral vascular disease, primarily intermittent claudication; currently being investigated for the treatment of acute coronary syndromes and for graft patency improvement in percutaneous coronary interventions with or without stenting

Usual Dosage Adults: Oral: 100 mg twice daily taken at least one-half hour before or 2 hours after breakfast and dinner; dosage should be reduced to 50 mg twice daily during concurrent therapy with inhibitors of CYP3A4 or CYP2C19

Dosage Forms Tablet: 50 mg, 100 mg

Ciloxan® [US/Can] *see* ciprofloxacin *on page 201*

cimetidine (sye MET i deen)

Sound-Alike/Look-Alike Issues

cimetidine may be confused with simethicone

U.S./Canadian Brand Names Apo-Cimetidine® [Can]; Gen-Cimetidine [Can]; Novo-Cimetidine [Can]; Nu-Cimet [Can]; PMS-Cimetidine [Can]; Tagamet® [US]; Tagamet® HB 200 [US-OTC/Can]

Therapeutic Category Histamine H_2 Antagonist

(Continued)

cimetidine *(Continued)*

Use Short-term treatment of active duodenal ulcers and benign gastric ulcers; long-term prophylaxis of duodenal ulcer; gastric hypersecretory states; gastroesophageal reflux; prevention of upper GI bleeding in critically-ill patients; labeled for OTC use for prevention or relief of heartburn, acid indigestion, or sour stomach

Usual Dosage

Children: Oral, I.M., I.V.: 20-40 mg/kg/day in divided doses every 6 hours

Children ≥12 years and Adults: Oral: Heartburn, acid indigestion, sour stomach (OTC labeling): 200 mg up to twice daily; may take 30 minutes prior to eating foods or beverages expected to cause heartburn or indigestion

Adults:

Short-term treatment of active ulcers:

Oral: 300 mg 4 times/day or 800 mg at bedtime or 400 mg twice daily for up to 8 weeks

I.M., I.V.: 300 mg every 6 hours or 37.5 mg/hour by continuous infusion; I.V. dosage should be adjusted to maintain an intragastric pH ≥5

Patients with an active bleed: Administer cimetidine as a continuous infusion (see above)

Duodenal ulcer prophylaxis: Oral: 400-800 mg at bedtime

Gastric hypersecretory conditions: Oral, I.M., I.V.: 300-600 mg every 6 hours; dosage not to exceed 2.4 g/day

Dosage Forms

Infusion, as hydrochloride [premixed in NS]: 300 mg (50 mL)

Injection, solution, as hydrochloride: 150 mg/mL (2 mL, 8 mL) [8 mL size contains benzyl alcohol]

Liquid, oral, as hydrochloride: 300 mg/5 mL (240 mL, 480 mL) [contains alcohol 2.8%; mint-peach flavor]

Tablet: 200 mg [OTC], 300 mg, 400 mg, 800 mg

Tagamet: 300 mg, 400 mg

Tagamet® HB 200: 200 mg

cinacalcet (sin a KAL cet)

Synonyms AMG 073; cinacalcet hydrochloride

U.S./Canadian Brand Names Sensipar™ [US]

Therapeutic Category Calcimimetic

Use Treatment of secondary hyperparathyroidism in dialysis patients; treatment of hypercalcemia in patients with parathyroid carcinoma

Usual Dosage Oral: Adults: **Do not titrate dose more frequently than every 2-4 weeks.**

Hyperparathyroidism: Initial: 30 mg once daily (maximum daily dose: 180 mg); increase dose incrementally (60 mg, 90 mg, 120 mg, 180 mg once daily) as necessary to maintain iPTH level between 150-300 pg/mL.

Parathyroid carcinoma: Initial: 30 mg twice daily (maximum daily dose: 360 mg daily as 90 mg 4 times/day); increase dose incrementally (60 mg twice daily, 90 mg twice daily, 90 mg 4 times/day) as necessary to normalize serum calcium levels.

Dosage Forms Tablet [film coated]: 30 mg, 60 mg, 90 mg

cinacalcet hydrochloride *see* cinacalcet *on this page*

cinoxacin (sin OKS a sin)

Therapeutic Category Quinolone

Use Urinary tract infections

Usual Dosage Children >12 years and Adults: Oral: 1 g/day in 2-4 doses

Dosage Forms Capsule: 500 mg

Cipralan® *(Discontinued)* *see page 1042*

Cipro® [US/Can] *see* ciprofloxacin *on next page*

Ciprodex® [US] *see* ciprofloxacin and dexamethasone *on page 203*

ciprofloxacin (sip roe FLOKS a sin)

Sound-Alike/Look-Alike Issues

ciprofloxacin may be confused with cephalexin
Ciloxan® may be confused with cinoxacin, Cytoxan®
Cipro® may be confused with Ceftin®

Synonyms ciprofloxacin hydrochloride

U.S./Canadian Brand Names Ciloxan® [US/Can]; Cipro® [US/Can]; Cipro® XL [Can]; Cipro® XR [US]

Therapeutic Category Antibiotic, Ophthalmic; Quinolone

Use

Children: Complicated urinary tract infections and pyelonephritis due to *E. coli.* **Note:** Although effective, ciprofloxacin is not the drug of first choice in children.

Children and adults: To reduce incidence or progression of disease following exposure to aerolized *Bacillus anthracis*. Ophthalmologically, for superficial ocular infections (corneal ulcers, conjunctivitis) due to susceptible strains

Adults: Treatment of the following infections when caused by susceptible bacteria: Urinary tract infections; acute uncomplicated cystitis in females; chronic bacterial prostatitis; lower respiratory tract infections (including acute exacerbations of chronic bronchitis); acute sinusitis; skin and skin structure infections; bone and joint infections; complicated intra-abdominal infections (in combination with metronidazole); infectious diarrhea; typhoid fever due to *Salmonella typhi* (eradication of chronic typhoid carrier state has not been proven); uncomplicated cervical and urethra gonorrhea (due to *N. gonorrhoeae*); nosocomial pneumonia; empirical therapy for febrile neutropenic patients (in combination with piperacillin)

Usual Dosage Note: Extended release tablets and immediate release formulations are not interchangeable. Unless otherwise specified, oral dosing reflects the use of immediate release formulations.

Children:

Oral:

Complicated urinary tract infection or pyelonephritis: Children 1-17 years: 20-30 mg/kg/day in 2 divided doses (every 12 hours) for 10-21 days; maximum: 1.5 g/day

Anthrax: Inhalational (postexposure prophylaxis): 15 mg/kg/dose every 12 hours for 60 days; maximum: 500 mg/dose Cutaneous (treatment, CDC guidelines): 10-15 mg/kg every 12 hours for 60 days (maximum: 1 g/day); amoxicillin 80 mg/kg/day divided every 8 hours is an option for completion of treatment after clinical improvement. **Note:** In the presence of systemic involvement, extensive edema, lesions on head/neck, refer to I.V. dosing for treatment of inhalational/gastrointestinal/oropharyngeal anthrax

I.V.:

Complicated urinary tract infection or pyelonephritis: Children 1-17 years: 6-10 mg/kg every 8 hours for 10-21 days (maximum: 400 mg/dose)

Anthrax: Inhalational (postexposure prophylaxis): 10 mg/kg/dose every 12 hours for 60 days; do **not** exceed 400 mg/dose (800 mg/day) Inhalational/gastrointestinal/oropharyngeal (treatment, CDC guidelines): Initial: 10-15 mg/kg every 12 hours for 60 days (maximum: 500 mg/dose); switch to oral therapy when clinically appropriate; refer to Adults dosing for notes on combined therapy and duration

Adults: Oral:

Urinary tract infection:

Acute uncomplicated: Immediate release formulation: 100 mg or 250 mg every 12 hours for 3 days

Acute uncomplicated pyelonephritis: Extended release formulation: 1000 mg every 24 hours for 7-14 days

Uncomplicated/acute cystitis: Extended release formulation: 500 mg every 24 hours for 3 days

Mild/moderate: Immediate release formulation: 250 mg every 12 hours for 7-14 days

(Continued)

ciprofloxacin *(Continued)*

Severe/complicated: Immediate release formulation: 500 mg every 12 hours for 7-14 days Extended release formulation: 1000 mg every 24 hours for 7-14 days

Lower respiratory tract, skin/skin structure infections: 500-750 mg twice daily for 7-14 days depending on severity and susceptibility

Bone/joint infections: 500-750 mg twice daily for 4-6 weeks, depending on severity and susceptibility

Infectious diarrhea: 500 mg every 12 hours for 5-7 days

Intra-abdominal (in combination with metronidazole): 500 mg every 12 hours for 7-14 days

Typhoid fever: 500 mg every 12 hours for 10 days

Urethral/cervical gonococcal infections: 250-500 mg as a single dose (CDC recommends concomitant doxycycline or azithromycin due to developing resistance; avoid use in Asian or Western Pacific travelers)

Disseminated gonococcal infection (CDC guidelines): 500 mg twice daily to complete 7 days of therapy (initial treatment with ceftriaxone 1 g I.M./I.V. daily for 24-48 hours after improvement begins)

Chancroid (CDC guidelines): 500 mg twice daily for 3 days

Sinusitis (acute): 500 mg every 12 hours for 10 days

Chronic bacterial prostatitis: 500 mg every 12 hours for 28 days

Anthrax:

Inhalational (postexposure prophylaxis): 500 mg every 12 hours for 60 days

Cutaneous (treatment, CDC guidelines): Immediate release formulation: 500 mg every 12 hours for 60 days. **Note:** In the presence of systemic involvement, extensive edema, lesions on head/neck, refer to I.V. dosing for treatment of inhalational/gastrointestinal/oropharyngeal anthrax

Adults: I.V.:

Bone/joint infections:

Mild to moderate: 400 mg every 12 hours for 4-6 weeks

Severe or complicated: 400 mg every 8 hours for 4-6 weeks

Lower respiratory tract, skin/skin structure infections:

Mild to moderate: 400 mg every 12 hours for 7-14 days

Severe or complicated: 400 mg every 8 hours for 7-14 days

Nosocomial pneumonia (mild to moderate to severe): 400 mg every 8 hours for 10-14 days

Prostatitis (chronic, bacterial): 400 mg every 12 hours for 28 days

Sinusitis (acute): 400 mg every 12 hours for 10 days

Urinary tract infection:

Mild to moderate: 200 mg every 12 hours for 7-14 days

Severe or complicated: 400 mg every 12 hours for 7-14 days

Febrile neutropenia (with piperacillin): 400 mg every 8 hours for 7-14 days

Intra-abdominal infection (with metronidazole): 400 mg every 12 hours for 7-14 days

Anthrax:

Inhalational (postexposure prophylaxis): 400 mg every 12 hours for 60 days

Inhalational/gastrointestinal/oropharyngeal (treatment, CDC guidelines): 400 mg every 12 hours. **Note:** Initial treatment should include two or more agents predicted to be effective (per CDC recommendations). Agents suggested for use in conjunction with ciprofloxacin or doxycycline include rifampin, vancomycin, imipenem, penicillin, ampicillin, chloramphenicol, clindamycin, and clarithromycin. May switch to oral antimicrobial therapy when clinically appropriate. Continue combined therapy for 60 days.

Ophthalmic:

Solution: Children >1 year and Adults:

Bacterial conjunctivitis: Instill 1-2 drops in eye(s) every 2 hours while awake for 2 days and 1-2 drops every 4 hours while awake for the next 5 days

Corneal ulcer: Instill 2 drops into affected eye every 15 minutes for the first 6 hours, then 2 drops into the affected eye every 30 minutes for the remainder of the first day. On day 2, instill 2 drops into the affected eye hourly. On days 3-14, instill 2 drops into affected eye every 4 hours. Treatment may continue after day 14 if re-epithelialization has not occurred.

Ointment: Children >2 years and Adults: Bacterial conjunctivitis: Apply a 1/2" ribbon into the conjunctival sac 3 times/day for the first 2 days, followed by a 1/2" ribbon applied twice daily for the next 5 days

Dosage Forms

Infusion, [premixed in D_5W] (Cipro®): 200 mg (100 mL); 400 mg (200 mL) [latex free]

Injection, solution (Cipro®): 10 mg/mL (20 mL, 40 mL, 120 mL)

Microcapsules for oral suspension (Cipro®): 250 mg/5 mL (100 mL); 500 mg/5 mL (100 mL) [strawberry flavor]

Ointment, ophthalmic, as hydrochloride (Ciloxan®): 3.33 mg/g [0.3% base] (3.5 g)

Solution, ophthalmic, as hydrochloride (Ciloxan®): 3.5 mg/mL [0.3% base] (2.5 mL, 5 mL, 10 mL) [contains benzalkonium chloride]

Tablet [film coated]: 250 mg, 500 mg, 750 mg

Cipro®: 100 mg, 250 mg, 500 mg, 750 mg

Tablet, extended release [film coated] (Cipro® XR): 500 mg [equivalent to ciprofloxacin hydrochloride 287.5 mg and ciprofloxacin base 212.6 mg]; 1000 mg [equivalent to ciprofloxacin hydrochloride 574.9 mg and ciprofloxacin base 425.2 mg]

ciprofloxacin and dexamethasone

(sip roe FLOKS a sin & deks a METH a sone)

Synonyms ciprofloxacin hydrochloride and dexamethasone; dexamethasone and ciprofloxacin

U.S./Canadian Brand Names Ciprodex® [US]

Therapeutic Category Antibiotic/Corticosteroid, Otic

Use Treatment of acute otitis media in pediatric patients with tympanostomy tubes or acute otitis externa in children and adults

Usual Dosage Otic:

Children: Acute otitis media in patients with tympanostomy tubes or acute otitis externa: Instill 4 drops into affected ear(s) twice daily for 7 days

Adults: Acute otitis externa: Instill 4 drops into affected ear(s) twice daily for 7 days

Dosage Forms Suspension, otic: Ciprofloxacin 0.3% and dexamethasone 0.1% (7.5 mL) [contains benzalkonium chloride]

ciprofloxacin and hydrocortisone

(sip roe FLOKS a sin & hye droe KOR ti sone)

Synonyms hydrocortisone and ciprofloxacin

U.S./Canadian Brand Names Cipro® HC Otic [US/Can]

Therapeutic Category Antibiotic/Corticosteroid, Otic

Use Treatment of acute otitis externa, sometimes known as "swimmer's ear"

Usual Dosage Children >1 year of age and Adults: Otic: The recommended dosage for all patients is three drops of the suspension in the affected ear twice daily for seven day; twice-daily dosing schedule is more convenient for patients than that of existing treatments with hydrocortisone, which are typically administered three or four times a day; a twice-daily dosage schedule may be especially helpful for parents and caregivers of young children

Dosage Forms Suspension, otic: Ciprofloxacin hydrochloride 0.2% and hydrocortisone 1% (10 mL) [contains benzyl alcohol]

ciprofloxacin hydrochloride *see* ciprofloxacin *on page 201*

ciprofloxacin hydrochloride and dexamethasone *see* ciprofloxacin and dexamethasone *on this page*

Cipro® HC Otic [US/Can] *see* ciprofloxacin and hydrocortisone *on this page*

Cipro® XL [Can] *see* ciprofloxacin *on page 201*

Cipro® XR [US] *see* ciprofloxacin *on page 201*

cisapride (SIS a pride)

Sound-Alike/Look-Alike Issues

Propulsid® may be confused with propranolol

U.S./Canadian Brand Names Propulsid® [US]

Therapeutic Category Gastrointestinal Agent, Prokinetic

Use Treatment of nocturnal symptoms of gastroesophageal reflux disease (GERD); has demonstrated effectiveness for gastroparesis, refractory constipation, and nonulcer dyspepsia

Usual Dosage Oral:

Children: 0.15-0.3 mg/kg/dose 3-4 times/day; maximum: 10 mg/dose

Adults: Initial: 10 mg 4 times/day at least 15 minutes before meals and at bedtime; in some patients the dosage will need to be increased to 20 mg to obtain a satisfactory result

Dosage Forms

Suspension, oral: 1 mg/mL (450 mL) [cherry cream flavor]

Tablet, scored: 10 mg, 20 mg

cisatracurium (sis a tra KYOO ree um)

Sound-Alike/Look-Alike Issues

Nimbex® may be confused with Revex®

Synonyms cisatracurium besylate

U.S./Canadian Brand Names Nimbex® [US/Can]

Therapeutic Category Skeletal Muscle Relaxant

Use Adjunct to general anesthesia to facilitate endotracheal intubation and to relax skeletal muscles during surgery; to facilitate mechanical ventilation in ICU patients; does not relieve pain or produce sedation

Usual Dosage I.V. (not to be used I.M.):

Operating room administration:

Children 2-12 years: Intubating doses: 0.1 mg over 5-15 seconds during either halothane or opioid anesthesia. (**Note:** When given during stable opioid/nitrous oxide/oxygen anesthesia, 0.1 mg/kg produces maximum neuromuscular block in an average of 2.8 minutes and clinically effective block for 28 minutes.)

Adults: Intubating doses: 0.15-0.2 mg/kg as component of propofol/nitrous oxide/oxygen induction-intubation technique. (**Note:** May produce generally good or excellent conditions for tracheal intubation in 1.5-2 minutes with clinically effective duration of action during propofol anesthesia of 55-61 minutes.); initial dose after succinylcholine for intubation: 0.1 mg/kg; maintenance dose: 0.03 mg/kg 40-60 minutes after initial dose, then at ~20-minute intervals based on clinical criteria

Children ≥2 years and Adults: Continuous infusion: After an initial bolus, a diluted solution can be given by continuous infusion for maintenance of neuromuscular blockade during extended surgery; adjust the rate of administration according to the patient's response as determined by peripheral nerve stimulation. An initial infusion rate of 3 mcg/kg/minute may be required to rapidly counteract the spontaneous recovery of neuromuscular function; thereafter, a rate of 1-2 mcg/kg/minute should be adequate to maintain continuous neuromuscular block in the 89% to 99% range in most pediatric and adult patients. Consider reduction of the infusion rate by 30% to 40% when administering during stable isoflurane, enflurane, sevoflurane, or desflurane anesthesia. Spontaneous recovery from neuromuscular blockade following discontinuation of infusion of cisatracurium may be expected to proceed at a rate comparable to that following single bolus administration.

Intensive care unit administration: Follow the principles for infusion in the operating room. At initial signs of recovery from bolus dose, begin the infusion at a dose of 3 mcg/kg/minute and adjust rates accordingly; dosage ranges of 0.5-10 mcg/kg/minute have been reported. If patient is allowed to recover from neuromuscular blockade, readministration of a bolus dose may be necessary to quickly re-establish neuromuscular block prior to reinstituting the infusion.

Dosage Forms

Injection, solution: 2 mg/mL (5 mL); 10 mg/mL (20 mL)

Injection, solution: 2 mg/mL (10 mL) [contains benzyl alcohol]

cisatracurium besylate *see* cisatracurium *on previous page*

cisplatin (SIS pla tin)

Sound-Alike/Look-Alike Issues
cisplatin may be confused with carboplatin
Platinol®-AQ may be confused with Paraplatin®, Patanol®, Plaquenil®

Synonyms CDDP

U.S./Canadian Brand Names Platinol®-AQ [US]

Therapeutic Category Antineoplastic Agent

Use Treatment of head and neck, breast, testicular, and ovarian cancer; Hodgkin and non-Hodgkin lymphoma; neuroblastoma; sarcomas, bladder, gastric, lung, esophageal, cervical, and prostate cancer; myeloma, melanoma, mesothelioma, small cell lung cancer, and osteosarcoma

Usual Dosage Refer to individual protocols. I.V.:

An estimated Cl_{cr} should be on all cisplatin chemotherapy orders along with other patient parameters (ie, patient's height, weight, and body surface area). Pharmacy and nursing staff should check the Cl_{cr} on the order and determine the appropriateness of cisplatin dosing.

The manufacturer recommends that subsequent cycles should only be given when serum creatinine <1.5 mg/dL, WBC ≥4,000/mm^3, platelets ≥100,000/mm^3, and BUN <25.

It is recommended that a 24-hour urine creatinine clearance be checked prior to a patient's first dose of cisplatin and periodically thereafter (ie, after every 2-3 cycles of cisplatin)

Pretreatment hydration with 1-2 L of chloride-containing fluid is recommended prior to cisplatin administration; adequate hydration and urinary output (>100 mL/hour) should be maintained for 24 hours after administration

If the dose prescribed is a reduced dose, then this should be indicated on the chemotherapy order

Children: Various dosage schedules range from 30-100 mg/m^2 once every 2-3 weeks; may also dose similar to adult dosing

Recurrent brain tumors: 60 mg/m^2 once daily for 2 consecutive days every 3-4 weeks

Adults:

Advanced bladder cancer: 50-70 mg/m^2 every 3-4 weeks

Head and neck cancer: 100-120 mg/m^2 every 3-4 weeks

Malignant pleural mesothelioma (in combination with pemetrexed): 75 mg/m^2 on day 1 of each 21-day cycle; see Pemetrexed monograph for additional details

Metastatic ovarian cancer: 75-100 mg/m^2 every 3 weeks

Intraperitoneal: Cisplatin has been administered intraperitoneal with systemic sodium thiosulfate for ovarian cancer; doses up to 90-270 mg/m^2 have been administered and retained for 4 hours before draining

Testicular cancer: 10-20 mg/m^2/day for 5 days repeated every 3-4 weeks

Dosage Forms
Injection, solution: 1 mg/mL (50 mL, 100 mL, 200 mL)
Platinol®-AQ: 1 mg/mL (50 mL, 100 mL)

13-*cis*-retinoic acid *see* isotretinoin *on page 489*

citalopram (sye TAL oh pram)

Sound-Alike/Look-Alike Issues
Celexa™ may be confused with Celebrex®, Cerebra®, Cerebyx®, Zyprexa®

Synonyms citalopram hydrobromide; nitalapram

U.S./Canadian Brand Names Celexa™ [US/Can]

Therapeutic Category Antidepressant

Use Treatment of depression
(Continued)

citalopram *(Continued)*

Usual Dosage Oral:

Adults: Depression: Initial: 20 mg/day, generally with an increase to 40 mg/day; doses of more than 40 mg are not usually necessary. Should a dose increase be necessary, it should occur in 20 mg increments at intervals of no less than 1 week. Maximum dose: 60 mg/day; reduce dosage in elderly or those with hepatic impairment.

Dosage Forms

Solution, oral: 10 mg/5 mL (240 mL) [alcohol free, sugar free; peppermint flavor]

Tablet: 10 mg, 20 mg, 40 mg

citalopram hydrobromide *see* citalopram *on previous page*

Citanest® Plain [US/Can] *see* prilocaine *on page 728*

Cithalith-S® Syrup ***(Discontinued)*** *see page 1042*

Citracal® Prenatal Rx [US] *see* vitamins (multiple/prenatal) *on page 927*

Citracal® [US-OTC] *see* calcium citrate *on page 147*

citrate of magnesia *see* magnesium citrate *on page 537*

citric acid and d-gluconic acid irrigant *see* citric acid, magnesium carbonate, and glucono-delta-lactone *on this page*

citric acid and potassium citrate *see* potassium citrate and citric acid *on page 714*

citric acid, magnesium carbonate, and glucono-delta-lactone

(SI trik AS id, mag NEE see um KAR bo nate, and GLOO kon o DEL ta LAK tone)

Sound-Alike/Look-Alike Issues

Renacidin® may be confused with Remicade®

Synonyms citric acid and d-gluconic acid irrigant; citric acid, magnesium hydroxycarbonate, D-gluconic acid, magnesium acid citrate, and calcium carbonate; hemiacidrin

U.S./Canadian Brand Names Renacidin® [US]

Therapeutic Category Irrigating Solution

Use Prevention of formation of calcifications of indwelling urinary tract catheters; treatment of renal and bladder calculi of the apatite or struvite type

Usual Dosage Adults:

Dissolution or prevention of calcifications: Irrigation (indwelling urethral catheters): 30-60 mL 2-3 times/day by means of a rubber syringe

Renal calculi: Irrigation: Infuse NS at 60 mL/hour and increase until pain, elevated pressure, or maximum flow rate of 120 mL/hour is reached. Begin flow of solution at maximum rate achieved with NS.

Bladder calculi: 30 mL instilled through urinary catheter; clamp for 30-60 minutes, then release and drain; repeat 4-6 times/day

Dosage Forms Solution, irrigation: Citric acid 6.602 g, magnesium carbonate 3.177 g, glucono-delta-lactone 0.198 g per 100 mL (500 mL) [contains benzoic acid]

citric acid, magnesium hydroxycarbonate, D-gluconic acid, magnesium acid citrate, and calcium carbonate *see* citric acid, magnesium carbonate, and glucono-delta-lactone *on this page*

citric acid, sodium citrate, and potassium citrate

(SIT rik AS id, SOW dee um SIT rate, & poe TASS ee um SIT rate)

Synonyms potassium citrate, citric acid, and sodium citrate; sodium citrate, citric acid, and potassium citrate

U.S./Canadian Brand Names Cytra-3 [US]; Polycitra® [US]; Polycitra®-LC [US]

Therapeutic Category Alkalinizing Agent

Use Conditions where long-term maintenance of an alkaline urine is desirable as in control and dissolution of uric acid and cystine calculi of the urinary tract

Usual Dosage Oral:
Children: 5-15 mL diluted in water after meals and at bedtime
Adults: 15-30 mL diluted in water after meals and at bedtime

Dosage Forms Note: Equivalent to potassium 1 mEq/mL, sodium 1 mEq/mL, and bicarbonate 2 mEq/mL
Solution, oral:
Cytra-3: Citric acid 334 mg, sodium citrate 500 mg, and potassium citrate 550 mg per 5 mL (480 mL) [alcohol free, sugar free; contains sodium benzoate; raspberry flavor]
Polycitra®-LC: Citric acid 334 mg, sodium citrate 500 mg, and potassium citrate 550 mg per 5 mL (480 mL) [alcohol free, sugar free]
Syrup, oral (Polycitra®): Citric acid 334 mg, sodium citrate 500 mg, and potassium citrate 550 mg per 5 mL (480 mL) [alcohol free]

Citro-Mag® [Can] *see* magnesium citrate *on page 537*

Citro-Nesia™ Solution *(Discontinued)* *see page 1042*

citrovorum factor *see* leucovorin *on page 509*

Citrucel® [US-OTC] *see* methylcellulose *on page 569*

CL-118,532 *see* triptorelin *on page 890*

CI-719 *see* gemfibrozil *on page 400*

CL-825 *see* pentostatin *on page 680*

CL-184116 *see* porfimer *on page 710*

Cla *see* clarithromycin *on this page*

cladribine (KLA dri been)

Sound-Alike/Look-Alike Issues
Leustatin™ may be confused with lovastatin

Synonyms 2-CdA; 2-chlorodeoxyadenosine

U.S./Canadian Brand Names Leustatin™ [US/Can]

Therapeutic Category Antineoplastic Agent

Use Treatment of hairy cell leukemia, chronic lymphocytic leukemia (CLL), chronic myelogenous leukemia (CML)

Usual Dosage Refer to individual protocols. I.V.:
Pediatrics: Acute leukemias: 6.2-7.5 mg/m^2/day continuous infusion for days 1-5; maximum tolerated dose was 8.9 mg/m^2/day.
Adults:
Hairy cell leukemia: Continuous infusion:
0.09-0.1 mg/kg/day days 1-7; may be repeated every 28-35 days **or**
3.4 mg/m^2/day SubQ days 1-7
Chronic lymphocytic leukemia: Continuous infusion:
0.1 mg/kg/day days 1-7 **or**
0.028-0.14 mg/kg/day as a 2-hour infusion days 1-5
Chronic myelogenous leukemia: 15 mg/m^2/day as a 1-hour infusion days 1-5; if no response increase dose to 20 mg/m^2/day in the second course.

Dosage Forms Injection, solution [preservative free]: 1 mg/mL (10 mL)

Claforan® [US/Can] *see* cefotaxime *on page 168*

Claravis™ [US] *see* isotretinoin *on page 489*

Clarinex® [US] *see* desloratadine *on page 251*

Claripel™ [US] *see* hydroquinone *on page 454*

clarithromycin (kla RITH roe mye sin)

Sound-Alike/Look-Alike Issues
clarithromycin may be confused with erythromycin

Synonyms Cla
(Continued)

clarithromycin *(Continued)*

U.S./Canadian Brand Names Biaxin® [US/Can]; Biaxin® XL [US/Can]; ratio-Clarithromycin [Can]

Therapeutic Category Macrolide (Antibiotic)

Use

Children:

Pharyngitis/tonsillitis, acute maxillary sinusitis, uncomplicated skin/skin structure infections, and mycobacterial infections due to the above organisms

Acute otitis media (*H. influenzae, M. catarrhalis,* or *S. pneumoniae*)

Prevention of disseminated mycobacterial infections due to MAC disease in patients with advanced HIV infection

Adults:

Pharyngitis/tonsillitis due to susceptible *S. pyogenes*

Acute maxillary sinusitis and acute exacerbation of chronic bronchitis due to susceptible *H. influenzae, M. catarrhalis*, or *S. pneumoniae*

Pneumonia due to susceptible *H. influenzae, Mycoplasma pneumoniae, S. pneumoniae*, or *Chlamydia pneumoniae* (TWAR);

Uncomplicated skin/skin structure infections due to susceptible *S. aureus, S. pyogenes*

Disseminated mycobacterial infections due to *M. avium* or *M. intracellulare*

Prevention of disseminated mycobacterial infections due to *M. avium* complex (MAC) disease (eg, patients with advanced HIV infection)

Duodenal ulcer disease due to *H. pylori* in regimens with other drugs including amoxicillin and lansoprazole or omeprazole, ranitidine bismuth citrate, bismuth subsalicylate, tetracycline, and/or an H_2 antagonist

Alternate antibiotic for prophylaxis of bacterial endocarditis in patients who are allergic to penicillin and undergoing surgical or dental procedures

Usual Dosage Oral:

Children ≥6 months: 15 mg/kg/day divided every 12 hours for 10 days

Mycobacterial infection (prevention and treatment): 7.5 mg/kg twice daily, up to 500 mg twice daily

Prophylaxis of bacterial endocarditis: 15 mg/kg 1 hour before procedure (maximum dose: 500 mg)

Adults:

Usual dose: 250-500 mg every 12 hours **or** 1000 mg (two 500 mg extended release tablets) once daily for for 7-14 days

Upper respiratory tract: 250-500 mg every 12 hours for 10-14 days

Pharyngitis/tonsillitis: 250 mg every 12 hours for 10 days

Acute maxillary sinusitis: 500 mg every 12 hours **or** 1000 mg (two 500 mg extended release tablets) once daily for 14 days

Lower respiratory tract: 250-500 mg every 12 hours for 7-14 days

Acute exacerbation of chronic bronchitis due to: *M. catarrhalis* and *S. pneumoniae*: 250 mg every 12 hours **or** 1000 mg (two 500 mg extended release tablets) once daily for 7-14 days *H. influenzae*: 500 mg every 12 hours for 7-14 days

Pneumonia due to: *C. pneumoniae, M. pneumoniae*, and *S. pneumoniae*: 250 mg every 12 hours for 7-14 days **or** 1000 mg (two 500 mg extended release tablets) once daily for 7 days *H. influenzae:* 250 mg every 12 hours for 7 days **or** 1000 mg (two 500 mg extended release tablets) once daily for 7 days

Mycobacterial infection (prevention and treatment): 500 mg twice daily (use with other antimycobacterial drugs, eg, ethambutol, clofazimine, or rifampin)

Prophylaxis of bacterial endocarditis: 500 mg 1 hour prior to procedure

Uncomplicated skin and skin structure: 250 mg every 12 hours for 7-14 days

Helicobacter pylori: Combination regimen with bismuth subsalicylate, tetracycline, clarithromycin, and an H_2-receptor antagonist; or combination of omeprazole and clarithromycin; 250 mg twice daily to 500 mg 3 times/day

Dosage Forms

Granules for oral suspension (Biaxin®): 125 mg/5 mL (50 mL, 100 mL); 250 mg/5 mL (50 mL, 100 mL) [fruit punch flavor]

Tablet [film coated] (Biaxin®): 250 mg, 500 mg

Tablet, extended release [film coated] (Biaxin® XL): 500 mg

clarithromycin, lansoprazole, and amoxicillin *see* lansoprazole, amoxicillin, and clarithromycin *on page 506*

Claritin® Allergic Decongestant [Can] *see* oxymetazoline *on page 658*

Claritin-D® 12-Hour [US-OTC] *see* loratadine and pseudoephedrine *on page 530*

Claritin-D® 24-Hour [US-OTC] *see* loratadine and pseudoephedrine *on page 530*

Claritin® Extra [Can] *see* loratadine and pseudoephedrine *on page 530*

Claritin® Hives Relief [US-OTC] *see* loratadine *on page 530*

Claritin® Kids [Can] *see* loratadine *on page 530*

Claritin® Liberator [Can] *see* loratadine and pseudoephedrine *on page 530*

Claritin® [US-OTC/Can] *see* loratadine *on page 530*

Clavulin® [Can] *see* amoxicillin and clavulanate potassium *on page 52*

Clear Away® Disc *(Discontinued)* *see page 1042*

Clear By Design® Gel *(Discontinued)* *see page 1042*

Clear Eyes® ACR [US-OTC] *see* naphazoline *on page 604*

Clear Eyes® [US-OTC] *see* naphazoline *on page 604*

Clearplex [US-OTC] *see* benzoyl peroxide *on page 109*

Clearsil® Maximum Strength *(Discontinued)* *see page 1042*

Clear Tussin® 30 *(Discontinued)* *see page 1042*

clemastine (KLEM as teen)

Synonyms clemastine fumarate

U.S./Canadian Brand Names Dayhist® Allergy [US-OTC]; Tavist® Allergy [US-OTC]

Therapeutic Category Antihistamine

Use Perennial and seasonal allergic rhinitis and other allergic symptoms including urticaria

Usual Dosage Oral:

Infants and Children <6 years: 0.05 mg/kg/day as **clemastine base** or 0.335-0.67 mg/day clemastine fumarate (0.25-0.5 mg base/day) divided into 2 or 3 doses; maximum daily dosage: 1.34 mg (1 mg base)

Children 6-12 years: 0.67-1.34 mg clemastine fumarate (0.5-1 mg base) twice daily; do not exceed 4.02 mg/day (3 mg/day base)

Children ≥12 years and Adults:

1.34 mg clemastine fumarate (1 mg base) twice daily to 2.68 mg (2 mg base) 3 times/day; do not exceed 8.04 mg/day (6 mg base)

OTC labeling: 1.34 mg clemastine fumarate (1 mg base) twice daily; do not exceed 2 mg base/24 hours

Dosage Forms

Syrup, as fumarate [prescription formulation]: 0.67 mg/5 mL (120 mL) [0.5 mg base/5 mL; contains alcohol 5.5%; citrus flavor]

Tablet, as fumarate: 1.34 mg [1 mg base; OTC], 2.68 mg [2 mg base; prescription formulation]

Dayhist® Allergy, Tavist® Allergy: 1.34 mg [1 mg base]

clemastine fumarate *see* clemastine *on this page*

Clenia™ [US] *see* sulfur and sulfacetamide *on page 834*

Cleocin® [US] *see* clindamycin *on next page*

Cleocin HCl® [US] *see* clindamycin *on next page*

Cleocin Pediatric® [US] *see* clindamycin *on next page*

Cleocin Phosphate® [US] *see* clindamycin *on this page*

Cleocin T® [US] *see* clindamycin *on this page*

clidinium and chlordiazepoxide (kli DI nee um & klor dye az e POKS ide)

Sound-Alike/Look-Alike Issues
Librax® may be confused with Librium®

Synonyms chlordiazepoxide and clidinium

U.S./Canadian Brand Names Apo-Chlorax® [Can]; Librax® [US/Can]

Therapeutic Category Anticholinergic Agent

Use Adjunct treatment of peptic ulcer; treatment of irritable bowel syndrome

Usual Dosage Oral: 1-2 capsules 3-4 times/day, before meals or food and at bedtime

Dosage Forms Capsule: Clidinium bromide 2.5 mg and chlordiazepoxide hydrochloride 5 mg

Climara® [US/Can] *see* estradiol *on page 324*

ClimaraPro™ [US] *see* estradiol and levonorgestrel *on page 327*

Clinac™ BPO [US] *see* benzoyl peroxide *on page 109*

Clindagel® [US] *see* clindamycin *on this page*

Clindamax™ [US] *see* clindamycin *on this page*

clindamycin (klin da MYE sin)

Sound-Alike/Look-Alike Issues
Cleocin® may be confused with bleomycin, Clinoril®, Lincocin®

Synonyms clindamycin hydrochloride; clindamycin palmitate; clindamycin phosphate

U.S./Canadian Brand Names Alti-Clindamycin [Can]; Apo-Clindamycin® [Can]; Cleocin® [US]; Cleocin HCl® [US]; Cleocin Pediatric® [US]; Cleocin Phosphate® [US]; Cleocin T® [US]; Clindagel® [US]; Clindamax™ [US]; Clindets® [US]; Clindoxyl® [Can]; Dalacin® C [Can]; Dalacin® T [Can]; Dalacin® Vaginal [Can]; Novo-Clindamycin [Can]

Therapeutic Category Acne Products; Antibiotic, Miscellaneous

Use Treatment against aerobic and anaerobic streptococci (except enterococci), most staphylococci, *Bacteroides* sp and *Actinomyces*; pelvic inflammatory disease (I.V.); topically in treatment of severe acne; vaginally for *Gardnerella vaginalis*

Usual Dosage Avoid in neonates (contains benzyl alcohol)
Infants and Children:
Oral: 8-20 mg/kg/day as hydrochloride; 8-25 mg/kg/day as palmitate in 3-4 divided doses; minimum dose of palmitate: 37.5 mg 3 times/day
I.M., I.V.:
<1 month: 15-20 mg/kg/day
>1 month: 20-40 mg/kg/day in 3-4 divided doses
Children ≥12 years and Adults: Topical: Apply a thin film twice daily
Adults:
Oral: 150-450 mg/dose every 6-8 hours; maximum dose: 1.8 g/day
I.M., I.V.: 1.2-1.8 g/day in 2-4 divided doses; maximum dose: 4.8 g/day
Pelvic inflammatory disease: I.V.: 900 mg every 8 hours with gentamicin 2 mg/kg, then 1.5 mg/kg every 8 hours; continue after discharge with doxycycline 100 mg twice daily to complete 14 days of total therapy

Dosage Forms Note: Strength is expressed as base
Capsule, as hydrochloride: 150 mg, 300 mg
Cleocin HCl®: 75 mg [contains tartrazine], 150 mg [contains tartrazine], 300 mg
Cream, vaginal, as phosphate (Cleocin®): 2% (40 g) [contains benzyl alcohol; packaged with 7 disposable applicators]
Gel, topical, as phosphate: 1% [10 mg/g] (30 g, 60 g)
Cleocin T®: 1% [10 mg/g] (30 g, 60 g)
Clindagel®: 1% [10 mg/g] (40 mL, 75 mL)
ClindaMax™: 1% (30 g, 60 g)

Granules for oral solution, as palmitate (Cleocin Pediatric®): 75 mg/5 mL (100 mL) [cherry flavor]
Infusion, as phosphate [premixed in D_5W] (Cleocin Phosphate®): 300 mg (50 mL); 600 mg (50 mL); 900 mg (50 mL)
Injection, solution, as phosphate (Cleocin Phosphate®): 150 mg/mL (2 mL, 4 mL, 6 mL, 60 mL) [contains benzyl alcohol and disodium edetate 0.5 mg]
Lotion, as phosphate (Cleocin T®, ClindaMax™): 1% [10 mg/mL] (60 mL)
Pledgets, topical: 1% (60s) [contains alcohol]
Clindets®: 1% (69s) [contains isopropyl alcohol 52%]
Cleocin T®: 1% (60s) [contains isopropyl alcohol 50%]
Solution, topical, as phosphate (Cleocin T®): 1% [10 mg/mL] (30 mL, 60 mL) [contains isopropyl alcohol 50%]
Suppository, vaginal, as phosphate (Cleocin®): 100 mg (3s)

clindamycin and benzoyl peroxide

(klin da MYE sin & BEN zoe il peer OKS ide)

Synonyms benzoyl peroxide and clindamycin; clindamycin phosphate and benzoyl peroxide

U.S./Canadian Brand Names BenzaClin® [US]; Duac™ [US]

Therapeutic Category Topical Skin Product; Topical Skin Product, Acne

Use Topical treatment of acne vulgaris

Usual Dosage Topical: Children ≥12 years and Adults: Apply to affected areas after skin has been cleansed and dried
BenzaClin®: Acne: Apply twice daily (morning and evening)
Duac™: Inflammatory acne: Apply once daily in the evening

Dosage Forms Gel, topical:
BenzaClin®: Clindamycin phosphate 1% and benzoyl peroxide 5% (25 g, 50 g)
Duac™: Clindamycin phosphate 1% and benzoyl peroxide 5% (45 g)

clindamycin hydrochloride *see* clindamycin *on previous page*

clindamycin palmitate *see* clindamycin *on previous page*

clindamycin phosphate *see* clindamycin *on previous page*

clindamycin phosphate and benzoyl peroxide *see* clindamycin and benzoyl peroxide *on this page*

Clindets® [US] *see* clindamycin *on previous page*

Clindex® *(Discontinued)* *see page 1042*

Clindoxyl® [Can] *see* clindamycin *on previous page*

Clinoril® [US] *see* sulindac *on page 835*

clioquinol (all products) *(Discontinued)* *see page 1042*

clioquinol and flumethasone *(Canada only)*

(klye ok KWIN ole & floo METH a sone)

Synonyms flumethasone and clioquinol; iodochlorhydroxyquin and flumethasone

U.S./Canadian Brand Names Locacorten® Vioform® [Can]

Therapeutic Category Antibiotic, Topical; Corticosteroid, Topical

Use Treatment of corticosteroid-responsive dermatoses complicated by infection with bacterial and/or fungal agents

Usual Dosage Children >2 years and Adults:
Otic solution (drops): Instill 2-3 drops into affected ear(s) 2 times/day; generally limit duration to 10 days
Topical: Apply in a thin layer to affected area 2-3 times/day; generally limit duration to 7 days

Dosage Forms
Cream, topical: Clioquinol 3% and flumethasone pivalate 0.02% (15 g, 50 g)
Solution, otic: Clioquinol 1% and flumethasone pivalate 0.02% (10 mL)

Clistin® Tablet *(Discontinued)* *see page 1042*

clobazam *(Canada only)* (KLOE ba zam)

U.S./Canadian Brand Names Alti-Clobazam [Can]; Apo-Clobazam® [Can]; Frisium® [Can]; Novo-Clobazam [Can]; PMS-Clobazam [Can]

Therapeutic Category Anticonvulsant; Antidepressant

Use Adjunctive treatment of epilepsy

Usual Dosage Oral:

Children:

<2 years: Initial 0.5-1 mg/kg/day

2-16 years: Initial: 5 mg/day; may be increased (no more frequently than every 5 days) to a maximum of 40 mg/day

Adults: Initial: 5-15 mg/day; dosage may be gradually adjusted (based on tolerance and seizure control) to a maximum of 80 mg/day

Note: Daily doses of up to 30 mg may be taken as a single dose at bedtime; higher doses should be divided.

Dosage Forms Tablet: 10 mg

clobetasol (kloe BAY ta sol)

Synonyms clobetasol propionate

U.S./Canadian Brand Names Clobevate® [US]; Clobex™ [US]; Cormax® [US]; Dermovate® [Can]; Embeline™ [US]; Embeline™ E [US]; Gen-Clobetasol [Can]; Novo-Clobetasol [Can]; Olux® [US]; Temovate® [US]; Temovate E® [US]

Therapeutic Category Corticosteroid, Topical

Use Short-term relief of inflammation of moderate to severe corticosteroid-responsive dermatoses (very high potency topical corticosteroid)

Usual Dosage Topical: Discontinue when control achieved; if improvement not seen within 2 weeks, reassessment of diagnosis may be necessary.

Children <12 years: Use is not recommended

Children ≥12 years and Adults:

Steroid-responsive dermatoses:

Cream, emollient cream, gel, lotion, ointment: Apply twice daily for up to 2 weeks (maximum dose: 50 g/week)

Foam, solution: Apply to affected scalp twice daily for up to 2 weeks (maximum dose: 50 g/week or 50 mL/week)

Mild to moderate plaque-type psoriasis of nonscalp areas: Foam: Apply to affected area twice daily for up to 2 weeks (maximum dose: 50 g/week); do not apply to face or intertriginous areas

Children ≥16 years and Adults: Moderate to severe plaque-type psoriasis: Emollient cream, lotion: Apply twice daily for up to 2 weeks, has been used for up to 4 weeks when application is <10% of body surface area; use with caution (maximum dose: 50 g/week)

Dosage Forms

Cream, as propionate: 0.05% (15 g, 30 g, 45 g, 60 g)

Cormax®: 0.05% (15 g, 30 g, 45 g)

Embeline™, Temovate®: 0.05% (15 g, 30 g, 45 g, 60 g)

Cream, as propionate [in emollient base]: 0.05% (15 g, 30 g, 60 g)

Embeline™ E, Temovate E®: 0.05% (15 g, 30 g, 60 g)

Foam, topical, as propionate [for scalp application] (Olux®): 0.05% (50 g, 100 g) [contains ethanol 60%]

Gel, as propionate (Clobevate®, Embeline™; Temovate®): 0.05% (15 g, 30 g, 60 g)

Lotion, as propionate (Clobex™): 0.05% (30 mL, 59 mL)

Ointment, as propionate: 0.05% (15 g, 30 g, 45 g, 60 g)

Cormax®: 0.05% (15 g, 45 g)

Embeline™, Temovate®: 0.05% (15 g, 30 g, 45 g, 60 g)

Solution, topical, as propionate [for scalp application] (Cormax®, Embeline™, Temovate®): 0.05% (25 mL, 50 mL) [contains isopropyl alcohol 40%]

clobetasol propionate *see* clobetasol *on previous page*

Clobevate® [US] *see* clobetasol *on previous page*

Clobex™ [US] *see* clobetasol *on previous page*

clocortolone (kloe KOR toe lone)

Sound-Alike/Look-Alike Issues
Cloderm® may be confused with Clocort®

Synonyms clocortolone pivalate

U.S./Canadian Brand Names Cloderm® [US/Can]

Therapeutic Category Corticosteroid, Topical

Use Inflammation of corticosteroid-responsive dermatoses (intermediate-potency topical corticosteroid)

Usual Dosage Adults: Apply sparingly and gently; rub into affected area from 1-4 times/day. Therapy should be discontinued when control is achieved; if no improvement is seen, reassessment of diagnosis may be necessary.

Dosage Forms Cream, as pivalate: 0.1% (15 g, 45 g, 90 g)

clocortolone pivalate *see* clocortolone *on this page*

Clocream® [US-OTC] *see* vitamin A and vitamin D *on page 915*

Cloderm® [US/Can] *see* clocortolone *on this page*

clodronate disodium *see* clodronate disodium *(Canada only)* *on this page*

clodronate disodium *(Canada only)* (KLOE droh nate dy SOW de um)

Synonyms clodronate disodium

U.S./Canadian Brand Names Bonefos® [Can]; Ostac® [Can]

Therapeutic Category Bisphosphonate Derivative

Use Management of hypercalcemia of malignancy

Usual Dosage

I.V.:

Multiple infusions: 300 mg/day; must be diluted (in 500 mL of dextrose 5% or sodium chloride 0.9%) and infused over 2-6 hours. Treatment should be continued until calcium returns to normal (usually 2-5 days); should not be prolonged beyond 10 days.

Single infusion: 1500 mg as a single dose; must be diluted (in 500 mL of dextrose 5% or sodium chloride 0.9%) and infused over at least 4 hours

Oral: Recommended daily maintenance dose following I.V. therapy: Range: 1600 mg (4 capsules) to 2400 mg (6 capsules) given in single or 2 divided doses; maximum recommended daily dose: 3200 mg (8 capsules). Should be taken at least 1 hour before or after food, because food may decrease the amount of clodronate absorbed by the body.

Dosage Forms

Injection, as disodium: 30 mg/mL (10 mL); 60 mg/mL (5 mL)

Capsule, as disodium: 400 mg

clofazimine (kloe FA zi meen)

Sound-Alike/Look-Alike Issues
clofazimine may be confused with clonazepam, clozapine

Synonyms clofazimine palmitate

U.S./Canadian Brand Names Lamprene® [US/Can]

Therapeutic Category Leprostatic Agent

Use Treatment of lepromatous leprosy including dapsone-resistant leprosy and lepromatous leprosy with erythema nodosum leprosum; multibacillary leprosy

Usual Dosage Oral:

Children: Leprosy: 1 mg/kg/day every 24 hours in combination with dapsone and rifampin

(Continued)

clofazimine *(Continued)*

Adults:

Dapsone-resistant leprosy: 100 mg/day in combination with one or more antileprosy drugs for 3 years; then alone 100 mg/day

Dapsone-sensitive multibacillary leprosy: 100 mg/day in combination with two or more antileprosy drugs for at least 2 years and continue until negative skin smears are obtained, then institute single drug therapy with appropriate agent

Erythema nodosum leprosum: 100-200 mg/day for up to 3 months or longer then taper dose to 100 mg/day when possible

Dosage Forms Capsule: 50 mg

clofazimine palmitate *see* clofazimine *on previous page*

Clomid® [US/Can] *see* clomiphene *on this page*

clomiphene (KLOE mi feen)

Sound-Alike/Look-Alike Issues

clomiphene may be confused with clomipramine, clonidine

Clomid® may be confused with clonidine

Serophene® may be confused with Sarafem™

Synonyms clomiphene citrate

Tall-Man clomi**PHENE**

U.S./Canadian Brand Names Clomid® [US/Can]; Milophene® [Can]; Serophene® [US/Can]

Therapeutic Category Ovulation Stimulator

Use Treatment of ovulatory failure in patients desiring pregnancy

Usual Dosage Adults: Oral:

Male (infertility): 25 mg/day for 25 days with 5 days rest, or 100 mg every Monday, Wednesday, Friday

Female (ovulatory failure): 50 mg/day for 5 days (first course); start the regimen on or about the fifth day of cycle. The dose should be increased only in those patients who do not ovulate in response to cyclic 50 mg Clomid®. A low dosage or duration of treatment course is particularly recommended if unusual sensitivity to pituitary gonadotropin is suspected, such as in patients with polycystic ovary syndrome.

If ovulation does not appear to occur after the first course of therapy, a second course of 100 mg/day (two 50 mg tablets given as a single daily dose) for 5 days should be given. This course may be started as early as 30 days after the previous one after precautions are taken to exclude the presence of pregnancy. Increasing the dosage or duration of therapy beyond 100 mg/day for 5 days is not recommended. The majority of patients who are going to ovulate will do so after the first course of therapy. If ovulation does not occur after 3 courses of therapy, further treatment is not recommended and the patient should be re-evaluated. If 3 ovulatory responses occur, but pregnancy has not been achieved, further treatment is not recommended. If menses does not occur after an ovulatory response, the patient should be reevaluated. Long-term cyclic therapy is not recommended beyond a total of about 6 cycles.

Dosage Forms Tablet, as citrate: 50 mg

clomiphene citrate *see* clomiphene *on this page*

clomipramine (kloe MI pra meen)

Sound-Alike/Look-Alike Issues

clomipramine may be confused with chlorpromazine, clomiphene, desipramine, Norpramin®

Anafranil® may be confused with alfentanil, enalapril, nafarelin

Synonyms clomipramine hydrochloride

Tall-Man clomi**PRAMINE**

U.S./Canadian Brand Names Anafranil® [US/Can]; Apo-Clomipramine® [Can]; CO Clomipramine [Can]; Gen-Clomipramine [Can]; Novo-Clopramine [Can]

Therapeutic Category Antidepressant, Tricyclic (Tertiary Amine)

Use Treatment of obsessive-compulsive disorder (OCD)

Usual Dosage Oral: Initial:

Children:

<10 years: Safety and efficacy have not been established.

≥10 years: OCD: 25 mg/day; gradually increase, as tolerated, to a maximum of 3 mg/kg/day or 200 mg/day (whichever is smaller)

Adults: OCD: 25 mg/day and gradually increase, as tolerated, to 100 mg/day the first 2 weeks, may then be increased to a total of 250 mg/day maximum

Dosage Forms Capsule, as hydrochloride: 25 mg, 50 mg, 75 mg

clomipramine hydrochloride *see* clomipramine *on previous page*

Clonapam [Can] *see* clonazepam *on this page*

clonazepam (kloe NA ze pam)

Sound-Alike/Look-Alike Issues

clonazepam may be confused with clofazimine, clonidine, clorazepate, Klonopin™, lorazepam

Klonopin® may be confused with clonazepam, clonidine

U.S./Canadian Brand Names Alti-Clonazepam [Can]; Apo-Clonazepam® [Can]; Clonapam [Can]; Gen-Clonazepam [Can]; Klonopin® [US/Can]; Novo-Clonazepam [Can]; Nu-Clonazepam [Can]; PMS-Clonazepam [Can]; Rho-Clonazepam [Can]; Rivotril® [Can]

Therapeutic Category Benzodiazepine

Controlled Substance C-IV

Use Alone or as an adjunct in the treatment of petit mal variant (Lennox-Gastaut), akinetic, and myoclonic seizures; petit mal (absence) seizures unresponsive to succimides; panic disorder with or without agoraphobia

Usual Dosage Oral:

Children <10 years or 30 kg: Seizure disorders:

Initial daily dose: 0.01-0.03 mg/kg/day (maximum: 0.05 mg/kg/day) given in 2-3 divided doses; increase by no more than 0.5 mg every third day until seizures are controlled or adverse effects seen

Usual maintenance dose: 0.1-0.2 mg/kg/day divided 3 times/day, not to exceed 0.2 mg/kg/day

Adults:

Seizure disorders:

Initial daily dose not to exceed 1.5 mg given in 3 divided doses; may increase by 0.5-1 mg every third day until seizures are controlled or adverse effects seen (maximum: 20 mg/day)

Usual maintenance dose: 0.05-0.2 mg/kg; do not exceed 20 mg/day

Panic disorder: 0.25 mg twice daily; increase in increments of 0.125-0.25 mg twice daily every 3 days; target dose: 1 mg/day (maximum: 4 mg/day)

Discontinuation of treatment: To discontinue, treatment should be withdrawn gradually. Decrease dose by 0.125 mg twice daily every 3 days until medication is completely withdrawn.

Dosage Forms

Tablet: 0.5 mg, 1 mg, 2 mg

Tablet, orally-disintegrating [wafer]: 0.125 mg, 0.25 mg, 0.5 mg, 1 mg, 2 mg

clonidine (KLOE ni deen)

Sound-Alike/Look-Alike Issues

clonidine may be confused with Clomid®, clomiphene, clonazepam, clozapine, Klonopin™, Loniten®, quinidine

Catapres® may be confused with Cataflam®, Cetapred®, Combipres®

Synonyms clonidine hydrochloride

(Continued)

clonidine *(Continued)*

U.S./Canadian Brand Names Apo-Clonidine® [Can]; Carapres® [Can]; Catapres® [US]; Catapres-TTS® [US]; Dixarit® [Can]; Duraclon™ [US]; Novo-Clonidine [Can]; Nu-Clonidine® [Can]

Therapeutic Category Alpha-Adrenergic Agonist

Use Management of mild to moderate hypertension; either used alone or in combination with other antihypertensives

Orphan drug: Duraclon™: For continuous epidural administration as adjunctive therapy with intraspinal opiates for treatment of cancer pain in patients tolerant to or unresponsive to intraspinal opiates

Usual Dosage

Children:

Oral:

Hypertension: Initial: 5-10 mcg/kg/day in divided doses every 8-12 hours; increase gradually at 5- to 7-day intervals to 25 mcg/kg/day in divided doses every 6 hours; maximum: 0.9 mg/day

Clonidine tolerance test (test of growth hormone release from pituitary): 0.15 mg/m^2 or 4 mcg/kg as single dose

Epidural infusion: Pain management: Reserved for patients with severe intractable pain, unresponsive to other analgesics or epidural or spinal opiates: Initial: 0.5 mcg/kg/hour; adjust with caution, based on clinical effect

Adults:

Oral:

Hypertension: Initial dose: 0.1 mg twice daily (maximum recommended dose: 2.4 mg/day); usual dose range (JNC 7): 0.1-0.8 mg/day in 2 divided doses

Nicotine withdrawal symptoms: 0.1 mg twice daily to maximum of 0.4 mg/day for 3-4 weeks

Transdermal: Hypertension: Apply once every 7 days; for initial therapy start with 0.1 mg and increase by 0.1 mg at 1- to 2-week intervals (dosages >0.6 mg do not improve efficacy); usual dose range (JNC 7): 0.1-0.3 mg once weekly

Epidural infusion: Pain management: Starting dose: 30 mcg/hour; titrate as required for relief of pain or presence of side effects; minimal experience with doses >40 mcg/hour; should be considered an adjunct to intraspinal opiate therapy

Dosage Forms

Injection, epidural solution, as hydrochloride [preservative free] (Duraclon™): 100 mcg/mL (10 mL); 500 mcg/mL (10 mL)

Patch, transdermal [once-weekly patch]:

Catapres-TTS®-1: 0.1 mg/24 hours (4s)

Catapres-TTS®-2: 0.2 mg/24 hours (4s)

Catapres-TTS®-3: 0.3 mg/24 hours (4s)

Tablet, as hydrochloride (Catapres®): 0.1 mg, 0.2 mg, 0.3 mg

clonidine and chlorthalidone (KLOE ni deen & klor THAL i done)

Synonyms chlorthalidone and clonidine

U.S./Canadian Brand Names Clorpres® [US]

Therapeutic Category Antihypertensive Agent, Combination

Use Management of mild to moderate hypertension

Usual Dosage Oral: 1 tablet 1-2 times/day; maximum: 0.6 mg clonidine and 30 mg chlorthalidone

Dosage Forms

Tablet:

0.1: Clonidine hydrochloride 0.1 mg and chlorthalidone 15 mg

0.2: Clonidine hydrochloride 0.2 mg and chlorthalidone 15 mg

0.3: Clonidine hydrochloride 0.3 mg and chlorthalidone 15 mg

clonidine hydrochloride *see* clonidine *on previous page*

clopidogrel (kloh PID oh grel)

Sound-Alike/Look-Alike Issues

Plavix® may be confused with Elavil®, Paxil®

Synonyms clopidogrel bisulfate

U.S./Canadian Brand Names Plavix® [US/Can]

Therapeutic Category Antiplatelet Agent

Use Reduce atherosclerotic events (myocardial infarction, stroke, vascular deaths) in patients with atherosclerosis documented by recent myocardial infarction (MI), recent stroke, or established peripheral arterial disease; prevention of thrombotic complications after coronary stenting; acute coronary syndrome (unstable angina or non-Q-wave MI)

Usual Dosage Oral: Adults:

Recent MI, recent stroke, or established arterial disease: 75 mg once daily

Acute coronary syndrome: Initial: 300 mg loading dose, followed by 75 mg once daily (in combination with aspirin 75-325 mg once daily). **Note:** A loading dose of 600 mg has been used in some investigations; limited research exists comparing the two doses.

Dosage Forms Tablet [film coated]: 75 mg

clopidogrel bisulfate *see* clopidogrel *on this page*

Clopixol® [Can] *see* zuclopenthixol *(Canada only) on page 944*

Clopixol-Acuphase® [Can] *see* zuclopenthixol *(Canada only) on page 944*

Clopixol® Depot [Can] *see* zuclopenthixol *(Canada only) on page 944*

Clopra® ***(Discontinued)*** *see page 1042*

clorazepate (klor AZ e pate)

Sound-Alike/Look-Alike Issues

clorazepate may be confused with clofibrate, clonazepam

Synonyms clorazepate dipotassium; tranxene T-Tab®

U.S./Canadian Brand Names Apo-Clorazepate® [Can]; Novo-Clopate [Can]; Tranxene® [US]; Tranxene® SD™ [US]; Tranxene® SD™-Half Strength [US]; T-Tab® [US]

Therapeutic Category Anticonvulsant; Benzodiazepine

Controlled Substance C-IV

Use Treatment of generalized anxiety disorder; management of ethanol withdrawal; adjunct anticonvulsant in management of partial seizures

Usual Dosage Oral:

Children 9-12 years: Anticonvulsant: Initial: 3.75-7.5 mg/dose twice daily; increase dose by 3.75 mg at weekly intervals, not to exceed 60 mg/day in 2-3 divided doses

Children >12 years and Adults: Anticonvulsant: Initial: Up to 7.5 mg/dose 2-3 times/day; increase dose by 7.5 mg at weekly intervals, not to exceed 90 mg/day

Adults:

Anxiety:

Regular release tablets (Tranxene® T-Tab®): 7.5-15 mg 2-4 times/day

Sustained release (Tranxene®-SD): 11.25 or 22.5 mg once daily at bedtime

Ethanol withdrawal: Initial: 30 mg, then 15 mg 2-4 times/day on first day; maximum daily dose: 90 mg; gradually decrease dose over subsequent days

Dosage Forms Tablet, as dipotassium: 3.75 mg, 7.5 mg, 15 mg

Tranxene®-SD™: 22.5 mg [once daily]

Tranxene®-SD™ Half Strength: 11.25 mg [once daily]

Tranxene® T-Tab®: 3.75 mg, 7.5 mg, 15 mg

clorazepate dipotassium *see* clorazepate *on this page*

Clorpactin® WCS-90 [US-OTC] *see* oxychlorosene *on page 655*

Clorpactin® XCB Powder ***(Discontinued)*** *see page 1042*

Clorpres® [US] *see* clonidine and chlorthalidone *on previous page*

Clotrimaderm [Can] *see* clotrimazole *on next page*

clotrimazole (kloe TRIM a zole)

Sound-Alike/Look-Alike Issues

clotrimazole may be confused with co-trimoxazole

Lotrimin® may be confused with Lotrisone®, Otrivin®

Mycelex® may be confused with Myoflex®

U.S./Canadian Brand Names Canesten® Topical [Can]; Canesten® Vaginal [Can]; Clotrimaderm [Can]; Cruex® Cream [US-OTC]; Gyne-Lotrimin® 3 [US-OTC]; Lotrimin® AF Athlete's Foot Cream [US-OTC]; Lotrimin® AF Athlete's Foot Solution [US-OTC]; Lotrimin® AF Jock Itch Cream [US-OTC]; Mycelex® [US]; Mycelex®-7 [US-OTC]; Mycelex® Twin Pack [US-OTC]; Trivagizole-3® [Can]

Therapeutic Category Antifungal Agent

Use Treatment of susceptible fungal infections, including oropharyngeal candidiasis, dermatophytoses, superficial mycoses, and cutaneous candidiasis, as well as vulvovaginal candidiasis; limited data suggest that clotrimazole troches may be effective for prophylaxis against oropharyngeal candidiasis in neutropenic patients

Usual Dosage

Children >3 years and Adults:

Oral:

Prophylaxis: 10 mg troche dissolved 3 times/day for the duration of chemotherapy or until steroids are reduced to maintenance levels

Treatment: 10 mg troche dissolved slowly 5 times/day for 14 consecutive days

Topical (cream, solution): Apply twice daily; if no improvement occurs after 4 weeks of therapy, reevaluate diagnosis

Children >12 years and Adults:

Vaginal:

Cream: 1%: Insert 1 applicatorful vaginal cream daily (preferably at bedtime) for 7 consecutive days 2%: Insert 1 applicatorful vaginal cream daily (preferably at bedtime) for 3 consecutive days

Tablet: Insert 100 mg/day for 7 days or 500 mg single dose

Topical (cream, solution): Apply to affected area twice daily (morning and evening) for 7 consecutive days

Dosage Forms

Combination pack (Mycelex®-7): Vaginal tablet 100 mg (7s) and vaginal cream 1% (7 g)

Cream, topical: 1% (15 g, 30 g, 45 g)

Cruex®: 1% (15 g)

Lotrimin® AF Athlete's Foot: 1% (12 g, 24 g)

Lotrimin® AF Jock Itch: 1% (12 g)

Cream, vaginal: 2% (21 g)

Mycelex®-7: 1% (45 g)

Solution, topical: 1% (10 mL, 30 mL)

Lotrimin® AF Athlete's Foot: 1% (10 mL)

Tablet, vaginal (Gyne-Lotrimin® 3): 200 mg (3s)

Troche (Mycelex®): 10 mg

clotrimazole and betamethasone *see* betamethasone and clotrimazole *on page 115*

cloxacillin (kloks a SIL in)

Synonyms cloxacillin sodium

U.S./Canadian Brand Names Apo-Cloxi® [Can]; Novo-Cloxin [Can]; Nu-Cloxi® [Can]; Riva-Cloxacillin [Can]

Therapeutic Category Penicillin

Use Treatment of susceptible bacterial infections, notably penicillinase-producing staphylococci causing respiratory tract, skin and skin structure, bone and joint, urinary tract infections

Usual Dosage Oral:

Children >1 month (<20 kg): 50-100 mg/kg/day in divided doses every 6 hours; up to a maximum of 4 g/day

Children (>20 kg) and Adults: 250-500 mg every 6 hours

Dosage Forms

Capsule, as sodium: 250 mg, 500 mg

Powder for oral suspension, as sodium: 125 mg/5 mL (100 mL, 200 mL)

cloxacillin sodium *see* cloxacillin *on previous page*

Cloxapen® *(Discontinued)* *see page 1042*

clozapine (KLOE za peen)

Sound-Alike/Look-Alike Issues

clozapine may be confused with clofazimine, clonidine

Clozaril® may be confused with Clinoril®, Colazal™

U.S./Canadian Brand Names Clozaril® [US/Can]; Fazaclo™ [US]; Gen-Clozapine [Can]; Rhoxal-clozapine [Can]

Therapeutic Category Antipsychotic Agent, Dibenzodiazepine

Use Treatment-refractory schizophrenia; to reduce risk of recurrent suicidal behavior in schizophrenia or schizoaffective disorder

Usual Dosage Oral: If dosing is interrupted for >48 hours, therapy must be reinitiated at 12.5-25 mg/day; may be increased more rapidly than with initial titration.

Adults: Schizophrenia or to reduce risk of suicidal behavior: Initial: 12.5 mg once or twice daily; increased, as tolerated, in increments of 25-50 mg/day to a target dose of 300-450 mg/day after 2-4 weeks, may require doses as high as 600-900 mg/day for the treatment of schizophrenia; median dose to reduce risk of suicidal behavior is ~300 mg/day (range 12.5-900 mg)

Note: In the event of planned termination of clozapine, gradual reduction in dose over a 1- to 2-week period is recommended. If conditions warrant abrupt discontinuation (leukopenia), monitor patient for psychosis and cholinergic rebound (headache, nausea, vomiting, diarrhea).

Dosage Forms

Tablet: 12.5 mg, 25 mg, 100 mg

Clozaril®: 25 mg, 100 mg

Tablet, orally-disintegrating (Fazaclo™): 25 mg [contains phenylalanine 1.75 mg; mint flavor], 100 mg [contains phenylalanine 6.96 mg; mint flavor]

Clozaril® [US/Can] *see* clozapine *on this page*

Clysodrast® *(Discontinued)* *see page 1042*

CMV-IGIV *see* cytomegalovirus immune globulin (intravenous-human) *on page 240*

CoActifed® [Can] *see* triprolidine, pseudoephedrine, and codeine *on page 890*

coagulant complex inhibitor *see* anti-inhibitor coagulant complex *on page 65*

coagulation factor VIIa *see* factor VIIa (recombinant) *on page 354*

coal tar (KOLE tar)

Sound-Alike/Look-Alike Issues

Pentrax® may be confused with Permax®

Tegrin® may be confused with Tegretol®

Synonyms crude coal tar; LCD; pix carbonis

U.S./Canadian Brand Names Balnetar® [US-OTC/Can]; Betatar® [US-OTC]; Cutar® [US-OTC]; DHS™ Targel [US-OTC]; DHS™ Tar [US-OTC]; Doak® Tar [US-OTC]; Estar® [US-OTC/Can]; Exorex® [US]; Ionil T® Plus [US-OTC]; Ionil T® [US-OTC]; MG217® Medicated Tar [US-OTC]; MG217® [US-OTC]; Neutrogena® T/Gel Extra Strength [US-OTC]; Neutrogena® T/Gel [US-OTC]; Oxipor® VHC [US-OTC]; Pentrax® [US-OTC]; Polytar® [US-OTC]; PsoriGel® [US-OTC]; Reme-T™ [US-OTC]; SpectroTar Skin Wash™ [Can]; Targel® [Can]; Tegrin® [US-OTC]; Zetar® [US-OTC]

Therapeutic Category Antipsoriatic Agent; Antiseborrheic Agent, Topical

Use Topically for controlling dandruff, seborrheic dermatitis, or psoriasis

(Continued)

coal tar *(Continued)*

Usual Dosage Topical:

Bath: Add appropriate amount to bath water; soak 5-20 minutes, then pat dry; use once daily to 3 days

Shampoo: Rub shampoo onto wet hair and scalp, rinse thoroughly; repeat; leave on 5 minutes; rinse thoroughly; apply twice weekly for the first 2 weeks then once weekly or more often if needed

Soap: Use on affected areas in place of regular soap. Work into a lather using warm water; massage into skin; rinse.

Skin: Apply to the affected area 1-4 times/day; decrease frequency to 2-3 times/week once condition has been controlled

Scalp psoriasis: Tar oil bath or coal tar solution may be painted sparingly to the lesions 3-12 hours before each shampoo

Psoriasis of the body, arms, legs: Apply at bedtime; if thick scales are present, use product with salicylic acid and apply several times during the day

Dosage Forms

Emulsion, topical (Cutar®): Coal tar solution 7.5% (180 mL, 3840 mL)

Gel, shampoo:

Betatar®: Coal tar solution 5% (240 mL) [green apple scent]

DHS™ Targel: Coal tar solution 2.9% (240 mL) [equivalent to 0.5% coal tar]

Gel, topical:

Estar®: Coal tar 5% (90 g)

PsoriGel®: Coal tar solution 7.5% (120 g)

Lotion, topical:

Doak® Tar: Coal tar distillate 5% (240 mL) [equivalent to coal tar 2%]

Exorex®: Coal tar 1% (240 mL)

MG217®: Coal tar solution 5% (120 mL) [equivalent to 1% coal tar; contains jojoba]

Oxipor® VHC: Coal tar solution 25% (60 mL, 120 mL)

Oil, topical:

Belnetar®: Water-dispersible emollient tar 2.5%, lanolin fraction, and mineral oil (225 mL) [for use in bath]

Doak® Tar: Coal tar distillate 2% (240 mL) [equivalent to coal tar 0.8%; for use in bath]

Ointment, topical (MG217®): Coal tar solution 10% (107 g, 430 g) [equivalent to 2% coal tar]

Shampoo:

DHS™ Tar: Coal tar solution 2.9% (120 mL, 240 mL, 480 mL) [equivalent to 0.5% coal tar]

Doak® Tar: Coal tar distillate 3% (240 mL) [equivalent to coal tar 1.2%]

Ionil T®: Coal tar 1% (240 mL, 480 mL, 960 mL)

Ionil T® Plus: Coal tar 2% (240 mL) [with conditioner]

MG217® Medicated Tar: Coal tar solution 15% (120 mL, 240 mL, 480 mL) [equivalent to 3% coal tar]

Neutrogena® T/Gel: Coal tar extract 2% (132 mL, 480 mL) [coal tar 0.5%]

Neutrogena® T/Gel Extra Strength: Coal tar extract 4% (132 mL) [coal tar 1%]

Pentrax®: Coal tar 5% (240 mL)

Polytar®: Coal tar 0.5% (177 mL, 355 mL)

Reme-T™: Coal tar distillate 5% (236 mL)

Tegrin®: Coal tar solution 7% (210 mL) [equivalent to 1% coal tar; available with or without conditioner]

Zetar®: Coal tar 1% (180 mL)

Soap (Polytar®): Coal tar 0.5% (113 g)

coal tar and salicylic acid (KOLE tar & sal i SIL ik AS id)

Synonyms salicylic acid and coal tar

U.S./Canadian Brand Names Sebcur/T® [Can]; Tarsum® [US-OTC]; X-Seb™ T [US-OTC]

Therapeutic Category Antipsoriatic Agent; Antiseborrheic Agent, Topical

Use Seborrheal dermatitis, dandruff, psoriasis

Usual Dosage Psoriasis: Scalp:
Gel: Apply directly to plaques; may leave in place for up to 1 hour. Apply water and work into a lather; rinse.
Shampoo: Apply to wet hair; massage into scalp; rinse.

Dosage Forms
Gel [shampoo] (Tarsum®): Coal tar solution 10% [equivalent to coal tar 2%] and salicylic acid (120 mL, 240 mL)
Shampoo, topical (X-Seb™ T): Coal tar solution 10% and salicylic acid (120 mL, 240 mL)

coal tar, lanolin, and mineral oil (KOLE tar, LAN oh lin, & MIN er al oyl)

Therapeutic Category Antipsoriatic Agent; Antiseborrheic Agent, Topical
Use Treatment of psoriasis, seborrheal dermatitis, atopic dermatitis, eczematoid dermatitis
Usual Dosage Add to bath water, soak for 5-20 minutes then pat dry
Dosage Forms Oil, bath: Water-dispersible emollient tar 2.5%, lanolin fraction, and mineral oil (225 mL)

Cobalasine® Injection *(Discontinued)* *see page 1042*

Cobex® *(Discontinued)* *see page 1042*

cocaine (koe KANE)

Synonyms cocaine hydrochloride
Therapeutic Category Local Anesthetic
Controlled Substance C-II
Use Topical anesthesia for mucous membranes
Usual Dosage Topical application (ear, nose, throat, bronchoscopy): Dosage depends on the area to be anesthetized, tissue vascularity, technique of anesthesia, and individual patient tolerance; the lowest dose necessary to produce adequate anesthesia should be used; concentrations of 1% to 10% are used (not to exceed 1 mg/kg). Use reduced dosages for children, elderly, or debilitated patients.

Dosage Forms
Powder, as hydrochloride: 1 g, 5 g, 25 g
Solution, topical, as hydrochloride: 4% [40 mg/mL] (4 mL, 10 mL); 10% [100 mg/mL] (4 mL, 10 mL)

cocaine hydrochloride *see* cocaine *on this page*

CO Clomipramine [Can] *see* clomipramine *on page 214*

Codafed® Expectorant [US] *see* guaifenesin, pseudoephedrine, and codeine *on page 422*

Codafed® Pediatric Expectorant [US] *see* guaifenesin, pseudoephedrine, and codeine *on page 422*

Codamine® *(Discontinued)* *see page 1042*

Codamine® Pediatric *(Discontinued)* *see page 1042*

Codehist® DH *(Discontinued)* *see page 1042*

codeine (KOE deen)

Sound-Alike/Look-Alike Issues
codeine may be confused with Cardene®, Cophene®, Cordran®, iodine, Lodine®
Synonyms codeine phosphate; codeine sulfate; methylmorphine
U.S./Canadian Brand Names Codeine Contin® [Can]
Therapeutic Category Analgesic, Narcotic; Antitussive
Controlled Substance C-II
Use Treatment of mild to moderate pain; antitussive in lower doses; dextromethorphan has equivalent antitussive activity but has much lower toxicity in accidental overdose
(Continued)

codeine *(Continued)*

Usual Dosage Note: These are guidelines and do not represent the maximum doses that may be required in all patients. Doses should be titrated to pain relief/prevention. Doses >1.5 mg/kg body weight are not recommended.

Analgesic:

Children: Oral, I.M., SubQ: 0.5-1 mg/kg/dose every 4-6 hours as needed; maximum: 60 mg/dose

Adults:

Oral: 30 mg every 4-6 hours as needed; patients with prior opiate exposure may require higher initial doses. Usual range: 15-120 mg every 4-6 hours as needed

Oral, controlled release formulation (Codeine Contin®, not available in U.S.): 50-300 mg every 12 hours. **Note:** A patient's codeine requirement should be established using prompt release formulations; conversion to long acting products may be considered when chronic, continuous treatment is required. Higher dosages should be reserved for use only in opioid-tolerant patients.

I.M., SubQ: 30 mg every 4-6 hours as needed; patients with prior opiate exposure may require higher initial doses. Usual range: 15-120 mg every 4-6 hours as needed; more frequent dosing may be needed

Antitussive: Oral (for nonproductive cough):

Children: 1-1.5 mg/kg/day in divided doses every 4-6 hours as needed: Alternative dose according to age:

2-6 years: 2.5-5 mg every 4-6 hours as needed; maximum: 30 mg/day

6-12 years: 5-10 mg every 4-6 hours as needed; maximum: 60 mg/day

Adults: 10-20 mg/dose every 4-6 hours as needed; maximum: 120 mg/day

Dosage Forms

Injection, as phosphate: 15 mg/mL (2 mL); 30 mg/mL (2 mL) [contains sodium metabisulfite]

Solution, oral, as phosphate: 15 mg/5 mL (5 mL, 500 mL) [strawberry flavor]

Tablet, controlled release (Codeine Contin®) [not available in U.S.]: 50 mg, 100 mg, 150 mg, 200 mg

Tablet, as phosphate: 30 mg, 60 mg

Tablet, as sulfate: 15 mg, 30 mg, 60 mg

codeine and acetaminophen *see* acetaminophen and codeine *on page 6*

codeine and aspirin *see* aspirin and codeine *on page 82*

codeine and butalbital compound *see* butalbital, aspirin, caffeine, and codeine *on page 139*

codeine and guaifenesin *see* guaifenesin and codeine *on page 416*

codeine and promethazine *see* promethazine and codeine *on page 735*

codeine, aspirin, and carisoprodol *see* carisoprodol, aspirin, and codeine *on page 162*

codeine, butalbital, aspirin, and caffeine *see* butalbital, aspirin, caffeine, and codeine *on page 139*

codeine, chlorpheniramine, and pseudoephedrine *see* chlorpheniramine, pseudoephedrine, and codeine *on page 193*

codeine, chlorpheniramine, phenylephrine, and potassium iodide *see* chlorpheniramine, phenylephrine, codeine, and potassium iodide *on page 193*

Codeine Contin® [Can] *see* codeine *on previous page*

codeine, guaifenesin, and pseudoephedrine *see* guaifenesin, pseudoephedrine, and codeine *on page 422*

codeine phosphate *see* codeine *on previous page*

codeine, promethazine, and phenylephrine *see* promethazine, phenylephrine, and codeine *on page 736*

codeine, pseudoephedrine, and triprolidine *see* triprolidine, pseudoephedrine, and codeine *on page 890*

codeine sulfate *see* codeine *on page 221*

Codiclear® DH [US] *see* hydrocodone and guaifenesin *on page 445*

Codimal-A® Injection *(Discontinued)* *see page 1042*

Codimal® Expectorant *(Discontinued)* *see page 1042*

cod liver oil *see* vitamin A and vitamin D *on page 915*

CO Fluoxetine [Can] *see* fluoxetine *on page 379*

Cogentin® [US/Can] *see* benztropine *on page 111*

Co-Gesic® [US] *see* hydrocodone and acetaminophen *on page 443*

Cognex® [US] *see* tacrine *on page 837*

Colace® [US-OTC/Can] *see* docusate *on page 285*

Colax-C® [Can] *see* docusate *on page 285*

Colazal® [US] *see* balsalazide *on page 100*

ColBenemid® *(Discontinued)* *see page 1042*

colchicine (KOL chi seen)

U.S./Canadian Brand Names ratio-Colchicine [Can]

Therapeutic Category Antigout Agent

Use Treatment of acute gouty arthritis attacks and prevention of recurrences of such attacks

Usual Dosage

Gouty arthritis: Adults:

Prophylaxis of acute attacks: Oral: 0.6 mg twice daily; initial and/or subsequent dosage may be decreased (ie, 0.6 mg once daily) in patients at risk of toxicity or in those who are intolerant (including weakness, loose stools, or diarrhea); range: 0.6 mg every other day to 0.6 mg 3 times/day

Acute attacks:

Oral: Initial: 0.6-1.2 mg, followed by 0.6 every 1-2 hours; some clinicians recommend a maximum of 3 doses; more aggressive approaches have recommended a maximum dose of up to 6 mg. Wait at least 3 days before initiating another course of therapy

I.V.: Initial: 1-2 mg, then 0.5 mg every 6 hours until response, not to exceed total dose of 4 mg. If pain recurs, it may be necessary to administer additional daily doses. The amount of colchicine administered intravenously in an acute treatment period (generally ~1 week) should not exceed a total dose of 4 mg. Do not administer more colchicine by any route for at least 7 days after a full course of I.V. therapy.

Note: Many experts would avoid use because of potential for serious, life-threatening complications. Should not be administered to patients with renal insufficiency, hepatobiliary obstruction, patients >70 years of age, or recent oral colchicine use. Should be reserved for hospitalized patients who are under the care of a physician experienced in the use of intravenous colchicine.

Surgery: Gouty arthritis, prophylaxis of recurrent attacks: Adults: Oral: 0.6 mg/day or every other day; patients who are to undergo surgical procedures may receive 0.6 mg 3 times/day for 3 days before and 3 days after surgery

Dosage Forms

Injection, solution: 0.5 mg/mL (2 mL)

Tablet: 0.6 mg

colchicine and probenecid (KOL chi seen & proe BEN e sid)

Synonyms probenecid and colchicine

Therapeutic Category Antigout Agent

Use Treatment of chronic gouty arthritis when complicated by frequent, recurrent acute attacks of gout

(Continued)

colchicine and probenecid *(Continued)*

Usual Dosage Adults: Oral: 1 tablet daily for 1 week, then 1 tablet twice daily thereafter

Dosage Forms Tablet: Colchicine 0.5 mg and probenecid 0.5 g

Cold & Allergy® Elixir *(Discontinued)* *see page 1042*

Coldlac-LA® *(Discontinued)* *see page 1042*

Coldloc® *(Discontinued)* *see page 1042*

Coldtuss DR [US] *see* chlorpheniramine, phenylephrine, and dextromethorphan *on page 191*

colesevelam (koh le SEV a lam)

U.S./Canadian Brand Names WelChol® [US/Can]

Therapeutic Category Antihyperlipidemic Agent, Miscellaneous; Bile Acid Sequestrant

Use Adjunctive therapy to diet and exercise in the management of elevated LDL in primary hypercholesterolemia (Fredrickson type IIa) when used alone or in combination with an HMG-CoA reductase inhibitor

Usual Dosage Adult: Oral:

Monotherapy: 3 tablets twice daily with meals or 6 tablets once daily with a meal; maximum dose: 7 tablets/day

Combination therapy with an HMG-CoA reductase inhibitor: 4-6 tablets daily; maximum dose: 6 tablets/day

Dosage Forms Tablet, as hydrochloride [film coated]: 625 mg

Colestid® [US/Can] *see* colestipol *on this page*

colestipol (koe LES ti pole)

Synonyms colestipol hydrochloride

U.S./Canadian Brand Names Colestid® [US/Can]

Therapeutic Category Antihyperlipidemic Agent, Miscellaneous

Use Adjunct in management of primary hypercholesterolemia; regression of arteriolosclerosis; relief of pruritus associated with elevated levels of bile acids; possibly used to decrease plasma half-life of digoxin in toxicity

Usual Dosage Adults: Oral:

Granules: 5-30 g/day given once or in divided doses 2-4 times/day; initial dose: 5 g 1-2 times/day; increase by 5 g at 1- to 2-month intervals

Tablets: 2-16 g/day; initial dose: 2 g 1-2 times/day; increase by 2 g at 1- to 2-month intervals

Dosage Forms

Granules, as hydrochloride:

5 g/7.5 g packet (30s, 90s) [unflavored]

5 g/7.5 g (300 g, 500 g) [unflavored]

5 g/7.5 g packet (60s) [contains phenylalanine 18.2 mg/7.5 g; orange flavor]

5 g/7.5 g (450 g) [contains phenylalanine 18.2 mg/7.5 g; orange flavor]

Tablet, as hydrochloride: 1 g

colestipol hydrochloride *see* colestipol *on this page*

colistimethate (koe lis ti METH ate)

Synonyms colistimethate sodium

U.S./Canadian Brand Names Coly-Mycin® M [US/Can]

Therapeutic Category Antibiotic, Miscellaneous

Use Treatment of infections due to sensitive strains of certain gram-negative bacilli which are resistant to other antibacterials or in patients allergic to other antibacterials

Usual Dosage Children and Adults:

I.M., I.V.: 2.5-5 mg/kg/day in 2-4 divided doses

Inhalation: 50-75 mg in NS (3-4 mL total) via nebulizer 2-3 times/day

Dosage Forms Injection, powder for reconstitution: 150 mg

colistimethate sodium *see* colistimethate *on previous page*

colistin, neomycin, hydrocortisone, and thonzonium *see* neomycin, colistin, hydrocortisone, and thonzonium *on page 610*

collagen *see* collagen hemostat *on this page*

collagen absorbable hemostat *see* collagen hemostat *on this page*

collagenase (KOL la je nase)

U.S./Canadian Brand Names Santyl® [US/Can]

Therapeutic Category Enzyme

Use Promotes debridement of necrotic tissue in dermal ulcers and severe burns

Orphan drug: Injection: Treatment of Peyronie disease; treatment of Dupytren disease

Usual Dosage Topical: Apply once daily (or more frequently if the dressing becomes soiled)

Dosage Forms Ointment (Santyl®): 250 units/g (15 g, 30 g)

collagen hemostat (KOL la jen HEE moe stat)

Sound-Alike/Look-Alike Issues

Avitene® may be confused with Ativan®

Synonyms collagen; collagen absorbable hemostat; MCH

U.S./Canadian Brand Names Avitene® [US]; Avitene® Flour [US]; Avitene® Ultrafoam [US]; Avitene® UltraWrap™ [US]; EndoAvitene® [US]; Helistat® [US]; Instat™ MCH [US]; SyringeAvitene™ [US]

Therapeutic Category Hemostatic Agent

Use Adjunct to hemostasis when control of bleeding by ligature is ineffective or impractical

Usual Dosage Apply dry directly to source of bleeding; remove excess material after ~10-15 minutes

Dosage Forms

Pad (Instat™) [bovine derived]: 1 inch x 2 inch (12s); 3 inch x 4 inch (12s)

Powder:

- Avitene® Flour [microfibrillar product, bovine derived]: 0.5 g, 1 g, 5 g
- Instat™ MCH [microfibrillar product, bovine derived]: 0.5 g, 1 g
- SyringeAvitene™ [microfibrillar product, bovine derived, prefilled syringe]: 1 g

Sheet:

- Avitene® [microfibrillar product, bovine derived, nonwoven web]: 35 mm x 35 mm (6s); 70 mm x 35 mm (6s, 12s); 70 mm x 70 mm (6s, 12s)
- EndoAvitene® [microfibrillar product, bovine derived, preloaded applicator]: 50 mm x 5 mm x 1 mm (6s); 50 mm x 5 mm x 1 mm (6s)

Sponge:

- Avitene® Ultrafoam™ [microfibrillar product, bovine derived]: 2 cm x 6.25 cm x 7 mm (12s); 8 cm x 6.25 cm x 1 cm (6s); 8 cm x 12.5 cm x 1 cm (6s); 8 cm x 12.5 cm x 3 mm (6s); 8 cm x 25 cm x 1 cm (6s)
- Avitene® UltraWrap™ [microfibrillar product, bovine derived]: 8 cm x 12.5 cm (6s)
- Helisat® [bovine derived]: 0.5 inch x 1 inch x 7 mm (18s) [packaged as 3 strips of 6 sponges]; 1 inch x 2 inch x 5 mm (10s); 3 inch x 4 inch x 5 inch (10s); 1 inch x 9 inch x 5 mm (4s)

collagen implants (KOL a jen im PLANTS)

U.S./Canadian Brand Names Soft Plug® [US]

Therapeutic Category Ophthalmic Agent, Miscellaneous

Use Relief of dry eyes; enhance the effect of ocular medications

Usual Dosage Implants inserted by physician

Dosage Forms

Implant, ophthalmic [bovine collagen]: 0.2 mm, 0.3 mm, 0.4 mm, 0.5 mm, 0.6 mm

- Soft Plug®: 0.2 mm, 0.3 mm, 0.4 mm

Colocort™ [US] *see* hydrocortisone (rectal) *on page 448*

Coly-Mycin® M [US/Can] *see* colistimethate *on page 224*

Coly-Mycin® S [US] *see* neomycin, colistin, hydrocortisone, and thonzonium *on page 610*

Coly-Mycin® S Oral ***(Discontinued)*** *see page 1042*

Colyte® [US/Can] *see* polyethylene glycol-electrolyte solution *on page 706*

Combantrin™ [Can] *see* pyrantel pamoate *on page 750*

CombiPatch® [US] *see* estradiol and norethindrone *on page 327*

Combipres® ***(Discontinued)*** *see page 1042*

Combivent® [US/Can] *see* ipratropium and albuterol *on page 483*

Combivir® [US/Can] *see* zidovudine and lamivudine *on page 939*

Comfort® Ophthalmic ***(Discontinued)*** *see page 1042*

Comfort® Tears Solution ***(Discontinued)*** *see page 1042*

Comhist® [US] *see* chlorpheniramine, phenylephrine, and phenyltoloxamine *on page 193*

Commit™ [US-OTC] *see* nicotine *on page 618*

Compazine® ***(Discontinued)*** *see page 1042*

Compazine® [Can] *see* prochlorperazine *on page 731*

compound E *see* cortisone acetate *on page 228*

compound F *see* hydrocortisone (systemic) *on page 449*

compound S *see* zidovudine *on page 939*

compound S, abacavir, and lamivudine *see* abacavir, lamivudine, and zidovudine *on page 2*

Compound W® One Step Wart Remover [US-OTC] *see* salicylic acid *on page 789*

Compound W® [US-OTC] *see* salicylic acid *on page 789*

Compoz® Nighttime Sleep Aid [US-OTC] *see* diphenhydramine *on page 277*

Compro™ [US] *see* prochlorperazine *on page 731*

Comtan® [US/Can] *see* entacapone *on page 310*

Comtrex® Maximum Strength Sinus and Nasal Decongestant [US-OTC] *see* acetaminophen, chlorpheniramine, and pseudoephedrine *on page 11*

Comtrex® Non-Drowsy Cold and Cough Relief [US-OTC] *see* acetaminophen, dextromethorphan, and pseudoephedrine *on page 12*

Comtrex® Sore Throat Maximum Strength [US-OTC] *see* acetaminophen *on page 5*

Comvax® [US] *see* *Haemophilus* B conjugate and hepatitis B vaccine *on page 426*

Conceptrol® [US-OTC] *see* nonoxynol 9 *on page 626*

Concerta® [US/Can] *see* methylphenidate *on page 571*

Condyline™ [Can] *see* podofilox *on page 704*

Condylox® [US] *see* podofilox *on page 704*

Conex® ***(Discontinued)*** *see page 1042*

Congess® Jr ***(Discontinued)*** *see page 1042*

Congess® Sr ***(Discontinued)*** *see page 1042*

Congest [Can] *see* estrogens (conjugated/equine) *on page 329*

Congestac® [US-OTC] *see* guaifenesin and pseudoephedrine *on page 419*

Congestant D® ***(Discontinued)*** *see page 1042*

Conray® [US] *see* radiological/contrast media (ionic) *on page 759*

Cortenema® *(Discontinued)* *see page 1042*

Corticool® [US] *see* hydrocortisone (topical) *on page 451*

corticotropin (kor ti koe TROE pin)

Synonyms ACTH; adrenocorticotropic hormone; corticotropin, repository

U.S./Canadian Brand Names H.P. Acthar® Gel [US]

Therapeutic Category Adrenal Corticosteroid

Use Acute exacerbations of multiple sclerosis; diagnostic aid in adrenocortical insufficiency, severe muscle weakness in myasthenia gravis

Cosyntropin is preferred over corticotropin for diagnostic test of adrenocortical insufficiency (cosyntropin is less allergenic and test is shorter in duration)

Usual Dosage

Children:

Antiinflammatory/immunosuppressant: I.M.: 0.8 units/kg/day or 25 units/m^2/day divided every 12-24 hours

Infantile spasms: Various regimens have been used. Some neurologists recommend low-dose ACTH (5-40 units/day) for short periods (1-6 weeks), while others recommend larger doses of ACTH (40-160 units/day) for long periods of treatment (3-12 months). Well designed comparative dosing studies are needed. Example of low dose regimen:

Initial: I.M.: 20 units/day for 2 weeks, if patient responds, taper and discontinue; if patient does not respond, increase dose to 30 units/day for 4 weeks then taper and discontinue

I.M. usual dose: 20-40 units/day or 5-8 units/kg/day in 1-2 divided doses; range: 5-160 units/day

Oral prednisone (2 mg/kg/day) was as effective as I.M. ACTH gel (20 units/day) in controlling infantile spasms

Adults: Acute exacerbation of multiple sclerosis: I.M.: 80-120 units/day for 2-3 weeks

Repository injection: I.M., SubQ: 40-80 units every 24-72 hours

Dosage Forms Injection, gelatin (H.P. Acthar® Gel): 80 units/mL (5 mL)

corticotropin, repository *see* corticotropin *on this page*

Cortifoam® [US/Can] *see* hydrocortisone (rectal) *on page 448*

Cortimyxin® [Can] *see* neomycin, polymyxin B, and hydrocortisone *on page 611*

cortisol *see* hydrocortisone (systemic) *on page 449*

cortisone acetate (KOR ti sone AS e tate)

Sound-Alike/Look-Alike Issues

cortisone may be confused with Cortizone®

Synonyms compound E

U.S./Canadian Brand Names Cortone® [Can]

Therapeutic Category Adrenal Corticosteroid

Use Management of adrenocortical insufficiency

Usual Dosage If possible, administer glucocorticoids before 9 AM to minimize adrenocortical suppression; dosing depends upon the condition being treated and the response of the patient; **Note:** Supplemental doses may be warranted during times of stress in the course of withdrawing therapy

Children:

Antiinflammatory or immunosuppressive: Oral: 2.5-10 mg/kg/day **or** 20-300 mg/m^2/day in divided doses every 6-8 hours

Physiologic replacement: Oral: 0.5-0.75 mg/kg/day **or** 20-25 mg/m^2/day in divided doses every 8 hours

Adults:

Antiinflammatory or immunosuppressive: Oral: 25-300 mg/day in divided doses every 12-24 hours

Physiologic replacement: Oral: 25-35 mg/day

Dosage Forms Tablet, as acetate: 25 mg

Cortisporin® Cream [US] *see* neomycin, polymyxin B, and hydrocortisone *on page 611*

Cortisporin® Ointment [US/Can] *see* bacitracin, neomycin, polymyxin B, and hydrocortisone *on page 98*

Cortisporin® Ophthalmic [US] *see* neomycin, polymyxin B, and hydrocortisone *on page 611*

Cortisporin® Otic [US/Can] *see* neomycin, polymyxin B, and hydrocortisone *on page 611*

Cortisporin®-TC [US] *see* neomycin, colistin, hydrocortisone, and thonzonium *on page 610*

Cortisporin® Topical Cream *(Discontinued)* *see page 1042*

Cortizone®-5 [US] *see* hydrocortisone (topical) *on page 451*

Cortizone®-10 [US] *see* hydrocortisone (rectal) *on page 448*

Cortizone®-10 Maximum Strength [US] *see* hydrocortisone (topical) *on page 451*

Cortizone®-10 Plus Maximum Strength [US] *see* hydrocortisone (topical) *on page 451*

Cortizone® 10 Quick Shot [US] *see* hydrocortisone (topical) *on page 451*

Cortizone® for Kids [US] *see* hydrocortisone (topical) *on page 451*

Cortone® *(Discontinued)* *see page 1042*

Cortone® [Can] *see* cortisone acetate *on previous page*

Cortrophin-Zinc® *(Discontinued)* *see page 1042*

Cortrosyn® [US/Can] *see* cosyntropin *on this page*

Corvert® [US] *see* ibutilide *on page 463*

Coryphen® Codeine [Can] *see* aspirin and codeine *on page 82*

Cosmegen® [US/Can] *see* dactinomycin *on page 241*

cosyntropin (koe sin TROE pin)

Sound-Alike/Look-Alike Issues

Cortrosyn® may be confused with Cotazym®

Synonyms synacthen; tetracosactide

U.S./Canadian Brand Names Cortrosyn® [US/Can]

Therapeutic Category Diagnostic Agent

Use Diagnostic test to differentiate primary adrenal from secondary (pituitary) adrenocortical insufficiency

Usual Dosage

Adrenocortical insufficiency: I.M., I.V. (over 2 minutes): Peak plasma cortisol concentrations usually occur 45-60 minutes after cosyntropin administration

Children <2 years: 0.125 mg

Children >2 years and Adults: 0.25-0.75 mg

When greater cortisol stimulation is needed, an I.V. infusion may be used:

Children >2 years and Adults: 0.25 mg administered at 0.04 mg/hour over 6 hours

Dosage Forms Injection, powder for reconstitution: 0.25 mg

Cotazym® *(Discontinued)* *see page 1042*

Cotazym® [Can] *see* pancrelipase *on page 663*

Cotazym-S® *(Discontinued)* *see page 1042*

CO Temazepam [Can] *see* temazepam *on page 843*

Cotrim® *(Discontinued)* *see page 1042*

Cotrim® DS *(Discontinued)* *see page 1042*

co-trimoxazole *see* sulfamethoxazole and trimethoprim *on page 831*

cromolyn sodium (KROE moe lin SOW dee um)

Sound-Alike/Look-Alike Issues

Intal® may be confused with Endal®

NasalCrom® may be confused with Nasacort®, Nasalide®

Synonyms cromoglycic acid; disodium cromoglycate; DSCG

U.S./Canadian Brand Names Apo-Cromolyn® [Can]; Crolom® [US]; Gastrocrom® [US]; Intal® [US/Can]; Nalcrom® [Can]; NasalCrom® [US-OTC]; Nu-Cromolyn [Can]; Opticrom® [US/Can]

Therapeutic Category Mast Cell Stabilizer

Use

Inhalation: May be used as an adjunct in the prophylaxis of allergic disorders, including asthma; prevention of exercise-induced bronchospasm

Nasal: Prevention and treatment of seasonal and perennial allergic rhinitis

Oral: Systemic mastocytosis

Ophthalmic: Treatment of vernal keratoconjunctivitis, vernal conjunctivitis, and vernal keratitis

Usual Dosage

Oral:

Systemic mastocytosis:

Children 2-12 years: 100 mg 4 times/day; not to exceed 40 mg/kg/day; given 1/2 hour prior to meals and at bedtime

Children >12 years and Adults: 200 mg 4 times/day; given 1/2 hour prior to meals and at bedtime; if control of symptoms is not seen within 2-3 weeks, dose may be increased to a maximum 40 mg/kg/day

Inhalation:

For chronic control of asthma, taper frequency to the lowest effective dose (ie, 4 times/day to 3 times/day to twice daily):

Nebulization solution: Children >2 years and Adults: Initial: 20 mg 4 times/day; usual dose: 20 mg 3-4 times/day

Metered spray:

Children 5-12 years: Initial: 2 inhalations 4 times/day; usual dose: 1-2 inhalations 3-4 times/day

Children ≥12 years and Adults: Initial: 2 inhalations 4 times/day; usual dose: 2-4 inhalations 3-4 times/day

Prevention of allergen- or exercise-induced bronchospasm: Administer 10-15 minutes prior to exercise or allergen exposure but no longer than 1 hour before:

Nebulization solution: Children >2 years and Adults: Single dose of 20 mg

Metered spray: Children >5 years and Adults: Single dose of 2 inhalations

Ophthalmic: Children >4 years and Adults: 1-2 drops in each eye 4-6 times/day

Nasal: Allergic rhinitis (treatment and prophylaxis): Children ≥2 years and Adults: 1 spray into each nostril 3-4 times/day; may be increased to 6 times/day (symptomatic relief may require 2-4 weeks)

Dosage Forms

Aerosol, for oral inhalation, as sodium (Intal®): 800 mcg/inhalation (8.1 g) [112 metered inhalations; 56 doses], (14.2 g) [200 metered inhalations; 100 doses]

Solution for nebulization, as sodium (Intal®): 20 mg/2 mL (60s, 120s)

Solution, intranasal spray, as sodium (NasalCrom®): 40 mg/mL (13 mL, 26 mL) [5.2 mg/inhalation; contains benzalkonium chloride]

Solution, ophthalmic, as sodium (Crolom®, Opticrom®): 4% (10 mL) [contains benzalkonium chloride]

Solution, oral, as sodium (Gastrocrom®): 100 mg/5 mL (96s)

Crosseal™ [US] *see* fibrin sealant kit *on page 367*

crotaline antivenin, polyvalent *see* antivenin *(Crotalidae)* polyvalent *on page 67*

crotamiton (kroe TAM i tonn)

Sound-Alike/Look-Alike Issues

Eurax® may be confused with Efudex®, Eulexin®, Evoxac™, Serax®, Urex®

U.S./Canadian Brand Names Eurax® [US]

Therapeutic Category Scabicides/Pediculicides

Use Treatment of scabies (*Sarcoptes scabiei*) and symptomatic treatment of pruritus

Usual Dosage Topical:

Scabicide: Children and Adults: Wash thoroughly and scrub away loose scales, then towel dry; apply a thin layer and massage drug onto skin of the entire body from the neck to the toes (with special attention to skin folds, creases, and interdigital spaces). Repeat application in 24 hours. Take a cleansing bath 48 hours after the final application. Treatment may be repeated after 7-10 days if live mites are still present.

Pruritus: Massage into affected areas until medication is completely absorbed; repeat as necessary

Dosage Forms

Cream: 10% (60 g)

Lotion: 10% (60 mL, 480 mL)

crude coal tar *see* coal tar *on page 219*

Cruex® Cream [US-OTC] *see* clotrimazole *on page 218*

Cryselle™ [US] *see* ethinyl estradiol and norgestrel *on page 347*

crystalline penicillin *see* penicillin G (parenteral/aqueous) *on page 676*

Crystamine® *(Discontinued)* *see page 1042*

Crysti 1000® *(Discontinued)* *see page 1042*

Crysticillin® A.S. *(Discontinued)* *see page 1042*

Crystodigin® *(Discontinued)* *see page 1042*

CsA *see* cyclosporine *on page 235*

CSP *see* cellulose sodium phosphate *on page 175*

CTM *see* chlorpheniramine *on page 187*

CTX *see* cyclophosphamide *on page 234*

Cubicin™ [US] *see* daptomycin *on page 245*

Cuprimine® [US/Can] *see* penicillamine *on page 674*

Curosurf® [US/Can] *see* poractant alfa *on page 710*

Cutar® [US-OTC] *see* coal tar *on page 219*

Cutivate™ [US] *see* fluticasone (topical) *on page 384*

CyA *see* cyclosporine *on page 235*

Cyanide Antidote Package *see* sodium nitrite, sodium thiosulfate, and amyl nitrite *on page 813*

cyanocobalamin (sye an oh koe BAL a min)

Synonyms vitamin B_{12}

U.S./Canadian Brand Names Nascobal® [US]; Scheinpharm B12 [Can]; Twelve Resin-K® [US]

Therapeutic Category Vitamin, Water Soluble

Use Treatment of pernicious anemia; vitamin B_{12} deficiency; increased B_{12} requirements due to pregnancy, thyrotoxicosis, hemorrhage, malignancy, liver or kidney disease

Usual Dosage

Recommended daily allowance (RDA):

Children: 0.3-2 mcg

Adults: 2 mcg

Nutritional deficiency:

Intranasal gel: 500 mcg once weekly

Oral: 25-250 mcg/day

Anemias: I.M. or deep SubQ (oral is not generally recommended due to poor absorption and I.V. is not recommended due to more rapid elimination):

Pernicious anemia, congenital (if evidence of neurologic involvement): 1000 mcg/day for at least 2 weeks; maintenance: 50-100 mcg/month or 100 mcg for 6-7 days; if there is clinical improvement, give 100 mcg every other day for 7 doses, then every 3-4 days for 2-3 weeks; follow with 100 mcg/month for life. Administer with folic acid if needed (1 mg/day for 1 month concomitantly)

Children: 30-50 mcg/day for 2 or more weeks (to a total dose of 1000-5000 mcg), then follow with 100 mcg/month as maintenance dosage

Adults: 100 mcg/day for 6-7 days; if improvement, administer same dose on alternate days for 7 doses; then every 3-4 days for 2-3 weeks; once hematologic values have returned to normal, maintenance dosage: 100 mcg/month. **Note:** Use only parenteral therapy as oral therapy is not dependable.

Hematologic remission (without evidence of nervous system involvement): Intranasal gel: 500 mcg once weekly

Vitamin B_{12} deficiency:

Children:

Neurologic signs: 100 mcg/day for 10-15 days (total dose of 1-1.5 mg), then once or twice weekly for several months; may taper to 60 mcg every month

Hematologic signs: 10-50 mcg/day for 5-10 days, followed by 100-250 mcg/dose every 2-4 weeks

Adults: Initial: 30 mcg/day for 5-10 days; maintenance: 100-200 mcg/month

Schilling test: I.M.: 1000 mcg

Dosage Forms

Gel, intranasal (Nascobal®): 500 mcg/0.1 mL (2.3 mL)

Injection, solution: 1000 mcg/mL (1 mL, 10 mL, 30 mL) [products may contain benzyl alcohol]

Lozenge [OTC]: 100 mcg, 250 mcg, 500 mcg

Tablet [OTC]: 50 mcg, 100 mcg, 250 mcg, 500 mcg, 1000 mcg, 5000 mcg

Twelve Resin-K: 1000 mcg [may be used as oral, sublingual, or buccal]

Tablet, extended release [OTC]: 1500 mcg

Tablet, sublingual [OTC]: 2500 mcg

cyanocobalamin, folic acid, and pyridoxine *see* folic acid, cyanocobalamin, and pyridoxine *on page 386*

Cyanoject® *(Discontinued)* *see page 1042*

cyclandelate (sye KLAN de late)

Therapeutic Category Vasodilator, Peripheral

Use Considered as "possibly effective" for adjunctive therapy in peripheral vascular disease and possibly senility due to cerebrovascular disease or multi-infarct dementia; migraine prophylaxis, vertigo, tinnitus, and visual disturbances secondary to cerebrovascular insufficiency and diabetic peripheral polyneuropathy

Usual Dosage Adults: Oral: Initial: 1.2-1.6 g/day in divided doses before meals and at bedtime until response; maintenance therapy: 400-800 mg/day in 2-4 divided doses; start with lowest dose in elderly due to hypotensive potential; decrease dose by 200 mg decrements to achieve minimal maintenance dose; improvement can usually be seen over weeks of therapy and prolonged use; short courses of therapy are usually ineffective and not recommended

Dosage Forms Capsule: 200 mg, 400 mg

Cyclen® [Can] *see* ethinyl estradiol and norgestimate *on page 346*

Cyclessa® [US] *see* ethinyl estradiol and desogestrel *on page 335*

cyclobenzaprine (sye kloe BEN za preen)

Sound-Alike/Look-Alike Issues

cyclobenzaprine may be confused with cycloserine, cyproheptadine

Flexeril® may be confused with Floxin®

Synonyms cyclobenzaprine hydrochloride

U.S./Canadian Brand Names Apo-Cyclobenzaprine® [Can]; Flexeril® [US/Can]; Flexitec [Can]; Gen-Cyclobenzaprine [Can]; Novo-Cycloprine [Can]; Nu-Cyclobenzaprine [Can]

Therapeutic Category Skeletal Muscle Relaxant

Use Treatment of muscle spasm associated with acute painful musculoskeletal conditions

Usual Dosage Oral: **Note:** Do not use longer than 2-3 weeks

Adults: Initial: 5 mg 3 times/day; may increase to 10 mg 3 times/day if needed

Dosage Forms

Tablet, as hydrochloride: 10 mg

Flexeril®: 5 mg, 10 mg [film coated]

cyclobenzaprine hydrochloride *see* cyclobenzaprine *on this page*

Cyclocort® [US/Can] *see* amcinonide *on page 42*

Cyclogyl® [US/Can] *see* cyclopentolate *on next page*

Cyclomen® [Can] *see* danazol *on page 243*

Cyclomydril® [US] *see* cyclopentolate and phenylephrine *on next page*

cyclopentolate (sye kloe PEN toe late)

Synonyms cyclopentolate hydrochloride

U.S./Canadian Brand Names Cyclogyl® [US/Can]; Cylate® [US]; Diopentolate® [Can]

Therapeutic Category Anticholinergic Agent

Use Diagnostic procedures requiring mydriasis and cycloplegia

Usual Dosage Ophthalmic:

Neonates and Infants: **Note:** Cyclopentolate and phenylephrine combination formulation is the preferred agent for use in neonates and infants due to lower cyclopentolate concentration and reduced risk for systemic reactions

Children: Instill 1 drop of 0.5%, 1%, or 2% in eye followed by 1 drop of 0.5% or 1% in 5 minutes, if necessary

Adults: Instill 1 drop of 1% followed by another drop in 5 minutes; 2% solution in heavily pigmented iris

Dosage Forms

Solution, ophthalmic, as hydrochloride: 1% (2 mL, 15 mL)

AK-Pentolate® [DSC], Cylate®: 1% (2 mL, 15 mL) [contains benzalkonium chloride]

Cyclogyl®: 0.5% (15 mL); 1% (2 mL, 5 mL, 15 mL); 2% (2 mL, 5 mL, 15 mL) [contains benzalkonium chloride]

cyclopentolate and phenylephrine (sye kloe PEN toe late & fen il EF rin)

Synonyms phenylephrine and cyclopentolate

U.S./Canadian Brand Names Cyclomydril® [US]

Therapeutic Category Anticholinergic/Adrenergic Agonist

Use Induce mydriasis greater than that produced with cyclopentolate HCl alone

Usual Dosage Ophthalmic: Neonates, Infants, Children, and Adults: Instill 1 drop into the eye every 5-10 minutes, for up to 3 doses, approximately 40-50 minutes before the examination

Dosage Forms Solution, ophthalmic: Cyclopentolate hydrochloride 0.2% and phenylephrine hydrochloride 1% (2 mL, 5 mL) [contains benzalkonium chloride]

cyclopentolate hydrochloride *see* cyclopentolate *on this page*

cyclophosphamide (sye kloe FOS fa mide)

Sound-Alike/Look-Alike Issues

cyclophosphamide may be confused with cyclosporine

Cytoxan® may be confused with cefoxitin, Centoxin®, Ciloxan®, cytarabine, CytoGam®, Cytosar®, Cytosar-U®, Cytotec®

Synonyms CPM; CTX; CYT; NSC-26271

U.S./Canadian Brand Names Cytoxan® [US/Can]; Procytox® [Can]

Therapeutic Category Antineoplastic Agent

Use

Oncologic: Treatment of Hodgkin and non-Hodgkin lymphoma, Burkitt lymphoma, chronic lymphocytic leukemia (CLL), chronic myelocytic leukemia (CML), acute myelocytic leukemia (AML), acute lymphocytic leukemia (ALL), mycosis fungoides, multiple myeloma, neuroblastoma, retinoblastoma, rhabdomyosarcoma, Ewing sarcoma; breast, testicular, endometrial, ovarian, and lung cancers, and in conditioning regimens for bone marrow transplantation

Nononcologic: Prophylaxis of rejection for kidney, heart, liver, and bone marrow transplants, severe rheumatoid disorders, nephrotic syndrome, Wegener granulomatosis, idiopathic pulmonary hemosideroses, myasthenia gravis, multiple sclerosis, systemic lupus erythematosus, lupus nephritis, autoimmune hemolytic anemia, idiopathic thrombocytic purpura (ITP), macroglobulinemia, and antibody-induced pure red cell aplasia

Usual Dosage Refer to individual protocols.

Patients who are heavily pretreated with cytotoxic radiation or chemotherapy, or who have compromised bone marrow function may require a 33% to 50% reduction in initial dose.

Children:

SLE: I.V.: 500-750 mg/m^2 every month; maximum dose: 1 g/m^2

JRA/vasculitis: I.V.: 10 mg/kg every 2 weeks
Children and Adults:
Oral: 50-100 mg/m^2/day as continuous therapy or 400-1000 mg/m^2 in divided doses over 4-5 days as intermittent therapy
I.V.:
Single doses: 400-1800 mg/m^2 (30-50 mg/kg) per treatment course (1-5 days) which can be repeated at 2-4 week intervals
Continuous daily doses: 60-120 mg/m^2 (1-2.5 mg/kg) per day
Autologous BMT: IVPB: 50 mg/kg/dose x 4 days or 60 mg/kg/dose for 2 days; total dose is usually divided over 2-4 days
Nephrotic syndrome: Oral: 2-3 mg/kg/day every day for up to 12 weeks when corticosteroids are unsuccessful

Dosage Forms
Injection, powder for reconstitution: Cytoxan®: 500 mg, 1 g, 2 g [contains mannitol 75 mg per cyclophosphamide 100 mg]
Tablet (Cytoxan®): 25 mg, 50 mg

cycloserine (sye kloe SER een)

Sound-Alike/Look-Alike Issues
cycloserine may be confused with cyclobenzaprine, cyclosporine

Tall-Man cyclo**SERINE**

U.S./Canadian Brand Names Seromycin® [US]

Therapeutic Category Antibiotic, Miscellaneous

Use Adjunctive treatment in pulmonary or extrapulmonary tuberculosis

Usual Dosage Some of the neurotoxic effects may be relieved or prevented by the concomitant administration of pyridoxine
Tuberculosis: Oral:
Children: 10-20 mg/kg/day in 2 divided doses up to 1000 mg/day for 18-24 months
Adults: Initial: 250 mg every 12 hours for 14 days, then administer 500 mg to 1 g/day in 2 divided doses for 18-24 months (maximum daily dose: 1 g)

Dosage Forms Capsule: 250 mg

Cyclospasmol® ***(Discontinued)*** *see page 1042*

cyclosporin A *see* cyclosporine *on this page*

cyclosporine (SYE kloe spor een)

Sound-Alike/Look-Alike Issues
cyclosporine may be confused with cyclophosphamide, Cyklokapron®, cycloserine
Gengraf® may be confused with Prograf®
Neoral® may be confused with Neurontin®, Nizoral®
Sandimmune® may be confused with Sandostatin®

Synonyms CsA; CyA; cyclosporin A

Tall-Man cyclo**SPORINE**

U.S./Canadian Brand Names Apo-Cyclosporine® [Can]; Gengraf® [US]; Neoral® [US/Can]; Restasis™ [US]; Rhoxal-cyclosporine [Can]; Sandimmune® [US]; Sandimmune® I.V. [Can]

Therapeutic Category Immunosuppressant Agent

Use Prophylaxis of organ rejection in kidney, liver, and heart transplants, has been used with azathioprine and/or corticosteroids; severe, active rheumatoid arthritis (RA) not responsive to methotrexate alone; severe, recalcitrant plaque psoriasis in nonimmunocompromised adults unresponsive to or unable to tolerate other systemic therapy

Ophthalmic emulsion (Restasis™): Increase tear production when suppressed tear production is presumed to be due to keratoconjunctivitis sicca-associated ocular inflammation (in patients not already using topical antiinflammatory drugs or punctal plugs)

Usual Dosage Note: Neoral® and Sandimmune® are not bioequivalent and cannot be used interchangeably
(Continued)

cyclosporine *(Continued)*

Children: Transplant: Refer to adult dosing; children may require, and are able to tolerate, larger doses than adults.

Adults:

Newly-transplanted patients: Adjunct therapy with corticosteroids is recommended. Initial dose should be given 4-12 hours prior to transplant or may be given postoperatively; adjust initial dose to achieve desired plasma concentration

Oral: Dose is dependent upon type of transplant and formulation:

Cyclosporine (modified): Renal: 9 ± 3 mg/kg/day, divided twice daily Liver: 8 ± 4 mg/kg/day, divided twice daily Heart: 7 ± 3 mg/kg/day, divided twice daily

Cyclosporine (non-modified): Initial dose: 15 mg/kg/day as a single dose (range 14-18 mg/kg); lower doses of 10-14 mg/kg/day have been used for renal transplants. Continue initial dose daily for 1-2 weeks; taper by 5% per week to a maintenance dose of 5-10 mg/kg/day; some renal transplant patients may be dosed as low as 3 mg/kg/day **Note:** When using the non-modified formulation, cyclosporine levels may increase in liver transplant patients when the T-tube is closed; dose may need decreased

I.V.: Cyclosporine (non-modified): Initial dose: 5-6 mg/kg/day as a single dose ($^1/_3$ the oral dose), infused over 2-6 hours; use should be limited to patients unable to take capsules or oral solution; patients should be switched to an oral dosage form as soon as possible

Conversion to cyclosporine (modified) from cyclosporine (non-modified): Start with daily dose previously used and adjust to obtain preconversion cyclosporine trough concentration. Plasma concentrations should be monitored every 4-7 days and dose adjusted as necessary, until desired trough level is obtained. When transferring patients with previously poor absorption of cyclosporine (non-modified), monitor trough levels at least twice weekly (especially if initial dose exceeds 10 mg/kg/day); high plasma levels are likely to occur.

Rheumatoid arthritis: Oral: Cyclosporine (modified): Initial dose: 2.5 mg/kg/day, divided twice daily; salicylates, NSAIDs, and oral glucocorticoids may be continued (refer to Drug Interactions); dose may be increased by 0.5-0.75 mg/kg/day if insufficient response is seen after 8 weeks of treatment; additional dosage increases may be made again at 12 weeks (maximum dose: 4 mg/kg/day). Discontinue if no benefit is seen by 16 weeks of therapy.

Note: Increase the frequency of blood pressure monitoring after each alteration in dosage of cyclosporine. Cyclosporine dosage should be decreased by 25% to 50% in patients with no history of hypertension who develop sustained hypertension during therapy and, if hypertension persists, treatment with cyclosporine should be discontinued.

Psoriasis: Oral: Cyclosporine (modified): Initial dose: 2.5 mg/kg/day, divided twice daily; dose may be increased by 0.5 mg/kg/day if insufficient response is seen after 4 weeks of treatment. Additional dosage increases may be made every 2 weeks if needed (maximum dose: 4 mg/kg/day). Discontinue if no benefit is seen by 6 weeks of therapy. Once patients are adequately controlled, the dose should be decreased to the lowest effective dose. Doses lower than 2.5 mg/kg/day may be effective. Treatment longer than 1 year is not recommended.

Note: Increase the frequency of blood pressure monitoring after each alteration in dosage of cyclosporine. Cyclosporine dosage should be decreased by 25% to 50% in patients with no history of hypertension who develop sustained hypertension during therapy and, if hypertension persists, treatment with cyclosporine should be discontinued.

Focal segmental glomerulosclerosis: Initial: 3 mg/kg/day divided every 12 hours

Autoimmune diseases: 1-3 mg/kg/day

Keratoconjunctivitis sicca: Ophthalmic: Children ≥16 years and Adults: Instill 1 drop in each eye every 12 hours

Dosage Forms

Capsule, soft gel, modified: 25 mg, 100 mg [contains castor oil, ethanol]

Gengraf®: 25 mg, 100 mg [contains ethanol, castor oil, propylene glycol]

Neoral®: 25 mg, 100 mg [contains dehydrated ethanol, corn oil, castor oil, propylene glycol]

Capsule, soft gel, non-modified (Sandimmune®): 25 mg, 100 mg [contains dehydrated ethanol, corn oil]

Emulsion, ophthalmic [preservative free, single-use vial] (Restasis™): 0.05% (0.4 mL) [contains glycerin, castor oil, polysorbate 80, carbomer 1342; 32 vials/box]

Injection, solution, non-modified (Sandimmune®): 50 mg/mL (5 mL) [contains Cremophor® EL (polyoxyethylated castor oil), ethanol]

Solution, oral, modified:

Gengraf®: 100 mg/mL (50 mL) [contains castor oil, propylene glycol]

Neoral®: 100 mg/mL (50 mL) [contains dehydrated ethanol, corn oil, castor oil, propylene glycol]

Solution, oral, non-modified (Sandimmune®): 100 mg/mL (50 mL) [contains olive oil, ethanol]

Cycofed® Pediatric *(Discontinued)* *see page 1042*

Cycrin® 10 mg Tablet *(Discontinued)* *see page 1042*

Cyklokapron® [US/Can] *see* tranexamic acid *on page 876*

Cylate® [US] *see* cyclopentolate *on page 234*

Cylert® [US] *see* pemoline *on page 673*

Cylex® [US-OTC] *see* benzocaine *on page 107*

Cyomin® *(Discontinued)* *see page 1042*

cyproheptadine (si proe HEP ta deen)

Sound-Alike/Look-Alike Issues

cyproheptadine may be confused with cyclobenzaprine

Periactin may be confused with Perative®, Percodan®, Persantine®

Synonyms cyproheptadine hydrochloride

U.S./Canadian Brand Names Periactin® [Can]

Therapeutic Category Antihistamine

Use Perennial and seasonal allergic rhinitis and other allergic symptoms including urticaria

Usual Dosage Oral:

Children:

Allergic conditions: 0.25 mg/kg/day or 8 mg/m^2/day in 2-3 divided doses **or**

2-6 years: 2 mg every 8-12 hours (not to exceed 12 mg/day)

7-14 years: 4 mg every 8-12 hours (not to exceed 16 mg/day)

Migraine headaches: 4 mg 2-3 times/day

Children ≥12 years and Adults: Spasticity associated with spinal cord damage: 4 mg at bedtime; increase by a 4 mg dose every 3-4 days; average daily dose: 16 mg in divided doses; not to exceed 36 mg/day

Children >13 years and Adults: Appetite stimulation (anorexia nervosa): 2 mg 4 times/day; may be increased gradually over a 3-week period to 8 mg 4 times/day

Adults:

Allergic conditions: 4-20 mg/day divided every 8 hours (not to exceed 0.5 mg/kg/day)

Cluster headaches: 4 mg 4 times/day

Migraine headaches: 4-8 mg 3 times/day

Dosage Forms

Syrup, as hydrochloride: 2 mg/5 mL (473 mL) [contains alcohol 5%; mint flavor]

Tablet, as hydrochloride: 4 mg

cyproheptadine hydrochloride *see* cyproheptadine *on this page*

cyproterone acetate *see* cyproterone *(Canada only) on next page*

cyproterone and ethinyl estradiol *(Canada only)*

(sye PROE ter one & ETH in il es tra DYE ole)

Synonyms ethinyl estradiol and cyproterone acetate

U.S./Canadian Brand Names Diane®-35 [Can]

Therapeutic Category Acne Products; Estrogen and Androgen Combination

Use Treatment of females with severe acne, unresponsive to other therapies, with associated symptoms of androgenization (including mild hirsutism or seborrhea). **Should not be used solely for contraception;** however, will provide reliable contraception if taken as recommended for approved indications.

Usual Dosage Oral: Adults: Female: Acne: One tablet daily for 21 days, followed by 7 days off; first cycle should begin on the first day of menstrual flow. Discontinue therapy 3-4 cycles after symptoms have resolved.

Dosage Forms Tablet: Cyproterone acetate 2 mg and ethinyl estradiol 0.35 mg [orange tablets] (21s)

cyproterone *(Canada only)* (sye PROE ter one)

Synonyms cyproterone acetate

U.S./Canadian Brand Names Alti-CPA [Can]; Androcur® [Can]; Androcur® Depot [Can]; Gen-Cyproterone [Can]

Therapeutic Category Antiandrogen; Progestin

Use Palliative treatment of advanced prostate carcinoma

Usual Dosage Adults: Males: Prostatic carcinoma (palliative treatment):

Oral: 200-300 mg/day in 2-3 divided doses; following orchiectomy, reduce dose to 100-200 mg/day; should be taken with meals

I.M. (depot): 300 mg (3 mL) once weekly; reduce dose in orchiectomized patients to 300 mg every 2 weeks

Dosage Forms

Injection, solution, as acetate (Androcur® Depot): 100 mg/mL (3 mL) [contains benzyl benzoate and castor oil]

Tablet, as acetate (Androcur®): 50 mg

Cystadane® [US/Can] *see* betaine anhydrous *on page 114*

Cystagon® [US] *see* cysteamine *on this page*

cysteamine (sis TEE a meen)

Synonyms cysteamine bitartrate

U.S./Canadian Brand Names Cystagon® [US]

Therapeutic Category Urinary Tract Product

Use Orphan drug: Treatment of nephropathic cystinosis

Usual Dosage Oral: Initiate therapy with 1/4 to 1/6 of maintenance dose; titrate slowly upward over 4-6 weeks. **Note:** Dosage may be increased if cystine levels are <1 nmol/1/2 cystine/mg protein, although intolerance and incidence of adverse events may be increased.

Children <12 years: Maintenance: 1.3 g/m^2/day or 60 mg/kg/day divided into 4 doses (maximum dose: 1.95 g/m^2/day or 90 mg/kg/day)

Children >12 years and Adults (>110 lb): 2 g/day in 4 divided doses; maximum dose: 1.95 g/m^2/day or 90 mg/kg/day

Dosage Forms Capsule: 50 mg, 150 mg

cysteamine bitartrate *see* cysteamine *on this page*

cysteine (SIS teen)

Synonyms cysteine hydrochloride

Therapeutic Category Nutritional Supplement

Use Supplement to crystalline amino acid solutions, in particular the specialized pediatric formulas (eg, Aminosyn® PF, TrophAmine®) to meet the intravenous amino acid nutritional requirements of infants receiving parenteral nutrition (PN)

Usual Dosage Neonates and Infants: I.V.: Added as a fixed ratio to crystalline amino acid solution: 40 mg cysteine per g of amino acids; dosage will vary with the daily amino acid dosage (eg, 0.5-2.5 g/kg/day amino acids would result in 20-100 mg/kg/day cysteine); individual doses of cysteine of 0.8-1 mmol/kg/day have also been added directly to the daily PN solution; the duration of treatment relates to the need for PN; patients on chronic PN therapy have received cysteine until 6 months of age and in some cases until 2 years of age

Dosage Forms Injection, solution, as hydrochloride: 50 mg/mL (10 mL, 50 mL)

cysteine hydrochloride *see* cysteine *on previous page*

Cystografin® [US] *see* radiological/contrast media (ionic) *on page 759*

Cystospaz® [US/Can] *see* hyoscyamine *on page 459*

Cystospaz-M® [US] *see* hyoscyamine *on page 459*

CYT *see* cyclophosphamide *on page 234*

Cytadren® [US] *see* aminoglutethimide *on page 45*

cytarabine (sye TARE a been)

Sound-Alike/Look-Alike Issues

cytarabine may be confused with Cytadren®, Cytosar®, Cytoxan®, vidarabine

Cytosar-U® may be confused with cytarabine, Cytovene®, Cytoxan®, Neosar®

Synonyms arabinosylcytosine; ara-C; cytarabine hydrochloride; cytosine arabinosine hydrochloride; NSC-63878

U.S./Canadian Brand Names Cytosar® [Can]; Cytosar-U® [US]

Therapeutic Category Antineoplastic Agent

Use Cytarabine is one of the most active agents in leukemia; also active against lymphoma, meningeal leukemia, and meningeal lymphoma; has little use in the treatment of solid tumors

Usual Dosage I.V. bolus, IVPB, and CIV doses of cytarabine are very different. Bolus doses are relatively well tolerated since the drug is rapidly metabolized; but are associated with greater neurotoxicity. Continuous infusion uniformly results in myelosuppression. Refer to individual protocols. Children and Adults:

Remission induction:

I.V.: 100-200 mg/m²/day for 5-10 days; a second course, beginning 2-4 weeks after the initial therapy, may be required in some patients.

I.T.: 5-75 mg/m² every 2-7 days until CNS findings normalize; or age-based dosing:

<1 year: 20 mg

1-2 years: 30 mg

2-3 years: 50 mg

>3 years: 75 mg

Remission maintenance:

I.V.: 70-200 mg/m²/day for 2-5 days at monthly intervals

I.M., SubQ: 1-1.5 mg/kg single dose for maintenance at 1- to 4-week intervals

High-dose therapies:

Doses as high as 1-3 g/m² have been used for refractory or secondary leukemias or refractory non-Hodgkin lymphoma.

Doses of 1-3 g/m² every 12 hours for up to 12 doses have been used

Bone marrow transplant: 1.5 g/m² continuous infusion over 48 hours

Hemodialysis: Supplemental dose is not necessary.

Peritoneal dialysis: Supplemental dose is not necessary.

Dosage Forms

Injection, powder for reconstitution: 100 mg, 500 mg, 1 g, 2 g

Injection, solution: 20 mg/mL (5 mL, 25 mL, 50 mL); 100 mg/mL (20 mL)

cytarabine hydrochloride *see* cytarabine *on this page*

cytarabine (liposomal) (sye TARE a been lip po SOE mal)

Sound-Alike/Look-Alike Issues
cytarabine may be confused with Cytadren®, Cytosar®, Cytoxan®, vidarabine
DepoCyt™ may be confused with Depoject®

U.S./Canadian Brand Names DepoCyt™ [US/Can]

Therapeutic Category Antineoplastic Agent, Antimetabolite (Purine)

Use Treatment of neoplastic (lymphomatous) meningitis

Usual Dosage Adults:
Induction: 50 mg intrathecally every 14 days for a total of 2 doses (weeks 1 and 3)
Consolidation: 50 mg intrathecally every 14 days for 3 doses (weeks 5, 7, and 9), followed by an additional dose at week 13
Maintenance: 50 mg intrathecally every 28 days for 4 doses (weeks 17, 21, 25, and 29)
If drug-related neurotoxicity develops, the dose should be reduced to 25 mg. If toxicity persists, treatment with liposomal cytarabine should be discontinued.
Note: Patients should be started on dexamethasone 4 mg twice daily (oral or I.V.) for 5 days, beginning on the day of liposomal cytarabine injection

Dosage Forms Injection, suspension: 10 mg/mL (5 mL) [preservative free]

CytoGam® [US] *see* cytomegalovirus immune globulin (intravenous-human) *on this page*

cytomegalovirus immune globulin (intravenous-human)

(sye toe meg a low VYE rus i MYUN GLOB yoo lin in tra VEE nus-HYU man)

Sound-Alike/Look-Alike Issues
CytoGam® may be confused with Cytoxan®, Gamimune® N

Synonyms CMV-IGIV

U.S./Canadian Brand Names CytoGam® [US]

Therapeutic Category Immune Globulin

Use Prophylaxis of cytomegalovirus (CMV) disease associated with kidney, lung, liver, pancreas, and heart transplants; concomitant use with ganciclovir should be considered in organ transplants (other than kidney) from CMV seropositive donors to CMV seronegative recipients

Usual Dosage I.V.: Adults:
Kidney transplant:
Initial dose (within 72 hours of transplant): 150 mg/kg/dose
2-, 4-, 6-, and 8 weeks after transplant: 100 mg/kg/dose
12 and 16 weeks after transplant: 50 mg/kg/dose
Liver, lung, pancreas, or heart transplant:
Initial dose (within 72 hours of transplant): 150 mg/kg/dose
2-, 4-, 6-, and 8 weeks after transplant: 150 mg/kg/dose
12 and 16 weeks after transplant: 100 mg/kg/dose
Severe CMV pneumonia: Various regimens have been used, including 400 mg/kg CMV-IGIV in combination with ganciclovir on days 1, 2, 7, or 8, followed by 200 mg/kg CMV-IGIV on days 14 and 21

Dosage Forms Injection, solution [preservative free]: 50 mg ± 10 mg/mL (50 mL) [contains human albumin and sucrose]

Cytomel® [US/Can] *see* liothyronine *on page 523*

Cytosar® [Can] *see* cytarabine *on previous page*

Cytosar-U® [US] *see* cytarabine *on previous page*

cytosine arabinosine hydrochloride *see* cytarabine *on previous page*

Cytotec® [US/Can] *see* misoprostol *on page 585*

Cytovene® [US/Can] *see* ganciclovir *on page 396*

Cytoxan® [US/Can] *see* cyclophosphamide *on page 234*

Cytra-3 [US] *see* citric acid, sodium citrate, and potassium citrate *on page 206*

Cytra-K [US] *see* potassium citrate and citric acid *on page 714*

D2E7 *see* adalimumab *on page 20*

D_3 *see* cholecalciferol *on page 196*

D-3-mercaptovaline *see* penicillamine *on page 674*

d4T *see* stavudine *on page 823*

dacarbazine (da KAR ba zeen)

Sound-Alike/Look-Alike Issues
dacarbazine may be confused with Dicarbosil®, procarbazine

Synonyms DIC; dimethyl triazeno imidazol carboxamide; DTIC; imidazol carboxamide dimethyltriazene; imidazole carboxamide; WR-139007

U.S./Canadian Brand Names DTIC® [Can]; DTIC-Dome® [US]

Therapeutic Category Antineoplastic Agent

Use Treatment of malignant melanoma, Hodgkin disease, soft-tissue sarcomas, fibrosarcomas, rhabdomyosarcoma, islet cell carcinoma, medullary carcinoma of the thyroid, and neuroblastoma

Usual Dosage Refer to individual protocols. Some dosage regimens include:
Intra-arterial: 50-400 mg/m^2 for 5-10 days
I.V.:
Hodgkin disease, ABVD: 375 mg/m^2 days 1 and 15 every 4 weeks **or** 100 mg/m^2/day for 5 days
Metastatic melanoma (alone or in combination with other agents): 150-250 mg/m^2 days 1-5 every 3-4 weeks
Metastatic melanoma: 850 mg/m^2 every 3 weeks
High dose: Bone marrow/blood cell transplantation: I.V.: 1-3 g/m^2; maximum dose as a single agent: 3.38 g/m^2; generally combined with other high-dose chemotherapeutic drugs

Dosage Forms Injection, powder for reconstitution: 100 mg, 200 mg, 500 mg
DTIC-Dome®: 200 mg

daclizumab (da KLIK si mab)

U.S./Canadian Brand Names Zenapax® [US/Can]

Therapeutic Category Immunosuppressant Agent

Use Part of an immunosuppressive regimen (including cyclosporine and corticosteroids) for the prophylaxis of acute organ rejection in patients receiving renal transplant

Usual Dosage Daclizumab is used adjunctively with other immunosuppressants (eg, cyclosporine, corticosteroids, mycophenolate mofetil, and azathioprine): I.V.:
Children: Use same weight-based dose as adults
Adults:
Immunoprophylaxis against acute renal allograft rejection: 1 mg/kg infused over 15 minutes within 24 hours before transplantation (day 0), then every 14 days for 4 additional doses

Dosage Forms Injection, solution [preservative free]: 5 mg/mL (5 mL)

Dacodyl® ***(Discontinued)*** *see page 1042*

DACT *see* dactinomycin *on this page*

dactinomycin (dak ti noe MYE sin)

Sound-Alike/Look-Alike Issues
dactinomycin may be confused with daunorubicin
actinomycin may be confused with Achromycin®

Synonyms act-D; actinomycin; actinomycin CI; actinomycin D; DACT; NSC-3053

U.S./Canadian Brand Names Cosmegen® [US/Can]

Therapeutic Category Antineoplastic Agent

Use Treatment of testicular tumors, melanoma, choriocarcinoma, Wilms tumor, neuroblastoma, retinoblastoma, rhabdomyosarcoma, uterine sarcomas, Ewing sarcoma, Kaposi sarcoma, sarcoma botryoides, and soft tissue sarcoma
(Continued)

dactinomycin *(Continued)*

Usual Dosage Refer to individual protocols: I.V.:

Note: Medication orders for dactinomycin are commonly written in MICROgrams (eg, 150 mcg) although many regimens list the dose in MILLIgrams (eg, mg/kg or mg/m²). One-time doses for >1000 mcg, or multiple-day doses for >500 mcg/day are not common. Some practitioners recommend calculation of the dosage for obese or edematous patients on the basis of body surface area in an effort to relate dosage to lean body mass.

Children >6 months: 15 mcg/kg/day **or** 400-600 mcg/m²/day for 5 days every 3-6 weeks

Adults: 2.5 mg/m² in divided doses over 1 week, repeated every 2 weeks **or**
0.75-2 mg/m² every 1-4 weeks **or**
400-600 mcg/m²/day for 5 days, repeated every 3-6 weeks

Dosage Forms Injection, powder for reconstitution: 0.5 mg [contains mannitol 20 mg]

DAD *see* mitoxantrone *on page 586*

Dairyaid® [Can] *see* lactase *on page 500*

Dakin's Solution [US] *see* sodium hypochlorite solution *on page 813*

Dakrina® Ophthalmic Solution *(Discontinued)* *see page 1042*

Dalacin® C [Can] *see* clindamycin *on page 210*

Dalacin® T [Can] *see* clindamycin *on page 210*

Dalacin® Vaginal [Can] *see* clindamycin *on page 210*

Dalgan® *(Discontinued)* *see page 1042*

Dallergy® [US] *see* chlorpheniramine, phenylephrine, and methscopolamine *on page 192*

Dallergy-D® Syrup *(Discontinued)* *see page 1042*

Dallergy-JR® [US] *see* chlorpheniramine and phenylephrine *on page 188*

Dalmane® [US/Can] *see* flurazepam *on page 381*

***d*-alpha tocopherol** *see* vitamin E *on page 918*

dalteparin (dal TE pa rin)

U.S./Canadian Brand Names Fragmin® [US/Can]

Therapeutic Category Anticoagulant (Other)

Use Prevention of deep vein thrombosis which may lead to pulmonary embolism, in patients requiring abdominal surgery who are at risk for thromboembolism complications (eg, patients >40 years of age, obesity, patients with malignancy, history of deep vein thrombosis or pulmonary embolism, and surgical procedures requiring general anesthesia and lasting >30 minutes); prevention of DVT in patients undergoing hip-replacement surgery; patients immobile during an acute illness; acute treatment of unstable angina or non-Q-wave myocardial infarction; prevention of ischemic complications in patients on concurrent aspirin therapy

Usual Dosage Adults: SubQ:

Abdominal surgery:

Low-to-moderate DVT risk: 2500 int. units 1-2 hours prior to surgery, then once daily for 5-10 days postoperatively

High DVT risk: 5000 int. units 1-2 hours prior to surgery and then once daily for 5-10 days postoperatively

Patients undergoing total hip surgery: **Note:** Three treatment options are currently available. Dose is given for 5-10 days, although up to 14 days of treatment have been tolerated in clinical trials:

Postoperative start:

Initial: 2500 int. units 4-8 hours* after surgery

Maintenance: 5000 int. units once daily; start at least 6 hours after postsurgical dose

Preoperative (starting day of surgery):

Initial: 2500 int. units within 2 hours before surgery

Adjustment: 2500 int. units 4-8 hours* after surgery
Maintenance: 5000 int. units once daily; start at least 6 hours after postsurgical dose
Preoperative (starting evening prior to surgery):
Initial: 5000 int. units 10-14 hours before surgery
Adjustment: 5000 int. units 4-8 hours* after surgery
Maintenance: 5000 int. units once daily, allowing 24 hours between doses.
***Dose may be delayed if hemostasis is not yet achieved.**

Unstable angina or non-Q-wave myocardial infarction: 120 int. units/kg body weight (maximum dose: 10,000 int. units) every 12 hours for 5-8 days with concurrent aspirin therapy. Discontinue dalteparin once patient is clinically stable.

Immobility during acute illness: 5000 int. units once daily

Dosage Forms

Injection, solution [multidose vial]: Antifactor Xa 10,000 int. units per 1 mL (9.5 mL) [contains benzyl alcohol]; antifactor Xa 25,000 units per 1 mL (3.8 mL) [contains benzyl alcohol]

Injection, solution [preservative free; prefilled syringe]: Antifactor Xa 2500 int. units per 0.2 mL (0.2 mL); antifactor Xa 5000 int. units per 0.2 mL (0.2 mL); antifactor Xa 7500 int. units per 0.3 mL (0.3 mL); antifactor Xa 10,000 int. units per 1 mL (1 mL)

Damason-P® [US] *see* hydrocodone and aspirin *on page 445*

D-Amp® *(Discontinued)* *see page 1042*

danaparoid (da NAP a roid)

Synonyms danaparoid sodium

U.S./Canadian Brand Names Orgaran® [Can]

Therapeutic Category Anticoagulant (Other)

Use Prevention of postoperative deep vein thrombosis following elective hip replacement surgery

Usual Dosage SubQ:

Children: Safety and effectiveness have not been established.

Adults: Prevention of DVT following hip replacement: SubQ: 750 anti-Xa units twice daily; beginning 1-4 hours before surgery and then not sooner than 2 hours after surgery and every 12 hours until the risk of DVT has diminished. The average duration of therapy is 7-10 days.

Dosage Forms Injection, solution, as sodium 750 anti-Xa units/0.6 mL (0.6 mL) [prefilled syringe or ampul; contains sodium sulfite]

danaparoid sodium *see* danaparoid *on this page*

danazol (DA na zole)

Sound-Alike/Look-Alike Issues

danazol may be confused with Dantrium®
Danocrine® may be confused with Dacriose®

U.S./Canadian Brand Names Cyclomen® [Can]; Danocrine® [US/Can]

Therapeutic Category Androgen

Use Treatment of endometriosis, fibrocystic breast disease, and hereditary angioedema

Usual Dosage Adults: Oral:

Female: Endometriosis: Initial: 200-400 mg/day in 2 divided doses for mild disease; individualize dosage. Usual maintenance dose: 800 mg/day in 2 divided doses to achieve amenorrhea and rapid response to painful symptoms. Continue therapy uninterrupted for 3-6 months (up to 9 months).

Female: Fibrocystic breast disease: Range: 100-400 mg/day in 2 divided doses

Male/Female: Hereditary angioedema: Initial: 200 mg 2-3 times/day; after favorable response, decrease the dosage by 50% or less at intervals of 1-3 months or longer if the frequency of attacks dictates. If an attack occurs, increase the dosage by up to 200 mg/day.

Dosage Forms Capsule: 50 mg, 100 mg, 200 mg

Danex® Shampoo *(Discontinued)* *see page 1042*

Danocrine® [US/Can] *see* danazol *on previous page*

Dantrium® [US/Can] *see* dantrolene *on this page*

dantrolene (DAN troe leen)

Sound-Alike/Look-Alike Issues

Dantrium® may be confused with danazol, Daraprim®

Synonyms dantrolene sodium

U.S./Canadian Brand Names Dantrium® [US/Can]

Therapeutic Category Skeletal Muscle Relaxant

Use Treatment of spasticity associated with spinal cord injury, stroke, cerebral palsy, or multiple sclerosis; treatment of malignant hyperthermia

Usual Dosage

Spasticity: Oral:

Children: Initial: 0.5 mg/kg/dose twice daily, increase frequency to 3-4 times/day at 4- to 7-day intervals, then increase dose by 0.5 mg/kg to a maximum of 3 mg/kg/dose 2-4 times/day up to 400 mg/day

Adults: 25 mg/day to start, increase frequency to 2-4 times/day, then increase dose by 25 mg every 4-7 days to a maximum of 100 mg 2-4 times/day or 400 mg/day

Malignant hyperthermia: Children and Adults:

Preoperative prophylaxis:

Oral: 4-8 mg/kg/day in 4 divided doses, begin 1-2 days prior to surgery with last dose 3-4 hours prior to surgery

I.V.: 2.5 mg/kg ~1¼ hours prior to anesthesia and infused over 1 hour with additional doses as needed and individualized

Crisis: I.V.: 2.5 mg/kg; may repeat dose up to cumulative dose of 10 mg/kg; if physiologic and metabolic abnormalities reappear, repeat regimen

Postcrisis follow-up: Oral: 4-8 mg/kg/day in 4 divided doses for 1-3 days; I.V. dantrolene may be used when oral therapy is not practical; individualize dosage beginning with 1 mg/kg or more as the clinical situation dictates

Dosage Forms

Capsule, as sodium: 25 mg, 50 mg, 100 mg

Injection, powder for reconstitution, as sodium: 20 mg [contains mannitol 3 g]

dantrolene sodium *see* dantrolene *on this page*

Dapacin® Cold Capsule *(Discontinued)* *see page 1042*

dapcin *see* daptomycin *on next page*

dapiprazole (DA pi pray zole)

Synonyms dapiprazole hydrochloride

U.S./Canadian Brand Names Rēv-Eyes™ [US]

Therapeutic Category Alpha-Adrenergic Blocking Agent

Use Reverse dilation due to drugs (adrenergic or parasympathomimetic) after eye exams

Usual Dosage Adults: Ophthalmic: Instill 2 drops followed 5 minutes later by an additional 2 drops into the conjunctiva of each eye; should not be used more frequently than once a week in the same patient

Dosage Forms Powder, ophthalmic, as hydrochloride: 25 mg [contains benzalkonium chloride; 0.5% solution when mixed with supplied diluent]

dapiprazole hydrochloride *see* dapiprazole *on this page*

dapsone (DAP sone)

Sound-Alike/Look-Alike Issues

dapsone may be confused with Diprosone®

Synonyms diaminodiphenylsulfone

Therapeutic Category Sulfone

Use Treatment of leprosy and dermatitis herpetiformis (infections caused by *Mycobacterium leprae*)

Usual Dosage Oral:

Leprosy:

Children: 1-2 mg/kg/24 hours, up to a maximum of 100 mg/day

Adults: 50-100 mg/day for 3-10 years

Dermatitis herpetiformis: Adults: Start at 50 mg/day, increase to 300 mg/day, or higher to achieve full control, reduce dosage to minimum level as soon as possible

Dosage Forms Tablet: 25 mg, 100 mg

Daptacel™ [US] *see* diphtheria, tetanus toxoids, and acellular pertussis vaccine *on page 280*

daptomycin (DAP toe mye sin)

Synonyms cidecin; dapcin; LY146032

U.S./Canadian Brand Names Cubicin™ [US]

Therapeutic Category Antibiotic, Cyclic Lipopeptide

Use Treatment of complicated skin and skin structure infections caused by susceptible aerobic Gram-positive organisms

Usual Dosage I.V.: Adults: Skin and soft tissue: 4 mg/kg once daily for 7-14 days

Dosage Forms Injection, powder for reconstitution: 250 mg, 500 mg

Daranide® [US/Can] *see* dichlorphenamide *on page 266*

Daraprim® [US/Can] *see* pyrimethamine *on page 753*

darbepoetin alfa (dar be POE e tin AL fa)

Synonyms erythropoiesis stimulating protein

U.S./Canadian Brand Names Aranesp® [US/Can]

Therapeutic Category Colony-Stimulating Factor; Growth Factor; Recombinant Human Erythropoietin

Use Treatment of anemia associated with chronic renal failure (CRF), including patients on dialysis (ESRD) and patients not on dialysis; anemia associated with chemotherapy for nonmyeloid malignancies

Usual Dosage Adults:

Anemia associated with CRF: I.V., SubQ:

Manufacturer recommended dosing: Initial: 0.45 mcg/kg once weekly; titrate to response; some patients may respond to doses given once every 2 weeks

Dosage Forms

Injection, solution, with human albumin 2.5 mg/mL [preservative free, single-dose vial]: 25 mcg/mL (1 mL); 40 mcg/mL (1 mL); 60 mcg/mL (1 mL); 100 mcg/mL (1 mL); 150 mcg/0.75 mL (0.75 mL); 200 mcg/mL (1 mL); 300 mcg/mL (1 mL)

Injection, solution, with human albumin 2.5 mg/mL [preservative free, prefilled syringe]: 25 mcg/0.42 mL (0.42 mL); 40 mcg/0.4 mL (0.4 mL); 60 mcg/0.3 mL (0.3 mL); 100 mcg/0.5 mL (0.5 mL); 200 mcg/0.4 mL (0.4 mL); 300 mcg/0.6 mL (0.6 mL); 500 mcg/mL (1 mL)

Darbid® Tablet *(Discontinued)* *see page 1042*

Daricon® *(Discontinued)* *see page 1042*

Darvocet A500™ [US] *see* propoxyphene and acetaminophen *on page 740*

Darvocet-N® 50 [US/Can] *see* propoxyphene and acetaminophen *on page 740*

Darvocet-N® 100 [US/Can] *see* propoxyphene and acetaminophen *on page 740*

Darvon® [US] *see* propoxyphene *on page 739*

Darvon® 32 mg Capsule *(Discontinued)* *see page 1042*

Darvon-N® [US/Can] *see* propoxyphene *on page 739*

Darvon-N® Oral Suspension *(Discontinued)* *see page 1042*

Datril® Extra Strength *(Discontinued)* *see page 1042*

daunomycin *see* daunorubicin hydrochloride *on this page*

daunorubicin citrate (liposomal)

(daw noe ROO bi sin SI trate lip po SOE mal)

Sound-Alike/Look-Alike Issues

daunorubicin citrate (liposomal) may be confused with dactinomycin, doxorubicin, daunorubicin

DaunoXome® may be confused with Doxil®

Tall-Man **DAUNO**rubicin citrate (liposomal)

U.S./Canadian Brand Names DaunoXome® [US]

Therapeutic Category Antineoplastic Agent

Use First-line cytotoxic therapy for advanced HIV-associated Kaposi sarcoma

Usual Dosage Refer to individual protocols. Adults: I.V.:

20-40 mg/m^2 every 2 weeks

100 mg/m^2 every 3 weeks

Dosage Forms Injection, solution [preservative free]: 2 mg/mL (25 mL) [contains sucrose 2125 mg/25 mL]

daunorubicin hydrochloride (daw noe ROO bi sin hye droe KLOR ide)

Sound-Alike/Look-Alike Issues

daunorubicin may be confused with dactinomycin, doxorubicin, idarubicin

Synonyms daunomycin; DNR; NSC-82151; rubidomycin hydrochloride

Tall-Man **DAUNO**rubicin hydrochloride

U.S./Canadian Brand Names Cerubidine® [US/Can]

Therapeutic Category Antineoplastic Agent

Use Treatment of acute lymphocytic (ALL) and nonlymphocytic (ANLL) leukemias

Usual Dosage Refer to individual protocols: I.V.:

Children:

ALL combination therapy: Remission induction: 25-45 mg/m^2 on day 1 every week for 4 cycles **or** 30-45 mg/m^2/day for 3 days

AML combination therapy: Induction: I.V. continuous infusion: 30-60 mg/m^2/day on days 1-3 of cycle

Note: In children <2 years or <0.5 m^2, daunorubicin should be based on weight - mg/kg: 1 mg/kg per protocol with frequency dependent on regimen employed

Cumulative dose should not exceed 300 mg/m^2 in children >2 years; maximum cumulative doses for younger children are unknown.

Adults:

Range: 30-60 mg/m^2/day for 3-5 days, repeat dose in 3-4 weeks

AML: Single agent induction: 60 mg/m^2/day for 3 days; repeat every 3-4 weeks

AML: Combination therapy induction: 45 mg/m^2/day for 3 days of the first course of induction therapy; subsequent courses: Every day for 2 days

ALL combination therapy: 45 mg/m^2/day for 3 days

Cumulative dose should not exceed 400-600 mg/m^2

Dosage Forms

Injection, powder for reconstitution: 20 mg, 50 mg

Cerubidine®: 20 mg

Injection, solution: 5 mg/mL (4 mL, 10 mL)

DaunoXome® [US] *see* daunorubicin citrate (liposomal) *on this page*

DAVA *see* vindesine *on page 912*

Dayhist® Allergy [US-OTC] *see* clemastine *on page 209*

Daypro® [US/Can] *see* oxaprozin *on page 652*

Dayto Himbin® *(Discontinued)* *see page 1042*

1-Day™ [US-OTC] *see* tioconazole *on page 865*

DC 240® Softgel® *(Discontinued)* *see page 1042*

deferoxamine (de fer OKS a meen)

Sound-Alike/Look-Alike Issues

deferoxamine may be confused with cefuroxime

Desferal® may be confused with desflurane, DexFerrum®, Disophrol®

Synonyms deferoxamine mesylate

U.S./Canadian Brand Names Desferal® [US/Can]; PMS-Deferoxamine [Can]

Therapeutic Category Antidote

Use Acute iron intoxication when serum iron is >450-500 mcg/dL or when clinical signs of significant iron toxicity exist; chronic iron overload secondary to multiple transfusions; iron overload secondary to congenital anemias; hemochromatosis

Usual Dosage

Children and Adults:

Acute iron toxicity: I.V. route is used when severe toxicity is evidenced by systemic symptoms (coma, shock, metabolic acidosis, or severe gastrointestinal bleeding) or potentially severe intoxications (serum iron level >500 mcg/dL). When severe symptoms are not present, the I.M. route may be preferred; however, the use of deferoxamine in situations where the serum iron concentration is <500 mcg/dL or when severe toxicity is not evident is a subject of some clinical debate.

(Continued)

deferoxamine *(Continued)*

Dose: For the first 1000 mg, infuse at 15 mg/kg/hour (although rates up to 40-50 mg/kg/hour have been given in patients with massive iron intoxication); may be followed by 500 mg every 4 hours for up to 2 doses; subsequent doses of 500 mg have been administered every 4-12 hours Maximum recommended dose: 6 g/day (however, doses as high as 16-37 g have been administered)

Children:

Chronic iron overload: SubQ: 20-40 mg/kg/day over 8-12 hours (via a portable, controlled infusion device)

Adults: Chronic iron overload:

I.M.: 500-1000 mg/day; in addition, 2000 mg should be given with each unit of blood transfused (administer separately from blood)

I.V.: 2 g after each unit of blood infusion at 15 mg/kg/hour

SubQ: 1-2 g every day over 8-24 hours

Dosage Forms Injection, powder for reconstitution, as mesylate: 500 mg, 2 g

deferoxamine mesylate *see* deferoxamine *on previous page*

Deficol® *(Discontinued)* *see page 1042*

Definity® [US/Can] *see* perflutren lipid microspheres *on page 681*

Degest® 2 Ophthalmic *(Discontinued)* *see page 1042*

Dehist® *(Discontinued)* *see page 1042*

Dehistine [US] *see* chlorpheniramine, phenylephrine, and methscopolamine *on page 192*

Dehydral® [Can] *see* methenamine *on page 563*

dehydrobenzperidol *see* droperidol *on page 297*

Deladumone® *(Discontinued)* *see page 1042*

Del Aqua® [US] *see* benzoyl peroxide *on page 109*

Delatest® Injection *(Discontinued)* *see page 1042*

Delatestryl® [US/Can] *see* testosterone *on page 848*

delavirdine (de la VIR deen)

Synonyms U-90152S

U.S./Canadian Brand Names Rescriptor® [US/Can]

Therapeutic Category Antiviral Agent

Use Treatment of HIV-1 infection in combination with at least two additional antiretroviral agents

Usual Dosage Adults: Oral: 400 mg 3 times/day

Dosage Forms Tablet, as mesylate: 100 mg, 200 mg

Delestrogen® [US/Can] *see* estradiol *on page 324*

Delfen® [US-OTC] *see* nonoxynol 9 *on page 626*

Del-Mycin® Topical *(Discontinued)* *see page 1042*

Delsym® [US-OTC] *see* dextromethorphan *on page 261*

delta-9-tetrahydro-cannabinol *see* dronabinol *on page 297*

delta-9 THC *see* dronabinol *on page 297*

Delta-Cortef® *(Discontinued)* *see page 1042*

deltacortisone *see* prednisone *on page 725*

Delta-D® [US] *see* cholecalciferol *on page 196*

deltadehydrocortisone *see* prednisone *on page 725*

deltahydrocortisone *see* prednisolone (systemic) *on page 724*

Deltalin® Capsule *(Discontinued)* *see page 1042*

Deltasone® [US] *see* prednisone *on page 725*

Delta-Tritex® Topical *(Discontinued)* *see page 1042*

Del-Vi-A® *(Discontinued)* *see page 1042*

Demadex® [US] *see* torsemide *on page 872*

Demazin® Syrup *(Discontinued)* *see page 1042*

demeclocycline (dem e kloe SYE kleen)

Synonyms demeclocycline hydrochloride; demethylchlortetracycline

U.S./Canadian Brand Names Declomycin® [US/Can]

Therapeutic Category Tetracycline Derivative

Use Treatment of susceptible bacterial infections (acne, gonorrhea, pertussis and urinary tract infections) caused by both gram-negative and gram-positive organisms

Usual Dosage Oral:

Children ≥8 years: 8-12 mg/kg/day divided every 6-12 hours

Adults: 150 mg 4 times/day or 300 mg twice daily

Dosage Forms Tablet, as hydrochloride: 150 mg, 300 mg

demeclocycline hydrochloride *see* demeclocycline *on this page*

Demerol® [US/Can] *see* meperidine *on page 553*

4-demethoxydaunorubicin *see* idarubicin *on page 464*

demethylchlortetracycline *see* demeclocycline *on this page*

Demser® [US/Can] *see* metyrosine *on page 577*

Demulen® [US] *see* ethinyl estradiol and ethynodiol diacetate *on page 338*

Demulen® 30 [Can] *see* ethinyl estradiol and ethynodiol diacetate *on page 338*

Denavir™ [US] *see* penciclovir *on page 674*

denileukin diftitox (de ne LU kin DIFT e tox)

U.S./Canadian Brand Names ONTAK® [US]

Therapeutic Category Antineoplastic Agent, Miscellaneous

Use Treatment of persistent or recurrent cutaneous T-cell lymphoma whose malignant cells express the CD25 component of the IL-2 receptor

Usual Dosage Adults: I.V.: A treatment cycle consists of 9 or 18 mcg/kg/day for 5 consecutive days administered every 21 days. The optimal duration of therapy has not been determined. Only 2% of patients who failed to demonstrate a response (at least a 25% decrease in tumor burden) prior to the fourth cycle responded to subsequent treatment.

Dosage Forms Injection, solution [frozen]: 150 mcg/mL (2 mL)

Dent's Ear Wax [US-OTC] *see* carbamide peroxide *on page 155*

deoxycoformycin *see* pentostatin *on page 680*

2′-deoxycoformycin *see* pentostatin *on page 680*

Depacon® [US] *see* valproic acid and derivatives *on page 901*

Depakene® [US/Can] *see* valproic acid and derivatives *on page 901*

Depakote® Delayed Release [US] *see* valproic acid and derivatives *on page 901*

Depakote® ER [US] *see* valproic acid and derivatives *on page 901*

Depakote® Sprinkle® [US] *see* valproic acid and derivatives *on page 901*

depAndrogyn® *(Discontinued)* *see page 1042*

depAndro® Injection *(Discontinued)* *see page 1042*

Depen® [US/Can] *see* penicillamine *on page 674*

depGynogen® Injection *(Discontinued)* *see page 1042*

depMedalone® Injection *(Discontinued)* *see page 1042*

DepoCyt™ [US/Can] *see* cytarabine (liposomal) *on page 240*

DepoDur™ [US] *see* morphine sulfate *on page 591*

Depo®-Estradiol [US/Can] *see* estradiol *on page 324*

Depoject® Injection *(Discontinued)* *see page 1042*

Depo-Medrol® [US/Can] *see* methylprednisolone *on page 572*

Deponit® Patch *(Discontinued)* *see page 1042*

Depo-Provera® [US/Can] *see* medroxyprogesterone acetate *on page 548*

Depo-Provera® 100 mg/mL *(Discontinued)* *see page 1042*

Depo-Provera® Contraceptive [US] *see* medroxyprogesterone acetate *on page 548*

Depotest® 100 [Can] *see* testosterone *on page 848*

Depo-Testadiol® *(Discontinued)* *see page 1042*

Depotest® Injection *(Discontinued)* *see page 1042*

Depotestogen® *(Discontinued)* *see page 1042*

Depo®-Testosterone [US] *see* testosterone *on page 848*

deprenyl *see* selegiline *on page 798*

Deprol® *(Discontinued)* *see page 1042*

dequalinium *(Canada only)* (de kwal LI ne um)

Therapeutic Category Antibacterial, Topical; Antifungal Agent, Topical

Use Treatment of mouth and throat infections

Usual Dosage Adults:

Lozenge: One lozenge sucked slowly every 2-3 hours

Oral paint: Apply freely to infected area, every 2-3 hours, or as directed by physician

Dosage Forms

Lozenge, as chloride: 0.25 mg (20s)

Oral paint, as chloride: 0.5% (25 mL)

Dermaflex® Gel *(Discontinued)* *see page 1042*

Dermarest® Dri-Cort [US] *see* hydrocortisone (topical) *on page 451*

Dermasept Antifungal [US-OTC] *see* tolnaftate *on page 870*

Derma-Smoothe/FS® [US/Can] *see* fluocinolone *on page 374*

Dermatop® [US/Can] *see* prednicarbate *on page 723*

Dermatophytin-O *(Discontinued)* *see page 1042*

Dermazene® [US] *see* iodoquinol and hydrocortisone *on page 481*

Dermazin™ [Can] *see* silver sulfadiazine *on page 804*

Dermazole [Can] *see* miconazole *on page 578*

Dermovate® [Can] *see* clobetasol *on page 212*

Dermoxyl® Gel *(Discontinued)* *see page 1042*

Dermtex® HC [US] *see* hydrocortisone (topical) *on page 451*

desacetyl vinblastine amide sulfate *see* vindesine *on page 912*

deserpidine and methyclothiazide *see* methyclothiazide and deserpidine *on page 568*

Desferal® [US/Can] *see* deferoxamine *on page 247*

desflurane (des FLOO rane)

Sound-Alike/Look-Alike Issues

desflurane may be confused with Desferal®

U.S./Canadian Brand Names Suprane® [US/Can]
Therapeutic Category General Anesthetic
Use Maintenance of general anesthesia; not recommended for induction of general anesthesia due to its airway irritant properties and unpleasant odor
Usual Dosage
Children: Maintenance: Surgical levels of anesthesia (MAC) range between 5.2% to 10%
Adults: The minimum alveolar concentration (MAC), the concentration at which 50% of patients do not respond to surgical incision, ranges from 6.0% (45 years of age) to 7.3% (25 years of age). The concentration at which amnesia and loss of awareness occur (MAC - awake) is 2.4%.
Dosage Forms Liquid, for inhalation: 240 mL

desiccated thyroid *see* thyroid *on page 860*

desipramine (des IP ra meen)

Sound-Alike/Look-Alike Issues
desipramine may be confused with clomipramine, deserpidine, diphenhydramine, disopyramide, imipramine, nortriptyline
Norpramin® may be confused with clomipramine, imipramine, Norpace®, nortriptyline, Tenormin®
Synonyms desipramine hydrochloride; desmethylimipramine hydrochloride
U.S./Canadian Brand Names Alti-Desipramine [Can]; Apo-Desipramine® [Can]; Norpramin® [US/Can]; Novo-Desipramine [Can]; Nu-Desipramine [Can]; PMS-Desipramine
Therapeutic Category Antidepressant, Tricyclic (Secondary Amine)
Use Treatment of depression
Usual Dosage Oral (dose is generally administered at bedtime):
Children 6-12 years: Depression: 10-30 mg/day or 1-3 mg/kg/day in divided doses; do not exceed 5 mg/kg/day
Adolescents: Depression: Initial: 25-50 mg/day; gradually increase to 100 mg/day in single or divided doses (maximum: 150 mg/day)
Adults:
Depression: Initial: 75 mg/day in divided doses; increase gradually to 150-200 mg/day in divided or single dose (maximum: 300 mg/day)
Dosage Forms Tablet, as hydrochloride: 10 mg, 25 mg, 50 mg, 75 mg, 100 mg, 150 mg

desipramine hydrochloride *see* desipramine *on this page*

Desitin® Creamy [US-OTC] *see* zinc oxide *on page 940*

Desitin® [US-OTC] *see* zinc oxide *on page 940*

desloratadine (des lor AT a deen)

U.S./Canadian Brand Names Aerius® [Can]; Clarinex® [US]
Therapeutic Category Antihistamine, Nonsedating
Use Relief of nasal and non-nasal symptoms of seasonal allergic rhinitis (SAR) and perennial allergic rhinitis (PAR); treatment of chronic idiopathic urticaria (CIU)
Usual Dosage Oral:
Children:
6-11 months: 1 mg once daily
12 months to 5 years: 1.25 mg once daily
6-11 years: 2.5 mg once daily
Children ≥12 years and Adults: 5 mg once daily
Dosage Forms
Syrup (Clarinex®): 0.5 mg/mL (480 mL) [bubblegum flavor]
Tablet (Clarinex®): 5 mg
Tablet, orally-disintegrating (Clarinex® RediTabs®): 5 mg [contains phenylalanine 1.75 mg/tablet; tutti-frutti flavor]

desmethylimipramine hydrochloride *see* desipramine *on previous page*

desmopressin acetate (des moe PRES in AS e tate)

Synonyms 1-deamino-8-D-arginine vasopressin

U.S./Canadian Brand Names Apo-Desmopressin® [Can]; DDAVP® [US/Can]; Minirin® [Can]; Octostim® [Can]; Stimate™ [US]

Therapeutic Category Vasopressin Analog, Synthetic

Use Treatment of diabetes insipidus; control of bleeding in hemophilia A, and mild-to-moderate classic von Willebrand disease (type I); primary nocturnal enuresis

Usual Dosage

Children:

Diabetes insipidus:

Intranasal (using 100 mcg/mL nasal solution): 3 months to 12 years: Initial: 5 mcg/day (0.05 mL/day) divided 1-2 times/day; range: 5-30 mcg/day (0.05-0.3 mL/day) divided 1-2 times/day; adjust morning and evening doses separately for an adequate diurnal rhythm of water turnover; doses <10 mcg should be administered using the rhinal tube system

Oral: ≥4 years: Initial: 0.05 mg twice daily; total daily dose should be increased or decreased as needed to obtain adequate antidiuresis (range: 0.1-1.2 mg divided 2-3 times/day)

Hemophilia A and von Willebrand disease (type I):

I.V.: >3 months: 0.3 mcg/kg by slow infusion; may repeat dose if needed; begin 30 minutes before procedure

Intranasal: ≥11 months: Refer to adult dosing.

Nocturnal enuresis:

Intranasal (using 100 mcg/mL nasal solution): ≥6 years: Initial: 20 mcg (0.2 mL) at bedtime; range: 10-40 mcg; it is recommended that $1/2$ of the dose be given in each nostril

Oral: 0.2 mg at bedtime; dose may be titrated up to 0.6 mg to achieve desired response. Patients previously on intranasal therapy can begin oral tablets 24 hours after the last intranasal dose.

Children ≥12 years and Adults:

Diabetes insipidus:

I.V., SubQ: 2-4 mcg/day (0.5-1 mL) in 2 divided doses or $1/10$ of the maintenance intranasal dose

Intranasal (using 100 mcg/mL nasal solution): 10-40 mcg/day (0.1-0.4 mL) divided 1-3 times/day; adjust morning and evening doses separately for an adequate diurnal rhythm of water turnover. **Note:** The nasal spray pump can only deliver doses of 10 mcg (0.1 mL) or multiples of 10 mcg (0.1 mL); if doses other than this are needed, the rhinal tube delivery system is preferred.

Oral: Initial: 0.05 mg twice daily; total daily dose should be increased or decreased as needed to obtain adequate antidiuresis (range: 0.1-1.2 mg divided 2-3 times/day)

Hemophilia A and mild to moderate von Willebrand disease (type I):

I.V.: 0.3 mcg/kg by slow infusion, begin 30 minutes before procedure

Intranasal: Using high concentration spray (1.5 mg/mL): <50 kg: 150 mcg (1 spray); >50 kg: 300 mcg (1 spray each nostril); repeat use is determined by the patient's clinical condition and laboratory work; if using preoperatively, administer 2 hours before surgery

Dosage Forms

Injection, solution, as acetate (DDAVP®): 4 mcg/mL (1 mL, 10 mL)

Solution, intranasal, as acetate (DDAVP®): 100 mcg/mL (2.5 mL) [with rhinal tube]

Solution, intranasal spray, as acetate:

DDAVP®: 100 mcg/mL (5 mL) [delivers 10 mcg/spray]

Stimate™: 1.5 mg/mL (2.5 mL) [delivers 150 mcg/spray]

Tablet, as acetate (DDAVP®): 0.1 mg, 0.2 mg

Desocort® [Can] *see* desonide *on next page*

Desogen® [US] *see* ethinyl estradiol and desogestrel *on page 335*

desonide (DES oh nide)

U.S./Canadian Brand Names Desocort® [Can]; DesOwen® [US]; LoKara™ [US]; PMS-Desonide [Can]; Tridesilon® [US]

Therapeutic Category Corticosteroid, Topical

Use Adjunctive therapy for inflammation in acute and chronic corticosteroid responsive dermatosis (low potency corticosteroid)

Usual Dosage Corticosteroid responsive dermatoses: Topical: Apply 2-4 times/day sparingly. Therapy should be discontinued when control is achieved; if no improvement is seen, reassessment of diagnosis may be necessary.

Dosage Forms

Cream, topical: 0.05% (15 g, 60 g)
 DesOwen®: 0.05% (15 g, 60 g, 90 g)
 Tridesilon®: 0.05% (15 g)
Lotion, topical (DesOwen®, LoKara™): 0.05% (60 mL, 120 mL)
Ointment, topical: 0.05% (15 g, 60 g)
 DesOwen®: 0.05% (15 g, 60 g)
 Tridesilon®: 0.05% (15 g)

DesOwen® [US] *see* desonide *on this page*

Desoxi® [Can] *see* desoximetasone *on this page*

desoximetasone (des oks i MET a sone)

Sound-Alike/Look-Alike Issues

desoximetasone may be confused with dexamethasone
Topicort® may be confused with Topic®

U.S./Canadian Brand Names Desoxi® [Can]; Taro-Desoximetasone [Can]; Topicort® [US/Can]; Topicort®-LP [US]

Therapeutic Category Corticosteroid, Topical

Use Relieves inflammation and pruritic symptoms of corticosteroid-responsive dermatosis (intermediate- to high-potency topical corticosteroid)

Usual Dosage Desoximetasone is a potent fluorinated topical corticosteroid. Therapy should be discontinued when control is achieved; if no improvement is seen, reassessment of diagnosis may be necessary.

Cream, gel: Children and Adults: Apply a thin film to affected area twice daily
Ointment: Children ≥10 years and Adults: Apply a thin film to affected area twice daily

Dosage Forms

Cream, topical: 0.25% (15 g, 60 g); 0.05% (15 g, 60 g)
 Topicort®: 0.25% (15 g, 60 g)
 Topicort®-LP: 0.05% (15 g, 60 g)
Gel, topical (Topicort®): 0.05% (15 g, 60 g) [contains alcohol 20%]
Ointment, topical (Topicort®): 0.25% (15 g, 60 g)

desoxyephedrine hydrochloride *see* methamphetamine *on page 562*

Desoxyn® [US/Can] *see* methamphetamine *on page 562*

desoxyphenobarbital *see* primidone *on page 728*

Despec® Liquid *(Discontinued)* *see page 1042*

Desquam-E™ [US] *see* benzoyl peroxide *on page 109*

Desquam-X® [US/Can] *see* benzoyl peroxide *on page 109*

Desquam-X® Wash *(Discontinued)* *see page 1042*

Desyrel® [US/Can] *see* trazodone *on page 877*

Detane® [US-OTC] *see* benzocaine *on page 107*

Detrol® [US/Can] *see* tolterodine *on page 870*

Detrol® LA [US] *see* tolterodine *on page 870*

Detussin® Expectorant *(Discontinued)* *see page 1042*

Dex4 Glucose [US-OTC] *see* glucose (instant) *on page 408*

Dexacen-4® *(Discontinued)* *see page 1042*

Dexacen® LA-8 *(Discontinued)* *see page 1042*

Dexacidin® [US] *see* neomycin, polymyxin B, and dexamethasone *on page 611*

Dexacine™ [US] *see* neomycin, polymyxin B, and dexamethasone *on page 611*

Dexalone® [US-OTC] *see* dextromethorphan *on page 261*

dexamethasone and ciprofloxacin *see* ciprofloxacin and dexamethasone *on page 203*

dexamethasone and neomycin *see* neomycin and dexamethasone *on page 610*

dexamethasone and tobramycin *see* tobramycin and dexamethasone *on page 868*

Dexamethasone Intensol® [US] *see* dexamethasone (systemic) *on this page*

dexamethasone, neomycin, and polymyxin B *see* neomycin, polymyxin B, and dexamethasone *on page 611*

dexamethasone (ophthalmic) (deks a METH a sone op THAL mik)

Sound-Alike/Look-Alike Issues

Maxidex® may be confused with Maxzide®

U.S./Canadian Brand Names Maxidex® [US/Can]

Therapeutic Category Adrenal Corticosteroid

Use Systemically and locally for chronic swelling; allergic, hematologic, neoplastic, and autoimmune diseases; may be used in management of cerebral edema, septic shock, as a diagnostic agent, antiemetic

Usual Dosage Ophthalmic:

Ointment: Apply thin coating into conjunctival sac 3-4 times/day; gradually taper dose to discontinue

Suspension: Instill 2 drops into conjunctival sac every hour during the day and every other hour during the night; gradually reduce dose to every 3-4 hours, then to 3-4 times/day

Dosage Forms

Ointment, ophthalmic, as sodium phosphate: 0.05% (3.5 g)

Solution, ophthalmic, as sodium phosphate: 0.1% (5 mL)

Suspension, ophthalmic (Maxidex®): 0.1% (5 mL, 15 mL)

dexamethasone sodium phosphate *see* dexamethasone (systemic) *on this page*

dexamethasone (systemic) (deks a METH a sone sis TEM ik)

Sound-Alike/Look-Alike Issues

dexamethasone may be confused with desoximetasone

Decadron® may be confused with Percodan®

Synonyms dexamethasone sodium phosphate

U.S./Canadian Brand Names Decadron® [US/Can]; Dexamethasone Intensol® [US]; DexPak® TaperPak® [US]; Diodex® [Can]; PMS-Dexamethasone [Can]

Therapeutic Category Adrenal Corticosteroid

Use Systemically and locally for chronic swelling; allergic, hematologic, neoplastic, and autoimmune diseases; may be used in management of cerebral edema, septic shock, as a diagnostic agent, antiemetic

Usual Dosage

Children:

Antiemetic (prior to chemotherapy): I.V. (should be given as sodium phosphate): 10 $mg/m^2/dose$ (maximum: 20 mg) for first dose then 5 $mg/m^2/dose$ every 6 hours as needed

Anti-inflammatory immunosuppressant: Oral, I.M., I.V. (injections should be given as sodium phosphate): 0.08-0.3 mg/kg/day **or** 2.5-10 mg/m^2/day in divided doses every 6-12 hours

Extubation or airway edema: Oral, I.M., I.V. (injections should be given as sodium phosphate): 0.5-2 mg/kg/day in divided doses every 6 hours beginning 24 hours prior to extubation and continuing for 4-6 doses afterwards

Cerebral edema: I.V. (should be given as sodium phosphate): Loading dose: 1-2 mg/kg/dose as a single dose; maintenance: 1-1.5 mg/kg/day (maximum: 16 mg/day) in divided doses every 4-6 hours for 5 days then taper for 5 days, then discontinue

Bacterial meningitis in infants and children >2 months: I.V. (should be given as sodium phosphate): 0.6 mg/kg/day in 4 divided doses every 6 hours for the first 4 days of antibiotic treatment; start dexamethasone at the time of the first dose of antibiotic

Physiologic replacement: Oral, I.M., I.V.: 0.03-0.15 mg/kg/day **or** 0.6-0.75 mg/m^2/day in divided doses every 6-12 hours

Adults:

Antiemetic:

Prophylaxis: Oral, I.V.: 10-20 mg 15-30 minutes before treatment on each treatment day

Continuous infusion regimen: Oral or I.V.: 10 mg every 12 hours on each treatment day

Mildly emetogenic therapy: Oral, I.M., I.V.: 4 mg every 4-6 hours

Delayed nausea/vomiting: Oral:

8 mg every 12 hours for 2 days; then
4 mg every 12 hours for 2 days **or**
20 mg 1 hour before chemotherapy; then
10 mg 12 hours after chemotherapy; then
8 mg every 12 hours for 4 doses; then
4 mg every 12 hours for 4 doses

Anti-inflammatory:

Oral, I.M., I.V. (injections should be given as sodium phosphate): 0.75-9 mg/day in divided doses every 6-12 hours

I.M. (as acetate): 8-16 mg; may repeat in 1-3 weeks

Intralesional (as acetate): 0.8-1.6 mg

Intra-articular/soft tissue (as acetate): 4-16 mg; may repeat in 1-3 weeks

Intra-articular, intralesional, or soft tissue (as sodium phosphate): 0.4-6 mg/day

Chemotherapy: Oral, I.V.: 40 mg every day for 4 days, repeated every 4 weeks (VAD regimen)

Cerebral edema: I.V. 10 mg stat, 4 mg I.M./I.V. (should be given as sodium phosphate) every 6 hours until response is maximized, then switch to oral regimen, then taper off if appropriate; dosage may be reduced after 24 days and gradually discontinued over 5-7 days

Dexamethasone suppression test (depression indicator) or diagnosis for Cushing's syndrome (unlabeled uses): Oral: 1 mg at 11 PM, draw blood at 8 AM the following day for plasma cortisol determination

Physiological replacement: Oral, I.M., I.V. (should be given as sodium phosphate): 0.03-0.15 mg/kg/day **or** 0.6-0.75 mg/m^2/day in divided doses every 6-12 hours

Treatment of shock:

Addisonian crisis/shock (ie, adrenal insufficiency/responsive to steroid therapy): I.V. (given as sodium phosphate): 4-10 mg as a single dose, which may be repeated if necessary

Unresponsive shock (ie, unresponsive to steroid therapy): I.V. (given as sodium phosphate): 1-6 mg/kg as a single I.V. dose or up to 40 mg initially followed by repeat doses every 2-6 hours while shock persists

Dosage Forms

Elixir, as base: 0.5 mg/5 mL (240 mL) [contains alcohol 5%; raspberry flavor]

Injection, solution, as sodium phosphate: 4 mg/mL (1 mL, 5 mL, 10 mL, 25 mL, 30 mL); 10 mg/mL (1 mL, 10 mL)

Solution, oral: 0.5 mg/5 mL (500 mL) [cherry flavor]

(Continued)

dexamethasone (systemic) *(Continued)*

Solution, oral concentrate (Dexamethasone Intensol®): 1 mg/mL (30 mL) [contains alcohol 30%]

Tablet: 0.25 mg, 0.5 mg, 0.75 mg, 1 mg, 1.5 mg, 2 mg, 4 mg, 6 mg [some 0.5 mg tablets may contain tartrazine]

Decadron®: 0.5 mg, 0.75 mg, 4 mg

DexPak® TaperPak®: 1.5 mg [51 tablets on taper dose card]

Dexatrim® Pre-Meal *(Discontinued)* *see page 1042*

dexbrompheniramine and pseudoephedrine

(deks brom fen EER a meen & soo doe e FED rin)

Synonyms pseudoephedrine and dexbrompheniramine

U.S./Canadian Brand Names Drixoral® [Can]; Drixoral® Cold & Allergy [US-OTC]

Therapeutic Category Antihistamine/Decongestant Combination

Use Relief of symptoms of upper respiratory mucosal congestion in seasonal and perennial nasal allergies, acute rhinitis, rhinosinusitis and eustachian tube blockage

Usual Dosage Children >12 years and Adults: Oral: 1 timed release tablet every 12 hours, may require 1 tablet every 8 hours

Dosage Forms Tablet, sustained action (Drixoral® Cold & Allergy): Dexbrompheniramine maleate 6 mg and pseudoephedrine sulfate 120 mg

Dexchlor® *(Discontinued)* *see page 1042*

dexchlorpheniramine (deks klor fen EER a meen)

Synonyms dexchlorpheniramine maleate

Therapeutic Category Antihistamine

Use Perennial and seasonal allergic rhinitis and other allergic symptoms including urticaria

Usual Dosage Oral:

Children:

2-5 years: 0.5 mg every 4-6 hours (do not use timed release)

6-11 years: 1 mg every 4-6 hours or 4 mg timed release at bedtime

Adults: 2 mg every 4-6 hours or 4-6 mg timed release at bedtime or every 8-10 hours

Dosage Forms

Syrup, as maleate: 2 mg/5 mL (480 mL, 3840 mL) [contains alcohol 6%; orange flavor]

Tablet, sustained action, as maleate: 4 mg, 6 mg

dexchlorpheniramine maleate *see* dexchlorpheniramine *on this page*

dexchlorpheniramine tannate and pseudoephedrine tannate *see* chlorpheniramine and pseudoephedrine *on page 189*

Dexedrine® [US/Can] *see* dextroamphetamine *on page 259*

Dexedrine® Elixir *(Discontinued)* *see page 1042*

Dexferrum® [US] *see* iron dextran complex *on page 485*

Dexiron™ [Can] *see* iron dextran complex *on page 485*

dexmedetomidine (deks MED e toe mi deen)

Sound-Alike/Look-Alike Issues

Precedex™ may be confused with Peridex®

Synonyms dexmedetomidine hydrochloride

U.S./Canadian Brand Names Precedex™ [US/Can]

Therapeutic Category Alpha-Adrenergic Agonist - Central-Acting (Alpha$_2$-Agonists); Sedative

Use Sedation of initially intubated and mechanically ventilated patients during treatment in an intensive care setting; duration of infusion should not exceed 24 hours

Usual Dosage Individualized and titrated to desired clinical effect

Adults: I.V.: Solution must be diluted prior to administration. Initial: Loading infusion of 1 mcg/kg over 10 minutes, followed by a maintenance infusion of 0.2-0.7 mcg/kg/hour; not indicated for infusions lasting >24 hours

Dosage Forms Injection, solution [preservative free]: 100 mcg/mL (2 mL)

dexmedetomidine hydrochloride *see* dexmedetomidine *on previous page*

dexmethylphenidate (dex meth il FEN i date)

Synonyms dexmethylphenidate hydrochloride

U.S./Canadian Brand Names Focalin™ [US]

Therapeutic Category Central Nervous System Stimulant, Nonamphetamine

Controlled Substance C-II

Use Treatment of attention-deficit/hyperactivity disorder (ADHD)

Usual Dosage Oral: Children ≥6 years and Adults: Treatment of ADHD: Initial: 2.5 mg twice daily in patients not currently taking methylphenidate; dosage may be adjusted in 2.5-5 mg increments at weekly intervals (maximum dose: 20 mg/day); doses should be taken at least 4 hours apart

When switching from methylphenidate to dexmethylphenidate, the starting dose of dexmethylphenidate should be half that of methylphenidate (maximum dose: 20 mg/day)

Safety and efficacy for long-term use of dexmethylphenidate have not yet been established. Patients should be reevaluated at appropriate intervals to assess continued need of the medication.

Dose reductions and discontinuation: Reduce dose or discontinue in patients with paradoxical aggravation. Discontinue if no improvement is seen after one month of treatment.

Dosage Forms Tablet, as hydrochloride: 2.5 mg, 5 mg, 10 mg

dexmethylphenidate hydrochloride *see* dexmethylphenidate *on this page*

DexPak® TaperPak® [US] *see* dexamethasone (systemic) *on page 254*

dexpanthenol (deks PAN the nole)

Synonyms pantothenyl alcohol

U.S./Canadian Brand Names Panthoderm® [US-OTC]

Therapeutic Category Gastrointestinal Agent, Stimulant

Use Prophylactic use to minimize paralytic ileus; treatment of postoperative distention; topical to relieve itching and to aid healing of minor dermatoses

Usual Dosage

Children and Adults: Relief of itching and aid in skin healing: Topical: Apply to affected area 1-2 times/day

Adults:

Prevention of postoperative ileus: I.M.: 250-500 mg stat, repeat in 2 hours, followed by doses every 6 hours until danger passes

Paralytic ileus: I.M.: 500 mg stat, repeat in 2 hours, followed by doses every 6 hours, if needed

Dosage Forms

Cream, topical (Panthoderm®): 2% (30 g, 60 g)

Injection, solution: 250 mg/mL (2 mL)

Dex PC [US] *see* chlorpheniramine, phenylephrine, and dextromethorphan *on page 191*

dexrazoxane (deks ray ZOKS ane)

Sound-Alike/Look-Alike Issues

Zinecard® may be confused with Gemzar®

Synonyms ICRF-187

U.S./Canadian Brand Names Zinecard® [US/Can]

Therapeutic Category Cardiovascular Agent, Other

(Continued)

dexrazoxane *(Continued)*

Use Reduction of the incidence and severity of cardiomyopathy associated with doxorubicin administration in women with metastatic breast cancer who have received a cumulative doxorubicin dose of 300 mg/m^2 and who would benefit from continuing therapy with doxorubicin. It is not recommended for use with the initiation of doxorubicin therapy.

Usual Dosage Adults: I.V.: A 10:1 ratio of dexrazoxane:doxorubicin (500 mg/m^2 dexrazoxane: 50 mg/m^2 doxorubicin)

Dosage Forms Injection, powder for reconstitution: 250 mg, 500 mg [10 mg/mL when reconstituted]

dextran (DEKS tran)

Sound-Alike/Look-Alike Issues

dextran may be confused with Dexatrim®, Dexedrine®

Synonyms dextran 40; dextran 70; dextran, high molecular weight; dextran, low molecular weight

U.S./Canadian Brand Names Gentran® [US/Can]; LMD® [US]

Therapeutic Category Plasma Volume Expander

Use Blood volume expander used in treatment of shock or impending shock when blood or blood products are not available; dextran 40 is also used as a priming fluid in cardiopulmonary bypass and for prophylaxis of venous thrombosis and pulmonary embolism in surgical procedures associated with a high risk of thromboembolic complications

Usual Dosage I.V. (requires an infusion pump): Dose and infusion rate are dependent upon the patient's fluid status and must be individualized:

Volume expansion/shock:

Children: Total dose should not exceed 20 mL/kg during first 24 hours

Adults: 500-1000 mL at a rate of 20-40 mL/minute; maximum daily dose: 20 mL/kg for first 24 hours; 10 mL/kg/day thereafter; therapy should not be continued beyond 5 days

Pump prime (Dextran 40): Varies with the volume of the pump oxygenator; generally, the 10% solution is added in a dose of 1-2 g/kg

Prophylaxis of venous thrombosis/pulmonary embolism (Dextran 40): Begin during surgical procedure and give 50-100 g on the day of surgery; an additional 50 g (500 mL) should be administered every 2-3 days during the period of risk (up to 2 weeks postoperatively); usual maximum infusion rate for nonemergency use: 4 mL/minute

Dosage Forms

Infusion [premixed in D_5W; high molecular weight]: 6% Dextran 70 (500 mL)

Infusion [premixed in D_5W; low molecular weight] (Gentran, LMD®): 10% Dextran 40 (500 mL)

Infusion [premixed in $D_{10}W$; high molecular weight]: 32% Dextran 70 (500 mL)

Infusion [premixed in NS; high molecular weight] (Gentran®): 6% Dextran 70 (500 mL)

Infusion [premixed in NS; low molecular weight] (Gentran, LMD®): 10% Dextran (500 mL)

dextran 1 (DEKS tran won)

U.S./Canadian Brand Names Promit® [US]

Therapeutic Category Plasma Volume Expander

Use Prophylaxis of serious anaphylactic reactions to I.V. infusion of dextran

Usual Dosage I.V. (time between dextran 1 and dextran solution should not exceed 15 minutes):

Children: 0.3 mL/kg 1-2 minutes before I.V. infusion of dextran

Adults: 20 mL 1-2 minutes before I.V. infusion of dextran

Dosage Forms Injection, solution: 150 mg/mL (20 mL)

dextran 40 *see* dextran *on this page*

dextran 70 *see* dextran *on previous page*

dextran, high molecular weight *see* dextran *on previous page*

dextran, low molecular weight *see* dextran *on previous page*

dextroamphetamine (deks troe am FET a meen)

Sound-Alike/Look-Alike Issues

Dexedrine® may be confused with Dextran®, Excedrin®

Synonyms dextroamphetamine sulfate

U.S./Canadian Brand Names Dexedrine® [US/Can]; Dextrostat® [US]

Therapeutic Category Amphetamine

Controlled Substance C-II

Use Narcolepsy; attention deficit/hyperactivity disorder (ADHD)

Usual Dosage Oral:

Children:

Narcolepsy: 6-12 years: Initial: 5 mg/day; may increase at 5 mg increments in weekly intervals until side effects appear (maximum dose: 60 mg/day)

ADHD:

3-5 years: Initial: 2.5 mg/day given every morning; increase by 2.5 mg/day in weekly intervals until optimal response is obtained; usual range: 0.1-0.5 mg/kg/dose every morning with maximum of 40 mg/day

≥6 years: 5 mg once or twice daily; increase in increments of 5 mg/day at weekly intervals until optimal response is obtained; usual range: 0.1-0.5 mg/kg/dose every morning (5-20 mg/day) with maximum of 40 mg/day

Children >12 years and Adults:

Narcolepsy: Initial: 10 mg/day, may increase at 10 mg increments in weekly intervals until side effects appear; maximum: 60 mg/day

Dosage Forms

Capsule, sustained release, as sulfate: 5 mg, 10 mg, 15 mg

Dexedrine® Spansule®: 5 mg, 10 mg, 15 mg

Tablet, as sulfate: 5 mg, 10 mg

Dexedrine®: 5 mg [contains tartrazine]

Dextrostat®: 5 mg, 10 mg [contains tartrazine]

dextroamphetamine and amphetamine

(deks troe am FET a meen & am FET a meen)

Sound-Alike/Look-Alike Issues

Adderall® may be confused with Inderal®

Synonyms amphetamine and dextroamphetamine

U.S./Canadian Brand Names Adderall® [US]; Adderall XR™ [US]

Therapeutic Category Amphetamine

Controlled Substance C-II

Use Attention deficit/hyperactivity disorder (ADHD); narcolepsy

Usual Dosage Oral: **Note:** Use lowest effective individualized dose; administer first dose as soon as awake

ADHD:

Children: <3 years: Not recommended

Children: 3-5 years (Adderall®): Initial 2.5 mg/day given every morning; increase daily dose in 2.5 mg increments at weekly intervals until optimal response is obtained (maximum dose: 40 mg/day given in 1-3 divided doses); use intervals of 4-6 hours between additional doses

Children: ≥6 years:

Adderall®: Initial: 5 mg 1-2 times/day; increase daily dose in 5 mg increments at weekly intervals until optimal response is obtained (usual maximum dose: 40 mg/day given in 1-3 divided doses); use intervals of 4-6 hours between additional doses

Adderall XR™: 5-10 mg once daily in the morning; if needed, may increase daily dose in 5-10 mg increments at weekly intervals (maximum dose: 30 mg/day)

(Continued)

dextroamphetamine and amphetamine *(Continued)*

Adults: Adderall XR™: Initial: 20 mg once daily in the morning; higher doses (up to 60 mg once daily) have been evaluated; however, there is not adequate evidence that higher doses afforded additional benefit,

Narcolepsy: Adderall®:

Children: 6-12 years: Initial: 5 mg/day; increase daily dose in 5 mg at weekly intervals until optimal response is obtained (maximum dose: 60 mg/day given in 1-3 divided doses)

Children >12 years and Adults: Initial: 10 mg/day; increase daily dose in 10 mg increments at weekly intervals until optimal response is obtained (maximum dose: 60 mg/day given in 1-3 divided doses)

Dosage Forms

Capsule, extended release (Adderall XR™):

5 mg [dextroamphetamine sulfate 1.25 mg, dextroamphetamine saccharate 1.25 mg, amphetamine aspartate monohydrate 1.25 mg, amphetamine sulfate 1.25 mg] (equivalent to amphetamine base 3.1 mg)

10 mg [dextroamphetamine sulfate 2.5 mg, dextroamphetamine saccharate 2.5 mg, amphetamine aspartate monohydrate 2.5 mg, amphetamine sulfate 2.5 mg] (equivalent to amphetamine base 6.3 mg)

15 mg [dextroamphetamine sulfate 3.75 mg, dextroamphetamine saccharate 3.75 mg, amphetamine aspartate monohydrate 3.75 mg, amphetamine sulfate 3.75 mg] (equivalent to amphetamine base 9.4 mg)

20 mg [dextroamphetamine sulfate 5 mg, dextroamphetamine saccharate 5 mg, amphetamine aspartate monohydrate 5 mg, amphetamine sulfate 5 mg] (equivalent to amphetamine base 12.5 mg)

25 mg [dextroamphetamine sulfate 6.25 mg, dextroamphetamine saccharate 6.25 mg, amphetamine aspartate monohydrate 6.25 mg, amphetamine sulfate 6.25 mg] (equivalent to amphetamine base 15.6 mg)

30 mg [dextroamphetamine sulfate 7.5 mg, dextroamphetamine saccharate 7.5 mg, amphetamine aspartate monohydrate 7.5 mg, amphetamine sulfate 7.5 mg] (equivalent to amphetamine base 18.8 mg)

Tablet (Adderall®):

5 mg [dextroamphetamine sulfate 1.25 mg, dextroamphetamine saccharate 1.25 mg, amphetamine aspartate 1.25 mg, amphetamine sulfate 1.25 mg] (equivalent to amphetamine base 3.13 mg)

7.5 mg [dextroamphetamine 1.875 mg, dextroamphetamine saccharate 1.875 mg, amphetamine aspartate 1.875 mg, amphetamine sulfate 1.875 mg] (equivalent to amphetamine base 4.7 mg)

10 mg [dextroamphetamine sulfate 2.5 mg, dextroamphetamine saccharate 2.5 mg, amphetamine aspartate 2.5 mg, amphetamine sulfate 2.5 mg] (equivalent to amphetamine base 6.3 mg)

12.5 mg [dextroamphetamine sulfate 3.125 mg, dextroamphetamine saccharate 3.125 mg, amphetamine aspartate 3.125 mg, amphetamine sulfate 3.125 mg] (equivalent to amphetamine base 7.8 mg)

15 mg [dextroamphetamine sulfate 3.75 mg, dextroamphetamine saccharate 3.75 mg, amphetamine aspartate 3.75 mg, amphetamine sulfate 3.75 mg] (equivalent to amphetamine base 9.4 mg)

20 mg [dextroamphetamine sulfate 5 mg, dextroamphetamine saccharate 5 mg, amphetamine aspartate 5 mg, amphetamine sulfate 5 mg] (equivalent to amphetamine base 12.6 mg)

30 mg [dextroamphetamine sulfate 7.5 mg, dextroamphetamine saccharate 7.5 mg, amphetamine aspartate 7.5 mg, amphetamine sulfate 7.5 mg] (equivalent to amphetamine base 18.8 mg)

dextroamphetamine sulfate *see* dextroamphetamine *on previous page*

dextromethorphan (deks troe meth OR fan)

Sound-Alike/Look-Alike Issues

Benylin® may be confused with Benadryl®, Ventolin®

Delsym® may be confused with Delfen®, Desyrel®

U.S./Canadian Brand Names Babee® Cof Syrup [US-OTC]; Benylin® Adult [US-OTC]; Benylin® Pediatric [US-OTC]; Creomulsion® Cough [US-OTC]; Creomulsion® for Children [US-OTC]; Creo-Terpin® [US-OTC]; Delsym® [US-OTC]; Dexalone® [US-OTC]; ElixSure™ Cough [US-OTC]; Hold® DM [US-OTC]; PediaCare® Infants' Long-Acting Cough [US-OTC]; Robitussin® CoughGels™ [US-OTC]; Robitussin® Honey Cough [US-OTC]; Robitussin® Maximum Strength Cough [US-OTC]; Robitussin® Pediatric Cough [US-OTC]; Robitussin® Pediatric [US-OTC]; Scot-Tussin DM® Cough Chasers [US-OTC]; Silphen DM® [US-OTC]; Simply Cough® [US-OTC]; Vicks® 44® Cough Relief [US-OTC]

Therapeutic Category Antitussive

Use Symptomatic relief of coughs caused by minor viral upper respiratory tract infections or inhaled irritants; most effective for a chronic nonproductive cough

Usual Dosage Oral:

Children:

<2 years: Use only as directed by a physician

2-6 years (syrup): 2.5-7.5 mg every 4-8 hours; extended release is 15 mg twice daily (maximum: 30 mg/24 hours)

6-12 years: 5-10 mg every 4 hours or 15 mg every 6-8 hours; extended release is 30 mg twice daily (maximum: 60 mg/24 hours)

Children >12 years and Adults: 10-20 mg every 4 hours or 30 mg every 6-8 hours; extended release: 60 mg twice daily; maximum: 120 mg/day

Dosage Forms

Gelcap, as hydrobromide:

Dexalone®: 30 mg

Robitussin® CoughGels™: 15 mg [contains coconut oil]

Liquid, as hydrobromide:

Creo-Terpin®: 10 mg/15 mL (120 mL) [contains alcohol 25% and tartrazine]

Simply Cough®: 5 mg/5 mL (120 mL) [contains sodium benzoate; cherry berry flavor]

Vicks® 44® Cough Relief: 10 mg/5 mL (120 mL) [contains alcohol, sodium 10 mg/5 mL, sodium benzoate]

Liquid, oral drops, as hydrobromide (PediaCare® Infants' Long-Acting Cough): 7.5 mg/0.8 mL (15 mL) [alcohol free, dye free; contains sodium benzoate; grape flavor]

Lozenge, as hydrobromide:

Hold® DM: 5 mg (10s) [cherry or original flavor]

Scot-Tussin DM® Cough Chasers: 5 mg (20s)

Suspension, extended release, as hydrobromide (Delsym®): 30 mg/5 mL (89 mL, 148 mL) [contains alcohol 0.26%, sodium 5 mg/5 mL; orange flavor]

Syrup, as hydrobromide:

Babee® Cof Syrup: 7.5 mg/5 mL (120 mL) [alcohol free, dye free; cherry flavor]

Benylin® Adult: 15 mg/5 mL (120 mL) [alcohol free, sugar free; contains sodium benzoate; raspberry flavor]

Benylin® Pediatric: 7.5 mg/mL (120 mL) [alcohol free, sugar free; contains sodium benzoate; grape flavor]

Creomulsion® Cough: 20 mg/15 mL (120 mL) [alcohol free; contains sodium benzoate]

Creomulsion® for Children: 5 mg/5 mL (120 mL) [alcohol free; contains sodium benzoate; cherry flavor]

ElixSure™ Cough: 7.5 mg/5 mL (120 mL) [cherry bubblegum flavor]

Robitussin® Honey Cough: 10 mg/5 mL (120 mL) [alcohol free; contains sodium benzoate]

Robitussin® Maximum Strength Cough: 15 mg/5 mL (120 mL, 240 mL) [contains alcohol, sodium benzoate]

Robitussin® Pediatric Cough: 7.5 mg/5mL (120 mL) [alcohol free; contains sodium benzoate; fruit punch flavor]

Silphen DM®: 10 mg/5 mL (120 mL) [strawberry flavor]

dextromethorphan, acetaminophen, and pseudoephedrine *see* acetaminophen, dextromethorphan, and pseudoephedrine *on page 12*

dextromethorphan and guaifenesin *see* guaifenesin and dextromethorphan *on page 416*

dextromethorphan and promethazine *see* promethazine and dextromethorphan *on page 736*

dextromethorphan and pseudoephedrine *see* pseudoephedrine and dextromethorphan *on page 746*

dextromethorphan, carbinoxamine, and pseudoephedrine *see* carbinoxamine, pseudoephedrine, and dextromethorphan *on page 159*

dextromethorphan, chlorpheniramine, and phenylephrine *see* chlorpheniramine, phenylephrine, and dextromethorphan *on page 191*

dextromethorphan, guaifenesin, and pseudoephedrine *see* guaifenesin, pseudoephedrine, and dextromethorphan *on page 422*

dextromethorphan, pseudoephedrine, and carbinoxamine *see* carbinoxamine, pseudoephedrine, and dextromethorphan *on page 159*

dextropropoxyphene *see* propoxyphene *on page 739*

dextrose and tetracaine *see* tetracaine and dextrose *on page 851*

dextrose, levulose and phosphoric acid *see* fructose, dextrose, and phosphoric acid *on page 392*

Dextrostat® [US] *see* dextroamphetamine *on page 259*

Dey-Dose® Isoproterenol *(Discontinued)* *see page 1042*

Dey-Dose® Metaproterenol *(Discontinued)* *see page 1042*

Dey-Lute® Isoetharine *(Discontinued)* *see page 1042*

DFMO *see* eflornithine *on page 305*

DHAD *see* mitoxantrone *on page 586*

DHAQ *see* mitoxantrone *on page 586*

DHC® *(Discontinued)* *see page 1042*

DHC Plus® *(Discontinued)* *see page 1042*

DHE *see* dihydroergotamine *on page 271*

D.H.E. 45® [US] *see* dihydroergotamine *on page 271*

DHPG sodium *see* ganciclovir *on page 396*

DHS™ Sal [US-OTC] *see* salicylic acid *on page 789*

DHS™ Targel [US-OTC] *see* coal tar *on page 219*

DHS™ Tar [US-OTC] *see* coal tar *on page 219*

DHS™ Zinc [US-OTC] *see* pyrithione zinc *on page 754*

DHT™ [US] *see* dihydrotachysterol *on page 272*

DHT™ Intensol™ [US] *see* dihydrotachysterol *on page 272*

Diaβeta® [US/Can] *see* glyburide *on page 409*

Diabetic Tussin® Allergy Relief [US-OTC] *see* chlorpheniramine *on page 187*

Diabetic Tussin C® [US] *see* guaifenesin and codeine *on page 416*

Diabetic Tussin® DM Maximum Strength [US-OTC] *see* guaifenesin and dextromethorphan *on page 416*

Diabetic Tussin® DM [US-OTC] *see* guaifenesin and dextromethorphan *on page 416*

Diabetic Tussin® EX [US-OTC] *see* guaifenesin *on page 415*

Diabinese® [US] *see* chlorpropamide *on page 195*

Dialose® Capsule ***(Discontinued)*** *see page 1042*

Dialose® Plus Capsule ***(Discontinued)*** *see page 1042*

Dialose® Tablet ***(Discontinued)*** *see page 1042*

Dialume® ***(Discontinued)*** *see page 1042*

Diamicron® [Can] *see* gliclazide *(Canada only) on page 405*

Diamicron® MR [Can] *see* gliclazide *(Canada only) on page 405*

Diamine T.D.® ***(Discontinued)*** *see page 1042*

diaminocyclohexane oxalatoplatinum *see* oxaliplatin *on page 652*

diaminodiphenylsulfone *see* dapsone *on page 244*

Diamox® [Can] *see* acetazolamide *on page 14*

Diamox® 250 mg Tablet ***(Discontinued)*** *see page 1042*

Diamox® Sequels® [US] *see* acetazolamide *on page 14*

Diane®-35 [Can] *see* cyproterone and ethinyl estradiol *(Canada only) on page 238*

Diaparene® Cradol® ***(Discontinued)*** *see page 1042*

Diapid® Nasal Spray ***(Discontinued)*** *see page 1042*

Diar-aid® ***(Discontinued)*** *see page 1042*

Diarr-Eze [Can] *see* loperamide *on page 528*

Diasorb® ***(Discontinued)*** *see page 1042*

Diastat® [US/Can] *see* diazepam *on this page*

diatrizoate meglumine *see* radiological/contrast media (ionic) *on page 759*

diatrizoate meglumine and diatrizoate sodium *see* radiological/contrast media (ionic) *on page 759*

diatrizoate meglumine and iodipamide meglumine *see* radiological/contrast media (ionic) *on page 759*

diatrizoate sodium *see* radiological/contrast media (ionic) *on page 759*

Diatx™ [US] *see* vitamin B complex combinations *on page 915*

DiatxFe™ [US] *see* vitamin B complex combinations *on page 915*

Diazemuls® [Can] *see* diazepam *on this page*

Diazemuls® Injection ***(Discontinued)*** *see page 1042*

diazepam (dye AZ e pam)

Sound-Alike/Look-Alike Issues
diazepam may be confused with diazoxide, Ditropan®, lorazepam
Valium® may be confused with Valcyte™

U.S./Canadian Brand Names Apo-Diazepam® [Can]; Diastat® [US/Can]; Diazemuls® [Can]; Diazepam Intensol® [US]; Valium® [US/Can]

Therapeutic Category Benzodiazepine

Controlled Substance C-IV

Use Management of anxiety disorders, ethanol withdrawal symptoms; skeletal muscle relaxant; treatment of convulsive disorders

Orphan drug: Viscous solution for rectal administration: Management of selected, refractory epilepsy patients on stable regimens of antiepileptic drugs (AEDs) requiring intermittent use of diazepam to control episodes of increased seizure activity

Usual Dosage Oral absorption is more reliable than I.M.

Children:

Conscious sedation for procedures: Oral: 0.2-0.3 mg/kg (maximum: 10 mg) 45-60 minutes prior to procedure

Sedation/muscle relaxant/anxiety:

Oral: 0.12-0.8 mg/kg/day in divided doses every 6-8 hours

(Continued)

diazepam *(Continued)*

I.M., I.V.: 0.04-0.3 mg/kg/dose every 2-4 hours to a maximum of 0.6 mg/kg within an 8-hour period if needed

Status epilepticus:

Infants 30 days to 5 years: I.V.: 0.05-0.3 mg/kg/dose given over 2-3 minutes, every 15-30 minutes to a maximum total dose of 5 mg; repeat in 2-4 hours as needed **or** 0.2-0.5 mg/dose every 2-5 minutes to a maximum total dose of 5 mg

>5 years: I.V.: 0.05-0.3 mg/kg/dose given over 2-3 minutes every 15-30 minutes to a maximum total dose of 10 mg; repeat in 2-4 hours as needed **or** 1 mg/dose given over 2-3 minutes, every 2-5 minutes to a maximum total dose of 10 mg

Rectal: 0.5 mg/kg, then 0.25 mg/kg in 10 minutes if needed

Anticonvulsant (acute treatment): Rectal gel formulation:

Infants <6 months: Not recommended

Children <2 years: Safety and efficacy have not been studied

Children 2-5 years: 0.5 mg/kg

Children 6-11 years: 0.3 mg/kg

Children ≥12 years and Adults: 0.2 mg/kg

Note: Dosage should be rounded upward to the next available dose, 2.5, 5, 10, 15, and 20 mg/dose; dose may be repeated in 4-12 hours if needed; do not use more than 5 times per month or more than once every 5 days

Adolescents: Conscious sedation for procedures:

Oral: 10 mg

I.V.: 5 mg, may repeat with ½ dose if needed

Adults:

Anxiety/sedation/skeletal muscle relaxant:

Oral: 2-10 mg 2-4 times/day

I.M., I.V.: 2-10 mg, may repeat in 3-4 hours if needed

Sedation in the ICU patient: I.V.: 0.03-0.1 mg/kg every 30 minutes to 6 hours

Status epilepticus: I.V.: 5-10 mg every 10-20 minutes, up to 30 mg in an 8-hour period; may repeat in 2-4 hours if necessary

Rapid tranquilization of agitated patient (administer every 30-60 minutes): Oral: 5-10 mg; average total dose for tranquilization: 20-60 mg

Dosage Forms

Gel, rectal (Diastat®):

Adult rectal tip [6 cm]: 5 mg/mL (15 mg, 20 mg) [contains ethyl alcohol, sodium benzoate, benzyl alcohol; twin pack]

Pediatric rectal tip [4.4 cm]: 5 mg/mL (2.5 mg, 5 mg) [contains ethyl alcohol, sodium benzoate, benzyl alcohol; twin pack]

Universal rectal tip [for pediatric and adult use; 4.4 cm]: 5 mg/mL (10 mg) [contains ethyl alcohol, sodium benzoate, benzyl alcohol; twin pack]

Injection, solution: 5 mg/mL (2 mL, 10 mL) [may contain benzyl alcohol, sodium benzoate, benzoic acid]

Solution, oral: 5 mg/5 mL (5 mL, 500 mL) [wintergreen-spice flavor]

Solution, oral concentrate (Diazepam Intensol®): 5 mg/mL (30 mL)

Tablet (Valium®): 2 mg, 5 mg, 10 mg

Diazepam Intensol® [US] *see* diazepam *on previous page*

diazoxide (dye az OKS ide)

Sound-Alike/Look-Alike Issues

diazoxide may be confused with diazepam, Dyazide®

Hyperstat® may be confused with Nitrostat®

U.S./Canadian Brand Names Hyperstat® [US]; Hyperstat® I.V. [Can]; Proglycem® [US/Can]

Therapeutic Category Antihypertensive Agent; Antihypoglycemic Agent

Use

Oral: Hypoglycemia related to islet cell adenoma, carcinoma, hyperplasia, or adenomatosis, nesidioblastosis, leucine sensitivity, or extrapancreatic malignancy

I.V.: Severe hypertension

Usual Dosage

Hypertension: Children and Adults: I.V.: 1-3 mg/kg up to a maximum of 150 mg in a single injection; repeat dose in 5-15 minutes until blood pressure adequately reduced; repeat administration at intervals of 4-24 hours; monitor the blood pressure closely; do not use longer than 10 days

Hyperinsulinemic hypoglycemia: Oral: **Note:** Use lower dose listed as initial dose

Newborns and Infants: 8-15 mg/kg/day in divided doses every 8-12 hours

Children and Adults: 3-8 mg/kg/day in divided doses every 8-12 hours

Dosage Forms

Capsule (Proglycem®): 50 mg [not available in the U.S.]

Injection, solution (Hyperstat®): 15 mg/mL (20 mL)

Suspension, oral (Proglycem®): 50 mg/mL (30 mL) [contains alcohol 7.25%; chocolate-mint flavor]

Dibent® Injection *(Discontinued)* *see page 1042*

Dibenzyline® [US/Can] *see* phenoxybenzamine *on page 688*

dibucaine (DYE byoo kane)

U.S./Canadian Brand Names Nupercainal® [US-OTC]

Therapeutic Category Local Anesthetic

Use Fast, temporary relief of pain and itching due to hemorrhoids, minor burns

Usual Dosage Children and Adults: Topical: Apply gently to the affected areas; no more than 30 g for adults or 7.5 g for children should be used in any 24-hour period

Dosage Forms Ointment: 1% (30 g, 454 g)

Nupercainal®: 1% (30 g, 60g) [contains sodium bisulfite]

dibucaine and hydrocortisone (DYE byoo kane & hye droe KOR ti sone)

Synonyms hydrocortisone and dibucaine

Therapeutic Category Anesthetic/Corticosteroid

Use Relief of the inflammatory and pruritic manifestations of corticosteroid-responsive dermatoses and for external anal itching

Usual Dosage Topical: Apply to affected areas 2-4 times/day

Dosage Forms Cream: Dibucaine 5% and hydrocortisone 5%

DIC *see* dacarbazine *on page 241*

Dicarbosil® *(Discontinued)* *see page 1042*

Dicetel® [Can] *see* pinaverium *(Canada only) on page 696*

dichloralphenazone, acetaminophen, and isometheptene *see* acetaminophen, isometheptene, and dichloralphenazone *on page 13*

dichloralphenazone, isometheptene, and acetaminophen *see* acetaminophen, isometheptene, and dichloralphenazone *on page 13*

6,7-dichloro-1,5-dihydroimidazo [2,1b] quinazolin-2(3H)-one monohydrochloride *see* anagrelide *on page 58*

dichlorodifluoromethane and trichloromonofluoromethane

(dye klor oh dye flor oh METH ane & tri klor oh mon oh flor oh METH ane)

Synonyms trichloromonofluoromethane and dichlorodifluoromethane

U.S./Canadian Brand Names Fluori-Methane® [US]

Therapeutic Category Analgesic, Topical

Use Management of pain associated with injections

Usual Dosage Invert bottle over treatment area approximately 12" away from site of application; open dispenseal spring valve completely, allowing liquid to flow in a stream from the bottle. The rate of spraying is approximately 10 cm/second and should be continued until entire muscle has been covered.

(Continued)

dichlorodifluoromethane and trichloromonofluoromethane *(Continued)*

Dosage Forms Aerosol, topical: Dichlorodifluoromethane 15% and trichloromonofluoromethane 85% (103 mL) [contains chlorofluorocarbons]

dichlorotetrafluoroethane and ethyl chloride *see* ethyl chloride and dichlorotetrafluoroethane *on page 349*

dichlorphenamide (dye klor FEN a mide)

Sound-Alike/Look-Alike Issues

Daranide® may be confused with Daraprim®

Synonyms diclofenamide

U.S./Canadian Brand Names Daranide® [US/Can]

Therapeutic Category Carbonic Anhydrase Inhibitor

Use Adjunct in treatment of open-angle glaucoma and perioperative treatment for angle-closure glaucoma

Usual Dosage Adults: Oral: 100-200 mg to start followed by 100 mg every 12 hours until desired response is obtained; maintenance dose: 25-50 mg 1-3 times/day

Dosage Forms Tablet: 50 mg

dichysterol *see* dihydrotachysterol *on page 272*

diclofenac (dye KLOE fen ak)

Sound-Alike/Look-Alike Issues

diclofenac may be confused with Diflucan®, Duphalac®

Cataflam® may be confused with Catapres®

Voltaren® may be confused with tramadol, Ultram®, Verelan®

Synonyms diclofenac potassium; diclofenac sodium

U.S./Canadian Brand Names Apo-Diclo® [Can]; Apo-Diclo Rapide® [Can]; Apo-Diclo SR® [Can]; Cataflam® [US/Can]; Diclotec [Can]; Novo-Difenac® [Can]; Novo-Difenac-K [Can]; Novo-Difenac® SR [Can]; Nu-Diclo [Can]; Nu-Diclo-SR [Can]; Pennsaid® [Can]; PMS-Diclofenac [Can]; PMS-Diclofenac SR [Can]; Riva-Diclofenac [Can]; Riva-Diclofenac-K [Can]; Solaraze™ [US]; Voltaren® [US/Can]; Voltaren Ophthalmic® [US]; Voltaren Rapide® [Can]; Voltaren®-XR [US]; Voltare Ophtha® [Can]

Therapeutic Category Analgesic, Nonnarcotic; Nonsteroidal Antiinflammatory Drug (NSAID)

Use

Immediate release: Ankylosing spondylitis; primary dysmenorrhea; acute and chronic treatment of rheumatoid arthritis, osteoarthritis

Delayed-release tablets: Acute and chronic treatment of rheumatoid arthritis, osteoarthritis, ankylosing spondylitis

Extended-release tablets: Chronic treatment of osteoarthritis, rheumatoid arthritis

Ophthalmic solution: Postoperative inflammation following cataract extraction; temporary relief of pain and photophobia in patients undergoing corneal refractive surgery

Topical gel: Actinic keratosis (AK) in conjunction with sun avoidance

Usual Dosage Adults:

Oral:

Analgesia/primary dysmenorrhea: Starting dose: 50 mg 3 times/day; maximum dose: 150 mg/day

Rheumatoid arthritis: 150-200 mg/day in 2-4 divided doses (100 mg/day of sustained release product)

Osteoarthritis: 100-150 mg/day in 2-3 divided doses (100-200 mg/day of sustained release product)

Ankylosing spondylitis: 100-125 mg/day in 4-5 divided doses

Ophthalmic:

Cataract surgery: Instill 1 drop into affected eye 4 times/day beginning 24 hours after cataract surgery and continuing for 2 weeks

Corneal refractive surgery: Instill 1-2 drops into affected eye within the hour prior to surgery, within 15 minutes following surgery, and then continue for 4 times/day, up to 3 days

Topical: Apply gel to lesion area twice daily for 60-90 days

Dosage Forms

Gel, as sodium (Solaraze™): 30 mg/g (50 g)

Solution, ophthalmic, as sodium (Voltaren Ophthalmic®): 0.1% (2.5 mL, 5 mL)

Tablet, as potassium (Cataflam®): 50 mg

Tablet, delayed release, enteric coated, as sodium (Voltaren®): 25 mg, 50 mg, 75 mg

Tablet, extended release, as sodium (Voltaren®-XR): 100 mg

diclofenac and misoprostol (dye KLOE fen ak & mye soe PROST ole)

Synonyms misoprostol and diclofenac

U.S./Canadian Brand Names Arthrotec® [US/Can]

Therapeutic Category Analgesic, Nonnarcotic; Prostaglandin

Use The diclofenac component is indicated for the treatment of osteoarthritis and rheumatoid arthritis; the misoprostol component is indicated for the prophylaxis of NSAID-induced gastric and duodenal ulceration

Usual Dosage Oral: Adults:

Arthrotec® 50:

Osteoarthritis: 1 tablet 2-3 times/day

Rheumatoid arthritis: 1 tablet 3-4 times/day

For both regimens, if not tolerated by patient, the dose may be reduced to 1 tablet twice daily

Arthrotec® 75:

Patients who cannot tolerate full daily Arthrotec® 50 regimens: 1 tablet twice daily

Note: The use of these tablets may not be as effective at preventing GI ulceration

Dosage Forms Tablet: Diclofenac sodium 50 mg and misoprostol 200 mcg; diclofenac sodium 75 mg and misoprostol 200 mcg

diclofenac potassium *see* diclofenac *on previous page*

diclofenac sodium *see* diclofenac *on previous page*

diclofenamide *see* dichlorphenamide *on previous page*

Diclotec [Can] *see* diclofenac *on previous page*

dicloxacillin (dye kloks a SIL in)

Synonyms dicloxacillin sodium

U.S./Canadian Brand Names Dycil® [Can]; Pathocil® [Can]

Therapeutic Category Penicillin

Use Treatment of systemic infections such as pneumonia, skin and soft tissue infections, and osteomyelitis caused by penicillinase-producing staphylococci

Usual Dosage Oral:

Use in newborns not recommended

Children <40 kg: 12.5-25 mg/kg/day divided every 6 hours; doses of 50-100 mg/kg/day in divided doses every 6 hours have been used for therapy of osteomyelitis

Children >40 kg and Adults: 125-250 mg every 6 hours

Dosage Forms Capsule: 250 mg, 500 mg

dicloxacillin sodium *see* dicloxacillin *on this page*

dicumarol (all products) ***(Discontinued)*** *see page 1042*

dicyclomine (dye SYE kloe meen)

Sound-Alike/Look-Alike Issues

dicyclomine may be confused with diphenhydramine, doxycycline, dyclonine

Bentyl® may be confused with Aventyl®, Benadryl®, Bontril®, Cantil®, Proventil®, Trental®

Synonyms dicyclomine hydrochloride; dicycloverine hydrochloride

(Continued)

dicyclomine *(Continued)*

U.S./Canadian Brand Names Bentyl® [US]; Bentylol® [Can]; Formulex® [Can]; Lomine [Can]

Therapeutic Category Anticholinergic Agent

Use Treatment of functional disturbances of GI motility such as irritable bowel syndrome

Usual Dosage

Oral:

Infants >6 months: 5 mg/dose 3-4 times/day

Children: 10 mg/dose 3-4 times/day

Adults: Begin with 80 mg/day in 4 equally divided doses, then increase up to 160 mg/day

I.M. **(should not be used I.V.)**: Adults: 80 mg/day in 4 divided doses (20 mg/dose)

Dosage Forms

Capsule, as hydrochloride: 10 mg

Injection, solution, as hydrochloride: 10 mg/mL (2 mL)

Syrup, as hydrochloride: 10 mg/5 mL (480 mL)

Tablet, as hydrochloride: 20 mg

dicyclomine hydrochloride *see* dicyclomine *on previous page*

dicycloverine hydrochloride *see* dicyclomine *on previous page*

didanosine (dye DAN oh seen)

Sound-Alike/Look-Alike Issues

Videx® may be confused with Lidex®

Synonyms ddI; dideoxyinosine

U.S./Canadian Brand Names Videx® [US/Can]; Videx® EC [US/Can]

Therapeutic Category Antiviral Agent

Use Treatment of HIV infection; always to be used in combination with at least two other antiretroviral agents

Usual Dosage Treatment of HIV infection: Oral (administer on an empty stomach):

Children:

2 weeks to 8 months: 100 mg/m^2 twice daily

>8 months: 120 mg/m^2 twice daily; dosing range: 90-150 mg/m^2 twice daily; patients with CNS disease may require higher dose

Children <1 year should receive 1 tablet per dose and children >1 year should receive 2-4 tablets per dose for adequate buffering and absorption; tablets should be chewed or dispersed

Adolescents and Adults: Dosing based on patient weight:

Note: Preferred dosing frequency is twice daily for didanosine tablets/oral solution

Chewable tablets, powder for oral solution:

<60 kg: 125 mg twice daily or 250 mg once daily

≥60 kg: 200 mg twice daily or 400 mg once daily

Note: Adults should receive 2-4 tablets per dose for adequate buffering and absorption; tablets should be chewed or dispersed

Delayed release capsule (Videx® EC):

<60 kg: 250 mg once daily

≥60 kg; 400 mg once daily

Dosing adjustment with tenofovir (didanosine tablets or delayed release capsules; based on tenofovir product labeling):

<60 kg: 200 mg once daily

≥60 kg: 250 mg once daily

Dosage Forms

Capsule, delayed release (Videx® EC): 125 mg, 200 mg, 250 mg, 400 mg

Powder for oral solution, pediatric (Videx®): 2 g, 4 g [makes 10 mg/mL solution after final mixing]

Tablet, buffered, chewable/dispersible (Videx®): 25 mg, 50 mg, 100 mg, 150 mg, 200 mg [all strengths contain phenylalanine 36.5 mg/tablet; orange flavor]

dideoxycytidine *see* zalcitabine *on page 937*

dideoxyinosine *see* didanosine *on previous page*

Didrex® [US/Can] *see* benzphetamine *on page 111*

Didronel® [US/Can] *see* etidronate disodium *on page 350*

diethylpropion (dye eth il PROE pee on)

Synonyms amfepramone; diethylpropion hydrochloride

U.S./Canadian Brand Names Tenuate® Dospan® [US/Can]; Tenuate® [US/Can]

Therapeutic Category Anorexiant

Controlled Substance C-IV

Use Short-term adjunct in a regimen of weight reduction based on exercise, behavioral modification, and caloric reduction in the management of exogenous obesity for patients with an initial body mass index ≥30 kg/m^2 or ≥27 kg/m^2 in the presence of other risk factors (diabetes, hypertension)

Usual Dosage Adults: Oral:

Tablet: 25 mg 3 times/day before meals or food

Tablet, controlled release: 75 mg at midmorning

Dosage Forms

Tablet, as hydrochloride (Tenuate®): 25 mg

Tablet, controlled release, as hydrochloride (Tenuate® Dospan®): 75 mg

diethylpropion hydrochloride *see* diethylpropion *on this page*

difenoxin and atropine (dye fen OKS in & A troe peen)

Synonyms atropine and difenoxin

U.S./Canadian Brand Names Motofen® [US]

Therapeutic Category Antidiarrheal

Controlled Substance C-IV

Use Treatment of diarrhea

Usual Dosage Adults: Oral: Initial: 2 tablets, then 1 tablet after each loose stool; 1 tablet every 3-4 hours, up to 8 tablets in a 24-hour period; if no improvement after 48 hours, continued administration is not indicated

Dosage Forms Tablet: Difenoxin hydrochloride 1 mg and atropine sulfate 0.025 mg

Differin® [US/Can] *see* adapalene *on page 20*

diflorasone (dye FLOR a sone)

Sound-Alike/Look-Alike Issues

Psorcon® may be confused with Proscar®, ProSom®, Psorion®

Synonyms diflorasone diacetate

U.S./Canadian Brand Names ApexiCon™ [US]; ApexiCon™ E [US]; Florone® [US/Can]; Psorcon® [US/Can]; Psorcon® E™ [US]

Therapeutic Category Corticosteroid, Topical

Use Relieves inflammation and pruritic symptoms of corticosteroid-responsive dermatosis (high to very high potency topical corticosteroid)

Psorcon®: Very high potency topical corticosteroid

Usual Dosage Topical: Apply ointment sparingly 1-3 times/day; apply cream sparingly 2-4 times/day. Therapy should be discontinued when control is achieved; if no improvement is seen, reassessment of diagnosis may be necessary.

Dosage Forms [DSC] = Discontinued product

Cream, as diacetate: 0.05% (15 g, 30 g, 60 g)

ApexiCon™ E, Florone®: 0.05% (30 g, 60 g)

Psorcon® e™: 0.05% (15 g, 30 g, 60 g)

Ointment, as diacetate: 0.05% (15 g, 30 g, 60 g)

ApexiCon™: 0.05% (30 g, 60 g)

Psorcon®: 0.05% (60 g)

Psorcon® e™: 0.05% (15 g, 30 g, 60 g)

diflorasone diacetate *see* diflorasone *on previous page*

Diflucan® [US/Can] *see* fluconazole *on page 371*

diflunisal (dye FLOO ni sal)

Sound-Alike/Look-Alike Issues

Dolobid® may be confused with Slo-Bid®

U.S./Canadian Brand Names Apo-Diflunisal® [Can]; Dolobid® [US]; Novo-Diflunisal [Can]; Nu-Diflunisal [Can]

Therapeutic Category Analgesic, Nonnarcotic; Nonsteroidal Antiinflammatory Drug (NSAID)

Use Management of inflammatory disorders usually including rheumatoid arthritis and osteoarthritis; can be used as an analgesic for treatment of mild to moderate pain

Usual Dosage Adults: Oral:

Osteoarthritis: 500-750 mg/day in divided doses

Pain: Initial: 500-1000 mg followed by 250-500 mg every 8-12 hours; maximum daily dose: 1.5 g

Inflammatory condition: 500-1000 mg/day in 2 divided doses; maximum daily dose: 1.5 g

Dosage Forms Tablet: 250 mg, 500 mg

Digepepsin® ***(Discontinued)*** *see page 1042*

Digibind® [US/Can] *see* digoxin immune Fab *on next page*

DigiFab™ [US] *see* digoxin immune Fab *on next page*

Digitek® [US] *see* digoxin *on this page*

digoxin (di JOKS in)

Sound-Alike/Look-Alike Issues

digoxin may be confused with Desoxyn®, doxepin

Lanoxin® may be confused with Lasix®, Levoxyl®, Levsinex®, Lomotil®, Lonox®, Mefoxin®, Xanax®

U.S./Canadian Brand Names Digitek® [US]; Digoxin CSD [Can]; Lanoxicaps® [US/Can]; Lanoxin® [US/Can]; Novo-Digoxin [Can]

Therapeutic Category Antiarrhythmic Agent, Miscellaneous; Cardiac Glycoside

Use Treatment of congestive heart failure and to slow the ventricular rate in tachyarrhythmias such as atrial fibrillation, atrial flutter, and supraventricular tachycardia (paroxysmal atrial tachycardia); cardiogenic shock

Usual Dosage Adults (based on lean body weight and normal renal function for age. Decrease dose in patients with decreased renal function)

Total digitalizing dose: Administer 1/2 as initial dose, then administer 1/4 of the total digitalizing dose (TDD) in each of 2 subsequent doses at 8- to 12-hour intervals; obtain ECG 6 hours after each dose to assess potential toxicity

Oral: 0.75-1.5 mg

I.M., I.V.: 0.5-1 mg

Daily maintenance dose:

Oral: 0.125-0.5 mg

I.M., I.V.: 0.1-0.4 mg

Dosage Forms

Capsule (Lanoxicaps®): 50 mcg, 100 mcg, 200 mcg [contains ethyl alcohol]

Elixir: 50 mcg/mL (2.5 mL, 5 mL, 60 mL) [contains alcohol 10%; lime flavor]

Lanoxin® (pediatric): 50 mcg/mL (60 mL) [contains alcohol 10%; lime flavor]

Injection: 250 mcg/mL (1 mL, 2 mL) [contains alcohol 10% and propylene glycol 40%]

Lanoxin®: 250 mcg/mL (2 mL) [contains alcohol 10% and propylene glycol 40%]

Injection, pediatric: 100 mcg/mL (1 mL) [contains alcohol 10% and propylene glycol 40%]

Tablet: 125 mcg, 250 mcg, 500 mcg

Digitek®, Lanoxin®: 125 mcg, 250 mcg

Digoxin CSD [Can] *see* digoxin *on previous page*

digoxin immune Fab (di JOKS in i MYUN fab)

Synonyms antidigoxin fab fragments, ovine

U.S./Canadian Brand Names Digibind® [US/Can]; DigiFab™ [US]

Therapeutic Category Antidote

Use Treatment of life-threatening or potentially life-threatening digoxin intoxication, including:

- acute digoxin ingestion (ie, >10 mg in adults or >4 mg in children)
- chronic ingestions leading to steady-state digoxin concentrations >6 ng/mL in adults or >4 ng/mL in children
- manifestations of digoxin toxicity due to overdose (life-threatening ventricular arrhythmias, progressive bradycardia, second- or third-degree heart block not responsive to atropine, serum potassium >5 mEq/L in adults or >6 mEq in children)

Usual Dosage Each vial of Digibind® 38 mg or DigiFab™ 40 mg will bind ~0.5 mg of digoxin or digitoxin.

Estimation of the dose is based on the body burden of digitalis. This may be calculated if the amount ingested is known or the postdistribution serum drug level is known (round dose to the nearest whole vial).

Fab dose based on serum drug level postdistribution:

Digoxin: No. of vials = level (ng/mL) x body weight (kg) divided by 100

Digitoxin: No. of vials = digitoxin (ng/mL) x body weight (kg) divided by 1000

If neither amount ingested nor drug level are known, dose empirically as follows:

For acute toxicity: 20 vials, administered in 2 divided doses to decrease the possibility of a febrile reaction, and to avoid fluid overload in small children.

For chronic toxicity: 6 vials; for infants and small children (≤20kg), a single vial may be sufficient

Dosage Forms Injection, powder for reconstitution:

Digibind®: 38 mg

DigiFab™: 40 mg

dihematoporphyrin ether *see* porfimer *on page 710*

Dihistine® DH [US] *see* chlorpheniramine, pseudoephedrine, and codeine *on page 193*

Dihistine® Expectorant [US] *see* guaifenesin, pseudoephedrine, and codeine *on page 422*

dihydrocodeine, aspirin, and caffeine

(dye hye droe KOE deen, AS pir in, & KAF een)

Sound-Alike/Look-Alike Issues

Synalgos®-DC may be confused with Synagis®

U.S./Canadian Brand Names Synalgos®-DC [US]

Therapeutic Category Analgesic, Narcotic

Controlled Substance C-III

Use Management of mild to moderate pain that requires relaxation

Usual Dosage Adults: Oral: 1-2 capsules every 4-6 hours as needed for pain

Dosage Forms Capsule (Synalgos®-DC): Dihydrocodeine bitartrate 16 mg, aspirin 356.4 mg, and caffeine 30 mg

dihydroergotamine (dye hye droe er GOT a meen)

Synonyms DHE; dihydroergotamine mesylate

U.S./Canadian Brand Names D.H.E. 45® [US]; Migranal® [US/Can]

Therapeutic Category Ergot Alkaloid and Derivative

Use Treatment of migraine headache with or without aura; injection also indicated for treatment of cluster headaches

(Continued)

dihydroergotamine *(Continued)*

Usual Dosage Adults:

I.M., SubQ: 1 mg at first sign of headache; repeat hourly to a maximum dose of 3 mg total; maximum dose: 6 mg/week

I.V.: 1 mg at first sign of headache; repeat hourly up to a maximum dose of 2 mg total; maximum dose: 6 mg/week

Intranasal: 1 spray (0.5 mg) of nasal spray should be administered into each nostril; if needed, repeat after 15 minutes, up to a total of 4 sprays. **Note:** Do not exceed 3 mg (6 sprays) in a 24-hour period and no more than 8 sprays in a week.

Dosage Forms

Injection, solution, as mesylate (D.H.E. 45®): 1 mg/mL (1 mL) [contains ethanol 94%]

Solution, intranasal spray, as mesylate (Migranal®): 4 mg/mL [0.5 mg/spray] (1 mL) [contains caffeine 10 mg/mL]

dihydroergotamine mesylate *see* dihydroergotamine *on previous page*

dihydroergotoxine *see* ergoloid mesylates *on page 318*

dihydrogenated ergot alkaloids *see* ergoloid mesylates *on page 318*

dihydrohydroxycodeinone *see* oxycodone *on page 656*

dihydromorphinone *see* hydromorphone *on page 453*

dihydrotachysterol (dye hye droe tak IS ter ole)

Synonyms dichysterol

U.S./Canadian Brand Names DHT™ [US]; DHT™ Intensol™ [US]; Hytakerol® [US/Can]

Therapeutic Category Vitamin D Analog

Use Treatment of hypocalcemia associated with hypoparathyroidism; prophylaxis of hypocalcemic tetany following thyroid surgery

Usual Dosage Oral:

Hypoparathyroidism:

Infants and young Children: Initial: 1-5 mg/day for 4 days, then 0.1-0.5 mg/day

Older Children and Adults: Initial: 0.8-2.4 mg/day for several days followed by maintenance doses of 0.2-1 mg/day

Nutritional rickets: 0.5 mg as a single dose or 13-50 mcg/day until healing occurs

Renal osteodystrophy: Maintenance: 0.25-0.6 mg/24 hours adjusted as necessary to achieve normal serum calcium levels and promote bone healing

Dosage Forms

Capsule (Hytakerol®): 0.125 mg [contains sesame oil]

Solution, oral concentrate (DHT™ Intensol™): 0.2 mg/mL (30 mL) [contains alcohol 20%]

Tablet (DHT™): 0.125 mg, 0.2 mg, 0.4 mg

dihydroxyanthracenedione dihydrochloride *see* mitoxantrone *on page 586*

1,25 dihydroxycholecalciferol *see* calcitriol *on page 143*

dihydroxydeoxynorvinkaleukoblastine *see* vinorelbine *on page 912*

dihydroxypropyl theophylline *see* dyphylline *on page 301*

Dihyrex® Injection *(Discontinued)* *see page 1042*

diiodohydroxyquin *see* iodoquinol *on page 481*

Dilacor® XR [US] *see* diltiazem *on next page*

Dilantin® [US/Can] *see* phenytoin *on page 691*

Dilantin-30® Pediatric Suspension *(Discontinued)* *see page 1042*

Dilantin® With Phenobarbital *(Discontinued)* *see page 1042*

Dilatrate®-SR [US] *see* isosorbide dinitrate *on page 488*

Dilaudid® [US/Can] *see* hydromorphone *on page 453*

Dilaudid® 1 mg & 3 mg Tablet *(Discontinued)* *see page 1042*

Dilaudid® Cough Syrup *(Discontinued)* *see page 1042*

Dilaudid-HP® [US/Can] *see* hydromorphone *on page 453*

Dilaudid-HP-Plus® [Can] *see* hydromorphone *on page 453*

Dilaudid® Sterile Powder [Can] *see* hydromorphone *on page 453*

Dilaudid-XP® [Can] *see* hydromorphone *on page 453*

Dilocaine® Injection *(Discontinued)* *see page 1042*

Dilomine® Injection *(Discontinued)* *see page 1042*

Dilor® [US/Can] *see* dyphylline *on page 301*

Diltia XT® [US] *see* diltiazem *on this page*

diltiazem (dil TYE a zem)

Sound-Alike/Look-Alike Issues

diltiazem may be confused with Dilantin®

Cardizem® may be confused with Cardene®, Cardene SR®, Cardizem CD®, Cardizem SR®, cardiem

Cartia XT™ may be confused with Procardia XL®

Tiazac® may be confused with Tigan®, Ziac®

Synonyms diltiazem hydrochloride

U.S./Canadian Brand Names Alti-Diltiazem CD [Can]; Apo-Diltiaz® [Can]; Apo-Diltiaz CD® [Can]; Apo-Diltiaz SR® [Can]; Cardizem® [US/Can]; Cardizem® CD [US/Can]; Cardizem® LA [US]; Cardizem® SR [Can]; Cartia XT™ [US]; Dilacor® XR [US]; Diltia XT® [US]; Gen-Diltiazem [Can]; Gen-Diltiazem SR [Can]; Med-Diltiazem [Can]; Novo-Diltazem [Can]; Novo-Diltazem SR [Can]; Novo-Diltiazem-CD [Can]; Nu-Diltiaz [Can]; Nu-Diltiaz-CD [Can]; ratio-Diltiazem CD [Can]; Rhoxal-diltiazem CD [Can]; Rhoxal-diltiazem SR [Can]; Syn-Diltiazem® [Can]; Taztia XT™ [US]; Tiazac® [US/Can]

Therapeutic Category Calcium Channel Blocker

Use

Oral: Essential hypertension; chronic stable angina or angina from coronary artery spasm

Injection: Atrial fibrillation or atrial flutter; paroxysmal supraventricular tachycardia (PSVT)

Usual Dosage Adults:

Oral:

Angina:

Capsule, extended release (Cardizem® CD, Cartia XT™, Dilacor XR®, Diltia XT™, Tiazac®): Initial: 120-180 mg once daily (maximum dose: 480 mg/day)

Tablet, extended release (Cardizem® LA): 180 mg once daily; may increase at 7- to 14-day intervals (maximum recommended dose: 360 mg/day)

Tablet, immediate release (Cardizem®): Usual starting dose: 30 mg 4 times/day; usual range: 180-360 mg/day

Hypertension:

Capsule, extended release (Cardizem® CD, Cartia XT™, Dilacor XR®, Diltia XT™, Tiazac®): Initial: 180-240 mg once daily; dose adjustment may be made after 14 days; usual dose range (JNC 7): 180-420 mg/day; Tiazac®: usual dose range: 120-540 mg/day

Capsule, sustained release (Cardizem® SR): Initial: 60-120 mg twice daily; dose adjustment may be made after 14 days; usual range: 240-360 mg/day

Tablet, extended release (Cardizem® LA): Initial: 180-240 mg once daily; dose adjustment may be made after 14 days; usual dose range (JNC 7): 120-540 mg/day

I.V.: Atrial fibrillation, atrial flutter, PSVT:

Initial bolus dose: 0.25 mg/kg actual body weight over 2 minutes (average adult dose: 20 mg)

Repeat bolus dose (may be administered after 15 minutes if the response is inadequate.): 0.35 mg/kg actual body weight over 2 minutes (average adult dose: 25 mg)

Continuous infusion (requires an infusion pump; infusions >24 hours or infusion rates >15 mg/hour are not recommended.): Initial infusion rate of 10 mg/hour; rate may be

(Continued)

diltiazem *(Continued)*

increased in 5 mg/hour increments up to 15 mg/hour as needed; some patients may respond to an initial rate of 5 mg/hour.

If diltiazem injection is administered by continuous infusion for >24 hours, the possibility of decreased diltiazem clearance, prolonged elimination half-life, and increased diltiazem and/or diltiazem metabolite plasma concentrations should be considered.

Conversion from I.V. diltiazem to oral diltiazem: Start oral approximately 3 hours after bolus dose.

Oral dose (mg/day) is approximately equal to [rate (mg/hour) x 3 + 3] x 10.

3 mg/hour = 120 mg/day
5 mg/hour = 180 mg/day
7 mg/hour = 240 mg/day
11 mg/hour = 360 mg/day

Dosage Forms [DSC] = Discontinued product

Capsule, extended release, as hydrochloride [once-daily dosing]: 120 mg, 180 mg, 240 mg, 300 mg

Cardizem® CD: 120 mg, 180 mg, 240 mg, 300 mg, 360 mg
Cartia XT™: 120 mg, 180 mg, 240 mg, 300 mg
Dilacor® XR, Diltia XT®: 120 mg, 180 mg, 240 mg
Taztia XT™: 120 mg, 180 mg, 240 mg, 300 mg, 360 mg
Tiazac®: 120 mg, 180 mg, 240 mg, 300 mg, 360 mg, 420 mg

Capsule, sustained release, as hydrochloride [twice-daily dosing] (Cardizem® SR [DSC]): 60 mg, 90 mg, 120 mg

Injection, powder for reconstitution, as hydrochloride (Cardizem®): 25 mg

Injection, solution, as hydrochloride: 5 mg/mL (5 mL, 10 mL, 25 mL)

Tablet, as hydrochloride (Cardizem®): 30 mg, 60 mg, 90 mg, 120 mg

Tablet, extended release, as hydrochloride (Cardizem® LA): 120 mg, 180 mg, 240 mg, 300 mg, 360 mg, 420 mg

diltiazem hydrochloride *see* diltiazem *on previous page*

Dilusol® [Can] *see* alcohol (ethyl) *on page 27*

Dimaphen® Elixir *(Discontinued)* *see page 1042*

Dimaphen® Tablets *(Discontinued)* *see page 1042*

dimenhydrinate (dye men HYE dri nate)

Sound-Alike/Look-Alike Issues

dimenhydrinate may be confused with diphenhydramine

Tall-Man dimenhy**DRINATE**

U.S./Canadian Brand Names Apo-Dimenhydrinate® [Can]; Dramamine® [US-OTC]; Gravol® [Can]; Novo-Dimenate [Can]; TripTone® [US-OTC]

Therapeutic Category Antihistamine

Use Treatment and prevention of nausea, vertigo, and vomiting associated with motion sickness

Usual Dosage Oral:

Children:

2-5 years: 12.5-25 mg every 6-8 hours, maximum: 75 mg/day
6-12 years: 25-50 mg every 6-8 hours, maximum: 150 mg/day

Adults: 50-100 mg every 4-6 hours, not to exceed 400 mg/day

Dosage Forms

Caplet (TripTone®): 50 mg

Tablet (Dramamine®): 50 mg

Tablet, chewable (Dramamine®): 50 mg [contains phenylalanine 1.5 mg/tablet and tartrazine; orange flavor]

dimercaprol (dye mer KAP role)

Synonyms BAL; British anti-lewisite; dithioglycerol

U.S./Canadian Brand Names BAL in Oil® [US]

Therapeutic Category Chelating Agent

Use Antidote to gold, arsenic (except arsine), and mercury poisoning (except nonalkyl mercury); adjunct to edetate calcium disodium in lead poisoning; possibly effective for antimony, bismuth, chromium, copper, nickel, tungsten, or zinc

Usual Dosage Children and Adults: Deep I.M.:

Arsenic, mercury, and gold poisoning: 3 mg/kg every 4-6 hours for 2 days, then every 12 hours for 7-10 days or until recovery (initial dose may be up to 5 mg if severe poisoning)

Lead poisoning (in conjunction with calcium EDTA): For symptomatic acute encephalopathy or blood level >100 mcg/dL: 4-5 mg/kg every 4 hours for 3-5 days

Dosage Forms Injection, oil: 100 mg/mL (3 mL) [contains benzyl benzoate and peanut oil]

Dimetabs® Oral ***(Discontinued)*** *see page 1042*

Dimetane® ***(Discontinued)*** *see page 1042*

Dimetane®-DC ***(Discontinued)*** *see page 1042*

Dimetane® Decongestant Elixir ***(Discontinued)*** *see page 1042*

Dimetapp® 4-Hour Liqui-Gel Capsule ***(Discontinued)*** *see page 1042*

Dimetapp® 12-Hour Non-Drowsy Extentabs® [US-OTC] *see* pseudoephedrine *on page 745*

Dimetapp® Children's ND [US-OTC] *see* loratadine *on page 530*

Dimetapp® Cold and Congestion [US-OTC] *see* guaifenesin, pseudoephedrine, and dextromethorphan *on page 422*

Dimetapp® Decongestant [US-OTC] *see* pseudoephedrine *on page 745*

Dimetapp® Elixir ***(Discontinued)*** *see page 1042*

Dimetapp® Extentabs® ***(Discontinued)*** *see page 1042*

Dimetapp® Sinus Caplets ***(Discontinued)*** *see page 1042*

Dimetapp® Tablet ***(Discontinued)*** *see page 1042*

β,β-dimethylcysteine *see* penicillamine *on page 674*

dimethyl sulfoxide (dye meth il sul FOKS ide)

Synonyms DMSO

U.S./Canadian Brand Names Kemsol® [Can]; Rimso®-50 [US/Can]

Therapeutic Category Urinary Tract Product

Use Symptomatic relief of interstitial cystitis

Usual Dosage Instill 50 mL directly into bladder and allow to remain for 15 minutes; repeat every 2 weeks until maximum symptomatic relief is obtained

Dosage Forms Solution, intravesical: 50% [500 mg/mL] (50 mL)

dimethyl triazeno imidazol carboxamide *see* dacarbazine *on page 241*

Dinate® Injection ***(Discontinued)*** *see page 1042*

dinoprostone (dye noe PROST one)

Sound-Alike/Look-Alike Issues

Prepidil® may be confused with Bepridil®

Synonyms PGE_2; prostaglandin E_2

U.S./Canadian Brand Names Cervidil® [US/Can]; Prepidil® [US/Can]; Prostin E_2® [US/Can]

Therapeutic Category Prostaglandin

(Continued)

dinoprostone *(Continued)*

Use

Gel: Promote cervical ripening prior to labor induction; usage for gel include any patient undergoing induction of labor with an unripe cervix, most commonly for preeclampsia, eclampsia, postdates, diabetes, intrauterine growth retardation, and chronic hypertension

Suppositories: Terminate pregnancy from 12th through 28th week of gestation; evacuate uterus in cases of missed abortion or intrauterine fetal death; manage benign hydatidiform mole

Vaginal insert: Initiation and/or cervical ripening in patients at or near term in whom there is a medical or obstetrical indication for the induction of labor

Usual Dosage

Abortifacient: Insert 1 suppository high in vagina, repeat at 3- to 5-hour intervals until abortion occurs up to 240 mg (maximum dose); continued administration for longer than 2 days is not advisable

Cervical ripening:

- Gel:
  - Intracervical: 0.25-1 mg
  - Intravaginal: 2.5 mg
- Suppositories: Intracervical: 2-3 mg
- Vaginal Insert (Cervidil®): 10 mg (to be removed at the onset of active labor or after 12 hours)

Dosage Forms

Gel, endocervical (Prepidil®): 0.5 mg/3 g syringe [each package contains a 10 mm and 20 mm shielded catheter]

Insert, vaginal (Cervidil®): 10 mg [releases 0.3 mg/hour]

Suppository, vaginal (Prostin E_2®): 20 mg

Diocaine® [Can] *see* proparacaine *on page 738*

Diocarpine [Can] *see* pilocarpine *on page 694*

Diochloram® [Can] *see* chloramphenicol *on page 182*

Diocto C® *(Discontinued)* *see page 1042*

Diocto-K® *(Discontinued)* *see page 1042*

Diocto-K Plus® *(Discontinued)* *see page 1042*

Dioctolose Plus® *(Discontinued)* *see page 1042*

Diocto® [US-OTC] *see* docusate *on page 285*

dioctyl calcium sulfosuccinate *see* docusate *on page 285*

dioctyl sodium sulfosuccinate *see* docusate *on page 285*

Diodex® [Can] *see* dexamethasone (systemic) *on page 254*

Diodoquin® [Can] *see* iodoquinol *on page 481*

Diofluor™ [Can] *see* fluorescein sodium *on page 375*

Diogent® [Can] *see* gentamicin *on page 403*

Diomycin® [Can] *see* erythromycin *on page 320*

Dionephrine® [Can] *see* phenylephrine *on page 689*

Dionosil Oily® [US] *see* radiological/contrast media (ionic) *on page 759*

Diopentolate® [Can] *see* cyclopentolate *on page 234*

Diopred® [Can] *see* prednisolone (ophthalmic) *on page 723*

Dioptic's Atropine Solution [Can] *see* atropine *on page 88*

Dioptimyd® [Can] *see* sulfacetamide and prednisolone *on page 829*

Dioptrol® [Can] *see* neomycin, polymyxin B, and dexamethasone *on page 611*

Diosulf™ [Can] *see* sulfacetamide *on page 829*

Diotame® [US-OTC] *see* bismuth *on page 120*

Diotrope® [Can] *see* tropicamide *on page 892*

Dioval® Injection *(Discontinued)* *see page 1042*

Diovan® [US/Can] *see* valsartan *on page 902*

Diovan HCT® [US/Can] *see* valsartan and hydrochlorothiazide *on page 903*

Diovol® [Can] *see* aluminum hydroxide and magnesium hydroxide *on page 40*

Diovol® Ex [Can] *see* aluminum hydroxide and magnesium hydroxide *on page 40*

Diovol Plus® [Can] *see* aluminum hydroxide, magnesium hydroxide, and simethicone *on page 40*

Dipentum® [US/Can] *see* olsalazine *on page 643*

Diphenacen 50® Injection *(Discontinued)* *see page 1042*

Diphen® AF [US-OTC] *see* diphenhydramine *on this page*

Diphenatol® *(Discontinued)* *see page 1042*

Diphen® Cough [US-OTC] *see* diphenhydramine *on this page*

Diphenhist [US-OTC] *see* diphenhydramine *on this page*

diphenhydramine (dye fen HYE dra meen)

Sound-Alike/Look-Alike Issues

diphenhydramine may be confused with desipramine, dicyclomine, dimenhydrinate

Benadryl® may be confused with benazepril, Bentyl®, Benylin®, Caladryl®

Synonyms diphenhydramine hydrochloride

Tall-Man diphenhydr**AMINE**

U.S./Canadian Brand Names Aler-Dryl [US-OTC]; Allerdryl® [Can]; AllerMax® [US-OTC]; Allernix [Can]; Banophen® [US-OTC]; Benadryl® Allergy [US-OTC/Can]; Benadryl® Dye-Free Allergy [US-OTC]; Benadryl® Gel Extra Strength [US-OTC]; Benadryl® Gel [US-OTC]; Benadryl® Injection [US]; Compoz® Nighttime Sleep Aid [US-OTC]; Diphen® AF [US-OTC]; Diphen® Cough [US-OTC]; Diphenhist [US-OTC]; Diphen® [US-OTC]; Genahist® [US-OTC]; Hydramine® Cough [US-OTC]; Hydramine® [US-OTC]; Hyrexin-50® [US]; Nytol® Extra Strength [Can]; Nytol® Maximum Strength [US-OTC]; Nytol® [US-OTC/Can]; PMS-Diphenhydramine [Can]; Siladryl® Allergy [US-OTC]; Silphen® [US-OTC]; Simply Sleep® [Can]; Sleepinal® [US-OTC]; Sominex® Maximum Strength [US-OTC]; Sominex® [US-OTC]; Tusstat® [US]; Twilite® [US-OTC]; Unisom® Maximum Strength SleepGels® [US-OTC]

Therapeutic Category Antihistamine

Use Symptomatic relief of allergic symptoms caused by histamine release which include nasal allergies and allergic dermatosis; can be used for mild nighttime sedation; prevention of motion sickness and as an antitussive; has antinauseant and topical anesthetic properties; treatment of antipsychotic-induced extrapyramidal symptoms

Usual Dosage

Children:

Oral, I.M., I.V.:

Treatment of moderate to severe allergic reactions: 5 mg/kg/day or 150 mg/m^2/day in divided doses every 6-8 hours, not to exceed 300 mg/day

Minor allergic rhinitis or motion sickness: 2 to <6 years: 6.25 mg every 4-6 hours; maximum: 37.5 mg/day 6 to <12 years: 12.5-25 mg every 4-6 hours; maximum: 150 mg/day ≥12 years: 25-50 mg every 4-6 hours; maximum: 300 mg/day

Night-time sleep aid: 30 minutes before bedtime: 2 to <12 years: 1 mg/kg/dose; maximum: 50 mg/dose ≥12 years: 50 mg

Oral: Antitussive: 2 to <6 years: 6.25 mg every 4 hours; maximum 37.5 mg/day 6 to <12 years: 12.5 mg every 4 hours; maximum 75 mg/day ≥12 years: 25 mg every 4 hours; maximum 150 mg/day

I.M., I.V.: Treatment of dystonic reactions: 0.5-1 mg/kg/dose

(Continued)

diphenhydramine *(Continued)*

Adults:

Oral: 25-50 mg every 6-8 hours

Minor allergic rhinitis or motion sickness: 25-50 mg every 4-6 hours; maximum: 300 mg/day

Moderate to severe allergic reactions: 25-50 mg every 4 hours, not to exceed 400 mg/day

Nighttime sleep aid: 50 mg at bedtime

I.M., I.V.: 10-50 mg in a single dose every 2-4 hours, not to exceed 400 mg/day

Dystonic reaction: 50 mg in a single dose; may repeat in 20-30 minutes if necessary

Topical: For external application, not longer than 7 days

Dosage Forms

Capsule, as hydrochloride: 25 mg, 50 mg

Banophen®, Diphen®, Diphenhist®, Genahist®: 25 mg

Nytol® Maximum Strength, Sleepinal®: 50 mg

Elixir, as hydrochloride: 12.5 mg/5 mL (5 mL, 10 mL, 20 mL, 120 mL, 480 mL, 3780 mL)

Banophen®: 12.5 mg/5 mL (120 mL, 480 mL, 3840 mL)

Diphen AF: 12.5 mg/5 mL (120 mL, 240 mL, 480 mL, 3840 mL) [alcohol free; cherry flavor]

Genahist®: 12.5 mg/5 mL (120 mL)

Hydramine®: 12.5 mg/5 mL (120 mL) [alcohol free; cherry flavor]

Gel, topical, as hydrochloride:

Benadryl®: 1% (120 mL)

Benadryl® Extra Strength: 2% (120 mL)

Injection, solution, as hydrochloride: 10 mg/mL (30 mL); 50 mg/mL (1 mL, 10 mL)

Benadryl®: 50 mg/mL (1 mL, 10 mL)

Hyrexin®: 50 mg/mL (10 mL)

Liquid, as hydrochloride:

Benadryl® Allergy: 12.5 mg/5 mL (120 mL, 240 mL) [alcohol free; cherry flavor]

Benadryl® Dye-Free Allergy: 12.5 mg/5 mL (120 mL) [alcohol free, dye free, sugar free; bubblegum flavor]

Softgel, as hydrochloride:

Benadryl® Dye-Free Allergy: 25 mg [dye-free]

Unisom® Maximum Strength SleepGels®: 50 mg

Solution, oral, as hydrochloride:

AllerMax®: 12.5 mg/5 mL (120 mL)

Diphenhist®: 12.5 mg/5 mL (120 mL, 480 mL)

Solution, topical, as hydrochloride [spray]: 1% (60 mL); 2% (60 mL)

Syrup, as hydrochloride: 12.5 mg/5 mL (120 mL, 240 mL, 480 mL)

Diphen® Cough: 12.5 mg/5 mL (120 mL, 240 mL, 480 mL) [contains alcohol 5.1%; raspberry flavor]

Diphenhist®: 12.5 mg/5 mL (120 mL)

Hydramine® Cough: 12.5 mg/5 mL (120 mL, 480 mL) [contains alcohol 5%; fruit flavor]

Siladryl® Allergy, Silphen® Cough: 12.5 mg/5 mL (120 mL, 240 mL, 480 mL)

Tusstat®: 12.5 mg/5 mL (120 mL, 240 mL, 3840 mL)

Tablet, as hydrochloride: 25 mg, 50 mg

Aler-Dryl, AllerMax®, Compoz® Nighttime Sleep Aid, Sominex® Maximum Strength, Twilite®: 50 mg

Banophen®, Benadryl® Allergy, Diphenhist®, Genahist®, Nytol®, Sominex®: 25 mg

Tablet, chewable, as hydrochloride (Benadryl® Allergy): 12.5 mg [contains phenylalanine 4.2 mg/tablet; grape flavor]

diphenhydramine and acetaminophen *see* acetaminophen and diphenhydramine *on page 7*

diphenhydramine and pseudoephedrine

(dye fen HYE dra meen & soo doe e FED rin)

Synonyms pseudoephedrine and diphenhydramine

U.S./Canadian Brand Names Benadryl® Allergy and Sinus Fastmelt™ [US-OTC]; Benadryl® Allergy/Sinus [US-OTC]; Benadryl® Children's Allergy and Cold Fastmelt™ [US-OTC]; Benadryl® Children's Allergy and Sinus [US-OTC]

Therapeutic Category Antihistamine/Decongestant Combination

Use Relief of symptoms of upper respiratory mucosal congestion in seasonal and perennial nasal allergies, acute rhinitis, rhinosinusitis, and eustachian tube blockage

Usual Dosage Based on **pseudoephedrine** component:

Adults: Oral: 60 mg every 4-6 hours, maximum: 240 mg/day

Dosage Forms

Liquid (Benadryl® Children's Allergy and Sinus): Diphenhydramine hydrochloride 12.5 mg and pseudoephedrine hydrochloride 30 mg per 5 mL [contains sodium benzoate; alcohol free, sugar free; grape flavor]

Tablet: Benadryl® Allergy/Sinus: Diphenhydramine hydrochloride 25 mg and pseudoephedrine hydrochloride 60 mg

Tablet, quick-dissolving: Benadryl® Children's Allergy and Cold Fastmelt™, Benadryl® Allergy and Sinus Fastmelt™: Diphenhydramine citrate 19 mg [equivalent to diphenhydramine hydrochloride 12.5 mg] and pseudoephedrine 30 mg [contains phenylalanine 4.6 mg/tablet; cherry flavor]

diphenhydramine hydrochloride *see* diphenhydramine *on page 277*

diphenoxylate and atropine (dye fen OKS i late & A troe peen)

Sound-Alike/Look-Alike Issues

Lomotil® may be confused with Lamictal®, Lamisil®, lamotrigine, Lanoxin®, Lasix®, Ludiomil®

Lonox® may be confused with Lanoxin®, Loprox®

Synonyms atropine and diphenoxylate

U.S./Canadian Brand Names Lomotil® [US/Can]; Lonox® [US]

Therapeutic Category Antidiarrheal

Controlled Substance C-V

Use Treatment of diarrhea

Usual Dosage Oral:

Children (use with caution in young children due to variable responses): Liquid: 0.3-0.4 mg of diphenoxylate/kg/day in 2-4 divided doses **or**

<2 years: Not recommended

2-5 years: 2 mg of diphenoxylate 3 times/day

5-8 years: 2 mg of diphenoxylate 4 times/day

8-12 years: 2 mg of diphenoxylate 5 times/day

Adults: 15-20 mg/day of diphenoxylate in 3-4 divided doses; maintenance: 5-15 mg/day in 2-3 divided doses

Dosage Forms

Solution, oral: Diphenoxylate hydrochloride 2.5 mg and atropine sulfate 0.025 mg per 5 mL (5 mL, 10 mL, 60 mL)

Lomotil®: Diphenoxylate hydrochloride 2.5 mg and atropine sulfate 0.025 mg per 5 mL (60 mL) [contains alcohol 15%; cherry flavor]

Tablet (Lomotil®, Lonox®): Diphenoxylate hydrochloride 2.5 mg and atropine sulfate 0.025 mg

Diphen® [US-OTC] *see* diphenhydramine *on page 277*

Diphenylan Sodium® *(Discontinued)* *see page 1042*

diphenylhydantoin *see* phenytoin *on page 691*

diphtheria and tetanus toxoid (dif THEER ee a & TET a nus TOKS oyd)

Synonyms DT; Td; tetanus and diphtheria toxoid

U.S./Canadian Brand Names Decavac™ [US]

Therapeutic Category Toxoid

Use

Diphtheria and tetanus toxoids adsorbed for pediatric use (DT): Infants and children through 6 years of age: Active immunity against diphtheria and tetanus when pertussis vaccine is contraindicated

Tetanus and diphtheria toxoids adsorbed for adult use (Td) (Decavac™): Children ≥7 years of age and Adults: Active immunity against diphtheria and tetanus; tetanus prophylaxis in wound management

Usual Dosage I.M.:

Infants and Children ≤6 years (DT): Primary immunization:

6 weeks to 1 year: Three 0.5 mL doses at least 4 weeks apart; administer a reinforcing dose 6-12 months after the third injection

1-6 years: Two 0.5 mL doses at least 4 weeks apart; reinforcing dose 6-12 months after second injection; if final dose is given after seventh birthday, use adult preparation

4-6 years (booster immunization): 0.5 mL; not necessary if the fourth dose was given after fourth birthday; routinely administer booster doses at 10-year intervals with the adult preparation

Children ≥7 years and Adults:

Primary immunization: Patients previously not immunized should receive 2 primary doses of 0.5 mL each, given at an interval of 4-6 weeks; third (reinforcing) dose of 0.5 mL 6-12 months later

Booster immunization: 0.5 mL every 10 years; to be given to children 11-12 years of age if at least 5 years have elapsed since last dose of toxoid containing vaccine. Subsequent routine doses are not recommended more often than every 10 years.

Tetanus prophylaxis in wound management; use of tetanus toxoid (Td*) and/or tetanus immune globulin (TIG) depends upon the number of prior tetanus toxoid doses and type of wound.

Dosage Forms

Injection, suspension, adult: Diphtheria 2 Lf units and tetanus 5 Lf units per 0.5 mL (5 mL)

Decavac™: Diphtheria 2 Lf units and tetanus 5 Lf units per 0.5 mL (0.5 mL) [latex free prefilled syringe; contains thimerosal]

Injection, suspension, pediatric [preservative free]: Diphtheria 6.7 Lf units and tetanus 5 Lf units per 0.5 mL (0.5 mL)

diphtheria antitoxin (dif THEER ee a an tee TOKS in)

Therapeutic Category Antitoxin

Use Treatment of diphtheria (neutralizes unbound toxin, available from CDC)

Usual Dosage I.M. or slow I.V. infusion: Dosage varies; range: 20,000-120,000 units

Dosage Forms Injection: ≥500 units/mL (40 mL) [20,000 units/vial]

diphtheria CRM$_{197}$ protein *see* pneumococcal conjugate vaccine (7-valent) *on page 703*

diphtheria CRM$_{197}$ protein conjugate *see Haemophilus* B conjugate vaccine *on page 426*

diphtheria, tetanus toxoids, and acellular pertussis vaccine

(dif THEER ee a, TET a nus TOKS oyds, & ay CEL yoo lar per TUS sis vak SEEN)

Synonyms DTaP

U.S./Canadian Brand Names Adacel® [Can]; Daptacel™ [US]; Infanrix® [US]; Tripedia® [US]

Therapeutic Category Toxoid

Use Active immunization against diphtheria, tetanus, and pertussis from age 6 weeks through seventh birthday

Usual Dosage

Children 6 weeks to <7 years: I.M.: 0.5 mL

Primary series: Three doses, usually given at 2-, 4-, and 6 months of age; may be given as early as 6 weeks of age and repeated every 4-8 weeks; use same product for all 3 doses

Booster series:

Fourth dose: Given at ~15-20 months of age, but at least 6 months after third dose

Fifth dose: Given at 5-6 years of age, prior to starting school or kindergarten; if the fourth dose is given at ≥4 years of age, the fifth dose may be omitted

Children ≥7 years and Adults: Tetanus and diphtheria toxoids for adult use (Td) preparation is the preferred agent

Dosage Forms

Injection, suspension:

Daptacel™: Diphtheria 15 Lf units, tetanus 5 Lf units, and acellular pertussis vaccine 10 mcg per 0.5 mL (0.5 mL)

Infanrix®: Diphtheria 25 Lf units, tetanus 10 Lf units, and acellular pertussis vaccine 25 mcg per 0.5 mL (0.5 mL)

Tripedia®: Diphtheria 6.7 Lf units, tetanus 5 Lf units, and acellular pertussis vaccine 46.8 mcg per 0.5 mL (7.5 mL) [contains thimerosal]

Note: Tripedia® vaccine is also used to reconstitute ActHIB® to prepare TriHIBit® vaccine (diphtheria, tetanus toxoids, and acellular pertussis vaccine and *Haemophilus influenzae* b conjugate vaccine combination)

diphtheria, tetanus toxoids, and acellular pertussis vaccine and *Haemophilus* b conjugate vaccine

(dif THEER ee a, TET a nus TOKS oyds, & ay CEL yoo lar per TUS sis vak SEEN & hem OF fi lus bee KON joo gate vak SEEN)

Synonyms *Haemophilus influenzae* b conjugate vaccine and diphtheria, tetanus toxoids, and acellular pertussis vaccine

U.S./Canadian Brand Names TriHIBit® [US]

Therapeutic Category Toxoid; Vaccine, Inactivated Bacteria

Use Active immunization of children 15-18 months of age for prevention of diphtheria, tetanus, pertussis, and invasive disease caused by *H. influenzae* type b.

Usual Dosage Children >15 months of age: I.M.: 0.5 mL (as part of a general vaccination schedule; see individual vaccines). Vaccine should be used within 30 minutes of reconstitution.

Dosage Forms Injection, suspension: 5 Lf units tetanus toxoid, 6.7 Lf units diphtheria toxoid, 46.8 mcg pertussis antigens, and 10 mcg *H. influenzae* type b purified capsular polysaccharide per 0.5 mL (0.5 mL) [The combination of Tripedia® vaccine used to reconstitute ActHIB® forms TriHIBit®]

diphtheria toxoid conjugate *see Haemophilus* B conjugate vaccine *on page 426*

dipivalyl epinephrine *see* dipivefrin *on this page*

dipivefrin (dye PI ve frin)

Synonyms dipivalyl epinephrine; dipivefrin hydrochloride; DPE

U.S./Canadian Brand Names Apo-Dipivefrin® [Can]; Ophtho-Dipivefrin™ [Can]; PMS-Dipivefrin [Can]; Propine® [US/Can]

Therapeutic Category Adrenergic Agonist Agent

Use Reduces elevated intraocular pressure in chronic open-angle glaucoma; also used to treat ocular hypertension, low tension, and secondary glaucomas

Usual Dosage Adults: Ophthalmic: Instill 1 drop every 12 hours into the eyes

Dosage Forms Solution, ophthalmic, as hydrochloride: 0.1% (5 mL, 10 mL, 15 mL) [contains benzalkonium chloride]

dipivefrin hydrochloride *see* dipivefrin *on this page*

Diprivan® [US/Can] *see* propofol *on page 738*

Diprolene® [US] *see* betamethasone (topical) *on page 116*

Diprolene® AF [US] *see* betamethasone (topical) *on page 116*

Diprolene® Glycol [Can] *see* betamethasone (topical) *on page 116*

dipropylacetic acid *see* valproic acid and derivatives *on page 901*

Diprosone® ***(Discontinued)*** *see page 1042*

Diprosone® [Can] *see* betamethasone (topical) *on page 116*

dipyridamole (dye peer ID a mole)

Sound-Alike/Look-Alike Issues

dipyridamole may be confused with disopyramide

Persantine® may be confused with Periactin®, Permitil®

U.S./Canadian Brand Names Apo-Dipyridamole FC® [Can]; Novo-Dipiradol [Can]; Persantine® [US/Can]

Therapeutic Category Antiplatelet Agent; Vasodilator

Use

Oral: Used with warfarin to decrease thrombosis in patients after artificial heart valve replacement

I.V.: Diagnostic agent in CAD

Usual Dosage

Adults:

Oral: Adjunctive therapy for prophylaxis of thromboembolism with cardiac valve replacement: 75-100 mg 4 times/day

I.V.: Evaluation of coronary artery disease: 0.14 mg/kg/minute for 4 minutes; maximum dose: 60 mg

Dosage Forms

Injection, solution: 5 mg/mL (2 mL, 10 mL)

Tablet (Persantine®): 25 mg, 50 mg, 75 mg

dirithromycin (dye RITH roe mye sin)

Sound-Alike/Look-Alike Issues

Dynabac® may be confused with Dynacin®, DynaCirc®, Dynapen®

U.S./Canadian Brand Names Dynabac® [US]

Therapeutic Category Macrolide (Antibiotic)

Use Treatment of mild to moderate upper and lower respiratory tract infections due to *Moraxella catarrhalis, Streptococcus pneumoniae, Legionella pneumophila, H. influenzae*, or *S. pyogenes*, ie, acute exacerbation of chronic bronchitis, secondary bacterial infection of acute bronchitis, community-acquired pneumonia, pharyngitis/tonsillitis, and uncomplicated infections of the skin and skin structure due to *Staphylococcus aureus*

Usual Dosage Adults: Oral: 500 mg once daily for 5-14 days (14 days required for treatment of community-acquired pneumonia due to *Legionella*, *Mycoplasma*, or *S. pneumoniae*; 10 days is recommended for treatment of *S. pyogenes* pharyngitis/tonsillitis)

Dosage Forms Tablet, enteric coated: 250 mg

Disalcid® ***(Discontinued)*** *see page 1042*

disalicylic acid *see* salsalate *on page 793*

Disanthrol® ***(Discontinued)*** *see page 1042*

Disobrom® ***(Discontinued)*** *see page 1042*

disodium cromoglycate *see* cromolyn sodium *on page 230*

disodium thiosulfate pentahydrate *see* sodium thiosulfate *on page 817*

***d*-isoephedrine hydrochloride** *see* pseudoephedrine *on page 745*

Disonate® ***(Discontinued)*** *see page 1042*

disopyramide (dye soe PEER a mide)

Sound-Alike/Look-Alike Issues

disopyramide may be confused with desipramine, dipyridamole

Norpace® may be confused with Norpramin®

Synonyms disopyramide phosphate

U.S./Canadian Brand Names Norpace® CR [US]; Norpace® [US/Can]; Rythmodan® [Can]; Rythmodan®-LA [Can]

Therapeutic Category Antiarrhythmic Agent, Class I-A

Use Suppression and prevention of unifocal and multifocal atrial and premature, ventricular premature complexes, coupled ventricular tachycardia; effective in the conversion of atrial fibrillation, atrial flutter, and paroxysmal atrial tachycardia to normal sinus rhythm and prevention of the recurrence of these arrhythmias after conversion by other methods

Usual Dosage Oral:

Children:

<1 year: 10-30 mg/kg/24 hours in 4 divided doses

1-4 years: 10-20 mg/kg/24 hours in 4 divided doses

4-12 years: 10-15 mg/kg/24 hours in 4 divided doses

12-18 years: 6-15 mg/kg/24 hours in 4 divided doses

Adults:

<50 kg: 100 mg every 6 hours or 200 mg every 12 hours (controlled release)

>50 kg: 150 mg every 6 hours or 300 mg every 12 hours (controlled release); if no response, increase to 200 mg every 6 hours. Maximum dose required for patients with severe refractory ventricular tachycardia is 400 mg every 6 hours.

Dosage Forms

Capsule (Norpace®): 100 mg, 150 mg

Capsule, controlled release (Norpace® CR): 100 mg, 150 mg

disopyramide phosphate *see* disopyramide *on this page*

Disotate® *(Discontinued)* *see page 1042*

Di-Spaz® Injection *(Discontinued)* *see page 1042*

Di-Spaz® Oral *(Discontinued)* *see page 1042*

DisperMox™ [US] *see* amoxicillin *on page 51*

Dispos-a-Med® Isoproterenol *(Discontinued)* *see page 1042*

disulfiram (dye SUL fi ram)

Sound-Alike/Look-Alike Issues

disulfiram may be confused with Diflucan®

Antabuse® may be confused with Anturane®

U.S./Canadian Brand Names Antabuse® [US]

Therapeutic Category Aldehyde Dehydrogenase Inhibitor Agent

Use Management of chronic alcoholism

Usual Dosage Adults: Oral: Do not administer until the patient has abstained from ethanol for at least 12 hours

Initial: 500 mg/day as a single dose for 1-2 weeks; maximum daily dose is 500 mg

Average maintenance dose: 250 mg/day; range: 125-500 mg; duration of therapy is to continue until the patient is fully recovered socially and a basis for permanent self control has been established; maintenance therapy may be required for months or even years

Dosage Forms Tablet: 250 mg

Dital® *(Discontinued)* *see page 1042*

dithioglycerol *see* dimercaprol *on page 275*

dithranol *see* anthralin *on page 60*

Ditropan® [US/Can] *see* oxybutynin *on page 655*

Ditropan® XL [US/Can] *see* oxybutynin *on page 655*

Diucardin® *(Discontinued)* *see page 1042*

Diupress® *(Discontinued)* *see page 1042*

Diurigen® *(Discontinued)* *see page 1042*

Diuril® [US/Can] *see* chlorothiazide *on page 187*

divalproex sodium *see* valproic acid and derivatives *on page 901*

Dixarit® [Can] *see* clonidine *on page 215*

Dizac® Injectable Emulsion *(Discontinued)* *see page 1042*

Dizmiss® *(Discontinued)* *see page 1042*

Dizymes® Tablet *(Discontinued)* *see page 1042*

5071-1DL(6) *see* megestrol acetate *on page 549*

***dl*-alpha tocopherol** *see* vitamin E *on page 918*

***D*-mannitol** *see* mannitol *on page 542*

4-DMDR *see* idarubicin *on page 464*

D-Med® Injection *(Discontinued)* *see page 1042*

DMSA *see* succimer *on page 826*

DMSO *see* dimethyl sulfoxide *on page 275*

DNA-derived humanized monoclonal antibody *see* alemtuzumab *on page 29*

DNase *see* dornase alfa *on page 289*

DNR *see* daunorubicin hydrochloride *on page 246*

Doak® Tar [US-OTC] *see* coal tar *on page 219*

Doan's® Extra Strength [US-OTC] *see* magnesium salicylate *on page 539*

Doan's® [US-OTC] *see* magnesium salicylate *on page 539*

dobutamine (doe BYOO ta meen)

Sound-Alike/Look-Alike Issues
dobutamine may be confused with dopamine

Synonyms dobutamine hydrochloride

Tall-Man DOBUTamine

U.S./Canadian Brand Names Dobutrex® [Can]

Therapeutic Category Adrenergic Agonist Agent

Use Short-term management of patients with cardiac decompensation

Usual Dosage Administration requires the use of an infusion pump; I.V. infusion:

Neonates: 2-15 mcg/kg/minute, titrate to desired response

Children and Adults: 2.5-20 mcg/kg/minute; maximum: 40 mcg/kg/minute, titrate to desired response.

Dosage Forms

Infusion, as hydrochloride [premixed in dextrose]: 1 mg/mL (250 mL, 500 mL); 2 mg/mL (250 mL); 4 mg/mL (250 mL)

Injection, solution, as hydrochloride: 12.5 mg/mL (20 mL, 40 mL, 100 mL) [contains sodium bisulfite]

dobutamine hydrochloride *see* dobutamine *on this page*

Dobutrex® [Can] *see* dobutamine *on this page*

docetaxel (doe se TAKS el)

Sound-Alike/Look-Alike Issues
docetaxel may be confused with paclitaxel
Taxotere® may be confused with Taxol®

Synonyms NSC-628503; RP-6976

U.S./Canadian Brand Names Taxotere® [US/Can]

Therapeutic Category Antineoplastic Agent

Use Treatment of locally-advanced or metastatic breast cancer; adjuvant treatment of operable node-positive breast cancer (in combination with doxorubicin and cyclophosphamide); treatment of locally-advanced or metastatic nonsmall-cell lung cancer (NSCLC) in combination with cisplatin in treatment of patients who have not previously received chemotherapy for unresected NSCLC; treatment of prostate cancer (hormone refractory, metastatic)

Usual Dosage Refer to individual protocols. Children ≥16 years and Adults: I.V. infusion:

Breast cancer:

Locally-advanced or metastatic: 60-100 mg/m^2 every 3 weeks; patients initially started at 60 mg/m^2 who do not develop toxicity may tolerate higher doses

Operable, node-positive (adjuvant treatment): 75 mg/m^2 every 3 weeks for 6 courses

Nonsmall-cell lung cancer: I.V.: 75 mg/m^2 every 3 weeks

Prostate cancer: 75 mg/m^2 every 3 weeks; prednisone (5 mg twice daily) is administered continuously

Dosage Forms Injection, solution [concentrate]: 20 mg/0.5 mL (0.5 mL, 2 mL) [contains Polysorbate 80®; diluent contains ethanol 13%]

docosanol (doe KOE san ole)

Synonyms behenyl alcohol; *n*-docosanol

U.S./Canadian Brand Names Abreva® [US-OTC]

Therapeutic Category Antiviral Agent, Topical

Use Treatment of herpes simplex of the face or lips

Usual Dosage Children ≥12 years and Adults: Topical: Apply 5 times/day to affected area of face or lips. Start at first sign of cold sore or fever blister and continue until healed.

Dosage Forms Cream: 10% (2 g)

docusate (DOK yoo sate)

Sound-Alike/Look-Alike Issues

docusate may be confused with Doxinate®

Colace® may be confused with Calan®

Surfak® may be confused with Surbex®

Synonyms dioctyl calcium sulfosuccinate; dioctyl sodium sulfosuccinate; docusate calcium; docusate potassium; docusate sodium; DOSS; DSS

U.S./Canadian Brand Names Albert® Docusate [Can]; Apo-Docusate-Calcium® [Can]; Apo-Docusate-Sodium® [Can]; Colace® [US-OTC/Can]; Colax-C® [Can]; Diocto® [US-OTC]; Docusoft-S™ [US-OTC]; DOK™ [US-OTC]; DOS® [US-OTC]; D-S-S® [US-OTC]; Dulcolax® Stool Softener [US-OTC]; Enemeez® [US-OTC]; Fleet® Sof-Lax® [US-OTC]; Genasoft® [US-OTC]; Novo-Docusate Calcium [Can]; Novo-Docusate Sodium [Can]; Phillips'® Stool Softener Laxative [US-OTC]; PMS-Docusate Calcium [Can]; PMS-Docusate Sodium [Can]; Regulex® [Can]; Selax® [Can]; Silace [US-OTC]; Soflax™ [Can]; Surfak® [US-OTC]

Therapeutic Category Stool Softener

Use Stool softener in patients who should avoid straining during defecation and constipation associated with hard, dry stools; prophylaxis for straining (Valsalva) following myocardial infarction. A safe agent to be used in elderly; some evidence that doses <200 mg are ineffective; stool softeners are unnecessary if stool is well hydrated or "mushy" and soft; shown to be ineffective used long-term.

Usual Dosage Docusate salts are interchangeable; the amount of sodium or calcium per dosage unit is clinically insignificant

Infants and Children <3 years: Oral: 10-40 mg/day in 1-4 divided doses

Children: Oral:

3-6 years: 20-60 mg/day in 1-4 divided doses

6-12 years: 40-150 mg/day in 1-4 divided doses

Adolescents and Adults: Oral: 50-500 mg/day in 1-4 divided doses

(Continued)

docusate *(Continued)*

Older Children and Adults: Rectal: Add 50-100 mg of docusate liquid to enema fluid (saline or water); administer as retention or flushing enema

Dosage Forms

Capsule, as calcium (Surfak®): 240 mg

Capsule, as sodium: 100 mg, 250 mg

Colace®: 50 mg [contains sodium 3 mg], 100 mg [contains sodium 5 mg]

Docusoft-S™: 100 mg [contains sodium 5 mg]

DOK™, Genasoft®: 100 mg

DOS®, D-S-S®: 100 mg, 250 mg

Dulcolax® Stool Softener: 100 mg [contains sodium 5 mg]

Phillips'® Stool Softener Laxative: 100 mg [contains sodium 5.2 mg]

Enema, rectal, as sodium (Enemeez®): 283 mg/5 mL 5 mL

Gelcap, as sodium (Fleet® Sof-lax®): 100 mg

Liquid, as sodium: 150 mg/15 mL (480 mL)

Colace®: 150 mg/15 mL (30 mL) [contains sodium 1 mg/mL]

Diocto®: 150 mg/15 mL (480 mL) [vanilla flavor]

Silace: 150 mg/15 mL (480 mL) [lemon-vanilla flavor]

Syrup, as sodium: 60 mg/15 mL (480 mL)

Colace®, Diocto®: 60 mg/15 mL (480 mL) [alcohol free, sugar free; contains sodium 36 mg/5 mL]

Silace: 20 mg/5 mL (480 mL) [peppermint flavor]

docusate and senna (DOK yoo sate & SEN na)

Synonyms senna and docusate; senna-S

U.S./Canadian Brand Names Peri-Colace® *(reformulation)* [US-OTC]; Senokot-S® [US-OTC]

Therapeutic Category Laxative, Stimulant; Stool Softener

Use Short-term treatment of constipation

Usual Dosage Oral: Constipation: OTC ranges:

Children:

2-6 years: Initial: 4.3 mg sennosides plus 25 mg docusate (1/2 tablet) once daily (maximum: 1 tablet twice daily)

6-12 years: Initial: 8.6 sennosides plus 50 mg docusate (1 tablet) once daily (maximum: 2 tablets twice daily)

Children ≥12 years and Adults: Initial: 2 tablets (17.2 mg sennosides plus 100 mg docusate) once daily (maximum: 4 tablets twice daily)

Dosage Forms

Tablet: Docusate sodium 50 mg and sennosides 8.6 mg

Peri-Colace® (reformulation): Docusate sodium 50 mg and sennosides 8.6 mg

Senokot-S®: Docusate sodium 50 mg and sennosides 8.6 mg [sugar free; contains sodium 3 mg/tablet]

docusate calcium *see* docusate *on previous page*

docusate potassium *see* docusate *on previous page*

docusate sodium *see* docusate *on previous page*

Docusoft Plus™ ***(Discontinued)*** *see page 1042*

Docusoft-S™ [US-OTC] *see* docusate *on previous page*

dofetilide (doe FET il ide)

Synonyms UK-68-798

U.S./Canadian Brand Names Tikosyn™ [US/Can]

Therapeutic Category Antiarrhythmic Agent, Class III

Use Maintenance of normal sinus rhythm in patients with chronic atrial fibrillation/atrial flutter of longer than 1-week duration who have been converted to normal sinus rhythm; conversion of atrial fibrillation and atrial flutter to normal sinus rhythm

Usual Dosage Adults: Oral:

Note: QT or QT_c must be determined prior to first dose. If QT_c >440 msec (>500 msec in patients with ventricular conduction abnormalities), dofetilide is contraindicated

Initial: 500 mcg orally twice daily. Initial dosage must be adjusted in patients with estimated Cl_{cr} <60 mL/minute Dofetilide may be initiated at lower doses than recommended based on physician discretion.

Modification of dosage in response to initial dose: QT_c interval should be measured 2-3 hours after the initial dose. If the QT_c >15% of baseline, or if the QT_c is >500 msec (550 msec in patients with ventricular conduction abnormalities) dofetilide should be adjusted. If the starting dose is 500 mcg twice daily, then adjust to 250 mcg twice daily. If the starting dose was 250 mcg twice daily, then adjust to 125 mcg twice daily. If the starting dose was 125 mcg twice daily then adjust to 125 mcg every day.

Continued monitoring for doses 2-5: QT_c interval must be determined 2-3 hours after each subsequent dose of dofetilide for in-hospital doses 2-5. If the measured QT_c is >500 msec (550 msec in patients with ventricular conduction abnormalities) at any time, dofetilide should be discontinued.

Chronic therapy (following the 5th dose):

QT or QT_c and creatinine clearance should be evaluated every 3 months. If QT_c >500 msec (>550 msec in patients with ventricular conduction abnormalities), dofetilide should be discontinued.

Dosage Forms Capsule: 125 mcg, 250 mcg, 500 mcg

Doktors® Nasal Solution *(Discontinued)* *see page 1042*

DOK™ [US-OTC] *see* docusate *on page 285*

Dolacet® Forte *(Discontinued)* *see page 1042*

dolasetron (dol A se tron)

Sound-Alike/Look-Alike Issues

Anzemet® may be confused with Adlomet®

Synonyms dolasetron mesylate; MDL 73,147EF

U.S./Canadian Brand Names Anzemet® [US/Can]

Therapeutic Category Selective 5-HT_3 Receptor Antagonist

Use Prevention of nausea and vomiting associated with emetogenic cancer chemotherapy, including initial and repeat courses; prevention of postoperative nausea and vomiting and treatment of postoperative nausea and vomiting (injectable form only)

Generally **not** recommended for treatment of existing chemotherapy-induced emesis (CIE) or for prophylaxis of nausea from agents with a low emetogenic potential.

Usual Dosage

Children <2 years: Not recommended for use

Nausea and vomiting prophylaxis, chemotherapy-induced (including initial and repeat courses):

Children 2-16 years:

Oral: 1.8 mg/kg within 1 hour before chemotherapy; maximum: 100 mg/dose

I.V.: 1.8 mg/kg ~30 minutes before chemotherapy; maximum: 100 mg/dose

Adults:

Oral: 200 mg single dose

I.V.: 0.6-5 mg/kg as a single dose 50 mg 1-2 minute bolus 2.4-3 mg/kg 20-minute infusion

Prevention of postoperative nausea and vomiting:

Children 2-16 years:

Oral: 1.2 mg/kg within 2 hours before surgery; maximum: 100 mg/dose

I.V.: 0.35 mg/kg (maximum: 12.5 mg) ~15 minutes before stopping anesthesia

Adults:

Oral: 100 mg within 2 hours before surgery

I.V.: 12.5 mg ~15 minutes before stopping anesthesia

Treatment of postoperative nausea and vomiting: I.V. (only):

Children: 0.35 mg/kg (maximum: 12.5 mg) as soon as needed

Adults: 12.5 mg as soon as needed

(Continued)

dolasetron *(Continued)*

Dosage Forms

Injection, solution, as mesylate: 20 mg/mL (0.625 mL, 5 mL) [single-use ampuls and vial]; 20 mg/mL (25 mL) [multidose vial]

Tablet, as mesylate: 50 mg, 100 mg

dolasetron mesylate *see* dolasetron *on previous page*

Dolene® *(Discontinued)* *see page 1042*

Dolobid® [US] *see* diflunisal *on page 270*

Dolophine® [US/Can] *see* methadone *on page 562*

Dolorac™ *(Discontinued)* *see page 1042*

Dolorex® *(Discontinued)* *see page 1042*

Dom-Benzydamine [Can] *see* benzydamine *(Canada only) on page 112*

Dom-Domperidone [Can] *see* domperidone *(Canada only) on this page*

Domeboro® [US-OTC] *see* aluminum sulfate and calcium acetate *on page 41*

dome paste bandage *see* zinc gelatin *on page 940*

Dommanate® Injection *(Discontinued)* *see page 1042*

domperidone *(Canada only)* (dom PE ri done)

Synonyms domperidone maleate

U.S./Canadian Brand Names Alti-Domperidone [Can]; Apo-Domperidone® [Can]; Dom-Domperidone [Can]; FTP-Domperidone Maleate [Can]; Motilium® [Can]; Novo-Domperidone [Can]; Nu-Domperidone [Can]; ratio-Domperidone [Can]

Therapeutic Category Dopamine Antagonist

Use Symptomatic management of upper GI motility disorders associated with chronic and subacute gastritis and diabetic gastroparesis; prevention of GI symptoms associated with use of dopamine-agonist anti-Parkinson agents

Usual Dosage Oral: Adults:

GI motility disorders: 10 mg 3-4 times/day, 15-30 minutes before meals; severe/resistant cases: 20 mg 3-4 times/day, 15-30 minutes before meals

Nausea/vomiting associated with dopamine-agonist anti-Parkinson agents: 20 mg 3-4 times/day

Dosage Forms Tablet: 10 mg [domperidone maleate 12.72 mg]

domperidone maleate *see* domperidone *(Canada only) on this page*

Dom-Tiaprofenic® [Can] *see* tiaprofenic acid *(Canada only) on page 861*

donepezil (don EH pa zil)

Sound-Alike/Look-Alike Issues

Aricept® may be confused with Aciphex™, Ascriptin®

Synonyms E2020

U.S./Canadian Brand Names Aricept® [US/Can]

Therapeutic Category Acetylcholinesterase Inhibitor; Cholinergic Agent

Use Treatment of mild to moderate dementia of the Alzheimer type

Usual Dosage Oral: Adults: Dementia of Alzheimer type: Initial: 5 mg/day at bedtime; may increase to 10 mg/day at bedtime after 4-6 weeks

Dosage Forms Tablet, as hydrochloride: 5 mg, 10 mg

Donnamar® *(Discontinued)* *see page 1042*

Donnapectolin-PG® *(Discontinued)* *see page 1042*

Donnapine® *(Discontinued)* *see page 1042*

Donnatal® [US/Can] *see* hyoscyamine, atropine, scopolamine, and phenobarbital *on page 460*

Donnatal Extentabs® [US] *see* hyoscyamine, atropine, scopolamine, and phenobarbital *on page 460*

Donnazyme® *(Discontinued)* *see page 1042*

Donphen® Tablet *(Discontinued)* *see page 1042*

dopamine (DOE pa meen)

Sound-Alike/Look-Alike Issues
dopamine may be confused with dobutamine, Dopram®

Synonyms dopamine hydrochloride

Tall-Man DOPamine

U.S./Canadian Brand Names Intropin® [Can]

Therapeutic Category Adrenergic Agonist Agent

Use Adjunct in the treatment of shock (eg, MI, open heart surgery, renal failure, cardiac decompensation) which persists after adequate fluid volume replacement

Usual Dosage I.V. infusion (administration requires the use of an infusion pump):

Neonates: 1-20 mcg/kg/minute continuous infusion, titrate to desired response.

Children: 1-20 mcg/kg/minute, maximum: 50 mcg/kg/minute continuous infusion, titrate to desired response.

Adults: 1-5 mcg/kg/minute up to 20 mcg/kg/minute, titrate to desired response. Infusion may be increased by 1-4 mcg/kg/minute at 10- to 30-minute intervals until optimal response is obtained.

If dosages >20-30 mcg/kg/minute are needed, a more direct-acting pressor may be more beneficial (ie, epinephrine, norepinephrine).

The hemodynamic effects of dopamine are dose dependent:

Low-dose: 1-3 mcg/kg/minute, increased renal blood flow and urine output

Intermediate-dose: 3-10 mcg/kg/minute, increased renal blood flow, heart rate, cardiac contractility, and cardiac output

High-dose: >10 mcg/kg/minute, alpha-adrenergic effects begin to predominate, vasoconstriction, increased blood pressure

Dosage Forms

Infusion, as hydrochloride [premixed in D_5W]: 0.8 mg/mL (250 mL, 500 mL); 1.6 mg/mL (250 mL, 500 mL); 3.2 mg/mL (250 mL)

Injection, solution, as hydrochloride: 40 mg/mL (5 mL, 10 mL); 80 mg/mL (5 mL); 160 mg/mL (5 mL) [contains sodium metabisulfite]

dopamine hydrochloride *see* dopamine *on this page*

Dopar® *(Discontinued)* *see page 1042*

Dopastat® Injection *(Discontinued)* *see page 1042*

Dopram® [US] *see* doxapram *on page 291*

Doral® [US/Can] *see* quazepam *on page 755*

Doriden® Tablet *(Discontinued)* *see page 1042*

Dormarex® 2 Oral *(Discontinued)* *see page 1042*

dornase alfa (DOOR nase AL fa)

Synonyms DNase; recombinant human deoxyribonuclease

U.S./Canadian Brand Names Pulmozyme® [US/Can]

Therapeutic Category Enzyme

Use Management of cystic fibrosis patients to reduce the frequency of respiratory infections that require parenteral antibiotics, and to improve pulmonary function

Usual Dosage Inhalation:

Children >3 months to Adults: 2.5 mg once daily through selected nebulizers; experience in children <5 years is limited

Patients unable to inhale or exhale orally throughout the entire treatment period may use Pari-Baby™ nebulizer. Some patients may benefit from twice daily administration.

Dosage Forms Solution for nebulization: 1 mg/mL (2.5 mL)

Doryx® [US] *see* doxycycline *on page 294*

dorzolamide (dor ZOLE a mide)

Synonyms dorzolamide hydrochloride

U.S./Canadian Brand Names Trusopt® [US/Can]

Therapeutic Category Carbonic Anhydrase Inhibitor

Use Lowers intraocular pressure in patients with ocular hypertension or open-angle glaucoma

Usual Dosage Children and Adults: Reduction of intraocular pressure: Instill 1 drop in the affected eye(s) 3 times/day

Dosage Forms Solution, ophthalmic, as hydrochloride: 2% (5 mL, 10 mL) [contains benzalkonium chloride]

dorzolamide and timolol (dor ZOLE a mide & TYE moe lole)

Synonyms timolol and dorzolamide

Therapeutic Category Beta-Adrenergic Blocker; Carbonic Anhydrase Inhibitor

Use Lowers intraocular pressure to treat glaucoma in patients with ocular hypertension or open-angle glaucoma

Usual Dosage Adults: ophthalmic: One drop in eye(s) twice daily

Dosage Forms Solution, ophthalmic: Dorzolamide 2% and timolol 0.5% (5 mL, 10 mL) [contains benzalkonium chloride]

dorzolamide hydrochloride *see* dorzolamide *on this page*

DOSS *see* docusate *on page 285*

Dostinex® [US/Can] *see* cabergoline *on page 141*

DOS® [US-OTC] *see* docusate *on page 285*

Dovobet® [Can] *see* betamethasone and calcipotriol *(Canada only) on page 114*

Dovonex® [US] *see* calcipotriene *on page 142*

doxacurium (doks a KYOO ri um)

Sound-Alike/Look-Alike Issues

doxacurium may be confused with doxapram, doxorubicin

Synonyms doxacurium chloride

U.S./Canadian Brand Names Nuromax® [US/Can]

Therapeutic Category Skeletal Muscle Relaxant

Use Adjunct to general anesthesia to facilitate endotracheal intubation and to relax skeletal muscles during surgery; to facilitate mechanical ventilation in ICU patients; does not relieve pain or produce sedation; the characteristics of this agent make it especially useful in procedures requiring careful maintenance of hemodynamic stability for prolonged periods

Usual Dosage Administer I.V.; dose to effect; doses will vary due to interpatient variability; use ideal body weight for obese patients

Surgery:

- Children >2 years: Initial: 0.03-0.05 mg/kg followed by maintenance doses of 0.005-0.01 mg/kg after 30-45 minutes
- Adults: 0.05-0.08 mg/kg with thiopental/narcotic or 0.025 mg/kg after initial dose of succinylcholine for intubation; initial maintenance dose of 0.005-0.01 mg/kg after 100-160 minutes followed by repeat doses every 30-45 minutes

Pretreatment/priming: 10% of intubating dose given 3-5 minutes before initial dose

ICU: 0.05 mg/kg bolus followed by 0.025 mg/kg every 2-3 hours or 0.25-0.75 mcg/kg/minute once initial recovery from bolus dose observed

Dosage Forms Injection, solution, as chloride: 1 mg/mL (5 mL) [contains benzyl alcohol]

doxacurium chloride *see* doxacurium *on this page*

doxapram (DOKS a pram)

Sound-Alike/Look-Alike Issues

doxapram may be confused with doxacurium, doxazosin, doxepin, Doxinate®, doxorubicin

Dopram® may be confused with dopamine

Synonyms doxapram hydrochloride

U.S./Canadian Brand Names Dopram® [US]

Therapeutic Category Respiratory Stimulant

Use Respiratory and CNS stimulant for respiratory depression secondary to anesthesia, drug-induced CNS depression; acute hypercapnia secondary to COPD

Usual Dosage

Respiratory depression following anesthesia:

Intermittent injection: Initial: 0.5-1 mg/kg; may repeat at 5-minute intervals (only in patients who demonstrate initial response); maximum total dose: 2 mg/kg

I.V. infusion: Initial: 5 mg/minute until adequate response or adverse effects seen; decrease to 1-3 mg/minute; maximum total dose: 4 mg/kg

Drug-induced CNS depression:

Intermittent injection: Initial: 1-2 mg/kg, repeat after 5 minutes; may repeat at 1-2 hour intervals (until sustained consciousness); maximum: 3 g/day. May repeat in 24 hours if necessary.

I.V. infusion: Initial: Bolus dose of 2 mg/kg, repeat after 5 minutes. If no response, wait 1-2 hours and repeat. If some stimulation is noted, initiate infusion at 1-3 mg/minute (depending on size of patient/depth of CNS depression); suspend infusion if patient begins to awaken. Infusion should not be continued for >2 hours. May reinstitute infusion as described above, including bolus, after rest interval of 30 minutes to 2 hours; maximum: 3 g/day

Acute hypercapnia secondary to COPD: I.V. infusion: Initial: Initiate infusion at 1-2 mg/minute (depending on size of patient/depth of CNS depression); may increase to maximum rate of 3 mg/minute; infusion should not be continued for >2 hours. Monitor arterial blood gases prior to initiation of infusion and at 30-minute intervals during the infusion (to identify possible development of acidosis/CO_2 retention). Additional infusions are not recommended (per manufacturer).

Dosage Forms Injection, solution, as hydrochloride: 20 mg/mL (20 mL) [contains benzyl alcohol; vial stopper contains latex]

doxapram hydrochloride *see* doxapram *on this page*

doxazosin (doks AYE zoe sin)

Sound-Alike/Look-Alike Issues

doxazosin may be confused with doxapram, doxepin, doxorubicin

Cardura® may be confused with Cardene®, Cordarone®, Cordran®, Coumadin®, K-Dur®, Ridaura®

Synonyms doxazosin mesylate

U.S./Canadian Brand Names Alti-Doxazosin [Can]; Apo-Doxazosin® [Can]; Cardura® [US]; Cardura-1™ [Can]; Cardura-2™ [Can]; Cardura-4™ [Can]; Gen-Doxazosin [Can]; Novo-Doxazosin [Can]

Therapeutic Category Alpha-Adrenergic Blocking Agent

Use Treatment of hypertension alone or in conjunction with diuretics, cardiac glycosides, ACE inhibitors, or calcium antagonists (particularly appropriate for those with hypertension and other cardiovascular risk factors such as hypercholesterolemia and diabetes mellitus); treatment of urinary outflow obstruction and/or obstructive and irritative symptoms associated with benign prostatic hyperplasia (BPH), particularly useful in patients with troublesome symptoms who are unable or unwilling to undergo invasive procedures, but who require rapid symptomatic relief; can be used in combination with finasteride

(Continued)

doxazosin *(Continued)*

Usual Dosage Oral:

Adults: 1 mg once daily in morning or evening; may be increased to 2 mg once daily. Thereafter titrate upwards, if needed, over several weeks, balancing therapeutic benefit with doxazosin-induced postural hypotension

Hypertension: Maximum dose: 16 mg/day

BPH: Goal: 4-8 mg/day; maximum dose: 8 mg/day

Dosage Forms Tablet: 1 mg, 2 mg, 4 mg, 8 mg

doxazosin mesylate *see* doxazosin *on previous page*

doxepin (DOKS e pin)

Sound-Alike/Look-Alike Issues

doxepin may be confused with digoxin, doxapram, doxazosin, Doxidan®, doxycycline

Sinequan® may be confused with saquinavir, Serentil®, Seroquel®, Singulair®

Zonalon® may be confused with Zone-A Forte®

Synonyms doxepin hydrochloride

U.S./Canadian Brand Names Apo-Doxepin® [Can]; Novo-Doxepin [Can]; Prudoxin™ [US]; Sinequan® [US/Can]; Zonalon® [US/Can]

Therapeutic Category Antidepressant, Tricyclic (Tertiary Amine); Topical Skin Product

Use

Oral: Depression

Topical: Short-term (<8 days) management of moderate pruritus in adults with atopic dermatitis or lichen simplex chronicus

Usual Dosage

Oral (entire daily dose may be given at bedtime):

Chronic urticaria, angioedema, nocturnal pruritus: Adults and Elderly: 10-30 mg/day

Topical: Pruritus: Adults and Elderly: Apply a thin film 4 times/day with at least 3- to 4-hour interval between applications; not recommended for use >8 days. **Note:** Low-dose (25-50 mg) oral administration has also been used to treat pruritus, but systemic effects are increased.

Dosage Forms

Capsule, as hydrochloride (Sinequan®): 10 mg, 25 mg, 50 mg, 75 mg, 100 mg, 150 mg

Cream, as hydrochloride:

Prudoxin™: 5% (45 g) [contains benzyl alcohol]

Zonalon®: 5% (30 g, 45 g) [contains benzyl alcohol]

Solution, oral concentrate, as hydrochloride (Sinequan®): 10 mg/mL (120 mL)

doxepin hydrochloride *see* doxepin *on this page*

doxercalciferol (dox er kal si fe FEER ole)

Synonyms 1α-hydroxyergocalciferol

U.S./Canadian Brand Names Hectorol® [US/Can]

Therapeutic Category Vitamin D Analog

Use Treatment of secondary hyperparathyroidism in patients with chronic kidney disease

Usual Dosage

Oral:

Dialysis patients: Dose should be titrated to lower iPTH to 150-300 pg/mL; dose is adjusted at 8-week intervals (maximum dose: 20 mcg 3 times/week)

Initial dose: iPTH >400 pg/mL: 10 mcg 3 times/week at dialysis

Dose titration:

iPTH level decreased by 50% and >300 pg/mL: Dose can be increased to 12.5 mcg 3 times/week for 8 more weeks; this titration process can continue at 8-week intervals; each increase should be by 2.5 mcg/dose

iPTH level 150-300 pg/mL: Maintain current dose

iPTH level <100 pg/mL: Suspend doxercalciferol for 1 week; resume at a reduced dose; decrease each dose (not weekly dose) by at least 2.5 mcg

Predialysis patients: Dose should be titrated to lower iPTH to 35-70 pg/mL with stage 3 disease or to 70-110 pg/mL with stage 4 disease: Dose may be adjusted at 2-week intervals (maximum dose: 3.5 mcg/day)

Initial dose: 1 mcg/day

Dose titration:

iPTH level >70 pg/mL with stage 3 disease or >110 pg/mL with stage 4 disease: Increase dose by 0.5 mcg every 2 weeks as necessary

iPTH level 35-70 pg/mL with stage 3 disease or 70-110 pg/mL with stage 4 disease: Maintain current dose

iPTH level is <35 pg/mL with stage 3 disease or <70 pg/mL with stage 4 disease: Suspend doxercalciferol for 1 week, then resume at a reduced dose (at least 0.5 mcg lower)

I.V.:

Dialysis patients: Dose should be titrated to lower iPTH to 150-300 pg/mL; dose is adjusted at 8-week intervals (maximum dose: 18 mcg/week)

Initial dose: iPTH level >400 pg/mL: 4 mcg 3 times/week after dialysis, administered as a bolus dose

Dose titration:

iPTH level decreased by 50% and >300 pg/mL: Dose can be increased by 1-2 mcg at 8-week intervals, as necessary

iPTH level 150-300 pg/mL: Maintain the current dose

iPTH level <100 pg/mL: Suspend doxercalciferol for 1 week; resume at a reduced dose (at least 1 mcg lower)

Dosage Forms

Capsule: 0.5 mcg, 2.5 mcg [contains coconut oil]

Injection, solution: 2 mcg/mL (2 mL) [contains disodium edetate]

Doxidan® *(Discontinued)* *see page 1042*

Doxidan® *(reformulation)* [US-OTC] *see* bisacodyl *on page 120*

Doxil® [US] *see* doxorubicin (liposomal) *on next page*

Doxinate® Capsule *(Discontinued)* *see page 1042*

doxorubicin (doks oh ROO bi sin)

Sound-Alike/Look-Alike Issues

doxorubicin may be confused with dactinomycin, daunorubicin, doxacurium, doxapram, doxazosin, doxorubicin liposomal, idarubicin

Adriamycin PFS® may be confused with Achromycin®, Aredia®, Idamycin®

Rubex® may be confused with Robaxin®

Synonyms ADR; adria; doxorubicin hydrochloride; hydroxydaunomycin hydrochloride; hydroxyldaunorubicin hydrochloride; NSC-123127

Tall-Man **DOXO**rubicin

U.S./Canadian Brand Names Adriamycin® [Can]; Adriamycin PFS® [US]; Adriamycin RDF® [US]; Rubex® [US]

Therapeutic Category Antineoplastic Agent

Use Treatment of leukemias, lymphomas, multiple myeloma, osseous and nonosseous sarcomas, mesotheliomas, germ cell tumors of the ovary or testis, and carcinomas of the head and neck, thyroid, lung, breast, stomach, pancreas, liver, ovary, bladder, prostate, uterus, and neuroblastoma

Usual Dosage Refer to individual protocols. I.V.:

Children:

35-75 mg/m^2 as a single dose, repeat every 21 days **or**

20-30 mg/m^2 once weekly **or**

60-90 mg/m^2 given as a continuous infusion over 96 hours every 3-4 weeks

Adults: Usual or typical dose: 60-75 mg/m^2 as a single dose, repeat every 21 days **or** other dosage regimens like 20-30 mg/m^2/day for 2-3 days, repeat in 4 weeks **or** 20 mg/m^2 once weekly

(Continued)

doxorubicin *(Continued)*

The lower dose regimen should be given to patients with decreased bone marrow reserve, prior therapy or marrow infiltration with malignant cells

Dosage Forms

Injection, powder for reconstitution, as hydrochloride: 10 mg, 20 mg, 50 mg [contains lactose]

Adriamycin RDF®: 10 mg, 20 mg, 50 mg, 150 mg [contains lactose; rapid dissolution formula]

Rubex®: 50 mg, 100 mg [contains lactose]

Injection, solution, as hydrochloride [preservative free]: 2 mg/mL (5 mL, 10 mL, 25 mL, 100 mL)

Adriamycin PFS® [preservative free]: 2 mg/mL (5 mL, 10 mL, 25 mL, 37.5 mL, 100 mL)

doxorubicin hydrochloride *see* doxorubicin *on previous page*

doxorubicin hydrochloride (liposomal) *see* doxorubicin (liposomal) *on this page*

doxorubicin (liposomal) (doks oh ROO bi sin lip pah SOW mal)

Sound-Alike/Look-Alike Issues

doxorubicin (liposomal) may be confused with dactinomycin, daunorubicin, doxacurium, doxapram, doxazosin, doxorubicin, idarubicin

Doxil® may be confused with DaunoXome®, Doxy®, Paxil®

Synonyms doxorubicin hydrochloride (liposomal)

Tall-Man **DOXO**rubicin (liposomal)

U.S./Canadian Brand Names Caelyx® [Can]; Doxil® [US]

Therapeutic Category Antineoplastic Agent

Use Treatment of AIDS-related Kaposi sarcoma, breast cancer, ovarian cancer, solid tumors

Usual Dosage Refer to individual protocols.

I.V.: 20 mg/m^2 over 30 minutes, once every 3 weeks, for as long as patients respond satisfactorily and tolerate treatment.

AIDS-KS patients: I.V.: 20 mg/m^2/dose over 30 minutes once every 3 weeks for as long as patients respond satisfactorily and tolerate treatment

Breast cancer: I.V.: 20-80 mg/m^2/dose has been studied in a limited number of phase I/II trials

Ovarian cancer: I.V.: 50 mg/m^2/dose repeated every 4 weeks (minimum of 4 courses is recommended)

Solid tumors: I.V.: 50-60 mg/m^2/dose repeated every 3-4 weeks has been studied in a limited number of phase I/II trials

Dosage Forms Injection, solution, as hydrochloride: 2 mg/mL (10 mL, 25 mL)

Doxy-100® [US] *see* doxycycline *on this page*

Doxycin [Can] *see* doxycycline *on this page*

doxycycline (doks i SYE kleen)

Sound-Alike/Look-Alike Issues

doxycycline may be confused with dicyclomine, doxepin, doxylamine

Doxy-100® may be confused with Doxil®

Monodox® may be confused with Maalox®

Synonyms doxycycline calcium; doxycycline hyclate; doxycycline monohydrate

U.S./Canadian Brand Names Adoxa™ [US]; Apo-Doxy® [Can]; Apo-Doxy Tabs® [Can]; Doryx® [US]; Doxy-100® [US]; Doxycin [Can]; Doxytec [Can]; Monodox® [US]; Novo-Doxylin [Can]; Nu-Doxycycline [Can]; Periostat® [US]; Vibramycin® [US]; Vibra-Tabs® [US/Can]

Therapeutic Category Tetracycline Derivative

Use Principally in the treatment of infections caused by susceptible *Rickettsia*, *Chlamydia*, and *Mycoplasma*; alternative to mefloquine for malaria prophylaxis; treatment for syphilis, uncomplicated *Neisseria gonorrhoeae, Listeria, Actinomyces israelii,* and *Clostridium* infections in penicillin-allergic patients; used for community-acquired pneumonia and other common infections due to susceptible organisms; anthrax due to *Bacillus anthracis,* including inhalational anthrax (postexposure); treatment of infections caused by uncommon susceptible gram-negative and gram-positive organisms including *Borrelia recurrentis, Ureaplasma urealyticum, Haemophilus ducreyi, Yersinia pestis, Francisella tularensis, Vibrio cholerae, Campylobacter fetus, Brucella* spp, *Bartonella bacilliformis,* and *Calymmatobacterium granulomatis*

Usual Dosage

Children:

Anthrax: Doxycycline should be used in children if antibiotic susceptibility testing, exhaustion of drug supplies, or allergic reaction preclude use of penicillin or ciprofloxacin. For treatment, the consensus recommendation does not include a loading dose for doxycycline.

Inhalational (postexposure prophylaxis) (*MMWR*, 2001, 50:889-893): Oral, I.V. (use oral route when possible): ≤8 years: 2.2 mg/kg every 12 hours for 60 days >8 years and ≤45 kg: 2.2 mg/kg every 12 hours for 60 days >8 years and >45 kg: 100 mg every 12 hours for 60 days

Cutaneous (treatment): Oral: See dosing for "Inhalational (postexposure prophylaxis)" **Note:** In the presence of systemic involvement, extensive edema, and/or lesions on head/neck, doxycycline should initially be administered I.V.

Inhalational/gastrointestinal/oropharyngeal (treatment): I.V.: Refer to dosing for inhalational anthrax (postexposure prophylaxis); switch to oral therapy when clinically appropriate; refer to Adults dosing for "Note" on combined therapy and duration

Children ≥8 years (<45 kg): Susceptible infections: Oral, I.V.: 2-5 mg/kg/day in 1-2 divided doses, not to exceed 200 mg/day

Children >8 years (>45 kg) and Adults: Susceptible infections: Oral, I.V.: 100-200 mg/day in 1-2 divided doses

Acute gonococcal infection (PID) in combination with another antibiotic: 100 mg every 12 hours until improved, followed by 100 mg orally twice daily to complete 14 days

Community-acquired pneumonia: 100 mg twice daily

Lyme disease: Oral: 100 mg twice daily for 14-21 days

Early syphilis: 200 mg/day in divided doses for 14 days

Late syphilis: 200 mg/day in divided doses for 28 days

Uncomplicated chlamydial infections: 100 mg twice daily for ≥7 days

Endometritis, salpingitis, parametritis, or peritonitis: 100 mg I.V. twice daily with cefoxitin 2 g every 6 hours for 4 days and for ≥48 hours after patient improves; then continue with oral therapy 100 mg twice daily to complete a 10- to 14-day course of therapy

Adults:

Anthrax:

Inhalational (postexposure prophylaxis): Oral, I.V. (use oral route when possible): 100 mg every 12 hours for 60 days (*MMWR*, 2001, 50:889-93); **Note:** Preliminary recommendation, FDA review and update is anticipated.

Cutaneous (treatment): Oral: 100 mg every 12 hours for 60 days. **Note:** In the presence of systemic involvement, extensive edema, lesions on head/neck, refer to I.V. dosing for treatment of inhalational/gastrointestinal/oropharyngeal anthrax

Inhalational/gastrointestinal/oropharyngeal (treatment): I.V.: Initial: 100 mg every 12 hours; switch to oral therapy when clinically appropriate; some recommend initial loading dose of 200 mg, followed by 100 mg every 8-12 hours (*JAMA*, 1997, 278:399-411). **Note:** Initial treatment should include two or more agents predicted to be effective (per CDC recommendations). Agents suggested for use in conjunction with doxycycline or ciprofloxacin include rifampin, vancomycin, imipenem, penicillin, ampicillin, chloramphenicol, clindamycin, and clarithromycin. May switch to oral antimicrobial therapy when clinically appropriate. Continue combined therapy for 60 days

Dosage Forms

Capsule, as hyclate: 50 mg, 100 mg

Vibramycin®: 100 mg

Capsule, as monohydrate (Monodox®): 50 mg, 100 mg

(Continued)

doxycycline *(Continued)*

Capsule, coated pellets, as hyclate (Doryx®): 75 mg, 100 mg
Injection, powder for reconstitution, as hyclate (Doxy-100®): 100 mg
Powder for oral suspension, as monohydrate (Vibramycin®): 25 mg/5 mL (60 mL) [raspberry flavor]
Syrup, as calcium (Vibramycin®): 50 mg/5 mL (480 mL) [contains sodium metabisulfite; raspberry-apple flavor]
Tablet, as hyclate: 100 mg
Periostat®: 20 mg
Vibra-Tabs®: 100 mg
Tablet, as monohydrate (Adoxa™): 50 mg, 75 mg, 100 mg

doxycycline calcium *see* doxycycline *on page 294*

doxycycline hyclate *see* doxycycline *on page 294*

doxycycline monohydrate *see* doxycycline *on page 294*

doxylamine (dox IL a meen)

Therapeutic Category Antihistamine
Use Sleep aid; antihistamine for hypersensitivity reactions and antiemetic
Usual Dosage Oral: Children >12 years and Adults: 25 mg at bedtime
Dosage Forms Tablet, as succinate: 25 mg

Doxytec [Can] *see* doxycycline *on page 294*

DPA *see* valproic acid and derivatives *on page 901*

D-Pan® ***(Discontinued)*** *see page 1042*

DPE *see* dipivefrin *on page 281*

D-penicillamine *see* penicillamine *on page 674*

DPH *see* phenytoin *on page 691*

DPM™ [US-OTC] *see* urea *on page 897*

Dramamine® Injection ***(Discontinued)*** *see page 1042*

Dramamine® Less Drowsy Formula [US-OTC] *see* meclizine *on page 546*

Dramamine® [US-OTC] *see* dimenhydrinate *on page 274*

Dramilin® Injection ***(Discontinued)*** *see page 1042*

Dramocen® ***(Discontinued)*** *see page 1042*

Dramoject® ***(Discontinued)*** *see page 1042*

dried smallpox vaccine *see* smallpox vaccine *on page 808*

Drinex® ***(Discontinued)*** *see page 1042*

Drisdol® [US/Can] *see* ergocalciferol *on page 317*

Dristan® Long Lasting Nasal [Can] *see* oxymetazoline *on page 658*

Dristan® Long Lasting Nasal Solution ***(Discontinued)*** *see page 1042*

Dristan® N.D. [Can] *see* acetaminophen and pseudoephedrine *on page 9*

Dristan® N.D., Extra Strength [Can] *see* acetaminophen and pseudoephedrine *on page 9*

Dristan® Saline Spray ***(Discontinued)*** *see page 1042*

Dristan® Sinus Tablet [US-OTC/Can] *see* pseudoephedrine and ibuprofen *on page 747*

Drithocreme® [US] *see* anthralin *on page 60*

Drithocreme® HP 1% ***(Discontinued)*** *see page 1042*

Dritho-Scalp® [US] *see* anthralin *on page 60*

Drixoral® [Can] *see* dexbrompheniramine and pseudoephedrine *on page 256*

Drixoral® Cold & Allergy [US-OTC] *see* dexbrompheniramine and pseudoephedrine *on page 256*

Drixoral® Cough & Congestion Liquid Caps *(Discontinued)* *see page 1042*

Drixoral® Cough Liquid Caps *(Discontinued)* *see page 1042*

Drixoral® Nasal [Can] *see* oxymetazoline *on page 658*

Drixoral® ND [Can] *see* pseudoephedrine *on page 745*

Drixoral® Non-Drowsy *(Discontinued)* *see page 1042*

Drize®-R [US] *see* chlorpheniramine, phenylephrine, and methscopolamine *on page 192*

dronabinol (droe NAB i nol)

Sound-Alike/Look-Alike Issues

dronabinol may be confused with droperidol

Synonyms delta-9-tetrahydro-cannabinol; delta-9 THC; tetrahydrocannabinol; THC

U.S./Canadian Brand Names Marinol® [US/Can]

Therapeutic Category Antiemetic

Controlled Substance C-III

Use Chemotherapy-associated nausea and vomiting refractory to other antiemetic; AIDS- and cancer-related anorexia

Usual Dosage Refer to individual protocols. Oral:

Antiemetic:

Children: 5 mg/m^2 starting 6-8 hours before chemotherapy and every 4-6 hours after to be continued for 12 hours after chemotherapy is discontinued

Adults: 5 mg/m^2 1-3 hours before chemotherapy, then 5 mg/m^2/dose every 2-4 hours after chemotherapy for a total of 4-6 doses/day; increase doses in increments of 2.5 mg/m^2 to a maximum of 15 mg/m^2/dose.

Appetite stimulant: Initial: 2.5 mg twice daily (before lunch and dinner); titrate up to a maximum of 20 mg/day.

Dosage Forms Capsule, gelatin: 2.5 mg, 5 mg, 10 mg [contains sesame oil]

droperidol (droe PER i dole)

Sound-Alike/Look-Alike Issues

droperidol may be confused with dronabinol

Inapsine® may be confused with Nebcin®

Synonyms dehydrobenzperidol

U.S./Canadian Brand Names Inapsine® [US]

Therapeutic Category Antiemetic; Antipsychotic Agent, Butyrophenone

Use Antiemetic in surgical and diagnostic procedures; preoperative medication in patients when other treatments are ineffective or inappropriate

Usual Dosage Titrate carefully to desired effect

Children 2-12 years: Nausea and vomiting: I.M., I.V.: 0.05-0.06 mg/kg (maximum initial dose: 0.1 mg/kg); additional doses may be repeated to achieve effect; administer additional doses with caution

Adults: Nausea and vomiting: I.M., I.V.: Initial: 2.5 mg; additional doses of 1.25 mg may be administered to achieve desired effect; administer additional doses with caution

Dosage Forms Injection, solution: 2.5 mg/mL (1 mL, 2 mL)

drospirenone and ethinyl estradiol *see* ethinyl estradiol and drospirenone *on page 337*

drotrecogin alfa (droe tre KOE jin AL fa)

Synonyms activated protein C, human, recombinant; drotrecogin alfa, activated; protein C (activated), human, recombinant

U.S./Canadian Brand Names Xigris™ [US/Can]

Therapeutic Category Protein C (Activated)

(Continued)

drotrecogin alfa *(Continued)*

Use Reduction of mortality from severe sepsis (associated with organ dysfunction) in adults at high risk of death (eg, APACHE II score ≥25)

Usual Dosage I.V.: Adults: Sepsis: 24 mcg/kg/hour for a total of 96 hours; stop infusion **immediately** if clinically-important bleeding is identified

Dosage Forms Injection, powder for reconstitution [preservative free]: 5 mg [contains sucrose 31.8 mg], 20 mg [contains sucrose 124.9 mg]

drotrecogin alfa, activated *see* drotrecogin alfa *on previous page*

Droxia™ [US] *see* hydroxyurea *on page 457*

Dr. Scholl's® Callus Remover [US-OTC] *see* salicylic acid *on page 789*

Dr. Scholl's® Clear Away [US-OTC] *see* salicylic acid *on page 789*

Drug Products No Longer Available in the U.S. *see page 1042*

Dry Eye® Therapy Solution *(Discontinued)* *see page 1042*

Dryox® Gel *(Discontinued)* *see page 1042*

Dryox® Wash *(Discontinued)* *see page 1042*

Drysol™ [US] *see* aluminum chloride hexahydrate *on page 39*

Dryvax® [US] *see* smallpox vaccine *on page 808*

DSCG *see* cromolyn sodium *on page 230*

D-Ser(Bu^t)^6,Azgly^{10}-LHRH *see* goserelin *on page 413*

DSMC Plus® *(Discontinued)* *see page 1042*

DSS *see* docusate *on page 285*

D-S-S Plus® *(Discontinued)* *see page 1042*

D-S-S® [US-OTC] *see* docusate *on page 285*

DT *see* diphtheria and tetanus toxoid *on page 280*

DTaP *see* diphtheria, tetanus toxoids, and acellular pertussis vaccine *on page 280*

DTIC *see* dacarbazine *on page 241*

DTIC® [Can] *see* dacarbazine *on page 241*

DTIC-Dome® [US] *see* dacarbazine *on page 241*

DTO *see* opium tincture *on page 647*

D-Trp(6)-LHRH *see* triptorelin *on page 890*

Duac™ [US] *see* clindamycin and benzoyl peroxide *on page 211*

Duadacin® Capsule *(Discontinued)* *see page 1042*

Duet® [US] *see* vitamins (multiple/prenatal) *on page 927*

Duet® DHA [US] *see* vitamins (multiple/prenatal) *on page 927*

Dulcolax® Milk of Magnesia [US-OTC] *see* magnesium hydroxide *on page 537*

Dulcolax® Stool Softener [US-OTC] *see* docusate *on page 285*

Dulcolax® [US-OTC/Can] *see* bisacodyl *on page 120*

Dull-C® [US-OTC] *see* ascorbic acid *on page 79*

DuoCet™ *(Discontinued)* *see page 1042*

Duo-Cyp® *(Discontinued)* *see page 1042*

DuoFilm® [US-OTC/Can] *see* salicylic acid *on page 789*

Duoforte® 27 [Can] *see* salicylic acid *on page 789*

Duo-Medihaler® *(Discontinued)* *see page 1042*

Duonalc® [Can] *see* alcohol (ethyl) *on page 27*

Duonalc-E® Mild [Can] *see* alcohol (ethyl) *on page 27*
DuoNeb™ [US] *see* ipratropium and albuterol *on page 483*
DuoPlant® ***(Discontinued)*** *see page 1042*
Duo-Trach® Injection ***(Discontinued)*** *see page 1042*
Duotrate® ***(Discontinued)*** *see page 1042*
DuP 753 *see* losartan *on page 531*
Duphalac® ***(Discontinued)*** *see page 1042*
Durabolin® [Can] *see* nandrolone *on page 603*
Duracid® ***(Discontinued)*** *see page 1042*
Duraclon™ [US] *see* clonidine *on page 215*
Duract® ***(Discontinued)*** *see page 1042*
Duradyne DHC® ***(Discontinued)*** *see page 1042*
Duragesic® [US/Can] *see* fentanyl *on page 361*
Dura-Gest® ***(Discontinued)*** *see page 1042*
Duralith® [Can] *see* lithium *on page 525*
Duralone® Injection ***(Discontinued)*** *see page 1042*
Duramist® Plus [US-OTC] *see* oxymetazoline *on page 658*
Duramorph® [US] *see* morphine sulfate *on page 591*
Duranest® (plain and with epinephrine) ***(Discontinued)*** *see page 1042*
Duratest® Injection ***(Discontinued)*** *see page 1042*
Duratestrin® ***(Discontinued)*** *see page 1042*
Durathate® Injection ***(Discontinued)*** *see page 1042*
Duration® [US-OTC] *see* oxymetazoline *on page 658*
Duratuss® DM [US] *see* guaifenesin and dextromethorphan *on page 416*
Duratuss® HD [US] *see* hydrocodone, pseudoephedrine, and guaifenesin *on page 447*
Dura-Vent® ***(Discontinued)*** *see page 1042*
Dura-Vent®/DA ***(Discontinued)*** *see page 1042*
Duricef® [US/Can] *see* cefadroxil *on page 166*
Duricef® Oral Suspension 125 mg/5 mL ***(Discontinued)*** *see page 1042*
Durrax® Oral ***(Discontinued)*** *see page 1042*

dutasteride (doo TAS teer ide)

U.S./Canadian Brand Names Avodart™ [US]
Therapeutic Category Antineoplastic Agent, Anthracenedione
Use Treatment of symptomatic benign prostatic hyperplasia (BPH)
Usual Dosage Oral: Adults: Male: 0.5 mg once daily
Dosage Forms Capsule, softgel: 0.5 mg

Duvoid® ***(Discontinued)*** *see page 1042*
Duvoid® [Can] *see* bethanechol *on page 117*
DVA *see* vindesine *on page 912*
D-Vi-Sol® [Can] *see* cholecalciferol *on page 196*
DV® Vaginal Cream ***(Discontinued)*** *see page 1042*
DW286 *see* gemifloxacin *on page 400*
Dwelle® Ophthalmic Solution ***(Discontinued)*** *see page 1042*

d-xylose (dee-ZYE lose)

Synonyms wood sugar

Therapeutic Category Diagnostic Agent

Use Evaluating intestinal absorption and diagnosing malabsorptive states

Usual Dosage Oral:

Infants and young Children: 500 mg/kg as a 5% to 10% aqueous solution

Children: 5 g is dissolved in 250 mL water; additional fluids are permitted and are encouraged for children

Adults: 25 g dissolved in 200-300 mL water followed with an additional 200-400 mL water **or** 5 g dissolved in 200-300 mL water followed by an additional 200-400 mL water

Dosage Forms Powder for oral solution: 25 g

Dyazide® [US] *see* hydrochlorothiazide and triamterene *on page 443*

Dycil® [Can] *see* dicloxacillin *on page 267*

Dycill® *(Discontinued)* *see page 1042*

Dyclone® *(Discontinued)* *see page 1042*

dyclonine (DYE kloe neen)

Sound-Alike/Look-Alike Issues

dyclonine may be confused with dicyclomine

Synonyms dyclonine hydrochloride

U.S./Canadian Brand Names Cēpacol® Maximum Strength [US-OTC]; Sucrets® [US-OTC]

Therapeutic Category Local Anesthetic

Use Local anesthetic prior to laryngoscopy, bronchoscopy, or endotracheal intubation; use topically for temporary relief of pain associated with oral mucosa or anogenital lesions

Usual Dosage Use the lowest dose needed to provide effective anesthesia

Children and Adults:

Topical solution:

Mouth sores: 5-10 mL of 0.5% or 1% to oral mucosa (swab or swish and then spit) 3-4 times/day as needed; maximum single dose: 200 mg (40 mL of 0.5% solution or 20 mL of 1% solution)

Bronchoscopy: Use 2 mL of the 1% solution or 4 mL of the 0.5% solution sprayed onto the larynx and trachea every 5 minutes until the reflex has been abolished

Children >2 years and Adults: Lozenge: Slowly dissolve 1 lozenge in mouth every 2 hours as needed

Dosage Forms

Lozenge, as hydrochloride (Sucrets®): 1.2 mg, 2 mg, 3 mg [cherry, lemon, wintergreen, and assorted flavors]

Spray, oral, as hydrochloride (Cēpacol® Maximum Strength): 0.1% (120 mL) [cherry and menthol flavors]

dyclonine hydrochloride *see* dyclonine *on this page*

Dyflex-400® Tablet *(Discontinued)* *see page 1042*

Dymelor® *(Discontinued)* *see page 1042*

Dymenate® Injection *(Discontinued)* *see page 1042*

Dynabac® [US] *see* dirithromycin *on page 282*

Dynacin® [US] *see* minocycline *on page 583*

DynaCirc® [US/Can] *see* isradipine *on page 490*

DynaCirc® CR [US] *see* isradipine *on page 490*

Dyna-Hex® [US-OTC] *see* chlorhexidine gluconate *on page 183*

Dynapen® *(Discontinued)* *see page 1042*

Dynex [US] *see* guaifenesin and pseudoephedrine *on page 419*

dyphylline (DYE fi lin)

Synonyms dihydroxypropyl theophylline

U.S./Canadian Brand Names Dilor® [US/Can]; Lufyllin® [US/Can]

Therapeutic Category Theophylline Derivative

Use Bronchodilator in reversible airway obstruction due to asthma or COPD

Usual Dosage

Children: I.M.: 4.4-6.6 mg/kg/day in divided doses

Adults:

Oral: Up to 15 mg/kg 4 times/day, individualize dosage

I.M.: 250-500 mg, do not exceed total dosage of 15 mg/kg every 6 hours

Dosage Forms

Elixir: Lufyllin®: 100 mg/15 mL (473 mL) [contains alcohol 20%]

Injection, solution (Dilor®): 250 mg/mL (2 mL)

Tablet (Dilor®, Lufyllin®): 200 mg, 400 mg

Dyrenium® [US] *see* triamterene *on page 882*

Dyrexan-OD® ***(Discontinued)*** *see page 1042*

E_2C and MPA *see* estradiol cypionate and medroxyprogesterone acetate *on page 328*

7E3 *see* abciximab *on page 3*

E2020 *see* donepezil *on page 288*

Easprin® [US] *see* aspirin *on page 80*

echothiophate iodide (ek oh THYE oh fate EYE oh dide)

Synonyms ecostigmine iodide

U.S./Canadian Brand Names Phospholine Iodide® [US]

Therapeutic Category Cholinesterase Inhibitor

Use Used as miotic in treatment of open-angle glaucoma; may be useful in specific case of narrow-angle glaucoma; accommodative esotropia

Usual Dosage Adults:

Ophthalmic: Glaucoma: Instill 1 drop twice daily into eyes with 1 dose just prior to bedtime; some patients have been treated with 1 dose daily or every other day

Accommodative esotropia:

Diagnosis: Instill 1 drop of 0.125% once daily into both eyes at bedtime for 2-3 weeks

Treatment: Use lowest concentration and frequency which gives satisfactory response, with a maximum dose of 0.125% once daily, although more intensive therapy may be used for short periods of time

Dosage Forms Powder for reconstitution, ophthalmic: 6.25 mg [0.125%]

EC-Naprosyn® [US] *see* naproxen *on page 605*

E. coli **asparaginase** *see* asparaginase *on page 80*

econazole (e KONE a zole)

Synonyms econazole nitrate

U.S./Canadian Brand Names Ecostatin® [Can]; Spectazole® [US/Can]

Therapeutic Category Antifungal Agent

Use Topical treatment of tinea pedis (athlete's foot), tinea cruris (jock itch), tinea corporis (ringworm), tinea versicolor, and cutaneous candidiasis

Usual Dosage Children and Adults: Topical:

Tinea pedis, tinea cruris, tinea corporis, tinea versicolor: Apply sufficient amount to cover affected areas once daily

Cutaneous candidiasis: Apply sufficient quantity twice daily (morning and evening)

(Continued)

econazole *(Continued)*

Duration of treatment: Candidal infections and tinea cruris, versicolor, and corporis should be treated for 2 weeks and tinea pedis for 1 month; occasionally, longer treatment periods may be required

Dosage Forms Cream, topical, as nitrate: 1% (15 g, 30 g, 85 g)

econazole nitrate *see* econazole *on previous page*

Econopred® [US] *see* prednisolone (ophthalmic) *on page 723*

Econopred® Plus [US] *see* prednisolone (ophthalmic) *on page 723*

Ecostatin® [Can] *see* econazole *on previous page*

ecostigmine iodide *see* echothiophate iodide *on previous page*

Ecotrin® Low Strength [US-OTC] *see* aspirin *on page 80*

Ecotrin® Maximum Strength [US-OTC] *see* aspirin *on page 80*

Ecotrin® [US-OTC] *see* aspirin *on page 80*

Ectosone [Can] *see* betamethasone (topical) *on page 116*

Ed A-Hist® [US] *see* chlorpheniramine and phenylephrine *on page 188*

edathamil disodium *see* edetate disodium *on next page*

Edecrin® [US/Can] *see* ethacrynic acid *on page 334*

edetate calcium disodium (ED e tate KAL see um dye SOW dee um)

Synonyms calcium disodium edetate; calcium EDTA

U.S./Canadian Brand Names Calcium Disodium Versenate® [US]

Therapeutic Category Chelating Agent

Use Treatment of symptomatic acute and chronic lead poisoning or for symptomatic patients with high blood lead levels; used as an aid in the diagnosis of lead poisoning; possibly useful in poisoning by zinc, manganese, and certain heavy radioisotopes

Usual Dosage Several regimens have been recommended:

Diagnosis of lead poisoning: Mobilization test (not recommended by AAP guidelines): I.M., I.V.:

Children: 500 mg/m^2/dose (maximum dose: 1 g) as a single dose or divided into 2 doses

Adults: 500 mg/m^2/dose

Note: Urine is collected for 24 hours after first EDTA dose and analyzed for lead content; if the ratio of mcg of lead in urine to mg calcium EDTA given is >1, then test is considered positive; for convenience, an 8-hour urine collection may be done after a single 50 mg/kg I.M. (maximum dose: 1 g) or 500 mg/m^2 I.V. dose; a positive test occurs if the ratio of lead excretion to mg calcium EDTA >0.5-0.6.

Treatment of lead poisoning: Children and Adults (each regimen is specific for route):

Symptoms of lead encephalopathy and/or blood lead level >70 mcg/dL: Treat 5 days; give in conjunction with dimercaprol; wait a minimum of 2 days with no treatment before considering a repeat course:

I.M.: 250 mg/m^2/dose every 4 hours

I.V.: 50 mg/kg/day as 24-hour continuous I.V. infusion **or** 1-1.5 g/m^2 I.V. as either an 8- to 24-hour infusion or divided into 2 doses every 12 hours

Symptomatic lead poisoning **without** encephalopathy **or** asymptomatic with blood lead level >70 mcg/dL: Treat 3-5 days; treatment with dimercaprol is recommended until the blood lead level concentration <50 mcg/dL:

I.M.: 167 mg/m^2 every 4 hours

I.V.: 1 g/m^2 as an 8- to 24-hour infusion or divided every 12 hours

Asymptomatic **children** with blood lead level 45-69 mcg/dL: I.V.: 25 mg/kg/day for 5 days as an 8- to 24-hour infusion or divided into 2 doses every 12 hours

Depending upon the blood lead level, additional courses may be necessary; repeat at least 2-4 days and preferably 2-4 weeks apart

Adults with lead nephropathy: An alternative dosing regimen reflecting the reduction in renal clearance is based upon the serum creatinine. Refer to the following:

Dose of Ca EDTA based on serum creatinine:
S_{cr} ≤2 mg/dL: 1 g/m²/day for 5 days*
S_{cr} 2-3 mg/dL: 500 mg/m²/day for 5 days*
S_{cr} 3-4 mg/dL: 500 mg/m²/dose every 48 hours for 3 doses*
S_{cr} >4 mg/dL: 500 mg/m²/week*
*Repeat these regimens monthly until lead excretion is reduced toward normal.

Dosage Forms Injection, solution: 200 mg/mL (5 mL)

edetate disodium (ED e tate dye SOW dee um)

Synonyms edathamil disodium; EDTA; sodium edetate

U.S./Canadian Brand Names Endrate® [US]

Therapeutic Category Chelating Agent

Use Emergency treatment of hypercalcemia; control digitalis-induced cardiac dysrhythmias (ventricular arrhythmias)

Usual Dosage Hypercalcemia: I.V.:

Children: 40-70 mg/kg/day slow infusion over 3-4 hours or more to a maximum of 3 g/24 hours; administer for 5 days and allow 5 days between courses of therapy

Adults: 50 mg/kg/day over 3 or more hours to a maximum of 3 g/24 hours; a suggested regimen of 5 days followed by 2 days without drug and repeated courses up to 15 total doses

Digitalis-induced arrhythmias: Children and Adults: 15 mg/kg/hour (maximum dose: 60 mg/kg/day) as continuous infusion

Dosage Forms Injection, solution: 150 mg/mL (20 mL)

Edex® [US] *see* alprostadil *on page 35*

edrophonium (ed roe FOE nee um)

Synonyms edrophonium chloride

U.S./Canadian Brand Names Enlon® [US/Can]; Reversol® [US]

Therapeutic Category Cholinergic Agent

Use Diagnosis of myasthenia gravis; differentiation of cholinergic crises from myasthenia crises; reversal of nondepolarizing neuromuscular blockers; adjunct treatment of respiratory depression caused by curare overdose

Usual Dosage Usually administered I.V., however, if not possible, I.M. or SubQ may be used:

Infants:
- I.M.: 0.5-1 mg
- I.V.: Initial: 0.1 mg, followed by 0.4 mg if no response; total dose = 0.5 mg

Children:
- Diagnosis: Initial: 0.04 mg/kg over 1 minute followed by 0.16 mg/kg if no response, to a maximum total dose of 5 mg for children <34 kg, or 10 mg for children >34 kg **or**
- Alternative dosing (manufacturer's recommendation):
  - ≤34 kg: 1 mg; if no response after 45 seconds, repeat dosage in 1 mg increments every 30-45 seconds, up to a total of 5 mg
  - >34 kg: 2 mg; if no response after 45 seconds, repeat dosage in 1 mg increments every 30-45 seconds, up to a total of 10 mg
- I.M.:
  - <34 kg: 1 mg
  - >34 kg: 5 mg
- Titration of oral anticholinesterase therapy: 0.04 mg/kg once given 1 hour after oral intake of the drug being used in treatment; if strength improves, an increase in neostigmine or pyridostigmine dose is indicated

Adults:
- Diagnosis:
  - I.V.: 2 mg test dose administered over 15-30 seconds; 8 mg given 45 seconds later if no response is seen; test dose may be repeated after 30 minutes

(Continued)

edrophonium *(Continued)*

I.M.: Initial: 10 mg; if no cholinergic reaction occurs, administer 2 mg 30 minutes later to rule out false-negative reaction

Titration of oral anticholinesterase therapy: 1-2 mg given 1 hour after oral dose of anticholinesterase; if strength improves, an increase in neostigmine or pyridostigmine dose is indicated

Reversal of nondepolarizing neuromuscular blocking agents (neostigmine with atropine usually preferred): I.V.: 10 mg over 30-45 seconds; may repeat every 5-10 minutes up to 40 mg

Termination of paroxysmal atrial tachycardia: I.V. rapid injection: 5-10 mg

Differentiation of cholinergic from myasthenic crisis: I.V.: 1 mg; may repeat after 1 minute. **Note:** Intubation and controlled ventilation may be required if patient has cholinergic crisis

Dosage Forms Injection, solution, as chloride:

Enlon®: 10 mg/mL (15 mL) [contains sodium sulfite]

Reversol®: 10 mg/mL (10 mL) [contains sodium sulfite]

edrophonium chloride *see* edrophonium *on previous page*

ED-SPAZ® ***(Discontinued)*** *see page 1042*

EDTA *see* edetate disodium *on previous page*

E.E.S.® [US/Can] *see* erythromycin *on page 320*

efalizumab (e fa li ZOO mab)

Synonyms anti-CD11a; hu1124

U.S./Canadian Brand Names Raptiva™ [US]

Therapeutic Category Immunosuppressant Agent; Monoclonal Antibody

Use Treatment of chronic moderate-to-severe plaque psoriasis in patients who are candidates for systemic therapy or phototherapy

Usual Dosage SubQ: Adults: Psoriasis: Initial: 0.7 mg/kg, followed by weekly dose of 1 mg/kg (maximum: 200 mg/dose)

Dosage Forms Injection, powder for reconstitution: 150 mg [contains sucrose 123.2 mg/vial; delivers 125 mg/1.25 mL; packaged with prefilled syringe containing sterile water for injection]

efavirenz (e FAV e renz)

U.S./Canadian Brand Names Sustiva® [US/Can]

Therapeutic Category Nonnucleoside Reverse Transcriptase Inhibitor (NNRTI)

Use Treatment of HIV-1 infections in combination with at least two other antiretroviral agents

Usual Dosage Oral: Dosing at bedtime is recommended to limit central nervous system effects; should not be used as single-agent therapy

Children: Dosage is based on body weight

- 10 kg to <15 kg: 200 mg once daily
- 15 kg to <20 kg: 250 mg once daily
- 20 kg to <25 kg: 300 mg once daily
- 25 kg to <32.5 kg: 350 mg once daily
- 32.5 kg to <40 kg: 400 mg once daily
- ≥40 kg: 600 mg once daily

Adults: 600 mg once daily

Dosage Forms

Capsule: 50 mg, 100 mg, 200 mg

Tablet: 600 mg

Effer-K™ [US] *see* potassium bicarbonate and potassium citrate, effervescent *on page 712*

Effer-Syllium® ***(Discontinued)*** *see page 1042*

Effexor® [US/Can] *see* venlafaxine *on page 908*

Effexor® XR [US/Can] *see* venlafaxine *on page 908*

Eflone® ***(Discontinued)*** *see page 1042*

eflornithine (ee FLOR ni theen)

Sound-Alike/Look-Alike Issues

Vaniqa™ may be confused with Viagra®

Synonyms DFMO; eflornithine hydrochloride

U.S./Canadian Brand Names Vaniqa™ [US]

Therapeutic Category Antiprotozoal; Topical Skin Product

Use Cream: Females ≥12 years: Reduce unwanted hair from face and adjacent areas under the chin

Orphan status: Injection: Treatment of meningoencephalitic stage of *Trypanosoma brucei gambiense* infection (sleeping sickness)

Usual Dosage

Children ≥12 years and Adults: Females: Topical: Apply thin layer of cream to affected areas of face and adjacent chin twice daily, at least 8 hours apart

Adults: I.V. infusion: 100 mg/kg/dose given every 6 hours (over at least 45 minutes) for 14 days

Dosage Forms

Cream, topical, as hydrochloride: 13.9% (30 g)

Injection, solution, as hydrochloride: 200 mg/mL (100 mL) [orphan drug status]

eflornithine hydrochloride *see* eflornithine *on this page*

Efodine® ***(Discontinued)*** *see page 1042*

eformoterol and budesonide *see* budesonide and formoterol *(Canada only) on page 132*

Efudex® [US/Can] *see* fluorouracil *on page 378*

E-Gems® [US-OTC] *see* vitamin E *on page 918*

EHDP *see* etidronate disodium *on page 350*

Elase® (all products) ***(Discontinued)*** *see page 1042*

Elase®-Chloromycetin® Ointment ***(Discontinued)*** *see page 1042*

Elavil® ***(Discontinued)*** *see page 1042*

Eldepryl® [US/Can] *see* selegiline *on page 798*

Eldepryl® Tablet (only) ***(Discontinued)*** *see page 1042*

eldisine lilly 99094 *see* vindesine *on page 912*

Eldopaque Forte® [US] *see* hydroquinone *on page 454*

Eldopaque® [US-OTC/Can] *see* hydroquinone *on page 454*

Eldoquin® [US/Can] *see* hydroquinone *on page 454*

Eldoquin® Forte® [US] *see* hydroquinone *on page 454*

Eldoquin® Lotion ***(Discontinued)*** *see page 1042*

electrolyte lavage solution *see* polyethylene glycol-electrolyte solution *on page 706*

eletriptan (el e TRIP tan)

Synonyms eletriptan hydrobromide

U.S./Canadian Brand Names Relpax® [US]

Therapeutic Category Serotonin $5\text{-}HT_{1B,\ 1D}$ Receptor Agonist

Use Acute treatment of migraine, with or without aura

Usual Dosage Oral: Adults: Acute migraine: 20-40 mg; if the headache improves but returns, dose may be repeated after 2 hours have elapsed since first dose; maximum 80 mg/day.

(Continued)

eletriptan *(Continued)*

Note: If the first dose is ineffective, diagnosis needs to be re-evaluated. Safety of treating >3 headaches/month has not been established.

Dosage Forms Tablet, as hydrobromide [film coated]: 20 mg, 40 mg [as base]

eletriptan hydrobromide *see* eletriptan *on previous page*

Elidel® [US/Can] *see* pimecrolimus *on page 695*

Eligard® [US] *see* leuprolide acetate *on page 509*

Elimite® [US] *see* permethrin *on page 683*

elipten *see* aminoglutethimide *on page 45*

Elitek™ [US] *see* rasburicase *on page 764*

Elixomin® ***(Discontinued)*** *see page 1042*

Elixophyllin® [US] *see* theophylline *on page 854*

Elixophyllin-GG® [US] *see* theophylline and guaifenesin *on page 855*

Elixophyllin SR® ***(Discontinued)*** *see page 1042*

ElixSure™ Cough [US-OTC] *see* dextromethorphan *on page 261*

ElixSure™ Fever/Pain [US-OTC] *see* acetaminophen *on page 5*

Ellence® [US/Can] *see* epirubicin *on page 313*

Elmiron® [US/Can] *see* pentosan polysulfate sodium *on page 680*

Elocom® [Can] *see* mometasone furoate *on page 589*

Elocon® [US] *see* mometasone furoate *on page 589*

E-Lor® Tablet ***(Discontinued)*** *see page 1042*

Eloxatin™ [US] *see* oxaliplatin *on page 652*

Elspar® [US/Can] *see* asparaginase *on page 80*

Eltor® [Can] *see* pseudoephedrine *on page 745*

Eltroxin® [Can] *see* levothyroxine *on page 516*

Emadine® [US] *see* emedastine *on this page*

Embeline™ [US] *see* clobetasol *on page 212*

Embeline™ E [US] *see* clobetasol *on page 212*

Emcyt® [US/Can] *see* estramustine *on page 329*

Emecheck® ***(Discontinued)*** *see page 1042*

emedastine (em e DAS teen)

Synonyms emedastine difumarate

U.S./Canadian Brand Names Emadine® [US]

Therapeutic Category Antihistamine, H_1 Blocker, Ophthalmic

Use Treatment of allergic conjunctivitis

Usual Dosage Ophthalmic: Children ≥3 years and Adults: Instill 1 drop in affected eye up to 4 times/day

Dosage Forms Solution, ophthalmic, as difumarate: 0.05% (5 mL) [contains benzalkonium chloride]

emedastine difumarate *see* emedastine *on this page*

Emend® [US] *see* aprepitant *on page 74*

Emete-Con® Injection ***(Discontinued)*** *see page 1042*

emetine hydrochloride ***(Discontinued)*** *see page 1042*

Emetrol® [US-OTC] *see* fructose, dextrose, and phosphoric acid *on page 392*

Emitrip® ***(Discontinued)*** *see page 1042*

Emko® [US-OTC] *see* nonoxynol 9 *on page 626*

EMLA® [US/Can] *see* lidocaine and prilocaine *on page 520*

Emo-Cort® [Can] *see* hydrocortisone (rectal) *on page 448*

emtricitabine (em trye SYE ta been)

Synonyms BW524W91; coviracil; FTC

U.S./Canadian Brand Names Emtriva™ [US]

Therapeutic Category Antiretroviral Agent, Reverse Transcriptase Inhibitor (Nucleoside)

Use Treatment of HIV infection in combination with at least two other antiretroviral agents

Usual Dosage Oral: Adults: 200 mg once daily

Dosage Forms Capsule: 200 mg

emtricitabine and tenofovir (em trye SYE ta been & te NOE fo veer)

Synonyms tenofovir and emtricitabine

U.S./Canadian Brand Names Truvada™ [US]

Therapeutic Category Antiretroviral Agent, Reverse Transcriptase Inhibitor (Nucleoside); Antiretroviral Agent, Reverse Transcriptase Inhibitor (Nucleotide)

Use Treatment of HIV infection in combination with other antiretroviral agents

Usual Dosage Adults: Oral: One tablet (emtricitabine 200 mg and tenofovir 300 mg) once daily

Dosage Forms Tablet, film coated: Emtricitabine 200 mg and tenofovir disoproxil fumarate 300 mg

Emtriva™ [US] *see* emtricitabine *on this page*

Emulsoil® ***(Discontinued)*** *see page 1042*

E-Mycin® ***(Discontinued)*** *see page 1042*

E-Mycin-E® ***(Discontinued)*** *see page 1042*

ENA 713 *see* rivastigmine *on page 781*

enalapril (e NAL a pril)

Sound-Alike/Look-Alike Issues

enalapril may be confused with Anafranil®, Elavil®, Eldepryl®, nafarelin, ramipril

Synonyms enalaprilat; enalapril maleate

U.S./Canadian Brand Names Vasotec® [US/Can]

Therapeutic Category Angiotensin-Converting Enzyme (ACE) Inhibitor

Use Management of mild to severe hypertension; treatment of congestive heart failure, left ventricular dysfunction after myocardial infarction

Usual Dosage Use lower listed initial dose in patients with hyponatremia, hypovolemia, severe congestive heart failure, decreased renal function, or in those receiving diuretics.

Oral: **Enalapril**: Children 1 month to 16 years: Hypertension: Initial: 0.08 mg/kg (up to 5 mg) once daily; adjust dosage based on patient response; doses >0.58 mg/kg (40 mg) have not been evaluated in pediatric patients

Investigational: Congestive heart failure: Initial oral doses of **enalapril**: 0.1 mg/kg/day increasing as needed over 2 weeks to 0.5 mg/kg/day have been used in infants

Investigational: Neonatal hypertension: I.V. doses of **enalaprilat**: 5-10 mcg/kg/dose administered every 8-24 hours have been used; monitor patients carefully; select patients may require higher doses

Adults:

Oral: **Enalapril:**

Hypertension: 2.5-5 mg/day then increase as required, usually at 1- to 2-week intervals; usual dose range (JNC 7): 2.5-40 mg/day in 1-2 divided doses. **Note:** Initiate with 2.5 mg if patient is taking a diuretic which cannot be discontinued. May add a diuretic if blood pressure cannot be controlled with enalapril alone.

(Continued)

enalapril *(Continued)*

Heart failure: As standard therapy alone or with diuretics, beta-blockers, and digoxin, initiate with 2.5 mg once or twice daily (usual range: 5-20 mg/day in 2 divided doses; target: 40 mg). Titrate slowly at 1- to 2-week intervals.

Asymptomatic left ventricular dysfunction: 2.5 mg twice daily, titrated as tolerated to 20 mg/day

I.V.: **Enalaprilat:**

Hypertension: 1.25 mg/dose, given over 5 minutes every 6 hours; doses as high as 5 mg/dose every 6 hours have been tolerated for up to 36 hours. **Note:** If patients are concomitantly receiving diuretic therapy, begin with 0.625 mg I.V. over 5 minutes; if the effect is not adequate after 1 hour, repeat the dose and administer 1.25 mg at 6-hour intervals thereafter; if adequate, administer 0.625 mg I.V. every 6 hours.

Heart failure: Avoid I.V. administration in patients with unstable heart failure or those suffering acute myocardial infarction.

Conversion from I.V. to oral therapy if not concurrently on diuretics: 5 mg once daily; subsequent titration as needed; if concurrently receiving diuretics and responding to 0.625 mg I.V. every 6 hours, initiate with 2.5 mg/day.

Dosage Forms

Injection, solution, as enalaprilat: 1.25 mg/mL (1 mL, 2 mL) [contains benzyl alcohol]

Tablet, as maleate (Vasotec®): 2.5 mg, 5 mg, 10 mg, 20 mg

enalapril and felodipine (e NAL a pril & fe LOE di peen)

Synonyms felodipine and enalapril

U.S./Canadian Brand Names Lexxel® [US/Can]

Therapeutic Category Antihypertensive Agent, Combination

Use Treatment of hypertension, however, not indicated for initial treatment of hypertension; replacement therapy in patients receiving separate dosage forms (for patient convenience); when monotherapy with one component fails to achieve desired antihypertensive effect, or when dose-limiting adverse effects limit upward titration of monotherapy

Usual Dosage Adults: Oral: 1 tablet daily

Dosage Forms Tablet, extended release:

Enalapril maleate 5 mg and felodipine 2.5 mg

Enalapril maleate 5 mg and felodipine 5 mg

enalapril and hydrochlorothiazide

(e NAL a pril & hye droe klor oh THYE a zide)

Synonyms hydrochlorothiazide and enalapril

U.S./Canadian Brand Names Vaseretic® [US/Can]

Therapeutic Category Antihypertensive Agent, Combination

Use Treatment of hypertension

Usual Dosage Oral: Dose is individualized

Dosage Forms Tablet:

5-12.5: Enalapril maleate 5 mg and hydrochlorothiazide 12.5 mg

10-25: Enalapril maleate 10 mg and hydrochlorothiazide 25 mg

enalaprilat *see* enalapril *on previous page*

enalapril maleate *see* enalapril *on previous page*

Enbrel® [US/Can] *see* etanercept *on page 333*

Encare® [US-OTC] *see* nonoxynol 9 *on page 626*

Endal® [US] *see* guaifenesin and phenylephrine *on page 418*

Endantadine® [Can] *see* amantadine *on page 41*

Endep® 25 mg, 50 mg, 100 mg *(Discontinued)* *see page 1042*

EndoAvitene® [US] *see* collagen hemostat *on page 225*

Endocet® [US/Can] *see* oxycodone and acetaminophen *on page 656*

Endocodone® *(Discontinued)* *see page 1042*

Endodan® [US/Can] *see* oxycodone and aspirin *on page 657*

Endo®-Levodopa/Carbidopa [Can] *see* levodopa and carbidopa *on page 513*

Endolor® *(Discontinued)* *see page 1042*

Endrate® [US] *see* edetate disodium *on page 303*

Enduron® [US/Can] *see* methyclothiazide *on page 568*

Enduron® 2.5 mg Tablet *(Discontinued)* *see page 1042*

Enduronyl® [US/Can] *see* methyclothiazide and deserpidine *on page 568*

Enduronyl® Forte [US/Can] *see* methyclothiazide and deserpidine *on page 568*

Enecat® [US] *see* radiological/contrast media (ionic) *on page 759*

Enemeez® [US-OTC] *see* docusate *on page 285*

Ener-B® *(Discontinued)* *see page 1042*

enflurane (EN floo rane)

Sound-Alike/Look-Alike Issues
enflurane may be confused with isoflurane

U.S./Canadian Brand Names Ethrane® [US/Can]

Therapeutic Category General Anesthetic

Use Maintenance of general anesthesia; not recommended for induction of anesthesia due to airway irritant properties

Usual Dosage Minimum alveolar concentration (MAC), the concentration at which 50% of patients do not respond to surgical incision, is 1.6% for enflurane. The concentration at which amnesia and loss of awareness occur (MAC - awake) is 0.4%. MAC is reduced in the elderly.

Dosage Forms Liquid, for inhalation: >99.9% (125 mL [DSC], 250 mL)

enfuvirtide (en FYOO vir tide)

Synonyms T-20

U.S./Canadian Brand Names Fuzeon™ [US/Can]

Therapeutic Category Antiretroviral Agent, Fusion Protein Inhibitor

Controlled Substance Initial supplies of Fuzeon™ are available through a progressive distribution program. This program is set up to ensure that patients started on treatment will receive an uninterrupted supply until full distribution is available. During this period, all medication will be dispensed by a specialty pharmacy. To access the program, call 866-694-6670.

Use Treatment of HIV-1 infection in combination with other antiretroviral agents in treatment-experienced patients with evidence of HIV-1 replication despite ongoing antiretroviral therapy

Usual Dosage SubQ:
Children ≥6 years: 2 mg/kg twice daily (maximum dose: 90 mg twice daily)
Adults: 90 mg twice daily

Dosage Forms Injection, powder for reconstitution [single-use vial]: 108 mg [90 mg/mL following reconstitution; available in convenience kit of 60 vials, SWFI, syringes, alcohol wipes, patient instructions]

Engerix-B® [US/Can] *see* hepatitis B vaccine *on page 433*

enhanced-potency inactivated poliovirus vaccine *see* poliovirus vaccine (inactivated) *on page 705*

Enisyl® *(Discontinued)* *see page 1042*

Enkaid® *(Discontinued)* *see page 1042*

Enlon® [US/Can] *see* edrophonium *on page 303*

Enomine® *(Discontinued)* *see page 1042*

Enovid® *(Discontinued)* *see page 1042*

Enovil® *(Discontinued)* *see page 1042*

enoxaparin (ee noks a PA rin)

Sound-Alike/Look-Alike Issues

Lovenox® may be confused with Lotronex®

Synonyms enoxaparin sodium

U.S./Canadian Brand Names Lovenox® [US/Can]; Lovenox® HP [Can]

Therapeutic Category Anticoagulant (Other)

Use

DVT Treatment (acute): Inpatient treatment (patients with and without pulmonary embolism) and outpatient treatment (patients without pulmonary embolism)

DVT prophylaxis: Following hip or knee replacement surgery, abdominal surgery, or in medical patients with severely-restricted mobility during acute illness in patients at risk of thromboembolic complications

Note: High-risk patients include those with one or more of the following risk factors: >40 years of age, obesity, general anesthesia lasting >30 minutes, malignancy, history of deep vein thrombosis or pulmonary embolism

Unstable angina and non-Q-wave myocardial infarction (to prevent ischemic complications)

Usual Dosage Adults: S.C.: 30 mg twice daily

Dosage Forms

Injection, solution, as sodium [graduated prefilled syringe; preservative free]: 60 mg/0.6 mL (0.6 mL); 80 mg/0.8 mL (0.8 mL); 100 mg/mL (1 mL); 120 mg/0.8 mL (0.8 mL); 150 mg/mL (1 mL)

Injection, solution, as sodium [multidose vial]: 100 mg/mL (3 mL) [contains benzyl alcohol]

Injection, solution, as sodium [prefilled syringe; preservative free]: 30 mg/0.3 mL (0.3 mL); 40 mg/0.4 mL (0.4 mL)

enoxaparin sodium *see* enoxaparin *on this page*

Enpresse™ [US] *see* ethinyl estradiol and levonorgestrel *on page 339*

E.N.T.® *(Discontinued)* *see page 1042*

entacapone (en TA ka pone)

U.S./Canadian Brand Names Comtan® [US/Can]

Therapeutic Category Anti-Parkinson Agent; Reverse COMT Inhibitor

Use Adjunct to levodopa/carbidopa therapy in patients with idiopathic Parkinson disease who experience "wearing-off" symptoms at the end of a dosing interval

Usual Dosage Oral: Adults: 200 mg with each dose of levodopa/carbidopa, up to a maximum of 8 times/day (maximum daily dose: 1600 mg/day). To optimize therapy, the dosage of levodopa may need reduced or the dosing interval may need extended. Patients taking levodopa ≥800mg/day or who had moderate-to-severe dyskinesias prior to therapy required an average decrease of 25% in the daily levodopa dose.

Dosage Forms Tablet: 200 mg

entacapone, carbidopa, and levodopa *see* levodopa, carbidopa, and entacapone *on page 513*

Entertainer's Secret® [US-OTC] *see* saliva substitute *on page 792*

Entex® [US] *see* guaifenesin and phenylephrine *on page 418*

Entex® ER [US] *see* guaifenesin and phenylephrine *on page 418*

Entex® LA [US] *see* guaifenesin and phenylephrine *on page 418*

Entex® PSE [US] *see* guaifenesin and pseudoephedrine *on page 419*

Entocort® [Can] *see* budesonide *on page 131*

Entocort™ EC [US] *see* budesonide *on page 131*

Entozyme® ***(Discontinued)*** *see page 1042*

Entrobar® [US] *see* radiological/contrast media (ionic) *on page 759*

Entrophen® [Can] *see* aspirin *on page 80*

Entsol® [US-OTC] *see* sodium chloride *on page 810*

Entuss-D® Liquid ***(Discontinued)*** *see page 1042*

Enulose® [US] *see* lactulose *on page 502*

Enzone® [US] *see* pramoxine and hydrocortisone *on page 720*

Epaxal Berna® [Can] *see* hepatitis A vaccine *on page 432*

ephedrine (e FED rin)

Sound-Alike/Look-Alike Issues

ephedrine may be confused with Adrenalin®, Epifrin®, epinephrine

Synonyms ephedrine sulfate

U.S./Canadian Brand Names Pretz-D® [US-OTC]

Therapeutic Category Adrenergic Agonist Agent

Use Treatment of bronchial asthma, nasal congestion, acute bronchospasm, idiopathic orthostatic hypotension

Usual Dosage

Children:

Oral, SubQ: 3 mg/kg/day or 25-100 mg/m^2/day in 4-6 divided doses every 4-6 hours

I.M., slow I.V. push: 0.2-0.3 mg/kg/dose every 4-6 hours

Adults:

Oral: 25-50 mg every 3-4 hours as needed

I.M., SubQ: 25-50 mg, parenteral adult dose should not exceed 150 mg in 24 hours

I.V.: 5-25 mg/dose slow I.V. push repeated after 5-10 minutes as needed, then every 3-4 hours not to exceed 150 mg/24 hours

Nasal spray:

Children 6-12 years: 1-2 sprays into each nostril, not more frequently than every 4 hours

Children ≥12 years and Adults: 2-3 sprays into each nostril, not more frequently than every 4 hours

Dosage Forms

Capsule, as sulfate: 25 mg

Injection, solution, as sulfate: 50 mg/mL (1 mL, 10 mL)

Solution, intranasal spray, as sulfate (Pretz-D®): 0.25% (50 mL)

ephedrine, chlorpheniramine, phenylephrine, and carbetapentane *see* chlorpheniramine, ephedrine, phenylephrine, and carbetapentane *on page 190*

ephedrine sulfate *see* ephedrine *on this page*

Epi-C® [US] *see* radiological/contrast media (ionic) *on page 759*

epidermal thymocyte activating factor *see* aldesleukin *on page 28*

Epifoam® [US] *see* pramoxine and hydrocortisone *on page 720*

Epifrin® ***(Discontinued)*** *see page 1042*

E-Pilo-x® Ophthalmic ***(Discontinued)*** *see page 1042*

Epinal® ***(Discontinued)*** *see page 1042*

epinephrine (ep i NEF rin)

Sound-Alike/Look-Alike Issues

epinephrine may be confused with ephedrine

Adrenalin® may be confused with ephedrine

EpiPen® may be confused with Epifrin®

Synonyms adrenaline; epinephrine bitartrate; epinephrine hydrochlorid

(Continued)

epinephrine *(Continued)*

U.S./Canadian Brand Names Adrenalin® [US/Can]; EpiPen® [US/Can]; EpiPen® Jr [US/Can]; Primatene® Mist [US-OTC]; Vaponefrin® [Can]

Therapeutic Category Adrenergic Agonist Agent

Use Treatment of bronchospasms, anaphylactic reactions, cardiac arrest, management of open-angle (chronic simple) glaucoma; added to local anesthetics to decrease systemic absorption, increase duration of action, and decrease toxicity of the local anesthetic

Usual Dosage

Neonates: Cardiac arrest: I.V.: Intratracheal: 0.01-0.03 mg/kg (0.1-0.3 mL/kg of **1:10,000** solution) every 3-5 minutes as needed; dilute intratracheal doses to 1-2 mL with normal saline

Infants and Children:

Bronchodilator: SubQ: 10 mcg/kg (0.01 mL/kg of **1:1000**) (single doses not to exceed 0.5 mg) **or** suspension (1:200): 0.005 mL/kg/dose (0.025 mg/kg/dose) to a maximum of 0.15 mL (0.75 mg for single dose) every 8-12 hours

Bradycardia:

I.V.: 0.01 mg/kg (0.1 mL/kg of **1:10,000** solution) every 3-5 minutes as needed (maximum: 1 mg/10 mL)

Intratracheal: 0.1 mg/kg (0.1 mL/kg of **1:1000** solution every 3-5 minutes); doses as high as 0.2 mg/kg may be effective

Asystole or pulseless arrest:

I.V. or intraosseous: **First dose**: 0.01 mg/kg (0.1 mL/kg of a **1:10,000** solution); **subsequent doses**: 0.1 mg/kg (0.1 mL/kg of a **1:1000** solution); doses as high as 0.2 mg/kg may be effective; repeat every 3-5 minutes

Intratracheal: 0.1 mg/kg (0.1 mL/kg of a **1:1000** solution); doses as high as 0.2 mg/kg may be effective

Hypersensitivity reaction: SubQ: 0.01 mg/kg every 15 minutes for 2 doses then every 4 hours as needed (single doses not to exceed 0.5 mg)

Refractory hypotension (refractory to dopamine/dobutamine): Continuous I.V. infusions of 0.1-1 mcg/kg/minute; titrate dosage to desired effect

Nebulization: 0.25-0.5 mL of 2.25% **racemic epinephrine** solution diluted in 3 mL normal saline, or L-epinephrine at an equivalent dose; racemic epinephrine 10 mg = 5 mg L-epinephrine; use lower end of dosing range for younger infants

Intranasal: Children ≥6 years and Adults: Apply locally as drops or spray or with sterile swab

Adults:

Asystole:

I.V.: 1 mg every 3-5 minutes; if this approach fails, alternative regimens include:

Intermediate: 2-5 mg every 3-5 minutes

Escalating: 1 mg, 3 mg, 5 mg at 3-minute intervals

High: 0.1 mg/kg every 3-5 minutes

Intratracheal: 1 mg (although optimal dose is unknown, doses of 2-2.5 times the I.V. dose may be needed)

Bronchodilator: I.M., SubQ (**1:1000**): 0.1-0.5 mg every 10-15 minutes to 4 hours

Hypersensitivity reaction: I.M., SubQ: 0.3-0.5 mg every 15-20 minutes if condition requires; if hypotension is present: 0.1 mg I.V. slowly over 5-10 minutes followed by continuous infusion 1-10 mcg/minute

Symptomatic bradycardia or heart block (not responsive to atropine or pacing): I.V. infusion ... cg/minute; titrate to desired effect

... nsion (refractory to dopamine/dobutamine): Continuous I.V. infusion ... ange: 1-10 mcg/minute); titrate dosage to desired effect; severe ... n may require doses >10 mcg/minute (up to 0.1 mcg/kg/minute)

... 8-15 drops into nebulizer reservoirs; administer 1-3 inhalations 4-6

... 2 drops in eye(s) once or twice daily; when treating open-angle ... entration and dosage must be adjusted to the response of the

Dosage Forms
Aerosol for oral inhalation (Primatene® Mist): 0.22 mg/inhalation (15 mL, 22.5 mL) [contains CFCs]
Injection, solution [prefilled auto injector]:
EpiPen®: 0.3 mg/0.3 mL [1:1000] (2 mL) [contains sodium metabisulfite; available as single unit or in double-unit pack with training unit]
EpiPen® Jr: 0.15 mg/0.3 mL [1:2000] (2 mL) [contains sodium metabisulfite; available as single unit or in double-unit pack with training unit]
Injection, solution, as hydrochloride: 0.1 mg/mL [1:10,000] (10 mL); 1 mg/mL [1:1000] (1 mL) [products may contain sodium metabisulfite]
Adrenalin®: 1 mg/mL [1:1000] (1 mL, 30 mL) [contains sodium bisulfite]
Solution for oral inhalation, as hydrochloride: Adrenalin®: 1% [10 mg/mL, 1:100] (7.5 mL) [contains sodium bisulfite]
Solution, ophthalmic, as hydrochloride (Epifrin®): 0.5% (15 mL); 1% (15 mL); 2% (15 mL) [contains benzalkonium chloride and sodium metabisulfite] [DSC]

epinephrine and chlorpheniramine (ep i NEF rin & klor fen IR a meen)

Synonyms insect sting kit
U.S./Canadian Brand Names Ana-Kit® [US]
Therapeutic Category Antidote
Use Anaphylaxis emergency treatment of insect bites or stings by the sensitive patient that may occur within minutes of insect sting or exposure to an allergic substance
Usual Dosage Children and Adults: I.M. or SubQ:
Epinephrine:
<2 years: 0.05-0.1 mL
2-6 years: 0.15 mL
6-12 years: 0.2 mL
>12 years : 0.3 mL
Chlorpheniramine:
<6 years: 1 tablet
6-12 years: 2 tablets
>12 years: 4 tablets
Dosage Forms Kit: Epinephrine hydrochloride 1:1000 [prefilled syringe, delivers two 0.3 mL doses; contains sodium bisulfite] (1 mL), chlorpheniramine maleate chewable tablet 2 mg (4), sterile alcohol pads [isopropyl alcohol 70%] (2), tourniquet (1)

epinephrine and lidocaine *see* lidocaine and epinephrine *on page 520*
epinephrine and pilocarpine *see* pilocarpine and epinephrine *on page 695*
epinephrine bitartrate *see* epinephrine *on page 311*
epinephrine hydrochloride *see* epinephrine *on page 311*
EpiPen® [US/Can] *see* epinephrine *on page 311*
EpiPen® Jr [US/Can] *see* epinephrine *on page 311*
epipodophyllotoxin *see* etoposide *on page 351*
EpiQuin™ Micro [US] *see* hydroquinone *on page 454*

epirubicin (ep i ROO bi sin)

Sound-Alike/Look-Alike Issues
Ellence® may be confused with Elase®
Synonyms pidorubicin; pidorubicin hydrochloride
U.S./Canadian Brand Names Ellence® [US/Can]; Pharmorubicin® [Can]
Therapeutic Category Antineoplastic Agent, Anthracycline; Antineoplastic Agent, Antibiotic
Use Adjuvant therapy for primary breast cancer
Usual Dosage Adults: I.V.: 100-120 mg/m^2 once weekly every 3-4 weeks **or** 50-60 mg/m^2 days 1 and 8 every 3-4 weeks
(Continued)

epirubicin *(Continued)*

Breast cancer:

CEF-120: 60 mg/m^2 on days 1 and 8 every 28 days for 6 cycles

FEC-100: 100 mg/m^2 on day 1 every 21 days for 6 cycles

Dosage Forms Injection, solution [preservative free]: 2 mg/mL (25 mL, 100 mL)

Epitol® [US] *see* carbamazepine *on page 155*

Epival® ER [Can] *see* valproic acid and derivatives *on page 901*

Epival® I.V. [Can] *see* valproic acid and derivatives *on page 901*

Epivir® [US] *see* lamivudine *on page 502*

Epivir-HBV® [US] *see* lamivudine *on page 502*

eplerenone (e PLER en one)

U.S./Canadian Brand Names Inspra™ [US]

Therapeutic Category Antihypertensive Agent; Selective Aldosterone Blocker

Use Treatment of hypertension (may be used alone or in combination with other antihypertensive agents); treatment of CHF following acute MI

Usual Dosage Oral: Adults:

Hypertension: Initial: 50 mg once daily; may increase to 50 mg twice daily if response is not adequate; may take up to 4 weeks for full therapeutic response. Doses >100 mg/day are associated with increased risk of hyperkalemia and no greater therapeutic effect.

Concurrent use with moderate CYP3A4 inhibitors: Initial: 25 mg once daily

Congestive heart failure (post-MI): Initial: 25 mg once daily; dosage goal: titrate to 50 mg once daily within 4 weeks, as tolerated

Dosage adjustment per serum potassium concentrations for CHF:

<5.0 mEq/L: Increase dose from 25 mg every other day to 25 mg daily **or** Increase dose from 25 mg daily to 50 mg daily

5.0-5.4 mEq/L: No adjustment needed

5.5-5.9 mEq/L: Decrease dose from 50 mg daily to 25 mg daily **or** Decrease dose from 25 mg daily to 25 mg every other day **or** Decrease does from 25 mg every other day to withhold medication

≥6.0 mEq/L: Withhold medication until potassium <5.5 mEq/L, then restart at 25 mg every other day

Dosage Forms Tablet [film coated]: 25 mg, 50 mg

E.P. Mycin® Capsule *(Discontinued)* *see page 1042*

EPO *see* epoetin alfa *on this page*

epoetin alfa (e POE e tin AL fa)

Sound-Alike/Look-Alike Issues

Epogen® may be confused with Neupogen®.

Synonyms EPO; erythropoietin; *r*HuEPO-α

U.S./Canadian Brand Names Epogen® [US]; Eprex® [Can]; Procrit® [US]

Therapeutic Category Colony-Stimulating Factor

Use

Treatment of anemia related to zidovudine therapy in HIV-infected patients; in patients when the endogenous erythropoietin level is ≤500 mU/mL and the dose of zidovudine is ≤4200 mg/week

Treatment of anemia associated with chronic renal failure (CRF) including dialysis (end-stage renal disease, ESRD) and nondialysis patients. Prior to therapy, serum ferritin should be >100 ng/dL and transferrin saturation (serum iron/iron binding capacity x 100) of 20% to 30%; nondialysis patients should have a hematocrit <30%

Treatment of anemia in cancer patients on chemotherapy; in patients with nonmyeloid malignancies where anemia is caused by the effect of the concomitantly administered chemotherapy; to decrease the need for transfusions in patients who will be receiving chemotherapy for a minimum of 2 months

Reduction of allogeneic blood transfusion in surgery patients (with hemoglobin >10 g/dL up to 13 g/dL) scheduled to undergo elective, noncardiac, nonvascular surgery

Usual Dosage

Chronic renal failure patients: I.V., SubQ:

Children: Initial dose: 50 units/kg 3 times/week

Adults: Initial dose: 50-100 units/kg 3 times/week

Reduce dose when hemoglobin approaches 12 g/dL **or** hemoglobin increases 1 g/dL in any 2-week period.

Increase dose if hemoglobin does not increase by 2 g/dL after 8 weeks of therapy and hemoglobin is below suggested target range. Suggested target hemoglobin range: 10-12 g/dL

Maintenance dose: Individualize to target range

Dialysis patients: Median dose: Children: 167 units/kg/week **or** 76 units/kg 2-3 times/week Adults: 75 units/kg 3 times/week

Nondialysis patients: Children: Dosing range: 50-250 units/kg 1-3 times/week Adults: Median dose: 75-150 units/kg

Zidovudine-treated, HIV-infected patients (patients with erythropoietin levels >500 mU/mL are **unlikely** to respond): I.V., SubQ:

Children: Initial dose: Reported dosing range: 50-400 units/kg 2-3 times/week

Adults: 100 units/kg 3 times/week for 8 weeks

Increase dose by 50-100 units/kg 3 times/week if response is not satisfactory in terms of reducing transfusion requirements or increasing hemoglobin after 8 weeks of therapy

Evaluate response every 4-8 weeks thereafter and adjust the dose accordingly by 50-100 units/kg increments 3 times/week

If patient has not responded satisfactorily to a 300 unit/kg dose 3 times/week, a response to higher doses is unlikely

Stop dose if hemoglobin exceeds 13 g/dL and resume treatment at a 25% dose reduction when hemoglobin drops to 12 g/dL

Cancer patient on chemotherapy: Treatment of patients with erythropoietin levels >200 mU/mL is **not recommended**

Children: I.V., SubQ: Dosing range: 25-300 units/kg 3-7 times/week; commonly reported initial dose: 150 units/kg

Adults: SubQ:

Initial dose: 150 units/kg 3 times/week; commonly used doses range from 10,000 units 3 times/week to 40,000-60,000 units once weekly. **Dose adjustment:** If response is not satisfactory after a sufficient period of evaluation (8 weeks of 3 times/week and 4 weeks of once-weekly therapy), the dose may be increased up to 300 units/kg 3 times/week. If patient does not respond, a response to higher doses is unlikely. Stop dose if hemoglobin exceeds 13 g/dL and resume treatment at a 25% dose reduction when hemoglobin drops to 12 g/dL.

Surgery patients: Prior to initiating treatment, obtain a hemoglobin to establish that is >10 mg/dL or ≤13 mg/dL: Adults: SubQ: Initial dose: 300 units/kg/day for 10 days before surgery, on the day of surgery, and for 4 days after surgery

Alternative dose: 600 units/kg in once weekly doses (21, 14, and 7 days before surgery) plus a fourth dose on the day of surgery

Dosage Forms

Injection, solution [preservative free]: 2000 units/mL (1 mL); 3000 units/mL (1 mL); 4000 units/mL (1 mL); 10,000 units/mL (1 mL); 40,000 units/mL (1 mL) [contains human albumin]

Injection, solution [with preservative]: 10,000 units/mL (2 mL); 20,000 units/mL (1 mL) [contains human albumin and benzyl alcohol]

Epogen® [US] *see* epoetin alfa *on previous page*

epoprostenol (e poe PROST en ole)

Synonyms epoprostenol sodium; PGI_2; PGX; prostacyclin

U.S./Canadian Brand Names Flolan® [US/Can]

Therapeutic Category Platelet Inhibitor

Use **Orphan drug:** Treatment of primary pulmonary hypertension; treatment of secondary pulmonary hypertension due to intrinsic precapillary pulmonary vascular disease

Usual Dosage I.V.: The drug is administered by continuous intravenous infusion via a central venous catheter using an ambulatory infusion pump; during dose ranging it may be administered peripherally

Acute dose ranging: The initial infusion rate should be 2 ng/kg/minute by continuous I.V. and increased in increments of 2 ng/kg/minute every 15 minutes or longer until dose-limiting effects are elicited (such as chest pain, anxiety, dizziness, changes in heart rate, dyspnea, nausea, vomiting, headache, hypotension and/or flushing)

Continuous chronic infusion: Initial: 4 ng/kg/minute **less** than the maximum-tolerated infusion rate determined during acute dose ranging

If maximum-tolerated infusion rate is <5 ng/kg/minute, the chronic infusion rate should be 1/2 the maximum-tolerated acute infusion rate

Dosage Forms Injection, powder for reconstitution, as sodium: 0.5 mg, 1.5 mg [provided with 50 mL sterile diluent]

epoprostenol sodium *see* epoprostenol *on this page*

Eprex® [Can] *see* epoetin alfa *on page 314*

eprosartan (ep roe SAR tan)

U.S./Canadian Brand Names Teveten® [US/Can]

Therapeutic Category Angiotensin II Receptor Antagonist

Use Treatment of hypertension; may be used alone or in combination with other antihypertensives

Usual Dosage Adults: Oral: Dosage must be individualized; can administer once or twice daily with total daily doses of 400-800 mg. Usual starting dose is 600 mg once daily as monotherapy in patients who are euvolemic. Limited clinical experience with doses >800 mg.

Dosage Forms Tablet: 400 mg, 600 mg

eprosartan and HCTZ *see* eprosartan and hydrochlorothiazide *on this page*

eprosartan and hydrochlorothiazide

(ep roe SAR tan & hye droe klor oh THYE a zide)

Synonyms eprosartan and HCTZ; eprosartan mesylate and hydrochlorothiazide; hydrochlorothiazide and eprosartan

U.S./Canadian Brand Names Tevetan® HCT [US/Can]

Therapeutic Category Angiotensin II Antagonist Combination; Antihypertensive Agent, Combination; Diuretic, Thiazide

Use Treatment of hypertension (not indicated for initial treatment)

Usual Dosage Oral: Adults: Dose is individualized (combination substituted for individual components)

Usual recommended dose: Eprosartan 600 mg/hydrochlorothiazide 12.5 mg once daily (maximum dose: Eprosartan 600 mg/hydrochlorothiazide 25 mg once daily)

Dosage Forms

Tablet:

600 mg/12.5 mg: Eprosartan 600 mg and hydrochlorothiazide 12.5 mg

600 mg/25 mg: Eprosartan 600 mg and hydrochlorothiazide 25 mg

eprosartan mesylate and hydrochlorothiazide *see* eprosartan and hydrochlorothiazide *on this page*

epsilon aminocaproic acid *see* aminocaproic acid *on page 45*

epsom salts *see* magnesium sulfate *on page 539*

EPT *see* teniposide *on page 844*

eptacog alfa (activated) *see* factor VIIa (recombinant) *on page 354*

eptifibatide (ep TIF i ba tide)

Synonyms intrifiban

U.S./Canadian Brand Names Integrilin® [US/Can]

Therapeutic Category Antiplatelet Agent

Use Treatment of patients with acute coronary syndrome (UA/NQMI), including patients who are to be managed medically and those undergoing percutaneous coronary intervention (PCI including PTCA; intracoronary stenting)

Usual Dosage I.V.: Adults:

Acute coronary syndrome: Bolus of 180 mcg/kg (maximum: 22.6 mg) over 1-2 minutes, begun as soon as possible following diagnosis, followed by a continuous infusion of 2 mcg/kg/minute (maximum: 15 mg/hour) until hospital discharge or initiation of CABG surgery, up to 72 hours. Concurrent aspirin (160-325 mg initially and daily thereafter) and heparin therapy (target aPTT 50-70 seconds) are recommended.

Percutaneous coronary intervention (PCI) with or without stenting: Bolus of 180 mcg/kg (maximum: 22.6 mg) administered immediately before the initiation of PCI, followed by a continuous infusion of 2 mcg/kg/minute (maximum: 15 mg/hour). A second 180 mcg/kg bolus (maximum: 22.6 mg) should be administered 10 minutes after the first bolus. Infusion should be continued until hospital discharge or for up to 18-24 hours, whichever comes first; minimum of 12 hours of infusion is recommended. Concurrent aspirin (160-325 mg 1-24 hours before PCI and daily thereafter) and heparin therapy (ACT 200-300 seconds during PCI) are recommended. Heparin infusion after PCI is discouraged. In patients who undergo coronary artery bypass graft surgery, discontinue infusion prior to surgery.

Dosage Forms Injection, solution: 0.75 mg/mL (100 mL); 2 mg/mL (10 mL, 100 mL)

Epzicom™ [US] *see* abacavir and lamivudine *on page 2*

Equagesic® [US] *see* aspirin and meprobamate *on page 83*

Equalactin® [US-OTC] *see* polycarbophil *on page 706*

Equanil® *(Discontinued)* *see page 1042*

Equilet® *(Discontinued)* *see page 1042*

Erbitux™ [US] *see* cetuximab *on page 179*

Ercaf® *(Discontinued)* *see page 1042*

ergocalciferol (er goe kal SIF e role)

Sound-Alike/Look-Alike Issues

Calciferol™ may be confused with calcitriol

Drisdol® may be confused with Drysol®

Synonyms activated ergosterol; viosterol; vitamin D_2

U.S./Canadian Brand Names Calciferol™ [US]; Drisdol® [US/Can]; Ostoforte® [Can]

Therapeutic Category Vitamin D Analog

Use Treatment of refractory rickets, hypophosphatemia, hypoparathyroidism; dietary supplement

Usual Dosage Oral dosing is preferred; I.M. therapy required with GI, liver, or biliary disease associated with malabsorption

Dietary supplementation (each 1 mcg = 40 int. units):

Infants and Children: 5 mcg/day (200 int. units/day)

Adults:

18-50 years: 5 mcg/day (200 int. units/day)

51-70 years: 10 mcg/day (400 int. units/day)

Elderly >70 years: 15 mcg/day (600 int. units/day)

Renal failure:

Children: 100-1000 mcg/day (4000-40,000 int. units)

Adults: 500 mcg/day (20,000 int. units)

(Continued)

ergocalciferol *(Continued)*

Hypoparathyroidism:

Children: 1.25-5 mg/day (50,000-200,000 int. units) and calcium supplements

Adults: 625 mcg to 5 mg/day (25,000-200,000 int. units) and calcium supplements

Vitamin D-dependent rickets:

Children: 75-125 mcg/day (3000-5000 int. units); maximum: 1500 mcg/day

Adults: 250 mcg to 1.5 mg/day (10,000-60,000 int. units)

Nutritional rickets and osteomalacia:

Children and Adults (with normal absorption): 25-125 mcg/day (1000-5000 int. units)

Children with malabsorption: 250-625 mcg/day (10,000-25,000 int. units)

Adults with malabsorption: 250-7500 mcg (10,000-300,000 int. units)

Vitamin D-resistant rickets:

Children: Initial: 1000-2000 mcg/day (40,000-80,000 int. units) with phosphate supplements; daily dosage is increased at 3- to 4-month intervals in 250-500 mcg (10,000-20,000 int. units) increments

Adults: 250-1500 mcg/day (10,000-60,000 int. units) with phosphate supplements

Familial hypophosphatemia: 10,000-80,000 int. units daily plus 1-2 g/day elemental phosphorus

Osteoporosis prophylaxis: Adults:

51-70 years: 400 int. units/day

>70 years: 600 int. units/day

Maximum daily dose: 2000 int. units/day

Dosage Forms [DSC] = Discontinued product

Capsule (Drisdol®): 50,000 int. units [1.25 mg; contains tartrazine and soybean oil]

Injection, solution (Calciferol™): 500,000 int. units/mL [12.5 mg/mL] (1 mL) [contains sesame oil] [DSC]

Liquid, drops (Calciferol™, Drisdol®): 8000 int. units/mL [200 mcg/mL] (60 mL) [OTC]

ergoloid mesylates (ER goe loid MES i lates)

Synonyms dihydroergotoxine; dihydrogenated ergot alkaloids

U.S./Canadian Brand Names Hydergine® [Can]

Therapeutic Category Ergot Alkaloid and Derivative

Use Treatment of cerebrovascular insufficiency in primary progressive dementia, Alzheimer dementia, and senile onset

Usual Dosage Adults: Oral: 1 mg 3 times/day up to 4.5-12 mg/day; up to 6 months of therapy may be necessary

Dosage Forms

Tablet: 1 mg

Tablet, sublingual: 1 mg

Ergomar® [US] *see* ergotamine *on next page*

ergometrine maleate *see* ergonovine *on this page*

ergonovine (er goe NOE veen)

Synonyms ergometrine maleate; ergonovine maleate

Therapeutic Category Ergot Alkaloid and Derivative

Use Prevention and treatment of postpartum and postabortion hemorrhage caused by uterine atony or subinvolution

Usual Dosage Adults: I.M., I.V. (I.V. should be reserved for emergency use only): 0.2 mg, repeat dose in 2-4 hours as needed

Dosage Forms Injection, as maleate: 0.2 mg/mL (1 mL)

ergonovine maleate *see* ergonovine *on this page*

Ergostat® *(Discontinued)* *see page 1042*

ergotamine (er GOT a meen)

Synonyms ergotamine tartrate

U.S./Canadian Brand Names Ergomar® [US]

Therapeutic Category Ergot Alkaloid and Derivative

Use Abort or prevent vascular headaches, such as migraine, migraine variants, or so-called "histaminic cephalalgia"

Usual Dosage Sublingual: One tablet under tongue at first sign, then 1 tablet every 30 minutes if needed; maximum dose: 3 tablets/24 hours, 5 tablets/week

Dosage Forms Tablet, sublingual (Ergomar®): Ergotamine tartrate 2 mg

ergotamine tartrate *see* ergotamine *on this page*

Ergotamine Tartrate and Caffeine Cafatine® ***(Discontinued)*** *see page 1042*

ergotamine tartrate, belladonna, and phenobarbital *see* belladonna, phenobarbital, and ergotamine tartrate *on page 104*

Ergotrate® Maleate Injection ***(Discontinued)*** *see page 1042*

Eridium® ***(Discontinued)*** *see page 1042*

E•R•O [US-OTC] *see* carbamide peroxide *on page 155*

Errin™ [US] *see* norethindrone *on page 627*

Ertaczo™ [US] *see* sertaconazole *on page 801*

ertapenem (er ta PEN em)

Synonyms ertapenem sodium; L-749,345; MK0826

U.S./Canadian Brand Names Invanz® [US/Can]

Therapeutic Category Antibiotic, Carbapenem

Use Treatment of moderate-severe, complicated intra-abdominal infections, skin and skin structure infections, pyelonephritis, acute pelvic infections, and community-acquired pneumonia. Antibacterial coverage includes aerobic gram-positive organisms, aerobic gram-negative organisms, anaerobic organisms.

Note: Methicillin-resistant *Staphylococcus*, *Enterococcus* spp, penicillin-resistant strains of *Streptococcus pneumoniae,* beta-lactamase-positive strains of *Haemophilus influenzae* are **resistant** to ertapenem, as are most *Pseudomonas aeruginosa.*

Usual Dosage Adults: I.M., I.V.: **Note:** I.V. therapy may be administered for up to 14 days; I.M. for up to 7 days

Intra-abdominal infection: 1 g/day for 5-14 days

Skin and skin structure infections: 1 g/day for 7-14 days

Community-acquired pneumonia: 1 g/day; duration of total antibiotic treatment: 10-14 days

Urinary tract infections/pyelonephritis: 1 g/day; duration of total antibiotic treatment: 10-14 days

Acute pelvic infections: 1 g/day for 3-10 days

Dosage Forms Injection, powder for reconstitution: 1 g [contains sodium 137 mg/g]

ertapenem sodium *see* ertapenem *on this page*

***Erwinia* asparaginase** *see* asparaginase *on page 80*

Erybid™ [Can] *see* erythromycin *on next page*

Eryc® [US/Can] *see* erythromycin *on next page*

Eryderm® [US] *see* erythromycin *on next page*

Erygel® [US] *see* erythromycin *on next page*

EryPed® [US] *see* erythromycin *on next page*

Ery-Sol® Topical Solution ***(Discontinued)*** *see page 1042*

Ery-Tab® [US] *see* erythromycin *on next page*

Erythrocin® [US] *see* erythromycin *on next page*

Erythromid® [Can] *see* erythromycin *on this page*

erythromycin (er ith roe MYE sin sis TEM ik)

Sound-Alike/Look-Alike Issues

erythromycin may be confused with azithromycin, clarithromycin, Ethmozine®
Akne-Mycin® may be confused with AK-Mycin®
E.E.S.® may be confused with DES®
Eryc® may be confused with Emcyt®, Ery-Tab®
Ery-Tab® may be confused with Eryc®
Erythrocin® may be confused with Ethmozine®

Synonyms erythromycin base; erythromycin estolate; erythromycin ethylsuccinate; erythromycin gluceptate; erythromycin lactobionate; erythromycin stearate

U.S./Canadian Brand Names Akne-Mycin® [US]; Apo-Erythro Base® [Can]; Apo-Erythro E-C® [Can]; Apo-Erythro-ES® [Can]; Apo-Erythro-S® [Can]; A/T/S® [US]; Diomycin® [Can]; E.E.S.® [US/Can]; Erybid™ [Can]; Eryc® [US/Can]; Eryderm® [US]; Erygel® [US]; EryPed® [US]; Ery-Tab® [US]; Erythrocin® [US]; Erythromid® [Can]; Nu-Erythromycin-S [Can]; PCE® [US/Can]; PMS-Erythromycin [Can]; Romycin® [US]; Sans Acne® [Can]; Theramycin Z® [US]

Therapeutic Category Acne Products; Antibiotic, Ophthalmic; Antibiotic, Topical; Macrolide (Antibiotic)

Use

Systemic: Treatment of susceptible bacterial infections including *S. pyogenes*, some *S. pneumoniae*, some *S. aureus*, *M. pneumoniae*, *Legionella pneumophila*, diphtheria, pertussis, chancroid, *Chlamydia*, erythrasma, *N. gonorrhoeae*, *E. histolytica*, syphilis and nongonococcal urethritis, and *Campylobacter* gastroenteritis; used in conjunction with neomycin for decontaminating the bowel

Ophthalmic: Treatment of superficial eye infections involving the conjunctiva or cornea; neonatal ophthalmia

Topical: Treatment of acne vulgaris

Usual Dosage

Neonates: Ophthalmic: Prophylaxis of neonatal gonococcal or chlamydial conjunctivitis: 0.5-1 cm ribbon of ointment should be instilled into each conjunctival sac

Infants and Children (**Note:** 400 mg ethylsuccinate = 250 mg base, stearate, or estolate salts):

Oral: 30-50 mg/kg/day divided every 6-8 hours; may double doses in severe infections

Preop bowel preparation: 20 mg/kg erythromycin base at 1, 2, and 11 PM on the day before surgery combined with mechanical cleansing of the large intestine and oral neomycin

I.V.: Lactobionate: 20-40 mg/kg/day divided every 6 hours

Adults:

Oral:

Base: 250-500 mg every 6-12 hours

Ethylsuccinate: 400-800 mg every 6-12 hours

Preop bowel preparation: Oral: 1 g erythromycin base at 1, 2, and 11 PM on the day before surgery combined with mechanical cleansing of the large intestine and oral neomycin

I.V.: Lactobionate: 15-20 mg/kg/day divided every 6 hours or 500 mg to 1 g every 6 hours, or given as a continuous infusion over 24 hours (maximum: 4 g/24 hours)

Children and Adults:

Ophthalmic: Instill ½" (1.25 cm) 2-6 times/day depending on the severity of the infection

Topical: Apply over the affected area twice daily after the skin has been thoroughly washed and patted dry

Dialysis: Slightly dialyzable (5% to 20%); no supplemental dosage necessary in hemo or peritoneal dialysis or in continuous arteriovenous or venovenous hemofiltration

Dosage Forms [Can] = Canadian brand name

Capsule, delayed release, enteric-coated pellets, as base (Eryc®): 250 mg

Gel, topical: 2% (30 g, 60 g)

A/T/S®: 2% (30 g) [contains alcohol 92%]
Erygel®: 2% (30 g, 60 g) [contains alcohol 92%]
Granules for oral suspension, as ethylsuccinate (E.E.S.®): 200 mg/5 mL (100 mL, 200 mL) [cherry flavor]
Injection, powder for reconstitution, as lactobionate (Erythrocin®): 500 mg, 1 g
Ointment, ophthalmic: 0.5% [5 mg/g] (1 g, 3.5 g)
Romycin®: 0.5% [5 mg/g] (3.5 g)
Ointment, topical (Akne-Mycin®): 2% (25 g)
Powder for oral suspension, as ethylsuccinate (EryPed®): 200 mg/5 mL (100 mL, 200 mL) [fruit flavor]; 400 mg/5 mL (100 mL, 200 mL) [banana flavor]
Powder for oral suspension, as ethylsuccinate [drops] (EryPed®): 100 mg/2.5 mL (50 mL) [fruit flavor]
Solution, topical: 2% (60 mL)
A/T/S®: 2% (60 mL) [contains alcohol 66%]
Eryderm®, T-Stat® [DSC], Theramycin™ Z: 2% (60 mL) [contain alcohol]
Sans Acne® [Can]: 2% (60 mL) [contains ethyl alcohol 44%; not available in U.S.]
Staticin®: 1.5% (60 mL) [DSC]
Suspension, oral, as estolate: 125 mg/5 mL (480 mL); 250 mg/5 mL (480 mL)
Suspension, oral, as ethylsuccinate: 200 mg/5 mL (480 mL); 400 mg/5 mL (480 mL)
E.E.S.®: 200 mg/5 mL (100 mL, 480 mL) [fruit flavor]; 400 mg/5 mL (100 mL, 480 mL) [orange flavor]
Swab (T-Stat® [DSC]): 2% (60s)
Tablet, chewable, as ethylsuccinate (EryPed®): 200 mg [fruit flavor] [DSC]
Tablet, delayed release, enteric coated, as base (Ery-Tab®): 250 mg, 333 mg, 500 mg
Tablet [film coated], as base: 250 mg, 500 mg
Tablet [film coated], as ethylsuccinate (E.E.S.®): 400 mg
Tablet [film coated], as stearate: 250 mg
Erythrocin®: 250 mg, 500 mg
Tablet [polymer-coated particles], as base (PCE®): 333 mg, 500 mg

erythromycin and benzoyl peroxide

(er ith roe MYE sin & BEN zoe il per OKS ide)

Synonyms benzoyl peroxide and erythromycin

U.S./Canadian Brand Names Benzamycin® [US]; Benzamycin® Pak [US]

Therapeutic Category Acne Products

Use Topical control of acne vulgaris

Usual Dosage Apply twice daily, morning and evening

Dosage Forms

Gel, topical:
Benzamycin®: Erythromycin 30 mg and benzoyl peroxide 50 mg per g (47 g)
Benzamycin® Pak: Erythromycin 30 mg and benzoyl peroxide 50 mg per 0.8 g packet (60s) [supplied with diluent containing alcohol]

erythromycin and sulfisoxazole (er ith roe MYE sin & sul fi SOKS a zole)

Sound-Alike/Look-Alike Issues

Pediazole® may be confused with Pediapred®

Synonyms sulfisoxazole and erythromycin

U.S./Canadian Brand Names Pediazole® [US/Can]

Therapeutic Category Macrolide (Antibiotic); Sulfonamide

Use Treatment of susceptible bacterial infections of the upper and lower respiratory tract, otitis media in children caused by susceptible strains of *Haemophilus influenzae*, and many other infections in patients allergic to penicillin

Usual Dosage Oral (dosage recommendation is based on the product's erythromycin content):

Children ≥2 months: 50 mg/kg/day erythromycin and 150 mg/kg/day sulfisoxazole in divided doses every 6 hours; not to exceed 2 g erythromycin/day or 6 g sulfisoxazole/day for 10 days

Adults >45 kg: 400 mg erythromycin and 1200 mg sulfisoxazole every 6 hours

(Continued)

erythromycin and sulfisoxazole *(Continued)*

Dosage Forms Powder for oral suspension: Erythromycin ethylsuccinate 200 mg and sulfisoxazole acetyl 600 mg per 5 mL (100 mL, 150 mL, 200 mL) [strawberry-banana flavor]

erythromycin base *see* erythromycin *on page 320*

erythromycin estolate *see* erythromycin *on page 320*

erythromycin ethylsuccinate *see* erythromycin *on page 320*

erythromycin gluceptate *see* erythromycin *on page 320*

erythromycin lactobionate *see* erythromycin *on page 320*

erythromycin stearate *see* erythromycin *on page 320*

erythropoiesis stimulating protein *see* darbepoetin alfa *on page 245*

erythropoietin *see* epoetin alfa *on page 314*

escitalopram (es sye TAL oh pram)

Synonyms escitalopram oxalate; Lu-26-054; S-citalopram

U.S./Canadian Brand Names Lexapro™ [US]

Therapeutic Category Antidepressant, Selective Serotonin Reuptake Inhibitor

Use Treatment of major depressive disorder; generalized anxiety disorders (GAD)

Usual Dosage Oral: Adults: Depression, GAD: Initial: 10 mg/day; dose may be increased to 20 mg/day after at least 1 week

Dosage Forms

Solution, oral: 1 mg/mL (240 mL) [peppermint flavor]

Tablet: 5 mg, 10 mg, 20 mg

escitalopram oxalate *see* escitalopram *on this page*

Esclim® [US] *see* estradiol *on page 324*

Eserine® [Can] *see* physostigmine *on page 693*

eserine salicylate *see* physostigmine *on page 693*

Esgic® [US] *see* butalbital, acetaminophen, and caffeine *on page 138*

Esgic-Plus™ [US] *see* butalbital, acetaminophen, and caffeine *on page 138*

Esidrix® *(Discontinued)* *see page 1042*

Eskalith® [US] *see* lithium *on page 525*

Eskalith CR® [US] *see* lithium *on page 525*

esmolol (ES moe lol)

Sound-Alike/Look-Alike Issues

esmolol may be confused with Osmitrol®

Brevibloc® may be confused with bretylium, Brevital®, Bumex®, Buprenex®

Synonyms esmolol hydrochloride

U.S./Canadian Brand Names Brevibloc® [US/Can]

Therapeutic Category Antiarrhythmic Agent, Class II; Beta-Adrenergic Blocker

Use Treatment of supraventricular tachycardia and atrial fibrillation/flutter (primarily to control ventricular rate); treatment of tachycardia and/or hypertension (especially intraoperative or postoperative)

Usual Dosage I.V. infusion requires an infusion pump (must be adjusted to individual response and tolerance):

Children: A limited amount of information regarding esmolol use in pediatric patients is currently available. Some centers have utilized doses of 100-500 mcg/kg given over 1 minute for control of supraventricular tachycardias.

Loading doses of 500 mcg/kg/minute over 1 minute with maximal doses of 50-250 mcg/kg/minute (mean = 173) have been used in addition to nitroprusside to treat postoperative hypertension after coarctation of aorta repair.

Adults:

Intraoperative tachycardia and/or hypertension (immediate control): Initial bolus: 80 mg (~1 mg/kg) over 30 seconds, followed by a 150 mcg/kg/minute infusion, if necessary. Adjust infusion rate as needed to maintain desired heart rate and/or blood pressure, up to 300 mcg/kg/minute.

Supraventricular tachycardia or gradual control of postoperative tachycardia/hypertension: Loading dose: 500 mcg/kg over 1 minute; follow with a 50 mcg/kg/minute infusion for 4 minutes; response to this initial infusion rate may be a rough indication of the responsiveness of the ventricular rate.

Infusion may be continued at 50 mcg/kg/minute or, if the response is inadequate, titrated upward in 50 mcg/kg/minute increments (increased no more frequently than every 4 minutes) to a maximum of 200 mcg/kg/minute.

To achieve more rapid response, following the initial loading dose and 50 mcg/kg/minute infusion, rebolus with a second 500 mcg/kg loading dose over 1 minute, and increase the maintenance infusion to 100 mcg/kg/minute for 4 minutes. If necessary, a third (and final) 500 mcg/kg loading dose may be administered, prior to increasing to an infusion rate of 150 mcg/minute. After 4 minutes of the 150 mcg/kg/minute infusion, the infusion rate may be increased to a maximum rate of 200 mcg/kg/minute (without a bolus dose).

Usual dosage range (SVT): 50-200 mcg/kg/minute with average dose of 100 mcg/kg/minute. For control of postoperative hypertension, as many as one-third of patients may require higher doses (250-300 mcg/kg/minute) to control blood pressure; the safety of doses >300 mcg/kg/minute has not been studied.

Esmolol: Hemodynamic effects of beta-blockade return to baseline within 20-30 minutes after discontinuing esmolol infusions.

Guidelines for withdrawal of therapy:

Transfer to alternative antiarrhythmic drug (propranolol, digoxin, verapamil).

Infusion should be reduced by 50% 30 minutes following the first dose of the alternative agent.

Following the second dose of the alternative drug, patient's response should be monitored and if control is adequate for the first hours, esmolol may be discontinued.

Dosage Forms

Infusion [premixed in sodium chloride; preservative free] (Brevibloc®): 2000 mg (100 mL) [20 mg/mL; double strength]; 2500 mg (250 mL) [10 mg/mL]

Injection, solution, as hydrochloride: 10 mg/mL (10 mL) [premixed in sodium chloride]

Brevibloc®: 10 mg/mL (10 mL) [alcohol free; premixed in sodium chloride]; 20 mg/mL (5 mL) [alcohol free; double strength; premixed in sodium chloride]; 250 mg/mL (10 mL) [contains alcohol 25%; concentrate]

esmolol hydrochloride *see* esmolol *on previous page*

E-Solve-2® Topical *(Discontinued)* *see page 1042*

esomeprazole (es oh ME pray zol)

Synonyms esomeprazole magnesium

U.S./Canadian Brand Names Nexium® [US/Can]

Therapeutic Category Proton Pump Inhibitor

Use Short-term (4-8 weeks) treatment of erosive esophagitis; maintaining symptom resolution and healing of erosive esophagitis; treatment of symptomatic gastroesophageal reflux disease; as part of a multidrug regimen for *Helicobacter pylori* eradication in patients with duodenal ulcer disease (active or history of within the past 5 years)

Usual Dosage **Note:** Delayed-release capsules should be swallowed whole and taken at least 1 hour before eating

Children: Safety and efficacy have not been established in pediatric patients

Adults: Oral:

Erosive esophagitis (healing): 20-40 mg once daily for 4-8 weeks; maintenance: 20 mg once daily

Symptomatic GERD: 20 mg once daily for 4 weeks

Helicobacter pylori eradication: 40 mg once daily; requires combination therapy

Dosage Forms Capsule, delayed release: 20 mg, 40 mg

esomeprazole magnesium *see* esomeprazole *on previous page*

Esoterica® Regular [US-OTC] *see* hydroquinone *on page 454*

Especol® [US-OTC] *see* fructose, dextrose, and phosphoric acid *on page 392*

Estalis® [Can] *see* estradiol and norethindrone *on page 327*

Estalis-Sequi® [Can] *see* estradiol and norethindrone *on page 327*

Estar® [US-OTC/Can] *see* coal tar *on page 219*

estazolam (es TA zoe lam)

Sound-Alike/Look-Alike Issues
ProSom™ may be confused with PhosLo®, Proscar®, Pro-Sof® Plus, Prozac®, Psorcon®

U.S./Canadian Brand Names ProSom™ [US]

Therapeutic Category Benzodiazepine

Controlled Substance C-IV

Use Short-term management of insomnia

Usual Dosage Adults: Oral: 1 mg at bedtime, some patients may require 2 mg; start at doses of 0.5 mg in debilitated or small elderly patients

Dosage Forms Tablet: 1 mg, 2 mg

esterified estrogen and methyltestosterone *see* estrogens (esterified) and methyltestosterone *on page 332*

esterified estrogens *see* estrogens (esterified) *on page 331*

Estivin® II Ophthalmic *(Discontinued)* *see page 1042*

Estrace® [US/Can] *see* estradiol *on this page*

Estraderm® [US/Can] *see* estradiol *on this page*

estradiol (es tra DYE ole)

Sound-Alike/Look-Alike Issues
Alora® may be confused with Aldara™
Estraderm® may be confused with Testoderm®

Synonyms estradiol acetate; estradiol cypionate; estradiol hemihydrate; estradiol transdermal; estradiol valerate

U.S./Canadian Brand Names Alora® [US]; Climara® [US/Can]; Delestrogen® [US/Can]; Depo®-Estradiol [US/Can]; Esclim® [US]; Estrace® [US/Can]; Estraderm® [US/Can]; Estradot® [Can]; Estrasorb™ [US]; Estring® [US/Can]; EstroGel® [US/Can]; Femring™ [US]; Gynodiol® [US]; Menostar™ [US]; Oesclim® [Can]; Vagifem® [US/Can]; Vivelle® [US/Can]; Vivelle-Dot® [US]

Therapeutic Category Estrogen Derivative

Use Treatment of moderate to severe vasomotor symptoms associated with menopause; treatment of vulvar and vaginal atrophy; hypoestrogenism (due to hypogonadism, castration, or primary ovarian failure); prostatic cancer (palliation), breast cancer (palliation), osteoporosis (prophylaxis); abnormal uterine bleeding due to hormonal imbalance; postmenopausal urogenital symptoms of the lower urinary tract (urinary urgency, dysuria)

Usual Dosage All dosage needs to be adjusted based upon the patient's response

Oral:

Prostate cancer (androgen-dependent, inoperable, progressing): 10 mg 3 times/day for at least 3 months

Breast cancer (inoperable, progressing in appropriately selected patients): 10 mg 3 times/day for at least 3 months

Osteoporosis prophylaxis in postmenopausal females: 0.5 mg/day in a cyclic regimen (3 weeks on and 1 week off)

Female hypoestrogenism (due to hypogonadism, castration, or primary ovarian failure): 1-2 mg/day; titrate as necessary to control symptoms using minimal effective dose for maintenance therapy

Moderate to severe vasomotor symptoms associated with menopause: 1-2 mg/day, adjusted as necessary to limit symptoms; administration should be cyclic (3 weeks on, 1 week off). Patients should be re-evaluated at 3- to 6-month intervals to determine if treatment is still necessary.

I.M.:

Prostate cancer: Valerate: ≥30 mg or more every 1-2 weeks

Moderate to severe vasomotor symptoms associated with menopause:

Cypionate: 1-5 mg every 3-4 weeks

Valerate: 10-20 mg every 4 weeks

Female hypoestrogenism (due to hypogonadism):

Cypionate: 1.5-2 mg monthly

Valerate: 10-20 mg every 4 weeks

Topical:

Emulsion: Moderate to severe vasomotor symptoms associated with menopause: 3.84 g applied once daily in the morning

Gel: Moderate to severe vasomotor symptoms associated with menopause, vulvar and vaginal atrophy: 1.25 g/day applied at the same time each day

Transdermal: Indicated dose may be used continuously in patients without an intact uterus. May be given continuously or cyclically (3 weeks on, 1 week off) in patients with an intact uterus **(exception - Menostar™, see specific dosing instructions).** When changing patients from oral to transdermal therapy, start transdermal patch 1 week after discontinuing oral hormone (may begin sooner if symptoms reappear within 1 week):

Once-weekly patch:

Moderate to severe vasomotor symptoms associated with menopause (Climara®): Apply 0.025 mg/day patch once weekly. Adjust dose as necessary to control symptoms. Patients should be re-evaluated at 3- to 6-month intervals to determine if treatment is still necessary.

Osteoporosis prophylaxis in postmenopausal women: Climara®: Apply patch once weekly; minimum effective dose 0.025 mg/day; adjust response to therapy by biochemical markers and bone mineral density Menostar™: Apply patch once weekly. In women with a uterus, also administer a progestin for 14 days every 6-12 months

Twice-weekly patch:

Moderate to severe vasomotor symptoms associated with menopause, vulvar/vaginal atrophy, female hypogonadism: Titrate to lowest dose possible to control symptoms, adjusting initial dose after the first month of therapy; re-evaluate therapy at 3- to 6-month intervals to taper or discontinue medication: Alora®, Esclim®, Estraderm®, Vivelle-Dot®: Apply 0.05 mg patch twice weekly Vivelle®: Apply 0.0375 mg patch twice weekly

Prevention of osteoporosis in postmenopausal women: Alora®, Vivelle®, Vivelle-Dot®: Apply 0.025 mg patch twice weekly, increase dose as necessary Estraderm®: Apply 0.05 mg patch twice weekly

Vaginal cream: Vulvar and vaginal atrophy: Insert 2-4 g/day intravaginally for 2 weeks, then gradually reduce to 1/2 the initial dose for 2 weeks, followed by a maintenance dose of 1 g 1-3 times/week

Vaginal ring:

Postmenopausal vaginal atrophy, urogenital symptoms: Estring®: 2 mg intravaginally; following insertion, ring should remain in place for 90 days

Moderate to severe vasomotor symptoms associated with menopause; vulvar/vaginal atrophy: Femring™: 0.05 mg intravaginally; following insertion, ring should remain in place for 3 months; dose may be increased to 0.1 mg if needed

Vaginal tablets: Atrophic vaginitis: Vagifem®: Initial: Insert 1 tablet once daily for 2 weeks; maintenance: Insert 1 tablet twice weekly; attempts to discontinue or taper medication should be made at 3- to 6-month intervals

(Continued)

estradiol *(Continued)*

Dosage Forms

Cream, vaginal (Estrace®): 0.1 mg/g (12 g) [refill tube]: 0.1 mg/g (42.5 g) [tube with applicator]

Emulsion, topical, as hemihydrate (Estrasorb™): 2.5 mg/g (56s) [each pouch contains 4.35 mg estradiol hemihydrate; contents of two pouches delivers estradiol 0.05 mg/day]

Gel, topical (EstroGel®): 0.06% (80 g) [tube; delivers estradiol 0.75 mg/1.25 g; 64 doses], (93 g) [pump; delivers estradiol 0.75 mg/1.25 g; 64 doses]

Injection, oil, as cypionate (Depo®-Estradiol): 5 mg/mL (5 mL) [contains chlorobutanol; in cottonseed oil]

Injection, oil, as valerate (Delestrogen®):
- 10 mg/mL (5 mL) [contains chlorobutanol; in sesame oil]
- 20 mg/mL (5 mL) [contains benzyl alcohol; in castor oil]
- 40 mg/mL (5 mL) [contains benzyl alcohol; in castor oil]

Ring, vaginal, as base (Estring®): 2 mg [total estradiol 2 mg; releases 7.5 mcg/day over 90 days] (1s)

Ring, vaginal, as acetate (Femring™): 0.05 mg [total estradiol 12.4 mg; releases 0.05 mg/day over 3 months] (1s); 0.1 mg [total estradiol 24.8 mg; releases 0.1 mg/day over 3 months] (1s)

Tablet, oral, micronized: 0.5 mg, 1 mg, 2 mg
- Estrace®: 0.5 mg, 1 mg, 2 mg [2 mg tablets contain tartrazine]
- Gynodiol®: 0.5 mg, 1 mg, 1.5 mg, 2 mg

Tablet, vaginal, as base (Vagifem®): 25 mcg [contains lactose]

Transdermal system: 0.05 mg/24 hours (4s) [once-weekly patch]; 0.1 mg/24 hours (4s) [once-weekly patch]
- Alora® [twice-weekly patch]:
  - 0.025 mg/24 hours [9 cm^2, total estradiol 0.77 mg] (8s)
  - 0.05 mg/24 hours [18 cm^2, total estradiol 1.5 mg] (8s, 24s)
  - 0.075 mg/24 hours [27 cm^2, total estradiol 2.3 mg] (8s)
  - 0.1 mg/24 hours [36 cm^2, total estradiol 3.1 mg] (8s)
- Climara® [once-weekly patch]:
  - 0.025 mg/24 hours [6.5 cm^2, total estradiol 2.04 mg] (4s)
  - 0.0375 mg/24 hours [9.375 cm^2, total estradiol 2.85 mg] (4s)
  - 0.05 mg/24 hours [12.5 cm^2, total estradiol 3.8 mg] (4s)
  - 0.06 mg/24 hours [15 cm^2, total estradiol 4.55 mg] (4s)
  - 0.075 mg/24 hours [18.75 cm^2, total estradiol 5.7 mg] (4s)
  - 0.1 mg/24 hours [25 cm^2, total estradiol 7.6 mg] (4s)
- Esclim® [twice-weekly patch]:
  - 0.025 mg/day [11 cm^2, total estradiol 5 mg] (8s)
  - 0.0375 mg/day [16.5 cm^2, total estradiol 7.5 mg] (8s)
  - 0.05 mg/day [22 cm^2, total estradiol 10 mg] (8s)
  - 0.075 mg/day [33 cm^2, total estradiol 15 mg] (8s)
  - 0.1 mg/day [44 cm^2, total estradiol 20 mg] (8s)
- Estraderm® [twice-weekly patch]:
  - 0.05 mg/24 hours [10 cm^2, total estradiol 4 mg] (8s)
  - 0.1 mg/24 hours [20 cm^2, total estradiol 8 mg] (8s)
- Menostar™ [once-weekly patch]: 0.014 mg/24 hours [3.25 cm^2, total estradiol 1 mg] (4s)
- Vivelle® [twice-weekly patch]:
  - 0.025 mg/24 hours [7.25 cm^2, total estradiol 2.17 mg] (8s)
  - 0.0375 mg/24 hours [11 cm^2, total estradiol 3.28 mg] (8s)
  - 0.05 mg/24 hours [14.5 cm^2, total estradiol 4.33 mg] (8s)
  - 0.075 mg/24 hours [22 cm^2, total estradiol 6.57 mg] (8s)
  - 0.1 mg/24 hours [29 cm^2, total estradiol 8.66 mg] (8s)
- Vivelle-Dot® [twice-weekly patch]:
  - 0.0375 mg/day [3.75 cm^2, total estradiol 0.585 mg] (8s)
  - 0.05 mg/day [5 cm^2, total estradiol 0.78 mg] (8s)

0.075 mg/day [7.5 cm^2, total estradiol 1.17 mg] (8s)
0.1 mg/day [10 cm^2, total estradiol 1.56 mg] (8s)

estradiol acetate *see* estradiol *on page 324*

estradiol and levonorgestrel (es tra DYE ole & LEE voe nor jes trel)

Synonyms levonorgestrel and estradiol

U.S./Canadian Brand Names ClimaraPro™ [US]

Therapeutic Category Estrogen and Progestin Combination

Use Treatment of moderate to severe vasomotor symptoms associated with menopause in women with an intact uterus

Usual Dosage Topical: Adults: Treatment of moderate to severe vasomotor symptoms associated with menopause in females with an intact uterus:

Estradiol 0.045 mg/levonorgestrel 0.015 mg: Apply one patch weekly; patients should be re-evaluated at 3- to 6-month intervals to determine if treatment is still necessary

Dosage Forms Transdermal system: Estradiol 0.045 mg/24 hours and levonorgestrel 0.015 mg/24 hours (4s) [once-weekly patch; 22 cm^2; contains estradiol 4.4 mg and levonorgestrel 1.39 mg]

estradiol and NGM *see* estradiol and norgestimate *on next page*

estradiol and norethindrone (es tra DYE ole & nor eth IN drone)

Synonyms norethindrone and estradiol

U.S./Canadian Brand Names Activella™ [US]; CombiPatch® [US]; Estalis® [Can]; Estalis-Sequi® [Can]

Therapeutic Category Estrogen and Progestin Combination

Use Women with an intact uterus:

Tablet: Treatment of moderate to severe vasomotor symptoms associated with menopause; treatment of vulvar and vaginal atrophy; prophylaxis for postmenopausal osteoporosis

Transdermal patch: Treatment of moderate to severe vasomotor symptoms associated with menopause; treatment of vulvar and vaginal atrophy; treatment of hypoestrogenism due to hypogonadism, castration, or primary ovarian failure

Usual Dosage Adults:

Oral (Activella™): 1 tablet daily

Transdermal patch (CombiPatch®):

Continuous combined regimen: Apply one patch twice weekly

Continuous sequential regimen: Apply estradiol-only patch for first 14 days of cycle, followed by one CombiPatch™ applied twice weekly for the remaining 14 days of a 28-day cycle

Transdermal patch, combination pack (product-specific dosing for Canadian formulation):

Estalis®: Continuous combined regimen: Apply a new patch twice weekly during a 28-day cycle

Estalis-Sequi®: Continuous sequential regimen: Apply estradiol-only patch (Vivelle®) for first 14 days, followed by one Estalis® patch applied twice weekly during the last 14 days of a 28-day cycle

Note: In women previously receiving oral estrogens, initiate upon reappearance of menopausal symptoms following discontinuation of oral therapy.

Dosage Forms [Can] = Canadian brand name

Combination pack (Estalis-Sequi® [Can; not available in U.S.]):

140/50:

Transdermal system (Vivelle®): Estradiol 50 mcg per day (4s) [14.5 sq cm; total estradiol 4.33 mg]

Transdermal system (Estalis®): Norethindrone acetate 140 mcg and estradiol 50 mcg per day (4s) [9 sq cm; total norethindrone acetate 2.7 mg, total estradiol 0.62 mg; not available in U.S.]

(Continued)

estradiol and norethindrone *(Continued)*

250/50:

Transdermal system (Vivelle®): Estradiol 50 mcg per day (4s) [14.5 sq cm; total estradiol 4.33 mg]

Transdermal system (Estalis®): Norethindrone acetate 250 mcg and estradiol 50 mcg per day (4s) [16 sq cm; total norethindrone acetate 4.8 mg, total estradiol 0.51 mg; not available in U.S.]

Tablet (Activella®): Estradiol 1 mg and norethindrone acetate 0.5 mg (28s)

Transdermal system:

CombiPatch®:

0.05/0.14: Estradiol 0.05 mg and norethindrone acetate 0.14 mg per day (8s) [9 sq cm]

0.05/0.25: Estradiol 0.05 mg and norethindrone acetate 0.25 mg per day (8s) [16 sq cm]

Estalis® [Can]:

140/50: Norethindrone acetate 140 mcg and estradiol 50 mcg per day (8s) [9 sq cm; total norethindrone acetate 2.7 mg, total estradiol 0.62 mg; not available in U.S.]

250/50 Norethindrone acetate 250 mcg and estradiol 50 mcg per day (8s) [16 sq cm; total norethindrone acetate 4.8 mg, total estradiol 0.51 mg; not available in U.S.]

estradiol and norgestimate (es tra DYE ole & nor JES ti mate)

Synonyms estradiol and NGM; norgestimate and estradiol; ortho prefest

U.S./Canadian Brand Names Prefest™ [US]

Therapeutic Category Estrogen and Progestin Combination

Use Women with an intact uterus: Treatment of moderate to severe vasomotor symptoms associated with menopause; treatment of atrophic vaginitis; prevention of osteoporosis

Usual Dosage Oral: Adults: Females with an intact uterus:

Treatment of menopausal symptoms, atrophic vaginitis, prevention of osteoporosis: Treatment is cyclical and consists of the following: One tablet of estradiol 1 mg (pink tablet) once daily for 3 days, followed by 1 tablet of estradiol 1 mg and norgestimate 0.09 mg (white tablet) once daily for 3 days; repeat sequence continuously. **Note:** This dose may not be the lowest effective combination for these indications. In case of a missed tablet, restart therapy with next available tablet in sequence (taking only 1 tablet each day).

Dosage Forms Tablet: Estradiol 1 mg [15 pink tablets] and estradiol 1 mg and norgestimate 0.09 mg [15 white tablets] (supplied in blister card of 30)

estradiol cypionate *see* estradiol *on page 324*

estradiol cypionate and medroxyprogesterone acetate

(es tra DYE ole sip pe OH nate & me DROKS ee proe JES te rone AS e tate)

Synonyms E_2C and MPA; medroxyprogesterone acetate and estradiol cypionate

U.S./Canadian Brand Names Lunelle™ [US]

Therapeutic Category Contraceptive

Use Prevention of pregnancy

Usual Dosage Adults: Female: I.M.: 0.5 mL

First dose: Within first 5 days of menstrual period or within 5 days of a complete 1st trimester abortion; do not administer <4 weeks postpartum **if not breast-feeding** or <6 weeks postpartum **if breast-feeding**

Maintenance dose: Monthly, every 28-30 days following previous injection; do not exceed 33 days; pregnancy must be ruled out if >33 days have past between injections; bleeding episodes cannot be used to guide injection schedule; shortening schedule may lead to menstrual pattern changes

Switching from other forms of contraception: First injection should be given within 7 days of last active oral contraceptive pill; when switching from other methods, timing of injection should ensure continuous contraceptive coverage

Dosage Forms Injection, suspension: Estradiol cypionate 5 mg and medroxyprogesterone acetate 25 mg per 0.5 mL (0.5 mL)

estradiol hemihydrate *see* estradiol *on page 324*

estradiol transdermal *see* estradiol *on page 324*

estradiol valerate *see* estradiol *on page 324*

Estradot® [Can] *see* estradiol *on page 324*

Estradurin® Injection *(Discontinued)* *see page 1042*

Estra-L® Injection *(Discontinued)* *see page 1042*

estramustine (es tra MUS teen)

Sound-Alike/Look-Alike Issues

Emcyt® may be confused with Eryc®

Synonyms estramustine phosphate sodium; NSC-89199

U.S./Canadian Brand Names Emcyt® [US/Can]

Therapeutic Category Antineoplastic Agent

Use Palliative treatment of prostatic carcinoma (progressive or metastatic)

Usual Dosage Refer to individual protocols.

Oral: 10-16 mg/kg/day (14 mg/kg/day is most common) or 140 mg 4 times/day (some patients have been maintained for >3 years on therapy)

Dosage Forms Capsule, as phosphate sodium: 140 mg

estramustine phosphate sodium *see* estramustine *on this page*

Estrasorb™ [US] *see* estradiol *on page 324*

Estratab® *(Discontinued)* *see page 1042*

Estratab® [Can] *see* estrogens (esterified) *on page 331*

Estratest® [US/Can] *see* estrogens (esterified) and methyltestosterone *on page 332*

Estratest® H.S. [US] *see* estrogens (esterified) and methyltestosterone *on page 332*

Estring® [US/Can] *see* estradiol *on page 324*

Estro-Cyp® Injection *(Discontinued)* *see page 1042*

EstroGel® [US/Can] *see* estradiol *on page 324*

estrogenic substance aqueous *see* estrone *on page 332*

estrogenic substances, conjugated *see* estrogens (conjugated/equine) *on this page*

estrogens (conjugated A/synthetic)

(ES troe jenz KON joo gate ed aye/sin THET ik)

Sound-Alike/Look-Alike Issues

Cenestin® may be confused with Senexon®

U.S./Canadian Brand Names Cenestin® [US/Can]

Therapeutic Category Estrogen Derivative

Use Treatment of moderate to severe vasomotor symptoms of menopause; treatment of vulvar and vaginal atrophy

Usual Dosage The lowest dose that will control symptoms should be used; medication should be discontinued as soon as possible. Oral:

Adults:

Moderate to severe vasomotor symptoms: 0.45 mg/day; may be titrated up to 1.25 mg/day. Attempts to discontinue medication should be made at 3- to 6-month intervals.

Vulvar and vaginal atrophy: 0.3 mg/day

Dosage Forms Tablet: 0.3 mg, 0.45 mg, 0.625 mg, 0.9 mg, 1.25 mg

estrogens (conjugated/equine) (ES troe jenz KON joo gate ed/EE kwine)

Sound-Alike/Look-Alike Issues

Premarin® may be confused with Primaxin®, Provera®, Remeron®

(Continued)

estrogens (conjugated/equine) *(Continued)*

Synonyms CEE; estrogenic substances, conjugated

U.S./Canadian Brand Names C.E.S.® [Can]; Congest [Can]; Premarin® [US/Can]

Therapeutic Category Estrogen Derivative

Use Treatment of moderate to severe vasomotor symptoms associated with menopause; treatment of vulvar and vaginal atrophy; hypoestrogenism (due to hypogonadism, castration, or primary ovarian failure); prostatic cancer (palliation); breast cancer (palliation); osteoporosis (prophylaxis, postmenopausal women at significant risk only); abnormal uterine bleeding

Usual Dosage Adults:

Male: Androgen-dependent prostate cancer: Oral: 1.25-2.5 mg 3 times/day

Female:

Prevention of osteoporosis in postmenopausal women: Oral: Initial: 0.3 mg/day cyclically* or daily, depending on medical assessment of patient. Dose may be adjusted based on bone mineral density and clinical response. The lowest effective dose should be used.

Moderate to severe vasomotor symptoms associated with menopause: Oral: Initial: 0.3 mg/day, cyclically* or daily, depending on medical assessment of patient. The lowest dose that will control symptoms should be used. Medication should be discontinued as soon as possible.

Vulvar and vaginal atrophy:

Oral: Initial: 0.3 mg/day; the lowest dose that will control symptoms should be used. May be given cyclically* or daily, depending on medical assessment of patient. Medication should be discontinued as soon as possible.

Vaginal cream: Intravaginal: ½ to 2 g/day given cyclically*

Abnormal uterine bleeding:

Female hypogonadism: Oral: 0.3-0.625 mg/day given cyclically*; dose may be titrated in 6- to 12-month intervals; progestin treatment should be added to maintain bone mineral density once skeletal maturity is achieved.

Female castration, primary ovarian failure: Oral: 1.25 mg/day given cyclically*; adjust according to severity of symptoms and patient response. For maintenance, adjust to the lowest effective dose.

***Cyclic administration:** Either 3 weeks on, 1 week off **or** 25 days on, 5 days off

Male and Female:

Breast cancer palliation, metastatic disease in selected patients: Oral: 10 mg 3 times/day for at least 3 months

Dosage Forms

Cream, vaginal: 0.625 mg/g (42.5 g)

Injection, powder for reconstitution: 25 mg [diluent contains benzyl alcohol]

Tablet: 0.3 mg, 0.45 mg, 0.625 mg, 0.9 mg, 1.25 mg, 2.5 mg [DSC]

estrogens (conjugated/equine) and medroxyprogesterone

(ES troe jenz (KON joo gate ed/EE kwine) & me DROKS ee proe JES te rone)

Sound-Alike/Look-Alike Issues

Premphase® may be confused with Prempro™

Prempro™ may be confused with Premphase®

Synonyms medroxyprogesterone and estrogens (conjugated); MPA and estrogens (conjugated)

U.S./Canadian Brand Names Premphase® [US/Can]; Premplus® [Can]; Prempro™ [US/Can]

Therapeutic Category Estrogen and Progestin Combination

Use Women with an intact uterus: Treatment of moderate to severe vasomotor symptoms associated with menopause; treatment of atrophic vaginitis; osteoporosis (prophylaxis)

Usual Dosage Oral: Adults:

Treatment of moderate to severe vasomotor symptoms associated with menopause or treatment of atrophic vaginitis in females with an intact uterus. (The lowest dose that will control symptoms should be used; medication should be discontinued as soon as possible):

Premphase®: One maroon conjugated estrogen 0.625 mg tablet daily on days 1 through 14 and one light blue conjugated estrogen 0.625 mg/MPA 5 mg tablet daily on days 15 through 28; re-evaluate patients at 3- and 6-month intervals to determine if treatment is still necessary; monitor patients for signs of endometrial cancer; rule out malignancy if unexplained vaginal bleeding occurs

Prempro™: One conjugated estrogen 0.3 mg/MPA 1.5 mg tablet daily; reevaluate at 3- and 6-month intervals to determine if therapy is still needed; dose may be increased to a maximum of one conjugated estrogen 0.625 mg/MPA 5 mg tablet daily in patients with bleeding or spotting, once malignancy has been ruled out

Osteoporosis prophylaxis in females with an intact uterus:

Premphase®: One maroon conjugated estrogen 0.625 tablet daily on days 1 through 14 and one light blue conjugated estrogen 0.625 mg/MPA 5 mg tablet daily on days 15 through 28; monitor patients for signs of endometrial cancer; rule out malignancy if unexplained vaginal bleeding occurs

Prempro™: One conjugated estrogen 0.3 mg/MPA 1.5 mg tablet daily; dose may be increased to one conjugated estrogen 0.625 mg/MPA 5 mg tablet daily; in patients with bleeding or spotting, once malignancy has been ruled out

Dosage Forms Tablet:

Premphase® [therapy pack contains 2 separate tablet formulations]: Conjugated estrogens 0.625 mg [14 maroon tablets] and conjugated estrogen 0.625 mg/medroxyprogesterone acetate 5 mg [14 light blue tablets] (28s)

Prempro™:

0.3/1.5: Conjugated estrogens 0.3 mg and medroxyprogesterone acetate 1.5 mg (28s)

0.45/1.5: Conjugated estrogens 0.45 mg and medroxyprogesterone acetate 1.5 mg (28s)

0.625/2.5: Conjugated estrogens 0.625 mg and medroxyprogesterone acetate 2.5 mg (28s)

0.625/5: Conjugated estrogens 0.625 mg and medroxyprogesterone acetate 5 mg (28s)

estrogens (esterified) (ES troe jenz es TER i fied)

Sound-Alike/Look-Alike Issues

Estratab® may be confused with Estratest®, Estratest® H.S.

Synonyms esterified estrogens

U.S./Canadian Brand Names Estratab® [Can]; Menest® [US/Can]

Therapeutic Category Estrogen Derivative

Use Treatment of moderate to severe vasomotor symptoms associated with menopause; treatment of vulvar and vaginal atrophy; hypoestrogenism (due to hypogonadism, castration, or primary ovarian failure); prostatic cancer (palliation); breast cancer (palliation); osteoporosis (prophylaxis, in women at significant risk only)

Usual Dosage Oral: Adults:

Prostate cancer (palliation): 1.25-2.5 mg 3 times/day

Female hypogonadism: 2.5-7.5 mg of estrogen daily for 20 days followed by a 10-day rest period. Administer cyclically (3 weeks on and 1 week off). If bleeding does not occur by the end of the 10-day period, repeat the same dosing schedule; the number of courses is dependent upon the responsiveness of the endometrium. If bleeding occurs before the end of the 10-day period, begin an estrogen-progestin cyclic regimen of 2.5-7.5 mg esterified estrogens daily for 20 days. During the last 5 days of estrogen therapy, give an oral progestin. If bleeding occurs before regimen is concluded, discontinue therapy and resume on the fifth day of bleeding.

Moderate to severe vasomotor symptoms associated with menopause: 1.25 mg/day administered cyclically (3 weeks on and 1 week off). If patient has not menstruated within the last 2 months or more, cyclic administration is started arbitrary. If the patient is menstruating, cyclical administration is started on day 5 of the bleeding. For short-term use only and should be discontinued as soon as possible. Re-evaluate at 3- to 6-month intervals for tapering or discontinuation of therapy.

(Continued)

estrogens (esterified) *(Continued)*

Atopic vaginitis and kraurosis vulvae: 0.3 to ≥1.25 mg/day, depending on the tissue response of the individual patient. Administer cyclically. For short-term use only and should be discontinued as soon as possible. Re-evaluate at 3- to 6-month intervals for tapering or discontinuation of therapy.

Breast cancer (palliation): 10 mg 3 times/day for at least 3 months

Osteoporosis in postmenopausal women: Initial: 0.3 mg/day and increase to a maximum daily dose of 1.25 mg/day; initiate therapy as soon as possible after menopause; cyclically or daily, depending on medical assessment of patient. Monitor patients with an intact uterus for signs of endometrial cancer; rule out malignancy if unexplained vaginal bleeding occurs

Female castration and primary ovarian failure: 1.25 mg/day, cyclically. Adjust dosage upward or downward, according to the severity of symptoms and patient response. For maintenance, adjust dosage to lowest level that will provide effective control.

Dosage Forms Tablet: 0.3 mg, 0.625 mg, 1.25 mg, 2.5 mg

estrogens (esterified) and methyltestosterone

(ES troe jenz (es TER i fied) & meth il tes TOS te rone)

Sound-Alike/Look-Alike Issues

Estratest® may be confused with Eskalith®, Estratab®, Estratest® H.S.

Estratest® H.S. may be confused with Eskalith®, Estratab®, Estratest®

Synonyms esterified estrogen and methyltestosterone

U.S./Canadian Brand Names Estratest® [US/Can]; Estratest® H.S. [US]

Therapeutic Category Estrogen and Androgen Combination

Use Vasomotor symptoms of menopause

Usual Dosage Adults: Female: Oral: Lowest dose that will control symptoms should be chosen, normally given 3 weeks on and 1 week off

Dosage Forms Tablet:

Estratest®: Esterified estrogen 1.25 mg and methyltestosterone 2.5 mg [contains sodium benzoate]

Estratest® H.S.: Esterified estrogen 0.625 mg and methyltestosterone 1.25 mg [contains sodium benzoate]

Estroject-2® Injection ***(Discontinued)*** *see page 1042*

Estroject-L.A.® Injection ***(Discontinued)*** *see page 1042*

estrone (ES trone)

Synonyms estrogenic substance aqueous

Therapeutic Category Estrogen Derivative

Use Atrophic vaginitis; hypogonadism; primary ovarian failure; vasomotor symptoms of menopause; prostatic carcinoma; osteoporosis prophylactic

Usual Dosage Adults: I.M.:

Vasomotor symptoms, atrophic vaginitis: 0.1-0.5 mg 2-3 times/week

Primary ovarian failure, hypogonadism: 0.1-1 mg/week, up to 2 mg/week

Prostatic carcinoma: 2-4 mg 2-3 times/week

Dosage Forms Injection: 2 mg/mL (10 mL); 5 mg/mL (10 mL)

Estronol® Injection ***(Discontinued)*** *see page 1042*

estropipate (ES troe pih pate)

Synonyms ortho est; piperazine estrone sulfate

U.S./Canadian Brand Names Ogen® [US/Can]; Ortho-Est® [US]

Therapeutic Category Estrogen Derivative

Use Treatment of moderate to severe vasomotor symptoms associated with menopause; treatment of vulvar and vaginal atrophy; hypoestrogenism (due to hypogonadism, castration, or primary ovarian failure); osteoporosis (prophylaxis, in women at significant risk only)

Usual Dosage Adults:

Oral:

Moderate to severe vasomotor symptoms associated with menopause: Usual dosage range: 0.75-6 mg estropipate daily; use the lowest dose and regimen that will control symptoms, and discontinue as soon as possible. Attempt to discontinue or taper medication at 3- to 6-month intervals. If a patient with vasomotor symptoms has not menstruated within the last ≥2 months, start the cyclic administration arbitrarily. If the patient has menstruated, start cyclic administration on day 5 of bleeding.

Female hypogonadism: 1.5-9 mg estropipate daily for the first 3 weeks, followed by a rest period of 8-10 days; use the lowest dose and regimen that will control symptoms. Repeat if bleeding does not occur by the end of the rest period. The duration of therapy necessary to product the withdrawal bleeding will vary according to the responsiveness of the endometrium. If satisfactory withdrawal bleeding does not occur, give an oral progestin in addition to estrogen during the third week of the cycle.

Female castration or primary ovarian failure: 1.5-9 mg estropipate daily for the first 3 weeks of a theoretical cycle, followed by a rest period of 8-10 days; use the lowest dose and regimen that will control symptoms

Osteoporosis prophylaxis: 0.75 mg estropipate daily for 25 days of a 31-day cycle

Atrophic vaginitis or kraurosis vulvae: 0.75-6 mg estropipate daily; administer cyclically. Use the lowest dose and regimen that will control symptoms; discontinue as soon as possible.

Dosage Forms

Tablet: 0.625 mg [estropipate 0.75 mg]; 1.25 mg [estropipate 1.5 mg]; 2.5 mg [estropipate 3 mg]

Ogen®: 0.625 mg [estropipate 0.75 mg]; 1.25 mg [estropipate 1.5 mg]; 2.5 mg [estropipate 3 mg]

Ortho-Est®: 0.625 mg [estropipate 0.75 mg]; 1.25 mg [estropipate 1.5 mg]

Estrostep® 21 ***(Discontinued)*** *see page 1042*

Estrostep® Fe [US] *see* ethinyl estradiol and norethindrone *on page 342*

Estrovis® ***(Discontinued)*** *see page 1042*

ETAF *see* aldesleukin *on page 28*

etanercept (et a NER cept)

U.S./Canadian Brand Names Enbrel® [US/Can]

Therapeutic Category Antirheumatic, Disease Modifying

Use Treatment of moderately- to severely-active rheumatoid arthritis, moderately- to severely-active polyarticular juvenile arthritis, or psoriatic arthritis in patients who have had an inadequate response to one or more disease-modifying antirheumatic drugs (DMARDs); reduction in signs and symptoms of active ankylosing spondylitis (AS); treatment of chronic plaque psoriasis (moderate-to-severe)

Usual Dosage SubQ:

Children 4-17 years: Juvenile rheumatoid arthritis:

Once-weekly dosing: 0.8 mg/kg (maximum: 50 mg/dose) once weekly

Twice-weekly dosing: 0.4 mg/kg (maximum: 25 mg/dose) twice weekly (individual doses should be separated by 72-96 hours)

Adults:

Rheumatoid arthritis, psoriatic arthritis, ankylosing spondylitis:

Once-weekly dosing: 50 mg once weekly

Twice weekly dosing: 25 mg given twice weekly (individual doses should be separated by 72-96 hours)

Note: If the physician determines that it is appropriate, patients may self-inject after proper training in injection technique.

Plaque psoriasis:

Initial: 50 mg twice weekly, 3-4 days apart (starting doses of 25 or 50 mg once weekly have also been used successfully); maintain initial dose for 3 months

Maintenance dose: 50 mg weekly

(Continued)

etanercept *(Continued)*

Dosage Forms

Injection, powder for reconstitution: 25 mg [diluent contains benzyl alcohol; packaging may contain dry natural rubber (latex)]

Injection, solution: 50 mg/mL (0.98 mL) [prefilled syringe with 27-gauge 1/2 inch needle]

ethacrynate sodium *see* ethacrynic acid *on this page*

ethacrynic acid (eth a KRIN ik AS id)

Sound-Alike/Look-Alike Issues

Edecrin® may be confused with Eulexin®, Ecotrin®

Synonyms ethacrynate sodium

U.S./Canadian Brand Names Edecrin® [US/Can]

Therapeutic Category Diuretic, Loop

Use Management of edema associated with congestive heart failure; hepatic cirrhosis or renal disease; short-term management of ascites due to malignancy, idiopathic edema, and lymphedema

Usual Dosage I.V. formulation should be diluted in D_5W or NS (1 mg/mL) and infused over several minutes.

Children: Oral: 1 mg/kg/dose once daily; increase at intervals of 2-3 days as needed, to a maximum of 3 mg/kg/day.

Adults:

Oral: 50-200 mg/day in 1-2 divided doses; may increase in increments of 25-50 mg at intervals of several days; doses up to 200 mg twice daily may be required with severe, refractory edema.

I.V.: 0.5-1 mg/kg/dose (maximum: 100 mg/dose); repeat doses not routinely recommended; however, if indicated, repeat doses every 8-12 hours.

Dosage Forms

Injection, powder for reconstitution, as ethacrynate sodium: 50 mg

Tablet: 25 mg

ethambutol (e THAM byoo tole)

Sound-Alike/Look-Alike Issues

Myambutol® may be confused with Nembutal®

Synonyms ethambutol hydrochloride

U.S./Canadian Brand Names Etibi® [Can]; Myambutol® [US]

Therapeutic Category Antimycobacterial Agent

Use Treatment of tuberculosis and other mycobacterial diseases in conjunction with other antituberculosis agents

Usual Dosage Oral:

Ethambutol is generally not recommended in children whose visual acuity cannot be monitored. However, ethambutol should be considered for all children with organisms resistant to other drugs, when susceptibility to ethambutol has been demonstrated, or susceptibility is likely.

Note: A four-drug regimen (isoniazid, rifampin, pyrazinamide, and either streptomycin or ethambutol) is preferred for the initial, empiric treatment of TB. When the drug susceptibility results are available, the regimen should be altered as appropriate.

Children and Adults:

Daily therapy: 15-25 mg/kg/day (maximum: 2.5 g/day)

Directly observed therapy (DOT): Twice weekly: 50 mg/kg (maximum: 2.5 g)

DOT: 3 times/week: 25-30 mg/kg (maximum: 2.5 g)

Adults: Treatment of disseminated *Mycobacterium avium* complex (MAC) in patients with advanced HIV infection: 15 mg/kg ethambutol in combination with azithromycin 600 mg daily

Dosage Forms Tablet, as hydrochloride: 100 mg, 400 mg

ethambutol hydrochloride *see* ethambutol *on this page*

Ethamolin® [US] *see* ethanolamine oleate *on this page*

ethanoic acid *see* acetic acid *on page 15*

ethanol *see* alcohol (ethyl) *on page 27*

ethanolamine oleate (ETH a nol a meen OH lee ate)

Sound-Alike/Look-Alike Issues
Ethamolin® may be confused with ethanol
Synonyms monoethanolamine
U.S./Canadian Brand Names Ethamolin® [US]
Therapeutic Category Sclerosing Agent
Use **Orphan drug:** Sclerosing agent used for bleeding esophageal varices
Usual Dosage Adults: 1.5-5 mL per varix, up to 20 mL total or 0.4 mL/kg for a 50 kg patient; doses should be decreased in patients with severe hepatic dysfunction and should receive less than recommended maximum dose
Dosage Forms Injection, solution: 5% [50 mg/mL] (2 mL) [contains benzyl alcohol]

Ethaquin® ***(Discontinued)*** *see page 1042*

Ethatab® ***(Discontinued)*** *see page 1042*

ethaverine (eth AV er een)

Synonyms ethaverine hydrochloride
Therapeutic Category Vasodilator
Use Peripheral and cerebral vascular insufficiency associated with arterial spasm
Usual Dosage Adults: Oral: 100 mg 3 times/day
Dosage Forms Tablet, as hydrochloride: 100 mg

ethaverine hydrochloride *see* ethaverine *on this page*

ethinyl estradiol (ETH in il es tra DYE ole)

Therapeutic Category Estrogen Derivative
Use Atrophic vaginitis; hypogonadism; primary ovarian failure; vasomotor symptoms of menopause; prostatic carcinoma; osteoporosis prophylactic
Usual Dosage Adults: Oral:
Hypogonadism: 0.05 mg 1-3 times/day for 2 weeks
Prostatic carcinoma: 0.15-2 mg/day
Vasomotor symptoms: 0.02-0.05 mg for 21 days, off 7 days and repeat
Dosage Forms Tablet: 0.02 mg [contains tartrazine], 0.05 mg

ethinyl estradiol and cyproterone acetate *see* cyproterone and ethinyl estradiol *(Canada only) on page 238*

ethinyl estradiol and desogestrel

(ETH in il es tra DYE ole & des oh JES trel)

Sound-Alike/Look-Alike Issues
Ortho-Cept® may be confused with Ortho-Cyclen®
U.S./Canadian Brand Names Apri® [US]; Cyclessa® [US]; Desogen® [US]; Kariva™ [US]; Marvelon® [Can]; Mircette® [US]; Ortho-Cept® [US/Can]; Solia™ [US]; Velivet™ [US]
Therapeutic Category Contraceptive, Oral
Use Prevention of pregnancy
Usual Dosage Oral: Adults: Female: Contraception:
Schedule 1 (Sunday starter): Dose begins on first Sunday after onset of menstruation; if the menstrual period starts on Sunday, take first tablet that very same day. **With a Sunday start, an additional method of contraception should be used until after the first 7 days of consecutive administration.**
(Continued)

ethinyl estradiol and desogestrel *(Continued)*

For 21-tablet package: Dosage is 1 tablet daily for 21 consecutive days, followed by 7 days off of the medication; a new course begins on the 8th day after the last tablet is taken.

For 28-tablet package: Dosage is 1 tablet daily without interruption.

Schedule 2 (Day 1 starter): Dose starts on first day of menstrual cycle taking 1 tablet daily.

For 21-tablet package: Dosage is 1 tablet daily for 21 consecutive days, followed by 7 days off of the medication; a new course begins on the 8th day after the last tablet is taken.

For 28-tablet package: Dosage is 1 tablet daily without interruption.

If all doses have been taken on schedule and one menstrual period is missed, continue dosing cycle. If two consecutive menstrual periods are missed, pregnancy test is required before new dosing cycle is started.

Missed doses **monophasic formulations** (refer to package insert for complete information):

One dose missed: Take as soon as remembered or take 2 tablets next day

Two consecutive doses missed in the first 2 weeks: Take 2 tablets as soon as remembered or 2 tablets next 2 days. **An additional method of contraception should be used for 7 days after missed dose.**

Two consecutive doses missed in week 3 or three consecutive doses missed at any time:

Schedule 1 (Sunday starter): Continue to take 1 tablet daily until Sunday, then discard the rest of the pack, and a new pack is started that same day.

Schedule 2 (Day 1 starter): Current pack should be discarded, and a new pack started that same day. **An additional method of contraception should be used for 7 days after missed dose.**

Missed doses **biphasic/triphasic formulations** (refer to package insert for complete information):

One dose missed: Take as soon as remembered or take 2 tablets next day.

Two consecutive doses missed in week 1 or week 2 of the pack: Take 2 tablets as soon as remembered and 2 tablets the next day. Resume taking 1 tablet daily until the pack is empty. **An additional method of contraception should be used for 7 days after a missed dose.**

Two consecutive doses missed in week 3 of the pack; **an additional method of contraception must be used for 7 days after a missed dose**:

Schedule 1 (Sunday starter): Take 1 tablet every day until Sunday. Discard the remaining pack and start a new pack of pills on the same day.

Schedule 2 (Day 1 starter): Discard the remaining pack and start a new pack the same day.

Three or more consecutive doses missed; **an additional method of contraception must be used for 7 days after a missed dose**:

Schedule 1 (Sunday starter): Take 1 tablet every day until Sunday; on Sunday, discard the pack and start a new pack.

Schedule 2 (Day 1 starter): Discard the remaining pack and begin new pack of tablets starting on the same day.

Dosage Forms Tablet:

Low-dose formulation:

Kariva™:

Day 1-21: Ethinyl estradiol 0.02 mg and desogestrel 0.15 mg [21 white tablets]

Day 22-23: 2 inactive light green tablets

Day 24-28: Ethinyl estradiol 0.01 mg [5 light blue tablets] (28s)

Mircette®:

Day 1-21: Ethinyl estradiol 0.02 mg and desogestrel 0.15 mg [21 white tablets]

Day 22-23: 2 inactive green tablets

Day 24-28: Ethinyl estradiol 0.01 mg [5 yellow tablets] (28s)

Monophasic formulations:

Apri® 28: Ethinyl estradiol 0.03 mg and desogestrel 0.15 mg [21 rose tablets and 7 white inactive tablets] (28s)

Desogen®, Solia™: Ethinyl estradiol 0.03 mg and desogestrel 0.15 mg [21 white tablets and 7 green inactive tablets] (28s)

Ortho-Cept® 28: Ethinyl estradiol 0.03 mg and desogestrel 0.15 mg [21 orange tablets and 7 green inactive tablets] (28s)

Triphasic formulation:

Cyclessa®:

Day 1-7:Ethinyl estradiol 0.025 mg and desogestrel 0.1 mg [7 light yellow tablets]
Day 8-14: Ethinyl estradiol 0.025 mg and desogestrel 0.125 mg [7 orange tablets]
Day 14-21: Ethinyl estradiol 0.025 mg and desogestrel 0.15 mg [7 red tablets]
Day 21-28: 7 green inactive tablets (28s)

Velivet™:

Day 1-7: Ethinyl estradiol 0.025 mg and desogestrel 0.1 mg [7 beige tablets]
Day 8-14: Ethinyl estradiol 0.025 mg and desogestrel 0.125 mg [7 orange tablets]
Day 14-21: Ethinyl estradiol 0.025 mg and desogestrel 0.15 mg [7 pink tablets]
Day 21-28: 7 white inactive tablets (28s)

ethinyl estradiol and drospirenone

(ETH in il es tra DYE ole & droh SPYE re none)

Synonyms drospirenone and ethinyl estradiol

U.S./Canadian Brand Names Yasmin® [US]

Therapeutic Category Contraceptive

Use Prevention of pregnancy

Usual Dosage Oral: Adults: Female: Contraception: Dosage is 1 tablet daily for 28 consecutive days. Dose should be taken at the same time each day, either after the evening meal or at bedtime. Dosing may be started on the first day of menstrual period (Day 1 starter) or on the first Sunday after the onset of the menstrual period (Sunday starter).

Day 1 starter: Dose starts on first day of menstrual cycle taking 1 tablet daily.

Sunday starter: Dose begins on first Sunday after onset of menstruation; if the menstrual period starts on Sunday, take first tablet that very same day. **With a Sunday start, an additional method of contraception should be used until after the first 7 days of consecutive administration.**

If all doses have been taken on schedule and one menstrual period is missed, continue dosing cycle. If two consecutive menstrual periods are missed, pregnancy test is required before new dosing cycle is started.

If doses have been missed during the first 3 weeks and the menstrual period is missed, pregnancy should be ruled out prior to continuing treatment.

Missed doses (monophasic formulations) (refer to package insert for complete information):

One dose missed: Take as soon as remembered or take 2 tablets next day

Two consecutive doses missed in the first 2 weeks: Take 2 tablets as soon as remembered or 2 tablets next 2 days. **An additional method of contraception should be used for 7 days after missed dose.**

Two consecutive doses missed in week 3 or three consecutive doses missed at any time: **An additional method of contraception must be used for 7 days after a missed dose.** Day 1 starter: Current pack should be discarded, and a new pack should be started that same day. Sunday starter: Continue dose of 1 tablet daily until Sunday, then discard the rest of the pack, and a new pack should be started that same day.

Any number of doses missed in week 4: Continue taking one pill each day until pack is empty; no back-up method of contraception is needed

Dosage Forms Tablet: Ethinyl estradiol 0.03 mg and drospirenone 3 mg [21 yellow active tablets and 7 white inactive tablets] (28s)

ethinyl estradiol and ethynodiol diacetate

(ETH in il es tra DYE ole & e thye noe DYE ole dye AS e tate)

Sound-Alike/Look-Alike Issues

Demulen® may be confused with Dalmane®, Demerol®

Synonyms ethynodiol diacetate and ethinyl estradiol

U.S./Canadian Brand Names Demulen® 30 [Can]; Demulen® [US]; Zovia™ [US]

Therapeutic Category Contraceptive, Oral

Use Prevention of pregnancy

Usual Dosage Oral: Adults: Female: Contraception:

Schedule 1 (Sunday starter): Dose begins on first Sunday after onset of menstruation; if the menstrual period starts on Sunday, take first tablet that very same day. **With a Sunday start, an additional method of contraception should be used until after the first 7 days of consecutive administration.**

For 21-tablet package: 1 tablet/day for 21 consecutive days, followed by 7 days off of the medication; a new course begins on the 8th day after the last tablet is taken.

For 28-tablet package: 1 tablet/day without interruption.

Schedule 2 (Day 1 starter): Dose starts on first day of menstrual cycle taking 1 tablet daily.

For 21-tablet package: 1 tablet/day for 21 consecutive days, followed by 7 days off of the medication; a new course begins on the 8th day after the last tablet is taken.

For 28-tablet package: 1 tablet/day without interruption.

If all doses have been taken on schedule and one menstrual period is missed, continue dosing cycle. If two consecutive menstrual periods are missed, pregnancy test is required before new dosing cycle is started.

Missed doses **monophasic formulations** (refer to package insert for complete information):

One dose missed: Take as soon as remembered or take 2 tablets next day

Two consecutive doses missed in the first 2 weeks: Take 2 tablets as soon as remembered or 2 tablets next 2 days. **An additional method of contraception should be used for 7 days after missed dose.**

Two consecutive doses missed in week 3 or three consecutive doses missed at any time: **An additional method of contraception should be used for 7 days after missed dose:**

Schedule 1 (Sunday starter): Continue dose of 1 tablet daily until Sunday, then discard the rest of the pack, and a new pack should be started that same day.

Schedule 2 (Day 1 starter): Current package should be discarded, and a new pack should be started that same day.

Dosage Forms [DSC] = Discontinued product

Tablet, monophasic formulations:

Demulen® 1/35-28: Ethinyl estradiol 0.035 mg and ethynodiol diacetate 1 mg [21 white tablets and 7 blue inactive tablets] (28s)

Demulen® 1/50-21: Ethinyl estradiol 0.05 mg and ethynodiol diacetate 1 mg [white tablets] (21s) [DSC]

Demulen® 1/50-28: Ethinyl estradiol 0.05 mg and ethynodiol diacetate 1 mg [21 white tablets and 7 pink inactive tablets] (28s) [DSC]

Zovia™ 1/35-28: Ethinyl estradiol 0.035 mg and ethynodiol diacetate 1 mg [21 light pink tablets and 7 white inactive tablets] (28s)

Zovia™ 1/50-28: Ethinyl estradiol 0.05 mg and ethynodiol diacetate 1 mg [21 pink tablets and 7 white inactive tablets] (28s)

ethinyl estradiol and etonogestrel

(ETH in il es tra DYE ole & et oh noe JES trel)

Synonyms etonogestrel and ethinyl estradiol

U.S./Canadian Brand Names NuvaRing® [US]

Therapeutic Category Contraceptive; Estrogen and Progestin Combination

Use Prevention of pregnancy

Usual Dosage Vaginal: Adults: Female: Contraception: One ring, inserted vaginally and left in place for 3 consecutive weeks, then removed for 1 week. A new ring is inserted 7

days after the last was removed (even if bleeding is not complete) and should be inserted at approximately the same time of day the ring was removed the previous week.

Initial treatment should begin as follows (pregnancy should always be ruled out first):

No hormonal contraceptive use in the past month: Using the first day of menstruation as "Day 1," insert the ring on or prior to "Day 5," even if bleeding is not complete. **An additional form of contraception should be used for the following 7 days.***

Switching from combination oral contraceptive: Ring should be inserted within 7 days after the last active tablet was taken and no later than the first day a new cycle of tablets would begin. Additional forms of contraception are not needed.

Switching from progestin-only contraceptive: **An additional form of contraception should be used for the following 7 days with any of the following.***

If previously using a progestin-only mini-pill, insert the ring on any day of the month; do not skip days between the last pill and insertion of the ring.

If previously using an implant, insert the ring on the same day of implant removal.

If previously using a progestin-containing IUD, insert the ring on day of IUD removal.

If previously using a progestin injection, insert the ring on the day the next injection would be given.

Following complete 1st trimester abortion: Insert ring within the first five days of abortion. If not inserted within five days, follow instructions for "No hormonal contraceptive use within the past month" and instruct patient to use a nonhormonal contraceptive in the interim.

Following delivery or 2nd trimester abortion: Insert ring 4 weeks postpartum (in women who are not breast-feeding) or following 2nd trimester abortion. **An additional form of contraception should be used for the following 7 days.***

If the ring is accidentally removed from the vagina at anytime during the 3-week period of use, it may be rinsed with cool or lukewarm water (not hot) and reinserted as soon as possible. If the ring is not reinserted within three hours, contraceptive effectiveness will be decreased. **An additional form of contraception should be used until the ring has been inserted for 7 continuous days.***

If the ring has been removed for longer than 1 week, pregnancy must be ruled out prior to restarting therapy. **An additional form of contraception should be used for the following 7 days.***

If the ring has been left in place for >3 weeks, a new ring should be inserted following a 1-week (ring-free) interval. Pregnancy must be ruled out prior to insertion and **an additional form of contraception should be used for the following 7 days.***

***Note:** Diaphragms may interfere with proper ring placement, and therefore, are not recommended for use as an additional form of contraception.

Dosage Forms Ring, intravaginal [3-week duration]: Ethinyl estradiol 0.015 mg/day and etonogestrel 0.12 mg/day (1s)

ethinyl estradiol and levonorgestrel

(ETH in il es tra DYE ole & LEE voe nor jes trel)

Sound-Alike/Look-Alike Issues

Alesse® may be confused with Aleve®
Nordette® may be confused with Nicorette®
PREVEN® may be confused with Prevnar®
Tri-Levlen® may be confused with Trilafon®
Triphasil® may be confused with Tri-Norinyl®

Synonyms levonorgestrel and ethinyl estradiol

U.S./Canadian Brand Names Alesse® [US/Can]; Aviane™ [US]; Enpresse™ [US]; Lessina™ [US]; Levlen® [US]; Levlite™ [US]; Levora® [US]; Min-Ovral® [Can]; Nordette® [US]; Portia™ [US]; PREVEN® [US]; Seasonale® [US]; Tri-Levlen® [US]; Triphasil® [US/Can]; Triquilar® [Can]; Trivora® [US]

Therapeutic Category Contraceptive, Oral

Use Prevention of pregnancy; postcoital contraception

(Continued)

ethinyl estradiol and levonorgestrel *(Continued)*

Usual Dosage Oral: Adults: Female:

Contraception, 28-day cycle:

Schedule 1 (Sunday starter): Dose begins on first Sunday after onset of menstruation; if the menstrual period starts on Sunday, take first tablet that very same day. With a Sunday start, an additional method of contraception should be used until after the first 7 days of consecutive administration:

For 21-tablet package: 1 tablet/day for 21 consecutive days, followed by 7 days off of the medication; a new course begins on the 8th day after the last tablet is taken

For 28-tablet package: 1 tablet/day without interruption

Schedule 2 (Day 1 starter): Dose starts on first day of menstrual cycle taking 1 tablet/day:

For 21-tablet package: 1 tablet/day for 21 consecutive days, followed by 7 days off of the medication; a new course begins on the 8th day after the last tablet is taken

For 28-tablet package: 1 tablet/day without interruption

If all doses have been taken on schedule and one menstrual period is missed, continue dosing cycle. If two consecutive menstrual periods are missed, pregnancy test is required before new dosing cycle is started.

Missed doses **monophasic formulations** (refer to package insert for complete information):

One dose missed: Take as soon as remembered or take 2 tablets next day

Two consecutive doses missed in the first 2 weeks: Take 2 tablets as soon as remembered or 2 tablets next 2 days. An additional method of contraception should be used for 7 days after missed dose.

Two consecutive doses missed in week 3 or three consecutive doses missed at any time: An additional method of contraception must be used for 7 days after a missed dose: Schedule 1 (Sunday starter): Continue dose of 1 tablet daily until Sunday, then discard the rest of the pack, and a new pack should be started that same day. Schedule 2 (Day 1 starter): Current pack should be discarded, and a new pack should be started that same day.

Missed doses **biphasic/triphasic formulations** (refer to package insert for complete information):

One dose missed: Take as soon as remembered or take 2 tablets next day.

Two consecutive doses missed in week 1 or week 2 of the pack: Take 2 tablets as soon as remembered and 2 tablets the next day. Resume taking 1 tablet daily until the pack is empty. An additional method of contraception should be used for 7 days after a missed dose.

Two consecutive doses missed in week 3 of the pack: An additional method of contraception must be used for 7 days after a missed dose. Schedule 1 (Sunday starter): Take 1 tablet every day until Sunday. Discard the remaining pack and start a new pack of pills on the same day. Schedule 2 (Day 1 starter): Discard the remaining pack and start a new pack the same day.

Three or more consecutive doses missed: An additional method of contraception must be used for 7 days after a missed dose. Schedule 1 (Sunday starter): Take 1 tablet every day until Sunday; on Sunday, discard the pack and start a new pack. Schedule 2 (Day 1 starter): Discard the remaining pack and begin new pack of tablets starting on the same day.

Contraception, 91-day cycle (Seasonale®): One active tablet/day for 84 consecutive days, followed by 1 inactive tablet/day for 7 days; if all doses have been taken on schedule and one menstrual period is missed, pregnancy should be ruled out prior to continuing therapy.

Missed doses:

One dose missed: Take as soon as remembered or take 2 tablets the next day

Two consecutive doses missed: Take 2 tablets as soon as remembered or 2 tablets the next 2 days. An additional nonhormonal method of contraception should be used for 7 consecutive days after the missed dose.

Three or more consecutive doses missed: Do not take the missed doses; continue taking 1 tablet/day until pack is complete. Bleeding may occur during the following week. An additional nonhormonal method of contraception should be used for 7 consecutive days after the missed dose.

Emergency contraception (PREVEN®): Initial: 2 tablets as soon as possible (but within 72 hours of unprotected intercourse), followed by a second dose of 2 tablets 12 hours later. Repeat dose or use antiemetic if vomiting occurs within 1 hour of dose.

Dosage Forms Tablet:

PREVEN®: Ethinyl estradiol 0.05 mg and levonorgestrel 0.25 mg (4s) [also available as a kit containing 4 tablets and a pregnancy test]

Low-dose formulations:

Alesse® 21: Ethinyl estradiol 0.02 mg and levonorgestrel 0.1 mg [pink tablets] (21s)

Alesse® 28: Ethinyl estradiol 0.02 mg and levonorgestrel 0.1 mg [21 pink tablets and 7 light green inactive tablets] (28s)

Aviane™ 28: Ethinyl estradiol 0.02 mg and levonorgestrel 0.1 mg [21 orange tablets and 7 light green inactive tablets] (28s)

Lessina™ 21: Ethinyl estradiol 0.02 mg and levonorgestrel 0.1 mg [pink tablets] (21s)

Lessina™ 28, Levlite™ 28: Ethinyl estradiol 0.02 mg and levonorgestrel 0.1 mg [21 pink tablets and 7 white inactive tablets] (28s)

Monophasic formulations:

Levlen® 21: Ethinyl estradiol 0.03 mg and levonorgestrel 0.15 mg [light orange tablets] (21s)

Levlen® 28: Ethinyl estradiol 0.03 mg and levonorgestrel 0.15 mg [21 light orange tablets and 7 pink inactive tablets] (28s)

Levora® 28: Ethinyl estradiol 0.03 mg and levonorgestrel 0.15 mg [21 white tablets and 7 peach inactive tablets] (28s)

Nordette® 21: Ethinyl estradiol 0.03 mg and levonorgestrel 0.15 mg [light orange tablets] (21s)

Nordette® 28: Ethinyl estradiol 0.03 mg and levonorgestrel 0.15 mg [21 light orange tablets and 7 pink inactive tablets] (28s)

Portia™ 21: Ethinyl estradiol 0.03 mg and levonorgestrel 0.15 mg [pink tablets] (21s)

Portia™ 28: Ethinyl estradiol 0.03 mg and levonorgestrel 0.15 mg [21 pink tablets and 7 white inactive tablets] (28s)

Seasonale®: Ethinyl estradiol 0.03 mg and levonorgestrel 0.15 mg [84 pink tablets and 7 white inactive tablets; extended cycle regimen]

Triphasic formulations:

Enpresse™:

Day 1-6: Ethinyl estradiol 0.03 mg and levonorgestrel 0.05 mg [6 pink tablets]

Day 7-11: Ethinyl estradiol 0.04 mg and levonorgestrel 0.075 mg [5 white tablets]

Day 12-21: Ethinyl estradiol 0.03 mg and levonorgestrel 0.125 mg [10 orange tablets]

Day 22-28: 7 light green inactive tablets (28s)

Tri-Levlen® 21, Triphasil® 21:

Day 1-6: Ethinyl estradiol 0.03 mg and levonorgestrel 0.05 mg [6 brown tablets]

Day 7-11: Ethinyl estradiol 0.04 mg and levonorgestrel 0.075 mg [5 white tablets]

Day 12-21: Ethinyl estradiol 0.03 mg and levonorgestrel 0.125 mg [10 light yellow tablets] (21s)

Tri-Levlen® 28, Triphasil® 28:

Day 1-6: Ethinyl estradiol 0.03 mg and levonorgestrel 0.05 mg [6 brown tablets]

Day 7-11: Ethinyl estradiol 0.04 mg and levonorgestrel 0.075 mg [5 white tablets]

Day 12-21: Ethinyl estradiol 0.03 mg and levonorgestrel 0.125 mg [10 light yellow tablets]

Day 22-28: 7 light green inactive tablets (28s)

Trivora® 28:

Day 1-6: Ethinyl estradiol 0.03 mg and levonorgestrel 0.05 mg [6 blue tablets]

Day 7-11: Ethinyl estradiol 0.04 mg and levonorgestrel 0.075 mg [5 white tablets]

Day 12-21: Ethinyl estradiol 0.03 mg and levonorgestrel 0.125 mg [10 pink tablets]

Day 22-28: 7 peach inactive tablets (28s)

ethinyl estradiol and NGM *see* ethinyl estradiol and norgestimate *on page 346*

ethinyl estradiol and norelgestromin

(ETH in il es tra DYE ole & nor el JES troe min)

Synonyms norelgestromin and ethinyl estradiol

U.S./Canadian Brand Names Evra® [Can]; Ortho Evra™ [US]

Therapeutic Category Contraceptive; Estrogen and Progestin Combination

Use Prevention of pregnancy

Usual Dosage Topical: Adults: Female:

Contraception: Apply one patch each week for 3 weeks (21 total days); followed by one week that is patch-free. Each patch should be applied on the same day each week ("patch change day") and only one patch should be worn at a time. No more than 7 days should pass during the patch-free interval.

Schedule 1 (Sunday starter): Dose begins on first Sunday after onset of menstruation; if the menstrual period starts on Sunday, apply one patch that very same day. **With a Sunday start, an additional method of contraception (nonhormonal) should be used until after the first 7 days of consecutive administration.** Each patch change will then occur on Sunday.

Schedule 2 (Day 1 starter): Dose starts on first day of menstrual cycle, applying one patch during the first 24 hours of menstrual cycle. No back-up method of contraception is needed as long as the patch is applied on the first day of cycle. Each patch change will then occur on that same day of the week.

Additional dosing considerations:

No bleeding during patch-free week/missed menstrual period: If patch has been applied as directed, continue treatment on usual "patch change day". If used correctly, no bleeding during patch-free week does not necessarily indicate pregnancy. However, if no withdrawal bleeding occurs for 2 consecutive cycles, pregnancy should be ruled out. If patch has not been applied as directed, and one menstrual period is missed, pregnancy should be ruled out prior to continuing treatment.

If a patch becomes partially or completely detached for <24 hours: Try to reapply to same place, or replace with a new patch immediately. Do not reapply if patch is no longer sticky, if it is sticking to itself or another surface, or if it has material sticking to it.

If a patch becomes partially or completely detached for >24 hours (or time period is unknown): Apply a new patch and use this day of the week as the new "patch change day" from this point on. **An additional method of contraception (nonhormonal) should be used until after the first 7 days of consecutive administration.**

Switching from oral contraceptives: Apply first patch on the first day of withdrawal bleeding. If there is no bleeding within 5 days of taking the last active tablet, pregnancy must first be ruled out. If patch is applied later than the first day of bleeding, **an additional method of contraception (nonhormonal) should be used until after the first 7 days of consecutive administration**

Use after childbirth: Therapy should not be started <4 weeks after childbirth. Pregnancy should be ruled out prior to treatment if menstrual periods have not restarted. **An additional method of contraception (nonhormonal) should be used until after the first 7 days of consecutive administration.**

Use after abortion or miscarriage: Therapy may be started immediately if abortion/miscarriage occur within the first trimester. If therapy is not started within 5 days, follow instructions for first time use. If abortion/miscarriage occur during the second trimester, therapy should not be started for at least 4 weeks. Follow directions for use after childbirth.

Dosage Forms Patch, transdermal: Ethinyl estradiol 0.75 mg and norelgestromin 6 mg [releases ethinyl estradiol 20 mcg and norelgestromin 150 mcg per day] (1s, 3s)

ethinyl estradiol and norethindrone

(ETH in il es tra DYE ole & nor eth IN drone)

Sound-Alike/Look-Alike Issues

femhrt® may be confused with Femara®
Modicon® may be confused with Mylicon®
Norinyl® may be confused with Nardil®
Tri-Norinyl® may be confused with Triphasil®

Synonyms norethindrone acetate and ethinyl estradiol

U.S./Canadian Brand Names Brevicon® [US]; Brevicon® 0.5/35 [Can]; Brevicon® 1/35 [Can]; Estrostep® Fe [US]; femhrt® [US/Can]; Junel™ [US]; Loestrin® [US/Can]; Loestrin® 1.5.30 [Can]; Loestrin® Fe [US]; Microgestin™ Fe [US]; Minestrin™ 1/20 [Can]; Modicon® [US]; Necon® 0.5/35 [US]; Necon® 1/35 [US]; Necon® 7/7/7 [US]; Necon® 10/11 [US]; Norinyl® 1+35 [US]; Nortrel™ [US]; Nortrel™ 7/7/7 [US]; Ortho® 0.5/35 [Can]; Ortho® 1/35 [Can]; Ortho® 7/7/7 [Can]; Ortho-Novum® [US]; Ovcon® [US]; Select™ 1/35 [Can]; Synphasic® [Can]; Tri-Norinyl® [US]

Therapeutic Category Contraceptive, Oral

Use Prevention of pregnancy; treatment of acne; moderate to severe vasomotor symptoms associated with menopause; prevention of osteoporosis (in women at significant risk only)

Usual Dosage Oral:

Adolescents ≥15 years and Adults: Female: Acne: Estrostep®: Refer to dosing for contraception

Adults: Female:

Moderate to severe vasomotor symptoms associated with menopause: femhrt® 1/5: 1 tablet daily; patients should be re-evaluated at 3- to 6-month intervals to determine if treatment is still necessary

Prevention of osteoporosis: femhrt® 1/5: 1 tablet daily

Contraception:

Schedule 1 (Sunday starter): Dose begins on first Sunday after onset of menstruation; if the menstrual period starts on Sunday, take first tablet that very same day. With a Sunday start, an additional method of contraception should be used until after the first 7 days of consecutive administration.

For 21-tablet package: Dosage is 1 tablet daily for 21 consecutive days, followed by 7 days off of the medication; a new course begins on the 8th day after the last tablet is taken.

For 28-tablet package: Dosage is 1 tablet daily without interruption.

Schedule 2 (Day 1 starter): Dose starts on first day of menstrual cycle taking 1 tablet daily.

For 21-tablet package: Dosage is 1 tablet daily for 21 consecutive days, followed by 7 days off of the medication; a new course begins on the 8th day after the last tablet is taken.

For 28-tablet package: Dosage is 1 tablet daily without interruption.

If all doses have been taken on schedule and one menstrual period is missed, continue dosing cycle. If two consecutive menstrual periods are missed, pregnancy test is required before new dosing cycle is started.

Missed doses **monophasic formulations** (refer to package insert for complete information):

One dose missed: Take as soon as remembered or take 2 tablets next day Two consecutive doses missed in the first 2 weeks: Take 2 tablets as soon as remembered or 2 tablets next 2 days. An additional method of contraception should be used for 7 days after missed dose.

Two consecutive doses missed in week 3 or three consecutive doses missed at any time: An additional method of contraception must be used for 7 days after a missed dose. Schedule 1 (Sunday starter): Continue dose of 1 tablet daily until Sunday, then discard the rest of the pack, and a new pack should be started that same day. Schedule 2 (Day 1 starter): Current pack should be discarded, and a new pack should be started that same day.

Missed doses **biphasic/triphasic formulations** (refer to package insert for complete information):

One dose missed: Take as soon as remembered or take 2 tablets next day.

Two consecutive doses missed in week 1 or week 2 of the pack: Take 2 tablets as soon as remembered and 2 tablets the next day. Resume taking 1 tablet daily until the pack is empty. An additional method of contraception should be used for 7 days after a missed dose.

(Continued)

ethinyl estradiol and norethindrone *(Continued)*

Two consecutive doses missed in week 3 of the pack: An additional method of contraception must be used for 7 days after a missed dose. Schedule 1 (Sunday Starter): Take 1 tablet every day until Sunday. Discard the remaining pack and start a new pack of pills on the same day. Schedule 2 (Day 1 starter): Discard the remaining pack and start a new pack the same day.

Three or more consecutive doses missed: An additional method of contraception must be used for 7 days after a missed dose. Schedule 1 (Sunday Starter): Take 1 tablet every day until Sunday; on Sunday, discard the pack and start a new pack. Schedule 2 (Day 1 Starter): Discard the remaining pack and begin new pack of tablets starting on the same day.

Dosage Forms

Tablet: femhrt® 1/5: Ethinyl estradiol 0.005 mg and norethindrone acetate 1 mg [white tablets]

Tablet, monophasic formulations:

Brevicon®: Ethinyl estradiol 0.035 mg and norethindrone 0.5 mg [21 blue tablets and 7 orange inactive tablets] (28s)

Junel™ 21 1/20: Ethinyl estradiol 0.02 mg and norethindrone acetate 1 mg [yellow tablets] (21s)

Junel™ 21 1.5/30: Ethinyl estradiol 0.03 mg and norethindrone acetate 1.5 mg [pink tablets] (21s)

Junel™ Fe 1/20: Ethinyl estradiol 0.02 mg and norethindrone acetate 1 mg [21 yellow tablets] and ferrous fumarate 75 mg [7 brown tablets] (28s)

Junel™ Fe 1.5/30: Ethinyl estradiol 0.03 mg and norethindrone acetate 1.5 mg [21 pink tablets] and ferrous fumarate 75 mg [7 brown tablets] (28s)

Loestrin® 21 1/20: Ethinyl estradiol 0.02 mg and norethindrone acetate 1 mg [white tablets] (21s)

Loestrin® 21 1.5/30: Ethinyl estradiol 0.03 mg and norethindrone acetate 1.5 mg [green tablets] (21s)

Loestrin® Fe 1/20, Microgestin™ Fe 1/20: Ethinyl estradiol 0.02 mg and norethindrone acetate 1 mg [21 white tablets] and ferrous fumarate 75 mg [7 brown tablets] (28s)

Loestrin® Fe 1.5/30, Microgestin™ Fe 1.5/30: Ethinyl estradiol 0.03 mg and norethindrone acetate 1.5 mg [21 green tablets] and ferrous fumarate 75 mg [7 brown tablets] (28s)

Modicon® 21: Ethinyl estradiol 0.035 mg and norethindrone 0.5 mg [white tablets] (21s)

Modicon® 28: Ethinyl estradiol 0.035 mg and norethindrone 0.5 mg [21 white tablets and 7 green inactive tablets] (28s)

Necon® 0.5/35-21: Ethinyl estradiol 0.035 mg and norethindrone 0.5 mg [light yellow tablets] (21s)

Necon® 0.5/35-28: Ethinyl estradiol 0.035 mg and norethindrone 0.5 mg [21 light yellow tablets and 7 white inactive tablets] (28s)

Necon® 1/35-21: Ethinyl estradiol 0.035 mg and norethindrone 1 mg [dark yellow tablets] (21s)

Necon® 1/35-28: Ethinyl estradiol 0.035 mg and norethindrone 1 mg [21 dark yellow tablets and 7 white inactive tablets] (28s)

Norinyl® 1+35: Ethinyl estradiol 0.035 mg and norethindrone 1 mg [21 yellow-green tablets and 7 orange inactive tablets] (28s)

Nortrel™ 0.5/35 mg:

Ethinyl estradiol 0.035 mg and norethindrone 0.5 mg [light yellow tablets] (21s)

Ethinyl estradiol 0.035 mg and norethindrone 0.5 mg [21 light yellow tablets and 7 white inactive tablets] (28s)

Nortrel™ 1/35 mg:

Ethinyl estradiol 0.035 mg and norethindrone 1 mg [yellow tablets] (21s)

Ethinyl estradiol 0.035 mg and norethindrone 1 mg [21 yellow tablets and 7 white inactive tablets] (28s)

Ortho-Novum® 1/35 21: Ethinyl estradiol 0.035 mg and norethindrone 1 mg [peach tablets] (21s)

Ortho-Novum® 1/35 28: Ethinyl estradiol 0.035 mg and norethindrone 1 mg [21 peach tablets and 7 green inactive tablets] (28s)
Ovcon® 35 21-day: Ethinyl estradiol 0.035 mg and norethindrone 0.4 mg [peach tablets] (21s)
Ovcon® 35 28-day: Ethinyl estradiol 0.035 mg and norethindrone 0.4 mg [21 peach tablets and 7 green inactive tablets] (28s)
Ovcon® 50: Ethinyl estradiol 0.05 mg and norethindrone 1 mg [21 yellow tablets and 7 green inactive tablets] (28s)

Tablet, biphasic formulations:
Necon® 10/11-21:
Day 1-10: Ethinyl estradiol 0.035 mg and norethindrone 0.5 mg [10 light yellow tablets]
Day 11-21: Ethinyl estradiol 0.035 mg and norethindrone 1 mg [11 dark yellow tablets] (21s)
Necon® 10/11-28:
Day 1-10: Ethinyl estradiol 0.035 mg and norethindrone 0.5 mg [10 light yellow tablets]
Day 11-21: Ethinyl estradiol 0.035 mg and norethindrone 1 mg [11 dark yellow tablets]
Day 22-28: 7 white inactive tablets (28s)
Ortho-Novum® 10/11-21:
Day 1-10: Ethinyl estradiol 0.035 mg and norethindrone 0.5 mg [10 white tablets]
Day 11-21: Ethinyl estradiol 0.035 mg and norethindrone 1 mg [11 peach tablets] (21s)
Ortho-Novum® 10/11-28:
Day 1-10: Ethinyl estradiol 0.035 mg and norethindrone 0.5 mg [10 white tablets]
Day 11-21: Ethinyl estradiol 0.035 mg and norethindrone 1 mg [11 peach tablets]
Day 22-28: 7 green inactive tablets (28s)

Tablet, triphasic formulations:
Estrostep® Fe:
Day 1-5: Ethinyl estradiol 0.02 mg and norethindrone acetate 1 mg [5 white triangular tablets]
Day 6-12: Ethinyl estradiol 0.03 mg and norethindrone acetate 1 mg [7 white square tablets]
Day 13-21: Ethinyl estradiol 0.035 mg and norethindrone acetate 1 mg [9 white round tablets]
Day 22-28: Ferrous fumarate 75 mg [7 brown tablets] (28s)
Necon® 7/7/7, Ortho-Novum® 7/7/7 28:
Day 1-7: Ethinyl estradiol 0.035 mg and norethindrone 0.5 mg [7 white tablets]
Day 8-14: Ethinyl estradiol 0.035 mg and norethindrone 0.75 mg [7 light peach tablets]
Day 15-21: Ethinyl estradiol 0.035 mg and norethindrone 1 mg [7 peach tablets]
Day 22-28: 7 green inactive tablets (28s)
Nortrel™ 7/7/7 21:
Day 1-7: Ethinyl estradiol 0.035 mg and norethindrone 0.5 mg [7 light yellow tablets]
Day 8-14: Ethinyl estradiol 0.035 mg and norethindrone 0.75 mg [7 blue tablets]
Day 15-21: Ethinyl estradiol 0.035 mg and norethindrone 1 mg [7 peach tablets] (21s)
Nortrel™ 7/7/7 28:
Day 1-7: Ethinyl estradiol 0.035 mg and norethindrone 0.5 mg [7 light yellow tablets]
Day 8-14: Ethinyl estradiol 0.035 mg and norethindrone 0.75 mg [7 blue tablets]
Day 15-21: Ethinyl estradiol 0.035 mg and norethindrone 1 mg [7 peach tablets]
Day 22-28: 7 white inactive tablets (28s)
Ortho-Novum® 7/7/7 21:
Day 1-7: Ethinyl estradiol 0.035 mg and norethindrone 0.5 mg [7 white tablets]
Day 8-14: Ethinyl estradiol 0.035 mg and norethindrone 0.75 mg [7 light peach tablets]
Day 15-21: Ethinyl estradiol 0.035 mg and norethindrone 1 mg [7 peach tablets] (21s)
Tri-Norinyl® 28:
Day 1-7: Ethinyl estradiol 0.035 mg and norethindrone 0.5 mg [7 blue tablets]
Day 8-16: Ethinyl estradiol 0.035 mg and norethindrone 1 mg [9 yellow-green tablets]
Day 17-21: Ethinyl estradiol 0.035 mg and norethindrone 0.5 mg [5 blue tablets]
Day 22-28: 7 orange inactive tablets (28s)
(Continued)

ethinyl estradiol and norethindrone *(Continued)*

Tablet, chewable: Monophasic formulations (Ovcon® 35 28-day): Ethinyl estradiol 0.035 mg and norethindrone 0.4 mg [21 white tablets and 7 green inactive tablets] (28s) [contains lactose; spearmint flavor]

ethinyl estradiol and norgestimate

(ETH in il es tra DYE ole & nor JES ti mate)

Sound-Alike/Look-Alike Issues

Ortho-Cyclen® may be confused with Ortho-Cept®

Synonyms ethinyl estradiol and NGM; norgestimate and ethinyl estradiol

U.S./Canadian Brand Names Cyclen® [Can]; MonoNessa™ [US]; Ortho-Cyclen® [US]; Ortho Tri-Cyclen® [US]; Ortho-Tri-Cyclen® Lo [US]; Previfem™ [US]; Sprintec™ [US]; Tri-Cyclen® [Can]; TriNessa™ [US]; Tri-Previfem™ [US]; Tri-Sprintec™ [US]

Therapeutic Category Contraceptive, Oral

Use Prevention of pregnancy; treatment of acne

Usual Dosage Oral:

Children ≥15 years and Adults: Female: Acne (Ortho Tri-Cyclen®): Refer to dosing for contraception

Adults: Female: Contraception:

Schedule 1 (Sunday starter): Dose begins on first Sunday after onset of menstruation; if the menstrual period starts on Sunday, take first tablet that very same day. **With a Sunday start, an additional method of contraception should be used until after the first 7 days of consecutive administration.**

For 21-tablet package: Dosage is 1 tablet daily for 21 consecutive days, followed by 7 days off of the medication; a new course begins on the 8th day after the last tablet is taken.

For 28-tablet package: Dosage is 1 tablet daily without interruption.

Schedule 2 (Day 1 starter): Dose starts on first day of menstrual cycle taking 1 tablet daily.

For 21-tablet package: Dosage is 1 tablet daily for 21 consecutive days, followed by 7 days off of the medication; a new course begins on the 8th day after the last tablet is taken.

For 28-tablet package: Dosage is 1 tablet daily without interruption.

If all doses have been taken on schedule and one menstrual period is missed, continue dosing cycle. If two consecutive menstrual periods are missed, pregnancy test is required before new dosing cycle is started.

Missed doses **monophasic formulations** (refer to package insert for complete information):

One dose missed: Take as soon as remembered or take 2 tablets next day

Two consecutive doses missed in the first 2 weeks: Take 2 tablets as soon as remembered or 2 tablets next 2 days. **An additional method of contraception should be used for 7 days after missed dose.**

Two consecutive doses missed in week 3 or three consecutive doses missed at any time: **An additional method of contraception must be used for 7 days after a missed dose:** Schedule 1 (Sunday starter): Continue dose of 1 tablet daily until Sunday, then discard the rest of the pack, and a new pack should be started that same day. Schedule 2 (Day 1 starter): Current pack should be discarded, and a new pack should be started that same day.

Missed doses **biphasic/triphasic formulations** (refer to package insert for complete information):

One dose missed: Take as soon as remembered or take 2 tablets next day.

Two consecutive doses missed in week 1 or week 2 of the pack: Take 2 tablets as soon as remembered and 2 tablets the next day. Resume taking 1 tablet daily until the pack is empty. **An additional method of contraception must be used for 7 days after a missed dose.**

Two consecutive doses missed in week 3 of the pack. **An additional method of contraception must be used for 7 days after a missed dose.** Schedule 1 (Sunday starter): Take 1 tablet every day until Sunday. Discard the remaining pack and start a new pack of pills on the same day. Schedule 2 (Day 1 starter): Discard the remaining pack and start a new pack the same day.

Three or more consecutive doses missed. **An additional method of contraception must be used for 7 days after a missed dose.** Schedule 1 (Sunday starter): Take 1 tablet every day until Sunday; on Sunday, discard the pack and start a new pack. Schedule 2 (Day 1 starter): Discard the remaining pack and begin new pack of tablets starting on the same day.

Dosage Forms Tablet:

Monophasic formulations:

MonoNessa™, Ortho-Cyclen®: Ethinyl estradiol 0.035 mg and norgestimate 0.25 mg [21 blue tablets and 7 green inactive tablets] (28s)

Previfem™: Ethinyl estradiol 0.035 mg and norgestimate 0.25 mg [21 blue tablets and 7 teal inactive tablets] (28s)

Sprintec™: Ethinyl estradiol 0.035 mg and norgestimate 0.25 mg [21 blue tablets and 7 white inactive tablets] (28s)

Triphasic formulations:

Ortho Tri-Cyclen®, TriNessa™:

Day 1-7: Ethinyl estradiol 0.035 mg and norgestimate 0.18 mg [7 white tablets]
Day 8-14: Ethinyl estradiol 0.035 mg and norgestimate 0.215 mg [7 light blue tablets]
Day 15-21: Ethinyl estradiol 0.035 mg and norgestimate 0.25 mg [7 blue tablets]
Day 22-28: 7 green inactive tablets (28s)

Tri-Previfem™:

Day 1-7: Ethinyl estradiol 0.035 mg and norgestimate 0.18 mg [7 white tablets]
Day 8-14: Ethinyl estradiol 0.035 mg and norgestimate 0.215 mg [7 light blue tablets]
Day 15-21: Ethinyl estradiol 0.035 mg and norgestimate 0.25 mg [7 blue tablets]
Day 22-28: 7 teal inactive tablets (28s)

Tri-Sprintec™:

Day 1-7: Ethinyl estradiol 0.035 mg and norgestimate 0.18 mg [7 gray tablets]
Day 8-14: Ethinyl estradiol 0.035 mg and norgestimate 0.215 mg [7 light blue tablets]
Day 15-21: Ethinyl estradiol 0.035 mg and norgestimate 0.25 mg [7 blue tablets]
Day 22-28: 7 white inactive tablets (28s)

Ortho Tri-Cyclen® Lo:

Day 1-7: Ethinyl estradiol 0.025 mg and norgestimate 0.18 mg [7 white tablets]
Day 8-14: Ethinyl estradiol 0.025 mg and norgestimate 0.215 mg [7 light blue tablets]
Day 15-21: Ethinyl estradiol 0.025 mg and norgestimate 0.25 mg [7 dark blue tablets]
Day 22-28: 7 green inactive tablets (28s)

ethinyl estradiol and norgestrel (ETH in il es tra DYE ole & nor JES trel)

Synonyms morning after pill; norgestrel and ethinyl estradiol

U.S./Canadian Brand Names Cryselle™ [US]; Lo/Ovral® [US]; Low-Ogestrel® [US]; Ogestrel®; Ovral® [Can]

Therapeutic Category Contraceptive, Oral

Use Prevention of pregnancy; postcoital contraceptive or "morning after" pill

Usual Dosage Oral: Adults: Female:

Contraception:

Schedule 1 (Sunday starter): Dose begins on first Sunday after onset of menstruation; if the menstrual period starts on Sunday, take first tablet that very same day. **With a Sunday start, an additional method of contraception should be used until after the first 7 days of consecutive administration.**

For 21-tablet package: Dosage is 1 tablet daily for 21 consecutive days, followed by 7 days off of the medication; a new course begins on the 8th day after the last tablet is taken.

For 28-tablet package: Dosage is 1 tablet daily without interruption.

Schedule 2 (Day 1 starter): Dose starts on first day of menstrual cycle taking 1 tablet daily.

For 21-tablet package: Dosage is 1 tablet daily for 21 consecutive days, followed by 7 days off of the medication; a new course begins on the 8th day after the last tablet is taken.

For 28-tablet package: Dosage is 1 tablet daily without interruption.

(Continued)

ethinyl estradiol and norgestrel *(Continued)*

If all doses have been taken on schedule and one menstrual period is missed, continue dosing cycle. If two consecutive menstrual periods are missed, pregnancy test is required before new dosing cycle is started.

Missed doses **monophasic formulations** (refer to package insert for complete information):

One dose missed: Take as soon as remembered or take 2 tablets next day

Two consecutive doses missed in the first 2 weeks: Take 2 tablets as soon as remembered or 2 tablets next 2 days. **An additional method of contraception should be used for 7 days after missed dose.**

Two consecutive doses missed in week 3 or three consecutive doses missed at any time:

Schedule 1 (Sunday starter): Continue to take 1 tablet daily until Sunday, then discard the rest of the pack, and a new pack is started that same day.

Schedule 2 (Day 1 starter): Current pack should be discarded, and a new pack started that same day. **An additional method of contraception should be used for 7 days after missed dose.**

Postcoital contraception:

Ethinyl estradiol 0.03 mg and norgestrel 0.3 mg formulation: 4 tablets within 72 hours of unprotected intercourse and 4 tablets 12 hours after first dose

Ethinyl estradiol 0.05 mg and norgestrel 0.5 mg formulation: 2 tablets within 72 hours of unprotected intercourse and 2 tablets 12 hours after first dose

Dosage Forms [DSC] = Discontinued product

Tablet, monophasic formulations:

Cryselle™: Ethinyl estradiol 0.03 mg and norgestrel 0.3 mg [21 white tablets and 7 light green inactive tablets] (28s)

Low-Ogestrel® 28: Ethinyl estradiol 0.03 mg and norgestrel 0.3 mg [21 white tablets and 7 peach inactive tablets] (28s)

Lo/Ovral® 28: Ethinyl estradiol 0.03 mg and norgestrel 0.3 mg [21 white tablets and 7 pink inactive tablets] (28s)

Ovral® 21: Ethinyl estradiol 0.05 mg and norgestrel 0.5 mg [white tablets] (21s) [DSC]

Ogestrel® 28: Ethinyl estradiol 0.05 mg and norgestrel 0.5 mg [21 white tablets and 7 peach inactive tablets] (28s)

Ovral® 28: Ethinyl estradiol 0.05 mg and norgestrel 0.5 mg [21 white tablets and 7 pink inactive tablets] (28s) [DSC]

ethiodized oil *see* radiological/contrast media (ionic) *on page 759*

Ethiodol® [US] *see* radiological/contrast media (ionic) *on page 759*

ethiofos *see* amifostine *on page 43*

ethionamide (e thye on AM ide)

U.S./Canadian Brand Names Trecator®-SC [US/Can]

Therapeutic Category Antimycobacterial Agent

Use Treatment of tuberculosis and other mycobacterial diseases, in conjunction with other antituberculosis agents, when first-line agents have failed or resistance has been demonstrated

Usual Dosage Oral:

Children: 15-20 mg/kg/day in 2 divided doses, not to exceed 1 g/day

Adults: 500-1000 mg/day in 1-3 divided doses

Dosage Forms Tablet, sugar coated: 250 mg

Ethmozine® [US/Can] *see* moricizine *on page 591*

ethopropazine *(Canada only)* (eth oh PROE pa zeen)

Therapeutic Category Anti-Parkinson Agent

Use Symptomatic treatment of drug induced extrapyramidal manifestations and of Parkinson disease of postencephalitic, arteriosclerotic or idiopathic etiology.

Usual Dosage Must be adapted to each individual. In drug induced extrapyramidal reactions 100 mg twice daily usually brings about good control of symptoms. In post encephalitic, arteriosclerotic or idiopathic parkinsonism, initiate treatment at a low dose of 50 mg 3 times a day and increase from 50 to 100 mg daily every 2 to 3 days until the optimum effect is obtained or the limit of tolerance is attained. Drowsiness and anticholinergic effects which may appear at the beginning of treatment generally subside after a few days. The normal daily dose usually ranges between 100 and 500 mg but it may reach 1 g or more per day in certain patients.

Dosage Forms Tablet, as hydrochloride: 50 mg

ethosuximide (eth oh SUKS i mide)

Sound-Alike/Look-Alike Issues

ethosuximide may be confused with methsuximide

Zarontin® may be confused with Xalatan®, Zantac®, Zaroxolyn®

U.S./Canadian Brand Names Zarontin® [US/Can]

Therapeutic Category Anticonvulsant

Use Management of absence (petit mal) seizures

Usual Dosage Oral:

Children 3-6 years: Initial: 250 mg/day (or 15 mg/kg/day) in 2 divided doses; increase every 4-7 days; usual maintenance dose: 15-40 mg/kg/day in 2 divided doses

Children >6 years and Adults: Initial: 250 mg twice daily; increase by 250 mg as needed every 4-7 days, up to 1.5 g/day in 2 divided doses; usual maintenance dose: 20-40 mg/kg/day in 2 divided doses

Dosage Forms

Capsule: 250 mg

Syrup: 250 mg/5 mL (473 mL) [contains sodium benzoate; raspberry flavor]

ethotoin (ETH oh toyn)

Synonyms ethylphenylhydantoin

U.S./Canadian Brand Names Peganone® [US/Can]

Therapeutic Category Hydantoin

Use Generalized tonic-clonic or complex-partial seizures

Usual Dosage Oral:

Children: 30-60 mg/kg/day or 250 mg twice daily, may be increased up to 2-3 g/day

Adults: 250 mg 4 times/day after meals, may be increased up to 3 g/day in divided doses 4 times/day

Dosage Forms Tablet: 250 mg

ethoxynaphthamido penicillin sodium *see* nafcillin *on page 600*

Ethrane® [US/Can] *see* enflurane *on page 309*

ethyl alcohol *see* alcohol (ethyl) *on page 27*

ethyl aminobenzoate *see* benzocaine *on page 107*

ethyl chloride (ETH il KLOR ide)

Synonyms chloroethane

U.S./Canadian Brand Names Gebauer's Ethyl Chloride® [US]

Therapeutic Category Local Anesthetic

Use Local anesthetic in minor operative procedures and to relieve pain caused by insect stings and burns, and irritation caused by myofascial and visceral pain syndromes

Usual Dosage Dosage varies with use

Dosage Forms Aerosol: 100% (103 mL) [available as a fine-point or medium spray]

ethyl chloride and dichlorotetrafluoroethane

(ETH il KLOR ide & dye klor oh te tra floo or oh ETH ane)

Synonyms dichlorotetrafluoroethane and ethyl chloride

U.S./Canadian Brand Names Fluro-Ethyl® [US]

(Continued)

ethyl chloride and dichlorotetrafluoroethane *(Continued)*

Therapeutic Category Local Anesthetic

Use Topical refrigerant anesthetic to control pain associated with minor surgical procedures, dermabrasion, injections, contusions, and minor strains

Usual Dosage Press gently on side of spray valve allowing the liquid to emerge as a fine mist approximately 2" to 4" from site of application

Dosage Forms Aerosol: Ethyl chloride 25% and dichlorotetrafluoroethane 75% (148 mL)

ethylphenylhydantoin *see* ethotoin *on previous page*

ethynodiol diacetate and ethinyl estradiol *see* ethinyl estradiol and ethynodiol diacetate *on page 338*

Ethyol® [US/Can] *see* amifostine *on page 43*

Etibi® [Can] *see* ethambutol *on page 334*

etidronate disodium (e ti DROE nate dye SOW dee um)

Sound-Alike/Look-Alike Issues

etidronate may be confused with etidocaine, etomidate, etretinate

Synonyms EHDP; sodium etidronate

U.S./Canadian Brand Names Didronel® [US/Can]; Gen-Etidronate [Can]

Therapeutic Category Bisphosphonate Derivative

Use Symptomatic treatment of Paget disease and heterotopic ossification due to spinal cord injury or after total hip replacement, hypercalcemia associated with malignancy

Usual Dosage Adults: Oral formulation should be taken on an empty stomach 2 hours before any meal.

Paget disease: Oral:

Initial: 5-10 mg/kg/day (not to exceed 6 months) or 11-20 mg/kg/day (not to exceed 3 months). Doses >10 mg/kg/day are **not** recommended.

Retreatment: Initiate only after etidronate-free period ≥90 days. Monitor patients every 3-6 months. Retreatment regimens are the same as for initial treatment.

Heterotopic ossification: Oral:

Caused by spinal cord injury: 20 mg/kg/day for 2 weeks, then 10 mg/kg/day for 10 weeks; total treatment period: 12 weeks

Complicating total hip replacement: 20 mg/kg/day for 1 month preoperatively then 20 mg/kg/day for 3 months postoperatively; total treatment period is 4 months

Hypercalcemia associated with malignancy:

I.V. (dilute dose in at least 250 mL NS): 7.5 mg/kg/day for 3 days; there should be at least 7 days between courses of treatment

Oral: Start 20 mg/kg/day on the last day of infusion and continue for 30-90 days

Dosage Forms

Injection, solution: 50 mg/mL (6 mL)

Tablet: 200 mg, 400 mg

etodolac (ee toe DOE lak)

Sound-Alike/Look-Alike Issues

Lodine® may be confused with codeine, iodine, Iopidine®, Lopid®

Synonyms etodolic acid

U.S./Canadian Brand Names Apo-Etodolac® [Can]; Lodine® [US/Can]; Lodine® XL [US]; Utradol™ [Can]

Therapeutic Category Analgesic, Nonnarcotic; Nonsteroidal Antiinflammatory Drug (NSAID)

Use Acute and long-term use in the management of signs and symptoms of osteoarthritis and management of pain; rheumatoid arthritis; juvenile rheumatoid arthritis

Usual Dosage Single dose of 76-100 mg is comparable to the analgesic effect of aspirin 650 mg; in patients ≥65 years, no substantial differences in the pharmacokinetics or side-effects profile were seen compared with the general population

Children 6-16 years: Oral: Juvenile rheumatoid arthritis (Lodine® XL):
20-30 kg: 400 mg once daily
31-45 kg: 600 mg once daily
46-60 kg: 800 mg once daily
>60 kg: 1000 mg once daily
Adults: Oral:
Acute pain: 200-400 mg every 6-8 hours, as needed, not to exceed total daily doses of 1200 mg; for patients weighing <60 kg, total daily dose should not exceed 20 mg/kg/day
Rheumatoid arthritis, osteoarthritis: Initial: 600-1200 mg/day given in divided doses: 400 mg 2 times/day; 300 mg 2 or 3 times/day; 500 mg 2 times/day; total daily dose should not exceed 1200 mg; for patients weighing <60 kg, total daily dose should not exceed 20 mg/kg/day
Lodine® XL: 400-1000 mg once daily

Dosage Forms [DSC] = Discontinued product
Capsule (Lodine®): 200 mg, 300 mg
Tablet: 400 mg, 500 mg
Lodine®: 400 mg, 500 mg [DSC]
Tablet, extended release (Lodine® XL): 400 mg, 500 mg, 600 mg

etodolic acid *see* etodolac *on previous page*

EtOH *see* alcohol (ethyl) *on page 27*

etomidate (e TOM i date)

Sound-Alike/Look-Alike Issues
etomidate may be confused with etidronate

U.S./Canadian Brand Names Amidate® [US/Can]

Therapeutic Category General Anesthetic

Use Induction and maintenance of general anesthesia

Usual Dosage Children >10 years and Adults: I.V.: Initial: 0.2-0.6 mg/kg over 30-60 seconds for induction of anesthesia; maintenance: 5-20 mcg/kg/minute

Dosage Forms Injection, solution: 2 mg/mL (10 mL, 20 mL) [contains propylene glycol 35% v/v]

etonogestrel and ethinyl estradiol *see* ethinyl estradiol and etonogestrel *on page 338*

Etopophos® [US] *see* etoposide phosphate *on next page*

etoposide (e toe POE side)

Sound-Alike/Look-Alike Issues
VePesid® may be confused with Versed®

Synonyms epipodophyllotoxin; VP-16; VP-16-213

U.S./Canadian Brand Names Toposar® [US]; VePesid® [US/Can]

Therapeutic Category Antineoplastic Agent

Use Treatment of lymphomas, ANLL, lung, testicular, bladder, and prostate carcinoma, hepatoma, rhabdomyosarcoma, uterine carcinoma, neuroblastoma, mycosis fungoides, Kaposi sarcoma, histiocytosis, gestational trophoblastic disease, Ewing sarcoma, Wilms tumor, and brain tumors

Usual Dosage Refer to individual protocols.
Children: I.V.: 60-120 mg/m²/day for 3-5 days every 3-6 weeks
AML:
Remission induction: 150 mg/m²/day for 2-3 days for 2-3 cycles
Intensification or consolidation: 250 mg/m²/day for 3 days, courses 2-5
Brain tumor: 150 mg/m²/day on days 2 and 3 of treatment course
Neuroblastoma: 100 mg/m²/day over 1 hour on days 1-5 of cycle; repeat cycle every 4 weeks
BMT conditioning regimen used in patients with rhabdomyosarcoma or neuroblastoma: I.V. continuous infusion: 160 mg/m²/day for 4 days
(Continued)

etoposide *(Continued)*

Conditioning regimen for allogenic BMT: 60 mg/kg/dose as a single dose

Adults:

Small cell lung cancer:

Oral: Twice the I.V. dose rounded to the nearest 50 mg given once daily if total dose ≤400 mg or in divided doses if >400 mg

I.V.: 35 mg/m^2/day for 4 days or 50 mg/m^2/day for 5 days every 3-4 weeks total dose ≤400 mg/day or in divided doses if >400 mg/day

IVPB: 60-100 mg/m^2/day for 3 days (with cisplatin)

CIV: 500 mg/m^2 over 24 hours every 3 weeks

Testicular cancer:

IVPB: 50-100 mg/m^2/day for 5 days repeated every 3-4 weeks

I.V.: 100 mg/m^2 every other day for 3 doses repeated every 3-4 weeks

BMT/relapsed leukemia: I.V.: 2.4-3.5 g/m^2 or 25-70 mg/kg administered over 4-36 hours

Dosage Forms

Capsule (VePesid®): 50 mg

Injection, solution: 20 mg/mL (5 mL, 25 mL, 50 mL) [contains benzyl alcohol]

Toposar®: 20 mg/mL (5 mL, 10 mL, 25 mL) [contains benzyl alcohol]

VePesid®: 20 mg/mL (5 mL, 7.5 mL, 25 mL, 50 mL) [contains benzyl alcohol

etoposide phosphate (e toe POE side FOS fate)

U.S./Canadian Brand Names Etopophos® [US]

Therapeutic Category Antineoplastic Agent

Use Treatment of refractory testicular tumors and small cell lung cancer

Usual Dosage Refer to individual protocols. Adults:

Small cell lung cancer: I.V. (in combination with other approved chemotherapeutic drugs): **Equivalent doses of etoposide phosphate to an etoposide dosage** range of 35 mg/m^2/day for 4 days to 50 mg/m^2/day for 5 days. Courses are repeated at 3- to 4-week intervals after adequate recovery from any toxicity.

Testicular cancer: I.V. (in combination with other approved chemotherapeutic agents): **Equivalent dose of etoposide phosphate to etoposide dosage** range of 50-100 mg/m^2/day on days 1-5 to 100 mg/m^2/day on days 1, 3, and 5. Courses are repeated at 3- to 4-week intervals after adequate recovery from any toxicity.

Dosage Forms Injection, powder for reconstitution, as base: 100 mg

Etrafon® [Can] *see* amitriptyline and perphenazine *on page 48*

ETS-2%® Topical *(Discontinued)* *see page 1042*

Eudal®-SR [US] *see* guaifenesin and pseudoephedrine *on page 419*

Euflex® [Can] *see* flutamide *on page 382*

Euglucon® [Can] *see* glyburide *on page 409*

Eulexin® [US/Can] *see* flutamide *on page 382*

Eurax® [US] *see* crotamiton *on page 231*

Euthroid® Tablet *(Discontinued)* *see page 1042*

Eutron® *(Discontinued)* *see page 1042*

Evac-Q-Mag® *(Discontinued)* *see page 1042*

Evac-U-Gen [US-OTC] *see* senna *on page 799*

Evalose® *(Discontinued)* *see page 1042*

Everone® 200 [Can] *see* testosterone *on page 848*

Everone® Injection *(Discontinued)* *see page 1042*

Evista® [US/Can] *see* raloxifene *on page 762*

Evoxac® [US/Can] *see* cevimeline *on page 179*

Evra® [Can] *see* ethinyl estradiol and norelgestromin *on page 342*

Exact® Acne Medication [US-OTC] *see* benzoyl peroxide *on page 109*

Excedrin® Extra Strength [US-OTC] *see* acetaminophen, aspirin, and caffeine *on page 10*

Excedrin® IB *(Discontinued)* *see page 1042*

Excedrin® Migraine [US-OTC] *see* acetaminophen, aspirin, and caffeine *on page 10*

Excedrin® P.M. [US-OTC] *see* acetaminophen and diphenhydramine *on page 7*

Exelderm® [US/Can] *see* sulconazole *on page 828*

Exelon® [US/Can] *see* rivastigmine *on page 781*

exemestane (ex e MES tane)

U.S./Canadian Brand Names Aromasin® [US/Can]

Therapeutic Category Antineoplastic Agent, Miscellaneous

Use Treatment of advanced breast cancer in postmenopausal women whose disease has progressed following tamoxifen therapy

Usual Dosage Adults: Oral: 25 mg once daily after a meal

Dosage Forms Tablet: 25 mg

Exidine® Scrub *(Discontinued)* *see page 1042*

ex-lax® Maximum Strength [US-OTC] *see* senna *on page 799*

ex-lax® [US-OTC] *see* senna *on page 799*

Exna® *(Discontinued)* *see page 1042*

Exorex® [US] *see* coal tar *on page 219*

Exosurf Neonatal® *(Discontinued)* *see page 1042*

Exsel® *(Discontinued)* *see page 1042*

Extendryl [US] *see* chlorpheniramine, phenylephrine, and methscopolamine *on page 192*

Extendryl JR [US] *see* chlorpheniramine, phenylephrine, and methscopolamine *on page 192*

Extendryl SR [US] *see* chlorpheniramine, phenylephrine, and methscopolamine *on page 192*

Extra Action Cough Syrup *(Discontinued)* *see page 1042*

Eye-Lube-A® Solution *(Discontinued)* *see page 1042*

Eye-Sed® Ophthalmic *(Discontinued)* *see page 1042*

Eye-Sine™ [US-OTC] *see* tetrahydrozoline *on page 852*

Eye-Stream® [Can] *see* balanced salt solution *on page 99*

EZ-Char™ [US-OTC] *see* charcoal *on page 180*

ezetimibe (ez ET i mibe)

Sound-Alike/Look-Alike Issues

Zetia™ may be confused with Zestril®

U.S./Canadian Brand Names Ezetrol® [Can]; Zetia™ [US]

Therapeutic Category Antilipemic Agent, 2-Azetidinone

Use Use in combination with dietary therapy for the treatment of primary hypercholesterolemia (as monotherapy or in combination with HMG-CoA reductase inhibitors); homozygous sitosterolemia; homozygous familial hypercholesterolemia (in combination with atorvastatin or simvastatin)

Usual Dosage Oral:

Hyperlipidemias: Children ≥10 years and Adults: 10 mg/day

Sitosterolemia: Adults: 10 mg/day

Dosage Forms Tablet: 10 mg [capsule shaped]

ezetimibe and simvastatin (ez ET i mibe & SIM va stat in)

U.S./Canadian Brand Names Vytorin™ [US]

Therapeutic Category Antilipemic Agent, 2-Azetidinone

Use Used in combination with dietary therapy for the Treatment of primary hypercholesterolemia and homozygous familial hypercholesterolemia

Usual Dosage Oral: Adults:

Homozygous familial hypercholesterolemia: Ezetimibe 10 mg and simvastatin 40 mg once daily or ezetimibe 10 mg and simvastatin 80 mg once daily in the evening

Hyperlipidemias: Initial: Ezetimibe 10 mg and simvastatin 20 mg once daily in the evening

Patients who require >55% reduction in LDL-C: Initial: Ezetimibe 10 mg and simvastatin 40 mg once daily

Dosage Forms Tablet:

10/10: Ezetimibe 10 mg and simvastatin 10 mg

10/20: Ezetimibe 10 mg and simvastatin 20 mg

10/40: Ezetimibe 10 mg and simvastatin 40 mg

10/80: Ezetimibe 10 mg and simvastatin 80 mg

Ezetrol® [Can] *see* ezetimibe *on previous page*

Ezide® ***(Discontinued)*** *see page 1042*

F_3T *see* trifluridine *on page 885*

Fabrazyme® [US] *see* agalsidase beta *on page 23*

Factive® [US] *see* gemifloxacin *on page 400*

factor VIIa (recombinant) (factor seven ay ree KOM be nant)

Sound-Alike/Look-Alike Issues

NovoSeven® may be confused with Novacet®

Synonyms coagulation factor VIIa; eptacog alfa (activated); rFVIIa

U.S./Canadian Brand Names Niastase® [Can]; NovoSeven® [US]

Therapeutic Category Antihemophilic Agent; Blood Product Derivative

Use Treatment of bleeding episodes in patients with hemophilia A or B when inhibitors to factor VIII or factor IX are present

Usual Dosage Children and Adults: I.V. administration only: 90 mcg/kg every 2 hours until hemostasis is achieved or until the treatment is judged ineffective. The dose and interval may be adjusted based upon the severity of bleeding and the degree of hemostasis achieved. The duration of therapy following hemostasis has not been fully established; for patients experiencing severe bleeds, dosing should be continued at 3-6 hour intervals after hemostasis has been achieved and the duration of dosing should be minimized.

In clinical trials, dosages have ranged from 35-120 mcg/kg and a decision on the final therapeutic dosages was reached within 8 hours in the majority of patients

Dosage Forms Injection, powder for reconstitution: 1.2 mg, 2.4 mg, 4.8 mg [preservative free, latex free; contains polysorbate 80]

factor IX (FAK ter nyne)

Synonyms factor IX purified; monoclonal antibody purified

U.S./Canadian Brand Names AlphaNine® SD [US]; BeneFix® [US/Can]; Immunine® VH [Can]; Mononine® [US/Can]

Therapeutic Category Antihemophilic Agent

Use Control bleeding in patients with factor IX deficiency (hemophilia B or Christmas disease)

Usual Dosage Dosage is expressed in units of factor IX activity and must be individualized.

I.V. only: **Formula for units required to raise blood level %:**

AlphaNine® SD, Mononine®: Children and Adults:

Number of Factor IX Units Required = body weight (in kg) x desired Factor IX level increase (% normal) x 1 unit/kg

For example, for a 100% level a patient who has an actual level of 20%: Number of Factor IX Units needed = 70 kg x 80% x 1 Unit/kg = 5600 Units

BeneFix®:

Children <15 years:

Number of Factor IX Units Required = body weight (in kg) x desired Factor IX level increase (% normal) x 1.4 units/kg

Adults:

Number of Factor IX Units Required = body weight (in kg) x desired Factor IX level increase (% normal) x 1.2 units/kg

Guidelines: As a general rule, the level of factor IX required for treatment of different conditions is listed below:

Minor spontaneous hemorrhage, prophylaxis:

Desired levels of factor IX for hemostasis: 15% to 25%

Initial loading dose to achieve desired level: 20-30 units/kg

Frequency of dosing: Every 12-24 hours if necessary

Duration of treatment: 1-2 days

Moderate hemorrhage:

Desired levels of factor IX for hemostasis: 25% to 50%

Initial loading dose to achieve desired level: 25-50 units/kg

Frequency of dosing: Every 12-24 hours

Duration of treatment: 2-7 days

Major hemorrhage:

Desired levels of factor IX for hemostasis: >50%

Initial loading dose to achieve desired level: 30-50 units/kg

Frequency of dosing: Every 12-24 hours, depending on half-life and measured factor IX levels (after 3-5 days, maintain at least 20% activity)

Duration of treatment: 7-10 days, depending upon nature of insult

Surgery:

Desired levels of factor IX for hemostasis: 50% to 100%

Initial loading dose to achieve desired level: 50-100 units/kg

Frequency of dosing: Every 12-24 hours, depending on half-life and measured factor IX levels

Duration of treatment: 7-10 days, depending upon nature of insult

Dosage Forms Injection, powder for reconstitution (**Note:** Exact potency labeled on each vial):

AlphaNine® SD [human derived; solvent detergent treated; virus filtered; contains nondetectable levels of factors II, VII, X; supplied with diluent]

BeneFix® [recombinant formulation; supplied with diluent]

Mononine® [human derived; monoclonal antibody purified; contains nondetectable levels of factors II, VII, X; supplied with diluent]

factor IX complex (human) (FAK ter nyne KOM pleks HYU man)

Synonyms prothrombin complex concentrate

U.S./Canadian Brand Names Bebulin® VH [US]; Profilnine® SD [US]; Proplex® T [US]

Therapeutic Category Antihemophilic Agent

Use

Control bleeding in patients with factor IX deficiency (hemophilia B or Christmas disease) **Note:** Factor IX concentrate containing **only** factor IX is also available and preferable for this indication.

Prevention/control of bleeding in hemophilia A patients with inhibitors to factor VIII

Prevention/control of bleeding in patients with factor VII deficiency

Emergency correction of the coagulopathy of warfarin excess in critical situations.

Usual Dosage Children and Adults: Dosage is expressed in units of factor IX activity and must be individualized.

(Continued)

factor IX complex (human) *(Continued)*

I.V. only: **Formula for units required to raise blood level %:**

Total blood volume (mL blood/kg) = 70 mL/kg (adults), 80 mL/kg (children)

Plasma volume = total blood volume (mL) x [1 - Hct (in decimals)]

For example, for a 70 kg adult with a Hct = 40%: Plasma volume = [70 kg x 70 mL/kg] x [1 - 0.4] = 2940 mL

To calculate number of units needed to increase level to desired range (highly individualized and dependent on patient's condition): Number of units = desired level increase [desired level - actual level] x plasma volume (in mL)

For example, for a 100% level in the above patient who has an actual level of 20%: Number of units needed = [1 (for a 100% level) - 0.2] x 2940 mL = 2352 units

As a general rule, the level of factor IX required for treatment of different conditions is listed below:

Minor Spontaneous Hemorrhage, Prophylaxis:

Desired levels of factor IX for hemostasis: 15% to 25%

Initial loading dose to achieve desired level: <20-30 units/kg

Frequency of dosing: Once; repeated in 24 hours if necessary

Duration of treatment: Once; repeated if necessary

Major Trauma or Surgery:

Desired levels of factor IX for hemostasis: 25% to 50%

Initial loading dose to achieve desired level: <75 units/kg

Frequency of dosing: Every 18-30 hours, depending on half-life and measured factor IX levels

Duration of treatment: Up to 10 days, depending upon nature of insult

Factor VIII inhibitor patients: 75 units/kg/dose; may be given every 6-12 hours

Anticoagulant overdosage: I.V.: 15 units/kg

Dosage Forms Injection, powder for reconstitution (**Note:** Exact potency labeled on each vial):

Bebulin® VH [single-dose vial; vapor heated; supplied with sterile water for injection]

Profilnine® SD [single-dose vial; solvent detergent treated]

Proplex® T [single-dose vial; heat treated; supplied with sterile water for injection]

factor IX purified *see* factor IX *on page 354*

factor VIII (human) *see* antihemophilic factor (human) *on page 62*

factor VIII (porcine) *see* antihemophilic factor (porcine) *on page 63*

factor VIII (recombinant) *see* antihemophilic factor (recombinant) *on page 63*

Factrel® [US] *see* gonadorelin *on page 412*

famciclovir (fam SYE kloe veer)

U.S./Canadian Brand Names Famvir® [US/Can]

Therapeutic Category Antiviral Agent

Use Management of acute herpes zoster (shingles) and recurrent episodes of genital herpes; treatment of recurrent herpes simplex in immunocompetent patients

Usual Dosage **Initiate therapy as soon as herpes zoster is diagnosed:** Adults: Oral:

Acute herpes zoster: 500 mg every 8 hours for 7 days

Recurrent herpes simplex in immunocompetent patients: 125 mg twice daily for 5 days

Genital herpes:

First episode: 250 mg 3 times/day for 7-10 days

Recurrent episodes: 125 mg twice daily for 5 days

Prophylaxis: 250 mg twice daily

Severe (hospitalized patients): 250 mg twice daily

Dosage Forms Tablet: 125 mg, 250 mg, 500 mg

famotidine (fa MOE ti deen)

U.S./Canadian Brand Names Apo-Famotidine® [Can]; Gen-Famotidine [Can]; Novo-Famotidine [Can]; Nu-Famotidine [Can]; Pepcid® [US/Can]; Pepcid® AC [US-OTC/Can];

Pepcid® I.V. [Can]; ratio-Famotidine [Can]; Rhoxal-famotidine [Can]; Riva-Famotidine [Can]

Therapeutic Category Histamine H_2 Antagonist

Use Therapy and treatment of duodenal ulcer, gastric ulcer, control gastric pH in critically-ill patients, symptomatic relief in gastritis, gastroesophageal reflux, active benign ulcer, and pathological hypersecretory conditions

OTC labeling: Relief of heartburn, acid indigestion, and sour stomach

Usual Dosage

Children: Treatment duration and dose should be individualized

Peptic ulcer: 1-16 years:

Oral: 0.5 mg/kg/day at bedtime or divided twice daily (maximum dose: 40 mg/day); doses of up to 1 mg/kg/day have been used in clinical studies

I.V.: 0.25 mg/kg every 12 hours (maximum dose: 40 mg/day); doses of up to 0.5 mg/kg have been used in clinical studies

GERD: Oral:

<3 months: 0.5 mg/kg once daily

3-12 months: 0.5 mg/kg twice daily

1-16 years: 1 mg/kg/day divided twice daily (maximum dose: 40 mg twice daily); doses of up to 2 mg/kg/day have been used in clinical studies

Children ≥12 years and Adults: Heartburn, indigestion, sour stomach: OTC labeling: Oral: 10-20 mg every 12 hours; dose may be taken 15-60 minutes before eating foods known to cause heartburn

Adults:

Duodenal ulcer: Oral: Acute therapy: 40 mg/day at bedtime for 4-8 weeks; maintenance therapy: 20 mg/day at bedtime

Gastric ulcer: Oral: Acute therapy: 40 mg/day at bedtime

Hypersecretory conditions: Oral: Initial: 20 mg every 6 hours, may increase in increments up to 160 mg every 6 hours

GERD: Oral: 20 mg twice daily for 6 weeks

Esophagitis and accompanying symptoms due to GERD: Oral: 20 mg or 40 mg twice daily for up to 12 weeks

Patients unable to take oral medication: I.V.: 20 mg every 12 hours

Dosage Forms

Gelcap (Pepcid® AC): 10 mg

Infusion [premixed in NS] (Pepcid®): 20 mg (50 mL)

Injection, solution: 10 mg/mL (4 mL, 20 mL, 50 mL) [contains benzyl alcohol]

Pepcid®: 10 mg/mL (4 mL, 20 mL)

Injection, solution [preservative free] (Pepcid®): 10 mg/mL (2 mL)

Powder for oral suspension (Pepcid®): 40 mg/5 mL (50 mL) [contains sodium benzoate; cherry-banana-mint flavor]

Tablet, chewable (Pepcid® AC): 10 mg [contains phenylalanine 1.4 mg/tablet; mint flavor]

Tablet: 10 mg [OTC], 20 mg, 40 mg

Pepcid®: 20 mg, 40 mg [film coated]

Pepcid® AC: 10 mg, 20 mg

famotidine, calcium carbonate, and magnesium hydroxide

(fa MOE ti deen, KAL see um KAR bun ate, & mag NEE zhum hye DROKS ide)

Synonyms calcium carbonate, magnesium hydroxide, and famotidine; magnesium hydroxide, famotidine, and calcium carbonate

U.S./Canadian Brand Names Pepcid® Complete [US-OTC/Can]

Therapeutic Category Antacid; Histamine H_2 Antagonist

Use Relief of heartburn due to acid indigestion

Usual Dosage Children ≥12 years and Adults: Relief of heartburn due to acid indigestion: Oral: Pepcid® Complete: 1 tablet as needed; no more than 2 tablets in 24 hours; do **not** swallow whole, chew tablet completely before swallowing; do not use for longer than 14 days

(Continued)

famotidine, calcium carbonate, and magnesium hydroxide *(Continued)*

Dosage Forms Tablet, chewable (Pepcid® Complete): Famotidine 10 mg, calcium carbonate 800 mg, and magnesium hydroxide 165 mg [berry blend and mint flavors]

Famvir® [US/Can] *see* famciclovir *on page 356*

Fansidar® [US] *see* sulfadoxine and pyrimethamine *on page 831*

Fareston® [US/Can] *see* toremifene *on page 872*

Faslodex® [US] *see* fulvestrant *on page 393*

Fastin® ***(Discontinued)*** *see page 1042*

fat emulsion (fat e MUL shun)

Synonyms intravenous fat emulsion

U.S./Canadian Brand Names Intralipid® [US/Can]; Liposyn® III [US]

Therapeutic Category Intravenous Nutritional Therapy

Use Source of calories and essential fatty acids for patients requiring parenteral nutrition of extended duration

Usual Dosage Fat emulsion should not exceed 60% of the total daily calories

Premature Infants: Initial dose: 0.25-0.5 g/kg/day, increase by 0.25-0.5 g/kg/day to a maximum of 3 g/kg/day depending on needs/nutritional goals; limit to 1 g/kg/day if on phototherapy; maximum rate of infusion: 0.15 g/kg/hour (0.75 mL/kg/hour of 20% solution)

Infants and Children: Initial dose: 0.5-1 g/kg/day, increase by 0.5 g/kg/day to a maximum of 3 g/kg/day depending on needs/nutritional goals; maximum rate of infusion: 0.25 g/kg/hour (1.25 mL/kg/hour of 20% solution)

Adolescents and Adults: Initial dose: 1 g/kg/day, increase by 0.5-1 g/kg/day to a maximum of 2.5 g/kg/day of 10% and 3 g/kg/day of 20% depending on needs/nutritional goals; maximum rate of infusion: 0.25 g/kg/hour (1.25 mL/kg/hour of 20% solution); do not exceed 50 mL/hour (20%) or 100 mL/hour (10%)

Prevention of essential fatty acid deficiency (8% to 10% of total caloric intake): 0.5-1 g/kg/24 hours

Children: 5-10 mL/kg/day at 0.1 mL/minute then up to 100 mL/hour

Adults: 500 mL (10%) twice weekly at rate of 1 mL/minute for 30 minutes, then increase to 42 mL/hour (500 mL over 12 hours)

Note: At the onset of therapy, the patient should be observed for any immediate allergic reactions such as dyspnea, cyanosis, and fever; slower initial rates of infusion may be used for the first 10-15 minutes of the infusion (eg, 0.1 mL/minute of 10% or 0.05 mL/minute of 20% solution)

Dosage Forms Injection, emulsion [soybean oil]:

Intralipid®: 10% [100 mg/mL] (100 mL, 250 mL, 500 mL); 20% [200 mg/mL] (50 mL, 100 mL, 250 mL, 500 mL, 1000 mL); 30% [300 mg/mL] (500 mL)

Liposyn® III: 10% [100 mg/mL] (200 mL, 500 mL); 20% [200 mg/mL] (200 mL, 500 mL); 30% [300 mg/mL] (500 mL)

Fazaclo™ [US] *see* clozapine *on page 219*

5-FC *see* flucytosine *on page 372*

FC1157a *see* toremifene *on page 872*

Fedahist® Expectorant ***(Discontinued)*** *see page 1042*

Fedahist® Expectorant Pediatric ***(Discontinued)*** *see page 1042*

Fedahist® Tablet ***(Discontinued)*** *see page 1042*

Feen-A-Mint® ***(Discontinued)*** *see page 1042*

Feiba VH® [US] *see* anti-inhibitor coagulant complex *on page 65*

Feiba VH Immuno® [Can] *see* anti-inhibitor coagulant complex *on page 65*

felbamate (FEL ba mate)

U.S./Canadian Brand Names Felbatol® [US]

Therapeutic Category Anticonvulsant

Use Not as a first-line antiepileptic treatment; only in those patients who respond inadequately to alternative treatments and whose epilepsy is so severe that a substantial risk of aplastic anemia and/or liver failure is deemed acceptable in light of the benefits conferred by its use. Patient must be fully advised of risk and provide signed written informed consent. Felbamate can be used as either monotherapy or adjunctive therapy in the treatment of partial seizures (with and without generalization) and in adults with epilepsy.

Orphan drug: Adjunctive therapy in the treatment of partial and generalized seizures associated with Lennox-Gastaut syndrome in children

Usual Dosage Anticonvulsant:

Monotherapy: Children >14 years and Adults:

Initial: 1200 mg/day in divided doses 3 or 4 times/day; titrate previously untreated patients under close clinical supervision, increasing the dosage in 600 mg increments every 2 weeks to 2400 mg/day based on clinical response and thereafter to 3600 mg/day as clinically indicated

Conversion to monotherapy: Initiate at 1200 mg/day in divided doses 3 or 4 times/day, reduce the dosage of the concomitant anticonvulsant(s) by 20% to 33% at the initiation of felbamate therapy; at week 2, increase the felbamate dosage to 2400 mg/day while reducing the dosage of the other anticonvulsant(s) up to an additional 33% of their original dosage; at week 3, increase the felbamate dosage up to 3600 mg/day and continue to reduce the dosage of the other anticonvulsant(s) as clinically indicated

Adjunctive therapy: Children with Lennox-Gastaut and ages 2-14 years:

Week 1:

Felbamate: 15 mg/kg/day divided 3-4 times/day

Concomitant anticonvulsant(s): Reduce original dosage by 20% to 30%

Week 2:

Felbamate: 30 mg/kg/day divided 3-4 times/day

Concomitant anticonvulsant(s): Reduce original dosage up to an additional 33%

Week 3:

Felbamate: 45 mg/kg/day divided 3-4 times/day

Concomitant anticonvulsant(s): Reduce dosage as clinically indicated

Adjunctive therapy: Children >14 years and Adults:

Week 1:

Felbamate: 1200 mg/day initial dose

Concomitant anticonvulsant(s): Reduce original dosage by 20% to 33%

Week 2:

Felbamate: 2400 mg/day (therapeutic range)

Concomitant anticonvulsant(s): Reduce original dosage by up to an additional 33%

Week 3:

Felbamate: 3600 mg/day (therapeutic range)

Concomitant anticonvulsant(s): Reduce original dosage as clinically indicated

Dosage Forms

Suspension, oral: 600 mg/5 mL (240 mL, 960 mL)

Tablet: 400 mg, 600 mg

Felbatol® [US] *see* felbamate *on this page*

Feldene® [US/Can] *see* piroxicam *on page 698*

felodipine (fe LOE di peen)

Sound-Alike/Look-Alike Issues

Plendil® may be confused with Isordil®, pindolol, Pletal®, Prilosec®, Prinivil®

U.S./Canadian Brand Names Plendil® [US/Can]; Renedil® [Can]

Therapeutic Category Calcium Channel Blocker

Use Treatment of hypertension

(Continued)

felodipine *(Continued)*

Usual Dosage

Adults: Oral: 2.5-10 mg once daily; usual initial dose: 5 mg; increase by 5 mg at 2-week intervals, as needed; maximum: 10 mg

Usual dose range (JNC 7) for hypertension: 2.5-20 mg once daily

Dosage Forms Tablet, extended release: 2.5 mg, 5 mg, 10 mg

felodipine and enalapril *see* enalapril and felodipine *on page 308*

Femara® [US/Can] *see* letrozole *on page 508*

FemCare® *(Discontinued)* *see page 1042*

Femcet® *(Discontinued)* *see page 1042*

Femguard® *(Discontinued)* *see page 1042*

femhrt® [US/Can] *see* ethinyl estradiol and norethindrone *on page 342*

Femilax™ [US-OTC] *see* bisacodyl *on page 120*

Femiron® [US-OTC] *see* ferrous fumarate *on page 363*

Femizol-M™ [US-OTC] *see* miconazole *on page 578*

Fem-Prin® [US-OTC] *see* acetaminophen, aspirin, and caffeine *on page 10*

Femring™ [US] *see* estradiol *on page 324*

Femstat® *(Discontinued)* *see page 1042*

Femstat® One [Can] *see* butoconazole *on page 139*

Fenesin™ DM [US] *see* guaifenesin and dextromethorphan *on page 416*

fenofibrate (fen oh FYE brate)

Synonyms procetofene; proctofene

U.S./Canadian Brand Names Apo-Fenofibrate® [Can]; Apo-Feno-Micro® [Can]; Gen-Fenofibrat Micro [Can]; Lipidil Micro® [Can]; Lipidil Supra® [Can]; Lofibra™ [US]; Novo-Fenofibrate [Can]; Nu-Fenofibrate [Can]; PMS-Fenofibrate Micro [Can]; TriCor® [US/Can]

Therapeutic Category Antihyperlipidemic Agent, Miscellaneous

Use Adjunct to dietary therapy for the treatment of adults with very high elevations of serum triglyceride levels (types IV and V hyperlipidemia) who are at risk of pancreatitis and who do not respond adequately to a determined dietary effort; adjunct to dietary therapy for the reduction of low density lipoprotein cholesterol (LDL-C), total cholesterol (total-C), triglycerides, and apolipoprotein B (apo B) in adult patients with primary hypercholesterolemia or mixed dyslipidemia (Fredrickson types IIa and IIb)

Usual Dosage Oral: Adults:

Hypertriglyceridemia: Initial:

Capsule: 67 mg/day with meals, up to 200 mg/day

Tablet: 54 mg/day with meals, up to 160 mg/day

Hypercholesterolemia or mixed hyperlipidemia: Initial:

Capsule: 200 mg/day with meals

Tablet: 160 mg/day with meals

Dosage Forms

Capsule [micronized] (Lofibra™): 67 mg, 134 mg, 200 mg [contains lactose]

Tablet (TriCor®): 54 mg, 160 mg [contains lactose]

fenoldopam (fe NOL doe pam)

Synonyms fenoldopam mesylate

U.S./Canadian Brand Names Corlopam® [US/Can]

Therapeutic Category Antihypertensive Agent

Use Treatment of severe hypertension (up to 48 hours in adults), including in patients with renal compromise; short-term (up to 4 hours) blood pressure reduction in pediatric patients

Usual Dosage I.V.: Hypertension, severe:
Children: Initial: 0.2 mcg/kg/minute; may be increased to dosages of 0.3-0.5 mcg/kg/minute every 20-30 minutes (maximum dose: 0.8 mcg/kg/minute); limited to short-term (4 hours) use
Adults: Initial: 0.1-0.3 mcg/kg/minute (lower initial doses may be associated with less reflex tachycardia); may be increased in increments of 0.05-0.1 mcg/kg/minute every 15 minutes until target blood pressure is reached; the maximal infusion rate reported in clinical studies was 1.6 mcg/kg/minute
Dosage Forms Injection, solution: 10 mg/mL (1 mL, 2 mL) [contains sodium metabisulfite and propylene glycol]

fenoldopam mesylate *see* fenoldopam *on previous page*

fenoprofen (fen oh PROE fen)

Sound-Alike/Look-Alike Issues
fenoprofen may be confused with flurbiprofen
Nalfon® may be confused with Naldecon®
Synonyms fenoprofen calcium
U.S./Canadian Brand Names Nalfon® [US/Can]
Therapeutic Category Analgesic, Nonnarcotic; Nonsteroidal Antiinflammatory Drug (NSAID)
Use Symptomatic treatment of acute and chronic rheumatoid arthritis and osteoarthritis; relief of mild to moderate pain
Usual Dosage Adults: Oral:
Rheumatoid arthritis: 300-600 mg 3-4 times/day up to 3.2 g/day
Mild to moderate pain: 200 mg every 4-6 hours as needed
Dosage Forms
Capsule, as calcium (Nalfon®): 200 mg, 300 mg
Tablet, as calcium: 600 mg

fenoprofen calcium *see* fenoprofen *on this page*

fenoterol *(Canada only)* (fen oh TER ole)

Synonyms fenoterol hydrobromide
U.S./Canadian Brand Names Berotec® [Can]
Therapeutic Category $Beta_2$-Adrenergic Agonist Agent
Use Treatment and prevention of symptoms of reversible obstructive pulmonary disease (including asthma and acute bronchospasm), chronic bronchitis, emphysema
Usual Dosage Inhalation: Children ≥12 years of age and Adults:
MDI:
Acute treatment: 1 puff initially; may repeat in 5 minutes; if relief is not evident, additional doses and/or other therapy may be necessary
Intermittent/long-term treatment: 1-2 puffs 3-4 times/day (maximum of 8 puffs/24 hours)
Solution: 0.5-1 mg (up to maximum of 2.5 mg)
Dosage Forms
Aerosol for inhalation, as hydrobromide: MDI: 100 mcg/dose [200 doses]
Solution for inhalation, as hydrobromide: 0.625 mg/mL (2 mL); 0.25 mg/mL (2 mL)

fenoterol hydrobromide *see* fenoterol *(Canada only)* *on this page*

fentanyl (FEN ta nil)

Sound-Alike/Look-Alike Issues
fentanyl may be confused with alfentanil, sufentanil
Sublimaze® may be confused with Sufenta®
Synonyms fentanyl citrate
U.S./Canadian Brand Names Actiq® [US/Can]; Duragesic® [US/Can]; Sublimaze® [US]
Therapeutic Category Analgesic, Narcotic; General Anesthetic
(Continued)

fentanyl *(Continued)*

Controlled Substance C-II

Use Sedation, relief of pain, preoperative medication, adjunct to general or regional anesthesia, management of chronic pain (transdermal product)

Actiq® is indicated only for management of breakthrough cancer pain in patients who are tolerant to and currently receiving opioid therapy for persistent cancer pain.

Usual Dosage Doses should be titrated to appropriate effects; wide range of doses, dependent upon desired degree of analgesia/anesthesia

Children:

Sedation for minor procedures/analgesia: I.M., I.V.:

1-3 years: 2-3 mcg/kg/dose; may repeat after 30-60 minutes as required

3-12 years: 1-2 mcg/kg/dose; may repeat at 30- to 60-minute intervals as required. **Note:** Children 18-36 months of age may require 2-3 mcg/kg/dose

Continuous sedation/analgesia: Initial I.V. bolus: 1-2 mcg/kg then 1 mcg/kg/hour; titrate upward; usual: 1-3 mcg/kg/hour

Transdermal: Not recommended

Children <12 years and Adults:

Sedation for minor procedures/analgesia: 0.5-1 mcg/kg/dose; higher doses are used for major procedures

Preoperative sedation, adjunct to regional anesthesia, postoperative pain: I.M., I.V.: 50-100 mcg/dose

Adjunct to general anesthesia: I.M., I.V.: 2-50 mcg/kg

General anesthesia without additional anesthetic agents: I.V. 50-100 mcg/kg with O_2 and skeletal muscle relaxant

Transdermal: Initial: 25 mcg/hour system; if currently receiving opiates, convert to fentanyl equivalent and administer equianalgesic dosage (see package insert for further information)

Dosage Forms

Infusion [premixed in NS]: 0.05 mg (10 mL); 1 mg (100 mL); 1.25 mg (250 mL); 2 mg (100 mL); 2.5 mg (250 mL)

Injection, solution, as citrate [preservative free]: 0.05 mg/mL (2 mL, 5 mL, 10 mL, 20 mL, 30 mL, 50 mL)

Sublimaze®: 0.05 mg/mL (2 mL, 5 mL, 10 mL, 20 mL)

Lozenge, oral transmucosal, as citrate (Actiq®): 200 mcg, 400 mcg, 600 mcg, 800 mcg, 1200 mcg, 1600 mcg [mounted on a plastic radiopaque handle; raspberry flavor]

Transdermal system (Duragesic®): 25 mcg/hour [10 cm^2] (5s); 50 mcg/hour [20 cm^2] (5s); 75 mcg/hour [30 cm^2]; 100 mcg/hour [40 cm^2] (5s)

fentanyl citrate *see* fentanyl *on previous page*

Fentanyl Oralet® *(Discontinued)* *see page 1042*

Feosol® Elixir *(Discontinued)* *see page 1042*

Feosol® [US-OTC] *see* ferrous sulfate *on page 364*

Feostat® [US-OTC] *see* ferrous fumarate *on next page*

Ferancee® *(Discontinued)* *see page 1042*

Feratab® [US-OTC] *see* ferrous sulfate *on page 364*

Fer-Gen-Sol [US-OTC] *see* ferrous sulfate *on page 364*

Fergon Plus® *(Discontinued)* *see page 1042*

Fergon® [US-OTC] *see* ferrous gluconate *on page 364*

Feridex I.V.® [US] *see* ferumoxides *on page 366*

Fer-in-Sol® Capsule *(Discontinued)* *see page 1042*

Fer-In-Sol® Syrup *(Discontinued)* *see page 1042*

Fer-In-Sol® [US-OTC/Can] *see* ferrous sulfate *on page 364*

Fer-Iron® [US-OTC] *see* ferrous sulfate *on page 364*

Fermalac [Can] *see* Lactobacillus *on page 501*

Fermalox® *(Discontinued)* *see page 1042*

Ferndex® *(Discontinued)* *see page 1042*

Ferodan™ [Can] *see* ferrous sulfate *on next page*

Fero-Grad 500® [US-OTC] *see* ferrous sulfate and ascorbic acid *on page 365*

Fero-Gradumet® *(Discontinued)* *see page 1042*

Ferospace® *(Discontinued)* *see page 1042*

Ferralet® *(Discontinued)* *see page 1042*

Ferralyn® Lanacaps® *(Discontinued)* *see page 1042*

Ferra-TD® *(Discontinued)* *see page 1042*

Ferretts [US-OTC] *see* ferrous fumarate *on this page*

ferric gluconate (FER ik GLOO koe nate)

Sound-Alike/Look-Alike Issues

Ferrlecit® may be confused with Ferralet®

Synonyms sodium ferric gluconate

U.S./Canadian Brand Names Ferrlecit® [US]

Therapeutic Category Iron Salt

Use Repletion of total body iron content in patients with iron-deficiency anemia who are undergoing hemodialysis in conjunction with erythropoietin therapy

Usual Dosage I.V.: Repletion of iron in hemodialysis patients:

Children ≥6 years: 1.5 mg/kg (maximum: 125 mg/dose) diluted in NS 25 mL, administered over 60 minutes at 8 sequential dialysis sessions

Adults: **Note:** A test dose of 2 mL diluted in NS 50 mL administered over 60 minutes was previously recommended (not in current manufacturer labeling).

125 mg elemental iron per 10 mL (either by I.V. infusion or slow I.V. injection). Most patients will require a cumulative dose of 1 g elemental iron over approximately 8 sequential dialysis treatments to achieve a favorable response.

Dosage Forms Injection, solution: Elemental iron 12.5 mg/mL (5 mL) [contains benzyl alcohol and sucrose 20%]

Ferrlecit® [US] *see* ferric gluconate *on this page*

Ferro-Sequels® [US-OTC] *see* ferrous fumarate *on this page*

ferrous fumarate (FER us FYOO ma rate)

Sound-Alike/Look-Alike Issues

Feostat® may be confused with Feosol®

Synonyms iron fumarate

U.S./Canadian Brand Names Femiron® [US-OTC]; Feostat® [US-OTC]; Ferretts [US-OTC]; Ferro-Sequels® [US-OTC]; Hemocyte® [US-OTC]; Ircon® [US-OTC]; Nephro-Fer® [US-OTC]; Palafer® [Can]

Therapeutic Category Electrolyte Supplement, Oral

Use Prevention and treatment of iron-deficiency anemias

Usual Dosage Oral **(dose expressed in terms of elemental iron):**

Children:

Severe iron-deficiency anemia: 4-6 mg Fe/kg/day in 3 divided doses

Mild to moderate iron deficiency anemia: 3 mg Fe/kg/day in 1-2 divided doses

Prophylaxis: 1-2 mg Fe/kg/day

Adults:

Iron deficiency: 60-100 mg twice daily up to 60 mg 2 times/day

Prophylaxis: 60-100 mg/day

To avoid GI upset, start with a single daily dose and increase by 1 tablet/day each week or as tolerated until desired daily dose is achieved

(Continued)

ferrous fumarate *(Continued)*

Dosage Forms

Tablet: 324 mg [elemental iron 106 mg]
Femiron®: 63 mg [elemental iron 20 mg]
Ferretts: 325 mg [elemental iron 106 mg]
Hemocyte®: 324 mg [elemental iron 106 mg]
Ircon®: 200 mg [elemental iron 66 mg]
Nephro-Fer®: 350 mg [elemental iron 115 mg; contains tartrazine]
Tablet, chewable (Feostat®): 100 mg [elemental iron 33 mg; chocolate flavor]
Tablet, timed release (Ferro-Sequels®): 150 mg [elemental iron 50 mg; contains docusate sodium and sodium benzoate]

ferrous gluconate (FER us GLOO koe nate)

Synonyms iron gluconate

U.S./Canadian Brand Names Apo-Ferrous Gluconate® [Can]; Fergon® [US-OTC]; Novo-Ferrogluc [Can]

Therapeutic Category Electrolyte Supplement, Oral

Use Prevention and treatment of iron-deficiency anemias

Usual Dosage Oral **(dose expressed in terms of elemental iron):**

Children:
Severe iron-deficiency anemia: 4-6 mg Fe/kg/day in 3 divided doses
Mild to moderate iron deficiency anemia: 3 mg Fe/kg/day in 1-2 divided doses
Prophylaxis: 1-2 mg Fe/kg/day

Adults:
Iron deficiency: 60 mg twice daily up to 60 mg 4 times/day
Prophylaxis: 60 mg/day

Dosage Forms

Tablet: 246 mg [elemental iron 28 mg]; 300 mg [elemental iron 34 mg]; 325 mg [elemental iron 36 mg]
Fergon®: 240 mg [elemental iron 27 mg]

ferrous sulfate (FER us SUL fate)

Sound-Alike/Look-Alike Issues

Feosol® may be confused with Feostat®, Fer-In-Sol®
Fer-In-Sol® may be confused with Feosol®
Slow FE® may be confused with Slow-K®

Synonyms $FeSO_4$; iron sulfate

U.S./Canadian Brand Names Apo-Ferrous Sulfate® [Can]; Feosol® [US-OTC]; Feratab® [US-OTC]; Fer-Gen-Sol [US-OTC]; Fer-In-Sol® [US-OTC/Can]; Fer-Iron® [US-OTC]; Ferodan™ [Can]; Slow FE® [US-OTC]

Therapeutic Category Electrolyte Supplement, Oral

Use Prevention and treatment of iron-deficiency anemias

Usual Dosage Oral:

Children **(dose expressed in terms of elemental iron)**:
Severe iron-deficiency anemia: 4-6 mg Fe/kg/day in 3 divided doses
Mild to moderate iron deficiency anemia: 3 mg Fe/kg/day in 1-2 divided doses
Prophylaxis: 1-2 mg Fe/kg/day up to a maximum of 15 mg/day

Adults **(dose expressed in terms of ferrous sulfate)**:
Iron deficiency: 300 mg twice daily up to 300 mg 4 times/day or 250 mg (extended release) 1-2 times/day
Prophylaxis: 300 mg/day

Dosage Forms

Elixir: 220 mg/5 mL (480 mL) [elemental iron 44 mg/5 mL; contains alcohol]
Liquid, oral drops: 75 mg/0.6 mL (50 mL) [elemental iron 15 mg/0.6 mL]
Fer-Gen-Sol: 75 mg/0.6 mL (50 mL) [elemental iron 15 mg/0.6 mL]
Fer-In-Sol®: 75 mg/0.6 mL (50 mL) [elemental iron 15 mg/0.6 mL; contains alcohol 0.2% and sodium bisulfite]

Fer-Iron: 75 mg/0.6 mL (50 mL) [elemental iron 15 mg/0.6 mL]
Tablet: 324 mg [elemental iron 65 mg]; 325 mg [elemental iron 65 mg]
Feratab®: 300 mg [elemental iron 60 mg]
Tablet, exsiccated (Feosol®): 200 mg [elemental iron 65 mg]
Tablet, exsiccated, timed release (Slow FE®): 160 mg [elemental iron 50 mg]

ferrous sulfate and ascorbic acid (FER us SUL fate & a SKOR bik AS id)

Synonyms ascorbic acid and ferrous sulfate; iron sulfate and vitamin C
U.S./Canadian Brand Names Fero-Grad 500® [US-OTC]
Therapeutic Category Vitamin
Use Treatment of iron deficiency in nonpregnant adults; treatment and prevention of iron deficiency in pregnant adults
Usual Dosage Adults: Oral: 1 tablet daily
Dosage Forms [DSC] = Discontinued product
Capsule, extended release (Vitelle™ Irospan®): Ferrous sulfate [elemental iron 65 mg] and ascorbic acid 150 mg [DSC]
Tablet, controlled release (Fero-Grad 500®): Ferrous sulfate 525 mg [elemental iron 105 mg] and ascorbic acid 500 mg
Tablet, extended release (Vitelle™ Irospan®): Ferrous sulfate [elemental iron 65 mg] and ascorbic acid 150 mg [DSC]

ferrous sulfate, ascorbic acid, and vitamin B-complex

(FER us SUL fate, a SKOR bik AS id, & VYE ta min bee-KOM pleks)
Therapeutic Category Vitamin
Use Treatment of conditions of iron deficiency with an increased need for B complex vitamins and vitamin C
Usual Dosage Oral:
Children 1-3 years: 5 mL twice daily after meals
Children >4 years and Adults: 10 mL 3 times/day after meals
Dosage Forms Liquid (components all per 15 mL):
Iberet®-Liquid:
Ascorbic acid: 112.5 mg
B_1: 4.5 mg
B_2: 4.5 mg
B_3: 22.5 mg
B_5: 7.5 mg
B_6: 3.75 mg
B_{12}: 18.75 mg
Ferrous sulfate: 78.75 mg
Iberet®-Liquid 500:
Ascorbic acid: 375 mg
B_1: 4.5 mg
B_2: 4.5 mg
B_3: 22.5 mg
B_5: 7.5 mg
B_6: 3.75 mg
B_{12}: 18.75 mg
Ferrous sulfate: 78.75 mg

ferrous sulfate, ascorbic acid, vitamin B-complex, and folic acid

(FER us SUL fate, a SKOR bik AS id, VYE ta min bee-KOM pleks, & FOE lik AS id)
Therapeutic Category Vitamin
Use Treatment of iron deficiency and prevention of concomitant folic acid deficiency where there is an associated deficient intake or increased need for B complex vitamins
Usual Dosage Adults: Oral: 1 tablet daily
(Continued)

ferrous sulfate, ascorbic acid, vitamin B-complex, and folic acid *(Continued)*

Dosage Forms

Tablet, controlled release:

Ascorbic acid: 500 mg

B_1: 6 mg

B_2: 6 mg

B_3: 30 mg

B_5: 10 mg

B_6: 5 mg

B_{12}: 25 mcg

Ferrous sulfate: 105 mg

Folic acid: 800 mcg

ferumoxides (fer yoo MOX ides)

Sound-Alike/Look-Alike Issues

Feridex I.V.® may be confused with Fertinex®

U.S./Canadian Brand Names Feridex I.V.® [US]

Therapeutic Category Radiopaque Agents

Use For I.V. administration as an adjunct to MRI (in adult patients) to enhance the T2 weighted images used in the detection and evaluation of lesions of the liver

Usual Dosage Adults: 0.56 mg of iron (0.05 mL Feridex I.V.®)/kg body weight diluted in 100 mL of 5% dextrose and infused over 30 minutes; a 5-micron filter is recommended; do not administer undiluted

Dosage Forms Injection, solution: Iron 11.2 mg/mL (5 mL) [contains mannitol 61.3 mg/mL]

$FeSO_4$ *see* ferrous sulfate *on page 364*

Fe-Tinic™ 150 [US-OTC] *see* polysaccharide-iron complex *on page 709*

FeverALL® [US-OTC] *see* acetaminophen *on page 5*

fexofenadine (feks oh FEN a deen)

Sound-Alike/Look-Alike Issues

Allegra® may be confused with Viagra®

Synonyms fexofenadine hydrochloride

U.S./Canadian Brand Names Allegra® [US/Can]

Therapeutic Category Antihistamine

Use Relief of symptoms associated with seasonal allergic rhinitis; treatment of chronic idiopathic urticaria

Usual Dosage Oral:

Children 6-11 years: 30 mg twice daily

Children ≥12 years and Adults:

Seasonal allergic rhinitis: 60 mg twice daily **or** 180 mg once daily

Chronic idiopathic urticaria: 60 mg twice daily

Dosage Forms Tablet, as hydrochloride: 30 mg, 60 mg, 180 mg

fexofenadine and pseudoephedrine

(feks oh FEN a deen & soo doe e FED rin)

Sound-Alike/Look-Alike Issues

Allegra-D® may be confused with Viagra®

Synonyms pseudoephedrine and fexofenadine

U.S./Canadian Brand Names Allegra-D® [US/Can]

Therapeutic Category Antihistamine/Decongestant Combination

Use Relief of symptoms associated with seasonal allergic rhinitis in adults and children ≥12 years of age

Usual Dosage Oral: Children ≥12 years and Adults: One tablet twice daily; it is recommended that the administration with food should be avoided.

Dosage Forms Tablet, extended release: Fexofenadine hydrochloride 60 mg and pseudoephedrine hydrochloride 120 mg

fexofenadine hydrochloride *see* fexofenadine *on previous page*

Fiberall® [US] *see* psyllium *on page 749*

FiberCon® [US-OTC] *see* polycarbophil *on page 706*

FiberEase™ [US-OTC] *see* methylcellulose *on page 569*

Fiber-Lax® [US-OTC] *see* polycarbophil *on page 706*

FiberNorm™ [US-OTC] *see* polycarbophil *on page 706*

fibrin sealant kit (FI brin SEEL ent kit)

Synonyms FS

U.S./Canadian Brand Names Crosseal™ [US]; Tisseel® VH [US/Can]

Therapeutic Category Hemostatic Agent

Use

Crosseal™: Adjunct to hemostasis in liver surgery

Tisseel® VH: Adjunct to hemostasis in cardiopulmonary bypass surgery and splenic injury (due to blunt or penetrating trauma to the abdomen) when the control of bleeding by conventional surgical techniques is ineffective or impractical; adjunctive sealant for closure of colostomies; hemostatic agent in heparinized patients undergoing cardiopulmonary bypass

Usual Dosage Adjunct to hemostasis: Apply topically; actual dose is based on size of surface to be covered:

Crosseal™: Children and Adults: To cover a layer of 1 mm thickness:

Maximum area to be sealed: 20 cm^2

Required size of Crosseal™ kit: 1 mL

Maximum area to be sealed: 40 cm^2

Required size of Crosseal™ kit: 2 mL

Maximum area to be sealed: 100 cm^2

Required size of Crosseal™ kit: 5 mL

Note: If hemostatic effect is not complete, apply a second layer.

Tisseel® VH: Adults:

Maximum area to be sealed: 4 cm^2

Required size of Tisseel® VH kit: 0.5 mL

Maximum area to be sealed: 8 cm^2

Required size of Tisseel® VH kit: 1 mL

Maximum area to be sealed: 16 cm^2

Required size of Tisseel® VH kit: 2 mL

Maximum area to be sealed: 40 cm^2

Required size of Tisseel® VH kit: 5 mL

Apply in thin layers to avoid excess formation of granulation tissue and slow absorption of the sealant. Following application, hold the sealed parts in the desired position for 3-5 minutes. To prevent sealant from adhering to gloves or surgical instruments, wet them with saline prior to contact.

Dosage Forms

Crosseal™ Kit: Each kit contains: Fibrinogen 40-60 mg/mL [human; also contains tranexamic acid]; thrombin 800-1200 int. units/mL [human; also contains human albumin and mannitol]; spray application device (1 mL, 2 mL, 5 mL)

Tisseel® VH Kit: Following reconstitution, each kit contains: Fibrinogen 75-115 mg/mL [sealer protein concentrate, human]; aprotinin 3000 KIU/mL [fibrinolysis inhibitor solution, bovine]; thrombin 500 int. units/mL [human]; calcium chloride solution 40 micromoles/mL (0.5 mL, 1 mL, 2 mL, 5 mL)

filgrastim (fil GRA stim)

Sound-Alike/Look-Alike Issues

Neupogen® may be confused with Epogen®, Neumega®, Nutramigen®

Synonyms G-CSF; granulocyte colony stimulating factor

U.S./Canadian Brand Names Neupogen® [US/Can]

Therapeutic Category Colony-Stimulating Factor

Use Stimulation of granulocyte production in patients with malignancies, including myeloid malignancies; receiving myelosuppressive therapy associated with a significant risk of neutropenia; severe chronic neutropenia (SCN); receiving bone marrow transplantation (BMT); undergoing peripheral blood progenitor cell (PBPC) collection

Usual Dosage Refer to individual protocols.

Dosing, even in morbidly obese patients, should be based on actual body weight. Rounding doses to the nearest vial size often enhances patient convenience and reduces costs without compromising clinical response.

Myelosuppressive therapy: 5 mcg/kg/day - doses may be increased by 5 mcg/kg according to the duration and severity of the neutropenia.

Bone marrow transplantation: 5-10 mcg/kg/day - doses may be increased by 5 mcg/kg according to the duration and severity of neutropenia; recommended steps based on neutrophil response:

When ANC >1000/mm^3 for 3 consecutive days: Reduce filgrastim dose to 5 mcg/kg/day

If ANC remains >1000/mm^3 for 3 more consecutive days: Discontinue filgrastim

If ANC decreases to <1000/mm^3: Resume at 5 mcg/kg/day

If ANC decreases <1000/mm^3 during the 5 mcg/kg/day dose, increase filgrastim to 10 mcg/kg/day and follow the above steps

Peripheral blood progenitor cell (PBPC) collection: 10 mcg/kg/day **or** 5-8 mcg/kg twice daily in donors. The optimal timing and duration of growth factor stimulation has not been determined.

Severe chronic neutropenia:

Congenital: 6 mcg/kg twice daily

Idiopathic/cyclic: 5 mcg/kg/day

Not removed by hemodialysis

Dosage Forms

Injection, solution [preservative free]: 300 mcg/mL (1 mL, 1.6 mL) [vial; contains sodium 0.035 mg/mL and sorbitol]

Injection, solution [preservative free]: 600 mcg/mL (0.5 mL, 0.8 mL) [prefilled Singleject® syringe; contains sodium 0.035 mg/mL and sorbitol]

Finacea™ [US] *see* azelaic acid *on page 93*

finasteride (fi NAS teer ide)

Sound-Alike/Look-Alike Issues

Proscar® may be confused with ProSom®, Prozac®, Psorcon®

U.S./Canadian Brand Names Propecia® [US/Can]; Proscar® [US/Can]

Therapeutic Category Antiandrogen

Use

Propecia®: Treatment of male pattern hair loss in **men only**. Safety and efficacy were demonstrated in men between 18-41 years of age.

Proscar®: Treatment of symptomatic benign prostatic hyperplasia (BPH); can be used in combination with an alpha blocker, doxazosin

Usual Dosage Oral: Adults:

Male:

Benign prostatic hyperplasia (Proscar®): 5 mg/day as a single dose; clinical responses occur within 12 weeks to 6 months of initiation of therapy; long-term administration is recommended for maximal response

Male pattern baldness (Propecia®): 1 mg daily

Dosage Forms
Tablet [film coated]:
Propecia®: 1 mg
Proscar®: 5 mg

Fiorgen PF® ***(Discontinued)*** *see page 1042*

Fioricet® [US] *see* butalbital, acetaminophen, and caffeine *on page 138*

Fiorinal® [US/Can] *see* butalbital, aspirin, and caffeine *on page 138*

Fiorinal®-C 1/2 [Can] *see* butalbital, aspirin, caffeine, and codeine *on page 139*

Fiorinal®-C 1/4 [Can] *see* butalbital, aspirin, caffeine, and codeine *on page 139*

Fiorinal® With Codeine [US] *see* butalbital, aspirin, caffeine, and codeine *on page 139*

Fiorital® ***(Discontinued)*** *see page 1042*

fisalamine *see* mesalamine *on page 556*

FK506 *see* tacrolimus *on page 837*

Flagyl® [US/Can] *see* metronidazole *on page 576*

Flagyl ER® [US] *see* metronidazole *on page 576*

Flamazine® [Can] *see* silver sulfadiazine *on page 804*

Flarex® [US/Can] *see* fluorometholone *on page 377*

Flatulex® [US-OTC] *see* simethicone *on page 804*

Flavorcee® ***(Discontinued)*** *see page 1042*

flavoxate (fla VOKS ate)

Sound-Alike/Look-Alike Issues
Urispas® may be confused with Urised®

Synonyms flavoxate hydrochloride

U.S./Canadian Brand Names Apo-Flavoxate® [Can]; Urispas® [US/Can]

Therapeutic Category Antispasmodic Agent, Urinary

Use Antispasmodic to provide symptomatic relief of dysuria, nocturia, suprapubic pain, urgency, and incontinence due to detrusor instability and hyper-reflexia in elderly with cystitis, urethritis, urethrocystitis, urethrotrigonitis, and prostatitis

Usual Dosage Children >12 years and Adults: Oral: 100-200 mg 3-4 times/day; reduce the dose when symptoms improve

Dosage Forms Tablet [film coated], as hydrochloride: 100 mg

flavoxate hydrochloride *see* flavoxate *on this page*

Flaxedil® ***(Discontinued)*** *see page 1042*

Flebogamma® [US] *see* immune globulin (intravenous) *on page 468*

flecainide (fle KAY nide)

Sound-Alike/Look-Alike Issues
flecainide may be confused with fluconazole
Tambocor™ may be confused with tamoxifen

Synonyms flecainide acetate

U.S./Canadian Brand Names Tambocor™ [US/Can]

Therapeutic Category Antiarrhythmic Agent, Class I-C

Use Prevention and suppression of documented life-threatening ventricular arrhythmias (eg, sustained ventricular tachycardia); controlling symptomatic, disabling supraventricular tachycardias in patients without structural heart disease in whom other agents fail

Usual Dosage Oral:
Children:
Initial: 3 mg/kg/day or 50-100 mg/m^2/day in 3 divided doses
(Continued)

flecainide *(Continued)*

Usual: 3-6 mg/kg/day or 100-150 mg/m^2/day in 3 divided doses; up to 11 mg/kg/day or 200 mg/m^2/day for uncontrolled patients with subtherapeutic levels

Adults:

Life-threatening ventricular arrhythmias:

Initial: 100 mg every 12 hours

Increase by 50-100 mg/day (given in 2 doses/day) every 4 days; maximum: 400 mg/day.

Use of higher initial doses and more rapid dosage adjustments have resulted in an increased incidence of proarrhythmic events and congestive heart failure, particularly during the first few days. Do not use a loading dose. Use very cautiously in patients with history of congestive heart failure or myocardial infarction.

Prevention of paroxysmal supraventricular arrhythmias in patients with disabling symptoms but no structural heart disease:

Initial: 50 mg every 12 hours

Increase by 50 mg twice daily at 4-day intervals; maximum: 300 mg/day.

Dosage Forms Tablet, as acetate: 50 mg, 100 mg, 150 mg

flecainide acetate *see* flecainide *on previous page*

Fleet® Babylax® [US-OTC] *see* glycerin *on page 410*

Fleet® Bisacodyl Enema [US-OTC] *see* bisacodyl *on page 120*

Fleet® Enema [US-OTC/Can] *see* sodium phosphates *on page 815*

Fleet® Flavored Castor Oil *(Discontinued)* *see page 1042*

Fleet® Glycerin Suppositories Maximum Strength [US-OTC] *see* glycerin *on page 410*

Fleet® Glycerin Suppositories [US-OTC] *see* glycerin *on page 410*

Fleet® Laxative *(Discontinued)* *see page 1042*

Fleet® Liquid Glycerin Suppositories [US-OTC] *see* glycerin *on page 410*

Fleet® Phospho®-Soda Accu-Prep™ [US-OTC] *see* sodium phosphates *on page 815*

Fleet® Phospho®-Soda Oral Laxative [Can] *see* sodium phosphates *on page 815*

Fleet® Phospho®-Soda [US-OTC] *see* sodium phosphates *on page 815*

Fleet® Sof-Lax® Overnight *(Discontinued)* *see page 1042*

Fleet® Sof-Lax® [US-OTC] *see* docusate *on page 285*

Fleet® Stimulant Laxative [US-OTC] *see* bisacodyl *on page 120*

Fletcher's® Castoria® [US-OTC] *see* senna *on page 799*

Flexaphen® *(Discontinued)* *see page 1042*

Flexeril® [US/Can] *see* cyclobenzaprine *on page 233*

Flexitec [Can] *see* cyclobenzaprine *on page 233*

Flintstones® Complete [US-OTC] *see* vitamins (multiple/pediatric) *on page 927*

Flintstones® Original [US-OTC] *see* vitamins (multiple/pediatric) *on page 927*

Flintstones® Plus Calcium [US-OTC] *see* vitamins (multiple/pediatric) *on page 927*

Flintstones® Plus Extra C [US-OTC] *see* vitamins (multiple/pediatric) *on page 927*

Flintstones® Plus Iron [US-OTC] *see* vitamins (multiple/pediatric) *on page 927*

Flo-Coat® [US] *see* radiological/contrast media (ionic) *on page 759*

floctafenine *(Canada only)* (flok ta FEN een)

Therapeutic Category Nonsteroidal Antiinflammatory Drug (NSAID), Oral

Use Short-term use in acute pain of mild and moderate severity

Usual Dosage Adults: Oral: 200-400 mg every 6-8 hours as required; maximum recommended daily dose: 1200 mg

Dosage Forms Tablet: 200 mg, 400 mg

Flolan® [US/Can] *see* epoprostenol *on page 316*

Flomax® [US/Can] *see* tamsulosin *on page 839*

Flonase® [US] *see* fluticasone (nasal) *on page 383*

Flonase® 9 g *(Discontinued)* *see page 1042*

Florazole ER® [Can] *see* metronidazole *on page 576*

Florical® [US-OTC] *see* calcium carbonate *on page 144*

Florinef® [US/Can] *see* fludrocortisone *on page 373*

Florone® [US/Can] *see* diflorasone *on page 269*

Florone E® *(Discontinued)* *see page 1042*

Floropryl® Ophthalmic *(Discontinued)* *see page 1042*

Flovent® *see* fluticasone (oral inhalation) *on page 383*

Flovent® Rotadisk® *see* fluticasone (oral inhalation) *on page 383*

Floxin® [US/Can] *see* ofloxacin *on page 640*

floxin otic singles *see* ofloxacin *on page 640*

floxuridine (floks YOOR i deen)

Sound-Alike/Look-Alike Issues

FUDR® may be confused with Fludara®

Synonyms fluorodeoxyuridine; 5-FUDR; NSC-27640

U.S./Canadian Brand Names FUDR® [US/Can]

Therapeutic Category Antineoplastic Agent

Use Management of hepatic metastases of colorectal and gastric cancers

Usual Dosage Refer to individual protocols.

Intra-arterial:
- 0.1-0.6 mg/kg/day
- 4-20 mg/day

I.V.:
- 0.15 mg/kg/day for 7-14 days
- 0.5-1 mg/kg/day for 6-15 days
- 30 mg/kg/day for 5 days, then 15 mg/kg/day every other day, up to 11 days

Dosage Forms Injection, powder for reconstitution: 500 mg

Fluanxol® [Can] *see* flupenthixol *(Canada only) on page 379*

flubenisolone *see* betamethasone (systemic) *on page 115*

Flucaine® [US] *see* proparacaine and fluorescein *on page 738*

fluconazole (floo KOE na zole)

Sound-Alike/Look-Alike Issues

fluconazole may be confused with flecainide

Diflucan® may be confused with diclofenac, Diprivan®, disulfiram

U.S./Canadian Brand Names Apo-Fluconazole® [Can]; Diflucan® [US/Can]; Gen-Fluconazole [Can]; Novo-Fluconazole [Can]

Therapeutic Category Antifungal Agent

Use Treatment of oral or vaginal candidiasis unresponsive to nystatin or clotrimazole; nonlife-threatening *Candida* infections (eg, cystitis, esophagitis); treatment of hepatosplenic candidiasis; treatment of other *Candida* infections in persons unable to tolerate

(Continued)

fluconazole *(Continued)*

amphotericin B; treatment of cryptococcal infections; secondary prophylaxis for cryptococcal meningitis in persons with AIDS; antifungal prophylaxis in allogeneic bone marrow transplant recipients

Oral fluconazole should be used in persons able to tolerate oral medications; parenteral fluconazole should be reserved for patients who are both unable to take oral medications and are unable to tolerate amphotericin B (eg, due to hypersensitivity or renal insufficiency)

Usual Dosage Daily dose of fluconazole is the same for oral and I.V. administration

Infants and Children: Oral, I.V.: Safety profile of fluconazole has been studied in 577 children, ages 1 day to 17 years; doses as high as 12 mg/kg/day once daily (equivalent to adult doses of 400 mg/day) have been used to treat candidiasis in immunocompromised children; 10-12 mg/kg/day doses once daily have been used prophylactically against fungal infections in pediatric bone marrow transplantation patients. Do not exceed 600 mg/day.

Adults:

Vaginal candidiasis: Oral: 150 mg single dose

Prophylaxis against fungal infections in bone marrow transplantation patients: Oral, I.V.: 400 mg/day once daily

Dosage Forms

Infusion [premixed in sodium chloride]: 2 mg/mL (100 mL, 200 mL)

Diflucan® [premixed in sodium chloride or dextrose] 2 mg/mL (100 mL, 200 mL)

Powder for oral suspension (Diflucan®): 10 mg/mL (35 mL); 40 mg/mL (35 mL) [contains sodium benzoate; orange flavor]

Tablet (Diflucan®): 50 mg, 100 mg, 150 mg, 200 mg

flucytosine (floo SYE toe seen)

Sound-Alike/Look-Alike Issues

flucytosine may be confused with fluorouracil

Ancobon® may be confused with Oncovin®

Synonyms 5-FC; 5-flurocytosine

U.S./Canadian Brand Names Ancobon® [US/Can]

Therapeutic Category Antifungal Agent

Use Adjunctive treatment of susceptible fungal infections (usually *Candida* or *Cryptococcus*); synergy with amphotericin B for certain fungal infections (*Cryptococcus* spp., *Candida* spp.)

Usual Dosage Children and Adults: Oral: 50-150 mg/kg/day in divided doses every 6 hours

Dosage Forms Capsule: 250 mg, 500 mg

Fludara® [US/Can] *see* fludarabine *on this page*

fludarabine (floo DARE a been)

Sound-Alike/Look-Alike Issues

fludarabine may be confused with Flumadine®

Fludara® may be confused with FUDR®

Synonyms fludarabine phosphate

U.S./Canadian Brand Names Fludara® [US/Can]

Therapeutic Category Antineoplastic Agent

Use Treatment of chronic lymphocytic leukemia (CLL) (including refractory CLL); non-Hodgkin lymphoma in adults

Usual Dosage I.V.: Adults:

Chronic lymphocytic leukemia: 25 mg/m^2/day for 5 days every 28 days

Non-Hodgkin lymphoma: Loading dose: 20 mg/m^2 followed by 30 mg/m^2/day for 48 hours

Dosage Forms Injection, powder for reconstitution, as phosphate: 50 mg

fludarabine phosphate *see* fludarabine *on previous page*

fludrocortisone (floo droe KOR ti sone)

Sound-Alike/Look-Alike Issues

Florinef® may be confused with Fiorinal®

Synonyms fludrocortisone acetate; fluohydrisone acetate; fluohydrocortisone acetate; 9α-fluorohydrocortisone acetate

U.S./Canadian Brand Names Florinef® [US/Can]

Therapeutic Category Adrenal Corticosteroid (Mineralocorticoid)

Use Partial replacement therapy for primary and secondary adrenocortical insufficiency in Addison disease; treatment of salt-losing adrenogenital syndrome

Usual Dosage Oral:

Infants and Children: 0.05-0.1 mg/day

Adults: 0.1-0.2 mg/day with ranges of 0.1 mg 3 times/week to 0.2 mg/day

Addison's disease: Initial: 0.1 mg/day; if transient hypertension develops, reduce the dose to 0.05 mg/day. Preferred administration with cortisone (10-37.5 mg/day) or hydrocortisone (10-30 mg/day).

Salt-losing adrenogenital syndrome: 0.1-0.2 mg/day

Dosage Forms Tablet, as acetate: 0.1 mg

fludrocortisone acetate *see* fludrocortisone *on this page*

Flumadine® [US/Can] *see* rimantadine *on page 778*

flumazenil (FLO may ze nil)

U.S./Canadian Brand Names Anexate® [Can]; Romazicon® [US/Can]

Therapeutic Category Antidote

Use Benzodiazepine antagonist; reverses sedative effects of benzodiazepines used in conscious sedation and general anesthesia; treatment of benzodiazepine overdose

Usual Dosage Reversal of conscious sedation or general anesthesia: 0.2 mg (2 mL) administered I.V. over 15 seconds; if desired effect is not achieved after 60 seconds, repeat in 0.2 mg (2 mL) increments every 60 seconds up to a total of 1 mg (10 mL); in event of resedation, repeat doses may be administered at 20-minute intervals with no more than 1 mg (10 mL) administered at any one time, with a maximum of 3 mg in any 1 hour

Dosage Forms Injection, solution: 0.1 mg/mL (5 mL, 10 mL) [contains edetate sodium]

flumethasone and clioquinol *see* clioquinol and flumethasone *(Canada only)* *on page 211*

FluMist™ [US] *see* influenza virus vaccine *on page 473*

flunarizine *(Canada only)* (floo NAR i zeen)

Therapeutic Category Calcium-Entry Blocker (Selective)

Use Prophylaxis of migraine with and without aura; the safety of flunarizine in long-term use (ie, >4 months) has not been systematically evaluated in controlled clinical trials. Flunarizine is not indicated in the treatment of acute migraine attacks.

Usual Dosage The usual adult dosage is 10 mg/day administered in the evening. Patients who experience side effects may be maintained on 5 mg at bedtime.

Duration of therapy: Clinical experience indicates that the onset of effect of flunarizine is gradual and maximum benefits may not be seen before the patient has completed several weeks of continuous treatment. Therapy, therefore, should not be discontinued for lack of response before an adequate time period has elapsed (ie, 6-8 weeks).

Dosage Forms Capsule, as hydrochloride: 5 mg

flunisolide (floo NIS oh lide)

Sound-Alike/Look-Alike Issues

flunisolide may be confused with Flumadine®, fluocinonide

Nasarel® may be confused with Nizoral®

(Continued)

flunisolide *(Continued)*

U.S./Canadian Brand Names AeroBid® [US]; AeroBid®-M [US]; Alti-Flunisolide [Can]; Apo-Flunisolide® [Can]; Nasalide® [Can]; Nasarel® [US]; Rhinalar® [Can]

Therapeutic Category Adrenal Corticosteroid

Use Steroid-dependent asthma; nasal solution is used for seasonal or perennial rhinitis

Usual Dosage

Children >6 years:

Oral inhalation: 2 inhalations twice daily (morning and evening) up to 4 inhalations/day

Nasal: 1 spray each nostril twice daily (morning and evening), not to exceed 4 sprays/day each nostril

Adults:

Oral inhalation: 2 inhalations twice daily (morning and evening) up to 8 inhalations/day maximum

Nasal: 2 sprays each nostril twice daily (morning and evening); maximum dose: 8 sprays/day in each nostril

Dosage Forms

Aerosol for oral inhalation:

AeroBid®: 250 mcg/actuation (7 g) [100 metered doses; contains CFCs]

AeroBid-M®: 250 mcg/actuation (7 g) [100 metered doses; contains CFCs; menthol flavor]

Solution, intranasal spray (Nasarel®): 25 mcg/actuation (25 mL) [200 sprays; contains benzalkonium chloride]

fluocinolone (floo oh SIN oh lone)

Sound-Alike/Look-Alike Issues

fluocinolone may be confused with fluocinonide

Synonyms fluocinolone acetonide

U.S./Canadian Brand Names Capex™ [US/Can]; Derma-Smoothe/FS® [US/Can]; Fluoderm [Can]; Synalar® [US/Can]

Therapeutic Category Corticosteroid, Topical

Use Relief of susceptible inflammatory dermatosis [low, medium, high potency topical corticosteroid]; psoriasis of the scalp; atopic dermatitis in children ≥2 years of age

Usual Dosage Topical:

Children ≥2 years: Atopic dermatitis (Derma-Smoothe/FS®): Moisten skin; apply to affected area twice daily; do not use for longer than 4 weeks

Children and Adults: Corticosteroid-responsive dermatoses: Cream, ointment, solution: Apply a thin layer to affected area 2-4 times/day; may use occlusive dressings to manage psoriasis or recalcitrant conditions

Adults:

Atopic dermatitis (Derma-Smoothe/FS®): Apply thin film to affected area 3 times/day

Scalp psoriasis (Derma-Smoothe/FS®): Massage thoroughly into wet or dampened hair/scalp; cover with shower cap. Leave on overnight (or for at least 4 hours). Remove by washing hair with shampoo and rinsing thoroughly.

Seborrheic dermatitis of the scalp (Capex™): Apply no more than 1 ounce to scalp once daily; work into lather and allow to remain on scalp for ~5 minutes. Remove from hair and scalp by rinsing thoroughly with water.

Dosage Forms

Cream, as acetonide: 0.01% (15 g, 60 g); 0.025% (15 g, 60 g)

Synalar®: 0.025% (15 g, 60 g)

Oil, as acetonide:

Derma-Smoothe/FS® [eczema oil]: 0.01% (120 mL) [contains peanut oil]

Derma-Smoothe/FS® [scalp oil]: 0.01% (120 mL) [contains peanut oil; packaged with shower caps]

Ointment, as acetonide (Synalar®): 0.025% (15 g, 60 g)

Shampoo, as acetonide (Capex™): 0.01% (120 mL)

Solution, as acetonide: 0.01% (60 mL)

Synalar®: 0.01% (20 mL, 60 mL)

fluocinolone acetonide *see* fluocinolone *on previous page*

fluocinolone, hydroquinone, and tretinoin

(floo oh SIN oh lone, HYE droe kwin one, & TRET i noyn)

Synonyms hydroquinone, fluocinolone acetonide, and tretinoin; tretinoin, fluocinolone acetonide, and hydroquinone

U.S./Canadian Brand Names Tri-Luma™ [US]

Therapeutic Category Corticosteroid, Topical; Depigmenting Agent; Retinoic Acid Derivative

Use Short-term treatment of moderate to severe melasma of the face

Usual Dosage Topical: Adults: Melasma: Apply a thin film once daily to hyperpigmented areas of melasma (including ½ inch of normal-appearing surrounding skin). Apply 30 minutes prior to bedtime; not indicated for use beyond 8 weeks. Do not use occlusive dressings.

Dosage Forms Cream, topical: Hydroquinone 4%, tretinoin 0.05%, fluocinolone acetonide 0.01% (30 g) [contains sodium metabisulfite]

fluocinonide (floo oh SIN oh nide)

Sound-Alike/Look-Alike Issues

fluocinonide may be confused with flunisolide, fluocinolone

Lidex® may be confused with Lasix®, Videx®, Wydase®

U.S./Canadian Brand Names Lidemol® [Can]; Lidex® [US/Can]; Lidex-E® [US]; Lyderm® [Can]; Lydonide [Can]; Tiamol® [Can]; Topsyn® [Can]

Therapeutic Category Corticosteroid, Topical

Use Antiinflammatory, antipruritic, relief of inflammatory and pruritic manifestations [high potency topical corticosteroid]

Usual Dosage Children and Adults: Topical: Apply thin layer to affected area 2-4 times/day depending on the severity of the condition. Therapy should be discontinued when control is achieved; if no improvement is seen, reassessment of diagnosis may be necessary.

Dosage Forms

Cream, anhydrous, emollient (Lidex®): 0.05% (15 g, 30 g, 60 g)
Cream, aqueous, emollient (Lidex-E®): 0.05% (15 g, 30 g, 60 g)
Gel (Lidex®): 0.05% (15 g, 30 g, 60 g)
Ointment (Lidex®): 0.05% (15 g, 30 g, 60 g)
Solution (Lidex®): 0.05% (20 mL [DSC], 60 mL) [contains alcohol 35%]

Fluoderm [Can] *see* fluocinolone *on previous page*

fluohydrisone acetate *see* fludrocortisone *on page 373*

fluohydrocortisone acetate *see* fludrocortisone *on page 373*

Fluonid® Topical *(Discontinued)* *see page 1042*

Fluoracaine® [US] *see* proparacaine and fluorescein *on page 738*

Fluor-A-Day [US-OTC/Can] *see* fluoride *on next page*

FluorCare® Neutral *(Discontinued)* *see page 1042*

fluorescein and proparacaine *see* proparacaine and fluorescein *on page 738*

fluorescein sodium (FLURE e seen SOW dee um)

Synonyms soluble fluorescein

U.S./Canadian Brand Names AK-Fluor [US]; Angiscein® [US]; Diofluor™ [Can]; Fluorescite® [US/Can]; Fluorets® [US/Can]; Fluor-I-Strip® [US]; Fluor-I-Strip-AT® [US]; Ful-Glo® [US]

Therapeutic Category Diagnostic Agent

Use Demonstrates defects of corneal epithelium; diagnostic aid in ophthalmic angiography

(Continued)

fluorescein sodium *(Continued)*

Usual Dosage

Ophthalmic:

Solution: Instill 1-2 drops of 2% solution and allow a few seconds for staining; wash out excess with sterile water or irrigating solution

Strips: Moisten strip with sterile water. Place moistened strip at the fornix into the lower cul-de-sac close to the punctum. For best results, patient should close lid tightly over strip until desired amount of staining is obtained. Patient should blink several times after application.

Removal of foreign bodies, sutures or tonometry (Fluress®): Instill 1 or 2 drops (single instillations) into each eye before operating

Deep ophthalmic anesthesia (Fluress®): Instill 2 drops into each eye every 90 seconds up to 3 doses

Injection: Prior to use, perform intradermal skin test; have epinephrine 1:1000, an antihistamine, and oxygen available

Children: 3.5 mg/lb (7.5 mg/kg) injected rapidly into antecubital vein

Adults: 500-750 mg injected rapidly into antecubital vein

Dosage Forms

Injection, solution:

AK-Fluor®, Fluorescite®: 10% (5 mL); 25% (2 mL)

Angiscein®: 10% (5 mL)

Strip, ophthalmic:

Fluorets®, Fluor-I-Strip-AT®: 1 mg

Fluor-I-Strip®: 9 mg

Ful-Glo®: 0.6 mg

Fluorescite® [US/Can] *see* fluorescein sodium *on previous page*

Fluorets® [US/Can] *see* fluorescein sodium *on previous page*

fluoride (FLOR ide)

Sound-Alike/Look-Alike Issues

Luride® may be confused with Lortab®

Phos-Flur® may be confused with PhosLo®

Thera-Flur-N® may be confused with Thera-Flu®

Synonyms acidulated phosphate fluoride; sodium fluoride; stannous fluoride

U.S./Canadian Brand Names Fluor-A-Day [US-OTC/Can]; Fluorigard® [US-OTC]; Fluorinse® [US]; Fluotic® [Can]; Flura-Drops® [US]; Flura-Loz® [US]; Gel-Kam® Rinse [US]; Gel-Kam® [US-OTC]; Lozi-Flur™ [US]; Luride® [US]; Luride® Lozi-Tab® [US]; NeutraCare® [US]; NeutraGard® [US-OTC]; Pediaflor® [US]; Pharmaflur® [US]; Pharmaflur® 1.1 [US]; Phos-Flur® [US]; Phos-Flur® Rinse [US-OTC]; PreviDent® [US]; PreviDent® 5000 Plus™ [US]; Stan-Gard® [US]; Stop® [US]; Thera-Flur-N® [US]

Therapeutic Category Mineral, Oral

Use Prevention of dental caries

Usual Dosage Oral: Dental rinse or gel:

Children 6-12 years: 5-10 mL rinse or apply to teeth and spit daily after brushing

Adults: 10 mL rinse or apply to teeth and spit daily after brushing

Dosage Forms

Cream, topical, as sodium (PreviDent® 5000 Plus™): 1.1% (51 g) [fluoride 2.5 mg/dose; fruit and spearmint flavors]

Gel-drops, as sodium fluoride (Thera-Flur-N®): 1.1% (24 mL) [fluoride 0.5%; neutral pH; no artificial color or flavor]

Gel, topical, as acidulated phosphate fluoride (Phos-Flur®): 1.1% (60 g) [fluoride 0.5%; cherry and mint flavors]

Gel, topical, as sodium fluoride:

NeutraCare®: 1.1% (60 g) [neutral pH; grape and mint flavors]

PreviDent®: 1.1% (60 g) [fluoride 2 mg/dose; berry, cherry, and mint flavors]

Gel, topical, as stannous fluoride:
Gel-Kam®: 0.4% (129 g) [bubblegum, cinnamon, fruit/berry, and mint flavors]
Stan-Gard®: 0.4% (122 g) [bubblegum, cherry, cinnamon, grape, mint, and raspberry flavors]
Stop®: 0.4% (120 g) [bubblegum, cinnamon, grape, and mint flavors]
Lozenge, as sodium:
Flura-Loz®: 2.2 mg [fluoride 1 mg; sugar free; raspberry flavor]
Fluor-A-Day: 2.2 mg [fluoride 1 mg; mint flavor]
Lozi-Flur™: 2.21 mg [fluoride 1 mg; cherry flavor]
Solution, oral drops, as sodium:
Flura-Drops®: 0.55 mg/drop (24 mL) [fluoride 0.25 mg/drop]
Luride®: 1.1 mg/mL (50 mL) [fluoride 0.5 mg/mL; sugar free]
Pediaflor®: 1.1 mg/mL (50 mL) [fluoride 0.5 mg/mL; contains alcohol <0.5%; sugar free; cherry flavor]
Solution, oral rinse, as sodium:
ACT®: 0.05% (530 mL) [fluoride 0.0226%; bubblegum flavor, cinnamon flavor (contains tartrazine)]
Fluorigard®: 0.05% (480 mL) [contains alcohol, sodium benzoate, and tartrazine; mint flavor]
Fluorinse®: 0.2% (480 mL) [alcohol free; cinnamon and mint flavors]
NeutraGard®: 0.05% (480 mL) [neutral pH; mint and tropical blast flavors]
Phos-Flur®: 0.44% (500 mL) [bubblegum, cherry, grape, and mint flavors]
PreviDent®: 0.2% (250 mL) [contains alcohol; mint flavor]
Solution, oral rinse concentrate, as stannous fluoride (Gel-Kam®): 0.63% (300 mL) [fluoride 7.1 mg/dose; cinnamon and mint flavors]
Tablet, chewable, as sodium:
Fluor-A-Day:
0.56 mg [fluoride 0.25 mg; raspberry flavor]
1.1 mg [fluoride 0.5 mg; raspberry flavor]
2.21 mg [fluoride 1 mg; raspberry flavor]
Luride® Lozi-Tabs®:
0.55 mg [fluoride 0.25 mg; sugar free; vanilla flavor]
1.1 mg [fluoride 0.5 mg; sugar free; grape flavor]
2.2 mg [fluoride 1 mg; sugar free; cherry flavor]
Pharmaflur®: 2.2 mg [fluoride 1 mg; dye free, sugar free; cherry flavor]
Pharmaflur® 1.1: 1.1 mg [fluoride 0.5 mg; dye free, sugar free; grape flavor]

Fluorigard® [US-OTC] *see* fluoride *on previous page*

Fluori-Methane® [US] *see* dichlorodifluoromethane and trichloromonofluoromethane *on page 265*

Fluorinse® [US] *see* fluoride *on previous page*

Fluor-I-Strip® [US] *see* fluorescein sodium *on page 375*

Fluor-I-Strip-AT® [US] *see* fluorescein sodium *on page 375*

Fluoritab® *(Discontinued)* *see page 1042*

fluorodeoxyuridine *see* floxuridine *on page 371*

9α-fluorohydrocortisone acetate *see* fludrocortisone *on page 373*

fluorometholone (flure oh METH oh lone)

U.S./Canadian Brand Names Flarex® [US/Can]; FML® [US/Can]; FML® Forte [US/Can]; PMS-Fluorometholone [Can]

Therapeutic Category Adrenal Corticosteroid

Use Treatment of steroid-responsive inflammatory conditions of the eye

Usual Dosage Children >2 years and Adults: Ophthalmic: Reevaluate therapy if improvement is not seen within 2 days; use care not to discontinue prematurely; in chronic conditions, gradually decrease dosing frequency prior to discontinuing treatment

(Continued)

fluorometholone *(Continued)*

Ointment: Apply small amount (~1/2 inch ribbon) to conjunctival sac every 4 hours in severe cases; 1-3 times/day in mild to moderate cases

Solution: Instill 1-2 drops into conjunctival sac every hour during day, every 2 hours at night until favorable response is obtained, then use 1 drop every 4 hours; for mild to moderate inflammation, instill 1-2 drops into conjunctival sac 2-4 times/day

Dosage Forms [DSC] = Discontinued product

Ointment, ophthalmic, as base (FML®): 0.1% (3.5 g)

Suspension, ophthalmic, as base: (5 mL, 10 mL, 15 mL)

Fluor-Op®: 0.1% (5 mL, 10 mL, 15 mL) [contains benzalkonium chloride and polyvinyl alcohol] [DSC]

FML®: 0.1% (5 mL, 10 mL, 15 mL) [contains benzalkonium chloride]

FML® Forte: 0.25% (2 mL, 5 mL, 10 mL, 15 mL) [contains benzalkonium chloride]

Suspension, ophthalmic, as acetate:

Eflone®: 0.1% (5 mL, 10 mL) [DSC]

Flarex®: 0.1% (5 mL, 10 mL) [contains benzalkonium chloride]

fluorometholone and sulfacetamide *see* sulfacetamide sodium and fluorometholone *on page 830*

Fluor-Op® *(Discontinued)* *see page 1042*

Fluoroplex® [US] *see* fluorouracil *on this page*

fluorouracil (flure oh YOOR a sil)

Sound-Alike/Look-Alike Issues

fluorouracil may be confused with flucytosine

Efudex® may be confused with Efidac®, Eurax®

Synonyms 5-fluorouracil; FU; 5-FU

U.S./Canadian Brand Names Adrucil® [US/Can]; Carac™ [US]; Efudex® [US/Can]; Fluoroplex® [US]

Therapeutic Category Antineoplastic Agent

Use Treatment of carcinomas of the breast, colon, head and neck, pancreas, rectum, or stomach; topically for the management of actinic or solar keratoses and superficial basal cell carcinomas

Usual Dosage Adults:

Refer to individual protocols:

I.V. bolus: 500-600 mg/m^2 every 3-4 weeks **or** 425 mg/m^2 on days 1-5 every 4 weeks

Continuous I.V. infusion: 1000 mg/m^2/day for 4-5 days every 3-4 weeks **or**

2300-2600 mg/m^2 on day 1 every week **or**

300-400 mg/m^2/day **or**

225 mg/m^2/day for 5-8 weeks (with radiation therapy)

Actinic keratoses: Topical:

Carac™: Apply thin film to lesions once daily for up to 4 weeks, as tolerated

Efudex®: Apply to lesions twice daily for 2-4 weeks; complete healing may not be evident for 1-2 months following treatment

Fluoroplex®: Apply to lesions twice daily for 2-6 weeks

Basal cell carcinoma: Topical: Efudex®: Apply to affected lesions twice daily for 3-6 weeks; treatment may be continued for up to 10-12 weeks

Dosage Forms

Cream, topical:

Carac™: 0.5% (30 g)

Efudex®: 5% (25 g)

Fluoroplex®: 1% (30 g) [contains benzyl alcohol]

Injection, solution: 50 mg/mL (10 mL, 20 mL, 50 mL, 100 mL)

Adrucil®: 50 mg/mL (10 mL, 50 mL, 100 mL)

Solution, topical (Efudex®): 2% (10 mL); 5% (10 mL)

5-fluorouracil *see* fluorouracil *on this page*

Fluothane® *(Discontinued)* *see page 1042*

Fluotic® [Can] *see* fluoride *on page 376*

fluoxetine (floo OKS e teen)

Sound-Alike/Look-Alike Issues
fluoxetine may be confused with fluvastatin
Prozac® may be confused with Prilosec®, Proscar®, ProSom®, ProStep®
Sarafem™ may be confused with Serophene®

Synonyms fluoxetine hydrochloride

U.S./Canadian Brand Names Alti-Fluoxetine [Can]; Apo-Fluoxetine® [Can]; CO Fluoxetine [Can]; FXT® [Can]; Gen-Fluoxetine [Can]; Novo-Fluoxetine [Can]; Nu-Fluoxetine [Can]; PMS-Fluoxetine [Can]; Prozac® [US/Can]; Prozac® Weekly™ [US]; Rhoxal-fluoxetine [Can]; Sarafem™ [US]

Therapeutic Category Antidepressant, Selective Serotonin Reuptake Inhibitor

Use Treatment of major depressive disorder; treatment of binge-eating and vomiting in patients with moderate-to-severe bulimia nervosa; obsessive-compulsive disorder (OCD); premenstrual dysphoric disorder (PMDD); panic disorder with or without agoraphobia

Usual Dosage Oral:
Children:
Depression: 8-18 years: 10-20 mg/day; lower-weight children can be started at 10 mg/day, may increase to 20 mg/day after 1 week if needed
OCD: 7-18 years: Initial: 10 mg/day; in adolescents and higher-weight children, dose may be increased to 20 mg/day after 2 weeks. Range: 10-60 mg/day
Usual dosage range:
Bulimia nervosa: 60-80 mg/day
Depression: 20-40 mg/day; patients maintained on Prozac® 20 mg/day may be changed to Prozac® Weekly™ 90 mg/week, starting dose 7 days after the last 20 mg/day dose
OCD: 40-80 mg/day
Panic disorder: Initial: 10 mg/day; after 1 week, increase to 20 mg/day; may increase after several weeks; doses >60 mg/day have not been evaluated
PMDD (Sarafem™): 20 mg/day continuously, **or** 20 mg/day starting 14 days prior to menstruation and through first full day of menses (repeat with each cycle)

Dosage Forms
Capsule, as hydrochloride: 10 mg, 20 mg, 40 mg
Prozac®: 10 mg, 20 mg, 40 mg
Sarafem™: 10 mg, 20 mg
Capsule, delayed release, as hydrochloride (Prozac® Weekly™): 90 mg
Solution, oral, as hydrochloride (Prozac®): 20 mg/5 mL (120 mL) [contains alcohol 0.23% and benzoic acid; mint flavor]
Tablet, as hydrochloride: 10 mg, 20 mg
Prozac® [scored]: 10 mg

fluoxetine and olanzapine *see* olanzapine and fluoxetine *on page 642*

fluoxetine hydrochloride *see* fluoxetine *on this page*

flupenthixol *(Canada only)* (floo pen THIKS ol)

Synonyms flupenthixol decanoate; flupenthixol dihydrochloride

U.S./Canadian Brand Names Fluanxol® [Can]

Therapeutic Category Antipsychotic Agent; Thioxanthene Derivative

Use Maintenance therapy of chronic schizophrenic patients whose main manifestations do **not** include excitement, agitation, or hyperactivity

Usual Dosage
I.M. (depot): Flupenthixol is administered by deep I.M. injection, preferably in the gluteus maximus, **NOT for I.V. use**; maintenance dosages are given at 2- to 3-week intervals
(Continued)

flupenthixol *(Canada only)* (Continued)

Patients not previously treated with long-acting depot neuroleptics should be given an initial test dose of 5-20 mg. An initial dose of 20 mg is usually well tolerated; however, a 5 mg test dose is recommended in elderly, frail, and cachectic patients, and in patients whose individual or family history suggests a predisposition to extrapyramidal reactions. In the subsequent 5-10 days, the therapeutic response and the appearance of extrapyramidal symptoms should be carefully monitored. Oral neuroleptic drugs may be continued, but dosage should be reduced during this overlapping period and eventually discontinued.

Oral: Initial: 1 mg 3 times/day; dose must be individualized. May be increased by 1 mg every 2-3 days based on tolerance and control of symptoms. Usual maintenance dosage: 3-6 mg/day in divided doses (doses ≥12 mg/day used in some patients).

Dosage Forms

Injection, solution, as decanoate [depot]: 20 mg/mL (10 mL); 100 mg/mL (2 mL)

Tablet, as dihydrochloride: 0.5 mg, 3 mg

flupenthixol decanoate *see* flupenthixol *(Canada only)* *on previous page*

flupenthixol dihydrochloride *see* flupenthixol *(Canada only)* *on previous page*

fluphenazine (floo FEN a zeen)

Sound-Alike/Look-Alike Issues

Prolixin® may be confused with Proloprim®

Synonyms fluphenazine decanoate

U.S./Canadian Brand Names Apo-Fluphenazine® [Can]; Apo-Fluphenzaine Decanoate® [Can]; Modecate® [Can]; Moditen® Enanthate [Can]; Moditen® HCl [Can]; PMS-Fluphenazine Decanoate [Can]; Prolixin Decanoate® [US]

Therapeutic Category Phenothiazine Derivative

Use Management of manifestations of psychotic disorders and schizophrenia; depot formulation may offer improved outcome in individuals with psychosis who are nonadherent with oral antipsychotics

Usual Dosage Adults: Psychoses:

Oral: 0.5-10 mg/day in divided doses at 6- to 8-hour intervals; some patients may require up to 40 mg/day

I.M.: 2.5-10 mg/day in divided doses at 6- to 8-hour intervals (parenteral dose is $^1/_3$ to $^1/_2$ the oral dose for the hydrochloride salts)

I.M. (decanoate): 12.5 mg every 2 weeks

Conversion from hydrochloride to decanoate I.M. 0.5 mL (12.5 mg) decanoate every 3 weeks is approximately equivalent to 10 mg hydrochloride/day

Dosage Forms [DSC] = Discontinued product

Elixir, as hydrochloride (Prolixin®): 2.5 mg/5 mL (60 mL) [contains alcohol 14% and sodium benzoate] [DSC]

Injection, oil, as decanoate: 25 mg/mL (5 mL) [may contain benzyl alcohol, sesame oil]

Prolixin Decanoate®: 25 mg/mL (5 mL) [contains benzyl alcohol, sesame oil]

Injection, solution, as hydrochloride (Prolixin® [DSC]): 2.5 mg/mL (10 mL)

Solution, oral concentrate, as hydrochloride (Prolixin®): 5 mg/mL (120 mL) [contains alcohol 14%] [DSC]

Tablet, as hydrochloride: 1 mg, 2.5 mg, 5 mg, 10 mg

Prolixin®: 1 mg, 2.5 mg, 5 mg [contains tartrazine], 10 mg [DSC]

fluphenazine decanoate *see* fluphenazine *on this page*

Flura® *(Discontinued)* *see* *page 1042*

Flura-Drops® [US] *see* fluoride *on page 376*

Flura-Loz® [US] *see* fluoride *on page 376*

flurandrenolide (flure an DREN oh lide)

Sound-Alike/Look-Alike Issues

Cordran® may be confused with Cardura®, codeine, Cordarone®

Synonyms flurandrenolone
U.S./Canadian Brand Names Cordran® SP [US]; Cordran® [US/Can]
Therapeutic Category Corticosteroid, Topical
Use Inflammation of corticosteroid-responsive dermatoses [medium potency topical corticosteroid]
Usual Dosage Topical: Therapy should be discontinued when control is achieved; if no improvement is seen, reassessment of diagnosis may be necessary.
Children:
Ointment, cream: Apply sparingly 1-2 times/day
Tape: Apply once daily
Adults: Cream, lotion, ointment: Apply sparingly 2-3 times/day
Dosage Forms
Cream, emulsified, as base (Cordran® SP): 0.025% (30 g, 60 g); 0.05% (15 g, 30 g, 60 g)
Lotion (Cordran®): 0.05% (15 mL, 60 mL)
Ointment (Cordran®): 0.025% (30 g, 60 g); 0.05% (15 g, 30 g, 60 g)
Tape, topical [roll] (Cordran®): 4 mcg/cm² (7.5 cm x 60 cm, 7.5 cm x 200 cm)

flurandrenolone *see* flurandrenolide *on previous page*

Flurate® Ophthalmic Solution *(Discontinued)* *see page 1042*

flurazepam (flure AZ e pam)

Sound-Alike/Look-Alike Issues
flurazepam may be confused with temazepam
Dalmane® may be confused with Demulen®, Dialume®
Synonyms flurazepam hydrochloride
U.S./Canadian Brand Names Apo-Flurazepam® [Can]; Dalmane® [US/Can]
Therapeutic Category Benzodiazepine
Controlled Substance C-IV
Use Short-term treatment of insomnia
Usual Dosage Oral: Insomnia:
Children:
≤15 years: Dose not established
>15 years: 15 mg at bedtime
Adults: 15-30 mg at bedtime
Dosage Forms Capsule, as hydrochloride: 15 mg, 30 mg

flurazepam hydrochloride *see* flurazepam *on this page*

flurbiprofen (flure BI proe fen)

Sound-Alike/Look-Alike Issues
flurbiprofen may be confused with fenoprofen
Ansaid® may be confused with Asacol®, Axid®
Ocufen® may be confused with Ocuflox®, Ocupress®
Synonyms flurbiprofen sodium
U.S./Canadian Brand Names Alti-Flurbiprofen [Can]; Ansaid® [US/Can]; Apo-Flurbiprofen® [Can]; Froben® [Can]; Froben-SR® [Can]; Novo-Flurprofen [Can]; Nu-Flurprofen [Can]; Ocufen® [US/Can]
Therapeutic Category Analgesic, Nonnarcotic; Nonsteroidal Antiinflammatory Drug (NSAID)
Use
Oral: Treatment of rheumatoid arthritis and osteoarthritis
Ophthalmic: Inhibition of intraoperative miosis
Usual Dosage
Oral:
Rheumatoid arthritis and osteoarthritis: 200-300 mg/day in 2-, 3-, or 4 divided doses; do not administer more than 100 mg for any single dose; maximum: 300 mg/day
Dental: Management of postoperative pain: 100 mg every 12 hours
(Continued)

flurbiprofen *(Continued)*

Ophthalmic: Instill 1 drop every 30 minutes, beginning 2 hours prior to surgery (total of 4 drops in each affected eye)

Dosage Forms

Solution, ophthalmic, as sodium (Ocufen®): 0.03% (2.5 mL) [contains thimerosal]
Tablet (Ansaid®): 50 mg, 100 mg

flurbiprofen sodium *see* flurbiprofen *on previous page*

5-flurocytosine *see* flucytosine *on page 372*

Fluro-Ethyl® [US] *see* ethyl chloride and dichlorotetrafluoroethane *on page 349*

Flurosyn® Topical *(Discontinued)* *see page 1042*

FluShield® *(Discontinued)* *see page 1042*

flutamide (FLOO ta mide)

Sound-Alike/Look-Alike Issues

flutamide may be confused with Flumadine®
Eulexin® may be confused with Edecrin®, Eurax®

Synonyms niftolid; 4′-nitro-3′-trifluoromethylisobutyrantide; NSC-147834; SCH 13521

U.S./Canadian Brand Names Apo-Flutamide® [Can]; Euflex® [Can]; Eulexin® [US/Can]; Novo-Flutamide [Can]; PMS-Flutamide [Can]

Therapeutic Category Antiandrogen

Use Treatment of metastatic prostatic carcinoma in combination therapy with LHRH agonist analogues

Usual Dosage Oral: Adults: Prostatic carcinoma: 250 mg 3 times/day

Dosage Forms Capsule: 125 mg

Flutex® Topical *(Discontinued)* *see page 1042*

fluticasone and salmeterol (floo TIK a sone & sal ME te role)

Sound-Alike/Look-Alike Issues

Advair Diskus® may be confused with Advicor®

Synonyms salmeterol and fluticasone

U.S./Canadian Brand Names Advair® Diskus® [US/Can]

Therapeutic Category Beta$_2$-Adrenergic Agonist Agent; Corticosteroid, Inhalant

Use Maintenance treatment of asthma in adults and children ≥4 years; **not** for use for relief of acute bronchospasm; maintenance treatment of COPD associated with chronic bronchitis

Usual Dosage Oral inhalation: **Note:** Do not use to transfer patients from systemic corticosteroid therapy.

COPD: Adults: Fluticasone 250 mcg/salmeterol 50 mcg twice daily, 12 hours apart

Asthma:

Children 4-11 years: Fluticasone 100 mg/salmeterol 50 mg twice daily, 12 hours apart

Children ≥12 and Adults: One inhalation twice daily, morning and evening, 12 hours apart

Note: Advair Diskus® is available in 3 strengths, initial dose prescribed should be based upon previous asthma therapy. Dose should be increased after 2 weeks if adequate response is not achieved. Patients should be titrated to lowest effective dose once stable. (Because each strength contains salmeterol 50 mcg/inhalation, dose adjustments should be made by changing inhaler strength. No more than 1 inhalation of any strength should be taken more than twice a day). Maximum dose: Fluticasone 500 mcg/salmeterol 50 mcg, one inhalation twice daily.

Patients not currently on inhaled corticosteroids: Fluticasone 100 mcg/salmeterol 50 mcg

Patients currently using inhaled beclomethasone dipropionate:

≤420 mcg/day: Fluticasone 100 mcg/salmeterol 50 mcg
462-840 mcg/day: Fluticasone 250 mcg/salmeterol 50 mcg

Patients currently using inhaled budesonide:
≤400 mcg/day: Fluticasone 100 mcg/salmeterol 50 mcg
800-1200 mcg/day: Fluticasone 250 mcg/salmeterol 50 mcg
1600 mcg/day: Fluticasone 500 mcg/salmeterol 50 mcg
Patients currently using inhaled flunisolide:
≤1000 mcg/day: Fluticasone 100 mcg/salmeterol 50 mcg
1250-2000 mcg/day: Fluticasone 250 mcg/salmeterol 50 mcg
Patients currently using inhaled fluticasone propionate aerosol:
≤176 mcg/day: Fluticasone 100 mcg/salmeterol 50 mcg
440 mcg/day: Fluticasone 250 mcg/salmeterol 50 mcg
660-880 mcg/day: Fluticasone 500 mcg/salmeterol 50 mcg
Patients currently using inhaled fluticasone propionate powder:
≤200 mcg/day: Fluticasone 100 mcg/salmeterol 50 mcg
500 mcg/day: Fluticasone 250 mcg/salmeterol 50 mcg
1000 mcg/day: Fluticasone 500 mcg/salmeterol 50 mcg
Patients currently using inhaled triamcinolone acetonide:
≤1000 mcg/day: Fluticasone 100 mcg/salmeterol 50 mcg
1100-1600 mcg/day: Fluticasone 250 mcg/salmeterol 50 mcg

Dosage Forms Powder for oral inhalation:
100/50: Fluticasone propionate 100 mcg and salmeterol xinafoate 50 mcg (28s, 60s) [contains lactose]
250/50: Fluticasone propionate 250 mcg and salmeterol xinafoate 50 mcg (28s, 60s) [contains lactose]
500/50: Fluticasone propionate 500 mcg and salmeterol xinafoate 50 mcg (28s, 60s) [contains lactose]

fluticasone (nasal) (floo TIK a sone NAY sal)

U.S./Canadian Brand Names Flonase® [US]

Therapeutic Category Adrenal Corticosteroid

Use Management of seasonal and perennial allergic rhinitis in patients ≥12 years of age

Usual Dosage
Adolescents:
Intranasal: Initial: 1 spray (50 mcg/spray) per nostril once daily. Patients not adequately responding or patients with more severe symptoms may use 2 sprays (100 mcg) per nostril. Depending on response, dosage may be reduced to 100 mcg daily. Total daily dosage should not exceed 4 sprays (200 mcg)/day.
Adults:
Intranasal: Initial: 2 sprays (50 mcg/spray) per nostril once daily. After the first few days, dosage may be reduced to 1 spray per nostril once daily for maintenance therapy. Maximum total daily dose should not exceed 4 sprays (200 mcg)/day.

Dosage Forms Nasal spray: 50 mcg/actuation (16 g = 120 actuations)

fluticasone (oral inhalation) (floo TIK a sone OR al in hil LA shun)

U.S./Canadian Brand Names Flovent®; Flovent® Rotadisk®

Therapeutic Category Adrenal Corticosteroid

Use Inhalation: Maintenance treatment of asthma as prophylactic therapy. It is also indicated for patients requiring oral corticosteroid therapy for asthma to assist in total discontinuation or reduction of total oral dose. NOT indicated for the relief of acute bronchospasm.

Usual Dosage Oral inhalation: If adequate response is not seen after 2 weeks of initial dosage, increase dosage; doses should be titrated to the lowest effective dose once asthma is controlled; Manufacturer recommendations:
Inhalation aerosol (Flovent®): Children ≥12 years and Adults:
Patients previously treated with bronchodilators only: Initial: 88 mcg twice daily; maximum dose: 440 mcg twice daily
Patients treated with an inhaled corticosteroid: Initial: 88-220 mcg twice daily; maximum dose: 440 mcg twice daily; may start doses above 88 mcg twice daily in
(Continued)

fluticasone (oral inhalation) *(Continued)*

poorly controlled patients or in those who previously required higher doses of inhaled corticosteroids

Patients previously treated with oral corticosteroids: Initial: 880 mcg twice daily; maximum dose: 880 mcg twice daily

Inhalation powder (Flovent® Rotadisk®):

Children 4-11 years: Patients previously treated with bronchodilators alone or inhaled corticosteroids: Initial: 50 mcg twice daily; maximum dose: 100 mcg twice daily; may start higher initial dose in poorly controlled patients or in those who previously required higher doses of inhaled corticosteroids

Adolescents and Adults:

Patients previously treated with bronchodilators alone: Initial: 100 mcg twice daily; maximum dose: 500 mcg twice daily

Patients previously treated with inhaled corticosteroids: Initial: 100-250 mcg twice daily; maximum dose: 500 mcg twice daily; may start doses above 100 mcg twice daily in poorly controlled patients or in those who previously required higher doses of inhaled corticosteroids

Patients previously treated with oral corticosteroids: Initial: 1000 mcg twice daily; maximum dose: 1000 mcg twice daily

Dosage Forms

Powder (in 4 blisters containing 15 Rotodisk® with inhalation device): 50 mcg, 100 mcg, 250 mcg

Spray, aerosol, oral inhalation (Flovent®): 44 mcg/actuation (7.9 g = 60 actuations or 13 g = 120 actuations), 110 mcg/actuation (13 g = 120 actuations); 220 mcg/actuation (13 g = 120 actuations)

fluticasone (topical) (floo TIK a sone TOP i kal)

U.S./Canadian Brand Names Cutivate™ [US]

Therapeutic Category Adrenal Corticosteroid; Corticosteroid, Topical

Use Relief of inflammation and pruritus associated with corticosteroid-responsive dermatoses [medium potency topical corticosteroid]

Usual Dosage Topical:

Children: Cutivate™ approved for use in patients ≥3 months of age

Adolescents and Adults: Apply sparingly in a thin film twice daily

Note: Therapy should be discontinued when control is achieved. If no improvement is seen, reassessment of diagnosis may be necessary.

Dosage Forms

Cream: 0.05% (15 g, 30 g, 60 g)

Ointment: 0.005% (15 g, 60 g)

fluvastatin (FLOO va sta tin)

Sound-Alike/Look-Alike Issues

fluvastatin may be confused with fluoxetine

U.S./Canadian Brand Names Lescol® [US/Can]; Lescol® XL [US]

Therapeutic Category HMG-CoA Reductase Inhibitor

Use To be used as a component of multiple risk factor intervention in patients at risk for atherosclerosis vascular disease due to hypercholesterolemia

Adjunct to dietary therapy to reduce elevated total cholesterol (total-C), LDL-C, triglyceride, and apolipoprotein B (apo-B) levels and to increase HDL-C in primary hypercholesterolemia and mixed dyslipidemia (Fredrickson types IIa and IIb); to slow the progression of coronary atherosclerosis in patients with coronary heart disease; reduce risk of coronary revascularization procedures in patients with coronary heart disease

Usual Dosage Adults: Oral:

Patients requiring ≥25% decrease in LDL-C: 40 mg capsule or 80 mg extended release tablet once daily in the evening; may also use 40 mg capsule twice daily

Patients requiring <25% decrease in LDL-C: 20 mg capsule once daily in the evening

Note: Dosing range: 20-80 mg/day; adjust dose based on response to therapy; maximum response occurs within 4-6 weeks

Dosage Forms

Capsule (Lescol®): 20 mg, 40 mg

Tablet, extended release (Lescol® XL): 80 mg

Fluviral S/F® [Can] *see* influenza virus vaccine *on page 473*

Fluvirin® [US] *see* influenza virus vaccine *on page 473*

fluvoxamine (floo VOKS ah meen)

Sound-Alike/Look-Alike Issues

Luvox® may be confused with Lasix®, Levoxyl®

U.S./Canadian Brand Names Alti-Fluvoxamine [Can]; Apo-Fluvoxamine® [Can]; Luvox® [Can]; Novo-Fluvoxamine [Can]; Nu-Fluvoxamine [Can]; PMS-Fluvoxamine [Can]; Rhoxal-fluvoxamine [Can]

Therapeutic Category Antidepressant, Selective Serotonin Reuptake Inhibitor

Use Treatment of obsessive-compulsive disorder (OCD) in children ≥8 years of age and adults

Usual Dosage Oral: **Note:** When total daily dose exceeds 50 mg, the dose should be given in 2 divided doses:

Children 8-17 years: Initial: 25 mg at bedtime; adjust in 25 mg increments at 4- to 7-day intervals, as tolerated, to maximum therapeutic benefit: Range: 50-200 mg/day

Maximum: Children: 8-11 years: 200 mg/day, adolescents: 300 mg/day; lower doses may be effective in female versus male patients

Adults: Initial: 50 mg at bedtime; adjust in 50 mg increments at 4- to 7-day intervals; usual dose range: 100-300 mg/day; divide total daily dose into 2 doses; administer larger portion at bedtime

Dosage Forms Tablet: 25 mg, 50 mg, 100 mg

Fluzone® [US/Can] *see* influenza virus vaccine *on page 473*

FML® [US/Can] *see* fluorometholone *on page 377*

FML® Forte [US/Can] *see* fluorometholone *on page 377*

FML-S® [US] *see* sulfacetamide sodium and fluorometholone *on page 830*

Focalin™ [US] *see* dexmethylphenidate *on page 257*

Foille® Medicated First Aid [US-OTC] *see* benzocaine *on page 107*

Foille® Plus [US-OTC] *see* benzocaine *on page 107*

Foille® [US-OTC] *see* benzocaine *on page 107*

folacin *see* folic acid *on this page*

folacin, vitamin B_{12}, and vitamin B_6 *see* folic acid, cyanocobalamin, and pyridoxine *on next page*

folate *see* folic acid *on this page*

Folbee [US] *see* folic acid, cyanocobalamin, and pyridoxine *on next page*

Folex® Injection *(Discontinued)* *see page 1042*

Folex® PFS™ *(Discontinued)* *see page 1042*

Folgard RX 2.2® [US] *see* folic acid, cyanocobalamin, and pyridoxine *on next page*

Folgard® [US-OTC] *see* folic acid, cyanocobalamin, and pyridoxine *on next page*

folic acid (FOE lik AS id)

Sound-Alike/Look-Alike Issues

folic acid may be confused with folinic acid

Synonyms folacin; folate; pteroylglutamic acid

U.S./Canadian Brand Names Apo-Folic® [Can]

(Continued)

folic acid *(Continued)*

Therapeutic Category Vitamin, Water Soluble

Use Treatment of megaloblastic and macrocytic anemias due to folate deficiency; dietary supplement to prevent neural tube defects

Usual Dosage

Infants: 0.1 mg/day

Children <4 years: Up to 0.3 mg/day

Children >4 years and Adults: 0.4 mg/day

Pregnant and lactating women: 0.8 mg/day

RDA:

Adult male: 0.15-0.2 mg/day

Adult female: 0.15-0.18 mg/day

Dosage Forms

Injection, solution, as sodium folate: 5 mg/mL (10 mL) [contains benzyl alcohol]

Tablet: 0.4 mg, 0.8 mg, 1 mg

folic acid, cyanocobalamin, and pyridoxine

(FOE lik AS id, sye an oh koe BAL a min, & peer i DOKS een)

Synonyms cyanocobalamin, folic acid, and pyridoxine; folacin, vitamin B_{12}, and vitamin B_6; pyridoxine, folic acid, and cyanocobalamin

U.S./Canadian Brand Names Folbee [US]; Folgard RX 2.2® [US]; Folgard® [US-OTC]; Foltx® [US]; Tricardio B [Can]

Therapeutic Category Vitamin

Use Nutritional supplement in end-stage renal failure, dialysis, hyperhomocysteinemia, homocystinuria, malabsorption syndromes, dietary deficiencies

Usual Dosage Oral: Adults: 1 tablet daily

Dosage Forms [DSC] = Discontinued product

Tablet: Folic acid 0.8 mg, cyanocobalamin 1000 mcg, and pyridoxine hydrochloride 50 mg

Folbee: Folic acid 2.5 mg, cyanocobalamin 1000 mcg, and pyridoxine hydrochloride 25 mg [dye free, lactose free, and sugar free]

Folgard®: Folic acid 0.8 mg, cyanocobalamin 115 mcg, and pyridoxine hydrochloride 10 mg

Folgard RX 2.2®: Folic acid 2.2 mg, cyanocobalamin 500 mcg, and pyridoxine hydrochloride 25 mg

Foltx®: Folic acid 2.5 mg, cyanocobalamin 1000 mcg, and pyridoxine hydrochloride 25 mg [DSC]; folic acid 2.5 mg, cyanocobalamin 2000 mcg, and pyridoxine hydrochloride 25 mg [new strength]

Tricardio B: Folic acid 0.4 mg, cyanocobalamin 250 mcg, and pyridoxine hydrochloride 25 mg

folinic acid *see* leucovorin *on page 509*

Follistim® [US] *see* follitropin beta *on this page*

follitropin alfa (foe li TRO pin AL fa)

Therapeutic Category Ovulation Stimulator

Use Induction of ovulation in the anovulatory infertile patient in whom the cause of infertility is functional and not caused by primary ovarian failure

Usual Dosage Adults (women): S.C.: Initial: 75 units/day for the first cycle; an incremental dose adjustment of up to 37.5 units may be considered after 14 days; treatment duration should not exceed 35 days unless an E2 rise indicates follicular development

Dosage Forms Injection: 37.5 FSH units, 75 FSH units, 150 FSH units

follitropin beta (foe li TRO pin BAY ta)

U.S./Canadian Brand Names Follistim® [US]

Therapeutic Category Ovulation Stimulator

Use The development of multiple follicles in infertility patients treated in Assisted Reproductive Technology (ART) program and for the induction of ovulation

Usual Dosage Adults (female): I.M./S.C.:

Ovulation: In general, a sequential treatment scheme is recommended. This usually starts with daily administration of 75 int. units (International Units) FSH activity. The starting dose is maintained for at least seven days. If there is no ovarian response, the daily dose is then gradually increased until follicle growth and/or plasma estradiol levels indicate an adequate pharmacodynamic response. A daily increase in estradiol levels of 40% to 100% is considered to be optimal. The daily dose is then maintained until preovulatory conditions are reached. Preovulatory conditions are reached when there ultrasonographic evidence of a dominant follicle of at least 18 mm in diameter and/or when plasma estradiol levels of 300-900 picograms/mL (1000-3000 pmol/L) are attained; usually, 7-14 days of treatment are sufficient to reach this state. The administration is then discontinued and ovulation can be induced by administering human chorionic gonadotropin (hCG). If the number of responding follicles is too high or estradiol levels increase too rapidly (ie, more than a daily doubling of estradiol for 2-3 consecutive days), the daily dose should be decreased. Since follicles of >14 mm may lead to pregnancies, multiple preovulatory follicles exceeding 14 mm carry the risk of multiple gestations. In that case, hCG should be withheld and pregnancy should be avoided in order to prevent multiple gestations.

ART: Various stimulation protocols are applied; starting dose of 150-225 units is recommended for at least the first four days; thereafter, the dose may be adjusted individually, based upon ovarian response. In clinical studies, it was shown that maintenance dosages ranging from 75-375 units for 6-12 days are sufficient, although longer treatment may be necessary. May be given either alone, or in combination with a GnRH agonist to prevent premature luteinization; in the latter case, a higher total treatment dose of Follistim® may be required. Ovarian response is monitored by ultrasonography and measurement of plasma estradiol levels; when ultrasonographic evaluation indicates the presence of at least three follicles of 16-20 mm, and there is evidence of a good estradiol (plasma levels of about 300-400 picogram/mL (1000-1300 pmol/L) for each follicle with a diameter >18 mm), the final phase of maturation of the follicles is induced by administration of hCG. Oocyte retrieval is performed 34-35 hours later.

Dosage Forms Injection: 75 FSH units

Follutein® *(Discontinued)* *see page 1042*

Foltx® [US] *see* folic acid, cyanocobalamin, and pyridoxine *on previous page*

Folvite® *(Discontinued)* *see page 1042*

fomepizole (foe ME pi zole)

Synonyms 4-methylpyrazole; 4-MP

U.S./Canadian Brand Names Antizol® [US]

Therapeutic Category Antidote

Use **Orphan drug:** Treatment of methanol or ethylene glycol poisoning alone or in combination with hemodialysis

Usual Dosage Adults: Ethylene glycol and methanol toxicity: I.V.: A loading dose of 15 mg/kg should be administered, followed by doses of 10 mg/kg every 12 hours for 4 doses, then 15 mg/kg every 12 hours thereafter until ethylene glycol levels have been reduced <20 mg/dL and patient is asymptomatic with normal pH

Dosage Forms Injection, solution [preservative free]: 1 g/mL (1.5 mL)

fomivirsen *(Canada only)* (foe MI vir sen)

Synonyms fomivirsen sodium

U.S./Canadian Brand Names Vitravene™ [Can]

Therapeutic Category Antiviral Agent, Ophthalmic

Use Local treatment of cytomegalovirus (CMV) retinitis in patients with acquired immunodeficiency syndrome who are intolerant or insufficiently responsive to other treatments for CMV retinitis or when other treatments for CMV retinitis are contraindicated

(Continued)

fomivirsen *(Canada only)* *(Continued)*

Usual Dosage Adults: Intravitreal injection: Induction: 330 mcg (0.05 mL) every other week for 2 doses, followed by maintenance dose of 330 mcg (0.05 mL) every 4 weeks

If progression occurs during maintenance, a repeat of the induction regimen may be attempted to establish resumed control. Unacceptable inflammation during therapy may be managed by temporary interruption, provided response has been established. Topical corticosteroids have been used to reduce inflammation.

Dosage Forms Injection, solution, intravitreal, as sodium: 6.6 mg/mL (0.25 mL)

fomivirsen sodium *see* fomivirsen *(Canada only)* *on previous page*

fondaparinux (fon da PARE i nuks)

Synonyms fondaparinux sodium

U.S./Canadian Brand Names Arixtra® [US/Can]

Therapeutic Category Factor Xa Inhibitor

Use Prophylaxis of deep vein thrombosis (DVT) in patients undergoing surgery for hip replacement, knee replacement, or hip fracture surgery (including extended prophylaxis following hip fracture surgery); treatment of acute pulmonary embolism (PE); treatment of acute DVT without PE

Usual Dosage SubQ:

DVT prophylaxis: Adults ≥50 kg: 2.5 mg once daily. **Note:** Initiate dose after hemostasis has been established, 6-8 hours postoperatively.

Usual duration: 5-9 days (up to 11 days) following hip replacement or knee replacement. Extended prophylaxis is recommended following hip fracture surgery (has been tolerated for up to 32 days).

Acute DVT/PE treatment: SubQ: Adults:

<50 kg: 5 mg once daily

50-100 kg: 7.5 mg once daily

>100 kg: 10 mg once daily

Dosage Forms Injection, solution, as sodium: 2.5 mg/0.5 mL (0.5 mL) [prefilled syringe]

fondaparinux sodium *see* fondaparinux *on this page*

Foradil® [Can] *see* formoterol *on this page*

Foradil® Aerolizer™ [US] *see* formoterol *on this page*

Forane® [US] *see* isoflurane *on page 486*

formoterol (for MOT ter ol)

Synonyms formoterol fumarate

U.S./Canadian Brand Names Foradil® [Can]; Foradil® Aerolizer™ [US]; Oxeze® Turbuhaler® [Can]

Therapeutic Category Beta$_2$-Adrenergic Agonist Agent

Use Maintenance treatment of asthma and prevention of bronchospasm in patients ≥5 years of age with reversible obstructive airway disease, including patients with symptoms of nocturnal asthma, who require regular treatment with inhaled, short-acting beta$_2$ agonists; maintenance treatment of bronchoconstriction in patients with COPD; prevention of exercise-induced bronchospasm in patients ≥5 years of age

Note: Oxeze® is also approved in Canada for acute relief of symptoms ("on demand" treatment) in patients ≥6 years of age.

Usual Dosage

Asthma maintenance treatment: Children ≥5 years and Adults: Inhalation: 12 mcg capsule every 12 hours

Oxeze® (CAN): **Note:** Not labeled for use in the U.S.: Children ≥6 years and Adults: Inhalation: 6 mcg or 12 mcg every 12 hours. Maximum dose: Children: 24 mcg/day; Adults: 48 mcg/day

Prevention of exercise-induced bronchospasm: Children ≥5 years and Adults: Inhalation: 12 mcg capsule at least 15 minutes before exercise on an "as needed" basis; additional doses should not be used for another 12 hours. **Note:** If already using for asthma maintenance then should not use additional doses for exercise-induced bronchospasm.

Oxeze® (CAN): **Note:** Not labeled for use in the U.S.: Children ≥6 years and Adults: Inhalation: 6 mcg or 12 mcg at least 15 minutes before exercise.

COPD maintenance treatment: Adults: Inhalation: 12 mcg capsule every 12 hours

Additional indication for Oxeze® (approved in Canada): Acute ("on demand") relief of bronchoconstriction: Children ≥12 years and Adults: 6 mcg or 12 mcg as a single dose (maximum dose: 72 mcg in any 24-hour period). The prolonged use of high dosages (48 mcg/day for ≥3 consecutive days) may be a sign of suboptimal control, and should prompt the re-evaluation of therapy.

Dosage Forms [Can] = Canadian brand name

Aerosol, oral (Oxeze® [Can]): 6 mcg/dose (60 doses), 12 mcg/dose (60 doses) [contains lactose 600 mcg/dose]

Powder for oral inhalation, as fumarate [capsule]: 12 mcg (12s, 60s) [contains lactose 25 mg]

formoterol fumarate *see* formoterol *on previous page*

formoterol fumarate dehydrate and budesonide *see* budesonide and formoterol *(Canada only) on page 132*

Formula EM [US-OTC] *see* fructose, dextrose, and phosphoric acid *on page 392*

Formula Q® *(Discontinued)* *see page 1042*

Formulation R™ [US-OTC] *see* phenylephrine *on page 689*

Formulex® [Can] *see* dicyclomine *on page 267*

5-formyl tetrahydrofolate *see* leucovorin *on page 509*

Fortamet™ [US] *see* metformin *on page 560*

Fortaz® [US/Can] *see* ceftazidime *on page 171*

Forteo™ [US] *see* teriparatide *on page 847*

Fortovase® [US/Can] *see* saquinavir *on page 794*

Fosamax® [US/Can] *see* alendronate *on page 30*

fosamprenavir (FOS am pren a veer)

Sound-Alike/Look-Alike Issues

Lexiva™ may be confused with Levitra®

Synonyms fosamprenavir calcium; GW433908G

U.S./Canadian Brand Names Lexiva™ [US]

Therapeutic Category Antiretroviral Agent, Protease Inhibitor

Use Treatment of HIV infections in combination with at least two other antiretroviral agents

Usual Dosage Oral: Adults: HIV infection:

Therapy-naive patients: 1400 mg twice daily (without ritonavir)

Dosage adjustments when administered in combination therapy:

Concurrent therapy with ritonavir: Adjustments necessary for both agents: Fosamprenavir 1400 mg plus ritonavir 200 mg once daily **or** Fosamprenavir 700 mg plus ritonavir 100 mg twice daily

Concurrent therapy with efavirenz and ritonavir: Fosamprenavir 1400 mg daily plus ritonavir 300 mg once daily; no dosage adjustment recommended for twice-daily regimen

Protease inhibitor-experienced patients: Fosamprenavir 700 mg plus ritonavir 100 mg twice daily. **Note:** Once-daily administration is not recommended in protease inhibitor-experienced patients.

Dosage Forms Tablet, as calcium: 700 mg

fosamprenavir calcium *see* fosamprenavir *on this page*

foscarnet (fos KAR net)

Synonyms PFA; phosphonoformate; phosphonoformic acid

U.S./Canadian Brand Names Foscavir® [US/Can]

Therapeutic Category Antiviral Agent

Use

Treatment of herpes virus infections suspected to be caused by acyclovir-resistant (HSV, VZV) or ganciclovir-resistant (CMV) strains; this occurs almost exclusively in immunocompromised persons (eg, with advanced AIDS) who have received prolonged treatment for a herpes virus infection

Treatment of CMV retinitis in persons with AIDS

Usual Dosage I.V.:

CMV retinitis:

Induction treatment: 60 mg/kg/dose every 8 hours **or** 100 mg/kg every 12 hours for 14-21 days

Maintenance therapy: 90-120 mg/kg/day as a single infusion

Acyclovir-resistant HSV induction treatment: 40 mg/kg/dose every 8-12 hours for 14-21 days

Dosage Forms Injection, solution: 24 mg/mL (250 mL, 500 mL)

Foscavir® [US/Can] *see* foscarnet *on this page*

fosfomycin (fos foe MYE sin)

Sound-Alike/Look-Alike Issues

Monurol™ may be confused with Monopril®

Synonyms fosfomycin tromethamine

U.S./Canadian Brand Names Monurol™ [US/Can]

Therapeutic Category Antibiotic, Miscellaneous

Use Single oral dose in the treatment of uncomplicated urinary tract infections in women due to susceptible strains of *E. coli* and *Enterococcus*; may have an advantage over other agents since it maintains high concentration in the urine for up to 48 hours

Usual Dosage Adults: Oral: Female: Uncomplicated UTI: Single dose of 3 g in 4 oz of water

Dosage Forms Powder, as tromethamine: 3 g

fosfomycin tromethamine *see* fosfomycin *on this page*

fosinopril (foe SIN oh pril)

Sound-Alike/Look-Alike Issues

fosinopril may be confused with lisinopril

Monopril® may be confused with Accupril®, minoxidil, moexipril, Monoket®, Monurol™, ramipril

Synonyms fosinopril sodium

U.S./Canadian Brand Names Monopril® [US/Can]

Therapeutic Category Angiotensin-Converting Enzyme (ACE) Inhibitor

Use Treatment of hypertension, either alone or in combination with other antihypertensive agents; treatment of congestive heart failure, left ventricular dysfunction after myocardial infarction

Usual Dosage Oral:

Children >50 kg: Hypertension: Initial: 5-10 mg once daily

Adults:

Hypertension: Initial: 10 mg/day; most patients are maintained on 20-40 mg/day. May need to divide the dose into two if trough effect is inadequate; discontinue the diuretic, if possible 2-3 days before initiation of therapy; resume diuretic therapy carefully, if needed.

Heart failure: Initial: 10 mg/day (5 mg if renal dysfunction present) and increase, as needed, to a maximum of 40 mg once daily over several weeks; usual dose: 20-40 mg/day. If hypotension, orthostasis, or azotemia occur during titration, consider decreasing concomitant diuretic dose, if any.

Dosage Forms Tablet, as sodium: 10 mg, 20 mg, 40 mg

fosinopril and hydrochlorothiazide

(foe SIN oh pril & hye droe klor oh THYE a zide)

Synonyms hydrochlorothiazide and fosinopril

U.S./Canadian Brand Names Monopril-HCT® [US/Can]

Therapeutic Category Angiotensin-Converting Enzyme (ACE) Inhibitor

Use Treatment of hypertension; not indicated for first-line treatment

Usual Dosage **Note:** A patient whose blood pressure is not adequately controlled with fosinopril or hydrochlorothiazide monotherapy may be switched to combination therapy; **not** for initial treatment. Oral:

Adults: Hypertension: Fosinopril 10-80 mg per day, hydrochlorothiazide 12.5-50 mg per day

Dosage Forms Tablet:

10/12.5: Fosinopril 10 mg and hydrochlorothiazide 12.5 mg
20/12.5: Fosinopril 20 mg and hydrochlorothiazide 12.5 mg

fosinopril sodium *see* fosinopril *on previous page*

fosphenytoin (FOS fen i toyn)

Sound-Alike/Look-Alike Issues

Cerebyx® may be confused with Celebrex®, Celexa®, Cerezyme®

Synonyms fosphenytoin sodium

U.S./Canadian Brand Names Cerebyx® [US/Can]

Therapeutic Category Hydantoin

Use Used for the control of generalized convulsive status epilepticus and prevention and treatment of seizures occurring during neurosurgery; indicated for short-term parenteral administration when other means of phenytoin administration are unavailable, inappropriate or deemed less advantageous (the safety and effectiveness of fosphenytoin in this use has not been systematically evaluated for more than 5 days)

Usual Dosage **The dose, concentration in solutions, and infusion rates for fosphenytoin are expressed as phenytoin sodium equivalents (PE); fosphenytoin should always be prescribed and dispensed in phenytoin sodium equivalents (PE)**

Adults:

Status epilepticus: I.V.: Loading dose: 15-20 mg PE/kg I.V. administered at 100-150 mg PE/minute

Nonemergent loading and maintenance dosing: I.V. or I.M.:

Loading dose: 10-20 mg PE/kg I.V. or I.M. (maximum I.V. rate: 150 mg PE/minute)

Initial daily maintenance dose: 4-6 mg PE/kg/day I.V. or I.M.

I.M. or I.V. substitution for oral phenytoin therapy: May be substituted for oral phenytoin sodium at the same total daily dose; however, Dilantin® capsules are ~90% bioavailable by the oral route; phenytoin, supplied as fosphenytoin, is 100% bioavailable by both the I.M. and I.V. routes; for this reason, plasma phenytoin concentrations may increase when I.M. or I.V. fosphenytoin is substituted for oral phenytoin sodium therapy; in clinical trials I.M. fosphenytoin was administered as a single daily dose utilizing either 1 or 2 injection sites; some patients may require more frequent dosing

Dosage Forms Injection, solution, as sodium: 75 mg/mL [equivalent to phenytoin sodium 50 mg/mL] (2 mL, 10 mL)

fosphenytoin sodium *see* fosphenytoin *on this page*

Fostex® 10% BPO [US-OTC] *see* benzoyl peroxide *on page 109*

Fragmin® [US/Can] *see* dalteparin *on page 242*

framycetin *(Canada only)* (fra mye CEE tin)

Therapeutic Category Antibiotic, Topical

Use Treatment of infected or potentially infected burns, wounds, ulcers, and graft sites

(Continued)

framycetin *(Canada only)* *(Continued)*

Usual Dosage A single layer to be applied directly to the wound and covered with an appropriate dressing. If exudative, dressings should be changed at least daily. In case of leg ulcers, cut dressing accurately to size of ulcer to decrease the risk of sensitization and to avoid contact with surrounding healthy skin.

Dosage Forms Dressing, gauze: 1% (10 cm x 10 cm, 10 cm x 30 cm)

Fraxiparine™ [Can] *see* nadroparin *(Canada only)* *on page 599*

Fraxiparine™ Forte [Can] *see* nadroparin *(Canada only)* *on page 599*

Freezone® [US-OTC] *see* salicylic acid *on page 789*

Frisium® [Can] *see* clobazam *(Canada only)* *on page 212*

Froben® [Can] *see* flurbiprofen *on page 381*

Froben-SR® [Can] *see* flurbiprofen *on page 381*

Frova® [US] *see* frovatriptan *on this page*

frovatriptan (froe va TRIP tan)

Synonyms frovatriptan succinate

U.S./Canadian Brand Names Frova® [US]

Therapeutic Category Antimigraine Agent; Serotonin 5-$HT_{1B, 1D}$ Receptor Agonist

Use Acute treatment of migraine with or without aura in adults

Usual Dosage Oral: Adults: Migraine: 2.5 mg; if headache recurs, a second dose may be given if first dose provided some relief and at least 2 hours have elapsed since the first dose (maximum daily dose: 7.5 mg)

Dosage Forms Tablet, as base: 2.5 mg

frovatriptan succinate *see* frovatriptan *on this page*

fructose, dextrose, and phosphoric acid

(FRUK tose, DEKS trose, & foss FOR ik AS id)

Sound-Alike/Look-Alike Issues

Emetrol® may be confused with emetine

Synonyms dextrose, levulose and phosphoric acid; levulose, dextrose and phosphoric acid; phosphorated carbohydrate solution; phosphoric acid, levulose and dextrose

U.S./Canadian Brand Names Emetrol® [US-OTC]; Especol® [US-OTC]; Formula EM [US-OTC]; Kalmz [US-OTC]; Nausea Relief [US-OTC]; Nausetrol® [US-OTC]

Therapeutic Category Antiemetic

Use Relief of nausea associated with upset stomach that occurs with intestinal flu, food indiscretions, and emotional upsets

Usual Dosage Oral:

Motion sickness and vomiting due to drug therapy: 5 mL doses for young children; 15 mL doses for older children and adults

Regurgitation in infants: 5 or 10 mL, 10-15 minutes before each feeding; in refractory cases: 10-15 mL, 30 minutes before each feeding

Vomiting due to psychogenic factors:

Children: 5-10 mL; repeat dose every 15 minutes until distress subsides; do not take for more than 1 hour

Adults: 15-30 mL; repeat dose every 15 minutes until distress subsides; do not take for more than 1 hour

Dosage Forms Liquid, oral: Fructose 1.87 g, dextrose 1.87 g, and phosphoric acid 21.5 mg per 5 mL (120 mL)

Emetrol®: Fructose 1.87 g, dextrose 1.87 g, and phosphoric acid 21.5 mg per 5 mL (120 mL, 240 mL) [cherry and lemon mint flavors]

Especol®: Fructose 1.87 g, dextrose 1.87 g, and phosphoric acid 21.5 mg per 5 mL (120 mL) [cherry and lemon-lime flavors]

Formula EM, Nausea Relief: Fructose 1.87 g, dextrose 1.87 g, and phosphoric acid 21.5 mg per 5 mL (120 mL)

Kalmz, Nausetrol®: Fructose 1.87 g, dextrose 1.87 g, and phosphoric acid 21.5 mg per 5 mL (120 mL) [cherry flavor]

frusemide *see* furosemide *on this page*

FS *see* fibrin sealant kit *on page 367*

FS Shampoo® Topical *(Discontinued)* *see page 1042*

FTC *see* emtricitabine *on page 307*

FTP-Domperidone Maleate [Can] *see* domperidone *(Canada only) on page 288*

FU *see* fluorouracil *on page 378*

5-FU *see* fluorouracil *on page 378*

Fucidin® [Can] *see* fusidic acid *(Canada only) on next page*

Fucithalmic® [Can] *see* fusidic acid *(Canada only) on next page*

FUDR® [US/Can] *see* floxuridine *on page 371*

5-FUDR *see* floxuridine *on page 371*

Ful-Glo® [US] *see* fluorescein sodium *on page 375*

fulvestrant (fool VES trant)

Synonyms ICI 182,780; zeneca 182,780; ZM-182,780

U.S./Canadian Brand Names Faslodex® [US]

Therapeutic Category Antineoplastic Agent, Estrogen Receptor Antagonist

Use Treatment of hormone receptor positive metastatic breast cancer in postmenopausal women with disease progression following antiestrogen therapy.

Usual Dosage I.M.: Adults (postmenopausal women): 250 mg at 1-month intervals

Dosage Forms Injection, solution: 50 mg/mL (2.5 mL, 5 mL) [prefilled syringe; contains alcohol, benzyl alcohol, benzyl stearate, castor oil]

Fulvicin-U/F® [Can] *see* griseofulvin *on page 414*

Fumasorb® *(Discontinued)* *see page 1042*

Fumerin® *(Discontinued)* *see page 1042*

Funduscein® Injection *(Discontinued)* *see page 1042*

Fungi-Guard [US-OTC] *see* tolnaftate *on page 870*

Fungi-Nail® [US-OTC] *see* undecylenic acid and derivatives *on page 896*

Fungizone® [US/Can] *see* amphotericin B (conventional) *on page 54*

Fungoid® Tincture [US-OTC] *see* miconazole *on page 578*

Fung-O® [US-OTC] *see* salicylic acid *on page 789*

Furacin® Topical *(Discontinued)* *see page 1042*

Furadantin® [US] *see* nitrofurantoin *on page 622*

Furalan® *(Discontinued)* *see page 1042*

Furamide® *(Discontinued)* *see page 1042*

Furan® *(Discontinued)* *see page 1042*

Furanite® *(Discontinued)* *see page 1042*

furazosin *see* prazosin *on page 722*

furosemide (fyoor OH se mide)

Sound-Alike/Look-Alike Issues

furosemide may be confused with torsemide

Lasix® may be confused with Esidrix®, Lanoxin®, Lidex®, Lomotil®, Luvox®, Luxiq™

Synonyms frusemide

(Continued)

furosemide *(Continued)*

U.S./Canadian Brand Names Apo-Furosemide® [Can]; Lasix® [US/Can]; Lasix® Special [Can]

Therapeutic Category Diuretic, Loop

Use Management of edema associated with congestive heart failure and hepatic or renal disease; alone or in combination with antihypertensives in treatment of hypertension

Usual Dosage

Infants and Children:

Oral: 1-2 mg/kg/dose increased in increments of 1 mg/kg/dose with each succeeding dose until a satisfactory effect is achieved to a maximum of 6 mg/kg/dose no more frequently than 6 hours.

I.M., I.V.: 1 mg/kg/dose, increasing by each succeeding dose at 1 mg/kg/dose at intervals of 6-12 hours until a satisfactory response up to 6 mg/kg/dose.

Adults:

Oral: 20-80 mg/dose initially increased in increments of 20-40 mg/dose at intervals of 6-8 hours; usual maintenance dose interval is twice daily or every day; may be titrated up to 600 mg/day with severe edematous states.

Hypertension (JNC 7): 20-80 mg/day in 2 divided doses

I.M., I.V.: 20-40 mg/dose, may be repeated in 1-2 hours as needed and increased by 20 mg/dose until the desired effect has been obtained. Usual dosing interval: 6-12 hours; for acute pulmonary edema, the usual dose is 40 mg I.V. over 1-2 minutes. If not adequate, may increase dose to 80 mg.

Continuous I.V. infusion: Initial I.V. bolus dose of 0.1 mg/kg followed by continuous I.V. infusion doses of 0.1 mg/kg/hour doubled every 2 hours to a maximum of 0.4 mg/kg/hour if urine output is <1 mL/kg/hour have been found to be effective and result in a lower daily requirement of furosemide than with intermittent dosing. Other studies have used a rate of ≤4 mg/minute as a continuous I.V. infusion.

Refractory heart failure: Oral, I.V.: Doses up to 8 g/day have been used.

Dosage Forms

Injection, solution: 10 mg/mL (2 mL, 4 mL, 8 mL, 10 mL)

Solution, oral: 10 mg/mL (60 mL, 120 mL) [orange flavor]; 40 mg/5 mL (5 mL, 500 mL) [pineapple-peach flavor]

Tablet (Lasix®): 20 mg, 40 mg, 80 mg

Furoxone® ***(Discontinued)*** *see page 1042*

fusidic acid *(Canada only)* (fyoo SI dik AS id)

Synonyms sodium fusidate

U.S./Canadian Brand Names Fucidin® [Can]; Fucithalmic® [Can]

Therapeutic Category Antifungal Agent, Systemic

Use

Systemic: Treatment of skin and soft tissue infections, or osteomyelitis, caused by susceptible organisms, including *Staphylococcus aureus* (penicillinase-producing or nonpenicillinase strains); may be used in the treatment of pneumonia, septicemia, endocarditis, burns, and cystic fibrosis caused by susceptible organisms when other antibiotics have failed

Topical: Treatment of primary and secondary skin infections caused by susceptible organisms

Ophthalmic: Treatment of superficial infections of the eye and conjunctiva caused by susceptible organisms

Usual Dosage

I.V.:

Children ≤12 years: 20 mg/kg/day in 3 divided doses

Children >12 years and Adults: 500 mg sodium fusidate 3 times/day

Ophthalmic: Children ≥2 years and Adults: Instill 1 drop in each eye every 12 hours for 7 days

Topical: Children and Adults: Apply to affected area 3-4 times/day until favorable results are achieved. If a gauze dressing is used, frequency of application may be reduced to 1-2 times/day.

Oral: Adults: 500 mg sodium fusidate 3 times/day. (**Note:** Oral dosage may be increased to 1000 mg 3 times/day in fulminating infections.)

Dosage Forms

Cream, as fusidic acid (Fucidin®): 2% (15 g, 30 g)

Injection, powder for reconstitution, as sodium fusidate (Fucidin®): 500 mg [packaged with 10 mL diluent/buffer solution]

Ointment, topical, as sodium fusidate (Fucinin®): 2% (15 g, 30 g) [contains lanolin]

Suspension, ophthalmic, as fusidic acid (Fucithalmic®): 10 mg/g [1%] (0.2 g) [unit-dose, without preservative]; (3 g, 5 g) [multidose, contains benzalkonium chloride]

Tablet [film coated], as sodium fusidate (Fucidin®): 250 mg

Fuzeon™ [US/Can] *see* enfuvirtide *on page 309*

FXT® [Can] *see* fluoxetine *on page 379*

G-1® *(Discontinued)* *see page 1042*

gabapentin (GA ba pen tin)

Sound-Alike/Look-Alike Issues

Neurontin® may be confused with Neoral®, Noroxin®

U.S./Canadian Brand Names Apo-Gabapentin® [Can]; Neurontin® [US/Can]; Novo-Gabapentin [Can]; Nu-Gabapentin [Can]; PMS-Gabapentin [Can]

Therapeutic Category Anticonvulsant

Use Adjunct for treatment of partial seizures with and without secondary generalized seizures in patients >12 years of age with epilepsy; adjunct for treatment of partial seizures in pediatric patients 3-12 years of age; management of postherpetic neuralgia (PHN) in adults

Usual Dosage Oral:

Children: Anticonvulsant:

3-12 years: Initial: 10-15 mg/kg/day in 3 divided doses; titrate to effective dose over ~3 days; dosages of up to 50 mg/kg/day have been tolerated in clinical studies

3-4 years: Effective dose: 40 mg/kg/day in 3 divided doses

≥5-12 years: Effective dose: 25-35 mg/kg/day in 3 divided doses

Note: If gabapentin is discontinued or if another anticonvulsant is added to therapy, it should be done slowly over a minimum of 1 week

Children >12 years and Adults:

Anticonvulsant: Initial: 300 mg 3 times/day; if necessary the dose may be increased using 300 mg or 400 mg capsules 3 times/day up to 1800 mg/day

Dosage range: 900-1800 mg administered in 3 divided doses at 8-hour intervals

Adults: Post-herpetic neuralgia: Day 1: 300 mg, Day 2: 300 mg twice daily, Day 3: 300 mg 3 times/day; dose may be titrated as needed for pain relief (range: 1800-3600 mg/day, daily doses >1800 mg do not generally show greater benefit)

Dosage Forms

Capsule: 100 mg, 300 mg, 400 mg

Solution, oral: 250 mg/5 mL (480 mL) [cool strawberry anise flavor]

Tablet: 600 mg, 800 mg

Gabitril® [US/Can] *see* tiagabine *on page 860*

gadopentetate dimeglumine *see* radiological/contrast media (ionic) *on page 759*

gadoteridol *see* radiological/contrast media (nonionic) *on page 761*

galantamine (ga LAN ta meen)

Sound-Alike/Look-Alike Issues

Reminyl® may be confused with Amaryl®

Synonyms galantamine hydrobromide

(Continued)

galantamine *(Continued)*

U.S./Canadian Brand Names Reminyl® [US/Can]

Therapeutic Category Acetylcholinesterase Inhibitor (Central)

Use Treatment of mild to moderate dementia of Alzheimer disease

Usual Dosage **Note:** Take with breakfast and dinner. If therapy is interrupted for ≥3 days, restart at the lowest dose and increase to current dose.

Oral: Adults: Mild to moderate dementia of Alzheimer: Initial: 4 mg twice a day for 4 weeks

If 8 mg per day tolerated, increase to 8 mg twice daily for ≥4 weeks

If 16 mg per day tolerated, increase to 12 mg twice daily

Range: 16-24 mg/day in 2 divided doses

Dosage Forms

Solution, oral, as hydrobromide: 4 mg/mL (100 mL) [with calibrated pipette]

Tablet, as hydrobromide: 4 mg, 8 mg, 12 mg

galantamine hydrobromide *see* galantamine *on previous page*

Gamastan® *(Discontinued)* *see page 1042*

Gamimune® N [US/Can] *see* immune globulin (intravenous) *on page 468*

gamma benzene hexachloride *see* lindane *on page 522*

Gammagard® Injection *(Discontinued)* *see page 1042*

Gammagard® S/D [US/Can] *see* immune globulin (intravenous) *on page 468*

gamma globulin *see* immune globulin (intramuscular) *on page 468*

gamma hydroxybutyric acid *see* sodium oxybate *on page 813*

gammaphos *see* amifostine *on page 43*

Gammar® *(Discontinued)* *see page 1042*

Gammar®-P I.V. [US] *see* immune globulin (intravenous) *on page 468*

Gamulin® Rh *(Discontinued)* *see page 1042*

Gamunex® [US/Can] *see* immune globulin (intravenous) *on page 468*

ganciclovir (gan SYE kloe veer)

Sound-Alike/Look-Alike Issues

Cytovene® may be confused with Cytosar®, Cytosar-U®

Synonyms DHPG sodium; GCV sodium; nordeoxyguanosine

U.S./Canadian Brand Names Cytovene® [US/Can]; Vitrasert® [US/Can]

Therapeutic Category Antiviral Agent

Use

Parenteral: Treatment of CMV retinitis in immunocompromised individuals, including patients with acquired immunodeficiency syndrome; prophylaxis of CMV infection in transplant patients

Oral: Alternative to the I.V. formulation for maintenance treatment of CMV retinitis in immunocompromised patients, including patients with AIDS, in whom retinitis is stable following appropriate induction therapy and for whom the risk of more rapid progression is balanced by the benefit associated with avoiding daily I.V. infusions.

Implant: Treatment of CMV retinitis

Usual Dosage

CMV retinitis: Slow I.V. infusion (dosing is based on total body weight):

Children >3 months and Adults:

Induction therapy: 5 mg/kg/dose every 12 hours for 14-21 days followed by maintenance therapy

Maintenance therapy: 5 mg/kg/day as a single daily dose for 7 days/week or 6 mg/kg/day for 5 days/week

CMV retinitis: Oral: 1000 mg 3 times/day with food **or** 500 mg 6 times/day with food

Prevention of CMV disease in patients with advanced HIV infection and normal renal function: Oral: 1000 mg 3 times/day with food

Prevention of CMV disease in transplant patients: Same initial and maintenance dose as CMV retinitis except duration of initial course is 7-14 days, duration of maintenance therapy is dependent on clinical condition and degree of immunosuppression

Intravitreal implant: One implant for 5- to 8-month period; following depletion of ganciclovir, as evidenced by progression of retinitis, implant may be removed and replaced

Dosage Forms

Capsule (Cytovene®): 250 mg, 500 mg

Implant, intravitreal (Vitrasert®): 4.5 mg [released gradually over 5-8 months]

Injection, powder for reconstitution, as sodium (Cytovene®): 500 mg

Ganidin NR [US] *see* guaifenesin *on page 415*

ganirelix (ga ni REL ix)

Synonyms ganirelix acetate

U.S./Canadian Brand Names Antagon® [US/Can]; Orgalutran® [Can]

Therapeutic Category Antigonadotropic Agent

Use Inhibits premature luteinizing hormone (LH) surges in women undergoing controlled ovarian hyperstimulation in fertility clinics.

Usual Dosage Adult: SubQ: 250 mcg/day during the mid-to-late phase after initiating follicle-stimulating hormone on day 2 or 3 of cycle. Treatment should be continued daily until the day of chorionic gonadotropin administration.

Dosage Forms Injection, solution, as acetate: 250 mcg/0.5 mL [prefilled glass syringe with 27-gauge x ½ inch needle]

ganirelix acetate *see* ganirelix *on this page*

Ganite™ *(Discontinued)* *see page 1042*

Gani-Tuss® NR [US] *see* guaifenesin and codeine *on page 416*

Gantanol® *(Discontinued)* *see page 1042*

Gantrisin® [US] *see* sulfisoxazole *on page 833*

Gantrisin® Ophthalmic *(Discontinued)* *see page 1042*

Gantrisin® Tablet *(Discontinued)* *see page 1042*

Garamycin® *(Discontinued)* *see page 1042*

Garamycin® [Can] *see* gentamicin *on page 403*

Gas-Ban DS® *(Discontinued)* *see page 1042*

Gastrocrom® [US] *see* cromolyn sodium *on page 230*

Gastrografin® [US] *see* radiological/contrast media (ionic) *on page 759*

Gastrosed™ *(Discontinued)* *see page 1042*

Gas-X® Extra Strength [US-OTC] *see* simethicone *on page 804*

Gas-X® [US-OTC] *see* simethicone *on page 804*

gatifloxacin (ga ti FLOKS a sin)

U.S./Canadian Brand Names Tequin® [US/Can]; Zymar™ [US]

Therapeutic Category Antibiotic, Quinolone

Use

Oral, I.V.: Treatment of the following infections when caused by susceptible bacteria: Acute bacterial exacerbation of chronic bronchitis; acute sinusitis; community-acquired pneumonia including pneumonia caused by multidrug-resistant *S. pneumoniae* (MDRSP); uncomplicated skin and skin structure infection; uncomplicated urinary tract infections (cystitis); complicated urinary tract infections; pyelonephritis; uncomplicated urethral and cervical gonorrhea; acute, uncomplicated rectal infections in women

Ophthalmic: Bacterial conjunctivitis

(Continued)

gatifloxacin *(Continued)*

Usual Dosage

Children ≥1 year and Adults: Ophthalmic: Bacterial conjunctivitis:

Days 1 and 2: Instill 1 drop into affected eye(s) every 2 hours while awake (maximum: 8 times/day)

Days 3-7: Instill 1 drop into affected eye(s) up to 4 times/day while awake

Adults: Oral, I.V.:

Acute bacterial exacerbation of chronic bronchitis: 400 mg every 24 hours for 5 days

Acute sinusitis: 400 mg every 24 hours for 10 days

Community-acquired pneumonia: 400 mg every 24 hours for 7-14 days

Uncomplicated skin/skin structure infections: 400 mg every 24 hours for 7-10 days

Uncomplicated urinary tract infections (cystitis): 400 mg single dose or 200 mg every 24 hours for 3 days

Complicated urinary tract infections: 400 mg every 24 hours for 7-10 days

Acute pyelonephritis: 400 mg every 24 hours for 7-10 days

Uncomplicated urethral gonorrhea in men, cervical or rectal gonorrhea in women: 400 mg single dose

Dosage Forms

Injection, infusion [premixed in D_5W] (Tequin®): 200 mg (100 mL); 400 mg (200 mL)

Injection, solution [preservative free] (Tequin®): 10 mg/mL (40 mL)

Powder for oral suspension (Tequin®): 200 mg/5 mL (25 mL, 50 mL, 75 mL, 100 mL) [contains phenylalanine 168 mg/5 mL; fruit flavor]

Solution, ophthalmic (Zymar™): 0.3% (5 mL) [contains benzalkonium chloride]

Tablet (Tequin®): 200 mg, 400 mg

Gaviscon® Extra Strength [US-OTC] *see* aluminum hydroxide and magnesium carbonate *on page 39*

Gaviscon® Liquid [US-OTC] *see* aluminum hydroxide and magnesium carbonate *on page 39*

G-CSF *see* filgrastim *on page 368*

G-CSF (PEG conjugate) *see* pegfilgrastim *on page 671*

GCV sodium *see* ganciclovir *on page 396*

Gebauer's Ethyl Chloride® [US] *see* ethyl chloride *on page 349*

Gee Gee® *(Discontinued)* *see page 1042*

gefitinib (ge FI tye nib)

Synonyms NSC-715055; ZD1839

U.S./Canadian Brand Names Iressa™ [US]

Therapeutic Category Antineoplastic, Tyrosine Kinase Inhibitor

Use Second-line treatment of nonsmall-cell lung cancer

Usual Dosage Oral: Adults: 250 mg/day; consider 500 mg/day in patients receiving effective CYP3A4 inducers (eg, rifampin, phenytoin)

Dosage Forms Tablet: 250 mg

gelatin (absorbable) (JEL a tin ab SORB a ble)

Synonyms absorbable gelatin sponge

U.S./Canadian Brand Names Gelfilm® [US]; Gelfoam® [US]

Therapeutic Category Hemostatic Agent

Use Adjunct to provide hemostasis in surgery; open prostatic surgery

Usual Dosage Hemostasis: Apply packs or sponges dry or saturated with sodium chloride. When applied dry, hold in place with moderate pressure. When applied wet, squeeze to remove air bubbles. The powder is applied as a paste prepared by adding approximately 4 mL of sterile saline solution to the powder.

Dosage Forms

Film, ophthalmic (Gelfilm®): 25 mm x 50 mm (6s)

Film, topical (Gelfilm®): 100 mm x 125 mm (1s)

Powder, topical (Gelfoam®): 1 g
Sponge, dental (Gelfoam®): Size 4 (12s)
Sponge, topical (Gelfoam®):
Size 50 (4s)
Size 100 (6s)
Size 200 (6s)
Size 2 cm (1s)
Size 6 cm (6s)
Size 12-7 mm (12s)

gelatin, pectin, and methylcellulose

(JEL a tin, PEK tin, & meth il SEL yoo lose)

Synonyms methylcellulose, gelatin, and pectin; pectin, gelatin, and methylcellulose
Therapeutic Category Protectant, Topical
Use Temporary relief from minor oral irritations
Usual Dosage Press small dabs into place until the involved area is coated with a thin film; do not try to spread onto area; may be used as often as needed
Dosage Forms Paste, oral: 5 g, 15 g

Gelclair™ [US] *see* maltodextrin *on page 541*

Gelfilm® [US] *see* gelatin (absorbable) *on previous page*

Gelfoam® [US] *see* gelatin (absorbable) *on previous page*

Gel-Kam® Rinse [US] *see* fluoride *on page 376*

Gel-Kam® [US-OTC] *see* fluoride *on page 376*

Gel-Tin® ***(Discontinued)*** *see page 1042*

Gelucast® [US] *see* zinc gelatin *on page 940*

Gelusil® [Can] *see* aluminum hydroxide and magnesium hydroxide *on page 40*

Gelusil® Extra Strength [Can] *see* aluminum hydroxide and magnesium hydroxide *on page 40*

Gelusil® Liquid ***(Discontinued)*** *see page 1042*

gemcitabine (jem SIT a been)

Sound-Alike/Look-Alike Issues
Gemzar® may be confused with Zinecard®
Synonyms gemcitabine hydrochloride
U.S./Canadian Brand Names Gemzar® [US/Can]
Therapeutic Category Antineoplastic Agent
Use
Adenocarcinoma of the pancreas; first-line therapy in locally-advanced (nonresectable stage II or stage III) or metastatic (stage IV) adenocarcinoma of the pancreas (indicated for patients previously treated with fluorouracil)
Breast cancer: First-line therapy in metastatic breast cancer after failure of an anthracycline-containing adjuvant therapy (unless contraindicated); used in combination with paclitaxel
Nonsmall-cell lung cancer: First-line therapy in locally-advanced (stage IIIA or IIIB) or metastatic (stage IV) nonsmall-cell lung cancer; used in combination with cisplatin
Usual Dosage Refer to individual protocols. **Note**: Prolongation of the infusion time >60 minutes has been shown to increase toxicity. I.V.:
Pancreatic cancer: Initial: 1000 mg/m^2 over 30 minutes once weekly for up to 7 weeks followed by 1 week rest; subsequent cycles once weekly for 3 consecutive weeks out of every 4 weeks. Patients who complete an entire cycle of therapy may have the dose in subsequent cycles increased by 25% as long as the absolute granulocyte count (AGC) nadir is >1500 x 10^6/L, platelet nadir is >100,000 x 10^6/L, and nonhematologic toxicity is less than WHO Grade 1. If the increased dose is tolerated (with the same parameters) the dose in subsequent cycles may again be increased by 20%.
(Continued)

gemcitabine *(Continued)*

Nonsmall-cell lung cancer in combination with cisplatin:
28-day cycle: 1000 mg/m² over 30 minutes on days 1, 8, 15; repeat every 28 days
or
21-day cycle: 1250 mg/m² over 30 minutes on days 1, 8; repeat every 21 days
Breast cancer in combination with paclitaxel: 1250 mg/m² over 30 minutes on days 1 and 8 of each 21-day cycle

Dosage Forms Injection, powder for reconstitution, as hydrochloride: 200 mg, 1 g

gemcitabine hydrochloride *see* gemcitabine *on previous page*

gemfibrozil (jem FI broe zil)

Sound-Alike/Look-Alike Issues
Lopid® may be confused with Levbid®, Lodine®, Lorabid®, Slo-bid™

Synonyms CI-719

U.S./Canadian Brand Names Apo-Gemfibrozil® [Can]; Gen-Gemfibrozil [Can]; Lopid® [US/Can]; Novo-Gemfibrozil [Can]; Nu-Gemfibrozil [Can]; PMS-Gemfibrozil [Can]

Therapeutic Category Antihyperlipidemic Agent, Miscellaneous

Use Treatment of hypertriglyceridemia in types IV and V hyperlipidemia for patients who are at greater risk for pancreatitis and who have not responded to dietary intervention

Usual Dosage Adults: Oral: 1200 mg/day in 2 divided doses, 30 minutes before breakfast and dinner

Dosage Forms Tablet [film coated]: 600 mg

gemifloxacin (je mi FLOKS a sin)

Synonyms DW286; gemifloxacin mesylate; LA 20304a; SB-265805

U.S./Canadian Brand Names Factive® [US]

Therapeutic Category Antibiotic, Quinolone

Use Treatment of acute exacerbation of chronic bronchitis; treatment of community-acquired pneumonia, including pneumonia caused by multidrug-resistant strains of *S. pneumoniae* (MDRSP)

Usual Dosage Oral: Adults: 320 mg once daily
Duration of therapy:
Acute exacerbations of chronic bronchitis: 5 days
Community-acquired pneumonia (mild to moderate severity): 7 days

Dosage Forms Tablet, as mesylate: 320 mg

gemifloxacin mesylate *see* gemifloxacin *on this page*

gemtuzumab ozogamicin (gem TUZ yu mab oh zog a MY sin)

U.S./Canadian Brand Names Mylotarg® [US/Can]

Therapeutic Category Antineoplastic Agent, Natural Source (Plant) Derivative

Use Treatment of acute myeloid leukemia (CD33 positive) in first relapse in patients who are ≥60 years of age and who are not considered candidates for cytotoxic chemotherapy.

Usual Dosage I.V.: Adults ≥60 years: 9 mg/m², infused over 2 hours. A full treatment course is a total of two doses administered with 14 days between doses. Full hematologic recovery is not necessary for administration of the second dose. There has been only limited experience with repeat courses of gemtuzumab ozogamicin.
Note: The patient should receive diphenhydramine 50 mg orally and acetaminophen 650-1000 mg orally 1 hour prior to administration of each dose. Acetaminophen dosage should be repeated as needed every 4 hours for two additional doses. Pretreatment with methylprednisolone may ameliorate infusion-related symptoms.

Dosage Forms Injection, powder for reconstitution: 5 mg

Gemzar® [US/Can] *see* gemcitabine *on previous page*

Genabid® ***(Discontinued)*** *see page 1042*

Gen-Acebutolol [Can] *see* acebutolol *on page 4*

Genaced™ [US-OTC] *see* acetaminophen, aspirin, and caffeine *on page 10*

Genac® [US-OTC] *see* triprolidine and pseudoephedrine *on page 889*

Gen-Acyclovir [Can] *see* acyclovir *on page 19*

Genagesic® *(Discontinued)* *see page 1042*

Genahist® [US-OTC] *see* diphenhydramine *on page 277*

Gen-Alprazolam [Can] *see* alprazolam *on page 35*

Genamin® Cold Syrup *(Discontinued)* *see page 1042*

Genamin® Expectorant *(Discontinued)* *see page 1042*

Gen-Amiodarone [Can] *see* amiodarone *on page 47*

Gen-Amoxicillin [Can] *see* amoxicillin *on page 51*

Genapap® Children [US-OTC] *see* acetaminophen *on page 5*

Genapap® Extra Strength [US-OTC] *see* acetaminophen *on page 5*

Genapap® Infant [US-OTC] *see* acetaminophen *on page 5*

Genapap™ Sinus Maximum Strength [US-OTC] *see* acetaminophen and pseudoephedrine *on page 9*

Genapap® [US-OTC] *see* acetaminophen *on page 5*

Genaphed® Plus [US-OTC] *see* chlorpheniramine and pseudoephedrine *on page 189*

Genaphed® [US-OTC] *see* pseudoephedrine *on page 745*

Genasal [US-OTC] *see* oxymetazoline *on page 658*

Genasoft® Plus *(Discontinued)* *see page 1042*

Genasoft® [US-OTC] *see* docusate *on page 285*

Genasyme® [US-OTC] *see* simethicone *on page 804*

Genatap® Elixir *(Discontinued)* *see page 1042*

Gen-Atenolol [Can] *see* atenolol *on page 85*

Genatuss® *(Discontinued)* *see page 1042*

Genatuss DM® [US-OTC] *see* guaifenesin and dextromethorphan *on page 416*

Gen-Azathioprine [Can] *see* azathioprine *on page 93*

Gen-Baclofen [Can] *see* baclofen *on page 98*

Gen-Beclo [Can] *see* beclomethasone *on page 102*

Gen-Bromazepam [Can] *see* bromazepam *(Canada only) on page 127*

Gen-Budesonide AQ [Can] *see* budesonide *on page 131*

Gen-Buspirone [Can] *see* buspirone *on page 137*

Gencalc® 600 *(Discontinued)* *see page 1042*

Gen-Captopril [Can] *see* captopril *on page 153*

Gen-Carbamazepine CR [Can] *see* carbamazepine *on page 155*

Gen-Cimetidine [Can] *see* cimetidine *on page 199*

Gen-Clobetasol [Can] *see* clobetasol *on page 212*

Gen-Clomipramine [Can] *see* clomipramine *on page 214*

Gen-Clonazepam [Can] *see* clonazepam *on page 215*

Gen-Clozapine [Can] *see* clozapine *on page 219*

Gen-Cyclobenzaprine [Can] *see* cyclobenzaprine *on page 233*

Gen-Cyproterone [Can] *see* cyproterone *(Canada only) on page 238*

Gen-Diltiazem [Can] *see* diltiazem *on page 273*

Gen-Diltiazem SR [Can] *see* diltiazem *on page 273*
Gen-Divalproex [Can] *see* valproic acid and derivatives *on page 901*
Gen-Doxazosin [Can] *see* doxazosin *on page 291*
Gen-D-phen® *(Discontinued)* *see page 1042*
Genebs® Extra Strength [US-OTC] *see* acetaminophen *on page 5*
Genebs® [US-OTC] *see* acetaminophen *on page 5*
Generlac® [US] *see* lactulose *on page 502*
Genesec® [US-OTC] *see* acetaminophen and phenyltoloxamine *on page 8*
Gen-Etidronate [Can] *see* etidronate disodium *on page 350*
Geneye® [US-OTC] *see* tetrahydrozoline *on page 852*
Gen-Famotidine [Can] *see* famotidine *on page 356*
Gen-Fenofibrat Micro [Can] *see* fenofibrate *on page 360*
Genfiber® [US-OTC] *see* psyllium *on page 749*
Gen-Fluconazole [Can] *see* fluconazole *on page 371*
Gen-Fluoxetine [Can] *see* fluoxetine *on page 379*
Gen-Gemfibrozil [Can] *see* gemfibrozil *on page 400*
Gen-Glybe [Can] *see* glyburide *on page 409*
Gengraf® [US] *see* cyclosporine *on page 235*
Gen-Hydroxyurea [Can] *see* hydroxyurea *on page 457*
Gen-Indapamide [Can] *see* indapamide *on page 470*
Gen-Ipratropium [Can] *see* ipratropium *on page 482*
Gen-K® *(Discontinued)* *see page 1042*
Gen-Lovastatin [Can] *see* lovastatin *on page 533*
Gen-Medroxy [Can] *see* medroxyprogesterone acetate *on page 548*
Gen-Metformin [Can] *see* metformin *on page 560*
Gen-Minocycline [Can] *see* minocycline *on page 583*
Gen-Nabumetone [Can] *see* nabumetone *on page 598*
Gen-Naproxen EC [Can] *see* naproxen *on page 605*
Gen-Nitro [Can] *see* nitroglycerin *on page 623*
Gen-Nizatidine [Can] *see* nizatidine *on page 625*
Gen-Nortriptyline [Can] *see* nortriptyline *on page 629*
Genoptic® [US] *see* gentamicin *on next page*
Genora® 0.5/35 *(Discontinued)* *see page 1042*
Genora® 1/35 *(Discontinued)* *see page 1042*
Genora® 1/50 *(Discontinued)* *see page 1042*
Genotropin® [US] *see* human growth hormone *on page 437*
Genotropin Miniquick® [US] *see* human growth hormone *on page 437*
Gen-Oxybutynin [Can] *see* oxybutynin *on page 655*
Gen-Pindolol [Can] *see* pindolol *on page 696*
Gen-Piroxicam [Can] *see* piroxicam *on page 698*
Genpril® [US-OTC] *see* ibuprofen *on page 462*
Gen-Propafenone [Can] *see* propafenone *on page 737*
Gen-Ranitidine [Can] *see* ranitidine hydrochloride *on page 763*
Gen-Salbutamol [Can] *see* albuterol *on page 25*

Gen-Selegiline [Can] *see* selegiline *on page 798*

Gen-Sertraline [Can] *see* sertraline *on page 801*

Gen-Simvastatin [Can] *see* simvastatin *on page 805*

Gen-Sotalol [Can] *see* sotalol *on page 819*

Gentacidin® *(Discontinued)* *see page 1042*

Gentak® [US] *see* gentamicin *on this page*

gentamicin (jen ta MYE sin)

Sound-Alike/Look-Alike Issues
gentamicin may be confused with kanamycin
Garamycin® may be confused with kanamycin, Terramycin®

Synonyms gentamicin sulfate

U.S./Canadian Brand Names Alcomicin® [Can]; Diogent® [Can]; Garamycin® [Can]; Genoptic® [US]; Gentak® [US]; Minim's Gentamicin 0.3% [Can]; SAB-Gentamicin [Can]

Therapeutic Category Aminoglycoside (Antibiotic); Antibiotic, Ophthalmic; Antibiotic, Topical

Use Treatment of susceptible bacterial infections, normally gram-negative organisms including *Pseudomonas*, *Proteus*, *Serratia*, and gram-positive *Staphylococcus*; treatment of bone infections, respiratory tract infections, skin and soft tissue infections, as well as abdominal and urinary tract infections, endocarditis, and septicemia; used topically to treat superficial infections of the skin or ophthalmic infections caused by susceptible bacteria; prevention of bacterial endocarditis prior to dental or surgical procedures

Usual Dosage Individualization is critical because of the low therapeutic index

Use of ideal body weight (IBW) for determining the mg/kg/dose appears to be more accurate than dosing on the basis of total body weight (TBW).

In morbid obesity, dosage requirement may best be estimated using a dosing weight of IBW + 0.4 (TBW - IBW)

Initial and periodic peak and trough plasma drug levels should be determined, particularly in critically ill patients with serious infections or in disease states known to significantly alter aminoglycoside pharmacokinetics (eg, cystic fibrosis, burns, or major surgery)

Newborns: Intrathecal: 1 mg every day

Infants >3 months: Intrathecal: 1-2 mg/day

Infants and Children <5 years: I.M., I.V.: 2.5 mg/kg/dose every 8 hours*
Cystic fibrosis: 2.5 mg/kg/dose every 6 hours

Children >5 years: I.M., I.V.: 1.5-2.5 mg/kg/dose every 8 hours*
Prevention of bacterial endocarditis: Dental, oral, upper respiratory procedures, GI/GU procedures: 2 mg/kg with ampicillin (50 mg/kg) 30 minutes prior to procedure

*Some patients may require larger or more frequent doses (eg, every 6 hours) if serum levels document the need (ie, cystic fibrosis or febrile granulocytopenic patients)

Adults: I.M., I.V.:
Severe life-threatening infections: 2-2.5 mg/kg/dose
Urinary tract infections: 1.5 mg/kg/dose
Synergy (for gram-positive infections): 1 mg/kg/dose
Prevention of bacterial endocarditis:
Dental, oral, or upper respiratory procedures: 1.5 mg/kg not to exceed 80 mg with ampicillin (1-2 g) 30 minutes prior to procedure
GI/GU surgery: 1.5 mg/kg not to exceed 80 mg with ampicillin (2 g) 30 minutes prior to procedure

Some clinicians suggest a daily dose of 4-7 mg/kg for all patients with normal renal function. This dose is at least as efficacious with similar, if not less, toxicity than conventional dosing.

Children and Adults:
Intrathecal: 4-8 mg/day
Ophthalmic:
Ointment: Instill ½" (1.25 cm) 2-3 times/day to every 3-4 hours

(Continued)

gentamicin *(Continued)*

Solution: Instill 1-2 drops every 2-4 hours, up to 2 drops every hour for severe infections

Topical: Apply 3-4 times/day to affected area

Dosage Forms [DSC] = Discontinued product

Cream, topical, as sulfate: 0.1% (15 g, 30 g)

Infusion, as sulfate [premixed in NS]: 40 mg (50 mL); 60 mg (50 mL, 100 mL); 70 mg (50 mL); 80 mg (50 mL, 100 mL); 90 mg (100 mL); 100 mg (50 mL, 100 mL); 120 mg (100 mL)

Injection, solution, as sulfate [ADD-Vantage® vial]: 10 mg/mL (6 mL, 8 mL, 10 mL)

Injection, solution, as sulfate: 40 mg/mL (2 mL, 20 mL) [may contain sodium metabisulfite]

Injection, solution, pediatric, as sulfate: 10 mg/mL (2 mL) [may contain sodium metabisulfite]

Injection, solution, pediatric, as sulfate [preservative free]: 10 mg/mL (2 mL)

Ointment, ophthalmic, as sulfate (Gentak®): 0.3% [3 mg/g] (3.5 g)

Ointment, topical, as sulfate: 0.1% (15 g, 30 g)

Solution, ophthalmic, as sulfate: 0.3% (5 mL, 15 mL) [contains benzalkonium chloride]

Genoptic®: 0.3% (1 mL) [contains benzalkonium chloride]

Gentacidin®: 0.3% (5 mL) [contains benzalkonium chloride] [DSC]

Gentak®: 0.3% (5 mL, 15 mL) [contains benzalkonium chloride]

gentamicin and prednisolone *see* prednisolone and gentamicin *on page 723*

gentamicin sulfate *see* gentamicin *on previous page*

Gen-Tamoxifen [Can] *see* tamoxifen *on page 839*

GenTeal® Mild [US-OTC] *see* hydroxypropyl methylcellulose *on page 457*

GenTeal® [US-OTC/Can] *see* hydroxypropyl methylcellulose *on page 457*

Gen-Temazepam [Can] *see* temazepam *on page 843*

Gen-Ticlopidine [Can] *see* ticlopidine *on page 862*

Gen-Timolol [Can] *see* timolol *on page 863*

Gentlax® [US-OTC] *see* bisacodyl *on page 120*

Gentran® [US/Can] *see* dextran *on page 258*

Gentrasul® *(Discontinued)* *see page 1042*

Gen-Trazodone [Can] *see* trazodone *on page 877*

Gen-Triazolam [Can] *see* triazolam *on page 883*

Gen-Verapamil [Can] *see* verapamil *on page 908*

Gen-Verapamil SR [Can] *see* verapamil *on page 908*

Gen-Warfarin [Can] *see* warfarin *on page 933*

Gen-Zopiclone [Can] *see* zopiclone *(Canada only) on page 944*

Geocillin® [US] *see* carbenicillin *on page 156*

Geodon® [US] *see* ziprasidone *on page 941*

Geref® *(Discontinued)* *see page 1042*

Geref® Diagnostic [US] *see* sermorelin acetate *on page 801*

Geridium® *(Discontinued)* *see page 1042*

Geri-Hydrolac™-12 [US-OTC] *see* lactic acid with ammonium hydroxide *on page 501*

Geri-Hydrolac™ [US-OTC] *see* lactic acid with ammonium hydroxide *on page 501*

Geritol® Tonic [US-OTC] *see* vitamins (multiple/oral) *on page 927*

german measles vaccine *see* rubella virus vaccine (live) *on page 788*

Gevrabon® [US-OTC] *see* vitamin B complex combinations *on page 915*

GF196960 *see* tadalafil *on page 838*

GG *see* guaifenesin *on page 415*

GG-Cen® ***(Discontinued)*** *see page 1042*

GHB *see* sodium oxybate *on page 813*

GI87084B *see* remifentanil *on page 767*

glargine, insulin *see* insulin preparations *on page 474*

glatiramer acetate (gla TIR a mer AS e tate)

Sound-Alike/Look-Alike Issues

Copaxone® may be confused with Compazine®

Synonyms copolymer-1

U.S./Canadian Brand Names Copaxone® [US/Can]

Therapeutic Category Biological, Miscellaneous

Use Treatment of relapsing-remitting type multiple sclerosis; studies indicate that it reduces the frequency of attacks and the severity of disability; appears to be most effective for patients with minimal disability

Usual Dosage Adults: SubQ: 20 mg daily

Dosage Forms Injection, solution [preservative free]: 20 mg/mL (1 mL) [prefilled syringe; contains mannitol; packaged with alcohol pads]

Glaucon® ***(Discontinued)*** *see page 1042*

Gleevec® [US/Can] *see* imatinib *on page 465*

Gliadel® [US] *see* carmustine *on page 162*

glibenclamide *see* glyburide *on page 409*

gliclazide *(Canada only)* (GLYE kla zide)

U.S./Canadian Brand Names Apo-Gliclazide® [Can]; Diamicron® [Can]; Diamicron® MR [Can]; Novo-Gliclazide [Can]

Therapeutic Category Antidiabetic Agent; Hypoglycemic Agent, Oral; Sulfonylurea Agent

Use Management of type 2 diabetes mellitus (noninsulin dependent, NIDDM)

Usual Dosage Oral: Adults:

Immediate release tablet: Initial: 80-160 mg/day; typical dose range 80-320 mg/day; dosage of ≥160 mg should be divided into 2 equal parts for twice-daily administration; maximum dose: 320 mg/day; should be taken with meals

Sustained release tablet: 30-120 mg once daily

Note: There is no fixed dosage regimen for the management of diabetes mellitus with gliclazide or any other hypoglycemic agent. Dose must be individualized based on frequent determinations of blood glucose during dose titration and throughout maintenance.

Dosage Forms

Tablet (Diamicron®): 80 mg

Tablet, sustained release (Diamicron® MR): 30 mg

glimepiride (GLYE me pye ride)

Sound-Alike/Look-Alike Issues

glimepiride may be confused with glipiZIDE

Amaryl® may be confused with Altace™, Amerge®, Reminyl®

U.S./Canadian Brand Names Amaryl® [US/Can]

Therapeutic Category Antidiabetic Agent, Oral

Use Management of type 2 diabetes mellitus (noninsulin dependent, NIDDM) as an adjunct to diet and exercise to lower blood glucose or in combination with metformin; use in combination with insulin to lower blood glucose in patients whose hyperglycemia

(Continued)

glimepiride *(Continued)*

cannot be controlled by diet and exercise in conjunction with an oral hypoglycemic agent

Usual Dosage Oral (allow several days between dose titrations):

Adults: Initial: 1-2 mg once daily, administered with breakfast or the first main meal; usual maintenance dose: 1-4 mg once daily; after a dose of 2 mg once daily, increase in increments of 2 mg at 1- to 2-week intervals based upon the patient's blood glucose response to a maximum of 8 mg once daily

Combination with insulin therapy (fasting glucose level for instituting combination therapy is in the range of >150 mg/dL in plasma or serum depending on the patient): initial recommended dose: 8 mg once daily with the first main meal

After starting with low-dose insulin, upward adjustments of insulin can be done approximately weekly as guided by frequent measurements of fasting blood glucose. Once stable, combination-therapy patients should monitor their capillary blood glucose on an ongoing basis, preferably daily.

Dosage Forms Tablet: 1 mg, 2 mg, 4 mg

glipizide (GLIP i zide)

Sound-Alike/Look-Alike Issues

glipizide may be confused with glimepiride, glyburide

Glucotrol® may be confused with Glucophage®, Glucotrol® XL, glyburide

Glucotrol® XL may be confused with Glucotrol®

Synonyms glydiazinamide

Tall-Man glipi**ZIDE**

U.S./Canadian Brand Names Glucotrol® [US]; Glucotrol® XL [US]

Therapeutic Category Antidiabetic Agent, Oral

Use Management of type 2 diabetes mellitus (noninsulin dependent, NIDDM)

Usual Dosage Oral (allow several days between dose titrations): Adults: Initial: 5 mg/day; adjust dosage at 2.5-5 mg daily increments as determined by blood glucose response at intervals of several days.

Immediate release tablet: Maximum recommended once-daily dose: 15 mg; maximum recommended total daily dose: 40 mg

Extended release tablet (Glucotrol® XL): Maximum recommended dose: 20 mg

When transferring from insulin to glipizide:

Current insulin requirement ≤20 units: Discontinue insulin and initiate glipizide at usual dose

Current insulin requirement >20 units: Decrease insulin by 50% and initiate glipizide at usual dose; gradually decrease insulin dose based on patient response. Several days should elapse between dosage changes.

Dosage Forms

Tablet (Glucotrol®): 5 mg, 10 mg

Tablet, extended release: 5 mg, 10 mg

(Glucotrol® XL): 2.5 mg, 5 mg, 10 mg

glipizide and metformin (GLIP i zide & met FOR min)

Synonyms glipizide and metformin hydrochloride; metformin and glipizide

U.S./Canadian Brand Names Metaglip™ [US]

Therapeutic Category Antidiabetic Agent (Biguanide); Antidiabetic Agent (Sulfonylurea)

Use Initial therapy for management of type 2 diabetes mellitus (noninsulin dependent, NIDDM) when hyperglycemia cannot be managed with diet and exercise alone. Second-line therapy for management of type 2 diabetes (NIDDM) when hyperglycemia cannot be managed with a sulfonylurea or metformin along with diet and exercise.

Usual Dosage Oral:

Adults:

Type 2 diabetes, first-line therapy: Initial: Glipizide 2.5 mg/metformin 250 mg once daily with a meal. Dose adjustment: Increase dose by 1 tablet/day every 2 weeks, up to a maximum of glipizide 10 mg/metformin 1000 mg daily

Patients with fasting plasma glucose (FPG) 280-320 mg/dL: Consider glipizide 2.5 mg/metformin 500 mg twice daily. Dose adjustment: Increase dose by 1 tablet/day every 2 weeks, up to a maximum of glipizide 10 mg/metformin 2000 mg daily in divided doses

Type 2 diabetes, second-line therapy: Glipizide 2.5 mg/metformin 500 mg **or** glipizide 5 mg/metformin 500 mg twice daily with morning and evening meals; starting dose should not exceed current daily dose of glipizide (or sulfonylurea equivalent) or metformin. Dose adjustment: Titrate dose in increments of no more than glipizide 5 mg/metformin 500 mg, up to a maximum dose of glipizide 20 mg/metformin 2000 mg daily.

Dosage Forms Tablet [film coated]:

2.5/250: Glipizide 2.5 mg and metformin 250 mg

2.5/500: Glipizide 2.5 mg and metformin 500 mg

5/500: Glipizide 5 mg and metformin 500 mg

glipizide and metformin hydrochloride *see* glipizide and metformin *on previous page*

glivec *see* imatinib *on page 465*

GlucaGen® [US] *see* glucagon *on this page*

GlucaGen® Diagnostic Kit [US] *see* glucagon *on this page*

glucagon (GLOO ka gon)

Sound-Alike/Look-Alike Issues

glucagon may be confused with Glaucon®

Synonyms glucagon hydrochloride

U.S./Canadian Brand Names GlucaGen® [US]; GlucaGen® Diagnostic Kit [US]; Glucagon Diagnostic Kit [US]; Glucagon Emergency Kit [US]

Therapeutic Category Antihypoglycemic Agent

Use Management of hypoglycemia; diagnostic aid in radiologic examinations to temporarily inhibit GI tract movement

Usual Dosage

Hypoglycemia or insulin shock therapy: I.M., I.V., SubQ:

Children <20 kg: 0.5 mg or 20-30 mcg/kg/dose; repeated in 20 minutes as needed

Children ≥20 kg and Adults: 1 mg; may repeat in 20 minutes as needed

Note: If patient fails to respond to glucagon, I.V. dextrose must be given.

Diagnostic aid: Adults: I.M., I.V.: 0.25-2 mg 10 minutes prior to procedure

Dosage Forms

Injection, powder for reconstitution, as hydrochloride:

GlucaGen®: 1 mg [equivalent to 1 unit; contains lactose 107 mg]

GlucaGen® Diagnostic Kit: 1 mg [equivalent to 1 unit; contains lactose 107 mg; packaged with sterile water]

Glucagon®: 1 mg [equivalent to 1 unit; contains lactose 49 mg]

Glucagon Diagnostic Kit, Glucagon Emergency Kit: 1 mg [equivalent to 1 unit; contains lactose 49 mg; packaged with diluent syringe containing glycerin 12 mg/mL and water for injection]

Glucagon Diagnostic Kit [US] *see* glucagon *on this page*

Glucagon Emergency Kit [US] *see* glucagon *on this page*

glucagon hydrochloride *see* glucagon *on this page*

glucocerebrosidase *see* alglucerase *on page 31*

GlucoNorm® [Can] *see* repaglinide *on page 768*

Glucophage® [US/Can] *see* metformin *on page 560*

Glucophage® XR [US] *see* metformin *on page 560*

glucose (instant) (GLOO kose IN stant)

Sound-Alike/Look-Alike Issues

GlutoseTM may be confused with Glutofac®

U.S./Canadian Brand Names B-DTM Glucose [US-OTC]; Dex4 Glucose [US-OTC]; GlutolTM [US-OTC]; GlutoseTM [US-OTC]; Insta-Glucose® [US-OTC]

Therapeutic Category Antihypoglycemic Agent

Use Management of hypoglycemia

Usual Dosage Adults: Oral: 10-20 g

Dosage Forms

Gel, oral:

GlutoseTM: 40% (15 g, 45 g)

Insta-Glucose®: 40% (30 g)

Solution, oral (GlutolTM): 55% [100 g dextrose/180 mL] (180 mL)

Tablet, chewable:

B-DTM Glucose: 5 g

Dex4 Glucose: 4 g

glucose polymers (GLOO kose POL i merz)

U.S./Canadian Brand Names Moducal® [US-OTC]; Polycose® [US-OTC]

Therapeutic Category Nutritional Supplement

Use Supplies calories for those persons not able to meet the caloric requirement with usual food intake

Usual Dosage Adults: Oral: Add to foods or beverages or mix in water

Dosage Forms

Liquid (Polycose®): 43% (126 mL)

Powder:

Moducal®: 368 g

Polycose®: 350 g

Glucotrol® [US] *see* glipizide *on page 406*

Glucotrol® XL [US] *see* glipizide *on page 406*

GlucovanceTM [US] *see* glyburide and metformin *on next page*

Glukor® *(Discontinued)* *see page 1042*

Glu-K® [US-OTC] *see* potassium gluconate *on page 715*

glulisine, insulin *see* insulin preparations *on page 474*

glutamic acid (gloo TAM ik AS id)

Synonyms glutamic acid hydrochloride

Therapeutic Category Gastrointestinal Agent, Miscellaneous

Use Treatment of hypochlorhydria and achlorhydria

Usual Dosage Adults: Oral:

Tablet/powder: 500-1000 mg/day before meals or food

Capsule: 1-3 capsules 3 times/day before meals

Dosage Forms

Capsule, as hydrochloride: 340 mg

Tablet: 500 mg

glutamic acid hydrochloride *see* glutamic acid *on this page*

GlutolTM [US-OTC] *see* glucose (instant) *on this page*

GlutoseTM [US-OTC] *see* glucose (instant) *on this page*

Glyate® *(Discontinued)* *see page 1042*

glybenclamide *see* glyburide *on next page*

glybenzcyclamide *see* glyburide *on this page*

glyburide (GLYE byoor ide)

Sound-Alike/Look-Alike Issues

glyburide may be confused with glipizide, Glucotrol®

DiaBeta® may be confused with Diabinese®, Zebeta®

Micronase® may be confused with microK®, miconazole, Micronor®

Synonyms glibenclamide; glybenclamide; glybenzcyclamide

Tall-Man gly**BURIDE**

U.S./Canadian Brand Names Albert® Glyburide [Can]; Apo-Glyburide® [Can]; Diaβeta® [US/Can]; Euglucon® [Can]; Gen-Glybe [Can]; Glynase® PresTab™ [US]; Micronase® [US]; Novo-Glyburide [Can]; Nu-Glyburide [Can]; PMS-Glyburide [Can]; ratio-Glyburide [Can]

Therapeutic Category Antidiabetic Agent, Oral

Use Management of type 2 diabetes mellitus (noninsulin dependent, NIDDM)

Usual Dosage Oral: Adults:

Initial: 2.5-5 mg/day, administered with breakfast or the first main meal of the day. In patients who are more sensitive to hypoglycemic drugs, start at 1.25 mg/day.

Increase in increments of no more than 2.5 mg/day at weekly intervals based on the patient's blood glucose response

Maintenance: 1.25-20 mg/day given as single or divided doses; maximum: 20 mg/day

Micronized tablets (Glynase™ PresTab™):

Initial: 1.5-3 mg/day, administered with breakfast or the first main meal of the day in patients who are more sensitive to hypoglycemic drugs, start at 0.75 mg/day. Increase in increments of no more than 1.5 mg/day in weekly intervals based on the patient's blood glucose response.

Maintenance: 0.75-12 mg/day given as a single dose or in divided doses. Some patients (especially those receiving >6 mg/day) may have a more satisfactory response with twice-daily dosing.

Dosage Forms

Tablet (Diaβeta®, Micronase®): 1.25 mg, 2.5 mg, 5 mg

Tablet, micronized (Glynase® PresTab®): 1.5 mg, 3 mg, 6 mg

glyburide and metformin (GLYE byoor ide & met FOR min)

Synonyms glyburide and metformin hydrochloride; metformin and glyburide

U.S./Canadian Brand Names Glucovance™ [US]

Therapeutic Category Antidiabetic Agent, Oral; Antidiabetic Agent (Sulfonylurea)

Use Initial therapy for management of type 2 diabetes mellitus (noninsulin dependent, NIDDM). Second-line therapy for management of type 2 diabetes (NIDDM) when hyperglycemia cannot be managed with a sulfonylurea or metformin; combination therapy with a thiazolidinedione may be required to achieve additional control.

Usual Dosage **Note:** Dose must be individualized. Dosages expressed as glyburide/metformin components.

Adults: Oral:

Initial therapy (no prior treatment with sulfonylurea or metformin): 1.25 mg/250 mg once daily with a meal; patients with Hb A_{1c} >9% or fasting plasma glucose (FPG) >200 mg/dL may start with 1.25 mg/250 mg twice daily

Dosage may be increased in increments of 1.25 mg/250 mg, at intervals of not less than 2 weeks; maximum daily dose: 10 mg/2000 mg (limited experience with higher doses)

Previously treated with a sulfonylurea or metformin alone: Initial: 2.5 mg/500 mg or 5 mg/500 mg twice daily; increase in increments no greater than 5 mg/500 mg; maximum daily dose: 20 mg/2000 mg

When switching patients previously on a sulfonylurea and metformin together, do not exceed the daily dose of glyburide (or glyburide equivalent) or metformin.

Note: May combine with a thiazolidinedione in patients with an inadequate response to glyburide/metformin therapy (risk of hypoglycemia may be increased).

(Continued)

glyburide and metformin *(Continued)*

Dosage Forms

Tablet [film coated]:

1.25 mg/250 mg: Glyburide 1.25 mg and metformin hydrochloride 250 mg
2.5 mg/500 mg: Glyburide 2.5 mg and metformin hydrochloride 500 mg
5 mg/500 mg: Glyburide 5 mg and metformin hydrochloride 500 mg

glyburide and metformin hydrochloride *see* glyburide and metformin *on previous page*

glycerin (GLIS er in)

Synonyms glycerol

U.S./Canadian Brand Names Bausch & Lomb® Computer Eye Drops [US-OTC]; Fleet® Babylax® [US-OTC]; Fleet® Glycerin Suppositories Maximum Strength [US-OTC]; Fleet® Glycerin Suppositories [US-OTC]; Fleet® Liquid Glycerin Suppositories [US-OTC]; Osmoglyn® [US]; Sani-Supp® [US-OTC]

Therapeutic Category Laxative; Ophthalmic Agent, Miscellaneous

Use Constipation; reduction of intraocular pressure; reduction of corneal edema; glycerin has been administered orally to reduce intracranial pressure

Usual Dosage

Constipation: Rectal:

Children <6 years: 1 infant suppository 1-2 times/day as needed or 2-5 mL as an enema

Children >6 years and Adults: 1 adult suppository 1-2 times/day as needed or 5-15 mL as an enema

Children and Adults:

Reduction of intraocular pressure: Oral: 1-1.8 g/kg 1-1½ hours preoperatively; additional doses may be administered at 5-hour intervals

Reduction of intracranial pressure: Oral: 1.5 g/kg/day divided every 4 hours; 1 g/kg/dose every 6 hours has also been used

Reduction of corneal edema: Ophthalmic solution: Instill 1-2 drops in eye(s) prior to examination OR for lubricant effect, instill 1-2 drops in eye(s) every 3-4 hours

Dosage Forms

Solution, ophthalmic, sterile (Bausch & Lomb® Computer Eye Drops): 1% (15 mL) [contains benzalkonium chloride]

Solution, oral (Osmoglyn®): 50% (220 mL) [lime flavor]

Solution, rectal:

Fleet® Babylax®: 2.3 g/2.3 mL (4 mL) [6 units per box]
Fleet® Liquid Glycerin Suppositories: 5.6 g/5.5 mL (7.5 mL) [4 units per box]

Suppository, rectal: 12s, 24s, 25s, 50s [pediatric and adult sizes]:

Fleet® Glycerin Suppositories: 1 g (12s) [pediatric size]; 2g (12s, 24s, 50s) [adult size]
Fleet® Glycerin Suppositories Maximum Strength: 3g (18s) [adult size]
Sani-Supp®: 82.5% (10s, 25s) [pediatric size]; 82.5% (10s, 25s, 50s) [adult size]

glycerin, lanolin, and peanut oil (GLIS er in, LAN oh lin, & PEE nut oyl)

Therapeutic Category Topical Skin Product

Use Nipple care of pregnant and nursing women

Usual Dosage Topical: Apply as often as needed

Dosage Forms Cream: 2 oz

glycerol *see* glycerin *on this page*

glycerol guaiacolate *see* guaifenesin *on page 415*

Glycerol-T® *(Discontinued)* *see page 1042*

glycerol triacetate *see* triacetin *on page 879*

glyceryl trinitrate *see* nitroglycerin *on page 623*

Glycofed® *(Discontinued)* *see page 1042*

GlycoLax™ [US] *see* polyethylene glycol-electrolyte solution *on page 706*

Glycon [Can] *see* metformin *on page 560*

glycopyrrolate (glye koe PYE roe late)

Synonyms glycopyrronium bromide

U.S./Canadian Brand Names Robinul® Forte [US]; Robinul® [US]

Therapeutic Category Anticholinergic Agent

Use Inhibit salivation and excessive secretions of the respiratory tract preoperatively; reversal of neuromuscular blockade; control of upper airway secretions; adjunct in treatment of peptic ulcer

Usual Dosage

Children:

Control of secretions:

Oral: 40-100 mcg/kg/dose 3-4 times/day

I.M., I.V.: 4-10 mcg/kg/dose every 3-4 hours; maximum: 0.2 mg/dose or 0.8 mg/24 hours

Intraoperative: I.V.: 4 mcg/kg not to exceed 0.1 mg; repeat at 2- to 3-minute intervals as needed

Preoperative: I.M.:

<2 years: 4.4-8.8 mcg/kg 30-60 minutes before procedure

>2 years: 4.4 mcg/kg 30-60 minutes before procedure

Children and Adults: Reverse neuromuscular blockade: I.V.: 0.2 mg for each 1 mg of neostigmine or 5 mg of pyridostigmine administered or 5-15 mcg/kg glycopyrrolate with 25-70 mcg/kg of neostigmine or 0.1-0.3 mg/kg of pyridostigmine (agents usually administered simultaneously, but glycopyrrolate may be administered first if bradycardia is present)

Adults:

Intraoperative: I.V.: 0.1 mg repeated as needed at 2- to 3-minute intervals

Preoperative: I.M.: 4.4 mcg/kg 30-60 minutes before procedure

Peptic ulcer:

Oral: 1-2 mg 2-3 times/day

I.M., I.V.: 0.1-0.2 mg 3-4 times/day

Dosage Forms

Injection, solution (Robinul®): 0.2 mg/mL (1 mL, 2 mL, 5 mL, 20 mL) [contains benzyl alcohol]

Tablet:

Robinul®: 1 mg

Robinul® Forte: 2 mg

glycopyrronium bromide *see* glycopyrrolate *on this page*

Glycotuss® ***(Discontinued)*** *see page 1042*

Glycotuss-dM® ***(Discontinued)*** *see page 1042*

glydiazinamide *see* glipizide *on page 406*

Glynase® PresTab™ [US] *see* glyburide *on page 409*

Gly-Oxide® [US-OTC] *see* carbamide peroxide *on page 155*

Glyquin® [US] *see* hydroquinone *on page 454*

Glyquin® XM [Can] *see* hydroquinone *on page 454*

Glyset® [US/Can] *see* miglitol *on page 582*

GM-CSF *see* sargramostim *on page 795*

G-myticin® ***(Discontinued)*** *see page 1042*

GnRH *see* gonadorelin *on next page*

Gold Bond® Antifungal [US-OTC] *see* tolnaftate *on page 870*

gold sodium thiomalate (gold SOW dee um thye oh MAL ate)

U.S./Canadian Brand Names Aurolate® [US]; Myochrysine® [Can]

Therapeutic Category Gold Compound

Use Treatment of progressive rheumatoid arthritis

Usual Dosage I.M.:

Children: Initial: Test dose of 10 mg is recommended, followed by 1 mg/kg/week for 20 weeks; maintenance: 1 mg/kg/dose at 2- to 4-week intervals thereafter for as long as therapy is clinically beneficial and toxicity does not develop. Administration for 2-4 months is usually required before clinical improvement is observed.

Adults: 10 mg first week; 25 mg second week; then 25-50 mg/week until 1 g cumulative dose has been given; if improvement occurs without adverse reactions, administer 25-50 mg every 2-3 weeks for 2-20 weeks, then every 3-4 weeks indefinitely

Dosage Forms Injection, solution: 50 mg/mL (1 mL, 10 mL) [contains benzyl alcohol]

GoLYTELY® [US] *see* polyethylene glycol-electrolyte solution *on page 706*

gonadorelin (goe nad oh REL in)

Sound-Alike/Look-Alike Issues

gonadorelin may be confused with gonadotropin, guanadrel

Factrel® may be confused with Sectral®

gonadotropin may be confused with gonadorelin

Synonyms GnRH; gonadorelin acetate; gonadorelin hydrochloride; gonadotropin releasing hormone; LHRH; LRH; luteinizing hormone releasing hormone

U.S./Canadian Brand Names Factrel® [US]; Lutrepulse™ [Can]

Therapeutic Category Diagnostic Agent; Gonadotropin

Use Evaluation of functional capacity and response of gonadotrophic hormones; evaluate abnormal gonadotropin regulation as in precocious puberty and delayed puberty.

Orphan drug: Lutrepulse®: Induction of ovulation in females with hypothalamic amenorrhea

Usual Dosage

Diagnostic test: Children >12 years and Female Adults: I.V., SubQ hydrochloride salt: 100 mcg administered in women during early phase of menstrual cycle (day 1-7)

Primary hypothalamic amenorrhea: Female Adults: Acetate: I.V.: 5 mcg every 90 minutes via Lutrepulse® pump kit at treatment intervals of 21 days (pump will pulsate every 90 minutes for 7 days)

Dosage Forms Injection, powder for reconstitution, as hydrochloride (Factrel®): 100 mcg [diluent contains benzyl alcohol]

gonadorelin acetate *see* gonadorelin *on this page*

gonadorelin hydrochloride *see* gonadorelin *on this page*

gonadotropin releasing hormone *see* gonadorelin *on this page*

Gonak™ [US-OTC] *see* hydroxypropyl methylcellulose *on page 457*

Gonic® *(Discontinued)* *see page 1042*

gonioscopic ophthalmic solution *see* hydroxypropyl methylcellulose *on page 457*

Goniosoft™ [US] *see* hydroxypropyl methylcellulose *on page 457*

Goniosol® *(Discontinued)* *see page 1042*

Goody's® Extra Strength Headache Powder [US-OTC] *see* acetaminophen, aspirin, and caffeine *on page 10*

Goody's® Extra Strength Pain Relief [US-OTC] *see* acetaminophen, aspirin, and caffeine *on page 10*

Goody's PM® Powder [US] *see* acetaminophen and diphenhydramine *on page 7*

Gordofilm® [US-OTC] *see* salicylic acid *on page 789*

Gormel® [US-OTC] *see* urea *on page 897*

goserelin (GOE se rel in)

Synonyms D-Ser(Bu^t)^6,Azgly^{10}-LHRH; goserelin acetate; ICI-118630; NSC-606864

U.S./Canadian Brand Names Zoladex® LA [Can]; Zoladex® [US/Can]

Therapeutic Category Gonadotropin-Releasing Hormone Analog

Use Palliative treatment of advanced breast cancer and carcinoma of the prostate; treatment of endometriosis, including pain relief and reduction of endometriotic lesions; endometrial thinning agent as part of treatment for dysfunctional uterine bleeding

Usual Dosage SubQ: Adults:

Prostate cancer:

Monthly implant: 3.6 mg injected into upper abdomen every 28 days

3-month implant: 10.8 mg injected into the upper abdominal wall every 12 weeks

Note: Treatment should begin 8 weeks prior to radiotherapy in Stage B2-C prostate cancer; treatment may continue indefinitely

Breast cancer, endometriosis, endometrial thinning: Monthly implant: 3.6 mg injected into upper abdomen every 28 days

Note: For breast cancer, treatment may continue indefinitely; for endometriosis, it is recommended that duration of treatment not exceed 6 months. Only 1-2 doses are recommended for endometrial thinning.

Dosage Forms

Injection, solution, 1-month implant [disposable syringe; single-dose]: 3.6 mg [with 16-gauge hypodermic needle]

Injection, solution, 3-month implant [disposable syringe; single-dose]: 10.8 mg [with 14-gauge hypodermic needle]

goserelin acetate *see* goserelin *on this page*

GP 47680 *see* oxcarbazepine *on page 653*

G-Phed [US] *see* guaifenesin and pseudoephedrine *on page 419*

GR38032R *see* ondansetron *on page 645*

gramicidin, neomycin, and polymyxin B *see* neomycin, polymyxin B, and gramicidin *on page 611*

granisetron (gra NI se tron)

Synonyms BRL 43694

U.S./Canadian Brand Names Kytril® [US/Can]

Therapeutic Category Selective 5-HT_3 Receptor Antagonist

Use Prophylaxis of chemotherapy-related emesis; prophylaxis of nausea and vomiting associated with radiation therapy, including total body irradiation and fractionated abdominal radiation; prophylaxis of postoperative nausea and vomiting (PONV)

Generally **not** recommended for treatment of existing chemotherapy-induced emesis (CIE) or for prophylaxis of nausea from agents with a low emetogenic potential.

Usual Dosage

Oral: Adults:

Prophylaxis of chemotherapy-related emesis: 2 mg once daily up to 1 hour before chemotherapy or 1 mg twice daily; the first 1 mg dose should be given up to 1 hour before chemotherapy.

Prophylaxis of radiation therapy-associated emesis: 2 mg once daily given 1 hour before radiation therapy.

I.V.:

Children ≥2 years and Adults: Prophylaxis of chemotherapy-related emesis:

Within U.S.: 10 mcg/kg/dose (or 1 mg/dose) administered IVPB over 5 minutes given within 30 minutes of chemotherapy: for some drugs (eg, carboplatin, cyclophosphamide) with a later onset of emetic action, 10 mcg/kg every 12 hours may be necessary.

Outside U.S.: 40 mcg/kg/dose (or 3 mg/dose); maximum: 9 mg/24 hours

Breakthrough: Repeat the dose 2-3 times within the first 24 hours as necessary **(not based on controlled trials, or generally recommended)**

(Continued)

granisetron *(Continued)*

Adults: PONV:

Prevention: 1 mg given undiluted over 30 seconds; administer before induction of anesthesia or before reversal of anesthesia

Treatment: 1 mg given undiluted over 30 seconds

Dosage Forms

Injection, solution: 1 mg/mL (4 mL) [contains benzyl alcohol]
Injection, solution [preservative free]: 1 mg/mL (1 mL)
Solution, oral: 2 mg/10 mL (30 mL) [contains sodium benzoate; orange flavor]
Tablet: 1 mg

Granulex® [US] *see* trypsin, balsam peru, and castor oil *on page 892*

granulocyte colony stimulating factor *see* filgrastim *on page 368*

granulocyte colony stimulating factor (PEG conjugate) *see* pegfilgrastim *on page 671*

granulocyte-macrophage colony stimulating factor *see* sargramostim *on page 795*

Gravol® [Can] *see* dimenhydrinate *on page 274*

Grifulvin® V [US] *see* griseofulvin *on this page*

Grifulvin® V Tablet 250 mg and 500 mg *(Discontinued)* *see page 1042*

Grisactin® *(Discontinued)* *see page 1042*

Grisactin® Ultra *(Discontinued)* *see page 1042*

griseofulvin (gri see oh FUL vin)

Sound-Alike/Look-Alike Issues

Fulvicin® may be confused with Furacin®

Synonyms griseofulvin microsize; griseofulvin ultramicrosize

U.S./Canadian Brand Names Fulvicin-U/F® [Can]; Grifulvin® V [US]; Gris-PEG® [US]

Therapeutic Category Antifungal Agent

Use Treatment of susceptible tinea infections of the skin, hair, and nails

Usual Dosage Oral:

Children >2 years:

Microsize: 10-20 mg/kg/day in single or 2 divided doses

Ultramicrosize: >2 years: 5-10 mg/kg/day in single or 2 divided doses

Adults:

Microsize: 500-1000 mg/day in single or divided doses

Ultramicrosize: 330-375 mg/day in single or divided doses; doses up to 750 mg/day have been used for infections more difficult to eradicate such as tinea unguium

Duration of therapy depends on the site of infection:

Tinea corporis: 2-4 weeks
Tinea capitis: 4-6 weeks or longer
Tinea pedis: 4-8 weeks
Tinea unguium: 3-6 months or longer

Dosage Forms

Suspension, oral, microsize (Grifulvin® V): 125 mg/5 mL (120 mL) [contains alcohol 0.2%]
Tablet, microsize (Grifulvin® V): 500 mg
Tablet, ultramicrosize: 125 mg, 250 mg, 330 mg
Gris-PEG®: 125 mg, 250 mg

griseofulvin microsize *see* griseofulvin *on this page*

griseofulvin ultramicrosize *see* griseofulvin *on this page*

Gris-PEG® [US] *see* griseofulvin *on this page*

growth hormone *see* human growth hormone *on page 437*

Guaifed® [US] *see* guaifenesin and phenylephrine *on page 418*

Guaifed-PD® [US] *see* guaifenesin and phenylephrine *on page 418*

guaifenesin (gwye FEN e sin)

Sound-Alike/Look-Alike Issues
guaifenesin may be confused with guanfacine
Mucinex® may be confused with Mucomyst®
Naldecon® may be confused with Nalfon®

Synonyms GG; glycerol guaiacolate

U.S./Canadian Brand Names Allfen Jr [US]; Balminil® Expectorant [Can]; Benylin® E Extra Strength [Can]; Diabetic Tussin® EX [US-OTC]; Ganidin NR [US]; Guiatuss™ [US-OTC]; Koffex Expectorant [Can]; Mucinex® [US-OTC]; Naldecon Senior EX® [US-OTC]; Organ-1 NR [US]; Organidin® NR [US]; Phanasin® Diabetic Choice [US-OTC]; Phanasin [US-OTC]; Q-Tussin [US-OTC]; Robitussin® [US-OTC/Can]; Scot-Tussin® Expectorant [US-OTC]; Siltussin DAS [US-OTC]; Siltussin SA [US-OTC]; Tussin [US-OTC]

Therapeutic Category Expectorant

Use Help loosen phlegm and thin bronchial secretions to make coughs more productive

Usual Dosage Oral:
Children:
6 months to 2 years: 25-50 mg every 4 hours, not to exceed 300 mg/day
2-5 years: 50-100 mg every 4 hours, not to exceed 600 mg/day
6-11 years: 100-200 mg every 4 hours, not to exceed 1.2 g/day
Children >12 years and Adults: 200-400 mg every 4 hours to a maximum of 2.4 g/day
Extended release tablet: 600-1200 mg every 12 hours, not to exceed 2.4 g/day

Dosage Forms [DSC] = Discontinued product
Caplet, sustained release (Touro Ex®): 575 mg [DSC]
Capsule, sustained release (Humibid® Pediatric [DSC]): 300 mg
Liquid: 100 mg/5 mL (120 mL, 480 mL)
Diabetic Tussin EX®: 100 mg/5 mL (120 mL) [alcohol free, sugar free, dye free; contains phenylalanine 8.4 mg/5 mL]
Ganidin NR: 100 mg/5 mL (480 mL) [raspberry flavor]
Iophen NR: 100 mg/5 mL (480 mL)
Naldecon Senior EX®: 200 mg/5 mL (120 mL) [alcohol free, sugar free; contains sodium benzoate]
Organidin NR®: 100 mg/5 mL (480 mL) [contains sodium benzoate; raspberry flavor]
Q-Tussin: 100 mg/5 mL (120 mL, 240 mL, 480 mL, 3840 mL) [alcohol free; cherry flavor]
Siltussin DAS: 100 mg/5 mL (120 mL) [alcohol free, dye free, sugar free; strawberry flavor]
Syrup: 100 mg/5 mL (120 mL, 480 mL)
Guiatuss™: 100 mg/5 mL (120 mL, 240 mL, 480 mL) [alcohol free; fruit-mint flavor]
Phanasin: 100 mg/5 mL (120 mL, 240 mL) [alcohol free, sugar free; mint flavor]
Phanasin® Diabetic Choice: 100 mg/5 mL (120 mL) [alcohol free, sugar free; mint flavor]
Robitussin®: 100 mg/5 mL (5 mL, 10 mL, 15 mL, 30 mL, 120 mL, 240 mL, 480 mL) [alcohol free; contains sodium benzoate]
Scot-Tussin® Expectorant: 100 mg/5 mL (120 mL) [alcohol free, dye free, sugar free; contains benzoic acid; grape flavor]
Siltussin SA: 100 mg/5 mL (120 mL, 240 mL, 480 mL) [alcohol free, sugar free; strawberry flavor]
Tussin: 100 mg/5 mL (120 mL, 240 mL)
Syrup, oral drops (Phanasin®): 50 mg/mL (50 mL) [alcohol free, sugar free; fruit flavor]
Tablet: 200 mg
Allfen Jr: 400 mg [dye free]
Organ-1 NR, Organidin® NR: 200 mg
Tablet, extended release (Mucinex®): 600 mg
Tablet, sustained release: 600 mg, 1200 mg [DSC]
Amibid LA [DSC], Humibid® LA [DSC], Liquibid® [DSC], Respa-GF® [DSC]: 600 mg
Liquibid® 1200 [DSC]: 1200 mg

guaifenesin and codeine (gwye FEN e sin & KOE deen)

Sound-Alike/Look-Alike Issues
Halotussin® may be confused with Halotestin®

Synonyms codeine and guaifenesin

U.S./Canadian Brand Names Brontex® [US]; Cheracol® [US]; Diabetic Tussin C® [US]; Gani-Tuss® NR [US]; Guiatuss AC® [US]; Halotussin AC [US]; Mytussin® AC [US]; Robafen® AC [US]; Romilar® AC [US]; Tussi-Organidin® NR [US]; Tussi-Organidin® S-NR [US]

Therapeutic Category Antitussive/Expectorant

Controlled Substance C-V

Use Temporary control of cough due to minor throat and bronchial irritation

Usual Dosage Oral:
Children:
2-6 years: 1-1.5 mg/kg codeine/day divided into 4 doses administered every 4-6 hours (maximum: 30 mg/24 hours)
6-12 years: 5 mL every 4 hours, not to exceed 30 mL/24 hours
Children >12 years and Adults: 5-10 mL every 6 hours not to exceed 60 mL/24 hours

Dosage Forms
Liquid: Guaifenesin 100 mg and codeine phosphate 10 mg per 5 mL (120 mL, 480 mL)
Brontex®: Guaifenesin 75 mg and codeine phosphate 2.5 mg per 5 mL (480 mL) [alcohol free; mint flavor]
Diabetic Tussin C®: Guaifenesin 200 mg and codeine phosphate 10 mg per 5 mL (480 mL) [contains phenylalanine 0.03 mcg/5 mL; cherry vanilla flavor]
Gani-Tuss® NR: Guaifenesin 100 mg and codeine phosphate 10 mg per 5 mL (480 mL) [sugar free, alcohol free; raspberry flavor]
Halotussin AC: Guaifenesin 100 mg and codeine phosphate 10 mg per 5 mL (120 mL, 480 mL, 3840 mL)
Tussi-Organidin® NR: Guaifenesin 100 mg and codeine phosphate 10 mg per 5 mL (480 mL) [contains sodium benzoate; raspberry flavor]
Tussi-Organidin® S-NR: Guaifenesin 100 mg and codeine phosphate 10 mg per 5 mL (120 mL) [contains sodium benzoate; raspberry flavor]
Syrup: Guaifenesin 100 mg and codeine phosphate 10 mg per 5 mL (120 mL, 480 mL)
Cheracol®: Guaifenesin 100 mg and codeine phosphate 10 mg per 5 mL (120 mL) [contains alcohol 4.75% and benzoic acid]
Guaituss AC®: Guaifenesin 100 mg and codeine phosphate 10 mg per 5 mL (120 mL, 480 mL) [contains alcohol; sugar free; fruit-mint flavor]
Mytussin® AC: Guaifenesin 100 mg and codeine phosphate 10 mg per 5 mL (120 mL, 480 mL, 3840 mL) [contains alcohol; sugar free; fruit flavor]
Robafen AC: Guaifenesin 100 mg and codeine phosphate 10 mg per 5 mL (120 mL, 480 mL)
Romilar® AC: Guaifenesin 100 mg and codeine phosphate 10 mg per 5 mL (480 mL) [contains phenylalanine; alcohol free, sugar free, dye free]
Tablet (Brontex®): Guaifenesin 300 mg and codeine phosphate 10 mg

guaifenesin and dextromethorphan
(gwye FEN e sin & deks troe meth OR fan)

Sound-Alike/Look-Alike Issues
Benylin® may be confused with Benadryl®, Ventolin®

Synonyms dextromethorphan and guaifenesin

U.S./Canadian Brand Names Aquatab® DM [US]; Balminil® DM E [Can]; Benylin® DM-E [Can]; Benylin® Expectorant [US-OTC]; Cheracol® D [US-OTC]; Cheracol® Plus [US-OTC]; Diabetic Tussin® DM Maximum Strength [US-OTC]; Diabetic Tussin® DM [US-OTC]; Duratuss® DM [US]; Fenesin™ DM [US]; Genatuss DM® [US-OTC]; Guaifenex® DM [US]; Guiatuss-DM® [US-OTC]; Humibid® DM [US]; Hydro-Tussin™ DM [US]; Koffex DM-Expectorant [Can]; Kolephrin® GG/DM [US-OTC]; Mytussin® DM [US-OTC]; Respa-DM® [US]; Robitussin® DM [US-OTC/Can]; Robitussin® Sugar Free Cough [US-OTC]; Safe Tussin® 30 [US-OTC]; Silexin® [US-OTC]; Tolu-Sed® DM [US-OTC]; Touro® DM

[US]; Tussi-Organidin® DM NR [US]; Vicks® 44E [US-OTC]; Vicks® Pediatric Formula 44E [US-OTC]; Z-Cof LA [US]

Therapeutic Category Antitussive/Expectorant

Use Temporary control of cough due to minor throat and bronchial irritation

Usual Dosage Oral: **Note:** Dosing based on dextromethorphan 10 mg/5 mL liquid/syrup or 30 mg tablet (adjust dose for alternate formulations).

Children:

2-6 years: 2.5 mL every 4 hours (maximum: 6 doses/24 hours)

6-12 years: 5 mL every 4 hours (maximum: 6 doses/24 hours) **or** 1 tablet every 12 hours (maximum: 2 tablets/24 hours)

≥12 years: See Adults dosing

Adults: 10 mL every 4 hours (maximum: 6 doses/24 hours) **or** 1-2 tablets every 12 hours (maximum: 4 tablets/24 hours)

Dosage Forms

Liquid: Guaifenesin 100 mg and dextromethorphan hydrobromide 10 mg per 5 mL (120 mL, 240 mL)

Diabetic Tussin® DM: Guaifenesin 100 mg and dextromethorphan hydrobromide 10 mg per 5 mL (120 mL) [alcohol free, sugar free, dye free; contains phenylalanine 8.4 mg/5 mL]

Diabetic Tussin® DM Maximum Strength: Guaifenesin 200 mg and dextromethorphan hydrobromide 10 mg per 5 mL (120 mL) [alcohol free, sugar free, dye free; contains phenylalanine 8.4 mg/5 mL]

Duratuss® DM: Guaifenesin 200 mg and dextromethorphan hydrobromide 20 mg per 5 mL (480 mL, 3840 mL) [contains alcohol 5%, sodium benzoate; fruit flavor]

Hydro-Tussin™ DM: Guaifenesin 200 mg and dextromethorphan hydrobromide 20 mg per 5 mL (480 mL) [alcohol free, sugar free]

Robitussin® Sugar Free Cough: Guaifenesin 100 mg and dextromethorphan hydrobromide 10 mg per 5 mL (120 mL) [alcohol free, sugar free]

Safe Tussin® 30: Guaifenesin 100 mg and dextromethorphan hydrobromide 15 mg per 5 mL (120 mL) [alcohol free, sugar free, dye free; mint flavor]

Tussi-Organidin® DM NR: Guaifenesin 100 mg and dextromethorphan hydrobromide 10 mg per 5 mL (120 mL, 480 mL) [contains sodium benzoate; raspberry flavor]

Vicks® 44E: Guaifenesin 200 mg and dextromethorphan hydrobromide 20 mg per 15 mL (120 mL, 235 mL) [contains sodium 31 mg/15 mL, alcohol, sodium benzoate]

Vicks® Pediatric Formula 44E: Guaifenesin 100 mg and dextromethorphan hydrobromide 10 mg per 15 mL (120 mL) [alcohol free; contains sodium 30 mg/15 mL, sodium benzoate; cherry flavor]

Syrup: Guaifenesin 100 mg and dextromethorphan hydrobromide 10 mg per 5 mL (120 mL, 240 mL, 480 mL)

Benylin® Expectorant: Guaifenesin 100 mg and dextromethorphan hydrobromide 5 mg per 5 mL (120 mL) [alcohol free, sugar free; contains sodium benzoate; raspberry flavor]

Cheracol® D: Guaifenesin 100 mg and dextromethorphan hydrobromide 10 mg per 5 mL (120 mL, 180 mL) [contains alcohol, benzoic acid]

Cheracol® Plus: Guaifenesin 100 mg and dextromethorphan hydrobromide 10 mg per 5 mL (120 mL)

Genatuss DM®: Guaifenesin 100 mg and dextromethorphan hydrobromide 10 mg per 5 mL (120 mL) [cherry flavor]

Guiatuss® DM: Guaifenesin 100 mg and dextromethorphan hydrobromide 10 mg per 5 mL (120 mL, 240 mL, 480 mL, 3840 mL) [alcohol free; fruit-mint flavor]

Kolephrin® GG/DM: Guaifenesin 150 mg and dextromethorphan hydrobromide 10 mg per 5 mL (120 mL) [alcohol free; cherry flavor]

Mytussin® DM: Guaifenesin 100 mg and dextromethorphan hydrobromide 10 mg per 5 mL (120 mL, 480 mL) [alcohol free; cherry flavor]

Robitussin®-DM: Guaifenesin 100 mg and dextromethorphan hydrobromide 10 mg per 5 mL (5 mL, 120 mL, 360 mL, 480 mL) [alcohol free]

Silexin®: Guaifenesin 100 mg and dextromethorphan hydrobromide 10 mg per 5 mL (45 mL, 480 mL)

(Continued)

guaifenesin and dextromethorphan *(Continued)*

Tolu-Sed®: Guaifenesin 100 mg and dextromethorphan hydrobromide 10 mg per 5 mL (120 mL)

Tablet (Silexin®): Guaifenesin 100 mg and dextromethorphan hydrobromide 10 mg

Tablet, extended release: Guaifenesin 600 mg and dextromethorphan hydrobromide 30 mg

Aquatab® DM: Guaifenesin 1200 mg and dextromethorphan hydrobromide 60 mg

Fenesin™ DM, Guaifenex® DM, Humibid® DM, Respa-DM®: Guaifenesin 600 mg and dextromethorphan hydrobromide 30 mg

Touro® DM: Guaifenesin 575 mg and dextromethorphan hydrobromide 30 mg

Tablet, long acting [scored] (Z-Cof LA): Guaifenesin 650 mg and dextromethorphan hydrobromide 30 mg

guaifenesin and hydrocodone *see* hydrocodone and guaifenesin *on page 445*

guaifenesin and phenylephrine (gwye FEN e sin & fen il EF rin)

Sound-Alike/Look-Alike Issues

Endal® may be confused with Depen®, Intal®

Entex® may be confused with Tenex®

Synonyms guaifenesin and phenylephrine tannate; phenylephrine hydrochloride and guaifenesin

U.S./Canadian Brand Names Aldex™ [US]; Amidal [US]; Ami-Tex LA [US]; Crantex ER [US]; Crantex LA [US]; Deconsal® II [US]; Endal® [US]; Entex® [US]; Entex® ER [US]; Entex® LA [US]; Guaifed® [US]; Guaifed-PD® [US]; Liquibid-D [US]; Liquibid-PD [US]; PhenaVent™ [US]; PhenaVent™ D [US]; PhenaVent™ Ped [US]; Prolex™-D [US]; Rescon GG [US]; Sil-Tex [US]; Sina-12X [US]; SINUvent® PE [US]

Therapeutic Category Cold Preparation

Use Temporary relief of nasal congestion, sinusitis, rhinitis and hay fever; temporary relief of cough associated with upper respiratory tract conditions, especially when associated with dry, nonproductive cough

Usual Dosage Oral:

Children 2-6 years:

Entex®, Rescon GG, Sil-Tex: 2.5 mL every 4-6 hours; maximum 10 mL/24 hours

Sina-12X suspension: 2.5-5 mL every 12 hours

Children 6-12 years:

Aldex™, Crantex LA, Liquibid-D, PhenaVent™ D, Sina-12X tablet: One-half tablet every 12 hours (maximum: 1 tablet/24 hours)

Deconsol® II: One capsule daily

Entex®, Rescon GG: 5 mL every 4-6 hours (maximum: 20 mL/24 hours)

Guaifed-PD®, PhenaVent™ Ped: One capsule every 12 hours

Liquibid-PD, SINUvent® PE: One tablet every 12 hours (maximum: 2 tablets/24 hours)

Prolex™D: One-half to 1 tablet every 12 hours

Sina-12X suspension: Refer to Adults dosing.

Children ≥12 years:

Aldex™, Crantex LA, Deconsol® II, Entex®, Entex® LA, Guaifed®, Guaifed-PD®, Liquibid-D, Liquibid-PD, PhenaVent™, PhenaVent™ D, PhenaVent™ Ped, Prolex™ D, Rescon GG, Sil-Tex, Sina-12X, SINUvent® PE: Refer to Adults dosing

Crantex ER, Entex® ER: One capsule every 12 hours

Adults:

Aldex™, Crantex LA, Liquibid-D, PhenaVent™ D: One tablet every 12 hours

Crantex ER, Entex® ER, Guaifed-PD®, PhenaVent™ Ped: 1-2 capsules every 12 hours

Deconsol® II: 1-2 capsules every 12 hours (maximum: 3 capsules/24 hours)

Endal®, Prolex™ D: 1-2 tablets every 12 hours

Entex®, Sil-Tex: 5-10 mL every 4-6 hours (maximum: 40 mL/24 hours)

Entex® LA, Guaifed®, PhenaVent™: One capsule every 12 hours (maximum: 2 capsules/24 hours)

Liquibid-PD, Sina-12X tablet: 1-2 tablets every 12 hours (maximum: 4 tablets/24 hours)

Rescon GG: 10 mL every 4-6 hours (maximum: 40 mL/24 hours)

Sina-12X suspension: 5-10 mL every 12 hours
SINUvent® PE: Two tablets every 12 hours

Dosage Forms

Capsule, variable release:
Crantex ER, Entex® ER: Guaifenesin 300 mg [immediate release] and phenylephrine hydrochloride 10 mg [extended release]
Deconsal® II: Guaifenesin 375 mg [immediate release] and phenylephrine hydrochloride 20 mg [extended release] [contains tartrazine]
Entex® LA: Guaifenesin 400 mg [immediate release] and phenylephrine hydrochloride 30 mg [extended release]
Guaifed®, PhenaVent™: Guaifenesin 400 mg [immediate release] and phenylephrine hydrochloride 15 mg [extended release]
Guaifed-PD®, PhenaVent™ Ped: Guaifenesin 200 mg [immediate release] and phenylephrine hydrochloride 7.5 mg [extended release]
Liquid: Guaifenesin 100 mg and phenylephrine hydrochloride 7.5 mg per 5 mL (480 mL)
Entex®, Sil-Tex: Guaifenesin 100 mg and phenylephrine hydrochloride 7.5 mg per 5 mL (480 mL) [alcohol free, dye-free, sugar free; punch flavor]
Rescon GG: Guaifenesin 100 mg and phenylephrine hydrochloride 5 mg per 5 mL (120 mL, 480 mL) [cherry orange-pineapple flavor]
Suspension (Sina-12X): Guaifenesin 100 mg and phenylephrine tannate 5 mg per 5 mL (120 mL) [contains benzoic acid; grape flavor]
Tablet:
Amidal: Guaifenesin 300 mg and phenylephrine hydrochloride 20 mg
Sina-12X: Guaifenesin 200 mg and phenylephrine tannate 25 mg
Tablet, extended release: Guaifenesin 600 mg and phenylephrine hydrochloride 20 mg; Guaifenesin 600 mg and phenylephrine hydrochloride 40 mg; Guaifenesin 1200 mg and phenylephrine hydrochloride 40 mg
Aldex™: Guaifenesin 650 mg and phenylephrine hydrochloride 25 mg
Ami-Tex LA: Guaifenesin 600 mg and phenylephrine hydrochloride 30 mg
Liquibid-D: Guaifenesin 600 mg and phenylephrine hydrochloride 40 mg
Liquibid-PD: Guaifenesin 275 mg and phenylephrine hydrochloride 25 mg
PhenaVent™ D: Guaifenesin 1200 mg and phenylephrine hydrochloride 40 mg
SINUvent® PE: Guaifenesin 600 mg and phenylephrine hydrochloride 15 mg
Tablet, sustained release: Guaifenesin 600 mg and phenylephrine hydrochloride 30 mg
Crantex-LA: Guaifenesin 600 mg and phenylephrine hydrochloride 30 mg [dye-free]
Prolex™D: Guaifenesin 600 mg and phenylephrine hydrochloride 20 mg [dye-free]
Tablet, timed release (Endal®): Guaifenesin 300 mg and phenylephrine hydrochloride 20 mg

guaifenesin and phenylephrine tannate *see* guaifenesin and phenylephrine *on previous page*

guaifenesin and pseudoephedrine (gwye FEN e sin & soo doe e FED rin)

Sound-Alike/Look-Alike Issues

Entex® may be confused with Tenex®

Synonyms pseudoephedrine and guaifenesin

U.S./Canadian Brand Names Ambifed-G [US]; Ami-Tex PSE [US]; Aquatab® D [US]; Congestac® [US-OTC]; Dynex [US]; Entex® PSE [US]; Eudal®-SR [US]; G-Phed [US]; Guaifenex® GP [US]; Guaifenex® PSE [US]; Guaifenex®-Rx [US]; Guaimax-D® [US]; Levall G [US]; Maxifed® [US]; Maxifed-G® [US]; Miraphen PSE [US]; Mucinex®-D [US]; Nasatab® LA [US]; Novahistex® Expectorant With Decongestant [Can]; PanMist® Jr. [US]; PanMist® LA [US]; PanMist® S [US]; Profen Forte® [US]; Profen® II [US]; Pseudoevent™ 400 [US]; Pseudo GG TR [US]; Pseudovent™ [US]; Pseudovent™-Ped [US]; Refenesen Plus [US-OTC]; Respaire®-60 SR [US]; Respaire®-120 SR [US]; Robitussin-PE® [US-OTC]; Robitussin® Severe Congestion [US-OTC]; Sudafed® Non-Drying Sinus [US-OTC]; Touro LA® [US]; Zephrex® [US]; Zephrex LA® [US]

Therapeutic Category Expectorant/Decongestant

Use Temporary relief of nasal congestion and to help loosen phlegm and thin bronchial secretions in the treatment of cough

(Continued)

guaifenesin and pseudoephedrine *(Continued)*

Usual Dosage Oral:

Children 2-6 years:

Guaifenex® PSE 60: One-half tablet every 12 hours (maximum: 1 tablet/12 hours)
Maxifed-G: One-third to 1/2 tablet every 12 hours (maximum: 1 tablet/12 hours)
PanMist® S: 2.5 mL 4 times/day (maximum: Pseudoephedrine 4 mg/kg/day)
Robitussin® PE: 2.5 mL every 4-6 hours (maximum: 4 doses/24 hours)

Children 6-12 years:

Ambifed-G, Dynex, Eudal-SR, Guaimax-D®, Guaifenex® PSE 80, Guaifenex® PSE 120, Maxifed, Miraphen PSE, Nasatab LA, PanMist® LA, Profen II®, Profen Forte®, Zephrex® LA: One-half caplet or tablet every 12 hours (maximum: 1 tablet/24 hours)
Congestac®: One-half caplet every 4-6 hours (maximum: 2 caplets/24 hours)
Guaifenex® PSE 60, PanMist®-Jr, Pseudovent™-Ped, Respaire®-60 SR: One tablet or capsule every 12 hours (maximum: 2 tablets or capsules every 24 hours)
Levall-G: One capsule every 24 hours
Maxifed-G: One-half to 1 tablet every 12 hours (maximum: 2 tablets/24 hours)
PanMist® S: 5 mL 4 times/day (maximum: Pseudoephedrine 4 mg/kg/day)
Robitussin® PE: 5 mL every 4-6 hours (maximum: 4 doses/24 hours)
Robitussin® Severe Congestion: One capsule every 4 hours (maximum: 4 doses/24 hours)
Zephrex®: One-half tablet every 6 hours

Children >12 years and Adults:

Ambifed-G, Aquatab® D, Dynex, Entex® PSE, Eudal- SR, G-Phed, Guaifenex® GP, Guaifenex® PSE 120, Guaimax-D®, Levall-G, Miraphen PSE, Mucinex®-D 1200/120, Nasatab LA, PanMist® LA, Profen Forte®, Pseudovent™, Respaire®-120 SR, Touro LA, Zephrex® LA: One tablet or capsule every 12 hours (maximum: 2 tablets or capsules in 24 hours)
Congestac®: One caplet every 4-6 hours (maximum: 4 caplets in 24 hours)
Guaifenex® PSE 60, Maxifed-G, Mucinex®-D 600/60, PanMist®-Jr, Pseudovent™-Ped, Respaire®-60 SR: 1-2 tablets or capsules every 12 hours (maximum: 4 tablets or capsules/24 hours)
Guaifenex® PSE 80, PanMist®-LA: One tablet every twelve hours (maximum: 3 tablets/24 hours)
Guaifenex® RX: 1-2 of the AM tablets every morning and 1-2 of the PM tablets 12 hours following morning dose
Maxifed, Profen II®: One to 1 1/2 tablets every 12 hours (maximum: 3 tablets/24 hours)
PanMist® S: Up to 10 mL 4 times/day
Robitussin® PE: 10 mL every 4-6 hours (maximum: 4 doses/24 hours)
Robitussin® Severe Congestion, Sudafed® Non-Drying Sinus: Two capsules every 4 hours (maximum: 4 doses/24 hours)
Zepthrex®: One tablet every 6 hours

Dosage Forms [DSC] = Discontinued product

Caplet (Congestac®, Refenesen Plus): Guaifenesin 400 mg and pseudoephedrine hydrochloride 60 mg
Caplet, long acting (Touro LA®): Guaifenesin 500 mg and pseudoephedrine hydrochloride 120 mg
Caplet, prolonged release (Ambifed-G): Guaifenesin 1000 mg and pseudoephedrine hydrochloride 60 mg
Capsule, extended release:
Respaire®-60 SR: Guaifenesin 200 mg and pseudoephedrine hydrochloride 60 mg
Respaire®-120 SR: Guaifenesin 250 mg and pseudoephedrine hydrochloride 120 mg
Capsule, liquicap (Sudafed® Non-Drying Sinus): Guaifenesin 200 mg and pseudoephedrine hydrochloride 30 mg
Capsule, softgel (Robitussin® Severe Congestion): Guaifenesin 200 mg and pseudoephedrine hydrochloride 30 mg
Capsule, variable release:
Entex® PSE: Guaifenesin 400 mg [immediate release] and pseudoephedrine hydrochloride 120 mg [extended release]

G-Phed: Guaifenesin 250 mg [immediate release] and pseudoephedrine hydrochloride 120 mg [prolonged release]

Levall G: Guaifenesin 400 mg [immediate release] and pseudoephedrine hydrochloride 90 mg [extended release]

Pseudovent™: Guaifenesin 250 mg [immediate release] and pseudoephedrine hydrochloride 120 mg [prolonged release]

Pseudovent™-Ped: Guaifenesin 300 mg [immediate release] and pseudoephedrine hydrochloride 60 mg [prolonged release]

Pseudovent™ 400: Guaifenesin 400 mg [immediate release] and pseudoephedrine hydrochloride 1200 mg [extended release]

Combination package (Guaifenex®-Rx) [14-day treatment package; each package contains]:

Tablet, extended release: Guaifenesin 600 mg and pseudoephedrine hydrochloride 60 mg (28s) [for AM dose]

Tablet, extended release: Guaifenesin 600 mg (28s) [for PM dose]

Syrup: Guaifenesin 200 mg and pseudoephedrine hydrochloride 40 mg per 5 mL (480 mL)

PanMist®-S: Guaifenesin 200 mg and pseudoephedrine hydrochloride 40 mg per 5 mL (480 mL) [alcohol free; grape flavor]

Robitussin-PE®: Guaifenesin 100 mg and pseudoephedrine hydrochloride 30 mg per 5 mL (120 mL, 240 mL) [alcohol free; contains sodium benzoate]

Tablet: Zephrex®: Guaifenesin 400 mg and pseudoephedrine hydrochloride 60 mg

Tablet, extended release: Guaifenesin 550 mg and pseudoephedrine hydrochloride 60 mg; guaifenesin 595 mg and pseudoephedrine hydrochloride 48 mg; guaifenesin 600 mg and pseudoephedrine hydrochloride 60 mg; guaifenesin 600 mg and pseudoephedrine hydrochloride 120 mg; guaifenesin 795 mg and pseudoephedrine hydrochloride 85 mg; guaifenesin 800 mg and pseudoephedrine hydrochloride 45 mg; guaifenesin 800 mg and pseudoephedrine hydrochloride 60 mg; guaifenesin 800 mg and pseudoephedrine hydrochloride 90 mg; guaifenesin 1200 mg and pseudoephedrine hydrochloride 50 mg; guaifenesin 1200 mg and pseudoephedrine hydrochloride 60 mg; guaifenesin 1200 mg and pseudoephedrine hydrochloride 75 mg; guaifenesin 1200 mg and pseudoephedrine hydrochloride 90 mg; guaifenesin 1200 mg and pseudoephedrine hydrochloride 120 mg

Amitex PSE, Guaimax-D®, Zephrex LA®: Guaifenesin 600 mg and pseudoephedrine hydrochloride 120 mg

Aquatab® D: Guaifenesin 1200 mg and pseudoephedrine hydrochloride 75 mg

Defen-LA®: Guaifenesin 600 mg and pseudoephedrine hydrochloride 60 mg [DSC]

Guaifenex® GP: Guaifenesin 1200 mg and pseudoephedrine hydrochloride 120 mg [dye free]

Guaifenex PSE® 60: Guaifenesin 600 mg and pseudoephedrine hydrochloride 60 mg

Guaifenex PSE® 80: Guaifenesin 800 mg and pseudoephedrine hydrochloride 80 mg

Maxifed®: Guaifenesin 700 mg and pseudoephedrine hydrochloride 80 mg

Maxifed-G®: Guaifenesin 550 mg and pseudoephedrine hydrochloride 60 mg

Mucinex®-D 600/60: Guaifenesin 600 mg and pseudoephedrine hydrochloride 60 mg

Mucinex®-D 1200/120: Guaifenesin 1200 mg and pseudoephedrine hydrochloride 120 mg

PanMist®-JR, Pseudo GG TR: Guaifenesin 595 mg and pseudoephedrine hydrochloride 48 mg

PanMist®-LA: Guaifenesin 795 mg and pseudoephedrine hydrochloride 85 mg

Profen II®: Guaifenesin 800 mg and pseudoephedrine hydrochloride 45 mg

Profen Forte®: Guaifenesin 800 mg and pseudoephedrine hydrochloride 90 mg

Tablet, long acting:

Dynex: Guaifenesin 1200 mg and pseudoephedrine hydrochloride 90 mg

Guaifenex PSE® 120: Guaifenesin 600 mg and pseudoephedrine hydrochloride 120 mg [dye free]

Miraphen PSE: Guaifenesin 600 mg and pseudoephedrine hydrochloride 120 mg

Tablet, sustained release (Nasatab® LA): Guaifenesin 500 mg and pseudoephedrine hydrochloride 120 mg

guaifenesin and theophylline *see* theophylline and guaifenesin *on page 855*

guaifenesin, hydrocodone, and pseudoephedrine *see* hydrocodone, pseudoephedrine, and guaifenesin *on page 447*

guaifenesin, pseudoephedrine, and codeine

(gwye FEN e sin, soo doe e FED rin, & KOE deen)

Sound-Alike/Look-Alike Issues

Halotussin® may be confused with Halotestin®

Synonyms codeine, guaifenesin, and pseudoephedrine; pseudoephedrine, guaifenesin, and codeine

U.S./Canadian Brand Names Benylin® 3.3 mg-D-E [Can]; Calmylin with Codeine [Can]; Cheratussin DAC [US]; Codafed® Expectorant [US]; Codafed® Pediatric Expectorant [US]; Dihistine® Expectorant [US]; Guiatuss™ DAC® [US]; Halotussin® DAC [US]; Mytussin® DAC [US]; Nucofed® Expectorant [US]; Nucofed® Pediatric Expectorant [US]; Nucotuss® [US]

Therapeutic Category Antitussive/Decongestant/Expectorant

Controlled Substance C-III; C-V

Use Temporarily relieves nasal congestion and controls cough due to minor throat and bronchial irritation; helps loosen phlegm and thin bronchial secretions to make coughs more productive

Usual Dosage Oral:

Children 6-12 years: 5 mL every 4 hours, not to exceed 40 mL/24 hours

Children >12 years and Adults: 10 mL every 4 hours, not to exceed 40 mL/24 hours

Dosage Forms [DSC] = Discontinued product

Liquid:

Cheratussin DAC: Guaifenesin 100 mg, pseudoephedrine hydrochloride 30 mg, and codeine phosphate 10 mg per 5 mL (480 mL) [sugar free]

Dihistine® Expectorant: Guaifenesin 100 mg, pseudoephedrine hydrochloride 30 mg, and codeine phosphate 10 mg per 5 mL (120 mL) [contains alcohol 7.5%; fruit flavor]

Halotussin DAC: Guaifenesin 100 mg, pseudoephedrine hydrochloride 30 mg, and codeine phosphate 10 mg per 5 mL (480 mL) [sugar free; cherry-raspberry flavor]

Syrup:

Codafed® Expectorant: Guaifenesin 200 mg, pseudoephedrine hydrochloride 60 mg, and codeine phosphate 20 mg per 5 mL (480 mL) [wintergreen flavor]

Codafed® Pediatric Expectorant: Guaifenesin 100 mg, pseudoephedrine hydrochloride 30 mg, and codeine phosphate 10 mg per 5 mL (480 mL) [strawberry flavor]

Guiatuss™ DAC: Guaifenesin 100 mg, pseudoephedrine hydrochloride 30 mg, and codeine phosphate 10 mg per 5 mL (480 mL) [may contain codeine]

Robitussin®-DAC [DSC]: Guaifenesin 100 mg, pseudoephedrine hydrochloride 30 mg, and codeine phosphate 10 mg per 5 mL

Mytussin® DAC: Guaifenesin 100 mg, pseudoephedrine hydrochloride 30 mg, and codeine phosphate 10 mg per 5 mL (120 mL, 480 mL) [sugar free; contains alcohol 1.7%; strawberry-raspberry flavor]

Nucofed® Expectorant, Nucotuss® Expectorant: Guaifenesin 200 mg, pseudoephedrine hydrochloride 60 mg, and codeine phosphate 20 mg per 5 mL (480 mL) [contains alcohol 12.5%; cherry flavor]

Nucofed® Pediatric Expectorant: Guaifenesin 100 mg, pseudoephedrine hydrochloride 30 mg, and codeine phosphate 10 mg per 5 mL (480 mL) [contains alcohol 6%; strawberry flavor]

guaifenesin, pseudoephedrine, and dextromethorphan

(gwye FEN e sin, soo doe e FED rin, & deks troe meth OR fan)

Synonyms dextromethorphan, guaifenesin, and pseudoephedrine; pseudoephedrine, dextromethorphan, and guaifenesin

U.S./Canadian Brand Names Ambifed-G DM [US]; Aquatab® C [US]; Balminil® DM + Decongestant + Expectorant [Can]; Benylin® DM-D-E [Can]; Dimetapp® Cold and

Congestion [US-OTC]; Guaifenex®-Rx DM [US]; Koffex DM + Decongestant + Expectorant [Can]; Maxifed® DM [US]; Novahistex® DM Decongestant Expectorant [Can]; Novahistine® DM Decongestant Expectorant [Can]; PanMist®-DM [US]; Profen Forte® DM [US]; Profen II DM® [US]; Pseudovent™ DM [US]; Relacon-DM [US]; Robitussin® CF [US-OTC]; Robitussin® Cold and Congestion [US-OTC]; Robitussin® Cough and Cold Infant [US-OTC]; Robitussin® Cough & Cold® [Can]; Touro™ CC [US]; Tri-Vent™ DM [US]; Z-Cof DM [US]

Therapeutic Category Cold Preparation

Use Temporarily relieves nasal congestion and controls cough due to minor throat and bronchial irritation; helps loosen phlegm and thin bronchial secretions to make coughs more productive

Usual Dosage Note: Also refer to specific product labeling.

Children 2-6 years:

Maxifed DM: $^1/_3$ to $^1/_2$ tablet every 12 hours, not to exceed 1 tablet/24 hours

PanMist® DM (syrup), Tri-Vent™ DM: 2.5 mL up to 3-4 times/day, not to exceed pseudoephedrine 4 mg/kg/day

Profen II DM (syrup): 1.25-2.5 mL every 4 hours, not to exceed 15 mL/24 hours

Robitussin® Pediatric Cough and Cold Infant: 2.5 mL every 4-6 hours, not to exceed 4 doses/24 hours

Touro CC: $^1/_2$ tablet every 12 hour, not to exceed 1 tablet/24 hours

Z-Cof DM: 2.5 mL 2-3 times/day, not to exceed 7.5 mL/24 hours

Children 6-12 years:

Ambifed-G DM, Profen Forte® DM, Profen II DM®: $^1/_2$ tablet every 12 hours not to exceed 1 tablet/24 hours

Dimetapp® Cold and Congestion, Robitussin® Cold and Congestion: 1 caplet every 4-6 hours, not to exceed 4 doses/24 hours

Maxifed DM: $^1/_2$ to 1 tablet every 12 hours, not to exceed 2 tablets/24 hours

PanMist® DM (syrup), Tri-Vent™ DM: 5 mL up to 3-4 times/day, not to exceed pseudoephedrine 4 mg/kg/day

PanMist® DM (tablet), Touro CC, Pseudovent™ DM: 1 tablet every 12 hours, not to exceed 2 tablets/24 hours

Profen II DM (syrup): 2.5-5 mL every 4 hours, not to exceed 30 mL/24 hours

Z-Cof DM: 5 mL 2-3 times/day, not to exceed 15 mL/24 hours

Children ≥12 years and Adults:

Ambifed-G DM, Aquatab® C, Profen Forte® DM: 1 tablet every 12 hours not to exceed 2 tablets/24 hours

Dimetapp® Cold and Congestion, Robitussin® Cold and Congestion: 2 caplets every 4-6 hours not to exceed 4 doses in 24 hours

Guaifenex®-Rx DM: 1-2 of the "AM" tablets in the morning and 1-2 of the "PM" tablets 12 hours later

Maxifed DM, PanMist® DM (tablet), Touro CC, Pseudovent™ DM: 1-2 tablets every 12 hours, not to exceed 4 tablets/24 hours

PanMist® DM (syrup), Tri-Vent™ DM: Up to 10 mL 3-4 times/day, not to exceed pseudoephedrine 240 mg/24 hours

Profen II DM (tablet): 1 to 1$^1/_2$ tablets every 12 hours, not to exceed 3 tablets/24 hours

Profen II DM (syrup): 5-10 mL every 4 hours, not to exceed 60 mL/24 hours

Z-Cof DM: 10 mL 2-3 times/day, not to exceed 30 mL/24 hours

Dosage Forms [DSC] = Discontinued product

Caplet (Dimetapp® Cold and Congestion, Robitussin® Cold and Congestion): Guaifenesin 200 mg, pseudoephedrine hydrochloride 30 mg, and dextromethorphan hydrobromide 10 mg

Caplet, prolonged release (Ambifed-G DM): Guaifenesin 1000 mg, pseudoephedrine hydrochloride 60 mg, and dextromethorphan hydrobromide 30 mg

Caplet, sustained release (Touro™ CC): Guaifenesin 575 mg, pseudoephedrine hydrochloride 60 mg, and dextromethorphan hydrobromide 30 mg [dye free]

Capsule, softgel (Robitussin® Cold and Congestion): Guaifenesin 200 mg, pseudoephedrine hydrochloride 30 mg, and dextromethorphan hydrobromide 10 mg

(Continued)

guaifenesin, pseudoephedrine, and dextromethorphan *(Continued)*

Combination package (Guaifenex®-Rx DM) [14 day treatment package]:
- Tablet, extended release: Guaifenesin 600 mg, and pseudoephedrine hydrochloride 60 mg (28s) [for AM dose]
- Tablet, extended release: Guaifenesin 600 mg, and dextromethorphan hydrobromide 30 mg (28s) [for PM dose]

Liquid: Guaifenesin 100 mg, pseudoephedrine hydrochloride 30 mg, and dextromethorphan hydrobromide 10 mg per 5 mL (120 mL)
- Profen II DM: Guaifenesin 200 mg, pseudoephedrine hydrochloride 15 mg, and dextromethorphan hydrobromide 10 mg per 5 mL (480 mL) [alcohol free, dye free, sugar free; cherry flavor]
- Relacon-DM: Guaifenesin 200 mg, pseudoephedrine hydrochloride 40 mg, and dextromethorphan hydrobromide 15 mg (480 mL) [grape flavor]

Liquid, oral drops (Robitussin® Cough and Cold Infant): Guaifenesin 100 mg, pseudoephedrine hydrochloride 15 mg, and dextromethorphan hydrobromide 5 mg per 2.5 mL (30 mL) [alcohol free; contains sodium benzoate]

Syrup: Guaifenesin 100 mg, pseudoephedrine hydrochloride 45 mg, and dextromethorphan hydrobromide 15 mg per 5 mL (480 mL)
- PanMist®-DM: Guaifenesin 100 mg, pseudoephedrine hydrochloride 40 mg, and dextromethorphan hydrobromide 15 mg per 5 mL (480 mL) [alcohol free, dye free, sugar free; strawberry flavor]
- Robitussin® CF: Guaifenesin 100 mg, pseudoephedrine hydrochloride 30 mg, and dextromethorphan hydrobromide 10 mg per 5 mL (120 mL, 240 mL, 360 mL) [alcohol free; contains sodium benzoate]
- Tri-Vent™ DM: Guaifenesin 100 mg, pseudoephedrine hydrochloride 40 mg, and dextromethorphan hydrobromide 15 mg per 5 mL (480 mL) [alcohol free, dye free, sugar free; strawberry flavor]

Tablet, extended release: Guaifenesin 800 mg, pseudoephedrine hydrochloride 60 mg, and dextromethorphan hydrobromide 30 mg; guaifenesin 1200 mg, pseudoephedrine hydrochloride 60 mg, and dextromethorphan hydrobromide 60 mg; guaifenesin 1200 mg, pseudoephedrine hydrochloride 120 mg, and dextromethorphan hydrobromide 60 mg; guaifenesin 800 mg, pseudoephedrine hydrochloride 90 mg, and dextromethorphan hydrobromide 60 mg; guaifenesin 550 mg, pseudoephedrine hydrochloride 60 mg, and dextromethorphan hydrobromide 30 mg; guaifenesin 595 mg, pseudoephedrine hydrochloride 48 mg, and dextromethorphan hydrobromide 32 mg; guaifenesin 600 mg, pseudoephedrine hydrochloride 60 mg, and dextromethorphan hydrobromide 30 mg
- Aquatab® C: Guaifenesin 1200 mg, pseudoephedrine hydrochloride 60 mg, and dextromethorphan hydrobromide 60 mg
- PanMist®-DM, PseudoventTM DM: Guaifenesin 595 mg, pseudoephedrine hydrochloride 48 mg, and dextromethorphan hydrobromide 32 mg
- Profen Forte® DM: Guaifenesin 800 mg, pseudoephedrine hydrochloride 90 mg, and dextromethorphan hydrobromide 60 mg
- Profen II DM®: Guaifenesin 800 mg, pseudoephedrine hydrochloride 45 mg, and dextromethorphan hydrobromide 30 mg
- Protuss®-DM [DSC]: Guaifenesin 600 mg, pseudoephedrine hydrochloride 60 mg, and dextromethorphan hydrobromide 30 mg

Tablet, sustained release (Maxifed® DM): Guaifenesin 550 mg, pseudoephedrine hydrochloride 60 mg, and dextromethorphan hydrobromide 30 mg [dye free]

Guaifenex® *(Discontinued)* *see page 1042*

Guaifenex® DM [US] *see* guaifenesin and dextromethorphan *on page 416*

Guaifenex® GP [US] *see* guaifenesin and pseudoephedrine *on page 419*

Guaifenex® PPA 75 *(Discontinued)* *see page 1042*

Guaifenex® PSE [US] *see* guaifenesin and pseudoephedrine *on page 419*

Guaifenex®-Rx [US] *see* guaifenesin and pseudoephedrine *on page 419*

Guaifenex®-Rx DM [US] *see* guaifenesin, pseudoephedrine, and dextromethorphan *on page 422*

Guaimax-D® [US] *see* guaifenesin and pseudoephedrine *on page 419*

Guaipax® ***(Discontinued)*** *see page 1042*

Guaitab® ***(Discontinued)*** *see page 1042*

Guaituss CF® ***(Discontinued)*** *see page 1042*

Guaivent® ***(Discontinued)*** *see page 1042*

guanabenz (GWAHN a benz)

Sound-Alike/Look-Alike Issues
guanabenz may be confused with guanadrel, guanfacine
Synonyms guanabenz acetate
U.S./Canadian Brand Names Wytensin® [Can]
Therapeutic Category Alpha-Adrenergic Agonist
Use Management of hypertension
Usual Dosage Adults: Oral: Initial: 4 mg twice daily; increase in increments of 4-8 mg/day every 1-2 weeks to a maximum of 32 mg twice daily.
Dosage Forms Tablet: 4 mg, 8 mg

guanabenz acetate *see* guanabenz *on this page*

guanfacine (GWAHN fa seen)

Sound-Alike/Look-Alike Issues
guanfacine may be confused with guaifenesin, guanabenz, guanidine
Tenex® may be confused with Entex®, Ten-K®, Xanax®
Synonyms guanfacine hydrochloride
U.S./Canadian Brand Names Tenex® [US/Can]
Therapeutic Category Alpha-Adrenergic Agonist
Use Management of hypertension
Usual Dosage Adults: Oral: Hypertension: 1 mg usually at bedtime, may increase if needed at 3- to 4-week intervals; usual dose range (JNC 7): 0.5-2 mg once daily
Dosage Forms Tablet: 1 mg, 2 mg

guanfacine hydrochloride *see* guanfacine *on this page*

guanidine (GWAHN i deen)

Sound-Alike/Look-Alike Issues
guanidine may be confused with guanfacine, guanethidine
Synonyms guanidine hydrochloride
Therapeutic Category Cholinergic Agent
Use Reduction of the symptoms of muscle weakness associated with the myasthenic syndrome of Eaton-Lambert, not for myasthenia gravis
Usual Dosage Adults: Oral: Eaton-Lambert syndrome: Initial: 10-15 mg/kg/day in 3-4 divided doses, gradually increase to 35 mg/kg/day or up to development of side effects
Dosage Forms Tablet, as hydrochloride: 125 mg

guanidine hydrochloride *see* guanidine *on this page*

GuiaCough® ***(Discontinued)*** *see page 1042*

GuiaCough® Expectorant ***(Discontinued)*** *see page 1042*

Guiatex® ***(Discontinued)*** *see page 1042*

Guiatuss AC® [US] *see* guaifenesin and codeine *on page 416*

Guiatuss™ DAC® [US] *see* guaifenesin, pseudoephedrine, and codeine *on page 422*

Guiatuss-DM® [US-OTC] *see* guaifenesin and dextromethorphan *on page 416*

Guiatuss™ [US-OTC] *see* guaifenesin *on page 415*

gum benjamin *see* benzoin *on page 109*

GVG *see* vigabatrin *(Canada only) on page 911*

GW433908G *see* fosamprenavir *on page 389*

G-well® *(Discontinued)* *see page 1042*

Gynazole-1® [US] *see* butoconazole *on page 139*

Gyne-Lotrimin® 3 [US-OTC] *see* clotrimazole *on page 218*

Gyne-Sulf® *(Discontinued)* *see page 1042*

Gynodiol® [US] *see* estradiol *on page 324*

Gynogen® Injection *(Discontinued)* *see page 1042*

Gynogen L.A.® Injection *(Discontinued)* *see page 1042*

Gynol II® [US-OTC] *see* nonoxynol 9 *on page 626*

Habitrol® [Can] *see* nicotine *on page 618*

Haemophilus B conjugate and hepatitis B vaccine

(hem OF fi lus bee KON joo gate & hep a TYE tis bee vak SEEN)

Sound-Alike/Look-Alike Issues

Comvax® may be confused with Recombivax®

Synonyms *Haemophilus* b (meningococcal protein conjugate) conjugate vaccine; Hib

U.S./Canadian Brand Names Comvax® [US]

Therapeutic Category Vaccine, Inactivated Virus

Use

Immunization against invasive disease caused by *H. influenzae* type b and against infection caused by all known subtypes of hepatitis B virus in infants 8 weeks to 15 months of age born of HB_sAg-negative mothers

Infants born of HB_sAg-positive mothers or mothers of unknown HB_sAg status should receive hepatitis B immune globulin and hepatitis B vaccine (recombinant) at birth and should complete the hepatitis B vaccination series given according to a particular schedule

Usual Dosage Infants (>8 weeks of age): I.M.: 0.5 mL at 2, 4, and 12-15 months of age (total of 3 doses)

If the recommended schedule cannot be followed, the interval between the first two doses should be at least 2 months and the interval between the second and third dose should be as close as possible to 8-11 months.

Modified Schedule: Children who receive one dose of hepatitis B vaccine at or shortly after birth may receive Comvax® on a schedule of 2, 4, and 12-15 months of age

Dosage Forms Injection, suspension [preservative free]: 7.5 mcg *Haemophilus* b PRP and 5 mcg HB_sAg/0.5 mL (0.5 mL)

Haemophilus B conjugate vaccine

(hem OF fi lus bee KON joo gate vak SEEN)

Synonyms diphtheria CRM_{197} protein conjugate; diphtheria toxoid conjugate; *Haemophilus* b oligosaccharide conjugate vaccine; *Haemophilus* b polysaccharide vaccine; HbCV; Hib polysaccharide conjugate; PRP-D

U.S./Canadian Brand Names ActHIB® [US/Can]; HibTITER® [US]; PedvaxHIB® [US/Can]

Therapeutic Category Vaccine, Inactivated Bacteria

Use Routine immunization of children 2 months to 5 years of age against invasive disease caused by *H. influenzae*

Unimmunized children ≥5 years of age with a chronic illness known to be associated with increased risk of *Haemophilus influenzae* type b disease, specifically, persons with anatomic or functional asplenia or sickle cell anemia or those who have undergone splenectomy, should receive Hib vaccine.

Haemophilus b conjugate vaccines are not indicated for prevention of bronchitis or other infections due to *H. influenzae* in adults; adults with specific dysfunction or certain complement deficiencies who are at especially high risk of *H. influenzae* type b infection (HIV-infected adults); patients with Hodgkin disease (vaccinated at least 2 weeks before the initiation of chemotherapy or 3 months after the end of chemotherapy)

Usual Dosage Children: I.M.: 0.5 mL as a single dose should be administered

Dosage Forms [DSC] = Discontinued product

Injection, powder for reconstitution (ActHIB®) [preservative free]: *Haemophilus* b capsular polysaccharide 10 mcg and tetanus toxoid 24 mcg per dose [may be reconstituted with provided diluent (forms solution), AvP DTP vaccine, or TriHIBit® (forms suspension)]

Injection, solution (HibTITER®): *Haemophilus* b saccharide 10 mcg and diphtheria CRM 197 protein 25 mcg per 0.5 mL (0.5 mL [preservative free], 5 mL [DSC; contains thimerosal])

Injection, suspension (PedvaxHIB®): *Haemophilus* b capsular polysaccharide 7.5 mcg and *Neisseria meningitidis* OMPC 125 mcg per 0.5 mL (0.5 mL) [contains aluminum 225 mcg/0.5 mL]

***Haemophilus* b (meningococcal protein conjugate) conjugate vaccine** *see* *Haemophilus* B conjugate and hepatitis B vaccine *on previous page*

***Haemophilus* b oligosaccharide conjugate vaccine** *see* *Haemophilus* B conjugate vaccine *on previous page*

***Haemophilus* b polysaccharide vaccine** *see* *Haemophilus* B conjugate vaccine *on previous page*

***Haemophilus influenzae* b conjugate vaccine and diphtheria, tetanus toxoids, and acellular pertussis vaccine** *see* diphtheria, tetanus toxoids, and acellular pertussis vaccine and *Haemophilus* b conjugate vaccine *on page 281*

halazone tablet *(Discontinued)* *see page 1042*

halcinonide (hal SIN oh nide)

Sound-Alike/Look-Alike Issues

halcinonide may be confused with Halcion®

Halog® may be confused with Haldol®, Mycolog®

U.S./Canadian Brand Names Halog® [US/Can]

Therapeutic Category Corticosteroid, Topical

Use Inflammation of corticosteroid-responsive dermatoses [high potency topical corticosteroid]

Usual Dosage Children and Adults: Topical: Steroid-responsive dermatoses: Apply sparingly 1-3 times/day, occlusive dressing may be used for severe or resistant dermatoses; a thin film is effective; do not overuse. Therapy should be discontinued when control is achieved; if no improvement is seen, reassessment of diagnosis may be necessary.

Dosage Forms [DSC] = Discontinued product

Cream (Halog®): 0.1% (15 g, 30 g, 60 g, 240 g)

Cream, emollient base (Halog®-E): 0.1% (30 g, 60 g) [DSC]

Ointment (Halog®): 0.1% (15 g, 30 g, 60 g, 240 g)

Solution, topical (Halog®): 0.1% (20 mL, 60 mL)

Halcion® [US/Can] *see* triazolam *on page 883*

Haldol® [US] *see* haloperidol *on next page*

Haldol® Decanoate [US] *see* haloperidol *on next page*

Haldrone® *(Discontinued)* *see page 1042*

Halenol® Tablet *(Discontinued)* *see page 1042*

Haley's M-O *see* magnesium hydroxide and mineral oil emulsion *on page 538*

Halfan® *(Discontinued)* *see page 1042*

HalfLytely® and Bisacodyl [US] *see* polyethylene glycol-electrolyte solution and bisacodyl *on page 707*

Halfprin® [US-OTC] *see* aspirin *on page 80*

halobetasol (hal oh BAY ta sol)

Sound-Alike/Look-Alike Issues

Ultravate® may be confused with Cutivate™

Synonyms halobetasol propionate

U.S./Canadian Brand Names Ultravate® [US/Can]

Therapeutic Category Corticosteroid, Topical

Use Relief of inflammatory and pruritic manifestations of corticosteroid-response dermatoses [super high potency topical corticosteroid]

Usual Dosage Children ≥12 years and Adults: Topical: Steroid-responsive dermatoses: Apply sparingly to skin twice daily, rub in gently and completely; treatment should not exceed 2 consecutive weeks and total dosage should not exceed 50 g/week. Therapy should be discontinued when control is achieved; if no improvement is seen, reassessment of diagnosis may be necessary.

Dosage Forms

Cream, as propionate: 0.05% (15 g, 50 g)

Ointment, as propionate: 0.05% (15 g, 50 g)

halobetasol propionate *see* halobetasol *on this page*

Halog® [US/Can] *see* halcinonide *on previous page*

Halog®-E *(Discontinued)* *see page 1042*

haloperidol (ha loe PER i dole)

Sound-Alike/Look-Alike Issues

haloperidol may be confused Halotestin®

Haldol® may be confused with Halcion®, Halenol®, Halog®, Halotestin®, Stadol®

Synonyms haloperidol decanoate; haloperidol lactate

U.S./Canadian Brand Names Apo-Haloperidol® [Can]; Apo-Haloperidol LA® [Can]; Haldol® [US]; Haldol® Decanoate [US]; Haloperidol-LA Omega [Can]; Haloperidol Long Acting [Can]; Novo-Peridol [Can]; Peridol [Can]; PMS-Haloperidol LA [Can]

Therapeutic Category Antipsychotic Agent, Butyrophenone

Use Management of schizophrenia; control of tics and vocal utterances of Tourette disorder in children and adults; severe behavioral problems in children

Usual Dosage

Children: 3-12 years (15-40 kg): Oral:

Initial: 0.05 mg/kg/day or 0.25-0.5 mg/day given in 2-3 divided doses; increase by 0.25-0.5 mg every 5-7 days; maximum: 0.15 mg/kg/day

Usual maintenance:

Agitation or hyperkinesia: 0.01-0.03 mg/kg/day once daily

Nonpsychotic disorders: 0.05-0.075 mg/kg/day in 2-3 divided doses

Psychotic disorders: 0.05-0.15 mg/kg/day in 2-3 divided doses

Children 6-12 years: Sedation/psychotic disorders: I.M. (as lactate): 1-3 mg/dose every 4-8 hours to a maximum of 0.15 mg/kg/day; change over to oral therapy as soon as able

Adults:

Psychosis:

Oral: 0.5-5 mg 2-3 times/day; usual maximum: 30 mg/day

I.M. (as lactate): 2-5 mg every 4-8 hours as needed

I.M. (as decanoate): Initial: 10-20 times the daily oral dose administered at 4-week intervals

Maintenance dose: 10-15 times initial oral dose; used to stabilize psychiatric symptoms

Dosage Forms Note: Strength expressed as base:
Injection, oil, as decanoate (Haldol® Decanoate): 50 mg/mL (1 mL, 5 mL); 100 mg/mL (1 mL, 5 mL) [contains benzyl alcohol, sesame oil]
Injection, solution, as lactate (Haldol®): 5 mg/mL (1 mL, 10 mL)
Solution, oral concentrate, as lactate: 2 mg/mL (15 mL, 120 mL)
Tablet: 0.5 mg, 1 mg, 2 mg, 5 mg, 10 mg, 20 mg

haloperidol decanoate *see* haloperidol *on previous page*

haloperidol lactate *see* haloperidol *on previous page*

Haloperidol-LA Omega [Can] *see* haloperidol *on previous page*

Haloperidol Long Acting [Can] *see* haloperidol *on previous page*

Halotex® ***(Discontinued)*** *see page 1042*

halothane (HA loe thane)

Sound-Alike/Look-Alike Issues
halothane may be confused with Halotestin®

Therapeutic Category General Anesthetic

Use Induction and maintenance of general anesthesia

Usual Dosage Minimum alveolar concentration (MAC), the concentration at which 50% of patients do not respond to surgical incision, is 0.74% for halothane. The concentration at which amnesia and loss of awareness occur (MAC - awake) is 0.41%. MAC is reduced in the elderly.

Dosage Forms Liquid: 125 mL, 250 mL

Halotussin® ***(Discontinued)*** *see page 1042*

Halotussin AC [US] *see* guaifenesin and codeine *on page 416*

Halotussin® DAC [US] *see* guaifenesin, pseudoephedrine, and codeine *on page 422*

Halotussin® DM ***(Discontinued)*** *see page 1042*

Halotussin® PE ***(Discontinued)*** *see page 1042*

Haltran® ***(Discontinued)*** *see page 1042*

hamamelis water *see* witch hazel *on page 934*

HandClens® [US-OTC] *see* benzalkonium chloride *on page 107*

Harmonyl® ***(Discontinued)*** *see page 1042*

Havrix® [US/Can] *see* hepatitis A vaccine *on page 432*

Hayfebrol® [US-OTC] *see* chlorpheniramine and pseudoephedrine *on page 189*

HbCV *see Haemophilus* B conjugate vaccine *on page 426*

H-BIG® ***(Discontinued)*** *see page 1042*

hbig *see* hepatitis B immune globulin *on page 433*

hBNP *see* nesiritide *on page 614*

HCG *see* chorionic gonadotropin (human) *on page 197*

HCTZ *see* hydrochlorothiazide *on page 441*

HCTZ and telmisartan *see* telmisartan and hydrochlorothiazide *on page 843*

HD 85® [US] *see* radiological/contrast media (ionic) *on page 759*

HD 200 Plus® [US] *see* radiological/contrast media (ionic) *on page 759*

HDA® Toothache [US-OTC] *see* benzocaine *on page 107*

HDCV *see* rabies virus vaccine *on page 759*

Head & Shoulders® Classic Clean 2-In-1 [US-OTC] *see* pyrithione zinc *on page 754*

Head & Shoulders® Classic Clean [US-OTC] *see* pyrithione zinc *on page 754*

Head & Shoulders® Dry Scalp Care [US-OTC] *see* pyrithione zinc *on page 754*

Head & Shoulders® Extra Fullness [US-OTC] *see* pyrithione zinc *on page 754*

Head & Shoulders® Intensive Treatment [US-OTC] *see* selenium sulfide *on page 799*

Head & Shoulders® Refresh [US-OTC] *see* pyrithione zinc *on page 754*

Head & Shoulders® Smooth & Silky 2-In-1 [US-OTC] *see* pyrithione zinc *on page 754*

Healon® ***(Discontinued)*** *see page 1042*

Healon®5 ***(Discontinued)*** *see page 1042*

Healon® GV ***(Discontinued)*** *see page 1042*

Hectorol® [US/Can] *see* doxercalciferol *on page 292*

Helidac® [US] *see* bismuth subsalicylate, metronidazole, and tetracycline *on page 121*

Helistat® [US] *see* collagen hemostat *on page 225*

Helixate® FS [US/Can] *see* antihemophilic factor (recombinant) *on page 63*

Hemabate® [US/Can] *see* carboprost tromethamine *on page 160*

HemFe® ***(Discontinued)*** *see page 1042*

hemiacidrin *see* citric acid, magnesium carbonate, and glucono-delta-lactone *on page 206*

hemin (HEE min)

U.S./Canadian Brand Names Panhematin® [US]

Therapeutic Category Blood Modifiers

Use Orphan drug: Treatment of recurrent attacks of acute intermittent porphyria (AIP) only after an appropriate period of alternate therapy has been tried

Usual Dosage I.V.: 1-4 mg/kg/day administered over 10-15 minutes for 3-14 days; may be repeated no earlier than every 12 hours; not to exceed 6 mg/kg in any 24-hour period

Dosage Forms Injection, powder for reconstitution [preservative free]: 313 mg [provides 7 mg/mL when reconstituted]

Hemocyte® [US-OTC] *see* ferrous fumarate *on page 363*

Hemofil® M [US/Can] *see* antihemophilic factor (human) *on page 62*

Hemril® HC [US] *see* hydrocortisone (rectal) *on page 448*

Hepalean® [Can] *see* heparin *on this page*

Hepalean® Leo [Can] *see* heparin *on this page*

Hepalean®-LOK [Can] *see* heparin *on this page*

heparin (HEP a rin)

Sound-Alike/Look-Alike Issues

heparin may be confused with Hespan®

Synonyms heparin calcium; heparin lock flush; heparin sodium

U.S./Canadian Brand Names Hepalean® [Can]; Hepalean® Leo [Can]; Hepalean®-LOK [Can]; Hep-Lock® [US]

Therapeutic Category Anticoagulant (Other)

Use Prophylaxis and treatment of thromboembolic disorders

Usual Dosage

Children:

Intermittent I.V.: Initial: 50-100 units/kg, then 50-100 units/kg every 4 hours

I.V. infusion: Initial: 50 units/kg, then 15-25 units/kg/hour; increase dose by 2-4 units/kg/hour every 6-8 hours as required

Adults:

Prophylaxis (low-dose heparin): SubQ: 5000 units every 8-12 hours

Intermittent I.V.: Initial: 10,000 units, then 50-70 units/kg (5000-10,000 units) every 4-6 hours

I.V. infusion (weight-based dosing per institutional nomogram recommended):

Acute coronary syndromes: MI: Fibrinolytic therapy: Alteplase or reteplase with first or second bolus: Concurrent bolus of 60 units/kg (maximum: 4000 units), then 12 units/kg/hour (maximum: 1000 units/hour) as continuous infusion. Check aPTT every 4-6 hours; adjust to target of 1.5-2 times the upper limit of control (50-70 seconds in clinical trials); usual range 10-30 units/kg/hour. Duration of heparin therapy depends on concurrent therapy and the specific patient risks for systemic or venous thromboembolism. Streptokinase: Heparin use optional depending on concurrent therapy and specific patient risks for systemic or venous thromboembolism (anterior MI, CHF, previous embolus, atrial fibrillation, LV thrombus): If heparin is administered, start when aPTT <2 times the upper limit of control; do not use a bolus, but initiate infusion adjusted to a target aPTT of 1.5-2 times the upper limit of control (50-70 seconds in clinical trials). If heparin is not administered by infusion, 7500-12,500 units SubQ every 12 hours (when aPTT <2 times the upper limit of control) is recommended. Percutaneous coronary intervention: Heparin bolus and infusion may be administered to an activated clotting time (ACT) of 300-350 seconds if no concurrent GPIIb/IIIa receptor antagonist is administered or 200-250 seconds if a GPIIb/IIIa receptor antagonist is administered. Treatment of unstable angina (high-risk and some intermediate-risk patients): Initial bolus of 60-70 units/kg (maximum: 5000 units), followed by an initial infusion of 12-15 units/kg/hour (maximum: 1000 units/hour). The American College of Chest Physicians consensus conference has recommended dosage adjustments to correspond to a therapeutic range equivalent to heparin levels of 0.3-0.7 units/mL by antifactor Xa determinations, which correlates with aPTT values between 60 and 80 seconds

Treatment of venous thromboembolism (DVT/PE): 80 units/kg I.V. push followed by continuous infusion of 18 units/kg/hour

Line flushing: When using daily flushes of heparin to maintain patency of single and double lumen central catheters, 10 units/mL is commonly used for younger infants (eg, <10 kg) while 100 units/mL is used for older infants, children, and adults. Capped PVC catheters and peripheral heparin locks require flushing more frequently (eg, every 6-8 hours). Volume of heparin flush is usually similar to volume of catheter (or slightly greater). Additional flushes should be given when stagnant blood is observed in catheter, after catheter is used for drug or blood administration, and after blood withdrawal from catheter.

Addition of heparin (0.5-3 unit/mL) to peripheral and central parenteral nutrition has not been shown to decrease catheter-related thrombosis. The final concentration of heparin used for TPN solutions may need to be decreased to 0.5 units/mL in small infants receiving larger amounts of volume in order to avoid approaching therapeutic amounts. Arterial lines are heparinized with a final concentration of 1 unit/mL.

Using a standard heparin solution (25,000 units/500 mL D_5W), the following infusion rates can be used to achieve the listed doses.

For a dose of: 400 units/hour: Infuse at 8 mL/hour 500 units/hour: Infuse at 10 mL/hour 600 units/hour: Infuse at 12 mL/hour 700 units/hour: Infuse at 14 mL/hour 800 units/hour: Infuse at 16 mL/hour 900 units/hour: Infuse at 18 mL/hour 1000 units/hour: Infuse at 20 mL/hour 1100 units/hour: Infuse at 22 mL/hour 1200 units/hour: Infuse at 24 mL/hour 1300 units/hour: Infuse at 26 mL/hour 1400 units/hour: Infuse at 28 mL/hour 1500 units/hour: Infuse at 30 mL/hour 1600 units/hour: Infuse at 32 mL/hour 1700 units/hour: Infuse at 34 mL/hour 1800 units/hour: Infuse at 36 mL/hour 1900 units/hour: Infuse at 38 mL/hour 2000 units/hour: Infuse at 40 mL/hour

Dosage Forms

Infusion, as sodium [premixed in NaCl 0.45%]: 12,500 units (250 mL); 25,000 units (250 mL, 500 mL)

(Continued)

heparin *(Continued)*

Infusion, as sodium [preservative free; premixed in D_5W; porcine intestinal mucosa source]: 10,000 units (100 mL); 12,500 units (250 mL); 20,000 units (500 mL); 25,000 units (250 mL, 500 mL) [contains sodium bisulfite]

Infusion, as sodium [preservative free; premixed in NaCl 0.9%; porcine intestinal mucosa source]: 1000 units (500 mL); 2000 units (1000 mL)

Injection, solution, as sodium [beef lung source; multidose vial]: 1000 units/mL (10 mL, 30 mL); 5000 units/mL (10 mL), 10,000 units/mL (1 mL, 4 mL) [contains benzyl alcohol]

Injection, solution, as sodium [lock flush preparation; porcine intestinal mucosa source; multidose vial]: 10 units/mL (1 mL, 10 mL, 30 mL); 100 units/mL (1 mL, 5 mL)

Injection, solution, as sodium [lock flush preparation; porcine intestinal mucosa source; multidose vial]: 10 units/mL (10 mL, 30 mL); 100 units/mL (10 mL, 30 mL) [contains benzyl alcohol]

Injection, solution, as sodium [lock flush preparation; porcine intestinal mucosa source; prefilled syringe]: 10 units/mL (1 mL, 2 mL, 2.5 mL, 3 mL, 5 mL); 100 units/mL (1 mL, 2 mL, 2.5 mL, 3 mL, 5 mL) [contains benzyl alcohol]

Injection, solution, as sodium [preservative free; lock flush preparation; porcine intestinal mucosa source; prefilled syringe]: 10 units/mL (1 mL, 2 mL, 3 mL, 5 mL, 10 mL); 100 units/mL (1 mL, 2 mL, 3 mL, 5 mL, 10 mL)

Injection, solution, as sodium [porcine intestinal mucosa source; multidose vial]: 10,000 units/mL (5 mL) [contains benzyl alcohol]

Injection, solution, as sodium [porcine intestinal mucosa source; prefilled syringe]: 1000 units/mL (1 mL); 2500 units/mL (1 mL); 5000 units/mL (0.5 mL, 1 mL); 7500 units/mL (1 mL); 10,000 units/mL (1mL); 20,000 units/mL (1 mL) [contains benzyl alcohol]

Injection, solution, as sodium [preservative free; porcine intestinal mucosa source; prefilled syringe]: 10,000 units/mL (0.25 mL, 0.5 mL, 0.75 mL, 1 mL)

Injection, solution, as sodium [preservative free; porcine intestinal mucosa source; vial]: 1000 units/mL (2 mL); 2000 units/mL (5 mL, 10 mL); 2500 units/mL (5 mL, 10 mL)

heparin calcium *see* heparin *on page 430*

heparin cofactor I *see* antithrombin III *on page 65*

heparin lock flush *see* heparin *on page 430*

heparin sodium *see* heparin *on page 430*

hepatitis A vaccine (hep a TYE tis aye vak SEEN)

U.S./Canadian Brand Names Avaxim® [Can]; Avaxim®-Pediatric [Can]; Epaxal Berna® [Can]; Havrix® [US/Can]; VAQTA® [US/Can]

Therapeutic Category Vaccine, Inactivated Virus

Use For populations desiring protection against hepatitis A or for populations at high risk of exposure to hepatitis A virus (travelers to developing countries, household and sexual contacts of persons infected with hepatitis A), child day care employees, patients with chronic liver disease, illicit drug users, male homosexuals, institutional workers (eg, institutions for the mentally and physically handicapped persons, prisons), and health-care workers who may be exposed to hepatitis A virus (eg, laboratory employees); protection lasts for approximately 15 years

Usual Dosage I.M.:

Havrix®:

Children 2-18 years: 720 ELISA units (administered as 2 injections of 360 ELISA units [0.5 mL]) 15-30 days prior to travel with a booster 6-12 months following primary immunization; the deltoid muscle should be used for I.M. injection

Adults: 1440 ELISA units (1 mL) 15-30 days prior to travel with a booster 6-12 months following primary immunization; injection should be in the deltoid

VAQTA®:

Children 2-17 years: 25 units (0.5 mL) with 25 units (0.5 mL) booster to be given 6-18 months after primary immunization

Adults: 50 units (1 mL) with 50 units (1 mL) booster to be given 6 months after primary immunization

Dosage Forms

Injection, suspension, adult [prefilled syringe; single-dose vial]:

Havrix®: Viral antigen 1440 ELISA units/mL (1 mL)

VAQTA®: HAV protein 50 units/mL (1 mL)

Injection, suspension, pediatric [prefilled syringe; single-dose vial] (Havrix®): Viral antigen 720 ELISA units/0.5 mL (0.5 mL)

Injection, suspension, pediatric/adolescent [prefilled syringe; single-dose vial] (VAQTA®): HAV protein 25 units/0.5 mL (0.5 mL)

hepatitis B immune globulin (hep a TYE tis bee i MYUN GLOB yoo lin)

Synonyms hbig

U.S./Canadian Brand Names BayHep B® [US/Can]; Nabi-HB® [US]

Therapeutic Category Immune Globulin

Use Provide prophylactic passive immunity to hepatitis B infection to those individuals exposed; newborns of mothers known to be hepatitis B surface antigen positive; hepatitis B immune globulin is not indicated for treatment of active hepatitis B infections and is ineffective in the treatment of chronic active hepatitis B infection

Usual Dosage I.M.:

Newborns: Hepatitis B: 0.5 mL as soon after birth as possible (within 12 hours); may repeat at 3 months in order for a higher rate of prevention of the carrier state to be achieved; at this time an active vaccination program with the vaccine may begin

Adults: Postexposure prophylaxis: 0.06 mL/kg as soon as possible after exposure (ie, within 24 hours of needlestick, ocular, or mucosal exposure or within 14 days of sexual exposure); usual dose: 3-5 mL; repeat at 28-30 days after exposure

Note: HBIG may be administered at the same time (but at a different site) or up to 1 month preceding hepatitis B vaccination without impairing the active immune response

Dosage Forms Note: Potency expressed in international units as compared to the WHO standard

Injection, solution [preservative free]:

BayHepB®: 217 int. units/mL (0.5 mL) [neonatal single-dose syringe]; (1 mL) [single-dose syringe or single-dose vial]; (5 mL) [single-dose vial]

Nabi-HB®: 208 int. units/mL (1 mL, 5 mL) [single-dose vial]

hepatitis B inactivated virus vaccine (plasma derived) *see* hepatitis B vaccine *on this page*

hepatitis B inactivated virus vaccine (recombinant DNA) *see* hepatitis B vaccine *on this page*

hepatitis B vaccine (hep a TYE tis bee vak SEEN)

Sound-Alike/Look-Alike Issues

Recombivax HB® may be confused with Comvax®

Synonyms hepatitis B inactivated virus vaccine (plasma derived); hepatitis B inactivated virus vaccine (recombinant DNA)

U.S./Canadian Brand Names Engerix-B® [US/Can]; Recombivax HB® [US/Can]

Therapeutic Category Vaccine, Inactivated Virus

Use I.M.:

Children:

≤11 years: 2.5 mcg doses

11-19 years: 5 mcg doses

Adults >20 years: 10 mcg doses

Usual Dosage I.M.:

Immunization regimen: Regimen consists of 3 doses (0, 1, and 6 months): First dose given on the elected date, second dose given 1 month later, third dose given 6 months after the first dose

Alternative dosing schedule for **Recombivax HB®:** Children 11-15 years (10 mcg/mL adult formulation): First dose of 1 mL given on the elected date, second dose given 4-6 months later

(Continued)

hepatitis B vaccine *(Continued)*

Alternative dosing schedules for **Engerix-B®:**

Children ≤10 years (10 mcg/0.5 mL formulation): High-risk children: 0.5 mL at 0, 1, 2, and 12 months; lower-risk children ages 5-10 who are candidates for an extended administration schedule may receive an alternative regimen of 0.5 mL at 0, 12, and 24 months. If booster dose is needed, revaccinate with 0.5 mL.

Adolescents 11-19 years (20 mcg/mL formulation): 1 mL at 0, 1, and 6 months. High-risk adolescents: 1 mL at 0, 1, 2, and 12 months; lower-risk adolescents 11-16 years who are candidates for an extended administration schedule may receive an alternative regimen of 0.5 mL (using the 10 mcg/0.5 mL) formulation at 0, 12, and 24 months. If booster dose is needed, revaccinate with 20 mcg.

Adults ≥20 years: High-risk adults (20 mcg/mL formulation): 1 mL at 0, 1, 2, and 12 months. If booster dose is needed, revaccinate with 1 mL.

Dosage Forms

Injection, suspension [recombinant DNA]:

Engerix-B®:

Adult: Hepatitis B surface antigen 20 mcg/mL (1 mL) [contains trace amounts of thimerosal]

Pediatric/adolescent: Hepatitis B surface antigen 10 mcg/0.5 mL (0.5 mL) [contains trace amounts of thimerosal]

Recombivax HB®:

Adult [preservative free]: Hepatitis B surface antigen 10 mcg/mL (1 mL, 3 mL)

Dialysis [preservative free]: Hepatitis B surface antigen 40 mcg/mL (1 mL)

Pediatric/adolescent [preservative free]: Hepatitis B surface antigen 5 mcg/0.5 mL (0.5 mL)

Hep-B-Gammagee® *(Discontinued)* *see page 1042*

Hep-Lock® [US] *see* heparin *on page 430*

Hepsera™ [US] *see* adefovir *on page 21*

Heptalac® *(Discontinued)* *see page 1042*

Heptovir® [Can] *see* lamivudine *on page 502*

Herceptin® [US/Can] *see* trastuzumab *on page 877*

Herplex® *(Discontinued)* *see page 1042*

HES *see* hetastarch *on this page*

Hespan® [US] *see* hetastarch *on this page*

hetastarch (HET a starch)

Sound-Alike/Look-Alike Issues

Hespan® may be confused with heparin

Synonyms HES; hydroxyethyl starch

U.S./Canadian Brand Names Hespan® [US]; Hextend® [US/Can]

Therapeutic Category Plasma Volume Expander

Use Blood volume expander used in treatment of hypovolemia

Hespan®: Adjunct in leukapheresis to improve harvesting and increasing the yield of granulocytes by centrifugal means

Usual Dosage I.V. infusion (requires an infusion pump):

Children: Safety and efficacy have not been established

Plasma volume expansion:

Adults: 500-1000 mL (up to 1500 mL/day) or 20 mL/kg/day (up to 1500 mL/day); larger volumes (15,000 mL/24 hours) have been used safely in small numbers of patients

Leukapheresis: 250-700 mL; **Note:** Citrate anticoagulant is added before use.

Dosage Forms

Infusion [premixed in lactated electrolyte injection] (Hextend®): 6% (500 mL)

Infusion, solution [premixed in NaCl 0.9%] (Hespan®): 6% (500 mL)

Hetrazan® *(Discontinued)* *see page 1042*

Hexabrix™ [US] *see* radiological/contrast media (ionic) *on page 759*

hexachlorocyclohexane *see* lindane *on page 522*

hexachlorophene (heks a KLOR oh feen)

Sound-Alike/Look-Alike Issues

pHisoHex® may be confused with Fostex®, pHisoDerm®

U.S./Canadian Brand Names pHisoHex® [US/Can]

Therapeutic Category Antibacterial, Topical

Use Surgical scrub and as a bacteriostatic skin cleanser; control an outbreak of gram-positive infection when other procedures have been unsuccessful

Usual Dosage Children and Adults: Topical: Apply 5 mL cleanser and water to area to be cleansed; lather and rinse thoroughly under running water

Dosage Forms Liquid, topical (pHisoHex®): 3% (150 mL, 500 mL, 3840 mL)

Hexalen® [US/Can] *see* altretamine *on page 38*

hexamethylenetetramine *see* methenamine *on page 563*

hexamethylmelamine *see* altretamine *on page 38*

Hexit™ [Can] *see* lindane *on page 522*

HEXM *see* altretamine *on page 38*

Hextend® [US/Can] *see* hetastarch *on previous page*

hexylresorcinol (heks il re ZOR si nole)

U.S./Canadian Brand Names Sucrets® Original [US-OTC]

Therapeutic Category Local Anesthetic

Use Minor antiseptic and local anesthetic for sore throat

Usual Dosage May be used as needed, allow to dissolve slowly in mouth

Dosage Forms

Lozenge: 2.4 mg

Sucrets® Original: 2.4 mg [mint flavor]

Hib *see Haemophilus* B conjugate and hepatitis B vaccine *on page 426*

Hibiclens® [US-OTC] *see* chlorhexidine gluconate *on page 183*

Hibidil® 1:2000 [Can] *see* chlorhexidine gluconate *on page 183*

Hibistat® [US-OTC] *see* chlorhexidine gluconate *on page 183*

Hib polysaccharide conjugate *see Haemophilus* B conjugate vaccine *on page 426*

HibTITER® [US] *see Haemophilus* B conjugate vaccine *on page 426*

Hiprex® [US/Can] *see* methenamine *on page 563*

hirulog *see* bivalirudin *on page 122*

Hismanal® *(Discontinued)* *see page 1042*

Histaject® *(Discontinued)* *see page 1042*

Histalet Forte® Tablet *(Discontinued)* *see page 1042*

Histalet® X *(Discontinued)* *see page 1042*

histamine (HIS ta meen)

Therapeutic Category Diagnostic Agent

Use To test the ability of the gastric mucosa to produce hydrochloric acid

Usual Dosage Adults: S.C.: Gastric acid test:

The patient fasts for 12 hours. A plastic duodenal tube is passed into the stomach, the gastric content withdrawn, and its acidity determined. Care should be taken to prevent the patient from swallowing salivary secretions during administration of the test results. The alkalinity of the saliva may interfere with the test results. Histamine phosphate 500 to 750 mcg is then injected.

(Continued)

histamine *(Continued)*

Gastric content is again removed after 5 minutes and at 15 minute intervals thereafter on 3 occasions

The volume and acidity of each specimen is determined. If no acidity is detected, a maximum histamine stimulation test can be performed using 40 mcg/kg histamine phosphate. Pulse rate and blood pressure should be determined immediately after histamine injection.

Dosage Forms Injection, as phosphate: 0.275 mg/mL (5 mL)

Histatab® Plus [US-OTC] *see* chlorpheniramine and phenylephrine *on page 188*

Hista-Vadrin® Tablet *(Discontinued)* *see page 1042*

Hista-Vent® DA [US] *see* chlorpheniramine, phenylephrine, and methscopolamine *on page 192*

Histerone® Injection *(Discontinued)* *see page 1042*

Histex™ [US] *see* chlorpheniramine and pseudoephedrine *on page 189*

Histex™ SR [US] *see* brompheniramine and pseudoephedrine *on page 129*

Histinex® D Liquid *(Discontinued)* *see page 1042*

Histolyn-CYL® *(Discontinued)* *see page 1042*

Histor-D® Syrup *(Discontinued)* *see page 1042*

Histor-D® Timecelles® *(Discontinued)* *see page 1042*

Histrodrix® *(Discontinued)* *see page 1042*

Histussin D® [US] *see* hydrocodone and pseudoephedrine *on page 446*

Hivid® [US/Can] *see* zalcitabine *on page 937*

HMM *see* altretamine *on page 38*

HMR 3647 *see* telithromycin *on page 842*

HMS Liquifilm® [US] *see* medrysone *on page 548*

HN_2 *see* mechlorethamine *on page 546*

Hold® DM [US-OTC] *see* dextromethorphan *on page 261*

homatropine (hoe MA troe peen)

Synonyms homatropine hydrobromide

U.S./Canadian Brand Names Isopto® Homatropine [US]

Therapeutic Category Anticholinergic Agent

Use Producing cycloplegia and mydriasis for refraction; treatment of acute inflammatory conditions of the uveal tract

Usual Dosage Ophthalmic:

Children:

Mydriasis and cycloplegia for refraction: Instill 1 drop of 2% solution immediately before the procedure; repeat at 10-minute intervals as needed

Uveitis: Instill 1 drop of 2% solution 2-3 times/day

Adults:

Mydriasis and cycloplegia for refraction: Instill 1-2 drops of 2% solution or 1 drop of 5% solution before the procedure; repeat at 5- to 10-minute intervals as needed; maximum of 3 doses for refraction

Uveitis: Instill 1-2 drops of 2% or 5% 2-3 times/day up to every 3-4 hours as needed

Dosage Forms Solution, ophthalmic, as hydrobromide: 2% (5 mL); 5% (5 mL, 15 mL) [contains benzalkonium chloride]

homatropine and hydrocodone *see* hydrocodone and homatropine *on page 446*

homatropine hydrobromide *see* homatropine *on this page*

horse antihuman thymocyte gamma globulin *see* antithymocyte globulin (equine) *on page 66*

H.P. Acthar® Gel [US] *see* corticotropin *on page 228*

Hp-PAC® [Can] *see* lansoprazole, amoxicillin, and clarithromycin *on page 506*

HTF919 *see* tegaserod *on page 842*

hu1124 *see* efalizumab *on page 304*

Humalog® [US/Can] *see* insulin preparations *on page 474*

Humalog® Mix 25™ [Can] *see* insulin preparations *on page 474*

Humalog® Mix 50/50 Insulin *(Discontinued)* *see page 1042*

Humalog® Mix 75/25™ [US] *see* insulin preparations *on page 474*

human antitumor necrosis factor-alpha *see* adalimumab *on page 20*

human diploid cell cultures rabies vaccine *see* rabies virus vaccine *on page 759*

human growth hormone (HYU man grothe HOR mone)

Sound-Alike/Look-Alike Issues

Protropin® may be confused with Proloprim®, protamine, Protopam®
somatrem may be confused with somatropin
somatropin may be confused with somatrem, sumatriptan

Synonyms growth hormone; somatrem; somatropin

U.S./Canadian Brand Names Genotropin® [US]; Genotropin Miniquick® [US]; Humatrope® [US/Can]; Norditropin® [US/Can]; Norditropin® Cartridges [US]; Nutropin® [US]; Nutropin AQ® [US/Can]; Nutropine® [Can]; Protropin® [US/Can]; Protropine® [Can]; Saizen® [US/Can]; Serostim® [US/Can]; Zorbtive™ [US]

Therapeutic Category Growth Hormone

Use

Children:

- Long-term treatment of growth failure due to lack of adequate endogenous growth hormone secretion (Genotropin®, Humatrope®, Norditropin®, Nutropin®, Nutropin AQ®, Nutropin Depot®, Protropin®, Saizen®)
- Long-term treatment of short stature associated with Turner syndrome (Humatrope®, Nutropin®, Nutropin AQ®)
- Treatment of Prader-Willi syndrome (Genotropin®)
- Treatment of growth failure associated with chronic renal insufficiency (CRI) up until the time of renal transplantation (Nutropin®, Nutropin AQ®)
- Long-term treatment of growth failure in children born small for gestational age who fail to manifest catch-up growth by 2 years of age (Genotropin®)
- Long-term treatment of idiopathic short stature (nongrowth hormone-deficient short stature) defined by height standard deviation score (SDS) less than or equal to -2.25 and growth rate not likely to attain normal adult height (Humatrope®)

Adults:

- AIDS-wasting or cachexia with concomitant antiviral therapy (Serostim®)
- Replacement of endogenous growth hormone in patients with adult growth hormone deficiency who meet both of the following criteria (Genotropin®, Humatrope®, Nutropin®, Nutropin AQ®, Saizen®):
  - Biochemical diagnosis of adult growth hormone deficiency by means of a subnormal response to a standard growth hormone stimulation test (peak growth hormone ≤5 mcg/L)
  - **and**
  - Adult-onset: Patients who have adult growth hormone deficiency whether alone or with multiple hormone deficiencies (hypopituitarism) as a result of pituitary disease, hypothalamic disease, surgery, radiation therapy, or trauma
  - **or**
  - Childhood-onset: Patients who were growth hormone deficient during childhood, confirmed as an adult before replacement therapy is initiated
- Treatment of short-bowel syndrome (Zorbtive™)

(Continued)

human growth hormone *(Continued)*

Usual Dosage

Children (individualize dose):

Growth hormone deficiency:

Somatrem: Protropin®: I.M., SubQ: Weekly dosage: 0.3 mg/kg divided into daily doses.

Somatropin: Genotropin®: SubQ: Weekly dosage: 0.16-0.24 mg/kg divided into 6-7 doses. Humatrope®: I.M., SubQ: Weekly dosage: 0.18 mg/kg; maximum replacement dose: 0.3 mg/kg/week; dosing should be divided into equal doses given 3 times/week on alternating days, 6 times/week, or daily. Norditropin®: SubQ: Weekly dosage: 0.024-0.034 mg/kg administered in the evening, divided into doses 6-7 times/week; cartridge and vial formulations are bioequivalent; cartridge formulation does not need to be reconstituted prior to use; cartridges must be administered using the corresponding color-coded NordiPen® injection pen. Nutropin Depot®: SubQ: Once-monthly injection: 1.5 mg/kg administered on the same day of each month; patients >15 kg will require more than 1 injection per dose. Twice-monthly injection: 0.75 mg/kg administered twice each month on the same days of each month (eg, days 1 and 15 of each month); patients >30 kg will require more than 1 injection per dose. Nutropin®, Nutropin® AQ: SubQ: Weekly dosage: 0.3 mg/kg divided into daily doses; pubertal patients: ≤0.7 mg/kg/week divided daily. Saizen®: I.M., SubQ: Weekly dosage: 0.06 mg/kg administered 3 times/week. **Note:** Therapy should be discontinued when patient has reached satisfactory adult height, when epiphyses have fused, or when the patient ceases to respond. Growth of 5 cm/year or more is expected, if growth rate does not exceed 2.5 cm in a 6-month period, double the dose for the next 6 months; if there is still no satisfactory response, discontinue therapy.

Chronic renal insufficiency (CRI): Nutropin®, Nutropin® AQ: SubQ: Weekly dosage: 0.35 mg/kg divided into daily injections; continue until the time of renal transplantation.

Dosage recommendations in patients treated for CRI who require dialysis: Hemodialysis: Administer dose at night prior to bedtime or at least 3-4 hours after hemodialysis to prevent hematoma formation from heparin. CCPD: Administer dose in the morning following dialysis. CAPD: Administer dose in the evening at the time of overnight exchange

Turner syndrome: Humatrope®, Nutropin®, Nutropin® AQ: SubQ: Weekly dosage: ≤0.375 mg/kg divided into equal doses 3-7 times per week

Prader-Willi syndrome: Genotropin®: SubQ: Weekly dosage: 0.24 mg/kg divided into 6-7 doses

Small for gestational age: Genotropin®: SubQ: Weekly dosage: 0.48 mg/kg divided into 6-7 doses

Idiopathic short stature: Humatrope®: SubQ: 0.37 mg/kg divided into equal doses 6-7 times per week

Adults:

Growth hormone deficiency: To minimize adverse events in older or overweight patients, reduced dosages may be necessary. During therapy, dosage should be decreased if required by the occurrence of side effects or excessive IGF-I levels.

Somatropin: Nutropin®, Nutropin® AQ: SubQ: ≤0.006 mg/kg/day; dose may be increased according to individual requirements, up to a maximum of 0.025 mg/kg/day in patients <35 years of age, or up to a maximum of 0.0125 mg/kg/day in patients ≥35 years of age. Humatrope®: SubQ: ≤0.006 mg/kg/day; dose may be increased according to individual requirements, up to a maximum of 0.0125 mg/kg/day. Genotropin®: SubQ: Weekly dosage: ≤0.04 mg/kg divided into 6-7 doses; dose may be increased at 4- to 8-week intervals according to individual requirements, to a maximum of 0.08 mg/kg/week. Saizen®: SubQ: ≤0.005 mg/kg/day; dose may be increased to not more than 0.01 mg/kg/day after 14 weeks, based on individual requirements.

AIDS-wasting or cachexia:

Serostim®: SubQ: Dose should be given once daily at bedtime; patients who continue to lose weight after 2 weeks should be re-evaluated for opportunistic infections or other clinical events; rotate injection sites to avoid lipodystrophy

Daily dose based on body weight: <35 kg: 0.1 mg/kg; 35-45 kg: 4 mg; 45-55 kg: 5 mg; >55 kg: 6 mg

Short-bowel syndrome (Zorbtive™): SubQ: 0.1 mg/kg once daily for 4 weeks (maximum: 8 mg/day)

Fluid retention (moderate) or arthralgias: Treat symptomatically or reduce dose by 50%

Severe toxicity: Discontinue therapy for up to 5 days; when symptoms resolve, restart at 50% of dose. If severe toxicity recurs or does not disappear within 5 days after discontinuation, permanently discontinue treatment.

Dosage Forms [DSC] = Discontinued product

Injection, powder for reconstitution [rDNA origin]:

Somatrem: Protropin® [diluent contains benzyl alcohol]: 5 mg [~15 int. units]; 10 mg [~30 int. units]

Somatropin:

Genotropin® [preservative free]: 1.5 mg [4 int. units/mL] [delivers 1.3 mg/mL]

Genotropin® [with preservative]: 5.8 mg [15 int. units/mL] [delivers 5 mg/mL] 13.8 mg [36 int. units/mL] [delivers 12 mg/mL]

Genotropin Miniquick® [preservative free]: 0.2 mg, 0.4 mg, 0.6 mg, 0.8 mg, 1 mg, 1.2 mg, 1.4 mg, 1.6 mg, 1.8 mg, 2 mg [each strength delivers 0.25 mL]

Humatrope®: 5 mg [~15 int. units], 6 mg [18 int. units], 12 mg [36 int. units], 24 mg [72 int. units]

Norditropin® [diluent contains benzyl alcohol]: 4 mg [~12 int. units]; 8 mg [~24 int. units]

Nutropin® [diluent contains benzyl alcohol]: 5 mg [~15 int. units]; 10 mg [~30 int. units]

Nutropin Depot® [preservative free]: 13.5 mg, 18 mg, 22.5 mg [DSC]

Saizen® [diluent contains benzyl alcohol]: 5 mg [~15 int. units]; 8.8 mg [~26.4 int. units]

Serostim®: 4 mg [12 int. units]; 5 mg [15 int. units]; 6 mg [18 int. units]

Zorbtive™: 4 mg [~12 int. units; packaged with diluent]; 5 mg [~15 int. units; packaged with diluent]; 6 mg [~18 int. units; packaged with diluent]; 8.8 mg [~26.4 int. units; packaged with diluent containing benzyl alcohol]

Injection, solution [rDNA origin]: Somatropin:

Norditropin®: 5 mg/1.5 mL (1.5 mL); 15 mg/1.5 mL (1.5 mL) [cartridge]

Nutropin AQ®: 5 mg/mL [~30 int. units/2 mL] (2 mL) [vial or cartridge]

humanized IgG1 anti-CD52 monoclonal antibody *see* alemtuzumab *on page 29*

human LFA-3/IgG(1) fusion protein *see* alefacept *on page 29*

human thyroid stimulating hormone *see* thyrotropin alpha *on page 860*

Humate-P® [US/Can] *see* antihemophilic factor (human) *on page 62*

Humatin® [US/Can] *see* paromomycin *on page 667*

Humatrope® [US/Can] *see* human growth hormone *on page 437*

Humegon™ *(Discontinued)* *see page 1042*

Humibid® DM [US] *see* guaifenesin and dextromethorphan *on page 416*

Humibid® LA *(Discontinued)* *see page 1042*

Humibid® Pediatric *(Discontinued)* *see page 1042*

Humibid® Sprinkle *(Discontinued)* *see page 1042*

Humira™ [US] *see* adalimumab *on page 20*

Humorsol® Ophthalmic *(Discontinued)* *see page 1042*

Humulin® [Can] *see* insulin preparations *on page 474*

Humulin® 50/50 [US] *see* insulin preparations *on page 474*

Humulin® 70/30 [US] *see* insulin preparations *on page 474*

Humulin® L [US] *see* insulin preparations *on page 474*

Humulin® N [US] *see* insulin preparations *on page 474*

Humulin® R [US] *see* insulin preparations *on page 474*

Humulin® R (Concentrated) U-500 [US] *see* insulin preparations *on page 474*

Humulin® U [US] *see* insulin preparations *on page 474*

Hurricaine® [US] *see* benzocaine *on page 107*

HXM *see* altretamine *on page 38*

hyaluronic acid *see* sodium hyaluronate *on page 812*

Hyate:C® [US] *see* antihemophilic factor (porcine) *on page 63*

hycamptamine *see* topotecan *on page 872*

Hycamtin® [US/Can] *see* topotecan *on page 872*

hycet™ [US] *see* hydrocodone and acetaminophen *on page 443*

HycoClear Tuss® ***(Discontinued)*** *see page 1042*

Hycodan® [US] *see* hydrocodone and homatropine *on page 446*

Hycomine® ***(Discontinued)*** *see page 1042*

Hycomine® Compound [US] *see* hydrocodone, chlorpheniramine, phenylephrine, acetaminophen, and caffeine *on page 446*

Hycomine® Pediatric ***(Discontinued)*** *see page 1042*

Hycort® [US] *see* hydrocortisone (rectal) *on page 448*

Hycosin [US] *see* hydrocodone and guaifenesin *on page 445*

Hycotuss® [US] *see* hydrocodone and guaifenesin *on page 445*

Hydeltra-T.B.A.® ***(Discontinued)*** *see page 1042*

Hydeltra-T.B.A.® [Can] *see* prednisolone (ophthalmic) *on page 723*

Hydergine® ***(Discontinued)*** *see page 1042*

Hydergine® [Can] *see* ergoloid mesylates *on page 318*

hydralazine (hye DRAL a zeen)

Sound-Alike/Look-Alike Issues
hydralazine may be confused with hydroxyzine

Synonyms hydralazine hydrochloride

Tall-Man hydr**ALAZINE**

U.S./Canadian Brand Names Apo-Hydralazine® [Can]; Apresoline® [Can]; Novo-Hylazin [Can]; Nu-Hydral [Can]

Therapeutic Category Vasodilator

Use Management of moderate to severe hypertension, congestive heart failure, hypertension secondary to pre-eclampsia/eclampsia; treatment of primary pulmonary hypertension

Usual Dosage

Children:

Oral: Initial: 0.75-1 mg/kg/day in 2-4 divided doses; increase over 3-4 weeks to maximum of 7.5 mg/kg/day in 2-4 divided doses; maximum daily dose: 200 mg/day

I.M., I.V.: 0.1-0.2 mg/kg/dose (not to exceed 20 mg) every 4-6 hours as needed, up to 1.7-3.5 mg/kg/day in 4-6 divided doses

Adults:

Oral: Hypertension:

Initial dose: 10 mg 4 times/day for first 2-4 days; increase to 25 mg 4 times/day for the balance of the first week

Increase by 10-25 mg/dose gradually to 50 mg 4 times/day (maximum: 300 mg/day); usual dose range (JNC 7): 25-100 mg/day in 2 divided doses

Oral: Congestive heart failure:

Initial dose: 10-25 mg 3-4 times/day

Adjustment: Dosage must be adjusted based on individual response

Target dose: 75 mg 4 times/day in combination with isosorbide dinitrate (40 mg 4 times/day)

Range: Typically 200-600 mg daily in 2-4 divided doses; dosages as high as 3 g/day have been used in some patients for symptomatic and hemodynamic improvement. Hydralazine 75 mg 4 times/day combined with isosorbide dinitrate 40 mg 4 times/day were shown in clinical trials to provide a mortality benefit in the treatment of CHF. Higher doses may be used for symptomatic and hemodynamic improvement following optimization of standard therapy.

I.M., I.V.:

Hypertension: Initial: 10-20 mg/dose every 4-6 hours as needed, may increase to 40 mg/dose; change to oral therapy as soon as possible.

Pre-eclampsia/eclampsia: 5 mg/dose then 5-10 mg every 20-30 minutes as needed.

Dosage Forms

Injection, solution, as hydrochloride: 20 mg/mL (1 mL)

Tablet, as hydrochloride: 10 mg, 25 mg, 50 mg, 100 mg

hydralazine and hydrochlorothiazide

(hye DRAL a zeen & hye droe klor oh THYE a zide)

Synonyms hydrochlorothiazide and hydralazine

Therapeutic Category Antihypertensive Agent, Combination

Use Management of moderate to severe hypertension and treatment of congestive heart failure

Usual Dosage Adults: Oral: Take as directed; not to exceed 50 mg hydrochlorothiazide per day

Dosage Forms Capsule:

25/25: Hydralazine hydrochloride 25 mg and hydrochlorothiazide 25 mg

50/50: Hydralazine hydrochloride 50 mg and hydrochlorothiazide 50 mg

100/50: Hydralazine hydrochloride 100 mg and hydrochlorothiazide 50 mg

hydralazine hydrochloride *see* hydralazine *on previous page*

hydralazine, hydrochlorothiazide, and reserpine

(hye DRAL a zeen, hye droe klor oh THYE a zide, & re SER peen)

Synonyms hydrochlorothiazide, hydralazine, and reserpine; reserpine, hydralazine, and hydrochlorothiazide

Therapeutic Category Antihypertensive Agent, Combination

Use Hypertensive disorders

Usual Dosage Adults: Oral: 1-2 tablets 3 times/day

Dosage Forms Tablet: Hydralazine 25 mg, hydrochlorothiazide 15 mg, and reserpine 0.1 mg

Hydramine® Cough [US-OTC] *see* diphenhydramine *on page 277*

Hydramine® [US-OTC] *see* diphenhydramine *on page 277*

Hydramyn® Syrup *(Discontinued)* *see page 1042*

Hydrate® *(Discontinued)* *see page 1042*

hydrated chloral *see* chloral hydrate *on page 181*

Hydrea® [US/Can] *see* hydroxyurea *on page 457*

Hydrisalic™ [US-OTC] *see* salicylic acid *on page 789*

Hydrobexan® Injection *(Discontinued)* *see page 1042*

Hydrocet® *(Discontinued)* *see page 1042*

hydrochlorothiazide (hye droe klor oh THYE a zide)

Sound-Alike/Look-Alike Issues

hydrochlorothiazide may be confused with hydroflumethiazide

Synonyms HCTZ

(Continued)

hydrochlorothiazide *(Continued)*

U.S./Canadian Brand Names Apo-Hydro® [Can]; Aquazide® H [US]; Microzide™ [US]; Novo-Hydrazide [Can]; Oretic® [US]

Therapeutic Category Diuretic, Thiazide

Use Management of mild to moderate hypertension; treatment of edema in congestive heart failure and nephrotic syndrome

Usual Dosage Oral (effect of drug may be decreased when used every day):

Children (in pediatric patients, chlorothiazide may be preferred over hydrochlorothiazide as there are more dosage formulations [eg, suspension] available):

<6 months: 2-3 mg/kg/day in 2 divided doses

>6 months: 2 mg/kg/day in 2 divided doses

Adults:

Edema: 25-100 mg/day in 1-2 doses; maximum: 200 mg/day

Hypertension: 12.5-50 mg/day; minimal increase in response and more electrolyte disturbances are seen with doses >50 mg/day

Dosage Forms [DSC] = Discontinued product

Capsule (Microzide™): 12.5 mg

Solution, oral [DSC]: 50 mg/5 mL (500 mL) [contains sodium benzoate; mint flavor]

Tablet: 25 mg, 50 mg

Aquazide® H, Oretic®: 50 mg

hydrochlorothiazide and amiloride *see* amiloride and hydrochlorothiazide *on page 45*

hydrochlorothiazide and benazepril *see* benazepril and hydrochlorothiazide *on page 105*

hydrochlorothiazide and bisoprolol *see* bisoprolol and hydrochlorothiazide *on page 122*

hydrochlorothiazide and captopril *see* captopril and hydrochlorothiazide *on page 154*

hydrochlorothiazide and enalapril *see* enalapril and hydrochlorothiazide *on page 308*

hydrochlorothiazide and eprosartan *see* eprosartan and hydrochlorothiazide *on page 316*

hydrochlorothiazide and fosinopril *see* fosinopril and hydrochlorothiazide *on page 391*

hydrochlorothiazide and hydralazine *see* hydralazine and hydrochlorothiazide *on previous page*

hydrochlorothiazide and irbesartan *see* irbesartan and hydrochlorothiazide *on page 484*

hydrochlorothiazide and lisinopril *see* lisinopril and hydrochlorothiazide *on page 525*

hydrochlorothiazide and losartan *see* losartan and hydrochlorothiazide *on page 532*

hydrochlorothiazide and methyldopa *see* methyldopa and hydrochlorothiazide *on page 569*

hydrochlorothiazide and moexipril *see* moexipril and hydrochlorothiazide *on page 588*

hydrochlorothiazide and olmesartan medoxomil *see* olmesartan and hydrochlorothiazide *on page 643*

hydrochlorothiazide and propranolol *see* propranolol and hydrochlorothiazide *on page 742*

hydrochlorothiazide and quinapril *see* quinapril and hydrochlorothiazide *on page 756*

hydrochlorothiazide and spironolactone

(hye droe klor oh THYE a zide & speer on oh LAK tone)

Sound-Alike/Look-Alike Issues

Aldactazide® may be confused with Aldactone®

Synonyms spironolactone and hydrochlorothiazide

U.S./Canadian Brand Names Aldactazide® [US]; Aldactazide 25® [Can]; Aldactazide 50® [Can]; Novo-Spirozine [Can]

Therapeutic Category Antihypertensive Agent, Combination

Use Management of mild to moderate hypertension; treatment of edema in congestive heart failure and nephrotic syndrome, and cirrhosis of the liver accompanied by edema and/or ascites

Usual Dosage Oral:

Children: 1.66-3.3 mg/kg/day (of spironolactone) in 2-4 divided doses

Adults:

Hydrochlorothiazide 25 mg and spironolactone 25 mg: $^1/_2$-8 tablets daily

Hydrochlorothiazide 50 mg and spironolactone 50 mg: $^1/_2$-4 tablets daily in 1-2 doses

Dosage Forms Tablet: Hydrochlorothiazide 25 mg and spironolactone 25 mg

Aldactazide®:

25/25: Hydrochlorothiazide 25 mg and spironolactone 25 mg

50/50: Hydrochlorothiazide 50 mg and spironolactone 50 mg

hydrochlorothiazide and telmisartan *see* telmisartan and hydrochlorothiazide *on page 843*

hydrochlorothiazide and triamterene

(hye droe klor oh THYE a zide & trye AM ter een)

Sound-Alike/Look-Alike Issues

Dyazide® may be confused with diazoxide, Dynacin®

Maxzide® may be confused with Maxidex®

Synonyms triamterene and hydrochlorothiazide

U.S./Canadian Brand Names Apo-Triazide® [Can]; Dyazide® [US]; Maxzide® [US]; Maxzide®-25 [US]; Novo-Triamzide [Can]; Nu-Triazide [Can]; Penta-Triamterene HCTZ [Can]; Riva-Zide [Can]

Therapeutic Category Antihypertensive Agent, Combination

Use Management of mild to moderate hypertension; treatment of edema in congestive heart failure and nephrotic syndrome

Usual Dosage Adults: Oral:

Hydrochlorothiazide 25 mg and triamterene 37.5 mg: 1-2 tablets/capsules once daily

Hydrochlorothiazide 50 mg and triamterene 75 mg: $^1/_2$-1 tablet daily

Dosage Forms

Capsule (Dyazide®): Hydrochlorothiazide 25 mg and triamterene 37.5 mg

Tablet:

Maxzide®: Hydrochlorothiazide 50 mg and triamterene 75 mg

Maxzide®-25: Hydrochlorothiazide 25 mg and triamterene 37.5 mg

hydrochlorothiazide and valsartan *see* valsartan and hydrochlorothiazide *on page 903*

hydrochlorothiazide, hydralazine, and reserpine *see* hydralazine, hydrochlorothiazide, and reserpine *on page 441*

Hydrocil® [US-OTC] *see* psyllium *on page 749*

Hydro Cobex® *(Discontinued)* *see page 1042*

hydrocodone and acetaminophen

(hye droe KOE done & a seet a MIN oh fen)

Sound-Alike/Look-Alike Issues

Lorcet® may be confused with Fioricet®

Lortab® may be confused with Cortef®, Lorabid®, Luride®

(Continued)

hydrocodone and acetaminophen *(Continued)*

Vicodin® may be confused with Hycodan®, Hycomine®, Indocin®, Uridon®
Zydone® may be confused with Vytone®

Synonyms acetaminophen and hydrocodone

U.S./Canadian Brand Names Anexsia® [US]; Bancap HC® [US]; Ceta-Plus® [US]; Co-Gesic® [US]; hycet™ [US]; Lorcet® 10/650 [US]; Lorcet®-HD [US]; Lorcet® Plus [US]; Lortab® [US]; Margesic® H [US]; Maxidone™ [US]; Norco® [US]; Stagesic® [US]; Vicodin® [US]; Vicodin® ES [US]; Vicodin® HP [US]; Zydone® [US]

Therapeutic Category Analgesic, Narcotic

Controlled Substance C-III

Use Relief of moderate to severe pain

Usual Dosage Oral (doses should be titrated to appropriate analgesic effect): Analgesic:

Children 2-13 years or <50 kg: Hydrocodone 0.135 mg/kg/dose every 4-6 hours; do not exceed 6 doses/day or the maximum recommended dose of acetaminophen

Children and Adults ≥50 kg: Average starting dose in opioid-naive patients: Hydrocodone 5-10 mg 4 times/day; the dosage of acetaminophen should be limited to ≤4 g/day (and possibly less in patients with hepatic impairment or ethanol use).

Dosage ranges (based on specific product labeling): Hydrocodone 2.5-10 mg every 4-6 hours; maximum: 60 mg hydrocodone/day (maximum dose of hydrocodone may be limited by the acetaminophen content of specific product)

Dosage Forms

Capsule (Bancap HC®, Ceta-Plus®, Lorcet®-HD, Margesic® H, Stagesic®): Hydrocodone bitartrate 5 mg and acetaminophen 500 mg

Elixir: Hydrocodone bitartrate 7.5 mg and acetaminophen 500 mg per 15 mL (480 mL)

Lortab®: Hydrocodone bitartrate 7.5 mg and acetaminophen 500 mg per 15 mL (480 mL) [contains alcohol 7%; tropical fruit punch flavor]

Solution, oral (hycet™): Hydrocodone bitartrate 7.5 mg and acetaminophen 325 mg per 15 mL (480 mL) [contains alcohol 7%; tropical fruit punch flavor]

Tablet:

Hydrocodone bitartrate 2.5 mg and acetaminophen 500 mg
Hydrocodone bitartrate 5 mg and acetaminophen 325 mg
Hydrocodone bitartrate 5 mg and acetaminophen 500 mg
Hydrocodone bitartrate 7.5 mg and acetaminophen 325 mg
Hydrocodone bitartrate 7.5 mg and acetaminophen 500 mg
Hydrocodone bitartrate 7.5 mg and acetaminophen 650 mg
Hydrocodone bitartrate 7.5 mg and acetaminophen 750 mg
Hydrocodone bitartrate 10 mg and acetaminophen 325 mg
Hydrocodone bitartrate 10 mg and acetaminophen 500 mg
Hydrocodone bitartrate 10 mg and acetaminophen 650 mg
Hydrocodone bitartrate 10 mg and acetaminophen 660 mg

Anexsia®:
5/500: Hydrocodone bitartrate 5 mg and acetaminophen 500 mg
7.5/650: Hydrocodone bitartrate 7.5 mg and acetaminophen 650 mg

Co-Gesic® 5/500: Hydrocodone bitartrate 5 mg and acetaminophen 500 mg

Lorcet® 10/650: Hydrocodone bitartrate 10 mg and acetaminophen 650 mg

Lorcet® Plus: Hydrocodone bitartrate 7.5 mg and acetaminophen 650 mg

Lortab®:
2.5/500: Hydrocodone bitartrate 2.5 mg and acetaminophen 500 mg
5/500: Hydrocodone bitartrate 5 mg and acetaminophen 500 mg
7.5/500: Hydrocodone bitartrate 7.5 mg and acetaminophen 500 mg
10/500: Hydrocodone bitartrate 10 mg and acetaminophen 500 mg

Maxidone™: Hydrocodone bitartrate 10 mg and acetaminophen 750 mg

Norco®:
Hydrocodone bitartrate 5 mg and acetaminophen 325 mg
Hydrocodone bitartrate 7.5 mg and acetaminophen 325 mg
Hydrocodone bitartrate 10 mg and acetaminophen 325 mg

Vicodin®: Hydrocodone bitartrate 5 mg and acetaminophen 500 mg

Vicodin® ES: Hydrocodone bitartrate 7.5 mg and acetaminophen 750 mg

Vicodin® HP: Hydrocodone bitartrate 10 mg and acetaminophen 660 mg
Zydone®:
Hydrocodone bitartrate 5 mg and acetaminophen 400 mg
Hydrocodone bitartrate 7.5 mg and acetaminophen 400 mg
Hydrocodone bitartrate 10 mg and acetaminophen 400 mg

hydrocodone and aspirin (hye droe KOE done & AS pir in)

Synonyms aspirin and hydrocodone
U.S./Canadian Brand Names Damason-P® [US]
Therapeutic Category Analgesic, Narcotic
Controlled Substance C-III
Use Relief of moderate to moderately severe pain
Usual Dosage Adults: Oral: 1-2 tablets every 4-6 hours as needed for pain
Dosage Forms Tablet: Hydrocodone bitartrate 5 mg and aspirin 500 mg

hydrocodone and chlorpheniramine

(hye droe KOE done & klor fen IR a meen)
Synonyms chlorpheniramine and hydrocodone
U.S./Canadian Brand Names Tussionex® [US]
Therapeutic Category Antihistamine/Antitussive
Controlled Substance C-III
Use Symptomatic relief of cough and allergy
Usual Dosage Oral:
Children 6-12 years: 2.5 mL every 12 hours; do not exceed 5 mL/24 hours
Adults: 5 mL every 12 hours; do not exceed 10 mL/24 hours
Dosage Forms Suspension, extended release: Hydrocodone polistirex (as bitartrate) 10 mg and chlorpheniramine polistirex (as maleate) 8 mg per 5 mL (480 mL)

hydrocodone and guaifenesin (hye droe KOE done & gwye FEN e sin)

Sound-Alike/Look-Alike Issues
Vicodin® may be confused with Hycodan®, Hycomine®, Indocin®, Uridon®
Synonyms guaifenesin and hydrocodone
U.S./Canadian Brand Names Codiclear® DH [US]; Hycosin [US]; Hycotuss® [US]; Kwelcof® [US]; Pneumotussin® [US]; Vicodin Tuss® [US]; Vitussin [US]
Therapeutic Category Antitussive/Expectorant
Controlled Substance C-III
Use Symptomatic relief of nonproductive coughs associated with upper and lower respiratory tract congestion
Usual Dosage Oral:
Children:
<2 years: 0.3 mg/kg/day (hydrocodone) in 4 divided doses
2-12 years: 2.5 mL every 4 hours, after meals and at bedtime
>12 years: 5 mL every 4 hours, after meals and at bedtime
Adults: 5 mL every 4 hours, after meals and at bedtime, not >30 mL in a 24-hour period
Dosage Forms
Liquid: Hydrocodone bitartrate 5 mg and guaifenesin 100 mg per 5 mL (480 mL, 960 mL) [may contain benzoic acid]
Codiclear® DH: Hydrocodone bitartrate 5 mg and guaifenesin 100 mg per 5 mL (120 mL, 480 mL) [alcohol free, dye free, sugar free]
Hycosin, Hycotuss®: Hydrocodone bitartrate 5 mg and guaifenesin 100 mg per 5 mL (480 mL) [contains alcohol 10%; butterscotch flavor]
Kwelcof®: Hydrocodone bitartrate 5 mg and guaifenesin 100 mg per 5 mL (480 mL)
Pneumotussin®: Hydrocodone bitartrate 2.5 mg and guaifenesin 200 mg per 5 mL (480 mL) [alcohol free, sugar free, dye free; cherry punch flavor]
Vicodin Tuss®, Vitussin: Hydrocodone bitartrate 5 mg and guaifenesin 100 mg per 5 mL (480 mL) [alcohol free, sugar free, dye free; cherry flavor]
Tablet (Pneumotussin®): Hydrocodone bitartrate 2.5 mg and guaifenesin 300 mg

hydrocodone and homatropine (hye droe KOE done & hoe MA troe peen)

Sound-Alike/Look-Alike Issues
Hycodan® may be confused with Hycomine®, Vicodin®

Synonyms homatropine and hydrocodone

U.S./Canadian Brand Names Hycodan® [US]; Hydromet® [US]; Hydropane® [US]; Tussigon® [US]

Therapeutic Category Antitussive

Controlled Substance C-III

Use Symptomatic relief of cough

Usual Dosage Oral (based on hydrocodone component):

Children: 0.6 mg/kg/day in 3-4 divided doses; do not administer more frequently than every 4 hours

A single dose should not exceed 1.25 mg in children <2 years of age, 5 mg in children 2-12 years, and 10 mg in children >12 years

Adults: 10 mg every 4-6 hours, a single dose should not exceed 15 mg; do not administer more frequently than every 4 hours

Dosage Forms

Syrup (Hycodan®, Hydromet®, Hydropane®): Hydrocodone bitartrate 5 mg and homatropine methylbromide 1.5 mg per 5 mL (480 mL) [cherry flavor]

Tablet (Hycodan®, Tussigon®): Hydrocodone bitartrate 5 mg and homatropine methylbromide 1.5 mg

hydrocodone and ibuprofen (hye droe KOE done & eye byoo PROE fen)

Synonyms ibuprofen and hydrocodone

U.S./Canadian Brand Names Vicoprofen® [US/Can]

Therapeutic Category Analgesic, Narcotic

Controlled Substance C-III

Use Short-term (generally <10 days) management of moderate to severe acute pain; is not indicated for treatment of such conditions as osteoarthritis or rheumatoid arthritis

Usual Dosage Adults: Oral: 1-2 tablets every 4-6 hours as needed for pain; maximum: 5 tablets/day

Dosage Forms

Tablet: Hydrocodone bitartrate 5 mg and ibuprofen 200 mg; hydrocodone bitartrate 7.5 mg and ibuprofen 200 mg

Vicoprofen®: Hydrocodone bitartrate 7.5 mg and ibuprofen 200 mg

hydrocodone and pseudoephedrine
(hye droe KOE done & soo doe e FED rin)

Synonyms pseudoephedrine and hydrocodone

U.S./Canadian Brand Names Histussin D® [US]; P-V Tussin Tablet [US]

Therapeutic Category Cough and Cold Combination

Use Symptomatic relief of cough due to colds, nasal congestion, and cough

Usual Dosage Oral: Adults: 5 mL 4 times/day

Dosage Forms

Syrup (Histussin D®): Hydrocodone bitartrate 5 mg and pseudoephedrine hydrochloride 60 mg per 5 mL (480 mL)

Tablet (P-V Tussin): Hydrocodone bitartrate 5 mg and pseudoephedrine hydrochloride 60 mg

hydrocodone, chlorpheniramine, phenylephrine, acetaminophen, and caffeine
(hye droe KOE done, klor fen IR a meen, fen il EF rin, a seet a MIN oh fen, & KAF een)

Sound-Alike/Look-Alike Issues
Hycomine® may be confused with Byclomine®, Hycamtin®, Hycodan®, Vicodin®

Synonyms acetaminophen, caffeine, hydrocodone, chlorpheniramine, and phenylephrine; caffeine, hydrocodone, chlorpheniramine, phenylephrine, and acetaminophen;

chlorpheniramine, hydrocodone, phenylephrine, acetaminophen, and caffeine; phenylephrine, hydrocodone, chlorpheniramine, acetaminophen, and caffeine

U.S./Canadian Brand Names Hycomine® Compound [US]

Therapeutic Category Antitussive

Use Symptomatic relief of cough and symptoms of upper respiratory infection

Usual Dosage Adults: Oral: 1 tablet every 4 hours, up to 4 times/day

Dosage Forms Tablet: Hydrocodone bitartrate 5 mg, chlorpheniramine maleate 2 mg, phenylephrine hydrochloride 10 mg, acetaminophen 250 mg, and caffeine 30 mg [cherry flavor]

Hydrocodone PA® Syrup ***(Discontinued)*** *see page 1042*

hydrocodone, pseudoephedrine, and guaifenesin

(hye droe KOE done, soo doe e FED rin, & gwye FEN e sin)

Synonyms guaifenesin, hydrocodone, and pseudoephedrine; pseudoephedrine, hydrocodone, and guaifenesin

U.S./Canadian Brand Names Duratuss® HD [US]; Hydro-Tussin™ HD [US]; Hydro-Tussin™ XP [US]; Pancof®-XP [US]; Su-Tuss®-HD [US]; Tussend® Expectorant [US]

Therapeutic Category Antitussive/Decongestant/Expectorant

Controlled Substance C-III

Use Symptomatic relief of irritating, nonproductive cough associated with respiratory conditions such as bronchitis, bronchial asthma, tracheobronchitis, and the common cold

Usual Dosage Adults: Oral: 5 mL every 4-6 hours

Dosage Forms

Elixir: Hydrocodone bitartrate 2.5 mg, pseudoephedrine hydrochloride 30 mg, and guaifenesin 100 mg per 5 mL (480 mL)

Duratuss® HD: Hydrocodone bitartrate 2.5 mg, pseudoephedrine hydrochloride 30 mg, and guaifenesin 100 mg per 5 mL (480 mL, 3785 mL) [contains alcohol; fruit punch flavor]

Su-Tuss® HD: Hydrocodone bitartrate 2.5 mg, pseudoephedrine hydrochloride 30 mg, and guaifenesin 100 mg per 5 mL (480 mL) [contains alcohol; fruit punch flavor]

Liquid: Hydrocodone bitartrate 2.5 mg, pseudoephedrine hydrochloride 30 mg, and guaifenesin 100 mg per 5 mL (480 mL)

Hydro-Tussin™ HD: Hydrocodone bitartrate 2.5 mg, pseudoephedrine hydrochloride 30 mg, and guaifenesin 100 mg per 5 mL [alcohol free; contains sodium benzoate]

Hydro-Tussin® XP: Hydrocodone bitartrate 3 mg, pseudoephedrine hydrochloride 15 mg, and guaifenesin 100 mg per 5 mL (480 mL) [alcohol free, dye free]

Pancof®-XP: Hydrocodone bitartrate 3 mg, pseudoephedrine hydrochloride 15 mg, and guaifenesin 100 mg per 5 mL (25 mL, 480 mL) [alcohol free, dye free]

Tussend® Expectorant: Hydrocodone bitartrate 2.5 mg, pseudoephedrine hydrochloride 30 mg, and guaifenesin 100 mg per 5 mL (480 mL) [contains alcohol; fruit punch flavor]

hydrocortisone acetate *see* hydrocortisone (systemic) *on page 449*

hydrocortisone, acetic acid, and propylene glycol diacetate *see* acetic acid, propylene glycol diacetate, and hydrocortisone *on page 15*

hydrocortisone and benzoyl peroxide *see* benzoyl peroxide and hydrocortisone *on page 111*

hydrocortisone and ciprofloxacin *see* ciprofloxacin and hydrocortisone *on page 203*

hydrocortisone and dibucaine *see* dibucaine and hydrocortisone *on page 265*

hydrocortisone and iodoquinol *see* iodoquinol and hydrocortisone *on page 481*

hydrocortisone and lidocaine *see* lidocaine and hydrocortisone *on page 520*

hydrocortisone and pramoxine *see* pramoxine and hydrocortisone *on page 720*

hydrocortisone and urea *see* urea and hydrocortisone *on page 898*

hydrocortisone, bacitracin, neomycin, and polymyxin B *see* bacitracin, neomycin, polymyxin B, and hydrocortisone *on page 98*

hydrocortisone buteprate *see* hydrocortisone (topical) *on page 451*

hydrocortisone butyrate *see* hydrocortisone (topical) *on page 451*

hydrocortisone cypionate *see* hydrocortisone (systemic) *on next page*

hydrocortisone, neomycin, and polymyxin B *see* neomycin, polymyxin B, and hydrocortisone *on page 611*

hydrocortisone, neomycin, colistin, and thonzonium *see* neomycin, colistin, hydrocortisone, and thonzonium *on page 610*

hydrocortisone, propylene glycol diacetate, and acetic acid *see* acetic acid, propylene glycol diacetate, and hydrocortisone *on page 15*

hydrocortisone (rectal) (hye droe KOR ti sone REK tal)

Sound-Alike/Look-Alike Issues

Anusol® may be confused with Anusol-HC®, Aplisol®, Aquasol®

Anusol-HC® may be confused with Anusol®

Proctocort® may be confused with ProctoCream®

ProctoCream® may be confused with Proctocort®

U.S./Canadian Brand Names Anucort™ HC [US]; Anusol-HC® Suppository [US]; Colocort™ [US]; Cortifoam® [US/Can]; Cortizone®-10 [US]; Emo-Cort® [Can]; Hemril® HC [US]; Hycort® [US]; Preparation H® Hydrocortisone [US]; Proctocort™ Rectal [US]; ProctoCream® HC [US]; ProctoCream® HC Cream [US]; Proctosol-HC® [US]

Therapeutic Category Adrenal Corticosteroid

Use Management of adrenocortical insufficiency; relief of inflammation of corticosteroid-responsive dermatoses (low and medium potency topical corticosteroid); adjunctive treatment of ulcerative colitis

Usual Dosage Dose should be based on severity of disease and patient response

Acute adrenal insufficiency: I.M., I.V.:

Infants and young Children: Succinate: 1-2 mg/kg/dose bolus, then 25-150 mg/day in divided doses every 6-8 hours

Older Children: Succinate: 1-2 mg/kg bolus then 150-250 mg/day in divided doses every 6-8 hours

Adults: Succinate: 100 mg I.V. bolus, then 300 mg/day in divided doses every 8 hours or as a continuous infusion for 48 hours; once patient is stable change to oral, 50 mg every 8 hours for 6 doses, then taper to 30-50 mg/day in divided doses

Chronic adrenal corticoid insufficiency: Adults: Oral: 20-30 mg/day

Antiinflammatory or immunosuppressive:

Infants and Children:

Oral: 2.5-10 mg/kg/day **or** 75-300 mg/m^2/day every 6-8 hours

I.M., I.V.: Succinate: 1-5 mg/kg/day **or** 30-150 mg/m^2/day divided every 12-24 hours

Adolescents and Adults: Oral, I.M., I.V.: Succinate: 15-240 mg every 12 hours

Congenital adrenal hyperplasia: Oral: Initial: 10-20 mg/m^2/day in 3 divided doses; a variety of dosing schedules have been used. **Note:** Inconsistencies have occurred with liquid formulations; tablets may provide more reliable levels. Doses must be individualized by monitoring growth, bone age, and hormonal levels. Mineralocorticoid and sodium supplementation may be required based upon electrolyte regulation and plasma renin activity.

Physiologic replacement: Children:

Oral: 0.5-0.75 mg/kg/day **or** 20-25 mg/m^2/day every 8 hours

I.M.: Succinate: 0.25-0.35 mg/kg/day **or** 12-15 mg/m^2/day once daily

Shock: I.M., I.V.: Succinate:
Children: Initial: 50 mg/kg, then repeated in 4 hours and/or every 24 hours as needed
Adolescents and Adults: 500 mg to 2 g every 2-6 hours
Status asthmaticus: Children and Adults: I.V.: Succinate: 1-2 mg/kg/dose every 6 hours for 24 hours, then maintenance of 0.5-1 mg/kg every 6 hours
Adults:
Rheumatic diseases:
Intralesional, intra-articular, soft tissue injection: Acetate: Large joints: 25 mg (up to 37.5 mg) Small joints: 10-25 mg
Tendon sheaths: 5-12.5 mg
Soft tissue infiltration: 25-50 mg (up to 75 mg)
Bursae: 25-37.5 mg
Ganglia: 12.5-25 mg
Stress dosing (surgery) in patients known to be adrenally-suppressed or on chronic systemic steroids: I.V.:
Minor stress (ie, inguinal herniorrhaphy): 25 mg/day for 1 day
Moderate stress (ie, joint replacement, cholecystectomy): 50-75 mg/day (25 mg every 8-12 hours) for 1-2 days
Major stress (pancreatoduodenectomy, esophagogastrectomy, cardiac surgery): 100-150 mg/day (50 mg every 8-12 hours) for 2-3 days
Dermatosis: Children >2 years and Adults: Topical: Apply to affected area 2-4 times/day (Buteprate: Apply once or twice daily). Therapy should be discontinued when control is achieved; if no improvement is seen, reassessment of diagnosis may be necessary.
Ulcerative colitis: Adults: Rectal: 10-100 mg 1-2 times/day for 2-3 weeks

Dosage Forms [DSC] = Discontinued product
Aerosol, rectal, as acetate (Cortifoam®): 10% (15 g) [90 mg/applicator]
Cream, rectal, as acetate (Nupercainal® Hydrocortisone Cream): 1% (30 g)
Cream, rectal, as base:
Cortizone®-10: 1% (30g) [contains aloe]
Preparation H® Hydrocortisone: 1% (27 g)
Anusol-HC®: 2.5% (30 g) [contains benzyl alcohol]
ProctoCream® HC: 2.5% (30 g) [contains benzyl alcohol]
Proctocort®: 1% (30 g)
Proctosol-HC®: 2.5% (30 g)
Ointment, topical, as acetate:
Anusol® HC-1: 1% (21 g)
Cortaid® Maximum Strength: 1% (15 g, 30 g)
Solution, rectal, as base (Colocort™): 100 mg/60 mL (7s) [packaged as single-dose enemas]
Suppository, rectal, as acetate: 25 mg (12s, 24s)
Anucort™ HC: 25 mg (12s, 24s, 100s)
Anusol-HC®: 25 mg (12s, 24s)
Hemril® HC: 25 mg (12s)
Proctocort®: 30 mg (12s, 24s)
Proctosol-HC®: 25 mg (12s, 24s)

hydrocortisone sodium phosphate *see* hydrocortisone (systemic) *on this page*

hydrocortisone sodium succinate *see* hydrocortisone (systemic) *on this page*

hydrocortisone (systemic) (hye droe KOR ti sone sis TEM ik)

Sound-Alike/Look-Alike Issues
hydrocortisone may be confused with hydrocodone, hydroxychloroquine
Cortef® may be confused with Lortab®

Synonyms compound F; cortisol; hydrocortisone acetate; hydrocortisone cypionate; hydrocortisone sodium phosphate; hydrocortisone sodium succinate

U.S./Canadian Brand Names A-HydroCort® [US]; Cortef® Tablet [US/Can]; Hydrocortone® Phosphate [US]; Solu-Cortef® [US/Can]

(Continued)

hydrocortisone (systemic) *(Continued)*

Therapeutic Category Adrenal Corticosteroid

Use Management of adrenocortical insufficiency; relief of inflammation of corticosteroid-responsive dermatoses (low and medium potency topical corticosteroid); adjunctive treatment of ulcerative colitis

Usual Dosage Dose should be based on severity of disease and patient response

Acute adrenal insufficiency: I.M., I.V.:

Infants and young Children: Succinate: 1-2 mg/kg/dose bolus, then 25-150 mg/day in divided doses every 6-8 hours

Older Children: Succinate: 1-2 mg/kg bolus then 150-250 mg/day in divided doses every 6-8 hours

Adults: Succinate: 100 mg I.V. bolus, then 300 mg/day in divided doses every 8 hours or as a continuous infusion for 48 hours; once patient is stable change to oral, 50 mg every 8 hours for 6 doses, then taper to 30-50 mg/day in divided doses

Chronic adrenal corticoid insufficiency: Adults: Oral: 20-30 mg/day

Antiinflammatory or immunosuppressive:

Infants and Children:

Oral: 2.5-10 mg/kg/day **or** 75-300 mg/m^2/day every 6-8 hours

I.M., I.V.: Succinate: 1-5 mg/kg/day **or** 30-150 mg/m^2/day divided every 12-24 hours

Adolescents and Adults: Oral, I.M., I.V.: Succinate: 15-240 mg every 12 hours

Congenital adrenal hyperplasia: Oral: Initial: 10-20 mg/m^2/day in 3 divided doses; a variety of dosing schedules have been used. **Note:** Inconsistencies have occurred with liquid formulations; tablets may provide more reliable levels. Doses must be individualized by monitoring growth, bone age, and hormonal levels. Mineralocorticoid and sodium supplementation may be required based upon electrolyte regulation and plasma renin activity.

Physiologic replacement: Children:

Oral: 0.5-0.75 mg/kg/day **or** 20-25 mg/m^2/day every 8 hours

I.M.: Succinate: 0.25-0.35 mg/kg/day **or** 12-15 mg/m^2/day once daily

Shock: I.M., I.V.: Succinate:

Children: Initial: 50 mg/kg, then repeated in 4 hours and/or every 24 hours as needed

Adolescents and Adults: 500 mg to 2 g every 2-6 hours

Status asthmaticus: Children and Adults: I.V.: Succinate: 1-2 mg/kg/dose every 6 hours for 24 hours, then maintenance of 0.5-1 mg/kg every 6 hours

Adults:

Rheumatic diseases:

Intralesional, intraarticular, soft tissue injection: Acetate: Large joints: 25 mg (up to 37.5 mg) Small joints: 10-25 mg

Tendon sheaths: 5-12.5 mg

Soft tissue infiltration: 25-50 mg (up to 75 mg)

Bursae: 25-37.5 mg

Ganglia: 12.5-25 mg

Stress dosing (surgery) in patients known to be adrenally-suppressed or on chronic systemic steroids: I.V.:

Minor stress (ie, inguinal herniorrhaphy): 25 mg/day for 1 day

Moderate stress (ie, joint replacement, cholecystectomy): 50-75 mg/day (25 mg every 8-12 hours) for 1-2 days

Major stress (pancreatoduodenectomy, esophagogastrectomy, cardiac surgery): 100-150 mg/day (50 mg every 8-12 hours) for 2-3 days

Dermatosis: Children >2 years and Adults: Topical: Apply to affected area 2-4 times/day (Buteprate: Apply once or twice daily). Therapy should be discontinued when control is achieved; if no improvement is seen, reassessment of diagnosis may be necessary.

Ulcerative colitis: Adults: Rectal: 10-100 mg 1-2 times/day for 2-3 weeks

Dosage Forms

Injection, powder for reconstitution, as sodium succinate:

A-Hydrocort®: 100 mg, 250 mg [diluent contains benzyl alcohol]

Solu-Cortef®: 100 mg, 250 mg, 500 mg, 1 g [diluent contains benzyl alcohol]

Injection, solution, as sodium phosphate (Hydrocortone® Phosphate): 50 mg/mL (2 mL) [contains sodium bisulfite]
Tablet, as base: 20 mg
Cortef®: 5 mg, 10 mg, 20 mg

hydrocortisone (topical) (hye droe KOR ti sone TOP i kal)

Sound-Alike/Look-Alike Issues
Hytone® may be confused with Vytone®

Synonyms hydrocortisone buteprate; hydrocortisone butyrate; hydrocortisone valerate; succinate

U.S./Canadian Brand Names Aquacort® [Can]; Aquanil™ HC [US]; CaldeCORT® [US]; Cetacort® [US]; Cortagel® Maximum Strength [US]; Cortaid® Intensive Therapy [US]; Cortaid® Maximum Strength [US]; Cortaid® Sensitive Skin With Aloe [US]; Corticool® [US]; Cortizone®-5 [US]; Cortizone®-10 Maximum Strength [US]; Cortizone®-10 Plus Maximum Strength [US]; Cortizone® 10 Quick Shot [US]; Cortizone® for Kids [US]; Dermarest® Dri-Cort [US]; Dermtex® HC [US]; Hytone® [US]; LactiCare-HC® [US]; Locoid® [US/Can]; Nupercainal® Hydrocortisone Cream [US]; Nutracort® [US]; Pandel® [US]; Post Peel Healing Balm [US]; Sarnol®-HC [US]; Summer's Eve® SpecialCare™ Medicated Anti-Itch Cream [US]; Texacort® [US]; Theracort® [US]; Westcort® [US/Can]

Therapeutic Category Corticosteroid, Topical

Use Management of adrenocortical insufficiency; relief of inflammation of corticosteroid-responsive dermatoses (low and medium potency topical corticosteroid); adjunctive treatment of ulcerative colitis

Usual Dosage Dose should be based on severity of disease and patient response
Acute adrenal insufficiency: I.M., I.V.:
Infants and young Children: Succinate: 1-2 mg/kg/dose bolus, then 25-150 mg/day in divided doses every 6-8 hours
Older Children: Succinate: 1-2 mg/kg bolus then 150-250 mg/day in divided doses every 6-8 hours
Adults: Succinate: 100 mg I.V. bolus, then 300 mg/day in divided doses every 8 hours or as a continuous infusion for 48 hours; once patient is stable change to oral, 50 mg every 8 hours for 6 doses, then taper to 30-50 mg/day in divided doses
Chronic adrenal corticoid insufficiency: Adults: Oral: 20-30 mg/day
Antiinflammatory or immunosuppressive:
Infants and Children:
Oral: 2.5-10 mg/kg/day **or** 75-300 mg/m^2/day every 6-8 hours
I.M., I.V.: Succinate: 1-5 mg/kg/day **or** 30-150 mg/m^2/day divided every 12-24 hours
Adolescents and Adults: Oral, I.M., I.V.: Succinate: 15-240 mg every 12 hours
Congenital adrenal hyperplasia: Oral: Initial: 10-20 mg/m^2/day in 3 divided doses; a variety of dosing schedules have been used. **Note:** Inconsistencies have occurred with liquid formulations; tablets may provide more reliable levels. Doses must be individualized by monitoring growth, bone age, and hormonal levels. Mineralocorticoid and sodium supplementation may be required based upon electrolyte regulation and plasma renin activity.
Physiologic replacement: Children:
Oral: 0.5-0.75 mg/kg/day **or** 20-25 mg/m^2/day every 8 hours
I.M.: Succinate: 0.25-0.35 mg/kg/day **or** 12-15 mg/m^2/day once daily
Shock: I.M., I.V.: Succinate:
Children: Initial: 50 mg/kg, then repeated in 4 hours and/or every 24 hours as needed
Adolescents and Adults: 500 mg to 2 g every 2-6 hours
Status asthmaticus: Children and Adults: I.V.: Succinate: 1-2 mg/kg/dose every 6 hours for 24 hours, then maintenance of 0.5-1 mg/kg every 6 hours
Adults:
Rheumatic diseases:
Intralesional, intra-articular, soft tissue injection: Acetate: Large joints: 25 mg (up to 37.5 mg) Small joints: 10-25 mg
Tendon sheaths: 5-12.5 mg
Soft tissue infiltration: 25-50 mg (up to 75 mg)
Bursae: 25-37.5 mg
(Continued)

hydrocortisone (topical) *(Continued)*

Ganglia: 12.5-25 mg

Stress dosing (surgery) in patients known to be adrenally-suppressed or on chronic systemic steroids: I.V.:

Minor stress (ie, inguinal herniorrhaphy): 25 mg/day for 1 day

Moderate stress (ie, joint replacement, cholecystectomy): 50-75 mg/day (25 mg every 8-12 hours) for 1-2 days

Major stress (pancreatoduodenectomy, esophagogastrectomy, cardiac surgery): 100-150 mg/day (50 mg every 8-12 hours) for 2-3 days

Dermatosis: Children >2 years and Adults: Topical: Apply to affected area 2-4 times/day (Buteprate: Apply once or twice daily). Therapy should be discontinued when control is achieved; if no improvement is seen, reassessment of diagnosis may be necessary.

Ulcerative colitis: Adults: Rectal: 10-100 mg 1-2 times/day for 2-3 weeks

Dosage Forms

Aerosol, topical spray, as base
- Cortizone® 10 Quick Shot: 1% (44 mL) [contains benzyl alcohol]
- Dermtex® HC: 1% (52 mL) [contains menthol 1%]

Cream, rectal, as acetate (Nupercainal® Hydrocortisone Cream): 1% (30 g)

Cream, rectal, as base:
- Cortizone®-10: 1% (30g) [contains aloe]
- Preparation H® Hydrocortisone: 1% (27 g)

Cream, topical, as acetate: 0.5% (30 g) [available with aloe]; 1% (30 g) [available with aloe]
- Cortaid® Maximum Strength: 1% (15 g, 30 g, 40 g)
- Cortaid® Sensitive Skin With Aloe: 0.5% (15 g) [contains aloe vera gel]

Cream, topical, as base: 0.5% (30 g); 1% (1.5 g, 30 g, 454 g); 2.5% (20 g, 30 g, 454 g)
- CaldeCORT®: 1% (15 g, 30 g)[contains aloe vera gel and benzyl alcohol]
- Cortaid® Intensive Therapy: 1% (60 g)
- Cortaid® Maximum Strength: 1% (15 g, 30 g, 40 g, 60 g) [contains aloe vera gel and benzyl alcohol]
- Cortizone®-5: 0.5% (30 g, 60 g) [contains aloe]
- Cortizone®-10 Maximum Strength: 1% (15 g, 30 g, 60 g) [contains aloe]
- Cortizone®-10 Plus Maximum Strength: 1% (30 g, 60 g) [contains vitamins A, D, E and aloe]
- Cortizone® for Kids: 0.5% (30 g) [contains aloe]
- Dermarest® Dri-Cort: 1% (15 g, 30 g)
- Hytone®: 2.5% (30 g, 60 g)
- Post Peel Healing Balm: 1% (23 g)
- Summer's Eve® SpecialCare™ Medicated Anti-Itch Cream: 1% (30 g)

Cream, topical, as butyrate (Locoid®, Locoid Lipocream®): 0.1% (15 g, 45 g)

Cream, topical, as probutate (Pandel®): 0.1% (15 g, 45 g, 80 g)

Cream, topical, as valerate (Westcort®): 0.2% (15 g, 45 g, 60 g)

Gel, topical, as base:
- Corticool®: 1% (45 g)
- Cortagel® Maximum Strength: 1% (15 g, 30 g) [contains aloe vera gel]

Lotion, topical, as base: 1% (120 mL); 2.5% (60 mL)
- Aquanil™ HC: 1% (120 mL)
- Cetacort®, Sarnol®-HC: 1% (60 mL)
- Hytone®: 1% (30 mL, 120 mL); 2.5% (60 mL)
- LactiCare-HC®: 1% (120 mL); 2.5% (60 mL, 120 mL)
- Nutracort®: 1% (60 mL, 120 mL); 2.5% (60 mL, 120 mL)
- Theracort®: 1% (120 mL)

Ointment, topical, as acetate: 1% (30 g) [available with aloe]
- Cortaid® Maximum Strength: 1% (15 g, 30 g)

Ointment, topical, as base: 0.5% (30 g); 1% (30 g, 454 g); 2.5% (20 g, 30 g, 454 g)
- Cortizone®-5: 0.5% (30 g) [contains aloe]
- Cortizone®-10 Maximum Strength: 1% (30 g, 60 g)
- Hytone®: 2.5% (30 g)

Ointment, topical, as base [in Orabase®]: 1% (25 g, 110 g, 454 g)
Ointment, topical, as butyrate (Locoid®): 0.1% (15 g, 45 g)
Ointment, topical, as valerate (Westcort®): 0.2% (15 g, 45 g, 60 g)
Solution, topical, as base (Texacort®): 1% (30 mL) [DSC]; 2.5% (30 mL) [contains alcohol]
Solution, topical, as butyrate (Locoid®): 0.1% (20 mL, 60 mL) [contains alcohol 50%]

hydrocortisone valerate *see* hydrocortisone (topical) *on page 451*

Hydrocortone® Acetate *(Discontinued)* *see page 1042*

Hydrocortone® Phosphate [US] *see* hydrocortisone (systemic) *on page 449*

Hydro-Crysti-12® *(Discontinued)* *see page 1042*

HydroDIURIL® *(Discontinued)* *see page 1042*

Hydrogesic® *(Discontinued)* *see page 1042*

Hydromet® [US] *see* hydrocodone and homatropine *on page 446*

Hydromorph Contin® [Can] *see* hydromorphone *on this page*

hydromorphone (hye droe MOR fone)

Sound-Alike/Look-Alike Issues

hydromorphone may be confused with morphine

Dilaudid® may be confused with Astramorph/PF™, Demerol®, Dilantin®, Duramorph®, Infumorph®

Synonyms dihydromorphinone; hydromorphone hydrochloride

U.S./Canadian Brand Names Dilaudid® [US/Can]; Dilaudid-HP® [US/Can]; Dilaudid-HP-Plus® [Can]; Dilaudid® Sterile Powder [Can]; Dilaudid-XP® [Can]; Hydromorph Contin® [Can]; Hydromorphone HP [Can]; PMS-Hydromorphone [Can]

Therapeutic Category Analgesic, Narcotic

Controlled Substance C-II

Use Management of moderate-to-severe pain

Usual Dosage

Acute pain (moderate to severe): **Note:** These are guidelines and do not represent the maximum doses that may be required in all patients. Doses should be titrated to pain relief/prevention.

Young Children ≥6 months and <50 kg:

Oral: 0.03-0.08 mg/kg/dose every 3-4 hours as needed

I.V.: 0.015 mg/kg/dose every 3-6 hours as needed

Older Children >50 kg and Adults:

Oral: Initial: Opiate-naive: 2-4 mg every 3-4 hours as needed; patients with prior opiate exposure may require higher initial doses; usual dosage range: 2-8 mg every 3-4 hours as needed

I.V.: Initial: Opiate-naive: 0.2-0.6 mg every 2-3 hours as needed; patients with prior opiate exposure may tolerate higher initial doses **Note:** More frequent dosing may be needed. Mechanically-ventilated patients (based on 70 kg patient): 0.7-2 mg every 1-2 hours as needed; infusion (based on 70 kg patient): 0.5-1 mg/hour

Patient-controlled analgesia (PCA): (Opiate-naive: Consider lower end of dosing range) Usual concentration: 0.2 mg/mL Demand dose: Usual: 0.1-0.2 mg; range: 0.05-0.5 mg Lockout interval: 5-15 minutes 4-hour limit: 4-6 mg

Epidural: Bolus dose: 1-1.5 mg Infusion concentration: 0.05-0.075 mg/mL Infusion rate: 0.04-0.4 mg/hour Demand dose: 0.15 mg Lockout interval: 30 minutes

I.M., SubQ: **Note:** I.M. use may result in variable absorption and a lag time to peak effect. Initial: Opiate-naive: 0.8-1 mg every 4-6 hours as needed; patients with prior opiate exposure may require higher initial doses; usual dosage range: 1-2 mg every 3-6 hours as needed

Rectal: 3 mg every 4-8 hours as needed

Chronic pain: Adults: Oral: **Note:** Patients taking opioids chronically may become tolerant and require doses higher than the usual dosage range to maintain the desired effect. Tolerance can be managed by appropriate dose titration. There is no optimal or

(Continued)

hydromorphone *(Continued)*

maximal dose for hydromorphone in chronic pain. The appropriate dose is one that relieves pain throughout its dosing interval without causing unmanageable side effects.

Controlled release formulation (Hydromorph Contin®, not available in U.S.): 3-30 mg every 12 hours. **Note:** A patient's hydromorphone requirement should be established using prompt release formulations; conversion to long acting products may be considered when chronic, continuous treatment is required. Higher dosages should be reserved for use only in opioid-tolerant patients.

Extended release formulation (Palladone™): For use only in opioid-tolerant patients requiring extended treatment of pain. Initial Palladone™ dose should be calculated using standard conversion estimates based on previous total daily opioid dose, rounding off to the most appropriate strength available. Doses should be administered once every 24 hours. Discontinue all previous around-the-clock opioids when treatment is initiated. Dose may be adjusted every 2 days as needed.

Conversion from transdermal fentanyl to oral Palladone™ (limited clinical experience): Initiate Palladone™ 18 hours after removal of patch; substitute Palladone™ 12 mg/day for each fentanyl 50 mcg/hour patch; monitor closely

Conversion from opioid combination drugs: Initial dose: Palladone™ 12 mg/day in patients receiving around-the-clock fixed combination-opioid analgesics with a total dose greater than or equal to oxycodone 45 mg/day, hydrocodone 45 mg/day, or codeine 300 mg/day

Dosage Forms [Can] = Canadian brand name

Capsule, controlled release (Hydromorph Contin®) [Can]: 3 mg, 6 mg, 12 mg, 18 mg, 24 mg, 30 mg [not available in U.S.]

Capsule, extended release, as hydrochloride (Pallidone™): 12 mg, 16 mg, 24 mg, 32 mg

Injection, powder for reconstitution, as hydrochloride (Dilaudid-HP®): 250 mg

Injection, solution, as hydrochloride: 1 mg/mL (1 mL); 2 mg/mL (1 mL, 20 mL); 4 mg/mL (1 mL); 10 mg/mL (1 mL, 5 mL, 10 mL)

Dilaudid®: 1 mg/mL (1 mL); 2 mg/mL (1 mL, 20 mL) [20 mL size contains edetate sodium; vial stopper contains latex]; 4 mg/mL (1 mL)

Dilaudid-HP®: 10 mg/mL (1 mL, 5 mL, 50 mL)

Liquid, oral, as hydrochloride (Dilaudid®): 1 mg/mL (480 mL) [may contain trace amounts of sodium bisulfite]

Suppository, rectal, as hydrochloride (Dilaudid®): 3 mg (6s)

Tablet, as hydrochloride (Dilaudid®): 2 mg, 4 mg, 8 mg (8 mg tablets may contain trace amounts of sodium bisulfite)

Hydromorphone HP [Can] *see* hydromorphone *on previous page*

hydromorphone hydrochloride *see* hydromorphone *on previous page*

Hydromox® ***(Discontinued)*** *see page 1042*

Hydropane® [US] *see* hydrocodone and homatropine *on page 446*

Hydro-Par® ***(Discontinued)*** *see page 1042*

Hydrophed® ***(Discontinued)*** *see page 1042*

Hydropres® ***(Discontinued)*** *see page 1042*

hydroquinol *see* hydroquinone *on this page*

hydroquinone (HYE droe kwin one)

Sound-Alike/Look-Alike Issues

Eldopaque Forte® may be confused with Eldoquin Forte®

Synonyms hydroquinol; quinol

U.S./Canadian Brand Names Alphaquin HP [US]; Alustra™ [US]; Claripel™ [US]; Eldopaque Forte® [US]; Eldopaque® [US-OTC/Can]; Eldoquin® [US/Can]; Eldoquin® Forte® [US]; EpiQuin™ Micro [US]; Esoterica® Regular [US-OTC]; Glyquin® [US]; Glyquin® XM [Can]; Lustra® [US/Can]; Lustra-AF™ [US]; Melanex® [US]; Melpaque HP® [US]; Melquin-3® [US]; Melquin HP® [US]; NeoStrata® AHA [US-OTC]; NeoStrata® HQ

[Can]; Nuquin HP® Cream [US]; Palmer's® Skin Success Fade Cream™ [US-OTC]; Solaquin Forte® [US/Can]; Solaquin® [US-OTC/Can]; Ultraquin™ [Can]

Therapeutic Category Topical Skin Product

Use Gradual bleaching of hyperpigmented skin conditions

Usual Dosage Children >12 years and Adults: Topical: Apply thin layer and rub in twice daily

Dosage Forms

Cream, topical: 4% (30 g) [may contain sodium metabisulfite]

Alphaquin HP, Alustra™: 4% (30 g)

Eldopaque®: 2% (15 g, 30 g)

Eldopaque Forte®, Eldoquin Forte®: 4% (30 g) [contains sodium metabisulfite]

EpiQuin™ Micro: 4% (30 g) [contains benzyl alcohol and sodium metabisulfite]

Esoterica® Regular: 2% (85 g) [contains sodium bisulfite]

Lustra®: 4% (30 g, 60 g) [contains sodium metabisulfite]

Melquin HP®: 4% (15 g, 30 g) [contains sodium metabisulfite]

Nuquin HP: 4% (15 g, 30 g, 60 g) [contains sodium metabisulfite]

Palmer's® Skin Success Fade Cream™: 2% (81 g, 132 g) [contains sodium sulfite; available in regular, oily skin, and dry skin formulas]

Cream, topical [with sunscreen]: 4% (30 g) [may contain sodium metabisulfite]

Claripel™: 4% (45 g) [contains sodium metabisulfite]

Glyquin®: 4% (30 g)

Solaquin®: 2% (30 g)

Solaquin Forte®: 4% (30 g) [contains sodium metabisulfite]

Lustra-AF™: 4% (30 g, 60 g) [contains sodium metabisulfite]

Melpaque HP®: 4% (15 g, 30 g) [contains sodium metabisulfite; sunblocking cream base]

Gel, topical (NeoStrata AHA): 2% (45 g) [contains sodium bisulfite and sodium sulfite]

Gel, topical [with sunscreen]:

Nuquin HP: 4% (15 g, 30 g) [contains sodium bisulfite]

Solaquin Forte®: 4% (30 g) [contains sodium metabisulfite]

Solution, topical (Melanex®, Melquin-3®): 3% (30 mL)

hydroquinone, fluocinolone acetonide, and tretinoin *see* fluocinolone, hydroquinone, and tretinoin *on page 375*

Hydrotropine® ***(Discontinued)*** *see page 1042*

Hydro-Tussin™-CBX [US] *see* carbinoxamine and pseudoephedrine *on page 157*

Hydro-Tussin™ DM [US] *see* guaifenesin and dextromethorphan *on page 416*

Hydro-Tussin™ HD [US] *see* hydrocodone, pseudoephedrine, and guaifenesin *on page 447*

Hydro-Tussin™ XP [US] *see* hydrocodone, pseudoephedrine, and guaifenesin *on page 447*

Hydroxacen® ***(Discontinued)*** *see page 1042*

4-hydroxybutyrate *see* sodium oxybate *on page 813*

hydroxycarbamide *see* hydroxyurea *on page 457*

hydroxychloroquine (hye droks ee KLOR oh kwin)

Sound-Alike/Look-Alike Issues

hydroxychloroquine may be confused with hydrocortisone

Plaquenil® may be confused with Platinol®

Synonyms hydroxychloroquine sulfate

U.S./Canadian Brand Names Apo-Hydroxyquine® [Can]; Plaquenil® [US/Can]

Therapeutic Category Aminoquinoline (Antimalarial)

Use Suppression and treatment of acute attacks of malaria; treatment of systemic lupus erythematosus and rheumatoid arthritis

(Continued)

hydroxychloroquine *(Continued)*

Usual Dosage Note: Hydroxychloroquine sulfate 200 mg is equivalent to 155 mg hydroxychloroquine base and 250 mg chloroquine phosphate. Oral:

Children:

Chemoprophylaxis of malaria: 5 mg/kg (base) once weekly; should not exceed the recommended adult dose; begin 2 weeks before exposure; continue for 4-6 weeks after leaving endemic area; if suppressive therapy is not begun prior to the exposure, double the initial dose and give in 2 doses, 6 hours apart

Acute attack: 10 mg/kg (base) initial dose; followed by 5 mg/kg at 6, 24, and 48 hours

JRA or SLE: 3-5 mg/kg/day divided 1-2 times/day; avoid exceeding 7 mg/kg/day

Adults:

Chemoprophylaxis of malaria: 310 mg base weekly on same day each week; begin 2 weeks before exposure; continue for 4-6 weeks after leaving endemic area; if suppressive therapy is not begun prior to the exposure, double the initial dose and give in 2 doses, 6 hours apart

Acute attack: 620 mg first dose day 1; 310 mg in 6 hours day 1; 310 mg in 1 dose day 2; and 310 mg in 1 dose on day 3

Rheumatoid arthritis: 310-465 mg/day to start taken with food or milk; increase dose until optimum response level is reached; usually after 4-12 weeks dose should be reduced by $^1/_2$ and a maintenance dose of 155-310 mg/day given

Lupus erythematosus: 310 mg every day or twice daily for several weeks depending on response; 155-310 mg/day for prolonged maintenance therapy

Dosage Forms Tablet, as sulfate: 200 mg [equivalent to 155 mg base]

hydroxychloroquine sulfate *see* hydroxychloroquine *on previous page*

hydroxydaunomycin hydrochloride *see* doxorubicin *on page 293*

1α-hydroxyergocalciferol *see* doxercalciferol *on page 292*

hydroxyethylcellulose *see* artificial tears *on page 78*

hydroxyethyl starch *see* hetastarch *on page 434*

hydroxyldaunorubicin hydrochloride *see* doxorubicin *on page 293*

hydroxyprogesterone caproate

(hye droks ee proe JES te rone KAP roe ate)

Therapeutic Category Progestin

Use Treatment of amenorrhea, abnormal uterine bleeding, submucous fibroids, endometriosis, uterine carcinoma, and testing of estrogen production

Usual Dosage Adults: I.M.:

Amenorrhea: 375 mg; if no bleeding, begin cyclic treatment with estradiol valerate

Endometriosis: Start cyclic therapy with estradiol valerate

Uterine carcinoma: 1 g one or more times/day (1-7 g/week) for up to 12 weeks

Test for endogenous estrogen production: 250 mg anytime; bleeding 7-14 days after injection indicate positive test

Dosage Forms Injection, as caproate (Hylutin®, Prodrox®): 250 mg/mL (5 mL)

hydroxypropyl cellulose (hye droks ee PROE pil SEL yoo lose)

U.S./Canadian Brand Names Lacrisert® [US/Can]

Therapeutic Category Ophthalmic Agent, Miscellaneous

Use Dry eyes (moderate to severe)

Usual Dosage Adults: Ophthalmic: Apply once daily into the inferior cul-de-sac beneath the base of tarsus, not in apposition to the cornea nor beneath the eyelid at the level of the tarsal plate

Dosage Forms Insert, ophthalmic [preservative free]: 5 mg

hydroxypropyl methylcellulose

(hye droks ee PROE pil meth il SEL yoo lose)

Sound-Alike/Look-Alike Issues

Isopto® Tears may be confused with Isoptin®

Synonyms gonioscopic ophthalmic solution; hypromellose

U.S./Canadian Brand Names Cellugel® [US]; GenTeal® Mild [US-OTC]; GenTeal® [US-OTC/Can]; Gonak™ [US-OTC]; Goniosoft™ [US]; Tears Again® MC [US-OTC]

Therapeutic Category Ophthalmic Agent, Miscellaneous

Use Relief of burning and minor irritation due to dry eyes; diagnostic agent in gonioscopic examination

Usual Dosage Adults: Dry eyes: Ophthalmic: Instill 1-2 drops in affected eye(s) as needed

Dosage Forms [DSC] = Discontinued product

Gel, ophthalmic (GenTeal®): 0.3% (10 mL)

Solution, ophthalmic: 0.4% (15 mL)

GenTeal®: 0.3% (15 mL, 25 mL)

GenTeal® Mild: 0.2% (15 mL, 25 mL)

Gonak™: 2.5% (15 mL)

Goniosoft™: 2.5% (15 mL)

Goniosol®: 2.5% (15 mL) [contains benzalkonium chloride] [DSC]

Isopto® Tears: 0.5% (15 mL) [contains benzalkonium chloride]

Tearisol®: 0.5% (15 mL) [contains benzalkonium chloride]

Tears Again® MC: 0.3% (15 mL)

Solution, ophthalmic [for injection] (Cellugel®): 2% (1 mL)

hydroxyurea (hye droks ee yoor EE a)

Sound-Alike/Look-Alike Issues

hydroxyurea may be confused with hydroxyzine

Synonyms hydroxycarbamide

U.S./Canadian Brand Names Droxia™ [US]; Gen-Hydroxyurea [Can]; Hydrea® [US/Can]; Mylocel™ [US]

Therapeutic Category Antineoplastic Agent

Use CML in chronic phase; radiosensitizing agent in the treatment of primary brain tumors, head and neck tumors, uterine cervix and nonsmall-cell lung cancer, and psoriasis; treatment of hematologic conditions such as essential thrombocythemia, polycythemia vera, hypereosinophilia, and hyperleukocytosis due to acute leukemia. Has shown activity against renal cell cancer, melanoma, ovarian cancer, head and neck cancer (excluding lip cancer), and prostate cancer.

Orphan drug: Droxia™: Sickle cell anemia: Specifically for patients >18 years of age who have had at least three "painful crises" in the previous year - to reduce frequency of these crises and the need for blood transfusions

Usual Dosage Oral (refer to individual protocols): All dosage should be based on ideal or actual body weight, whichever is less:

Children:

No FDA-approved dosage regimens have been established; dosages of 1500-3000 mg/m^2 as a single dose in combination with other agents every 4-6 weeks have been used in the treatment of pediatric astrocytoma, medulloblastoma, and primitive neuro-ectodermal tumors

CML: Initial: 10-20 mg/kg/day once daily; adjust dose according to hematologic response

Adults: Dose should always be titrated to patient response and WBC counts; usual oral doses range from 10-30 mg/kg/day or 500-3000 mg/day; if WBC count falls to <2500 cells/mm^3, or the platelet count to <100,000/mm^3, therapy should be stopped for at least 3 days and resumed when values rise toward normal

Solid tumors:

Intermittent therapy: 80 mg/kg as a single dose every third day

Continuous therapy: 20-30 mg/kg/day given as a single dose/day

(Continued)

hydroxyurea *(Continued)*

Concomitant therapy with irradiation: 80 mg/kg as a single dose every third day starting at least 7 days before initiation of irradiation

Resistant chronic myelocytic leukemia: Continuous therapy: 20-30 mg/kg as a single daily dose

Sickle cell anemia (moderate/severe disease): Initial: 15 mg/kg/day, increased by 5 mg/kg every 12 weeks if blood counts are in an acceptable range until the maximum tolerated dose of 35 mg/kg/day is achieved or the dose that does not produce toxic effects

Acceptable range: Neutrophils ≥2500 cells/mm³ Platelets ≥95,000/mm³ Hemoglobin >5.3 g/dL, and Reticulocytes ≥95,000/mm³ if the hemoglobin concentration is <9 g/dL

Toxic range: Neutrophils <2000 cells/mm³ Platelets <80,000/mm³ Hemoglobin <4.5 g/dL Reticulocytes <80,000/mm³ if the hemoglobin concentration is <9 g/dL Monitor for toxicity every 2 weeks; if toxicity occurs, stop treatment until the bone marrow recovers; restart at 2.5 mg/kg/day less than the dose at which toxicity occurs; if no toxicity occurs over the next 12 weeks, then the subsequent dose should be increased by 2.5 mg/kg/day; reduced dosage of hydroxyurea alternating with erythropoietin may decrease myelotoxicity and increase levels of fetal hemoglobin in patients who have not been helped by hydroxyurea alone

Dosage Forms

Capsule: 500 mg

Droxia™: 200 mg, 300 mg, 400 mg

Hydrea®: 500 mg

Tablet (Mylocel™): 1000 mg

hydroxyzine (hye DROKS i zeen)

Sound-Alike/Look-Alike Issues

hydroxyzine may be confused with hydralazine, hydroxyurea

Atarax® may be confused with amoxicillin, Ativan®

Vistaril® may be confused with Restoril®, Versed®, Zestril®

Synonyms hydroxyzine hydrochloride; hydroxyzine pamoate

Tall-Man hydro**OXY**zine

U.S./Canadian Brand Names Apo-Hydroxyzine® [Can]; Atarax® [US/Can]; Novo-Hydroxyzin [Can]; PMS-Hydroxyzine [Can]; Vistaril® [US/Can]

Therapeutic Category Antiemetic; Antihistamine

Use Treatment of anxiety; preoperative sedative; antipruritic

Usual Dosage

Children:

Oral: 0.6 mg/kg/dose every 6 hours

I.M.: 0.5-1.1 mg/kg/dose every 4-6 hours as needed

Adults:

Antiemetic: I.M.: 25-100 mg/dose every 4-6 hours as needed

Anxiety: Oral: 25-100 mg 4 times/day; maximum dose: 600 mg/day

Preoperative sedation:

Oral: 50-100 mg

I.M.: 25-100 mg

Management of pruritus: Oral: 25 mg 3-4 times/day

Dosage Forms [DSC] = Discontinued product

Capsule, as pamoate (Vistaril®): 25 mg, 50 mg, 100 mg

Injection, solution, as hydrochloride: 25 mg/mL (1 mL); 50 mg/mL (1 mL, 2 mL, 10 mL)

Vistaril® [DSC]: 50 mg/mL (10 mL) [contains benzyl alcohol]

Suspension, oral, as pamoate (Vistaril®): 25 mg/5 mL (120 mL, 480 mL) [lemon flavor]

Syrup, as hydrochloride: 10 mg/5 mL (120 mL, 480 mL)

Atarax®: 10 mg/5 mL (480 mL) [contains alcohol, sodium benzoate; mint flavor]

Tablet, as hydrochloride: 10 mg, 25 mg, 50 mg

Atarax®: 10 mg, 25 mg, 50 mg, 100 mg

hydroxyzine hydrochloride *see* hydroxyzine *on previous page*

hydroxyzine pamoate *see* hydroxyzine *on previous page*

Hygroton® *(Discontinued)* *see page 1042*

Hylorel® *(Discontinued)* *see page 1042*

hyoscine *see* scopolamine *on page 796*

hyoscyamine (hye oh SYE a meen)

Sound-Alike/Look-Alike Issues

Anaspaz® may be confused with Anaprox®, Antispas®
Levbid® may be confused with Lithobid®, Lopid®, Lorabid®
Levsinex® may be confused with Lanoxin®

Synonyms hyoscyamine sulfate; *l*-hyoscyamine sulfate

U.S./Canadian Brand Names Anaspaz® [US]; Cystospaz® [US/Can]; Cystospaz-M® [US]; Hyosine [US]; Levbid® [US]; Levsin® [US/Can]; Levsinex® [US]; Levsin/SL® [US]; NuLev™ [US]; Spacol [US]; Spacol T/S [US]; Symax SL [US]; Symax SR [US]

Therapeutic Category Anticholinergic Agent

Use

Oral: Adjunctive therapy for peptic ulcers, irritable bowel, neurogenic bladder/bowel; treatment of infant colic, GI tract disorders caused by spasm; to reduce rigidity, tremors, sialorrhea, and hyperhidrosis associated with parkinsonism; as a drying agent in acute rhinitis

Injection: Preoperative antimuscarinic to reduce secretions and block cardiac vagal inhibitory reflexes; to improve radiologic visibility of the kidneys; symptomatic relief of biliary and renal colic; reduce GI motility to facilitate diagnostic procedures (ie, endoscopy, hypotonic duodenography); reduce pain and hypersecretion in pancreatitis, certain cases of partial heart block associated with vagal activity; reversal of neuromuscular blockade

Usual Dosage

Oral: Children: Gastrointestinal disorders: Dose as listed, based on age and weight (kg) using 0.125 mg/mL drops; repeat dose every 4 hours as needed:

Children <2 years:

3.4 kg: 4 drops; maximum: 24 drops/24 hours
5 kg: 5 drops; maximum: 30 drops/24 hours
7 kg: 6 drops; maximum: 36 drops/24 hours
10 kg: 8 drops; maximum: 48 drops/24 hours

Oral, S.L.:

Children 2-12 years: Gastrointestinal disorders: Dose as listed, based on age and weight (kg); repeat dose every 4 hours as needed:

10 kg: 0.031-0.033 mg; maximum: 0.75 mg/24 hours
20 kg: 0.0625 mg; maximum: 0.75 mg/24 hours
40 kg: 0.0938 mg; maximum: 0.75 mg/24 hours
50 kg: 0.125 mg; maximum: 0.75 mg/24 hours

Children >12 years and Adults: Gastrointestinal disorders: 0.125-0.25 mg every 4 hours or as needed (before meals or food); maximum: 1.5 mg/24 hours

Cystospaz®: 0.15-0.3 mg up to 4 times/day

Oral (timed release): Children >12 years and Adults: Gastrointestinal disorders: 0.375-0.75 mg every 12 hours; maximum: 1.5 mg/24 hours

I.M., I.V., SubQ: Children >12 years and Adults: Gastrointestinal disorders: 0.25-0.5 mg; may repeat as needed up to 4 times/day, at 4-hour intervals

I.V.: Children >2 year and Adults: I.V.: Preanesthesia: 5 mcg/kg given 30-60 minutes prior to induction of anesthesia or at the time preoperative narcotics or sedatives are administered

I.V.: Adults: Diagnostic procedures: 0.25-0.5 mg given 5-10 minutes prior to procedure

To reduce drug-induced bradycardia during surgery: 0.125 mg; repeat as needed

To reverse neuromuscular blockade: 0.2 mg for every 1 mg neostigmine (or the physostigmine/pyridostigmine equivalent)

(Continued)

hyoscyamine *(Continued)*

Dosage Forms

Capsule, timed release, as sulfate (Cystospaz-M®, Levsinex®): 0.375 mg
Elixir, as sulfate: 0.125 mg/5 mL (480 mL)
Hyosine: 0.125 mg/5 mL (480 mL) [contains alcohol 20% and sodium benzoate; orange flavor]
Levsin®: 0.125 mg/5 mL (480 mL) [contains alcohol 20%; orange flavor]
Injection, solution, as sulfate (Levsin®): 0.5 mg/mL (1 mL)
Liquid, as sulfate (Spacol): 0.125 mg/5 mL (120 mL) [sugar free, alcohol free, simethicone based, bubblegum flavor]
Solution, oral drops, as sulfate: 0.125 mg/mL (15 mL)
Hyosine: 0.125 mg/mL (15 mL) [contains alcohol 5% and sodium benzoate; orange flavor]
Levsin®: 0.125 mg/mL (15 mL) [contains alcohol 5%; orange flavor]
Tablet (Cystospaz®): 0.15 mg
Tablet, as sulfate (Anaspaz®, Levsin®, Spacol): 0.125 mg
Tablet, extended release, as sulfate (Levbid®, Symax SR, Spacol T/S): 0.375 mg
Tablet, orally-disintegrating, as sulfate (NuLev™): 0.125 mg [contains phenylalanine 1.7 mg/tablet, mint flavor]
Tablet, sublingual, as sulfate: 0.125 mg
Levsin/SL®: 0.125 mg [peppermint flavor]
Symax SL: 0.125 mg

hyoscyamine, atropine, scopolamine, and phenobarbital

(hye oh SYE a meen, A troe peen, skoe POL a meen, & fee noe BAR bi tal)

Sound-Alike/Look-Alike Issues

Donnatal® may be confused with Donnagel®

Synonyms atropine, hyoscyamine, scopolamine, and phenobarbital; phenobarbital, hyoscyamine, atropine, and scopolamine; scopolamine, hyoscyamine, atropine, and phenobarbital

U.S./Canadian Brand Names Donnatal® [US/Can]; Donnatal Extentabs® [US]

Therapeutic Category Anticholinergic Agent

Use Adjunct in treatment of irritable bowel syndrome, acute enterocolitis, duodenal ulcer

Usual Dosage Oral:

Children: Donnatal® elixir: To be given every 4-6 hours; initial dose based on weight:
4.5 kg: 0.5 mL every 4 hours **or** 0.75 mL every 6 hours
10 kg: 1 mL every 4 hours **or** 1.5 mL every 6 hours
14 kg: 1.5 mL every 4 hours **or** 2 mL every 6 hours
23 kg: 2.5 mL every 4 hours **or** 3.8 mL every 6 hours
34 kg: 3.8 mL every 4 hours **or** 5 mL every 6 hours
≥45 kg: 5 mL every 4 hours **or** 7.5 mL every 6 hours
Adults:
Donnatal®: 1-2 tablets or 5-10 mL of elixir 3-4 times/day
Donnatal Extentabs®: 1 tablet every 12 hours; may increase to 1 tablet every 8 hours if needed

Dosage Forms

Elixir (Donnatal®): Hyoscyamine sulfate 0.1037 mg, atropine sulfate 0.0194 mg, scopolamine hydrobromide 0.0065 mg, and phenobarbital 16.2 mg per 5 mL (120 mL, 480 mL, 4000 mL) [contains alcohol 23%; citrus flavor]
Tablet (Donnatal®): Hyoscyamine sulfate 0.1037 mg, atropine sulfate 0.0194 mg, scopolamine hydrobromide 0.0065 mg, and phenobarbital 16.2 mg
Tablet, extended release (Donnatal Extentabs®): Hyoscyamine sulfate 0.3111 mg, atropine sulfate 0.0582 mg, scopolamine hydrobromide 0.0195 mg, and phenobarbital 48.6 mg

hyoscyamine, atropine, scopolamine, kaolin, and pectin ***(Discontinued)***
see page 1042

hyoscyamine sulfate *see* hyoscyamine *on previous page*

Hyosine [US] *see* hyoscyamine *on page 459*

Hy-Pam® Oral *(Discontinued)* *see page 1042*

Hypaque-Cysto® [US] *see* radiological/contrast media (ionic) *on page 759*

Hypaque® Meglumine [US] *see* radiological/contrast media (ionic) *on page 759*

Hypaque® Sodium [US] *see* radiological/contrast media (ionic) *on page 759*

Hyperab® *(Discontinued)* *see page 1042*

Hyperstat® [US] *see* diazoxide *on page 264*

Hyperstat® I.V. [Can] *see* diazoxide *on page 264*

Hyper-Tet® *(Discontinued)* *see page 1042*

Hy-Phen® *(Discontinued)* *see page 1042*

HypoTears PF [US-OTC] *see* artificial tears *on page 78*

HypoTears [US-OTC] *see* artificial tears *on page 78*

HypRho®-D *(Discontinued)* *see page 1042*

HypRho®-D Mini-Dose *(Discontinued)* *see page 1042*

Hyprogest® 250 *(Discontinued)* *see page 1042*

hypromellose *see* hydroxypropyl methylcellulose *on page 457*

Hyrexin-50® [US] *see* diphenhydramine *on page 277*

Hytakerol® [US/Can] *see* dihydrotachysterol *on page 272*

Hytinic® [US-OTC] *see* polysaccharide-iron complex *on page 709*

Hytone® [US] *see* hydrocortisone (topical) *on page 451*

Hytrin® [US/Can] *see* terazosin *on page 845*

Hyzaar® [US/Can] *see* losartan and hydrochlorothiazide *on page 532*

Hyzaar® DS [Can] *see* losartan and hydrochlorothiazide *on page 532*

Hyzine® *(Discontinued)* *see page 1042*

131 I anti-B1 antibody *see* tositumomab and iodine I 131 tositumomab *on page 873*

131 I-anti-B1 monoclonal antibody *see* tositumomab and iodine I 131 tositumomab *on page 873*

Iberet®-500 [US-OTC] *see* vitamins (multiple/oral) *on page 927*

Iberet-Folic-500® [US] *see* vitamins (multiple/oral) *on page 927*

Iberet® [US-OTC] *see* vitamins (multiple/oral) *on page 927*

ibidomide hydrochloride *see* labetalol *on page 499*

ibritumomab (ib ri TYOO mo mab)

Synonyms ibritumomab tiuxetan; In-111 zevalin; Y-90 zevalin

U.S./Canadian Brand Names Zevalin™ [US]

Therapeutic Category Antineoplastic Agent, Monoclonal Antibody; Radiopharmaceutical

Use Treatment of relapsed or refractory low-grade, follicular, or transformed B-cell non-Hodgkin lymphoma (including rituximab-refractory follicular non-Hodgkin lymphoma) as part of a therapeutic regimen with rituximab (Zevalin™ therapeutic regimen); **not to be used as single-agent therapy**; must be radiolabeled prior to use

Usual Dosage I.V.: Adults: Ibritumomab is administered **only** as part of the Zevalin™ therapeutic regimen (a combined treatment regimen with rituximab). The regimen consists of two steps:

Step 1:

Rituximab infusion: 250 mg/m^2 at an initial rate of 50 mg/hour. If hypersensitivity or infusion-related events do not occur, increase infusion in increments of 50 mg/hour every 30 minutes, to a maximum of 400 mg/hour. Infusions should be temporarily

(Continued)

ibritumomab *(Continued)*

slowed or interrupted if hypersensitivity or infusion-related events occur. The infusion may be resumed at one-half the previous rate upon improvement of symptoms.

In-111 ibritumomab infusion: Within 4 hours of the completion of rituximab infusion, inject 5 mCi (1.6 mg total antibody dose) over 10 minutes.

Biodistribution of In-111 ibritumomab should be assessed by imaging at 2-24 hours and at 48-72 hours postinjection. An optional third imaging may be performed 90-120 hours following injection. If biodistribution is not acceptable, the patient should not proceed to Step 2.

Step 2 (initiated 7-9 days following Step 1):

Rituximab infusion: 250 mg/m^2 at an initial rate of 100 mg/hour (50 mg/hour if infusion-related events occurred with the first infusion). If hypersensitivity or infusion-related events do not occur, increase infusion in increments of 100 mg/hour every 30 minutes, to a maximum of 400 mg/hour, as tolerated.

Y-90 ibritumomab infusion: Within 4 hours of the completion of rituximab infusion:

Platelet count >150,000 cells/mm^3: Inject 0.4 mCi/kg (14.8 MBq/kg actual body weight) over 10 minutes

Platelet count between 100,000-149,000 cells/mm^3: Inject 0.3 mCi/kg (11.1 MBq/kg actual body weight) over 10 minutes

Platelet count <100,000 cells/mm^3: Do **not** administer

Maximum dose: The prescribed, measured, and administered dose of Y-90 ibritumomab must not exceed 32 mCi (1184 MBq), regardless of the patient's body weight

Dosage Forms Each kit contains 4 vials for preparation of either In-111 or Y-90 conjugate (as indicated on container label)

Injection, solution: 1.6 mg/mL (2 mL) [supplied with sodium acetate solution, formulation buffer vial (includes albumin 750 mg), and an empty reaction vial]

ibritumomab tiuxetan *see* ibritumomab *on previous page*

Ibu-200 [US-OTC] *see* ibuprofen *on this page*

Ibuprin® *(Discontinued)* *see page 1042*

ibuprofen (eye byoo PROE fen)

Synonyms *p*-isobutylhydratropic acid

U.S./Canadian Brand Names Advil® Children's [US-OTC]; Advil® Infants' [US-OTC]; Advil® Junior [US-OTC]; Advil® Migraine [US-OTC]; Advil® [US-OTC/Can]; Apo-Ibuprofen® [Can]; Genpril® [US-OTC]; Ibu-200 [US-OTC]; I-Prin [US-OTC]; Menadol® [US-OTC]; Midol® Maximum Strength Cramp Formula [US-OTC]; Motrin® [US/Can]; Motrin® Children's [US-OTC/Can]; Motrin® IB [US-OTC/Can]; Motrin® Infants' [US-OTC]; Motrin® Junior Strength [US-OTC]; Motrin® Migraine Pain [US-OTC]; Novo-Profen® [Can]; Nu-Ibuprofen [Can]; Ultraprin [US-OTC]

Therapeutic Category Analgesic, Nonnarcotic; Antipyretic; Nonsteroidal Antiinflammatory Drug (NSAID)

Use Inflammatory diseases and rheumatoid disorders including juvenile rheumatoid arthritis, mild to moderate pain, fever, dysmenorrhea

Usual Dosage Oral:

Children:

Antipyretic: 6 months to 12 years: Temperature <102.5°F (39°C): 5 mg/kg/dose; temperature >102.5°F: 10 mg/kg/dose administered every 6-8 hours; maximum daily dose: 40 mg/kg/day

Juvenile rheumatoid arthritis: 30-50 mg/kg/day in 4 divided doses; start at lower end of dosing range and titrate upward; maximum: 2.4 g/day

Analgesic: 4-10 mg/kg/dose every 6-8 hours

Adults:

Inflammatory disease: 400-800 mg/dose 3-4 times/day; maximum dose: 3.2 g/day

Pain/fever/dysmenorrhea: 200-400 mg/dose every 4-6 hours; maximum daily dose: 1.2 g

Dosage Forms [DSC] = Discontinued product
Caplet: 200 mg [OTC]
Advil®: 200 mg [contains sodium benzoate]
Ibu-200, Menadol®, Motrin® IB, Motrin® Migraine Pain: 200 mg
Motrin® Junior Strength: 100 mg [contains tartrazine]
Capsule, liqui-gel:
Advil®: 200 mg
Advil® Migraine: 200 mg [solubilized ibuprofen]
Gelcap:
Advil®: 200 mg
Motrin® IB: 200 mg [contains benzyl alcohol]
Suspension, oral: 100 mg/5 mL (5 mL, 120 mL, 480 mL)
Advil® Children's: 100 mg/5 mL (60 mL, 120 mL) [contains sodium benzoate; blue raspberry, fruit, and grape flavors]
Motrin® Children's: 100 mg/5 mL (60 mL, 120 mL) [contains sodium benzoate; berry, dye-free berry, bubble gum, and grape flavors]
Suspension, oral drops: 40 mg/mL (15 mL)
Advil® Infants': 40 mg/mL (15 mL) [contains sodium benzoate; fruit and grape flavors]
Motrin® Infants': 40 mg/mL (15 mL, 30 mL) [contains sodium benzoate; berry and dye-free berry flavors]
Tablet: 200 mg [OTC], 400 mg, 600 mg, 800 mg
Advil®: 200 mg [contains sodium benzoate]
Advil® Junior: 100 mg [contains sodium benzoate; coated tablets]
Genpril®, Haltran® [DSC], I-Prin, Midol® Maximum Strength Cramp Formula, Motrin® IB, Proprinal, Ultraprin: 200 mg
Motrin®: 400 mg, 600 mg, 800 mg
Tablet, chewable:
Advil® Children's: 50 mg [contains phenylalanine 2.1 mg; fruit and grape flavors]
Advil® Junior: 100 mg [contains phenylalanine 2.1 mg; fruit and grape flavors]
Motrin® Children's: 50 mg [contains phenylalanine 1.4 mg; orange flavor]
Motrin® Junior Strength: 100 mg [contains phenylalanine 2.1 mg; grape and orange flavors]

ibuprofen and hydrocodone *see* hydrocodone and ibuprofen *on page 446*

ibuprofen and pseudoephedrine *see* pseudoephedrine and ibuprofen *on page 747*

ibutilide (i BYOO ti lide)

Synonyms ibutilide fumarate
U.S./Canadian Brand Names Corvert® [US]
Therapeutic Category Antiarrhythmic Agent, Class III
Use Acute termination of atrial fibrillation or flutter of recent onset; the effectiveness of ibutilide has not been determined in patients with arrhythmias >90 days in duration
Usual Dosage I.V.: Initial: Adults:
<60 kg: 0.01 mg/kg over 10 minutes
≥60 kg: 1 mg over 10 minutes
If the arrhythmia does not terminate within 10 minutes after the end of the initial infusion, a second infusion of equal strength may be infused over a 10-minute period
Dosage Forms Injection, solution, as fumarate: 0.1 mg/mL (10 mL)

ibutilide fumarate *see* ibutilide *on this page*

IC-Green® [US] *see* indocyanine green *on page 471*

ICI 182,780 *see* fulvestrant *on page 393*

ICI 204, 219 *see* zafirlukast *on page 936*

ICI-46474 *see* tamoxifen *on page 839*

ICI-118630 *see* goserelin *on page 413*

ICI-176334 *see* bicalutamide *on page 119*

ICI-D1033 *see* anastrozole *on page 59*

ICI-D1694 *see* raltitrexed *(Canada only) on page 762*

ICRF-187 *see* dexrazoxane *on page 257*

I.D.A. [US] *see* acetaminophen, isometheptene, and dichloralphenazone *on page 13*

Idamycin® [Can] *see* idarubicin *on this page*

Idamycin® *(Discontinued)* *see page 1042*

Idamycin PFS® [US] *see* idarubicin *on this page*

idarubicin (eye da ROO bi sin)

Sound-Alike/Look-Alike Issues
idarubicin may be confused with daunorubicin, doxorubicin
Idamycin PFS® may be confused with Adriamycin™

Synonyms 4-demethoxydaunorubicin; 4-DMDR; idarubicin hydrochloride; IDR; IMI 30; NSC-256439; SC 33428

U.S./Canadian Brand Names Idamycin® [Can]; Idamycin PFS® [US]

Therapeutic Category Antineoplastic Agent

Use Treatment of acute leukemias (AML, ANLL, ALL), accelerated phase or blast crisis of chronic myelogenous leukemia (CML), breast cancer

Usual Dosage Refer to individual protocols. I.V.:
Children:
Leukemia: 10-12 mg/m^2/day for 3 days every 3 weeks
Solid tumors: 5 mg/m^2/day for 3 days every 3 weeks
Adults:
Leukemia induction: 12 mg/m^2/day for 3 days
Leukemia consolidation: 10-12 mg/m^2/day for 2 days

Dosage Forms Injection, solution, as hydrochloride [preservative free] (Idamycin PFS®): 1 mg/mL (5 mL, 10 mL, 20 mL)

idarubicin hydrochloride *see* idarubicin *on this page*

IDEC-C2B8 *see* rituximab *on page 780*

IDR *see* idarubicin *on this page*

Ifex® [US/Can] *see* ifosfamide *on this page*

IFLrA *see* interferon alfa-2a *on page 476*

ifosfamide (eye FOSS fa mide)

Synonyms isophosphamide; NSC-109724; Z4942

U.S./Canadian Brand Names Ifex® [US/Can]

Therapeutic Category Antineoplastic Agent

Use Treatment of lung cancer, Hodgkin and non-Hodgkin lymphoma, breast cancer, acute and chronic lymphocytic leukemias, ovarian cancer, sarcomas, pancreatic and gastric carcinomas
Orphan drug: Treatment of testicular cancer

Usual Dosage Refer to individual protocols. To prevent bladder toxicity, ifosfamide should be given with the urinary protector mesna and hydration of at least 2 L of oral or I.V. fluid per day. I.V.:
Children:
1200-1800 mg/m^2/day for 3-5 days every 21-28 days **or**
5 g/m^2 once every 21-28 days **or**
3 g/m^2/day for 2 days every 21-28 days
Adults:
50 mg/kg/day or 700-2000 mg/m^2 for 5 days every 3-4 weeks
Alternatives: 2400 mg/m^2/day for 3 days or 5000 mg/m^2 as a single dose every 3-4 weeks

Dosage Forms Injection, powder for reconstitution: 1 g, 3 g [packaged with Mesnex® (mesna) 1 g]

IG *see* immune globulin (intramuscular) *on page 468*

IGIM *see* immune globulin (intramuscular) *on page 468*

IL-1Ra *see* anakinra *on page 59*

IL-2 *see* aldesleukin *on page 28*

IL-11 *see* oprelvekin *on page 647*

Iletin® II Pork [Can] *see* insulin preparations *on page 474*

Ilopan-Choline® Oral *(Discontinued)* *see page 1042*

Ilopan® Injection *(Discontinued)* *see page 1042*

Ilosone® Pulvules® *(Discontinued)* *see page 1042*

Ilozyme® *(Discontinued)* *see page 1042*

imatinib (eye MAT eh nib)

Synonyms CGP 57148B; glivec; imatinib mesylate; STI571

U.S./Canadian Brand Names Gleevec® [US/Can]

Therapeutic Category Antineoplastic, Tyrosine Kinase Inhibitor

Use Treatment of adult patients with Philadelphia chromosome-positive (Ph+) chronic myeloid leukemia (CML), including newly-diagnosed patients as well as patients in blast crisis, accelerated phase, or in chronic phase after failure of interferon-alpha therapy; treatment of pediatric patients with Ph+ CML (chronic phase) recurring following stem cell transplant or who are resistant to interferon-alpha therapy; treatment of Kit-positive (CD117) unresectable and/or (metastatic) malignant gastrointestinal stromal tumors (GIST)

Usual Dosage Oral:

Children ≥3 years: CML (chronic phase): 260 mg/m²/day; may be increased to 340 mg/m²/day in the event of disease progression, loss of previously achieved response, or failure to achieve response after at least 3 months of therapy and in the absence of severe adverse reaction. Dose may be given once daily or in 2 divided doses.

Adults:

CML:

Chronic phase: 400 mg once daily; may be increased to 600 mg daily in the event of disease progression, loss of previously achieved response, or failure to achieve response after at least 3 months of therapy and in the absence of severe adverse reaction

Accelerated phase or blast crisis: 600 mg once daily; may be increased to 800 mg daily (400 mg twice daily) in the event of disease progression, loss of previously achieved response, or failure to achieve response after at least 3 months of therapy and in the absence of severe adverse reaction

Gastrointestinal stromal tumors: 400-600 mg/day

Note: Dosage should be increased by at least 50% when used concurrently with a potent enzyme-inducing agent (ie, rifampin, phenytoin).

Dosage Forms Tablet: 100 mg, 400 mg

imatinib mesylate *see* imatinib *on this page*

IMC-C225 *see* cetuximab *on page 179*

Imdur® [US/Can] *see* isosorbide mononitrate *on page 489*

IMI 30 *see* idarubicin *on previous page*

imidazol carboxamide dimethyltriazene *see* dacarbazine *on page 241*

imidazole carboxamide *see* dacarbazine *on page 241*

imiglucerase (i mi GLOO ser ace)

Sound-Alike/Look-Alike Issues

Cerezyme® may be confused with Cerebyx®, Ceredase®

U.S./Canadian Brand Names Cerezyme® [US/Can]

Therapeutic Category Enzyme

Use Long-term enzyme replacement therapy for patients with Type 1 Gaucher disease

Usual Dosage I.V.: Children ≥2 years and Adults: Initial: 30-60 units/kg every 2 weeks; dosing is individualized based on disease severity. Dosing range: 2.5 units/kg 3 times/week up to as much as 60 units/kg administered as frequently as once a week or as infrequently as every 4 weeks. Average dose: 60 units/kg administered every 2 weeks

Dosage Forms Injection, powder for reconstitution [preservative free]: 200 units, 400 units

imipemide *see* imipenem and cilastatin *on this page*

imipenem and cilastatin (i mi PEN em & sye la STAT in)

Sound-Alike/Look-Alike Issues

Primaxin® may be confused with Premarin®, Primacor®

Synonyms imipemide

U.S./Canadian Brand Names Primaxin® [US/Can]

Therapeutic Category Carbapenem (Antibiotic)

Use Treatment of respiratory tract, urinary tract, intra-abdominal, gynecologic, bone and joint, skin structure, and polymicrobic infections as well as bacterial septicemia and endocarditis. Antibacterial activity includes resistant gram-negative bacilli (*Pseudomonas aeruginosa* and *Enterobacter* sp), gram-positive bacteria (methicillin-sensitive *Staphylococcus aureus* and *Streptococcus* sp) and anaerobes.

Note: I.M. administration is not intended for severe or life-threatening infections (eg, septicemia, endocarditis, shock)

Usual Dosage Dosage based on **imipenem** content:

Neonates: Non-CNS infections: I.V.:
- <1 week: 25 mg/kg every 12 hours
- 1-4 weeks: 25 mg/kg every 8 hours
- 4 weeks to 3 months: 25 mg/kg every 6 hours

Children: >3 months: Non-CNS infections: I.V.: 15-25 mg/kg every 6 hours
- Maximum dosage: Susceptible infections: 2 g/day; moderately susceptible organisms: 4 g/day

Children: Cystic fibrosis: I.V.: Doses up to 90 mg/kg/day have been used

Adults:
- Moderate infections:
  - I.M.: 750 mg every 12 hours
  - I.V.: Fully-susceptible organisms: 500 mg every 6-8 hours (1.5-2 g/day) Moderately-susceptible organisms: 500 mg every 6 hours or 1 g every 8 hours (2-3 g/day)
- Severe infections: I.V.: **Note:** I.M. administration is not intended for severe or life-threatening infections (eg, septicemia, endocarditis, shock):
  - Fully-susceptible organisms: 500 mg every 6 hours (2 g/day)
  - Moderately-susceptible organisms: 1 g every 6-8 hours (3-4 g/day)
  - Maximum daily dose should not exceed 50 mg/kg or 4 g/day, whichever is lower
- Urinary tract infection, uncomplicated: I.V.: 250 mg every 6 hours (1 g/day)
- Urinary tract infection, complicated: I.V.: 500 mg every 6 hours (2 g/day)
- Mild infections: **Note:** Rarely a suitable option in mild infections; normally reserved for moderate-severe cases:
  - I.M.: 500 mg every 12 hours; intra-abdominal infections: 750 mg every 12 hours
  - I.V.: Fully-susceptible organisms: 250 mg every 6 hours (1g/day) Moderately-susceptible organisms: 500 mg every 6 hours (2 g/day)

Dosage Forms

Injection, powder for reconstitution [I.M.]: Imipenem 500 mg and cilastatin 500 mg [contains sodium 32 mg (1.4 mEq)]

Injection, powder for reconstitution [I.V.]: Imipenem 250 mg and cilastatin 250 mg [contains sodium 18.8 mg (0.8 mEq)]; imipenem 500 mg and cilastatin 500 mg [contains sodium 37.5 mg (1.6 mEq)]

imipramine (im IP ra meen)

Sound-Alike/Look-Alike Issues

imipramine may be confused with amitriptyline, desipramine, Norpramin®

Synonyms imipramine hydrochloride; imipramine pamoate

U.S./Canadian Brand Names Apo-Imipramine® [Can]; Tofranil® [US/Can]; Tofranil-PM® [US]

Therapeutic Category Antidepressant, Tricyclic (Tertiary Amine)

Use Treatment of depression

Usual Dosage Oral:

Children:

Depression: 1.5 mg/kg/day with dosage increments of 1 mg/kg every 3-4 days to a maximum dose of 5 mg/kg/day in 1-4 divided doses; monitor carefully especially with doses ≥3.5 mg/kg/day

Enuresis: ≥6 years: Initial: 10-25 mg at bedtime, if inadequate response still seen after 1 week of therapy, increase by 25 mg/day; dose should not exceed 2.5 mg/kg/day or 50 mg at bedtime if 6-12 years of age or 75 mg at bedtime if ≥12 years of age

Adjunct in the treatment of cancer pain: Initial: 0.2-0.4 mg/kg at bedtime; dose may be increased by 50% every 2-3 days up to 1-3 mg/kg/dose at bedtime

Adolescents: Initial: 25-50 mg/day; increase gradually; maximum: 100 mg/day in single or divided doses

Adults: Initial: 25 mg 3-4 times/day, increase dose gradually, total dose may be given at bedtime; maximum: 300 mg/day

Dosage Forms

Capsule, as pamoate (Tofranil-PM®): 75 mg, 100 mg, 125 mg, 150 mg

Tablet, as hydrochloride (Tofranil®): 10 mg, 25 mg, 50 mg [generic tablets may contain sodium benzoate]

imipramine hydrochloride *see* imipramine *on this page*

imipramine pamoate *see* imipramine *on this page*

imiquimod (i mi KWI mod)

Sound-Alike/Look-Alike Issues

Aldara™ may be confused with Alora®

U.S./Canadian Brand Names Aldara™ [US/Can]

Therapeutic Category Immune Response Modifier

Use Treatment of external genital and perianal warts/condyloma acuminata in children ≥12 years of age and adults; nonhyperkeratotic, nonhypertrophic actinic keratosis; superficial basal cell carcinoma (SBCC)

Usual Dosage Topical:

Children ≥12 years and Adults: Perianal warts/condyloma acuminata: Apply 3 times/week prior to bedtime and leave on skin for 6-10 hours. Remove with mild soap and water. Examples of 3 times/week application schedules are: Monday, Wednesday, Friday; or Tuesday, Thursday, Saturday. Continue imiquimod treatment until there is total clearance of the genital/perianal warts for ≤16 weeks. A rest period of several days may be taken if required by the patient's discomfort or severity of the local skin reaction. Treatment may resume once the reaction subsides.

Adults:

Actinic keratosis: Apply twice weekly for 16 weeks to a treatment area on face or scalp; apply prior to bedtime and leave on skin for 8 hours. Remove with mild soap and water.

Superficial basal cell carcinoma: Apply once daily prior to bedtime, 5 days/week for 6 weeks. Treatment area should include a 1 cm margin of skin around the tumor. Leave on skin for 8 hours.

Dosage Forms Cream: 5% (12s) [contains benzyl alcohol; single-dose packets]

Imitrex® [US/Can] *see* sumatriptan succinate *on page 835*

ImmuCyst® [Can] *see* BCG vaccine *on page 101*

immune globulin (intramuscular)

(i MYUN GLOB yoo lin IN tra MUS kyoo ler)

Synonyms gamma globulin; IG; IGIM; immune serum globulin; ISG

U.S./Canadian Brand Names BayGam® [US/Can]

Therapeutic Category Immune Globulin

Use Household and sexual contacts of persons with hepatitis A, measles, varicella, and possibly rubella; travelers to high-risk areas outside tourist routes; staff, attendees, and parents of diapered attendees in day-care center outbreaks

For travelers, IG is not an alternative to careful selection of foods and water; immune globulin can interfere with the antibody response to parenterally administered live virus vaccines. Frequent travelers should be tested for hepatitis A antibody, immune hemolytic anemia, and neutropenia (with ITP, I.V. route is usually used).

Usual Dosage I.M.:

Hepatitis A:

Pre-exposure prophylaxis upon travel into endemic areas (hepatitis A vaccine preferred):

0.02 mL/kg for anticipated risk 1-3 months

0.06 mL/kg for anticipated risk >3 months

Repeat approximate dose every 4-6 months if exposure continues

Postexposure prophylaxis: 0.02 mL/kg given within 7 days of exposure

Measles:

Prophylaxis: 0.25 mL/kg/dose (maximum dose: 15 mL) given within 6 days of exposure followed by live attenuated measles vaccine in 3 months or at 15 months of age (whichever is later)

For patients with leukemia, lymphoma, immunodeficiency disorders, generalized malignancy, or receiving immunosuppressive therapy: 0.5 mL/kg (maximum dose: 15 mL)

Poliomyelitis: Prophylaxis: 0.3 mL/kg/dose as a single dose

Rubella: Prophylaxis: 0.55 mL/kg/dose within 72 hours of exposure

Varicella: Prophylaxis: 0.6-1.2 mL/kg (varicella zoster immune globulin preferred) within 72 hours of exposure

IgG deficiency: 1.3 mL/kg, then 0.66 mL/kg in 3-4 weeks

Hepatitis B: Prophylaxis: 0.06 mL/kg/dose (HBIG preferred)

Dosage Forms Injection, solution [preservative free]: 15% to 18% (2 mL, 10 mL)

immune globulin (intravenous) (i MYUN GLOB yoo lin IN tra VEE nus)

Sound-Alike/Look-Alike Issues

Gamimune® N may be confused with CytoGam®

Synonyms IVIG

U.S./Canadian Brand Names Carimune™ [US]; Flebogamma® [US]; Gamimune® N [US/Can]; Gammagard® S/D [US/Can]; Gammar®-P I.V. [US]; Gamunex® [US/Can]; Iveegam EN [US]; Iveegam Immuno® [Can]; Octagam® [US]; Panglobulin® [US]; Polygam® S/D [US]; Venoglobulin®-S [US]

Therapeutic Category Immune Globulin

Use

Treatment of primary immunodeficiency syndromes (congenital agammaglobulinemia, severe combined immunodeficiency syndromes [SCIDS], common variable immunodeficiency, X-linked immunodeficiency, Wiskott-Aldrich syndrome); idiopathic thrombocytopenic purpura (ITP); Kawasaki disease (in combination with aspirin)

Prevention of bacterial infection in B-cell chronic lymphocytic leukemia (CLL); pediatric HIV infection; bone marrow transplant (BMT)

Usual Dosage Approved doses and regimens may vary between brands; check manufacturer guidelines. **Note:** Some clinicians dose IVIG on ideal body weight or an adjusted ideal body weight in morbidly obese patients. The volume of distribution of IVIG preparations in healthy subjects is similar to that observed with endogenous IgG.

IVIG remains primarily in the intravascular space. Patients with congenital humoral immunodeficiencies appear to have about 70% of the IVIG available in the intravascular space.

Children and Adults: I.V.:

Primary immunodeficiency disorders: 200-400 mg/kg every 4 weeks or as per monitored serum IgG concentrations

Flebogamma®, Gamunex®, Octagam®: 300-600 mg/kg every 3-4 weeks; adjusted based on dosage and interval in conjunction with monitored serum IgG concentrations.

B-cell chronic lymphocytic leukemia (CLL): 400 mg/kg/dose every 3 weeks

Idiopathic thrombocytopenic purpura (ITP):

Acute: 400 mg/kg/day for 5 days or 1000 mg/kg/day for 1-2 days

Chronic: 400 mg/kg as needed to maintain platelet count >30,000/mm^3; may increase dose to 800 mg/kg (1000 mg/kg if needed)

Kawasaki disease: Initiate therapy within 10 days of disease onset: 2 g/kg as a single dose administered over 10 hours, or 400 mg/kg/day for 4 days. **Note:** Must be used in combination with aspirin: 80-100 mg/kg/day in 4 divided doses for 14 days; when fever subsides, dose aspirin at 3-5 mg/kg once daily for ≥6-8 weeks

Dosage Forms

Injection, powder for reconstitution [preservative free]:

Carimune™, Panglobulin®: 1 g, 3 g, 6 g, 12 g

Gammar®-P I.V.: 1 g, 2.5 g, 5 g, 10 g [stabilized with human albumin and sucrose]

Iveegam EN: 0.5 g, 1 g, 2.5 g, 5 g [stabilized with glucose]

Injection, powder for reconstitution [preservative free, solvent detergent treated] (Gammagard® S/D): 2.5 g, 5 g, 10 g [stabilized with human albumin, glycine, glucose, and polyethylene glycol]

Injection, solution [preservative free; solvent detergent-treated]:

Gamimune® N: 10% [100 mg/mL] (10 mL, 50 mL, 100 mL, 200 mL)

Octagam®: 5% [50 mg/mL] (20 mL, 50 mL, 100 mL, 200 mL) [sucrose free; contains sodium 30 mmol/L and maltose]

Venoglobulin®-S: 5% [50 mg/mL] (50 mL, 100 mL, 200 mL); 10% [100 mg/mL] (50 mL, 100 mL, 200 mL) [stabilized with human albumin]

Injection, solution [preservative free]:

Flebogamma®: 5% (10 mL, 50 mL, 100 mL, 200 mL) [PEG precipitated/chromatography purified]

Gamunex®: 10% (10 mL, 25 mL, 50 mL, 100 mL, 200 mL) [caprylate/chromatography purified]

immune serum globulin *see* immune globulin (intramuscular) *on previous page*

Immunine® VH [Can] *see* factor IX *on page 354*

Imodium® [Can] *see* loperamide *on page 528*

Imodium® A-D [US-OTC] *see* loperamide *on page 528*

Imogam® [US] *see* rabies immune globulin (human) *on page 759*

Imogam® Rabies Pasteurized [Can] *see* rabies immune globulin (human) *on page 759*

Imovane® [Can] *see* zopiclone *(Canada only) on page 944*

Imovax® Rabies [US/Can] *see* rabies virus vaccine *on page 759*

Imuran® [US/Can] *see* azathioprine *on page 93*

In-111 zevalin *see* ibritumomab *on page 461*

inamrinone (eye NAM ri none)

Sound-Alike/Look-Alike Issues

amrinone may be confused with amiodarone

Synonyms amrinone lactate

Therapeutic Category Adrenergic Agonist Agent

(Continued)

inamrinone *(Continued)*

Use Infrequently used as a last resort, short-term therapy in patients with intractable heart failure

Usual Dosage Dosage is based on clinical response (**Note:** Dose should not exceed 10 mg/kg/24 hours).

Infants, Children, and Adults: 0.75 mg/kg I.V. bolus over 2-3 minutes followed by maintenance infusion of 5-10 mcg/kg/minute; I.V. bolus may need to be repeated in 30 minutes.

Dosage Forms Injection, solution, as lactate: 5 mg/mL (20 mL) [contains sodium metabisulfite]

I-Naphline® Ophthalmic *(Discontinued)* *see page 1042*

Inapsine® [US] *see* droperidol *on page 297*

indapamide (in DAP a mide)

Sound-Alike/Look-Alike Issues

indapamide may be confused with Iopidine®

U.S./Canadian Brand Names Apo-Indapamide® [Can]; Gen-Indapamide [Can]; Lozide® [Can]; Lozol® [US/Can]; Novo-Indapamide [Can]; Nu-Indapamide [Can]; PMS-Indapamide [Can]

Therapeutic Category Diuretic, Miscellaneous

Use Management of mild to moderate hypertension; treatment of edema in congestive heart failure and nephrotic syndrome

Usual Dosage Adults: Oral:

Edema: 2.5-5 mg/day. **Note:** There is little therapeutic benefit to increasing the dose >5 mg/day; there is, however, an increased risk of electrolyte disturbances

Hypertension: 1.25 mg in the morning, may increase to 5 mg/day by increments of 1.25-2.5 mg; consider adding another antihypertensive and decreasing the dose if response is not adequate

Dosage Forms

Tablet: 1.25 mg, 2.5 mg

Lozol®: 1.25 mg

Inderal® [US/Can] *see* propranolol *on page 741*

Inderal® LA [US/Can] *see* propranolol *on page 741*

Inderide® [US] *see* propranolol and hydrochlorothiazide *on page 742*

indinavir (in DIN a veer)

Sound-Alike/Look-Alike Issues

indinavir may be confused with Denavir™

Synonyms indinavir sulfate

U.S./Canadian Brand Names Crixivan® [US/Can]

Therapeutic Category Antiviral Agent

Use Treatment of HIV infection; should always be used as part of a multidrug regimen (at least three antiretroviral agents)

Usual Dosage

Children (investigational): 500 mg/m^2 every 8 hours (patients with smaller BSA may require lower doses of 300-400 mg/m^2 every 8 hours)

Adults: Oral: 800 mg every 8 hours

Note: Dosage adjustments for indinavir when administered in combination therapy:

Delavirdine, itraconazole, or ketoconazole: Reduce indinavir dose to 600 mg every 8 hours

Efavirenz: Increase indinavir dose to 1000 mg every 8 hours

Lopinavir and ritonavir (Kaletra™): Indinavir 600 mg twice daily

Nevirapine: Increase indinavir dose to 1000 mg every 8 hours

Rifabutin: Reduce rifabutin to ½ the standard dose plus increase indinavir to 1000 mg every 8 hours

Ritonavir: Adjustments necessary for both agents: Ritonavir 100-200 mg twice daily plus indinavir 800 mg twice daily **or** Ritonavir 400 mg twice daily plus indinavir 400 mg twice daily

Dosage Forms Capsule: 100 mg, 200 mg, 333 mg, 400 mg

indinavir sulfate *see* indinavir *on previous page*

Indocid® [Can] *see* indomethacin *on this page*

Indocid® P.D.A. [Can] *see* indomethacin *on this page*

Indocin® [US/Can] *see* indomethacin *on this page*

Indocin® I.V. [US] *see* indomethacin *on this page*

Indocin® SR [US] *see* indomethacin *on this page*

indocyanine green (in doe SYE a neen green)

U.S./Canadian Brand Names IC-Green® [US]

Therapeutic Category Diagnostic Agent

Use Determining hepatic function, cardiac output and liver blood flow and for ophthalmic angiography

Usual Dosage

Angiography: Use 40 mg of dye in 2 mL of aqueous solvent, in some patients, half the volume (1 mL) has been found to produce angiograms of comparable resolution; immediately following the bolus dose of dye, a bolus of sodium chloride 0.9% is given; this regimen will deliver a spatially limited dye bolus of optimal concentration to the choroidal vasculature following I.V. injection

Determination of cardiac output: Dye is injected as rapidly as possible into the right atrium, right ventricle, or pulmonary artery through a cardiac catheter; the usual dose is 1.25 mg for infants, 2.5 mg for children, and 5 mg for adults; total dose should not exceed 2 mg/kg; the dye is diluted with sterile water for injection or sodium chloride 0.9% to make a final volume of 1 mL; doses are repeated periodically to obtain several dilution curves; the dye should be flushed from the catheter with sodium chloride 0.9% to prevent hemolysis

Dosage Forms Injection, powder for reconstitution: 25 mg [supplied with diluent]

Indo-Lemmon [Can] *see* indomethacin *on this page*

indometacin *see* indomethacin *on this page*

indomethacin (in doe METH a sin)

Sound-Alike/Look-Alike Issues

Indocin® may be confused with Imodium®, Lincocin®, Minocin®, Vicodin®

Synonyms indometacin; indomethacin sodium trihydrate

U.S./Canadian Brand Names Apo-Indomethacin® [Can]; Indocid® [Can]; Indocid® P.D.A. [Can]; Indocin® [US/Can]; Indocin® I.V. [US]; Indocin® SR [US]; Indo-Lemmon [Can]; Indotec [Can]; Novo-Methacin [Can]; Nu-Indo [Can]; Rhodacine® [Can]

Therapeutic Category Analgesic, Nonnarcotic; Nonsteroidal Antiinflammatory Drug (NSAID)

Use Management of inflammatory diseases and rheumatoid disorders; moderate pain; acute gouty arthritis, acute bursitis/tendonitis, moderate to severe osteoarthritis, rheumatoid arthritis, ankylosing spondylitis; I.V. form used as alternative to surgery for closure of patent ductus arteriosus in neonates

Usual Dosage

Patent ductus arteriosus:

Neonates: I.V.: Initial: 0.2 mg/kg, followed by 2 doses depending on postnatal age (PNA):

PNA **at time of first dose** <48 hours: 0.1 mg/kg at 12- to 24-hour intervals

PNA **at time of first dose** 2-7 days: 0.2 mg/kg at 12- to 24-hour intervals

PNA **at time of first dose** >7 days: 0.25 mg/kg at 12- to 24-hour intervals

(Continued)

indomethacin *(Continued)*

In general, may use 12-hour dosing interval if urine output >1 mL/kg/hour after prior dose; use 24-hour dosing interval if urine output is <1 mL/kg/hour but >0.6 mL/kg/hour; doses should be withheld if patient has oliguria (urine output <0.6 mL/kg/hour) or anuria

Inflammatory/rheumatoid disorders: Oral:

Children: 1-2 mg/kg/day in 2-4 divided doses; maximum dose: 4 mg/kg/day; not to exceed 150-200 mg/day

Adults: 25-50 mg/dose 2-3 times/day; maximum dose: 200 mg/day; extended release capsule should be given on a 1-2 times/day schedule; maximum dose for sustained release is 150 mg/day

Dosage Forms

Capsule (Indocin®): 25 mg, 50 mg

Capsule, sustained release (Indocin® SR): 75 mg

Injection, powder for reconstitution, as sodium trihydrate (Indocin® I.V.): 1 mg

Suspension, oral (Indocin®): 25 mg/5 mL (237 mL) [contains alcohol 1%; pineapple-coconut-mint flavor]

indomethacin sodium trihydrate *see* indomethacin *on previous page*

Indotec [Can] *see* indomethacin *on previous page*

INF-alpha 2 *see* interferon alfa-2b *on page 477*

Infanrix® [US] *see* diphtheria, tetanus toxoids, and acellular pertussis vaccine *on page 280*

Infants' Tylenol® Cold Plus Cough Concentrated Drops [US-OTC] *see* acetaminophen, dextromethorphan, and pseudoephedrine *on page 12*

Infants' Tylenol® Cold [US-OTC] *see* acetaminophen and pseudoephedrine *on page 9*

Infasurf® [US] *see* calfactant *on page 150*

INFeD® [US] *see* iron dextran complex *on page 485*

Infergen® [US/Can] *see* interferon alfacon-1 *on page 479*

Inflamase® Forte [US/Can] *see* prednisolone (ophthalmic) *on page 723*

Inflamase® Mild [US/Can] *see* prednisolone (ophthalmic) *on page 723*

infliximab (in FLIKS e mab)

Sound-Alike/Look-Alike Issues

Remicade® may be confused with Renacidin®

Synonyms infliximab, recombinant

U.S./Canadian Brand Names Remicade® [US/Can]

Therapeutic Category Monoclonal Antibody

Use

Crohn's disease: Induction and maintenance of remission in patients with moderate to severe disease who have an inadequate response to conventional therapy; to reduce the number of draining enterocutaneous and rectovaginal fistulas and to maintain fistula closure

Rheumatoid arthritis: Inhibits the progression of structural damage and improves physical function in patients with moderate to severe disease; used with methotrexate

Usual Dosage I.V.: Adults:

Crohn's disease:

Induction regimen: 5 mg/kg at 0, 2, and 6 weeks, followed by maintenance regimen

Maintenance regimen: 5 mg/kg every 8 weeks; dose may be increased to 10 mg/kg in patients who respond but then lose their response. If no response by week 14, consider discontinuing therapy.

Rheumatoid arthritis (in combination with methotrexate therapy): 3 mg/kg followed by an additional 3 mg/kg at 2- and 6 weeks after the first dose; then repeat every 8 weeks thereafter; doses have ranged from 3-10 mg/kg intravenous infusion repeated at 4-week intervals or 8-week intervals

Dosage adjustment with CHF: Weigh risk versus benefits for individual patient: NYHA Class III/IV: ≤5 mg/kg

Dosage Forms Injection, powder for reconstitution [preservative free]: 100 mg

infliximab, recombinant *see* infliximab *on previous page*

influenza virus vaccine (in floo EN za VYE rus vak SEEN)

Synonyms influenza virus vaccine (purified surface antigen); influenza virus vaccine (split-virus); influenza virus vaccine (trivalent, live)

U.S./Canadian Brand Names FluMist™ [US]; Fluviral S/F® [Can]; Fluvirin® [US]; Fluzone® [US/Can]; Vaxigrip® [Can]

Therapeutic Category Vaccine, Inactivated Virus

Use Provide active immunity to influenza virus strains contained in the vaccine

Groups at Increased Risk for Influenza-Related Complications:

- Persons ≥65 years of age
- Residents of nursing homes and other chronic-care facilities that house persons of any age with chronic medical conditions
- Adults and children with chronic disorders of the pulmonary or cardiovascular systems, including children with asthma
- Adults and children who have required regular medical follow-up or hospitalization during the preceding year because of chronic metabolic diseases (including diabetes mellitus), renal dysfunction, hemoglobinopathies, or immunosuppression (including immunosuppression caused by medications)
- Children and adolescents (6 months to 18 years of age) who are receiving long-term aspirin therapy and therefore, may be at risk for developing Reye's syndrome after influenza
- Women who will be pregnant during the influenza season
- Children 6-23 months of age

Vaccination is also recommended for persons 50-64 years of age, close contacts of children 0-23 months of age, and healthy persons who may transmit influenza to those at risk.

Usual Dosage Optimal time to receive vaccine is October-November, prior to exposure to influenza; however, vaccination can continue into December and later as long as vaccine is available.

I.M.:

Fluzone®:

Children 6-35 months: 0.25 mL/dose (1 or 2 doses per season; see **Note**)

Children 3-8 years: 0.5 mL/dose (1 or 2 doses per season; see **Note**)

Children ≥9 years and Adults: 0.5 mL/dose (1 dose per season)

Fluvirin®:

Children 4-8 years: 0.5 mL/dose (1 or 2 doses per season; see **Note**)

Children ≥9 years and Adults: 0.5 mL/dose (1 dose per season)

Note: Previously unvaccinated children <9 years should receive 2 doses, given >1 month apart in order to achieve satisfactory antibody response.

Intranasal (FluMist™):

Children 5-8 years, previously **not vaccinated** with influenza vaccine: 0.5 mL/dose (2 doses per season given 6-10 weeks apart)

Children 5-8 years, previously **vaccinated** with influenza vaccine: 0.5 mL/dose (1 dose per season)

Children ≥9 years and Adults ≤49 years: 0.5 mL/dose (1 dose per season)

Dosage Forms

Injection, solution, purified split-virus surface antigen [preservative free] (Fluvirin®): (0.5 mL) [prefilled syringe; contains thimerosal (trace amounts); manufactured using neomycin and polymyxin]; (5 mL) [multidose vial; contains thimerosal; manufactured using neomycin and polymyxin]

(Continued)

influenza virus vaccine *(Continued)*

Injection, suspension, purified split-virus:
Fluzone®: (0.5 mL) [prefilled syringe; contains thimerosal]; (5 mL) [vial; contains thimerosal]
Fluzone® [preservative free]: (0.25 mL) [prefilled syringe; contains thimerosal (trace amount)]
Solution, nasal spray, trivalent, live virus [preservative free] (FluMist™): (0.5 mL) [manufactured using eggs and gentamicin]

influenza virus vaccine (purified surface antigen) *see* influenza virus vaccine *on previous page*

influenza virus vaccine (split-virus) *see* influenza virus vaccine *on previous page*

influenza virus vaccine (trivalent, live) *see* influenza virus vaccine *on previous page*

Infufer® [Can] *see* iron dextran complex *on page 485*

Infumorph® [US] *see* morphine sulfate *on page 591*

Infuvite® Adult [US] *see* vitamins (multiple/injectable) *on page 919*

Infuvite® Pediatric [US] *see* vitamins (multiple/injectable) *on page 919*

INH *see* isoniazid *on page 487*

inhalation devices (in hal LAY shun deh VYE sez)

Therapeutic Category Inhalation, Miscellaneous

Use Improves the distribution and deposition in the lungs of aerosolized medication from metered dose inhalers (MDIs)

Dosage Forms
AeroChamber™, AeroChamber™ with mask (small, medium)
Inhalation kit (InspirEase™)
Replacement bags (InspirEase™)

Inhibace® [Can] *see* cilazapril *(Canada only) on page 199*

Innohep® [US/Can] *see* tinzaparin *on page 865*

InnoPran XL™ [US] *see* propranolol *on page 741*

Innovar® ***(Discontinued)*** *see page 1042*

Inocor® ***(Discontinued)*** *see page 1042*

INOmax® [US/Can] *see* nitric oxide *on page 622*

insect sting kit *see* epinephrine and chlorpheniramine *on page 313*

Inspra™ [US] *see* eplerenone *on page 314*

Insta-Glucose® [US-OTC] *see* glucose (instant) *on page 408*

Instat™ MCH [US] *see* collagen hemostat *on page 225*

insulin preparations (IN su lin prep a RAY shuns)

Sound-Alike/Look-Alike Issues
Humalog® may be confused with Humulin®
Humulin® may be confused with Humalog®
Lantus® may be confused with Lente®
Lente® may be confused with Lantus®
Novolin® may be confused with NovoLog®
Novolin® may be confused with NovoLog® Mix

Synonyms aspart, insulin; glargine, insulin; glulisine, insulin; lispro, insulin; NPH, insulin; regular, insulin

U.S./Canadian Brand Names Apidra™ [US]; Humalog® [US/Can]; Humalog® Mix 25™ [Can]; Humalog® Mix 75/25™ [US]; Humulin® [Can]; Humulin® 50/50 [US]; Humulin®

70/30 [US]; Humulin® L [US]; Humulin® N [US]; Humulin® R [US]; Humulin® R (Concentrated) U-500 [US]; Humulin® U [US]; Iletin® II Pork [Can]; Lantus® [US]; Novolin® 70/30 [US]; Novolin® ge [Can]; Novolin® N [US]; Novolin® R [US]; NovoLog® [US]; NovoLog® Mix 70/30 [US]; NovoRapid® [Can]; NPH Iletin® II [US]; Regular Iletin® II [US]

Therapeutic Category Antidiabetic Agent, Parenteral

Use Treatment of type 1 diabetes mellitus (insulin dependent, IDDM); type 2 diabetes mellitus (noninsulin dependent, NIDDM) unresponsive to treatment with diet and/or oral hypoglycemics; adjunct to parenteral nutrition

Usual Dosage Dose requires continuous medical supervision; may administer I.M., or SubQ; regular insulin may also be administered I.V.

Diabetes mellitus: The number and size of daily doses, time of administration, and diet and exercise require continuous medical supervision. In addition, specific formulations may require distinct administration procedures.

Children and Adults: 0.5-1 unit/kg/day in divided doses

Adolescents (growth spurts): 0.8-1.2 units/kg/day in divided doses

Adjust dose to maintain premeal and bedtime blood glucose of 80-140 mg/dL (children <5 years: 100-200 mg/dL)

Insulin glargine (Lantus®): SubQ:

Type 2 diabetes (patient not already on insulin): 10 units once daily, adjusted according to patient response (range in clinical study 2-100 units/day)

Patients already receiving insulin: In clinical studies, when changing to insulin glargine from once-daily NPH or Ultralente® insulin, the initial dose was not changed; when changing from twice-daily NPH to once-daily insulin glargine, the total daily dose was reduced by 20% and adjusted according to patient response

Diabetic ketoacidosis: Children and Adults: Regular insulin: I.V. loading dose: 0.1 unit/kg, then maintenance continuous infusion: 0.1 unit/kg/hour (range: 0.05-0.2 units/kg/hour depending upon the rate of decrease of serum glucose - too rapid decrease of serum glucose may lead to cerebral edema).

Optimum rate of decrease (serum glucose): 80-100 mg/dL/hour

Note: Newly-diagnosed patients with IDDM presenting in DKA and patients with blood sugars <800 mg/dL may be relatively "sensitive" to insulin and should receive loading and initial maintenance doses approximately 1/2 of those indicated above.

Dosage Forms [DSC] = Discontinued product

RAPID-ACTING:

Injection, solution, aspart, human:

NovoLog®: 100 units/mL (10 mL vial)

NovoLog® [InnoLet®]: 100 units/mL (3 mL prefilled syringe)

NovoLog® [PenFill®]: 100 units/mL (3 mL cartridge)

Injection, solution, lispro, human (Humalog®): 100 units/mL (1.5 mL cartridge [DSC], 3 mL disposable pen, 10 mL vial)

Injection, solution, glulisine (Apidra™): 100 units/mL (10 mL vial)

SHORT-ACTING:

Injection, solution, regular, human:

Humulin® R: 100 units/mL (10 mL vial)

Novolin® R: 100 units/mL (1.5 mL prefilled syringe, 10 mL vial)

Novolin® R [PenFill®]: 100 units/mL (1.5 mL cartridge, 3 mL cartridge)

Injection, solution, regular, human, buffered (Velosulin® BR) [DSC]: 100 units/mL (10 mL vial)

Injection, solution, regular, human, concentrate (Humulin® R U-500): 500 units/mL (20 mL vial)

Injection, solution, regular, purified pork (Regular Iletin® II): 100 units/mL (10 mL vial)

INTERMEDIATE-ACTING:

Injection, suspension, lente, human [zinc] (Humulin® L, Novolin® L [DSC]): 100 units/mL (10 mL vial)

Injection, suspension, lente, purified pork [zinc] (Lente® Iletin® II): 100 units/mL (10 mL vial) [DSC]

Injection, suspension, NPH, human [isophane]:

Humulin® N: 100 units/mL (3 mL disposable pen, 10 mL vial)

(Continued)

insulin preparations *(Continued)*

Novolin® N: 100 units/mL (1.5 mL prefilled syringe, 10 mL vial)
Novolin® N [PenFill®]: 100 units/mL (1.5 mL cartridge, 3 mL cartridge)
Injection, suspension, NPH, purified pork [isophane] (NPH Iletin® II): 100 units/mL (10 mL vial)

LONG-ACTING:
Injection, suspension, Ultralente®, human [zinc] (Humulin U Ultralente®): 100 units/mL (10 mL vial)
Injection, solution, glargine, human (Lantus®): 100 unit/mL (10 mL vial)

COMBINATION, INTERMEDIATE-ACTING:
Injection, aspart protamine human suspension 70% and rapid-acting aspart human solution 30% (NovoLog® Mix 70/30): 100 units/mL (3 mL cartridge, 3 mL prefilled syringe)
Injection, lispro protamine human suspension 75% and rapid-acting lispro human solution 25% (Humalog® Mix 75/25™): 100 units/mL (3 mL disposable pen, 10 mL vial)
Injection, NPH human insulin suspension 50% and short-acting regular human insulin solution 50% (Humulin® 50/50): 100 units/mL (10 mL vial)
Injection, NPH human insulin suspension 70% and short-acting regular human insulin solution 30%:
Humulin® 70/30: 100 units/mL (3 mL disposable pen, 10 mL vial)
Novolin® 70/30: 100 units/mL (1.5 mL prefilled syringe, 10 mL vial)
Novolin® 70/30 [PenFill®]: 100 units/mL (1.5 mL cartridge, 3 mL cartridge)

Intal® [US/Can] *see* cromolyn sodium *on page 230*
Intal® Inhalation Capsule *(Discontinued)* *see page 1042*
Integrilin® [US/Can] *see* eptifibatide *on page 317*
Intensol® Solution *(Discontinued)* *see page 1042*
Intercept™ *(Discontinued)* *see page 1042*
α-2-interferon *see* interferon alfa-2b *on next page*

interferon alfa-2a (in ter FEER on AL fa-too aye)

Sound-Alike/Look-Alike Issues
interferon alfa-2a may be confused with interferon alfa-2b
Roferon-A® may be confused with Rocephin®

Synonyms IFLrA; rIFN-A

U.S./Canadian Brand Names Roferon-A® [US/Can]

Therapeutic Category Biological Response Modulator

Use
Patients >18 years of age: Hairy cell leukemia, AIDS-related Kaposi sarcoma, chronic hepatitis C
Children and Adults: Chronic myelogenous leukemia (CML), Philadelphia chromosome positive, within 1 year of diagnosis (limited experience in children)

Usual Dosage Refer to individual protocols.
Children (limited data):
Chronic myelogenous leukemia (CML): I.M.: 2.5-5 million units/m^2/day; **Note:** In juveniles, higher dosages (30 million units/m^2/day) have been associated with severe adverse events, including death
Adults:
Hairy cell leukemia: SubQ, I.M.: 3 million units/day for 16-24 weeks, then 3 million units 3 times/week for up to 6-24 months
Chronic myelogenous leukemia (CML): SubQ, I.M.: 9 million units/day, continue treatment until disease progression
AIDS-related Kaposi sarcoma: SubQ, I.M.: 36 million units/day for 10-12 weeks, then 36 million units 3 times/week; to minimize adverse reactions, can use escalating dose (3-, 9-, then 18 million units each day for 3 days, then 36 million units daily thereafter).
Hepatitis C: SubQ, I.M.: 3 million units 3 times/week for 12 months

Dosage Forms Injection, solution, [single-dose prefilled syringe; SubQ use only]: 3 million units/0.5 mL (0.5 mL); 6 million units/0.5 mL (0.5 mL); 9 million units/0.5 mL (0.5 mL) [contains benzyl alcohol]

interferon alfa-2a (PEG conjugate) *see* peginterferon alfa-2a *on page 671*

interferon alfa-2b (in ter FEER on AL fa-too bee)

Sound-Alike/Look-Alike Issues

interferon alfa-2b may be confused with interferon alfa-2a

Synonyms INF-alpha 2; α-2-interferon; rLFN-α2

U.S./Canadian Brand Names Intron® A [US/Can]

Therapeutic Category Biological Response Modulator

Use

Patients ≥1 year of age: Chronic hepatitis B

Patients ≥18 years of age: Condyloma acuminata, chronic hepatitis C, hairy cell leukemia, malignant melanoma, AIDS-related Kaposi sarcoma, follicular non-Hodgkin lymphoma

Usual Dosage Refer to individual protocols.

Children 1-17 years: Chronic hepatitis B: SubQ: 3 million units/m^2 3 times/week for 1 week; then 6 million units/m^2 3 times/week; maximum: 10 million units 3 times/week; total duration of therapy 16-24 weeks

Adults:

Hairy cell leukemia: I.M., SubQ: 2 million units/m^2 3 times/week for 2-6 months

Lymphoma (follicular): SubQ: 5 million units 3 times/week for up to 18 months

Malignant melanoma: 20 million units/m^2 I.V. for 5 consecutive days per week for 4 weeks, then 10 million units/m^2 SubQ 3 times/week for 48 weeks

AIDS-related Kaposi sarcoma: I.M., SubQ: 30 million units/m^2 3 times/week

Chronic hepatitis B: I.M., SubQ: 5 million units/day or 10 million units 3 times/week for 16 weeks

Chronic hepatitis C: I.M., SubQ: 3 million units 3 times/week for 16 weeks. In patients with normalization of ALT at 16 weeks, continue treatment for 18-24 months; consider discontinuation if normalization does not occur at 16 weeks. **Note:** May be used in combination therapy with ribavirin in previously untreated patients or in patients who relapse following alpha interferon therapy; refer to Interferon Alfa-2b and Ribavirin Combination Pack monograph.

Condyloma acuminata: Intralesionally: 1 million units/lesion (maximum: 5 lesions/treatment) 3 times/week (on alternate days) for 3 weeks; may administer a second course at 12-16 weeks

Dosage Forms

Injection, powder for reconstitution: 10 million units; 18 million units; 50 million units [contains human albumin]

Injection, solution [multidose prefilled pen]:

Delivers 3 million units/0.2 mL (1.5 mL) [delivers 6 doses; 18 million units]

Delivers 5 million units/0.2 mL (1.5 mL) [delivers 6 doses; 30 million units]

Delivers 10 million units/0.2 mL (1.5 mL) [delivers 6 doses; 60 million units]

Injection, solution [multidose vial]: 6 million units/mL (3 mL); 10 million units/mL (2.5 mL)

Injection, solution [single-dose vial]: 10 million units/ mL (1 mL)

See also Interferon Alfa-2b and Ribavirin Combination Pack monograph.

interferon alfa-2b and ribavirin combination pack

(in ter FEER on AL fa-too bee & rye ba VYE rin com bi NAY shun pak)

Synonyms ribavirin and interferon alfa-2b combination pack

U.S./Canadian Brand Names Rebetron® [US/Can]

Therapeutic Category Antiviral Agent; Biological Response Modulator

Use Combination therapy for the treatment of chronic hepatitis C in patients with compensated liver disease previously untreated with alpha interferon or who have relapsed after alpha interferon therapy

(Continued)

interferon alfa-2b and ribavirin combination pack *(Continued)*

Usual Dosage

Children ≥3 years: Chronic hepatitis C: **Note:** Duration of therapy: genotype 1: 48 weeks; genotype 2 or 3: 24 weeks. Discontinue treatment in any patient if HCV-RNA is not below the limits of detection of the assay after 24 weeks of therapy. Combination therapy:

Intron® A: SubQ:

25-61 kg: 3 million int. units/m^2 3 times/week

>61 kg: Refer to Adults dosing

Rebetol®: Oral: **Note:** Oral solution should be used in children 3-5 years of age, children ≤25 kg, or those unable to swallow capsules.

Capsule/solution: 15 mg/kg/day in 2 divided doses (morning and evening)

Capsule dosing recommendations: 25-36 kg: 400 mg/day (200 mg morning and evening) 37-49 kg: 600 mg/day (200 mg in the morning and two 200 mg capsules in the evening) 50-61 kg: 800 mg/day (two 200 mg capsules morning and evening) >61 kg: Refer to Adults dosing

Adults: Chronic hepatitis C: Recommended dosage of combination therapy:

Intron® A: SubQ: 3 million int. units 3 times/week **and**

Rebetol® capsule: Oral:

≤75 kg (165 lb): 1000 mg/day (two 200 mg capsules in the morning and three 200 mg capsules in the evening)

>75 kg: 1200 mg/day (three 200 mg capsules in the morning and three 200 mg capsules in the evening)

Treatment duration recommendations:

Following relapse after alpha interferon monotherapy: 24 weeks

Previously untreated: 24-48 weeks (individualized based on response, tolerance, and baseline characteristics)

Consider discontinuing therapy in any patient not achieving HCV-RNA below the limit of assay detection by 24 weeks.

Dosage Forms

Combination package for patients ≤75 kg:

Injection, solution: Interferon alfa-2b (Intron® A): 3 million int. units/0.5 mL (0.5 mL) [6 vials (3 million int. units/vial), 6 syringes and alcohol swabs]
Capsules: Ribavirin (Rebetol®): 200 mg (70s)

Injection, solution: Interferon alfa-2b (Intron® A): 3 million int. units/0.5 mL (3.8 mL) [1 multidose vial (18 million int. units/vial), 6 syringes and alcohol swabs]
Capsules: Ribavirin (Rebetol®): 200 mg (70s)

Injection, solution: Interferon alfa-2b (Intron® A): 3 million int. units/0.2 mL (1.5 mL) [1 multidose pen (18 million int. units/pen), 6 needles and alcohol swabs]
Capsules: Ribavirin (Rebetol®): 200 mg (70s)

Combination package for patients >75 kg:

Injection, solution: Interferon alfa-2b (Intron® A): 3 million int. units/0.5 mL (0.5 mL) [6 vials (3 million int. units/vial), 6 syringes and alcohol swabs]
Capsules: Ribavirin (Rebetol®): 200 mg (84s)

Injection, solution: Interferon alfa-2b (Intron® A): 3 million int. units/0.5 mL (3.8 mL) [1 multidose vial (18 million int. units/vial), 6 syringes and alcohol swabs]
Capsules: Ribavirin (Rebetol®): 200 mg (84s)

Injection, solution: Interferon alfa-2b (Intron® A): 3 million int. units/0.2 mL (1.5 mL) [1 multidose pen (18 million int. units/pen), 6 needles and alcohol swabs]
Capsules: Ribavirin (Rebetol®): 200 mg (84s)

Combination package for Rebetol® dose reduction:

Injection, solution: Interferon alfa-2b (Intron® A): 3 million int. units/0.5 mL (0.5 mL) [6 vials (3 million int. units/vial), 6 syringes and alcohol swabs]
Capsules: Ribavirin (Rebetol®): 200 mg (42s)

Injection, solution: Interferon alfa-2b (Intron® A): 3 million int. units/0.5 mL (3.8 mL) [1 multidose vial (18 million int. units/vial), 6 syringes and alcohol swabs]
Capsules: Ribavirin (Rebetol®): 200 mg (42s)

Injection, solution: Interferon alfa-2b (Intron® A): 3 million int. units/0.2 mL (1.5 mL) [1 multidose pen (18 million int. units/pen), 6 needles and alcohol swabs]
Capsules: Ribavirin (Rebetol®): 200 mg (42s)

interferon alfa-2b (PEG conjugate) *see* peginterferon alfa-2b *on page 671*

interferon alfacon-1 (in ter FEER on AL fa con-one)

U.S./Canadian Brand Names Infergen® [US/Can]

Therapeutic Category Interferon

Use Treatment of chronic hepatitis C virus (HCV) infection in patients ≥18 years of age with compensated liver disease and anti-HCV serum antibodies or HCV RNA.

Usual Dosage Adults ≥18 years: SubQ:

Chronic HCV infection: 9 mcg 3 times/week for 24 weeks; allow 48 hours between doses

Patients who have previously tolerated interferon therapy but did not respond or relapsed: 15 mcg 3 times/week for 6 months

Dose reduction for toxicity: Dose should be held in patients who experience a severe adverse reaction, and treatment should be stopped or decreased if the reaction does not become tolerable.

Doses were reduced from 9 mcg to 7.5 mcg in the pivotal study.

For patients receiving 15 mcg/dose, doses were reduced in 3 mcg increments. Efficacy is decreased with doses <7.5 mcg

Dosage Forms Injection, solution [preservative free]: 30 mcg/mL (0.3 mL, 0.5 mL)

interferon alfa-n3 (in ter FEER on AL fa-en three)

Sound-Alike/Look-Alike Issues

Alferon® may be confused with Alkeran®

U.S./Canadian Brand Names Alferon® N [US/Can]

Therapeutic Category Biological Response Modulator

Use Patients ≥18 years of age: Intralesional treatment of refractory or recurring genital or venereal warts (condylomata acuminata)

Usual Dosage Adults: Inject 250,000 units (0.05 mL) in each wart twice weekly for a maximum of 8 weeks; therapy should not be repeated for at least 3 months after the initial 8-week course of therapy

Dosage Forms Injection, solution: 5 million int. units (1 mL) [contains albumin]

interferon beta-1a (in ter FEER on BAY-ta won aye)

Sound-Alike/Look-Alike Issues

Avonex® may be confused with Avelox®

Synonyms rIFN beta-1a

U.S./Canadian Brand Names Avonex® [US/Can]; Rebif® [US/Can]

Therapeutic Category Biological Response Modulator

Use Treatment of relapsing forms of multiple sclerosis (MS)

Usual Dosage Adults:

I.M. (Avonex®): 30 mcg once weekly

SubQ (Rebif®): Initial: 8.8 mcg 3 times/week, increasing over a 4-week period to the recommended dose of 44 mcg 3 times/week; doses should be separated by at least 48 hours

Dosage Forms

Injection, powder for reconstitution (Avonex®): 33 mcg [6.6 million units; provides 30 mcg/mL following reconstitution] [contains albumin; packaged with SWFI, alcohol wipes, and access pin and needle]

(Continued)

interferon beta-1a *(Continued)*

Injection, solution (Avonex®): 30 mcg/0.5 mL (0.5 mL) [albumin free; prefilled syringe; syringe cap contains latex; packaged with alcohol wipes, gauze pad, and adhesive bandages]

Injection, solution [preservative free] (Rebif®): 22 mcg/mL (0.5 mL); 44 mcg/mL (0.5 mL) [prefilled syringe; contains albumin]

interferon beta-1b (in ter FEER on BAY ta-won bee)

Synonyms rIFN beta-1b

U.S./Canadian Brand Names Betaseron® [US/Can]

Therapeutic Category Biological Response Modulator

Use Treatment of relapsing forms of multiple sclerosis (MS)

Usual Dosage SubQ:

Children <18 years: Not recommended

Adults: 0.25 mg (8 million units) every other day

Dosage Forms Injection, powder for reconstitution [preservative free]: 0.3 mg [9.6 million units] [contains albumin; packaged with prefilled syringe containing diluent]

interferon gamma-1b (in ter FEER on GAM ah-won bee)

U.S./Canadian Brand Names Actimmune® [US/Can]

Therapeutic Category Biological Response Modulator

Use Reduce frequency and severity of serious infections associated with chronic granulomatous disease; delay time to disease progression in patients with severe, malignant osteopetrosis

Usual Dosage If severe reactions occur, modify dose (50% reduction) or therapy should be discontinued until adverse reactions abate.

Chronic granulomatous disease: Children >1 year and Adults: SubQ:

BSA ≤0.5 m^2: 1.5 mcg/kg/dose 3 times/week

BSA >0.5 m^2: 50 mcg/m^2 (1 million int. units/m^2) 3 times/week

Severe, malignant osteopetrosis: Children >1 year: SubQ:

BSA ≤0.5 m^2: 1.5 mcg/kg/dose 3 times/week

BSA >0.5 m^2: 50 mcg/m^2 (1 million int. units/m^2) 3 times/week

Note: Previously expressed as 1.5 million units/m^2; 50 mcg is equivalent to 1 million int. units/m^2.

Dosage Forms Injection, solution [preservative free]: 100 mcg [2 million int. units] (0.5 mL)

Previously, 100 mcg was expressed as 3 million units. This is equivalent to 2 million int. units.

interleukin-1 receptor antagonist *see* anakinra *on page 59*

interleukin-2 *see* aldesleukin *on page 28*

interleukin-11 *see* oprelvekin *on page 647*

Intralipid® [US/Can] *see* fat emulsion *on page 358*

intravenous fat emulsion *see* fat emulsion *on page 358*

intrifiban *see* eptifibatide *on page 317*

Intron® A [US/Can] *see* interferon alfa-2b *on page 477*

Intropin® [Can] *see* dopamine *on page 289*

Intropin® *(Discontinued)* *see page 1042*

Invanz® [US/Can] *see* ertapenem *on page 319*

Inversine® [US/Can] *see* mecamylamine *on page 546*

Invirase® [US/Can] *see* saquinavir *on page 794*

iocetamic acid *see* radiological/contrast media (ionic) *on page 759*

iodamide meglumine *see* radiological/contrast media (ionic) *on page 759*

Iodex-p® *(Discontinued)* *see page 1042*

Iodex [US-OTC] *see* iodine *on this page*

iodine (EYE oh dyne)

Sound-Alike/Look-Alike Issues
iodine may be confused with codeine, Iopidine®, Lodine®

U.S./Canadian Brand Names Iodex [US-OTC]; Iodoflex™ [US]; Iodosorb® [US]

Therapeutic Category Topical Skin Product

Use Used topically as an antiseptic in the management of minor, superficial skin wounds and has been used to disinfect the skin preoperatively

Usual Dosage Apply topically as necessary to affected areas of skin

Dosage Forms
Dressing, topical [gel pad] (Iodoflex™): 0.9% (5 g, 10 g)
Gel, topical (Iodosorb®): 0.9% (40 g)
Ointment (Iodex): 4.7% (30 g, 720 g)
Tincture, topical: 2% (30 mL, 480 mL); 7% (30 mL, 480 mL)

iodine *see* trace metals *on page 874*

iodine I 131 tositumomab and tositumomab *see* tositumomab and iodine I 131 tositumomab *on page 873*

iodipamide meglumine *see* radiological/contrast media (ionic) *on page 759*

iodochlorhydroxyquin and flumethasone *see* clioquinol and flumethasone *(Canada only) on page 211*

Iodoflex™ [US] *see* iodine *on this page*

Iodo-Niacin® Tablet *(Discontinued)* *see page 1042*

Iodopen® [US] *see* trace metals *on page 874*

iodoquinol (eye oh doe KWIN ole)

Synonyms diiodohydroxyquin

U.S./Canadian Brand Names Diodoquin® [Can]; Yodoxin® [US]

Therapeutic Category Amebicide

Use Treatment of acute and chronic intestinal amebiasis; asymptomatic cyst passers; *Blastocystis hominis* infections; ineffective for amebic hepatitis or hepatic abscess

Usual Dosage Oral:
Children: 30-40 mg/kg/day (maximum: 650 mg/dose) in 3 divided doses for 20 days; not to exceed 1.95 g/day
Adults: 650 mg 3 times/day after meals for 20 days; not to exceed 1.95 g/day

Dosage Forms Tablet: 210 mg, 650 mg

iodoquinol and hydrocortisone

(eye oh doe KWIN ole & hye droe KOR ti sone)

Sound-Alike/Look-Alike Issues
Vytone® may be confused with Hytone®, Zydone®

Synonyms hydrocortisone and iodoquinol

U.S./Canadian Brand Names Dermazene® [US]; Vytone® [US]

Therapeutic Category Antifungal/Corticosteroid

Use Treatment of eczema; infectious dermatitis; chronic eczematoid otitis externa; mycotic dermatoses

Usual Dosage Apply 3-4 times/day

Dosage Forms Cream: Iodoquinol 1% and hydrocortisone acetate 1% (30 g)
Dermazene®: Iodoquinol 1% and hydrocortisone acetate 1% (30 g, 45 g)
Vytone®: Iodoquinol 1% and hydrocortisone acetate 1% (30 g)

Iodosorb® [US] *see* iodine *on this page*

iohexol *see* radiological/contrast media (nonionic) *on page 761*

Ionamin® [US/Can] *see* phentermine *on page 688*

Ionil® Plus [US-OTC] *see* salicylic acid *on page 789*

Ionil T® Plus [US-OTC] *see* coal tar *on page 219*

Ionil T® [US-OTC] *see* coal tar *on page 219*

Ionil® [US-OTC] *see* salicylic acid *on page 789*

iopamidol *see* radiological/contrast media (nonionic) *on page 761*

iopanoic acid *see* radiological/contrast media (ionic) *on page 759*

Iophen® ***(Discontinued)*** *see page 1042*

Iophen-C® ***(Discontinued)*** *see page 1042*

Iophen-DM® ***(Discontinued)*** *see page 1042*

Iophen NR ***(Discontinued)*** *see page 1042*

Iophylline® ***(Discontinued)*** *see page 1042*

Iopidine® [US/Can] *see* apraclonidine *on page 74*

Iosat™ [US-OTC] *see* potassium iodide *on page 715*

iothalamate meglumine and iothalamate sodium *see* radiological/contrast media (ionic) *on page 759*

iothalamate sodium *see* radiological/contrast media (ionic) *on page 759*

Iotuss® ***(Discontinued)*** *see page 1042*

Iotuss-DM® ***(Discontinued)*** *see page 1042*

ioversol *see* radiological/contrast media (nonionic) *on page 761*

ipecac syrup (IP e kak SIR up)

Synonyms syrup of ipecac

Therapeutic Category Antidote

Use Treatment of acute oral drug overdosage and in certain poisonings

Usual Dosage Oral:

Children:

6-12 months: 5-10 mL followed by 10-20 mL/kg of water; repeat dose one time if vomiting does not occur within 20 minutes

1-12 years: 15 mL followed by 10-20 mL/kg of water; repeat dose one time if vomiting does not occur within 20 minutes

If emesis does not occur within 30 minutes after second dose, ipecac must be removed from stomach by gastric lavage

Adults: 15-30 mL followed by 200-300 mL of water; repeat dose one time if vomiting does not occur within 20 minutes

Dosage Forms Syrup: 70 mg/mL (30 mL) [contains alcohol]

I-Pentolate® ***(Discontinued)*** *see page 1042*

I-Phrine® Ophthalmic Solution ***(Discontinued)*** *see page 1042*

I-Picamide® ***(Discontinued)*** *see page 1042*

ipodate calcium *see* radiological/contrast media (ionic) *on page 759*

ipodate sodium *see* radiological/contrast media (ionic) *on page 759*

IPOL® [US/Can] *see* poliovirus vaccine (inactivated) *on page 705*

ipratropium (i pra TROE pee um)

Sound-Alike/Look-Alike Issues

Atrovent® may be confused with Alupent®

Synonyms ipratropium bromide

U.S./Canadian Brand Names Alti-Ipratropium [Can]; Apo-Ipravent® [Can]; Atrovent® [US/Can]; Gen-Ipratropium [Can]; Novo-Ipramide [Can]; Nu-Ipratropium [Can]; PMS-Ipratropium [Can]

Therapeutic Category Anticholinergic Agent

Use Anticholinergic bronchodilator used in bronchospasm associated with COPD, bronchitis, and emphysema; symptomatic relief of rhinorrhea associated with the common cold and allergic and nonallergic rhinitis

Usual Dosage

Nebulization:

Infants and Children ≤12 years: 125-250 mcg 3 times/day

Children >12 years and Adults: 500 mcg (one unit-dose vial) 3-4 times/day with doses 6-8 hours apart

Oral inhalation: MDI:

Children 3-12 years: 1-2 inhalations 3 times/day, up to 6 inhalations/24 hours

Children >12 years and Adults: 2 inhalations 4 times/day, up to 12 inhalations/24 hours

Intranasal: Nasal spray:

Symptomatic relief of rhinorrhea associated with the common cold (safety and efficacy of use beyond 4 days in patients with the common cold have not been established):

Children 5-11 years: 0.06%: 2 sprays in each nostril 3 times/day

Children ≥5 years and Adults: 0.06%: 2 sprays in each nostril 3-4 times/day

Symptomatic relief of rhinorrhea associated with allergic/nonallergic rhinitis: Children ≥6 years and Adults: 0.03%: 2 sprays in each nostril 2-3 times/day

Dosage Forms

Solution for nebulization, as bromide: 0.02% (2.5 mL)

Solution for oral inhalation, as bromide: 18 mcg/actuation (14 g) [contains soya lecithin]

Solution, intranasal spray, as bromide: 0.03% (30 mL); 0.06% (15 mL)

ipratropium and albuterol (i pra TROE pee um & al BYOO ter ole)

Sound-Alike/Look-Alike Issues

Combivent® may be confused with Combivir®

Synonyms albuterol and ipratropium

U.S./Canadian Brand Names Combivent® [US/Can]; DuoNeb™ [US]

Therapeutic Category Bronchodilator

Use Treatment of COPD in those patients that are currently on a regular bronchodilator who continue to have bronchospasms and require a second bronchodilator

Usual Dosage Adults:

Inhalation: 2 inhalations 4 times/day (maximum: 12 inhalations/24 hours)

Inhalation via nebulization: Initial: 3 mL every 6 hours (maximum: 3 mL every 4 hours)

Dosage Forms

Aerosol for oral inhalation (Combivent®): Ipratropium bromide 18 mcg and albuterol sulfate 103 mcg per actuation [200 doses] (14.7 g) [contains soya lecithin]

Solution for oral inhalation (DuoNeb™): Ipratropium bromide 0.5 mg [0.017%] and albuterol base 2.5 mg [0.083%] per 3 mL vial (30s, 60s)

ipratropium bromide *see* ipratropium *on previous page*

I-Prin [US-OTC] *see* ibuprofen *on page 462*

iproveratril hydrochloride *see* verapamil *on page 908*

IPV *see* poliovirus vaccine (inactivated) *on page 705*

Iquix® [US] *see* levofloxacin *on page 514*

irbesartan (ir be SAR tan)

Sound-Alike/Look-Alike Issues

Avapro® may be confused with Anaprox®

U.S./Canadian Brand Names Avapro® [US/Can]

Therapeutic Category Angiotensin II Receptor Antagonist

Use Treatment of hypertension alone or in combination with other antihypertensives; treatment of diabetic nephropathy in patients with type 2 diabetes mellitus (noninsulin dependent, NIDDM) and hypertension

(Continued)

irbesartan *(Continued)*

Usual Dosage Oral:
Hypertension:
Children:
<6 years: Safety and efficacy have not been established.
≥6-12 years: Initial: 75 mg once daily; may be titrated to a maximum of 150 mg once daily
Children ≥13 years and Adults: 150 mg once daily; patients may be titrated to 300 mg once daily
Note: Starting dose in volume-depleted patients should be 75 mg
Nephropathy in patients with type 2 diabetes and hypertension: Adults: Target dose: 300 mg once daily

Dosage Forms Tablet: 75 mg, 150 mg, 300 mg

irbesartan and hydrochlorothiazide

(ir be SAR tan & hye droe klor oh THYE a zide)

Sound-Alike/Look-Alike Issues
Avalide® may be confused with Avandia®

Synonyms Avapro® HCT; hydrochlorothiazide and irbesartan

U.S./Canadian Brand Names Avalide® [US/Can]

Therapeutic Category Antihypertensive Agent, Combination

Use Combination therapy for the management of hypertension

Usual Dosage Dose must be individualized. A patient who is not controlled with either agent alone may be switched to the combination product. Mean effect increases with the dose of each component. The lowest dosage available is irbesartan 150 mg/hydrochlorothiazide 12.5 mg. Dose increases should be made not more frequently than every 2-4 weeks.

Dosage Forms
Tablet:
Irbesartan 150 mg and hydrochlorothiazide 12.5 mg
Irbesartan 300 mg and hydrochlorothiazide 12.5 mg

Ircon® [US-OTC] *see* ferrous fumarate *on page 363*

Iressa™ [US] *see* gefitinib *on page 398*

irinotecan (eye rye no TEE kan)

Synonyms camptothecin-11; CPT-11; NSC-616348

U.S./Canadian Brand Names Camptosar® [US/Can]

Therapeutic Category Antineoplastic Agent

Use Treatment of metastatic carcinoma of the colon or rectum

Usual Dosage Refer to individual protocols.
Single-agent therapy:
Weekly regimen: 125 mg/m^2 over 90 minutes on days 1, 8, 15, and 22, followed by a 2-week rest
Adjusted dose level -1: 100 mg/m^2
Adjusted dose level -2: 75 mg/m^2
Once-every-3-week regimen: 350 mg/m^2 over 90 minutes, once every 3 weeks
Adjusted dose level -1: 300 mg/m^2
Adjusted dose level -2: 250 mg/m^2
A reduction in the starting dose by one dose level may be considered for patients ≥65 years of age, prior pelvic/abdominal radiotherapy, performance status of 2, or increased bilirubin (dosing for patients with a bilirubin >2 mg/dL cannot be recommended based on lack of data per manufacturer)
Depending on the patient's ability to tolerate therapy, doses should be adjusted in increments of 25-50 mg/m^2. Irinotecan doses may range from 50-150 mg/m^2 for the weekly regimen; from 50-200 mg/m^2 for the once-every-3-week regimen

Combination therapy with fluorouracil and leucovorin: Six-week (42-day) cycle:
Regimen 1: 125 mg/m² over 90 minutes on days 1, 8, 15, and 22; to be given in combination with bolus leucovorin and fluorouracil (leucovorin administered immediately following irinotecan; fluorouracil immediately following leucovorin)
Adjusted dose level -1: 100 mg/m²
Adjusted dose level -2: 75 mg/m²
Regimen 2: 180 mg/m² over 90 minutes on days 1, 15, and 22; to be given in combination with infusional leucovorin and bolus/infusion fluorouracil (leucovorin administered immediately following irinotecan; fluorouracil immediately following leucovorin)
Adjusted dose level -1: 150 mg/m²
Adjusted dose level -2: 120 mg/m²

Note: For all regimens: It is recommended that new courses begin only after the granulocyte count recovers to ≥1500/mm³, the platelet count recovers to ≥100,000/mm³, and treatment-related diarrhea has fully resolved. Treatment should be delayed 1-2 weeks to allow for recovery from treatment-related toxicities. If the patient has not recovered after a 2-week delay, consideration should be given to discontinuing irinotecan.

Dosage Forms Injection, solution, as hydrochloride: 20 mg/mL (2 mL, 5 mL)

iron dextran complex (EYE ern DEKS tran KOM pleks)

Sound-Alike/Look-Alike Issues
Dexferrum® may be confused with Desferal®

U.S./Canadian Brand Names Dexferrum® [US]; Dexiron™ [Can]; INFeD® [US]; Infufer® [Can]

Therapeutic Category Electrolyte Supplement, Oral

Use Treatment of microcytic hypochromic anemia resulting from iron deficiency in patients in whom oral administration is infeasible or ineffective

Usual Dosage I.M. (Z-track method should be used for I.M. injection), I.V.:
A 0.5 mL test dose (0.25 mL in infants) should be given prior to starting iron dextran therapy; total dose should be divided into a daily schedule for I.M., total dose may be given as a single continuous infusion
Iron-deficiency anemia: Dose (mL) = 0.0476 x LBW (kg) x (normal hemoglobin - observed hemoglobin) + (1 mL/5 kg of LBW to maximum of 14 mL for iron stores)
LBW = Lean Body Weight
Iron replacement therapy for blood loss: Replacement iron (mg) = blood loss (mL) x hematocrit
Maximum daily dose (can administer total dose at one time I.V.):
Infants <5 kg: 25 mg iron (0.5 mL)
Children:
5-10 kg: 50 mg iron (1 mL)
10-50 kg: 100 mg iron (2 mL)
Adults >50 kg: 100 mg iron (2 mL)

Dosage Forms Note: Strength expressed as elemental iron
Injection, solution:
Dexferrum®: 50 mg/mL (1 mL, 2 mL)
INFeD®: 50 mg/mL (2 mL)

iron fumarate *see* ferrous fumarate *on page 363*

iron gluconate *see* ferrous gluconate *on page 364*

iron-polysaccharide complex *see* polysaccharide-iron complex *on page 709*

iron sucrose (EYE ern SOO krose)

U.S./Canadian Brand Names Venofer® [US/Can]

Therapeutic Category Iron Salt

Use Treatment of iron-deficiency anemia in patients undergoing chronic hemodialysis who are receiving supplemental erythropoietin therapy

(Continued)

iron sucrose *(Continued)*

Usual Dosage Doses expressed in mg of **elemental** iron

I.V.: Adults: Iron-deficiency anemia: 100 mg (5 mL of iron sucrose injection) administered 1-3 times/week during dialysis, to a total dose of 1000 mg (10 doses); administer no more than 3 times/week; may continue to administer at lowest dose necessary to maintain target hemoglobin, hematocrit, and iron storage parameters

Test dose: Product labeling does not indicate need for a test dose in product-naive patients; test doses were administered in some clinical trials as 50 mg (2.5 mL) in 50 mL 0.9% NaCl administered over 3-10 minutes

Dosage Forms Injection, solution [preservative free]: 20 mg of elemental iron/mL (5 mL)

iron sulfate *see* ferrous sulfate *on page 364*

iron sulfate and vitamin C *see* ferrous sulfate and ascorbic acid *on page 365*

ISD *see* isosorbide dinitrate *on page 488*

ISDN *see* isosorbide dinitrate *on page 488*

ISG *see* immune globulin (intramuscular) *on page 468*

Ismelin® *(Discontinued)* *see page 1042*

ISMN *see* isosorbide mononitrate *on page 489*

Ismo® [US] *see* isosorbide mononitrate *on page 489*

Ismotic® *(Discontinued)* *see page 1042*

isoamyl nitrite *see* amyl nitrite *on page 58*

isobamate *see* carisoprodol *on page 162*

Iso-Bid® *(Discontinued)* *see page 1042*

isocarboxazid (eye soe kar BOKS a zid)

U.S./Canadian Brand Names Marplan® [US]

Therapeutic Category Antidepressant, Monoamine Oxidase Inhibitor

Use Symptomatic treatment of atypical, nonendogenous or neurotic depression

Usual Dosage Adults: Oral: 10 mg 2-3 times/day; reduce to 10-20 mg/day in divided doses when condition improves

Dosage Forms Tablet: 10 mg

isoetharine (eye soe ETH a reen)

Therapeutic Category Adrenergic Agonist Agent

Use Bronchodilator used in asthma and for the reversible bronchospasm occurring with bronchitis and emphysema

Usual Dosage Treatments are usually not repeated more often than every 4 hours, except in severe cases, and may be repeated up to 5 times/day if necessary

Nebulizer: Children: 0.1-0.2 mg/kg/dose every 2-6 hours as needed; adult: 0.5 mL diluted in 2-3 mL normal saline or 4 inhalations of undiluted 1% solution

Dosage Forms Solution for oral inhalation, as hydrochloride: 1% (10 mL) [contains sodium sulfite and sodium bisulfite]

isoflurane (eye soe FLURE ane)

Sound-Alike/Look-Alike Issues

isoflurane may be confused with enflurane, isoflurophate

U.S./Canadian Brand Names Forane® [US]

Therapeutic Category General Anesthetic

Use Maintenance of general anesthesia

Usual Dosage Minimum alveolar concentration (MAC), the concentration at which 50% of patients do not respond to surgical incision, is 1.2% for isoflurane. The concentration at which amnesia and loss of awareness occur (MAC - awake) is 0.4%. MAC is reduced in the elderly.

Dosage Forms Solution: 100 mL, 250 mL

Isollyl® Improved *(Discontinued)* *see page 1042*

isometheptene, acetaminophen, and dichloralphenazone *see* acetaminophen, isometheptene, and dichloralphenazone *on page 13*

isometheptene, dichloralphenazone, and acetaminophen *see* acetaminophen, isometheptene, and dichloralphenazone *on page 13*

isoniazid (eye soe NYE a zid)

Synonyms INH; isonicotinic acid hydrazide

U.S./Canadian Brand Names Isotamine® [Can]; PMS-Isoniazid [Can]

Therapeutic Category Antitubercular Agent

Use Treatment of susceptible tuberculosis infections; prophylactically in those individuals exposed to tuberculosis

Usual Dosage Recommendations often change due to resistant strains and newly developed information; consult *MMWR* for current CDC recommendations: **Oral** (injectable is available for patients who are unable to either take or absorb oral therapy):

Note: A four-drug regimen (isoniazid, rifampin, pyrazinamide, and either streptomycin or ethambutol) is preferred for the initial, empiric treatment of TB. When the drug susceptibility results are available, the regimen should be altered as appropriate.

Infants and Children:

Prophylaxis: 10 mg/kg/day in 1-2 divided doses (maximum: 300 mg/day) 6 months in patients who do not have HIV infection and 12 months in patients who have HIV infection

Treatment:

Daily therapy: 10-20 mg/kg/day in 1-2 divided doses (maximum: 300 mg/day)

Directly observed therapy (DOT): Twice weekly therapy: 20-40 mg/kg (maximum: 900 mg/day); 3 times/week therapy: 20-40 mg/kg (maximum: 900 mg)

Adults:

Prophylaxis: 300 mg/day for 6 months in patients who do not have HIV infection and 12 months in patients who have HIV infection

Treatment:

Daily therapy: 5 mg/kg/day given daily (usual dose: 300 mg/day); 10 mg/kg/day in 1-2 divided doses in patients with disseminated disease

Directly observed therapy (DOT): Twice weekly therapy: 15 mg/kg (maximum: 900 mg); 3 times/week therapy: 15 mg/kg (maximum: 900 mg)

Note: Concomitant administration of 6-50 mg/day pyridoxine is recommended in malnourished patients or those prone to neuropathy (eg, alcoholics, diabetics)

Hemodialysis: Dialyzable (50% to 100%)

Administer dose postdialysis

Peritoneal dialysis effects: Dose for Cl_{cr} <10 mL/minute

Continuous arteriovenous or venovenous hemofiltration: Dose for Cl_{cr} <10 mL/minute

Dosage Forms

Injection, solution (Nydrazid®): 100 mg/mL (10 mL) [DSC]

Syrup: 50 mg/5 mL (473 mL) [orange flavor]

Tablet: 100 mg, 300 mg

isoniazid and rifampin *see* rifampin and isoniazid *on page 776*

isoniazid, rifampin, and pyrazinamide *see* rifampin, isoniazid, and pyrazinamide *on page 776*

isonicotinic acid hydrazide *see* isoniazid *on this page*

isonipecaine hydrochloride *see* meperidine *on page 553*

isophosphamide *see* ifosfamide *on page 464*

isoproterenol (eye soe proe TER e nole)

Sound-Alike/Look-Alike Issues

Isuprel® may be confused with Disophrol®, Ismelin®, Isordil®

(Continued)

isoproterenol *(Continued)*

Synonyms isoproterenol hydrochloride

U.S./Canadian Brand Names Isuprel® [US]

Therapeutic Category Adrenergic Agonist Agent

Use Ventricular arrhythmias due to AV nodal block; hemodynamically compromised bradyarrhythmias or atropine- and dopamine-resistant bradyarrhythmias (when transcutaneous/venous pacing is not available); temporary use in third-degree AV block until pacemaker insertion

Usual Dosage I.V.: Cardiac arrhythmias:

Children: Initial: 0.1 mcg/kg/minute (usual effective dose 0.2-2 mcg/kg/minute)

Adults: Initial: 2 mcg/minute; titrate to patient response (2-10 mcg/minute)

Dosage Forms Injection, solution, as hydrochloride: 0.02 mg/mL (10 mL); 0.2 mg/mL (1:5000) (1 mL, 5 mL) [contains sodium metabisulfite]

isoproterenol hydrochloride *see* isoproterenol *on previous page*

Isoptin® [Can] *see* verapamil *on page 908*

Isoptin® *(Discontinued)* *see page 1042*

Isoptin® I.V. [Can] *see* verapamil *on page 908*

Isoptin® SR [US/Can] *see* verapamil *on page 908*

Isopto® Atropine [US/Can] *see* atropine *on page 88*

Isopto® Carbachol [US/Can] *see* carbachol *on page 154*

Isopto® Carpine [US/Can] *see* pilocarpine *on page 694*

Isopto® Cetapred® *(Discontinued)* *see page 1042*

Isopto® Eserine [Can] *see* physostigmine *on page 693*

Isopto® Eserine *(Discontinued)* *see page 1042*

Isopto® Frin Ophthalmic Solution *(Discontinued)* *see page 1042*

Isopto® Homatropine [US] *see* homatropine *on page 436*

Isopto® Hyoscine [US] *see* scopolamine *on page 796*

Isopto® P-ES *(Discontinued)* *see page 1042*

Isopto® Plain Solution *(Discontinued)* *see page 1042*

Isopto® Tears [US] *see* artificial tears *on page 78*

Isordil® [US] *see* isosorbide dinitrate *on this page*

isosorbide dinitrate (eye soe SOR bide dye NYE trate)

Sound-Alike/Look-Alike Issues

Isordil® may be confused with Inderal®, Isuprel®

Synonyms ISD; ISDN

U.S./Canadian Brand Names Apo-ISDN® [Can]; Cedocard®-SR [Can]; Coronex® [Can]; Dilatrate®-SR [US]; Isordil® [US]; Novo-Sorbide [Can]; PMS-Isosorbide [Can]

Therapeutic Category Vasodilator

Use Prevention and treatment of angina pectoris; for congestive heart failure; to relieve pain, dysphagia, and spasm in esophageal spasm with GE reflux

Usual Dosage Adults (elderly should be given lowest recommended daily doses initially and titrate upward): Oral:

Angina: 5-40 mg 4 times/day or 40 mg every 8-12 hours in sustained-release dosage form

Congestive heart failure:

- Initial dose: 10 mg 3 times/day
- Target dose: 40 mg 3 times/day
- Maximum dose: 80 mg 3 times/day

Sublingual: 2.5-10 mg every 4-6 hours

Chewable tablet: 5-10 mg every 2-3 hours

Tolerance to nitrate effects develops with chronic exposure: Dose escalation does not overcome this effect. Tolerance can only be overcome by short periods of nitrate absence from the body. Short periods (10-12 hours) of nitrate withdrawal help minimize tolerance. General recommendations are to take the last dose of short-acting agents no later than 7 PM; administer 2-3 times/day rather than 4 times/day. Sustained release preparations could be administered at times to allow a 15- to 17-hour interval between first and last daily dose. Example: Administer sustained release at 8 AM and 2 PM for a twice daily regimen.

Dosage Forms
Capsule, sustained release (Dilatrate®-SR): 40 mg
Tablet: 5 mg, 10 mg, 20 mg, 30 mg,
Isordil®: 5 mg, 10 mg, 20 mg, 30 mg, 40 mg
Tablet, chewable: 5 mg, 10 mg
Tablet, sublingual (Isordil®): 2.5 mg, 5 mg, 10 mg

isosorbide mononitrate (eye soe SOR bide mon oh NYE trate)

Sound-Alike/Look-Alike Issues
Imdur® may be confused with Imuran®, Inderal LA®, K-Dur®
Monoket® may be confused with Monopril®

Synonyms ISMN

U.S./Canadian Brand Names Imdur® [US/Can]; Ismo® [US]; Monoket® [US]

Therapeutic Category Vasodilator

Use Long-acting metabolite of the vasodilator isosorbide dinitrate used for the prophylactic treatment of angina pectoris

Usual Dosage Adults and Geriatrics (start with lowest recommended dose): Oral:
Regular tablet: 5-10 mg twice daily with the two doses given 7 hours apart (eg, 8 AM and 3 PM) to decrease tolerance development; then titrate to 10 mg twice daily in first 2-3 days.
Extended release tablet: Initial: 30-60 mg given in morning as a single dose; titrate upward as needed, giving at least 3 days between increases; maximum daily single dose: 240 mg
Tolerance to nitrate effects develops with chronic exposure. Dose escalation does not overcome this effect. Tolerance can only be overcome by short periods of nitrate absence from the body. Short periods (10-12 hours) of nitrate withdrawal help minimize tolerance. Recommended dosage regimens incorporate this interval. General recommendations are to take the last dose of short-acting agents no later than 7 PM; administer 2 times/day rather than 4 times/day. Administer sustained release tablet once daily in the morning.

Dosage Forms
Tablet: 10 mg, 20 mg
Ismo®: 20 mg
Monoket®: 10 mg, 20 mg
Tablet, extended release (Imdur®): 30 mg, 60 mg, 120 mg

isosulfan blue *see* radiological/contrast media (ionic) *on page 759*

Isotamine® [Can] *see* isoniazid *on page 487*

isotretinoin (eye soe TRET i noyn)

Sound-Alike/Look-Alike Issues
Accutane® may be confused with Accolate®, Accupril®

Synonyms 13-*cis*-retinoic acid

U.S./Canadian Brand Names Accutane® [US/Can]; Amnesteem™ [US]; Claravis™ [US]; Isotrex® [Can]; Sotret® [US]

Therapeutic Category Retinoic Acid Derivative

Use Treatment of severe recalcitrant nodular acne unresponsive to conventional therapy

Usual Dosage Oral:
Children: Maintenance therapy for neuroblastoma (investigational): 100-250 mg/m^2/day in 2 divided doses
(Continued)

isotretinoin *(Continued)*

Children and Adults: Severe recalcitrant nodular acne: 0.5-2 mg/kg/day in 2 divided doses (dosages as low as 0.05 mg/kg/day have been reported to be beneficial) for 15-20 weeks or until the total cyst count decreases by 70%, whichever is sooner. A second course of therapy may be initiated after a period of ≥2 months off therapy.

Dosage Forms

Capsule:

Accutane®: 10 mg, 20 mg, 40 mg [contains soybean oil and parabens]
Amnesteem™: 10 mg, 20 mg, 40 mg [contains soybean oil]
Claravis™: 10 mg, 20 mg, 40 mg
Sotret®: 10 mg, 20 mg, 30 mg, 40 mg [contains soybean oil]

Isotrex® [Can] *see* isotretinoin *on previous page*

Isovex® *(Discontinued)* *see page 1042*

Isovue® [US] *see* radiological/contrast media (nonionic) *on page 761*

isoxsuprine (eye SOKS syoo preen)

Synonyms isoxsuprine hydrochloride

Therapeutic Category Vasodilator

Use Treatment of peripheral vascular diseases, such as arteriosclerosis obliterans and Raynaud disease

Usual Dosage Oral: Adults: 10-20 mg 3-4 times/day; start with lower dose in elderly due to potential hypotension

Dosage Forms Tablet, as hydrochloride: 10 mg, 20 mg

isoxsuprine hydrochloride *see* isoxsuprine *on this page*

isradipine (iz RA di peen)

Sound-Alike/Look-Alike Issues

DynaCirc® may be confused with Dynabac®, Dynacin®

U.S./Canadian Brand Names DynaCirc® CR [US]; DynaCirc® [US/Can]

Therapeutic Category Calcium Channel Blocker

Use Treatment of hypertension

Usual Dosage Oral: Adults: 2.5 mg twice daily; antihypertensive response occurs in 2-3 hours; maximal response in 2-4 weeks; increase dose at 2- to 4-week intervals at 2.5-5 mg increments; usual dose range (JNC 7): 2.5-10 mg/day in 2 divided doses. **Note:** Most patients show no improvement with doses >10 mg/day except adverse reaction rate increases; therefore, maximal dose in older adults should be 10 mg/day.

Dosage Forms

Capsule (DynaCirc®): 2.5 mg, 5 mg
Tablet, controlled release (DynaCirc® CR): 5 mg, 10 mg

Istalol™ [US] *see* timolol *on page 863*

Isuprel® [US] *see* isoproterenol *on page 487*

Isuprel® Glossets® *(Discontinued)* *see page 1042*

Itch-X® [US-OTC] *see* pramoxine *on page 720*

itraconazole (i tra KOE na zole)

Sound-Alike/Look-Alike Issues

Sporanox® may be confused with Suprax®

U.S./Canadian Brand Names Sporanox® [US/Can]

Therapeutic Category Antifungal Agent

Use Treatment of susceptible fungal infections in immunocompromised and immunocompetent patients including blastomycosis and histoplasmosis; indicated for aspergillosis, and onychomycosis of the toenail; treatment of onychomycosis of the fingernail without concomitant toenail infection via a pulse-type dosing regimen; has activity against *Aspergillus*, *Candida*, *Coccidioides*, *Cryptococcus*, *Sporothrix*, tinea unguium

Oral: Useful in superficial mycoses including dermatophytoses (eg, tinea capitis), pityriasis versicolor, sebopsoriasis, vaginal and chronic mucocutaneous candidiases; systemic mycoses including candidiasis, meningeal and disseminated cryptococcal infections, paracoccidioidomycosis, coccidioidomycoses; miscellaneous mycoses such as sporotrichosis, chromomycosis, leishmaniasis, fungal keratitis, alternariosis, zygomycosis

Oral solution: Treatment of oral and esophageal candidiasis

Intravenous solution: Indicated in the treatment of blastomycosis, histoplasmosis (nonmeningeal), and aspergillosis (in patients intolerant or refractory to amphotericin B therapy); empiric therapy of febrile neutropenic fever

Usual Dosage Note: Capsule: Absorption is best if taken with food, therefore, it is best to administer itraconazole after meals; Solution: Should be taken on an empty stomach.

Children: Efficacy and safety have not been established; a small number of patients 3-16 years of age have been treated with 100 mg/day for systemic fungal infections with no serious adverse effects reported. A dose of 5 mg/kg once daily was used in a pharmacokinetic study using the oral solution in patients 6 months-12 years; duration of study was 2 weeks.

Adults:

Oral:

Blastomycosis/histoplasmosis: 200 mg once daily, if no obvious improvement or there is evidence of progressive fungal disease, increase the dose in 100 mg increments to a maximum of 400 mg/day; doses >200 mg/day are given in 2 divided doses; length of therapy varies from 1 day to >6 months depending on the condition and mycological response

Aspergillosis: 200-400 mg/day

Onychomycosis: 200 mg once daily for 12 consecutive weeks

Life-threatening infections: Loading dose: 200 mg 3 times/day (600 mg/day) should be given for the first 3 days of therapy

Oropharyngeal candidiasis: Oral solution: 200 mg once daily for 1-2 weeks; in patients unresponsive or refractory to fluconazole: 100 mg twice daily (clinical response expected in 1-2 weeks)

Esophageal candidiasis: Oral solution: 100-200 mg once daily for a minimum of 3 weeks; continue dosing for 2 weeks after resolution of symptoms

I.V.: 200 mg twice daily for 4 doses, followed by 200 mg daily

Dosage Forms

Capsule: 100 mg

Injection, solution: 10 mg/mL (25 mL) [packaged in a kit containing sodium chloride 0.9% (50 mL); filtered infusion set (1)]

Solution, oral: 100 mg/10 mL (150 mL) [cherry flavor]

I-Tropine® *(Discontinued)* *see page 1042*

Iveegam EN [US] *see* immune globulin (intravenous) *on page 468*

Iveegam Immuno® [Can] *see* immune globulin (intravenous) *on page 468*

ivermectin (eye ver MEK tin)

U.S./Canadian Brand Names Stromectol® [US]

Therapeutic Category Antibiotic, Miscellaneous

Use Treatment of the following infections: Strongyloidiasis of the intestinal tract due to the nematode parasite *Strongyloides stercoralis*. Onchocerciasis due to the nematode parasite *Onchocerca volvulus*. Ivermectin is only active against the immature form of *Onchocerca volvulus*, and the intestinal forms of *Strongyloides stercoralis*.

Usual Dosage Oral: Children ≥15 kg and Adults:

Strongyloidiasis: 200 mcg/kg as a single dose; follow-up stool examinations

Onchocerciasis: 150 mcg/kg as a single dose; retreatment may be required every 3-12 months until the adult worms die

Dosage Forms Tablet [scored]: 3 mg

IVIG *see* immune globulin (intravenous) *on page 468*

IvyBlock® [US-OTC] *see* bentoquatam *on page 106*

Janimine® *(Discontinued)* *see page 1042*

Japanese encephalitis virus vaccine (inactivated)

(jap a NEESE en sef a LYE tis VYE rus vak SEEN in ak ti VAY ted)

U.S./Canadian Brand Names JE-VAX® [US/Can]

Therapeutic Category Vaccine, Inactivated Virus

Use Active immunization against Japanese encephalitis for persons 1 year of age and older who plan to spend 1 month or more in endemic areas in Asia, especially persons traveling during the transmission season or visiting rural areas; consider vaccination for shorter trips to epidemic areas or extensive outdoor activities in rural endemic areas; elderly (>55 years of age) individuals should be considered for vaccination, since they have increased risk of developing symptomatic illness after infection; those planning travel to or residence in endemic areas should consult the Travel Advisory Service (Central Campus) for specific advice

Usual Dosage U.S. recommended primary immunization schedule:

Children 1-3 years: SubQ: Three 0.5 mL doses given on days 0, 7, and 30; abbreviated schedules should be used only when necessary due to time constraints

Children >3 years and Adults: SubQ: Three 1 mL doses given on days 0, 7, and 30. Give third dose on day 14 when time does not permit waiting; 2 doses a week apart produce immunity in about 80% of recipients; the longest regimen yields highest titers after 6 months.

Booster dose: Give after 2 years, or according to current recommendation

Note: Travel should not commence for at least 10 days after the last dose of vaccine, to allow adequate antibody formation and recognition of any delayed adverse reaction

Advise concurrent use of other means to reduce the risk of mosquito exposure when possible, including bed nets, insect repellents, protective clothing, avoidance of travel in endemic areas, and avoidance of outdoor activity during twilight and evening periods

Dosage Forms Injection, powder for reconstitution: 1 mL, 10 mL

Jenamicin® *(Discontinued)* *see page 1042*

Jenest™-28 *(Discontinued)* *see page 1042*

JE-VAX® [US/Can] *see* Japanese encephalitis virus vaccine (inactivated) *on this page*

Jolivette™ [US] *see* norethindrone *on page 627*

Junel™ [US] *see* ethinyl estradiol and norethindrone *on page 342*

Just Tears® Solution *(Discontinued)* *see page 1042*

K+8 [US] *see* potassium chloride *on page 713*

K+10 [US] *see* potassium chloride *on page 713*

Kabikinase® *(Discontinued)* *see page 1042*

Kadian® [US/Can] *see* morphine sulfate *on page 591*

Kala® [US-OTC] *see* Lactobacillus *on page 501*

Kalcinate® *(Discontinued)* *see page 1042*

Kaletra™ [US/Can] *see* lopinavir and ritonavir *on page 529*

Kalmz [US-OTC] *see* fructose, dextrose, and phosphoric acid *on page 392*

kanamycin (kan a MYE sin)

Sound-Alike/Look-Alike Issues

kanamycin may be confused with Garamycin®, gentamicin

Synonyms kanamycin sulfate
U.S./Canadian Brand Names Kantrex® [US/Can]
Therapeutic Category Aminoglycoside (Antibiotic)
Use Treatment of serious infections caused by susceptible strains of *E. coli, Proteus species, Enterobacter aerogenes, Klebsiella pneumoniae, Serratia marcescens,* and *Acinetobacter* species; second-line treatment of *Mycobacterium tuberculosis*
Usual Dosage Note: Dosing should be based on ideal body weight
Children: Infections: I.M., I.V.: 15 mg/kg/day in divided doses every 8-12 hours
Adults:
Infections: I.M., I.V.: 5-7.5 mg/kg/dose in divided doses every 8-12 hours (<15 mg/kg/day)
Intraperitoneal: After contamination in surgery: 500 mg
Irrigating solution: 0.25%; maximum 1.5 g/day (via all administration routes)
Aerosol: 250 mg 2-4 times/day
Dosage Forms Injection, solution, as sulfate: 1 g/3 mL (3 mL) [contains sodium bisulfate]

kanamycin sulfate *see* kanamycin *on previous page*

Kank-A® [Can] *see* cetylpyridinium and benzocaine *on page 179*

Kantrex® [US/Can] *see* kanamycin *on previous page*

Kaochlor-Eff® ***(Discontinued)*** *see page 1042*

Kaochlor® SF ***(Discontinued)*** *see page 1042*

Kaodene® ***(Discontinued)*** *see page 1042*

Kaodene® NN [US-OTC] *see* kaolin and pectin *on this page*

kaolin and pectin (KAY oh lin & PEK tin)

Synonyms pectin and kaolin
U.S./Canadian Brand Names Kaodene® NN [US-OTC]; Kao-Spen® [US-OTC]; Kapectolin® [US-OTC]
Therapeutic Category Antidiarrheal
Use Treatment of uncomplicated diarrhea
Usual Dosage Oral:
Children:
<6 years: Do not use
6-12 years: 30-60 mL after each loose stool
Adults: 60-120 mL after each loose stool
Dosage Forms
Suspension, oral: Kaolin 967 mg and pectin 22 mg per 5 mL (30 mL, 180 mL)
Kaodene® NN: Kaolin 650 mg and pectin 32.4 mg per 5 mL (120 mL) [contains bismuth subsalicylate 2.8 mg/5 mL]
Kao-Spen®: Kaolin 860 mg and pectin 43 mg per 5 mL (3840 mL)
Kapectolin®: Kaolin 15 g and pectin 33 mg per 5 mL (120 mL, 240 mL, 480 mL)

Kaon® [US] *see* potassium gluconate *on page 715*

Kaon-Cl®-10 [US] *see* potassium chloride *on page 713*

Kaon-Cl® 20 [US] *see* potassium chloride *on page 713*

Kaopectate® [Can] *see* attapulgite *on page 90*

Kaopectate® Advanced Formula ***(Discontinued)*** *see page 1042*

Kaopectate® Extra Strength [US-OTC] *see* bismuth *on page 120*

Kaopectate® II ***(Discontinued)*** *see page 1042*

Kaopectate® Maximum Strength Caplets ***(Discontinued)*** *see page 1042*

Kaopectate® [US-OTC] *see* bismuth *on page 120*

Kao-Spen® [US-OTC] *see* kaolin and pectin *on this page*

Kapectolin PG® ***(Discontinued)*** *see page 1042*

Kapectolin® [US-OTC] *see* kaolin and pectin *on previous page*
Karidium® ***(Discontinued)*** *see page 1042*
Karigel® ***(Discontinued)*** *see page 1042*
Karigel®-N ***(Discontinued)*** *see page 1042*
Kariva™ [US] *see* ethinyl estradiol and desogestrel *on page 335*
Kasof® ***(Discontinued)*** *see page 1042*
Kato® Powder ***(Discontinued)*** *see page 1042*
Kaybovite-1000® ***(Discontinued)*** *see page 1042*
Kay Ciel® [US] *see* potassium chloride *on page 713*
Kayexalate® [US/Can] *see* sodium polystyrene sulfonate *on page 816*
K+ Care® [US] *see* potassium chloride *on page 713*
K+ Care® ET [US] *see* potassium bicarbonate *on page 711*
K-Citra® [Can] *see* potassium citrate *on page 714*
KCl *see* potassium chloride *on page 713*
K-Dur® [Can] *see* potassium chloride *on page 713*
K-Dur® 10 [US] *see* potassium chloride *on page 713*
K-Dur® 20 [US] *see* potassium chloride *on page 713*
Keflex® [US] *see* cephalexin *on page 176*
Keflin® ***(Discontinued)*** *see page 1042*
Keftab® [Can] *see* cephalexin *on page 176*
Kefurox® [Can] *see* cefuroxime *on page 173*
Kefurox® Injection ***(Discontinued)*** *see page 1042*
Kefzol® ***(Discontinued)*** *see page 1042*
K-Electrolyte® Effervescent ***(Discontinued)*** *see page 1042*
Kemadrin® [US] *see* procyclidine *on page 733*
Kemsol® [Can] *see* dimethyl sulfoxide *on page 275*
Kenacort® Oral ***(Discontinued)*** *see page 1042*
Kenaject® Injection ***(Discontinued)*** *see page 1042*
Kenalog® Injection [US/Can] *see* triamcinolone (systemic) *on page 881*
Kenalog® in Orabase® [US/Can] *see* triamcinolone (topical) *on page 882*
Kenalog® Topical [US/Can] *see* triamcinolone (topical) *on page 882*
Kenonel® Topical ***(Discontinued)*** *see page 1042*
keoxifene hydrochloride *see* raloxifene *on page 762*
Keppra® [US/Can] *see* levetiracetam *on page 511*
Keralyt® [US-OTC] *see* salicylic acid *on page 789*
Kerlac® [US] *see* urea *on page 897*
Kerlone® [US] *see* betaxolol *on page 117*
Kerr Insta-Char® [US-OTC] *see* charcoal *on page 180*
Kestrin® Injection ***(Discontinued)*** *see page 1042*
Ketalar® [US/Can] *see* ketamine *on this page*

ketamine (KEET a meen)

Sound-Alike/Look-Alike Issues
Ketalar® may be confused with Kenalog®
Synonyms ketamine hydrochloride
U.S./Canadian Brand Names Ketalar® [US/Can]

Therapeutic Category General Anesthetic

Controlled Substance C-III

Use Induction and maintenance of general anesthesia, especially when cardiovascular depression must be avoided (ie, hypotension, hypovolemia, cardiomyopathy, constrictive pericarditis); sedation; analgesia

Usual Dosage Used in combination with anticholinergic agents to decrease hypersalivation

Children:

Oral: 6-10 mg/kg for 1 dose (mixed in 0.2-0.3 mL/kg of cola or other beverage) given 30 minutes before the procedure

I.M.: 3-7 mg/kg

I.V.: Range: 0.5-2 mg/kg, use smaller doses (0.5-1 mg/kg) for sedation for minor procedures; usual induction dosage: 1-2 mg/kg

Continuous I.V. infusion: Sedation: 5-20 mcg/kg/minute

Adults:

I.M.: 3-8 mg/kg

I.V.: Range: 1-4.5 mg/kg; usual induction dosage: 1-2 mg/kg

Children and Adults: Maintenance: Supplemental doses of $^1/_3$ to $^1/_2$ of initial dose

Dosage Forms Injection, solution, as hydrochloride: 10 mg/mL (20 mL, 25 mL, 50 mL); 50 mg/mL (10 mL); 100 mg/mL (5 mL)

ketamine hydrochloride *see* ketamine *on previous page*

Ketek™ [US/Can] *see* telithromycin *on page 842*

ketoconazole (kee toe KOE na zole)

Sound-Alike/Look-Alike Issues

Nizoral® may be confused with Nasarel®, Neoral®, Nitrol®

U.S./Canadian Brand Names Apo-Ketoconazole® [Can]; Ketoderm® [Can]; Nizoral® [US/Can]; Nizoral® A-D [US-OTC]; Novo-Ketoconazole [Can]

Therapeutic Category Antifungal Agent

Use Treatment of susceptible fungal infections, including candidiasis, oral thrush, blastomycosis, histoplasmosis, paracoccidioidomycosis, coccidioidomycosis, chromomycosis, candiduria, chronic mucocutaneous candidiasis, as well as certain recalcitrant cutaneous dermatophytoses; used topically for treatment of tinea corporis, tinea cruris, tinea versicolor, and cutaneous candidiasis, seborrheic dermatitis

Usual Dosage Fungal infections:

Oral:

Children ≥2 years: 3.3-6.6 mg/kg/day as a single dose for 1-2 weeks for candidiasis, for at least 4 weeks in recalcitrant dermatophyte infections, and for up to 6 months for other systemic mycoses

Adults: 200-400 mg/day as a single daily dose for durations as stated above

Shampoo: Apply twice weekly for 4 weeks with at least 3 days between each shampoo

Topical: Rub gently into the affected area once daily to twice daily

Dosage Forms

Cream, topical: 2% (15 g, 30 g, 60 g)

Shampoo, topical (Nizoral® A-D): 1% (6 mL, 120 mL, 210 mL)

Tablet (Nizoral®): 200 mg

Ketoderm® [Can] *see* ketoconazole *on this page*

ketoprofen (kee toe PROE fen)

Sound-Alike/Look-Alike Issues

Oruvail® may be confused with Clinoril®, Elavil®

U.S./Canadian Brand Names Apo-Keto® [Can]; Apo-Keto-E® [Can]; Apo-Keto SR® [Can]; Novo-Keto [Can]; Novo-Keto-EC [Can]; Nu-Ketoprofen [Can]; Nu-Ketoprofen-E [Can]; Orudis® KT [US-OTC]; Orudis® SR [Can]; Oruvail® [US/Can]; Rhodis™ [Can]; Rhodis-EC™ [Can]; Rhodis SR™ [Can]

(Continued)

ketoprofen *(Continued)*

Therapeutic Category Analgesic, Nonnarcotic; Nonsteroidal Antiinflammatory Drug (NSAID)

Use Acute and long-term treatment of rheumatoid arthritis and osteoarthritis; primary dysmenorrhea; mild to moderate pain

Usual Dosage Oral:

Children ≥16 years and Adults:

Rheumatoid arthritis or osteoarthritis:

Capsule: 50-75 mg 3-4 times/day up to a maximum of 300 mg/day

Capsule, extended release: 200 mg once daily

Mild to moderate pain: Capsule: 25-50 mg every 6-8 hours up to a maximum of 300 mg/day

OTC labeling: 12.5 mg every 4-6 hours, up to a maximum of 6 tablets/24 hours

Dosage Forms

Capsule: 50 mg, 75 mg

Capsule, extended release (Oruvail®): 100 mg, 150 mg, 200 mg

Tablet (Orudis® KT): 12.5 mg [contains tartrazine and sodium benzoate]

ketorolac (KEE toe role ak)

Sound-Alike/Look-Alike Issues

Acular® may be confused with Acthar®, Ocular®

Toradol® may be confused with Inderal®, Tegretol®, Torecan®, tramadol

Synonyms ketorolac tromethamine

U.S./Canadian Brand Names Acular® [US/Can]; Acular LS™ [US]; Acular® P.F. [US]; Apo-Ketorolac® [Can]; Apo-Ketorolac Injectable® [Can]; Novo-Ketorolac [Can]; ratio-Ketorolac [Can]; Toradol® [US/Can]; Toradol® IM [Can]

Therapeutic Category Analgesic, Nonnarcotic; Nonsteroidal Antiinflammatory Drug (NSAID)

Use

Oral, injection: Short-term (≤5 days) management of moderately-severe acute pain requiring analgesia at the opioid level

Ophthalmic: Temporary relief of ocular itching due to seasonal allergic conjunctivitis; postoperative inflammation following cataract extraction; reduction of ocular pain and photophobia following incisional refractive surgery, reduction of ocular pain, burning and stinging following corneal refractive surgery

Usual Dosage

Children 2-16 years: **Do not exceed adult doses**

Single-dose treatment:

I.M.: 1 mg/kg (maximum: 30 mg)

I.V.: 0.5 mg/kg (maximum: 15 mg)

Adults (pain relief usually begins within 10 minutes with parenteral forms): **Note:** The maximum combined duration of treatment (for parenteral and oral) is 5 days; do not increase dose or frequency; supplement with low-dose opioids if needed for break-through pain.

I.M.: 60 mg as a single dose or 30 mg every 6 hours (maximum daily dose: 120 mg)

I.V.: 30 mg as a single dose or 30 mg every 6 hours (maximum daily dose: 120 mg)

Oral: 20 mg, followed by 10 mg every 4-6 hours; do not exceed 40 mg/day; oral dosing is intended to be a continuation of I.M. or I.V. therapy only

Ophthalmic: Children ≥3 years and Adults:

Allergic conjunctivitis (relief of ocular itching) (Acular®): Instill 1 drop (0.25 mg) 4 times/day for seasonal allergic conjunctivitis

Inflammation following cataract extraction (Acular®): Instill 1 drop (0.25 mg) to affected eye(s) 4 times/day beginning 24 hours after surgery; continue for 2 weeks

Pain and photophobia following incisional refractive surgery (Acular® PF): Instill 1 drop (0.25 mg) 4 times/day to affected eye for up to 3 days

Pain following corneal refractive surgery (Acular LS™): Instill 1 drop 4 times/day as needed to affected eye for up to 4 days

Dosage Forms
Injection, solution, as tromethamine (Toradol®): 15 mg/mL (1 mL); 30 mg/mL (1 mL, 2 mL) [contains alcohol]
Solution, ophthalmic, as tromethamine:
Acular®: 0.5% (3 mL, 5 mL, 10 mL) [contains benzalkonium chloride]
Acular LS™: 0.4% (5 mL) [contains benzalkonium chloride]
Acular® P.F. [preservative free]: 0.5% (0.4 mL)
Tablet, as tromethamine (Toradol®): 10 mg

ketorolac tromethamine *see* ketorolac *on previous page*

ketotifen (kee toe TYE fen)

Synonyms ketotifen fumarate
U.S./Canadian Brand Names Apo-Ketotifen® [Can]; Novo-Ketotifen [Can]; Zaditen® [Can]; Zaditor™ [US/Can]
Therapeutic Category Antihistamine, H_1 Blocker, Ophthalmic
Use Temporary prevention of eye itching due to allergic conjunctivitis
Usual Dosage Children ≥3 years and Adults: Ophthalmic: Instill 1 drop into the affected eye(s) twice daily, every 8-12 hours
Dosage Forms Solution, ophthalmic, as fumarate: 0.025% (5 mL) [contains benzalkonium chloride]

ketotifen fumarate *see* ketotifen *on this page*

Key-E® Kaps [US-OTC] *see* vitamin E *on page 918*

Key-E® [US-OTC] *see* vitamin E *on page 918*

Key-Pred® *(Discontinued)* *see page 1042*

Key-Pred-SP® *(Discontinued)* *see page 1042*

K-G® *(Discontinued)* *see page 1042*

K-Gen® Effervescent *(Discontinued)* *see page 1042*

KI *see* potassium iodide *on page 715*

K-Ide® *(Discontinued)* *see page 1042*

Kidkare Decongestant [US-OTC] *see* pseudoephedrine *on page 745*

Kidrolase® [Can] *see* asparaginase *on page 80*

Kinerase® *(Discontinued)* *see page 1042*

Kineret™ [US/Can] *see* anakinra *on page 59*

Kinesed® *(Discontinued)* *see page 1042*

Kinevac® [US] *see* sincalide *on page 806*

Kionex™ [US] *see* sodium polystyrene sulfonate *on page 816*

Klaron® [US] *see* sulfacetamide *on page 829*

Klean-Prep® [Can] *see* polyethylene glycol-electrolyte solution *on page 706*

K-Lease® *(Discontinued)* *see page 1042*

Klerist-D® Tablet *(Discontinued)* *see page 1042*

Klonopin® [US/Can] *see* clonazepam *on page 215*

K-Lor™ [US/Can] *see* potassium chloride *on page 713*

Klor-Con® [US] *see* potassium chloride *on page 713*

Klor-Con® 8 [US] *see* potassium chloride *on page 713*

Klor-Con® 10 [US] *see* potassium chloride *on page 713*

Klor-Con®/25 [US] *see* potassium chloride *on page 713*

Klor-Con®/EF [US] *see* potassium bicarbonate and potassium citrate, effervescent *on page 712*

Klor-Con® M [US] *see* potassium chloride *on page 713*

Klorominr® Oral *(Discontinued)* *see page 1042*

Klorvess® *(Discontinued)* *see page 1042*

Klorvess® Effervescent *(Discontinued)* *see page 1042*

Klotrix® [US] *see* potassium chloride *on page 713*

K-Lyte® [US/Can] *see* potassium bicarbonate and potassium citrate, effervescent *on page 712*

K-Lyte/Cl® [US] *see* potassium bicarbonate and potassium chloride, effervescent *on page 712*

K-Lyte/Cl® 50 [US] *see* potassium bicarbonate and potassium chloride, effervescent *on page 712*

K-Lyte® DS [US] *see* potassium bicarbonate and potassium citrate, effervescent *on page 712*

K-Lyte® Effervescent *(Discontinued)* *see page 1042*

K-Norm® *(Discontinued)* *see page 1042*

Koāte®-DVI [US] *see* antihemophilic factor (human) *on page 62*

Koate®-HP *(Discontinued)* *see page 1042*

Koāte®-HS Injection *(Discontinued)* *see page 1042*

Koāte®-HT Injection *(Discontinued)* *see page 1042*

Kodet SE [US-OTC] *see* pseudoephedrine *on page 745*

Koffex DM-D [Can] *see* pseudoephedrine and dextromethorphan *on page 746*

Koffex DM + Decongestant + Expectorant [Can] *see* guaifenesin, pseudoephedrine, and dextromethorphan *on page 422*

Koffex DM-Expectorant [Can] *see* guaifenesin and dextromethorphan *on page 416*

Koffex Expectorant [Can] *see* guaifenesin *on page 415*

Kogenate® [Can] *see* antihemophilic factor (recombinant) *on page 63*

Kogenate® *(Discontinued)* *see page 1042*

Kogenate® FS [US/Can] *see* antihemophilic factor (recombinant) *on page 63*

Kolephrin® GG/DM [US-OTC] *see* guaifenesin and dextromethorphan *on page 416*

Kolyum® Powder *(Discontinued)* *see page 1042*

Konakion [Can] *see* phytonadione *on page 693*

Konakion® Injection *(Discontinued)* *see page 1042*

Kondon's Nasal® *(Discontinued)* *see page 1042*

Konsyl-D® [US-OTC] *see* psyllium *on page 749*

Konsyl® Easy Mix [US-OTC] *see* psyllium *on page 749*

Konsyl® Orange [US-OTC] *see* psyllium *on page 749*

Konsyl® Tablets [US-OTC] *see* polycarbophil *on page 706*

Konsyl® [US-OTC] *see* psyllium *on page 749*

Konȳne-HT® Injection *(Discontinued)* *see page 1042*

K-Pek® *(Discontinued)* *see page 1042*

K-Phos® MF [US] *see* potassium phosphate and sodium phosphate *on page 717*

K-Phos® Neutral [US] *see* potassium phosphate and sodium phosphate *on page 717*

K-Phos® No. 2 [US] *see* potassium phosphate and sodium phosphate *on page 717*

K-Phos® Original [US] *see* potassium acid phosphate *on page 711*

KPN Prenatal [US] *see* vitamins (multiple/prenatal) *on page 927*

Kristalose™ [US] *see* lactulose *on page 502*

Kronofed-A® [US] *see* chlorpheniramine and pseudoephedrine *on page 189*

Kronofed-A®-Jr [US] *see* chlorpheniramine and pseudoephedrine *on page 189*

K-Tab® [US] *see* potassium chloride *on page 713*

Ku-Zyme® HP [US] *see* pancrelipase *on page 663*

Kwelcof® [US] *see* hydrocodone and guaifenesin *on page 445*

Kwell® *(Discontinued)* *see page 1042*

Kwellada-P™ [Can] *see* permethrin *on page 683*

Kytril® [US/Can] *see* granisetron *on page 413*

L-749,345 *see* ertapenem *on page 319*

L 754030 *see* aprepitant *on page 74*

LA-12® *(Discontinued)* *see page 1042*

LA 20304a *see* gemifloxacin *on page 400*

labetalol (la BET a lole)

Sound-Alike/Look-Alike Issues

labetalol may be confused with betaxolol, Hexadrol®, lamotrigine

Trandate® may be confused with tramadol, Trendar®, Trental®, Tridrate®

Synonyms ibidomide hydrochloride; labetalol hydrochloride

U.S./Canadian Brand Names Apo-Labetalol® [Can]; Normodyne® [US/Can]; Trandate® [US/Can]

Therapeutic Category Alpha-/Beta- Adrenergic Blocker

Use Treatment of mild to severe hypertension; I.V. for hypertensive emergencies

Usual Dosage Due to limited documentation of its use, labetalol should be initiated cautiously in pediatric patients with careful dosage adjustment and blood pressure monitoring.

Children:

Oral: Limited information regarding labetalol use in pediatric patients is currently available in literature. Some centers recommend initial oral doses of 4 mg/kg/day in 2 divided doses. Reported oral doses have started at 3 mg/kg/day and 20 mg/kg/day and have increased up to 40 mg/kg/day.

I.V., intermittent bolus doses of 0.3-1 mg/kg/dose have been reported.

For treatment of pediatric hypertensive emergencies, initial continuous infusions of 0.4-1 mg/kg/hour with a maximum of 3 mg/kg/hour have been used. Administration requires the use of an infusion pump.

Adults:

Oral: Initial: 100 mg twice daily, may increase as needed every 2-3 days by 100 mg until desired response is obtained; usual dose: 200-400 mg twice daily; may require up to 2.4 g/day.

Usual dose range (JNC 7): 200-800 mg/day in 2 divided doses

I.V.: 20 mg (0.25 mg/kg for an 80 kg patient) IVP over 2 minutes; may administer 40-80 mg at 10-minute intervals, up to 300 mg total dose.

I.V. infusion: Initial: 2 mg/minute; titrate to response up to 300 mg total dose, if needed. Administration requires the use of an infusion pump.

I.V. infusion (500 mg/250 mL D_5W) rates:

1 mg/minute: 30 mL/hour
2 mg/minute: 60 mL/hour
3 mg/minute: 90 mL/hour
4 mg/minute: 120 mL/hour
5 mg/minute: 150 mL/hour
6 mg/minute: 180 mL/hour

(Continued)

labetalol *(Continued)*

Dosage Forms

Injection, solution, as hydrochloride (Normodyne®): 5 mg/mL (20 mL, 40 mL)
Injection, solution, as hydrochloride [prefilled syringe]: 5 mg/mL (4 mL)
Normodyne®: 5 mg/mL (4 mL, 8 mL)
Tablet, as hydrochloride: 100 mg, 200 mg, 300 mg
Normodyne®: 100 mg, 200 mg, 300 mg
Trandate®: 100 mg, 200 mg [contains sodium benzoate], 300 mg

labetalol hydrochloride *see* labetalol *on previous page*

Lac-Hydrin® [US] *see* lactic acid with ammonium hydroxide *on next page*

Lac-Hydrin® Five [US-OTC] *see* lactic acid with ammonium hydroxide *on next page*

LAClotion™ [US] *see* lactic acid with ammonium hydroxide *on next page*

Lacril® Ophthalmic Solution *(Discontinued)* *see* *page 1042*

Lacrisert® [US/Can] *see* hydroxypropyl cellulose *on page 456*

Lactaid® Extra Strength [US-OTC] *see* lactase *on this page*

Lactaid® Ultra [US-OTC] *see* lactase *on this page*

Lactaid® [US-OTC] *see* lactase *on this page*

lactase (LAK tase)

U.S./Canadian Brand Names Dairyaid® [Can]; Lactaid® Extra Strength [US-OTC]; Lactaid® Ultra [US-OTC]; Lactaid® [US-OTC]; Lactrase® [US-OTC]

Therapeutic Category Nutritional Supplement

Use Help digest lactose in milk for patients with lactose intolerance

Usual Dosage Oral:

Capsule: 1-2 capsules taken with milk or meal; pretreat milk with 1-2 capsules/quart of milk
Liquid: 5-15 drops/quart of milk
Tablet: 1-3 tablets with meals

Dosage Forms

Caplet:
Lactaid®: 3000 FCC lactase units
Lactaid® Extra Strength: 4500 FCC lactase units
Lactaid® Ultra: 9000 FCC lactase units
Capsule (Lactrase®): 250 mg standardized enzyme lactase
Tablet, chewable (Lactaid® Ultra): 9000 FCC lactase units [vanilla twist flavor]

lactic acid (LAK tik AS id)

Synonyms sodium-PCA and lactic acid

U.S./Canadian Brand Names LactiCare® [US-OTC]; Lactinol® [US]; Lactinol-E® [US]

Therapeutic Category Topical Skin Product

Use Lubricate and moisturize the skin counteracting dryness and itching

Usual Dosage Adults: Lubricant/moisturizer: Topical: Apply twice daily

Dosage Forms

Cream: 10% (120 g) [contains vitamin E]
Lactinol-E®: 10% (120 g, 240 g) [contains vitamin E 3500 int. units/ounce]
Lotion: 10% (360 mL)
LactiCare®: 5% (222 mL, 340 mL) [contains sodium PCA]
Lactinol®: 10% (360 mL, 480 mL)

lactic acid and salicylic acid *see* salicylic acid and lactic acid *on page 791*

lactic acid with ammonium hydroxide

(LAK tik AS id with a MOE nee um hye DROKS ide)

Synonyms ammonium lactate

U.S./Canadian Brand Names AmLactin® [US-OTC]; Geri-Hydrolac™-12 [US-OTC]; Geri-Hydrolac™ [US-OTC]; Lac-Hydrin® [US]; Lac-Hydrin® Five [US-OTC]; LAClotion™ [US]

Therapeutic Category Topical Skin Product

Use Treatment of moderate to severe xerosis and ichthyosis vulgaris

Usual Dosage Children ≥2 years and Adults: Topical: Apply twice daily to affected area; rub in well

Dosage Forms

Cream, topical: Lactic acid 12% with ammonium hydroxide (280 g)

AmLactin®: Lactic acid 12% with ammonium hydroxide (140 g)

Lac-Hydrin®: Lactic acid 12% with ammonium hydroxide (280 g, 385 g)

Lotion, topical (Amlactin®, Lac-Hydrin®, LAClotion™): Lactic acid 12% with ammonium hydroxide (225 g, 400 g)

Geri-Hydrolac™, Lac-Hydrin® Five: Lactic acid 5% with ammonium hydroxide (120 mL, 240 mL)

Geri-Hydrolac™-12: Lactic acid 12% with ammonium hydroxide (120 mL, 240 mL)

LactiCare-HC® [US] *see* hydrocortisone (topical) *on page 451*

LactiCare® [US-OTC] *see* lactic acid *on previous page*

Lactinex® [US-OTC] *see* Lactobacillus *on this page*

Lactinol® [US] *see* lactic acid *on previous page*

Lactinol-E® [US] *see* lactic acid *on previous page*

Lactobacillus (lak toe ba SIL us)

Synonyms *Lactobacillus acidophilus*; *Lactobacillus acidophilus* and *Lactobacillus bulgaricus*; *Lactobacillus reuteri*

U.S./Canadian Brand Names Bacid® [US-OTC/Can]; Fermalac [Can]; Kala® [US-OTC]; Lactinex® [US-OTC]; Megadophilus® [US-OTC]; MoreDophilus® [US-OTC]; Probiotica® [US-OTC]; Superdophilus® [US-OTC]

Therapeutic Category Gastrointestinal Agent, Miscellaneous

Use Treatment of uncomplicated diarrhea particularly that caused by antibiotic therapy; re-establish normal physiologic and bacterial flora of the intestinal tract

Usual Dosage Children >2 years and Adults: Oral:

Capsules: 2 capsules 2-4 times/day

Granules: 1 packet added to or taken with cereal, food, milk, fruit juice, or water, 3-4 times/day

Powder: 1 teaspoonful daily with liquid

Tablet, chewable: 4 tablets 3-4 times/day; may follow each dose with a small amount of milk, fruit juice, or water

Probiotica®: 1 tablet/day; chew thoroughly before swallowing

Dosage Forms

Capsule: *Lactobacillus acidophilus* 100 million units

Bacid®: *Lactobacillus acidophilus* 500 million units

Megadophilus®, Superdophilus®: *Lactobacillus acidophilus* 2 billion units [available in dairy based or dairy free formulations]

Granules (Lactinex®): Mixed culture *L. acidophilus, L. bulgaricus* per 1 g packet (12s)

Powder:

Megadophilus®, Superdophilus®: *Lactobacillus acidophilus* 2 billion units per half-teaspoon (49 g) [available in dairy based or dairy free formulations]

MoreDophilus®: *Lactobacillus acidophilus* 12.4 billion units per teaspoon [carrot derived] (30 g, 120 g)

Tablet (Kala®): *Lactobacillus acidophilus* 200 million units [soy based]

Tablet, chewable:

Lactinex®: Mixed culture *L. acidophilus, L. bulgaricus*

Probiotica®: *L. reuteri* 100 million units (30s, 60s) [lemon flavor]

Lactobacillus acidophilus *see* Lactobacillus *on previous page*

Lactobacillus acidophilus* and *Lactobacillus bulgaricus *see* Lactobacillus *on previous page*

Lactobacillus reuteri *see* Lactobacillus *on previous page*

lactoflavin *see* riboflavin *on page 775*

Lactrase® [US-OTC] *see* lactase *on page 500*

lactulose (LAK tyoo lose)

Sound-Alike/Look-Alike Issues
lactulose may be confused with lactose

U.S./Canadian Brand Names Acilac [Can]; Apo-Lactulose® [Can]; Cholac® [US]; Constilac® [US]; Constulose® [US]; Enulose® [US]; Generlac® [US]; Kristalose™ [US]; Laxilose [Can]; PMS-Lactulose [Can]

Therapeutic Category Ammonium Detoxicant; Laxative

Use Adjunct in the prevention and treatment of portal-systemic encephalopathy; treatment of chronic constipation

Usual Dosage Diarrhea may indicate overdosage and responds to dose reduction

Prevention of portal systemic encephalopathy (PSE): Oral:
- Infants: 2.5-10 mL/day divided 3-4 times/day; adjust dosage to produce 2-3 stools/day
- Older Children: Daily dose of 40-90 mL divided 3-4 times/day; if initial dose causes diarrhea, then reduce it immediately; adjust dosage to produce 2-3 stools/day

Constipation: Oral:
- Children: 5 g/day (7.5 mL) after breakfast
- Adults: 15-30 mL/day increased to 60 mL/day in 1-2 divided doses if necessary

Acute PSE: Adults:
- Oral: 20-30 g (30-45 mL) every 1-2 hours to induce rapid laxation; adjust dosage daily to produce 2-3 soft stools; doses of 30-45 mL may be given hourly to cause rapid laxation, then reduce to recommended dose; usual daily dose: 60-100 g (90-150 mL) daily
- Rectal administration: 200 g (300 mL) diluted with 700 mL of H_2O or NS; administer rectally via rectal balloon catheter and retain 30-60 minutes every 4-6 hours

Dosage Forms

Crystals for reconstitution (Kristalose™): 10 g/packet (30s), 20 g/packet (30s)

Syrup: 10 g/15 mL (15 mL, 30 mL, 237 mL, 473 mL, 946 mL, 1000 mL, 1890 mL)
- Cholac®, Constilac®: 10 g/15 mL (30 mL, 240 mL, 480 mL, 960 mL, 1920 mL, 3875 mL)
- Constulose®: 10 g/15 mL (240 mL, 960 mL)
- Enulose®: 10 g/15 mL (480 mL, 1900 mL)
- Generlac: 10 g/15 mL (480 mL, 1920 mL)

Lactulose PSE® *(Discontinued)* *see page 1042*

ladakamycin *see* azacitidine *on page 92*

L-AmB *see* amphotericin B liposomal *on page 55*

Lamictal® [US/Can] *see* lamotrigine *on next page*

Lamisil® Oral *see* terbinafine (oral) *on page 845*

Lamisil® Topical *see* terbinafine (topical) *on page 846*

lamivudine (la MI vyoo deen)

Sound-Alike/Look-Alike Issues
lamivudine may be confused with lamotrigine
Epivir® may be confused with Combivir®

Synonyms 3TC

U.S./Canadian Brand Names Epivir® [US]; Epivir-HBV® [US]; Heptovir® [Can]; 3TC® [Can]

Therapeutic Category Antiviral Agent

Use

Epivir®: Treatment of HIV infection when antiretroviral therapy is warranted; should always be used as part of a multidrug regimen (at least three antiretroviral agents)

Epivir-HBV®: Treatment of chronic hepatitis B associated with evidence of hepatitis B viral replication and active liver inflammation

Usual Dosage Note: The formulation and dosage of Epivir-HBV® are not appropriate for patients infected with both HBV and HIV. Use with at least two other antiretroviral agents when treating HIV

Oral:

Children 3 months to 16 years: HIV: 4 mg/kg twice daily (maximum: 150 mg twice daily)

Children 2-17 years: Treatment of hepatitis B (Epivir-HBV®): 3 mg/kg once daily (maximum: 100 mg/day)

Adults:

HIV: 150 mg twice daily **or** 300 mg once daily; <50 kg: 2 mg/kg twice daily

Treatment of hepatitis B (Epivir-HBV®): 100 mg/day

Dosage Forms

Solution, oral:

Epivir®: 10 mg/mL (240 mL) [strawberry-banana flavor]

Epivir-HBV®: 5 mg/mL (240 mL) [strawberry-banana flavor]

Tablet:

Epivir®: 150 mg, 300 mg

Epivir-HBV®: 100 mg

lamivudine, abacavir, and zidovudine *see* abacavir, lamivudine, and zidovudine *on page 2*

lamivudine and abacavir *see* abacavir and lamivudine *on page 2*

lamivudine and zidovudine *see* zidovudine and lamivudine *on page 939*

lamotrigine (la MOE tri jeen)

Sound-Alike/Look-Alike Issues

lamotrigine may be confused with labetalol, Lamisil®, lamivudine, Lomotil®, Ludiomil®

Lamictal® may be confused with Lamisil®, Lomotil®, Ludiomil®

Synonyms BW-430C; LTG

U.S./Canadian Brand Names Apo-Lamotrigine® [Can]; Lamictal® [US/Can]; PMS-Lamotrigine [Can]; ratio-Lamotrigine [Can]

Therapeutic Category Anticonvulsant

Use Adjunctive therapy in the treatment of generalized seizures of Lennox-Gastaut syndrome and partial seizures in adults and children ≥2 years of age; conversion to monotherapy in adults with partial seizures who are receiving treatment with valproate or a single enzyme-inducing antiepileptic drug; maintenance treatment of bipolar disorder

Usual Dosage Note: Only whole tablets should be used for dosing, round calculated dose down to the nearest whole tablet: Oral:

Children 2-12 years: Lennox-Gastaut (adjunctive) or partial seizures (adjunctive): **Note:** Children 2-6 years will likely require maintenance doses at the higher end of recommended range:

Patients receiving AED regimens containing valproic acid:

Weeks 1 and 2: 0.15 mg/kg/day in 1-2 divided doses; round dose down to the nearest whole tablet. For patients >6.7 kg and <14 kg, dosing should be 2 mg every other day.

Weeks 3 and 4: 0.3 mg/kg/day in 1-2 divided doses; round dose down to the nearest whole tablet; may use combinations of 2 mg and 5 mg tablets. For patients >6.7 kg and <14 kg, dosing should be 2 mg/day.

Maintenance dose: Titrate dose to effect; after week 4, increase dose every 1-2 weeks by a calculated increment; calculate increment as 0.3 mg/kg/day rounded down to the

(Continued)

lamotrigine *(Continued)*

nearest whole tablet; add this amount to the previously administered daily dose; usual maintenance: 1-5 mg/kg/day in 1-2 divided doses; maximum: 200 mg/day given in 1-2 divided doses

Patients receiving enzyme-inducing AED regimens without valproic acid:

Weeks 1 and 2: 0.6 mg/kg/day in 2 divided doses; round dose down to the nearest whole tablet

Weeks 3 and 4: 1.2 mg/kg/day in 2 divided doses; round dose down to the nearest whole tablet

Maintenance dose: Titrate dose to effect; after week 4, increase dose every 1-2 weeks by a calculated increment; calculate increment as 1.2 mg/kg/day rounded down to the nearest whole tablet; add this amount to the previously administered daily dose; usual maintenance: 5-15 mg/kg/day in 2 divided doses; maximum: 400 mg/day

Children >12 years: Lennox-Gastaut (adjunctive) or partial seizures (adjunctive): Refer to Adults dosing

Children ≥16 years: Conversion from single enzyme-inducing AED regimen to monotherapy: Refer to Adults dosing

Adults:

Lennox-Gastaut (adjunctive) or treatment of partial seizures (adjunctive):

Patients receiving AED regimens containing valproic acid: Initial dose: 25 mg every other day for 2 weeks, then 25 mg every day for 2 weeks. Dose may be increased by 25-50 mg every day for 1-2 weeks in order to achieve maintenance dose. Maintenance dose: 100-400 mg/day in 1-2 divided doses (usual range 100-200 mg/day).

Patients receiving enzyme-inducing AED regimens without valproic acid: Initial dose: 50 mg/day for 2 weeks, then 100 mg in 2 doses for 2 weeks; thereafter, daily dose can be increased by 100 mg every 1-2 weeks to be given in 2 divided doses. Usual maintenance dose: 300-500 mg/day in 2 divided doses; doses as high as 700 mg/day have been reported

Conversion to monotherapy (partial seizures in patients ≥16 years of age):

Adjunctive therapy with valproate: Initiate and titrate as per recommendations to a lamotrigine dose of 200 mg/day. Then taper valproate dose in decrements of not more than 500 mg/day at intervals of one week (or longer) to a valproate dosage of 500 mg/day; this dosage should be maintained for one week. The lamotrigine dosage should then be increased to 300 mg/day while valproate is decreased to 250 mg/day; this dosage should be maintained for one week. Valproate may then be discontinued, while the lamotrigine dose is increased by 100 mg/day at weekly intervals to achieve a lamotrigine maintenance dose of 500 mg/day.

Adjunctive therapy with enzyme-inducing AED: Initiate and titrate as per recommendations to a lamotrigine dose of 500 mg/day. Concomitant enzyme-inducing AED should then be withdrawn by 20% decrements each week over a 4-week period. Patients should be monitored for rash.

Adjunctive therapy with nonenzyme-inducing AED: No specific guidelines available

Bipolar disorder: 25 mg/day for 2 weeks, followed by 50 mg/day for 2 weeks, followed by 100 mg/day for 1 week; thereafter, daily dosage may be increased to 200 mg/day

Patients receiving valproic acid: Initial: 25 mg every other day for 2 weeks, followed by 25 mg/day for 2 weeks, followed by 50 mg/day for 1 week, followed by 100 mg/day (target dose) thereafter. **Note:** If valproate is discontinued, increase daily lamotrigine dose in 50 mg increments at weekly intervals until daily dosage of 200 mg is attained.

Patients receiving enzyme-inducing drugs (eg, carbamazepine): Initial: 50 mg/day for 2 weeks, followed by 100 mg/day (in divided doses) for 2 weeks, followed by 200 mg/day (in divided doses) for 1 week, followed by 300 mg/day (in divided doses) for 1 week. May increase to 400 mg/day (in divided doses) during week 7 and thereafter. **Note:** If carbamazepine (or other enzyme-inducing drug) is discontinued, decrease daily lamotrigine dose in 100 mg increments at weekly intervals until daily dosage of 200 mg is attained.

Discontinuing therapy: Children and Adults: Decrease dose by ~50% per week, over at least 2 weeks unless safety concerns require a more rapid withdrawal.

Restarting therapy after discontinuation: If lamotrigine has been withheld for >5 half-lives, consider restarting according to initial dosing recommendations.

Dosage Forms

Tablet: 25 mg, 100 mg, 150 mg, 200 mg [contains lactose]

Tablet, dispersible/chewable: 2 mg, 5 mg, 25 mg [black currant flavor]

Lamprene® [US/Can] *see* clofazimine *on page 213*

Lamprene® 100 mg *(Discontinued)* *see page 1042*

Lanacane® [US-OTC] *see* benzocaine *on page 107*

Lanaphilic® [US-OTC] *see* urea *on page 897*

Laniazid® Tablet *(Discontinued)* *see page 1042*

lanolin, cetyl alcohol, glycerin, petrolatum, and mineral oil

(LAN oh lin, SEE til AL koe hol, GLIS er in, pe troe LAY tum, & MIN er al oyl)

Synonyms mineral oil, petrolatum, lanolin, cetyl alcohol, and glycerin

U.S./Canadian Brand Names Lubriderm® Fragrance Free [US-OTC]; Lubriderm® [US-OTC]

Therapeutic Category Topical Skin Product

Use Treatment of dry skin

Usual Dosage Topical: Apply to skin as necessary

Dosage Forms

Lotion, topical [bottle]: 180 mL, 300 mL, 480 mL

Lotion, topical [tube]: 100 mL

Lanorinal® *(Discontinued)* *see page 1042*

Lanoxicaps® [US/Can] *see* digoxin *on page 270*

Lanoxin® [US/Can] *see* digoxin *on page 270*

lansoprazole (lan SOE pra zole)

Sound-Alike/Look-Alike Issues

Prevacid® may be confused with Pravachol®, Prevpac™, Prilosec®, Prinivil®

U.S./Canadian Brand Names Prevacid® [US/Can]; Prevacid® SoluTab™ [US]

Therapeutic Category Gastric Acid Secretion Inhibitor

Use

Oral: Short-term treatment of active duodenal ulcers; maintenance treatment of healed duodenal ulcers; as part of a multidrug regimen for *H. pylori* eradication to reduce the risk of duodenal ulcer recurrence; short-term treatment of active benign gastric ulcer; treatment of NSAID-associated gastric ulcer; to reduce the risk of NSAID-associated gastric ulcer in patients with a history of gastric ulcer who require an NSAID; short-term treatment of symptomatic GERD; short-term treatment for all grades of erosive esophagitis; to maintain healing of erosive esophagitis; long-term treatment of pathological hypersecretory conditions, including Zollinger-Ellison syndrome

I.V.: Short-term treatment (≤7 days) of erosive esophagitis in adults unable to take oral medications

Usual Dosage

Children 1-11 years: GERD, erosive esophagitis: Oral:

≤30 kg: 15 mg once daily

>30 kg: 30 mg once daily

Note: Doses were increased in some pediatric patients if still symptomatic after 2 or more weeks of treatment (maximum dose: 30 mg twice daily)

Children 12-17 years: Oral:

Nonerosive GERD: 15 mg once daily for up to 8 weeks

Erosive esophagitis: 30 mg once daily for up to 8 weeks

Adults:

Duodenal ulcer: Oral: Short-term treatment: 15 mg once daily for 4 weeks; maintenance therapy: 15 mg once daily

(Continued)

lansoprazole *(Continued)*

Gastric ulcer: Oral: Short-term treatment: 30 mg once daily for up to 8 weeks

NSAID-associated gastric ulcer (healing): Oral: 30 mg once daily for 8 weeks; controlled studies did not extend past 8 weeks of therapy

NSAID-associated gastric ulcer (to reduce risk): Oral: 15 mg once daily for up to 12 weeks; controlled studies did not extend past 12 weeks of therapy

Symptomatic GERD: Oral: Short-term treatment: 15 mg once daily for up to 8 weeks

Erosive esophagitis:

Oral: Short-term treatment: 30 mg once daily for up to 8 weeks; continued treatment for an additional 8 weeks may be considered for recurrence or for patients that do not heal after the first 8 weeks of therapy; maintenance therapy: 15 mg once daily

I.V.: 30 mg once daily for up to 7 days; patients should be switched to an oral formulation as soon as they can take oral medications

Hypersecretory conditions: Oral: Initial: 60 mg once daily; adjust dose based upon patient response and to reduce acid secretion to <10 mEq/hour (5 mEq/hour in patients with prior gastric surgery); doses of 90 mg twice daily have been used; administer doses >120 mg/day in divided doses

Helicobacter pylori eradication: Oral: Currently accepted recommendations (may differ from product labeling): Dose varies with regimen: 30 mg once daily or 60 mg/day in 2 divided doses; requires combination therapy with antibiotics

Dosage Forms

Capsule, delayed release (Prevacid®): 15 mg, 30 mg

Granules, for oral suspension, delayed release (Prevacid®): 15 mg/packet (30s), 30 mg/packet (30s) [strawberry flavor]

Injection, powder for reconstitution (Prevacid®): 30 mg

Tablet, orally-disintegrating (Prevacid® SoluTab™): 15 mg [contains phenylalanine 2.5 mg; strawberry flavor]; 30 mg [contains phenylalanine 5.1 mg; strawberry flavor]

lansoprazole, amoxicillin, and clarithromycin

(lan SOE pra zole, a moks i SIL in, & kla RITH roe mye sin)

Sound-Alike/Look-Alike Issues

Prevpac® may be confused with Prevacid®

Synonyms amoxicillin, lansoprazole, and clarithromycin; clarithromycin, lansoprazole, and amoxicillin

U.S./Canadian Brand Names Hp-PAC® [Can]; Prevpac® [US/Can]

Therapeutic Category Antibiotic, Macrolide Combination; Antibiotic, Penicillin; Gastrointestinal Agent, Miscellaneous

Use Eradication of *H. pylori* to reduce the risk of recurrent duodenal ulcer

Usual Dosage Oral: Adults: Lansoprazole 30 mg, amoxicillin 1 g, and clarithromycin 500 mg taken together twice daily for 10 or 14 days

Dosage Forms Combination package (Prevpac®) [each administration card contains]:

Capsule (Trimox®): Amoxicillin 500 mg (4 capsules/day)

Capsule, delayed release (Prevacid®): Lansoprazole 30 mg (2 capsules/day)

Tablet (Biaxin®): Clarithromycin 500 mg (2 tablets/day)

lansoprazole and naproxen (lan SOE pra zole & na PROKS en)

Sound-Alike/Look-Alike Issues

Prevacid® may be confused with Pravachol®, Prevpac™, Prilosec®, Prinivil®

Synonyms NapraPAC™; naproxen and lansoprazole

U.S./Canadian Brand Names Prevacid® NapraPAC™ [US]

Therapeutic Category Gastric Acid Secretion Inhibitor; Nonsteroidal Antiinflammatory Drug (NSAID)

Use Reduction of the risk of NSAID-associated gastric ulcers in patients with history of gastric ulcer who require an NSAID for the treatment of rheumatoid arthritis, osteoarthritis, and ankylosing spondylitis

Usual Dosage Oral: Adults: Reduce NSAID-associated gastric ulcers during treatment for arthritis: Lansoprazole 15 mg once daily in the morning; naproxen 375 mg or 500 mg twice daily

Dosage Forms Combination package:

Prevacid® NapraPAC™ 375 [each administration card contains]:

Capsule, delayed release (Prevacid®): Lansoprazole 15 mg (7 capsules per card)

Tablet (Naprosyn®): Naproxen 375 mg (14 tablets per card)

Prevacid® NapraPAC™ 500 [each administration card contains]:

Capsule, delayed release (Prevacid®): Lansoprazole 15 mg (7 capsules per card)

Tablet (Naprosyn®): Naproxen 500 mg (14 tablets per card)

Lantus® [US] *see* insulin preparations *on page 474*

Lanvis® [Can] *see* thioguanine *on page 857*

Largactil® [Can] *see* chlorpromazine *on page 194*

Largon® ***(Discontinued)*** *see page 1042*

Lariam® [US/Can] *see* mefloquine *on page 549*

Larodopa® ***(Discontinued)*** *see page 1042*

laronidase (lair OH ni days)

Synonyms recombinant α-L-iduronidase (glycosaminoglycan α-L-iduronohydrolase)

U.S./Canadian Brand Names Aldurazyme® [US]

Therapeutic Category Enzyme

Use Treatment of Hurler and Hurler-Scheie forms of mucopolysaccharidosis I (MPS I); treatment of Scheie form of MPS I in patients with moderate to severe symptoms

Usual Dosage I.V.: Children ≥5 years and Adults: 0.58 mg/kg once weekly; dose should be rounded up to the nearest whole vial

Dosage Forms Injection, solution [preservative free]: 2.9 mg/5 mL (5 mL)

Lasan™ HP-1 Topical ***(Discontinued)*** *see page 1042*

Lasan™ Topical ***(Discontinued)*** *see page 1042*

Lasix® [US/Can] *see* furosemide *on page 393*

Lasix® Special [Can] *see* furosemide *on page 393*

L-asparaginase *see* asparaginase *on page 80*

Lassar's zinc paste *see* zinc oxide *on page 940*

latanoprost (la TAN oh prost)

Sound-Alike/Look-Alike Issues

Xalatan® may be confused with Travatan™, Zarontin®

U.S./Canadian Brand Names Xalatan® [US/Can]

Therapeutic Category Prostaglandin

Use Reduction of elevated intraocular pressure in patients with open-angle glaucoma or ocular hypertension

Usual Dosage Adults: Ophthalmic: 1 drop (1.5 mcg) in the affected eye(s) once daily in the evening; do not exceed the once daily dosage because it has been shown that more frequent administration may decrease the IOP lowering effect

Note: A medication delivery device (Xal-Ease™) is available for use with Xalatan®.

Dosage Forms Solution, ophthalmic: 0.005% (2.5 mL) [contains benzalkonium chloride]

Lavacol® [US-OTC] *see* alcohol (ethyl) *on page 27*

Laxilose [Can] *see* lactulose *on page 502*

***l*-bunolol hydrochloride** *see* levobunolol *on page 511*

L-carnitine *see* levocarnitine *on page 512*

LCD *see* coal tar *on page 219*

LCR *see* vincristine *on page 912*

L-deprenyl *see* selegiline *on page 798*

LDP-341 *see* bortezomib *on page 124*

Lectopam® [Can] *see* bromazepam *(Canada only)* *on page 127*

Ledercillin VK® *(Discontinued)* *see page 1042*

leflunomide (le FLU no mide)

U.S./Canadian Brand Names Arava® [US/Can]

Therapeutic Category Antiinflammatory Agent

Use Treatment of active rheumatoid arthritis; indicated to reduce signs and symptoms, and to retard structural damage and improve physical function

Usual Dosage Oral: Adults: Initial: 100 mg/day for 3 days, followed by 20 mg/day; dosage may be decreased to 10 mg/day in patients who have difficulty tolerating the 20 mg dose. Due to the long half-life of the active metabolite, plasma levels may require a prolonged period to decline after dosage reduction.

Dosage Forms Tablet: 10 mg, 20 mg

Legatrin PM® [US-OTC] *see* acetaminophen and diphenhydramine *on page 7*

Lente® Iletin® II *(Discontinued)* *see page 1042*

Lente® Insulin *(Discontinued)* *see page 1042*

Lente® L *(Discontinued)* *see page 1042*

lepirudin (leh puh ROO din)

Synonyms lepirudin (rDNA); recombinant hirudin

U.S./Canadian Brand Names Refludan® [US/Can]

Therapeutic Category Anticoagulant (Other)

Use Indicated for anticoagulation in patients with heparin-induced thrombocytopenia (HIT) and associated thromboembolic disease in order to prevent further thromboembolic complications

Usual Dosage Adults: Maximum dose: Do not exceed 0.21 mg/kg/hour unless an evaluation of coagulation abnormalities limiting response has been completed. **Dosing is weight-based, however, patients weighing >110 kg should not receive doses greater than the recommended dose for a patient weighing 110 kg (44 mg bolus and initial maximal infusion rate of 16.5 mg/hour).**

Heparin-induced thrombocytopenia: Bolus dose: 0.4 mg/kg IVP (over 15-20 seconds), followed by continuous infusion at 0.15 mg/kg/hour; bolus and infusion must be reduced in renal insufficiency

Concomitant use with thrombolytic therapy: Bolus dose: 0.2 mg/kg IVP (over 15-20 seconds), followed by continuous infusion at 0.1 mg/kg/hour

Dosage Forms Injection, powder for reconstitution: 50 mg

lepirudin (rDNA) *see* lepirudin *on this page*

Lescol® [US/Can] *see* fluvastatin *on page 384*

Lescol® XL [US] *see* fluvastatin *on page 384*

Lessina™ [US] *see* ethinyl estradiol and levonorgestrel *on page 339*

letrozole (LET roe zole)

Sound-Alike/Look-Alike Issues

Femara® may be confused with femhrt®

U.S./Canadian Brand Names Femara® [US/Can]

Therapeutic Category Antineoplastic Agent, Hormone (Antiestrogen)

Use First-line treatment of hormone receptor positive or hormone receptor unknown, locally advanced, or metastatic breast cancer in postmenopausal women; treatment of advanced breast cancer in postmenopausal women with disease progression following antiestrogen therapy

Usual Dosage Refer to individual protocols. Oral: Adults: Breast cancer: 2.5 mg once daily

Dosage Forms Tablet: 2.5 mg

leucovorin (loo koe VOR in)

Sound-Alike/Look-Alike Issues

leucovorin may be confused with Leukeran®, Leukine®

folinic acid may be confused with folic acid

Synonyms calcium leucovorin; citrovorum factor; folinic acid; 5-formyl tetrahydrofolate; leucovorin calcium

Therapeutic Category Folic Acid Derivative

Use Antidote for folic acid antagonists (methotrexate, trimethoprim, pyrimethamine); treatment of megaloblastic anemias when folate is deficient as in infancy, sprue, pregnancy, and nutritional deficiency when oral folate therapy is not possible; in combination with fluorouracil in the treatment of colon cancer

Usual Dosage Note: This drug should be given parenterally instead of orally in patients with GI toxicity, nausea, vomiting, and when individual doses are >25 mg.

Children and Adults:

Treatment of folic acid antagonist overdosage: Oral: 2-15 mg/day for 3 days or until blood counts are normal, **or** 5 mg every 3 days; doses of 6 mg/day are needed for patients with platelet counts <100,000/mm^3

Folate-deficient megaloblastic anemia: I.M.: 1 mg/day

Megaloblastic anemia secondary to congenital deficiency of dihydrofolate reductase: I.M.: 3-6 mg/day

Rescue dose: Initial: I.V.: 10 mg/m^2, then:

Oral, I.M., I.V., SubQ: 10-15 10 mg/m^2 every 6 hours until methotrexate level <0.05 μmol/mL; if methotrexate level remains >5 μmol/mL at 48-72 hours after the end of the methotrexate infusion, increase to 20-100 mg/m^2 every 6 hours until methotrexate level <0.05 μmol/mL

Investigational: Post I.T. methotrexate: Oral, I.V.: 12 mg/m^2 as a single dose

Dosage Forms

Injection, powder for reconstitution, as calcium: 50 mg, 100 mg, 200 mg, 350 mg, 500 mg

Injection, solution, as calcium: 10 mg/mL (50 mL)

Tablet, as calcium: 5 mg, 10 mg, 15 mg, 25 mg

leucovorin calcium *see* leucovorin *on this page*

Leukeran® [US/Can] *see* chlorambucil *on page 182*

Leukine™ [US/Can] *see* sargramostim *on page 795*

leuprolide acetate (loo PROE lide AS e tate)

Sound-Alike/Look-Alike Issues

Lupron® may be confused with Nuprin®

Synonyms abbott-43818; leuprorelin acetate; NSC-377526; TAP-144

U.S./Canadian Brand Names Eligard® [US]; Lupron® [US/Can]; Lupron Depot® [US/Can]; Lupron Depot-Ped® [US]; Viadur® [US/Can]

Therapeutic Category Antineoplastic Agent; Luteinizing Hormone-Releasing Hormone Analog

Use Palliative treatment of advanced prostate carcinoma; management of endometriosis as initial treatment and/or treatment of recurrent symptoms; preoperative treatment of anemia caused by uterine leiomyomata (fibroids); central precocious puberty

Usual Dosage

Children: Precocious puberty (consider discontinuing by age 11 for females and by age 12 for males):

SubQ (Lupron®): 20-45 mcg/kg/day; titrate dose upward by 10 mcg/kg/day if down-regulation is not achieved

I.M. (Lupron Depot-Ped®): 0.3 mg/kg/dose given every 28 days (minimum dose: 7.5 mg)

(Continued)

leuprolide acetate *(Continued)*

≤25 kg: 7.5 mg
>25-37.5 kg: 11.25 mg
>37.5 kg: 15 mg
Titrate dose upward in 3.75 mg every 4 weeks if down-regulation is not achieved.

Adults:

Advanced prostatic carcinoma:

SubQ: Eligard®: 7.5 mg monthly **or** 22.5 mg every 3 months **or** 30 mg every 4 months Lupron®: 1 mg/day Viadur®: 65 mg implanted subcutaneously every 12 months

I.M.: Lupron Depot®: 7.5 mg/dose given monthly (every 28-33 days) **or** Lupron Depot-3®: 22.5 mg every 3 months **or** Lupron Depot-4®: 30 mg every 4 months

Endometriosis: I.M.: Initial therapy may be with leuprolide alone or in combination with norethindrone; if retreatment for an additional 6 months is necessary, norethindrone should be used. Retreatment is not recommended for longer than one additional 6-month course.

Lupron Depot®: 3.75 mg/month for up to 6 months **or**

Lupron Depot-3®: 11.25 mg every 3 months for up to 2 doses (6 months total duration of treatment)

Uterine leiomyomata (fibroids): I.M. (in combination with iron):

Lupron Depot®: 3.75 mg/month for up to 3 months **or**

Lupron Depot-3®: 11.25 mg as a single injection

Dosage Forms

Implant (Viadur®): 65 mg [released over 12 months; packaged with administration kit]

Injection, solution, as acetate (Lupron®): 5 mg/mL (2.8 mL) [contains benzyl alcohol; packaged with syringes and alcohol swabs]

Injection, powder for reconstitution, as acetate [depot formulation; prefilled syringe]:

Eligard®:

7.5 mg [released over 1 month]
22.5 mg [released over 3 months]
30 mg [released over 4 months]

Lupron Depot®: 3.75 mg, 7.5 mg [released over 1 month; contains polysorbate 80]

Lupron Depot®-3 Month: 11.25 mg, 22.5 mg [released over 3 months; contains polysorbate 80]

Lupron Depot®-4 Month: 30 mg [released over 4 months; contains polysorbate 80]

Lupron Depot-Ped®: 7.5 mg, 11.25 mg, 15 mg [released over 1 month; contains polysorbate 80]

leuprorelin acetate *see* leuprolide acetate *on previous page*

leurocristine sulfate *see* vincristine *on page 912*

Leustatin™ [US/Can] *see* cladribine *on page 207*

levalbuterol (leve al BYOO ter ole)

Sound-Alike/Look-Alike Issues

Xopenex® may be confused with Xanax®

Synonyms R-albuterol

U.S./Canadian Brand Names Xopenex® [US/Can]

Therapeutic Category Adrenergic Agonist Agent; $Beta_2$-Adrenergic Agonist Agent; Bronchodilator

Use Treatment or prevention of bronchospasm in adults and adolescents ≥6 years of age with reversible obstructive airway disease

Usual Dosage

Children 6-11 years: 0.31 mg 3 times/day via nebulization (maximum dose: 0.63 mg 3 times/day)

Children >12 years and Adults: Inhalation: 0.63 mg 3 times/day at intervals of 6-8 hours, via nebulization. Dosage may be increased to 1.25 mg 3 times/day with close monitoring for adverse effects. Most patients gain optimal benefit from regular use

Dosage Forms
Solution for nebulization: 0.31 mg/3 mL (24s); 0.63 mg/3 mL (24s); 1.25 mg/3 mL (24s)
Solution for nebulization, concentrate: 1.25 mg/0.5 mL (30s)

Levall G [US] *see* guaifenesin and pseudoephedrine *on page 419*

Levaquin® [US/Can] *see* levofloxacin *on page 514*

levarterenol bitartrate *see* norepinephrine *on page 627*

Levate® [Can] *see* amitriptyline *on page 47*

Levatol® [US/Can] *see* penbutolol *on page 673*

Levbid® [US] *see* hyoscyamine *on page 459*

levetiracetam (lev e tir AS e tam)

U.S./Canadian Brand Names Keppra® [US/Can]

Therapeutic Category Anticonvulsant, Miscellaneous

Use Indicated as adjunctive therapy in the treatment of partial onset seizures in adults with epilepsy

Usual Dosage Oral: Children ≥16 years and Adults: Partial onset seizure: Initial: 500 mg twice daily; additional dosing increments may be given (1000 mg/day additional every 2 weeks) to a maximum recommended daily dose of 3000 mg

Dosage Forms
Solution, oral: 100 mg/mL (480 mL) [dye free; grape flavor]
Tablet: 250 mg, 500 mg, 750 mg

Levitra® [US] *see* vardenafil *on page 905*

Levlen® [US] *see* ethinyl estradiol and levonorgestrel *on page 339*

Levlite™ [US] *see* ethinyl estradiol and levonorgestrel *on page 339*

levobunolol (lee voe BYOO noe lole)

Sound-Alike/Look-Alike Issues
levobunolol may be confused with levocabastine
Betagan® may be confused with Betadine®

Synonyms *l*-bunolol hydrochloride; levobunolol hydrochloride

U.S./Canadian Brand Names Apo-Levobunolol® [Can]; Betagan® [US/Can]; Novo-Levobunolol [Can]; Optho-Bunolol® [Can]; PMS-Levobunolol [Can]

Therapeutic Category Beta-Adrenergic Blocker

Use To lower intraocular pressure in chronic open-angle glaucoma or ocular hypertension

Usual Dosage Adults: Ophthalmic: Instill 1 drop in the affected eye(s) 1-2 times/day

Dosage Forms
Solution, ophthalmic, as hydrochloride: 0.25% (5 mL, 10 mL); 0.5% (5 mL, 10 mL, 15 mL) [contains benzalkonium chloride and sodium metabisulfite]
Betagan®: 0.25% (5 mL, 10 mL); 0.5% (2 mL, 5 mL, 10 mL, 15 mL) [contains benzalkonium chloride and sodium metabisulfite]

levobunolol hydrochloride *see* levobunolol *on this page*

levobupivacaine (LEE voe byoo PIV a kane)

U.S./Canadian Brand Names Chirocaine® [Can]

Therapeutic Category Local Anesthetic, Amide Derivative; Local Anesthetic, Injectable

Use Production of local or regional anesthesia for surgery and obstetrics, and for postoperative pain management

Usual Dosage Adults: **Note:** Rapid injection of a large volume of local anesthetic solution should be avoided. Fractional (incremental) doses are recommended.

Maximum dosage: Epidural doses up to 375 mg have been administered incrementally to patients during a surgical procedure

(Continued)

levobupivacaine *(Continued)*

Intraoperative block and postoperative pain: 695 mg in 24 hours
Postoperative epidural infusion over 24 hours: 570 mg
Single-fractionated injection for brachial plexus block: 300 mg

Dosage Forms [DSC] = Discontinued product
Injection, solution [preservative free]: 2.5 mg/mL (10 mL, 30 mL); 5 mg/mL (10 mL, 30 mL); 7.5 mg/mL (10 mL, 30 mL) [DSC]

levocabastine (LEE voe kab as teen)

Sound-Alike/Look-Alike Issues
levocabastine may be confused with levobunolol, levocarnitine
Livostin® may be confused with lovastatin

Synonyms levocabastine hydrochloride

U.S./Canadian Brand Names Livostin® [US/Can]

Therapeutic Category Antihistamine

Use Treatment of allergic conjunctivitis

Usual Dosage Children ≥12 years and Adults: Instill 1 drop in affected eye(s) 4 times/day for up to 2 weeks

Dosage Forms Suspension, ophthalmic, as hydrochloride: 0.05% (5 mL, 10 mL) [contains benzalkonium chloride]

levocabastine hydrochloride *see* levocabastine *on this page*

levocarnitine (lee voe KAR ni teen)

Sound-Alike/Look-Alike Issues
levocarnitine may be confused with levocabastine

Synonyms L-carnitine

U.S./Canadian Brand Names Carnitor® [US/Can]

Therapeutic Category Dietary Supplement

Use Orphan drug:
Oral: Primary systemic carnitine deficiency; acute and chronic treatment of patients with an inborn error of metabolism which results in secondary carnitine deficiency
I.V.: Acute and chronic treatment of patients with an inborn error of metabolism which results in secondary carnitine deficiency; prevention and treatment of carnitine deficiency in patients with end-stage renal disease (ESRD) who are undergoing hemodialysis.

Usual Dosage
Oral:
Infants/Children: Initial: 50 mg/kg/day; titrate to 50-100 mg/kg/day in divided doses with a maximum dose of 3 g/day
Adults: 990 mg (oral tablets) 2-3 times/day or 1-3 g/day (oral solution)
I.V.:
Metabolic disorders: 50 mg/kg as a slow 2- to 3-minute I.V. bolus or by I.V. infusion
Severe metabolic crisis:
A loading dose of 50 mg/kg over 2-3 minutes followed by an equivalent dose over the following 24 hours administered as every 3 hours or every 4 hours (never less than every 6 hours either by infusion or by intravenous injection)
All subsequent daily doses are recommended to be in the range of 50 mg/kg or as therapy may require
The highest dose administered has been 300 mg/kg
It is recommended that a plasma carnitine concentration be obtained prior to beginning parenteral therapy accompanied by weekly and monthly monitoring
ESRD patients on hemodialysis:
Predialysis levocarnitine concentrations below normal (40-50 μmol/L): 10-20 mg/kg dry body weight as a slow 2- to 3-minute bolus after each dialysis session
Dosage adjustments should be guided by predialysis trough levocarnitine concentrations and downward dose adjustments (to 5 mg/kg after dialysis) may be made as early as every 3rd or 4th week of therapy

Note: Safety and efficacy of oral carnitine have not been established in ESRD. Chronic administration of high oral doses to patients with severely compromised renal function or ESRD patients on dialysis may result in accumulation of metabolites.

Dosage Forms

Capsule: 250 mg

Injection, solution (Carnitor®): 200 mg/mL (5 mL)

Solution, oral (Carnitor®): 100 mg/mL (118 mL) [cherry flavor]

Tablet: 500 mg

Carnitor®: 330 mg

levodopa ***(Discontinued)*** *see page 1042*

levodopa and benserazide *see* benserazide and levodopa *(Canada only) on page 106*

levodopa and carbidopa (lee voe DOE pa & kar bi DOE pa)

Synonyms carbidopa and levodopa

U.S./Canadian Brand Names Apo-Levocarb® [Can]; Endo®-Levodopa/Carbidopa [Can]; Novo-Levocarbidopa [Can]; Nu-Levocarb [Can]; Sinemet® [US/Can]; Sinemet® CR [US/Can]

Therapeutic Category Anti-Parkinson Agent; Dopaminergic Agent (Anti-Parkinson)

Use Idiopathic Parkinson disease; postencephalitic parkinsonism; symptomatic parkinsonism

Usual Dosage Oral: Adults: Parkinson disease:

Immediate release tablet:

Initial: Carbidopa 25 mg/levodopa 100 mg 3 times/day

Dosage adjustment: Alternate tablet strengths may be substituted according to individual carbidopa/levodopa requirements. Increase by 1 tablet every other day as necessary, except when using the carbidopa 25 mg/levodopa 250 mg tablets where increases should be made using $^1/_2$-1 tablet every 1-2 days. Use of more than 1 dosage strength or dosing 4 times/day may be required (maximum: 8 tablets of any strength/day or 200 mg of carbidopa and 2000 mg of levodopa)

Sustained release tablet:

Initial: Carbidopa 50 mg/levodopa 200 mg 2 times/day, at intervals not <6 hours

Dosage adjustment: May adjust every 3 days; intervals should be between 4-8 hours during the waking day (maximum: 8 tablets/day)

Dosage Forms

Tablet immediate release (Sinemet®):

10/100: Carbidopa 10 mg and levodopa 100 mg

25/100: Carbidopa 25 mg and levodopa 100 mg

25/250: Carbidopa 25 mg and levodopa 250 mg

Tablet, immediate release, orally-disintegrating (Parcopa™):

10/100: Carbidopa 10 mg and levodopa 100 mg [contains phenylalanine 3.4 mg/tablet; mint flavor]

25/100: Carbidopa 25 mg and levodopa 100 mg [contains phenylalanine 3.4 mg/tablet; mint flavor]

25/250: Carbidopa 25 mg and levodopa 250 mg [contains phenylalanine 8.4 mg/tablet; mint flavor]

Tablet, sustained release (Sinemet® CR):

Carbidopa 25 mg and levodopa 100 mg

Carbidopa 50 mg and levodopa 200 mg

levodopa, carbidopa, and entacapone

(lee voe DOE pa, kar bi DOE pa, & en TA ka pone)

Synonyms carbidopa, levodopa, and entacapone; entacapone, carbidopa, and levodopa

U.S./Canadian Brand Names Stalevo™ [US]

Therapeutic Category Anti-Parkinson Agent, COMT Inhibitor; Anti-Parkinson Agent (Dopamine Agonist)

(Continued)

levodopa, carbidopa, and entacapone *(Continued)*

Use Treatment of idiopathic Parkinson disease

Usual Dosage Oral: Adults: Parkinson disease:

Note: All strengths of Stalevo™ contain a carbidopa/levodopa ratio of 1:4 plus entacapone 200 mg.

Dose should be individualized based on therapeutic response; doses may be adjusted by changing strength or adjusting interval. Fractionated doses are not recommended and only 1 tablet should be given at each dosing interval; maximum dose: 8 tablets/day (equivalent to entacapone 1600 mg/day)

Patients previously treated with carbidopa/levodopa immediate release tablets (ratio of 1:4):

With current entacapone therapy: May switch directly to corresponding strength of combination tablet. No data available on transferring patients from controlled release preparations or products with a 1:10 ratio of carbidopa/levodopa.

Without entacapone therapy:

If current levodopa dose is >600 mg/day: Levodopa dose reduction may be required when adding entacapone to therapy; therefore, titrate dose using individual products first (carbidopa/levodopa immediate release with a ratio of 1:4 plus entacapone 200 mg); then transfer to combination product once stabilized.

If current levodopa dose is <600 mg without dyskinesias: May transfer to corresponding dose of combination product; monitor, dose reduction of levodopa may be required.

Dosage Forms Tablet [film coated]:

50: Carbidopa 12.5 mg, levodopa 50 mg, and entacapone 200 mg

100: Carbidopa 25 mg, levodopa 100 mg, and entacapone 200 mg

150: Carbidopa 37.5 mg, levodopa 150 mg, and entacapone 200 mg

Levo-Dromoran® [US] *see* levorphanol *on next page*

levofloxacin (lee voe FLOKS a sin)

U.S./Canadian Brand Names Iquix® [US]; Levaquin® [US/Can]; Quixin™ [US]

Therapeutic Category Antibiotic, Ophthalmic; Antibiotic, Quinolone

Use

Systemic: Treatment of mild, moderate, or severe infections caused by susceptible organisms. Includes the treatment of community-acquired pneumonia, including multidrug resistant strains of *S. pneumoniae* (MDRSP); nosocomial pneumonia; chronic bronchitis (acute bacterial exacerbation); acute maxillary sinusitis; urinary tract infection (uncomplicated or complicated), including acute pyelonephritis caused by *E. coli*; prostatitis (chronic bacterial); skin or skin structure infections (uncomplicated or complicated)

Ophthalmic: Treatment of bacterial conjunctivitis caused by susceptible organisms (Quixin™ 0.5% ophthalmic solution); treatment of corneal ulcer caused by susceptible organisms (Iquix® 1.5% ophthalmic solution)

Usual Dosage

Oral, I.V. (infuse I.V. solution over 60 minutes): Adults:

Note: Sequential therapy (intravenous to oral) may be instituted based on prescriber's discretion.

Chronic bronchitis (acute bacterial exacerbation): 500 mg every 24 hours for at least 7 days

Maxillary sinusitis (acute): 500 mg every 24 hours for 10-14 days

Pneumonia:

Community-acquired: 500 mg every 24 hours for 7-14 days or 750 mg every 24 hours for 5 days (efficacy of 5-day regimen for MDRSP not established)

Nosocomial: 750 mg every 24 hours for 7-14 days

Prostatitis (chronic bacterial): 500 mg every 24 hours for 28 days

Skin infections:

Uncomplicated: 500 mg every 24 hours for 7-10 days

Complicated: 750 mg every 24 hours for 7-14 days

Urinary tract infections:

Uncomplicated: 250 mg once daily for 3 days

Complicated, including acute pyelonephritis: 250 mg every 24 hours for 10 days

Ophthalmic:

Conjunctivitis (0.5% ophthalmic solution): Children ≥1 year and Adults:

Treatment day 1 and day 2: Instill 1-2 drops into affected eye(s) every 2 hours while awake, up to 8 times/day

Treatment day 3 through day 7: Instill 1-2 drops into affected eye(s) every 4 hours while awake, up to 4 times/day

Corneal ulceration (1.5% ophthalmic solution): Children ≥6 years and Adults:

Treatment day 1 through day 3: Instill 1-2 drops into affected eye(s) every 30 minutes to 2 hours while awake and ~4-6 hours after retiring.

Treatment day 4 to treatment completion: Instill 1-2 drops into affected eye(s) every 1-4 hours while awake.

Dosage Forms

Infusion [premixed in D_5W] (Levaquin®): 5 mg/mL (50 mL, 100 mL, 150 mL)

Injection, solution [preservative free] (Levaquin®): 25 mg/mL (20 mL, 30 mL)

Solution, ophthalmic:

Iquix®: 1.5% (5 mL)

Quixin™: 0.5% (5 mL) [contains benzalkonium chloride]

Tablet (Levaquin®): 250 mg, 500 mg, 750 mg

levomepromazine *see* methotrimeprazine *(Canada only)* *on page 566*

levonorgestrel (LEE voe nor jes trel)

Synonyms LNg 20

U.S./Canadian Brand Names Mirena® [US]; Norplant® Implant [Can]; Plan B® [US/Can]

Therapeutic Category Contraceptive, Implant (Progestin); Contraceptive, Progestin Only

Use Prevention of pregnancy

Usual Dosage Adults: Females:

Long-term prevention of pregnancy: Intrauterine system: To be inserted into uterine cavity; should be inserted within 7 days of onset of menstruation or immediately after 1st trimester abortion; releases 20 mcg levonorgestrel/day over 5 years. May be removed and replaced with a new unit at anytime during menstrual cycle; do not leave any one system in place for >5 years

Emergency contraception: Oral tablet: One 0.75 mg tablet as soon as possible within 72 hours of unprotected sexual intercourse; a second 0.75 mg tablet should be taken 12 hours after the first dose; may be used at any time during menstrual cycle

Dosage Forms

Intrauterine device (Mirena®): 52 mg levonorgestrel/unit [releases levonorgestrel 20 mcg/day]

Tablet (Plan B®): 0.75 mg

levonorgestrel and estradiol *see* estradiol and levonorgestrel *on page 327*

levonorgestrel and ethinyl estradiol *see* ethinyl estradiol and levonorgestrel *on page 339*

Levophed® [US/Can] *see* norepinephrine *on page 627*

Levora® [US] *see* ethinyl estradiol and levonorgestrel *on page 339*

levorphanol (lee VOR fa nole)

Synonyms levorphanol tartrate

U.S./Canadian Brand Names Levo-Dromoran® [US]

Therapeutic Category Analgesic, Narcotic

Controlled Substance C-II

(Continued)

levorphanol *(Continued)*

Use Relief of moderate to severe pain; also used parenterally for preoperative sedation and an adjunct to nitrous oxide/oxygen anesthesia; 2 mg levorphanol produces analgesia comparable to that produced by 10 mg of morphine

Usual Dosage Adults: **Note:** These are guidelines and do not represent the maximum doses that may be required in all patients. Doses should be titrated to pain relief/ prevention.

Acute pain (moderate to severe):

Oral: Initial: Opiate-naive: 2 mg every 6-8 hours as needed; patients with prior opiate exposure may require higher initial doses; usual dosage range: 2-4 mg every 6-8 hours as needed

I.M., SubQ: Initial: Opiate-naive: 1 mg every 6-8 hours as needed; patients with prior opiate exposure may require higher initial doses; usual dosage range: 1-2 mg every 6-8 hours as needed

Slow I.V.: Initial: Opiate-naive: Up to 1 mg/dose every 3-6 hours as needed; patients with prior opiate exposure may require higher initial doses

Chronic pain: Patients taking opioids chronically may become tolerant and require doses higher than the usual dosage range to maintain the desired effect. Tolerance can be managed by appropriate dose titration. There is no optimal or maximal dose for levorphanol in chronic pain. The appropriate dose is one that relieves pain throughout its dosing interval without causing unmanageable side effects.

Premedication: I.M., SubQ: 1-2 mg/dose 60-90 minutes prior to surgery; older or debilitated patients usually require less drug

Dosage Forms

Injection, solution, as tartrate: 2 mg/mL (1 mL, 10 mL)

Tablet, as tartrate: 2 mg

levorphanol tartrate *see* levorphanol *on previous page*

Levo-T™ *(Discontinued)* *see page 1042*

Levothroid® [US] *see* levothyroxine *on this page*

levothyroxine (lee voe thye ROKS een)

Sound-Alike/Look-Alike Issues

levothyroxine may be confused with liothyronine

Levoxyl® may be confused with Lanoxin®, Luvox®

Synthroid® may be confused with Symmetrel®

Synonyms levothyroxine sodium; *L*-thyroxine sodium; T_4

U.S./Canadian Brand Names Eltroxin® [Can]; Levothroid® [US]; Levoxyl® [US]; Novothyrox [US]; Synthroid® [US/Can]; Unithroid® [US]

Therapeutic Category Thyroid Product

Use Replacement or supplemental therapy in hypothyroidism; pituitary TSH suppression

Usual Dosage Doses should be adjusted based on clinical response and laboratory parameters.

Oral:

Children: Hypothyroidism:

Newborns: Initial: 10-15 mcg/kg/day. Lower doses of 25 mcg/day should be considered in newborns at risk for cardiac failure. Newborns with T_4 levels <5 mcg/dL should be started at 50 mcg/day. Adjust dose at 4- to 6-week intervals.

Infants and Children: Dose based on body weight and age as listed below. Children with severe or chronic hypothyroidism should be started at 25 mcg/day; adjust dose by 25 mcg every 2-4 weeks. In older children, hyperactivity may be decreased by starting with $^1/_4$ of the recommended dose and increasing by $^1/_4$ dose each week until the full replacement dose is reached. Refer to adult dosing once growth and puberty are complete. 0-3 months: 10-15 mcg/kg/day 3-6 months: 8-10 mcg/kg/day 6-12 months: 6-8 mcg/kg/day 1-5 years: 5-6 mcg/kg/day 6-12 years: 4-5 mcg/kg/day >12 years: 2-3 mcg/kg/day

Adults:

Hypothyroidism: 1.7 mcg/kg/day in otherwise healthy adults <50 years old, children in whom growth and puberty are complete, and older adults who have been recently treated for hyperthyroidism or who have been hypothyroid for only a few months. Titrate dose every 6 weeks. Average starting dose ~100 mcg; usual doses are ≤200 mcg/day; doses ≥300 mcg/day are rare (consider poor compliance, malabsorption, and/or drug interactions). **Note:** For patients >50 years or patients with cardiac disease, refer to Elderly dosing.

Severe hypothyroidism: Initial: 12.5-25 mcg/day; adjust dose by 25 mcg/day every 2-4 weeks as appropriate; **Note:** Oral agents are not recommended for myxedema (see I.V. dosing).

Subclinical hypothyroidism (if treated): 1 mcg/kg/day

TSH suppression: Well-differentiated thyroid cancer: Highly individualized; Doses >2 mcg/kg/day may be needed to suppress TSH to <0.1 mU/L. Benign nodules and nontoxic multinodular goiter: Goal TSH suppression: 0.1-0.3 mU/L

Elderly: Hypothyroidism:

>50 years without cardiac disease **or** <50 years with cardiac disease: Initial: 25-50 mcg/day; adjust dose at 6- to 8-week intervals as needed

>50 years with cardiac disease: Initial: 12.5-25 mcg/day; adjust dose by 12.5-25 mcg increments at 4- to 6-week intervals

Note: Elderly patients may require <1 mcg/kg/day

I.M., I.V.: Children, Adults, Elderly: Hypothyroidism: 50% of the oral dose

I.V.:

Adults: Myxedema coma or stupor: 200-500 mcg, then 100-300 mcg the next day if necessary; smaller doses should be considered in patients with cardiovascular disease

Elderly: Myxedema coma: Refer to Adults dosing; lower doses may be needed

Dosage Forms

Injection, powder for reconstitution, as sodium (Synthroid®): 0.2 mg, 0.5 mg

Tablet, as sodium:

Levothroid®, Levoxyl®, Synthroid®: 25 mcg, 50 mcg, 75 mcg, 88 mcg, 100 mcg, 112 mcg, 125 mcg, 137 mcg, 150 mcg, 175 mcg, 200 mcg, 300 mcg

Novothyrox: 25 mcg, 50 mcg, 75 mcg, 88 mcg, 100 mcg, 112 mcg, 125 mcg, 137 mcg, 150 mcg, 175 mcg, 200 mcg, 300 mcg [dye free]

Unithroid®: 25 mcg, 50 mcg, 75 mcg, 88 mcg, 100 mcg, 112 mcg, 125 mcg, 150 mcg, 175 mcg, 200 mcg, 300 mcg

levothyroxine sodium *see* levothyroxine *on previous page*

Levoxyl® [US] *see* levothyroxine *on previous page*

Levsin® [US/Can] *see* hyoscyamine *on page 459*

Levsinex® [US] *see* hyoscyamine *on page 459*

Levsin/SL® [US] *see* hyoscyamine *on page 459*

Levulan® [Can] *see* aminolevulinic acid *on page 45*

Levulan® Kerastick™ [US] *see* aminolevulinic acid *on page 45*

levulose, dextrose and phosphoric acid *see* fructose, dextrose, and phosphoric acid *on page 392*

Lexapro™ [US] *see* escitalopram *on page 322*

Lexiva™ [US] *see* fosamprenavir *on page 389*

Lexxel® [US/Can] *see* enalapril and felodipine *on page 308*

LFA-3/IgG(1) fusion protein, human *see* alefacept *on page 29*

LHRH *see* gonadorelin *on page 412*

***l*-hyoscyamine sulfate** *see* hyoscyamine *on page 459*

Librax® [US/Can] *see* clidinium and chlordiazepoxide *on page 210*

Libritabs® (all products) *(Discontinued)* *see page 1042*

Librium® [US] *see* chlordiazepoxide *on page 183*

Lice-Enz® Shampoo *(Discontinued)* *see* *page 1042*

LidaMantle® [US] *see* lidocaine *on this page*

LidaMantle® HC [US] *see* lidocaine and hydrocortisone *on page 520*

Lidemol® [Can] *see* fluocinonide *on page 375*

Lidex® [US/Can] *see* fluocinonide *on page 375*

Lidex-E® [US] *see* fluocinonide *on page 375*

lidocaine (LYE doe kane)

Synonyms lidocaine hydrochloride; lignocaine hydrochloride

U.S./Canadian Brand Names Anestacon® [US]; Band-Aid® Hurt-Free™ Antiseptic Wash [US-OTC]; Betacaine® [Can]; Burnamycin [US-OTC]; Burn Jel [US-OTC]; Burn-O-Jel [US-OTC]; LidaMantle® [US]; Lidodan™ [Can]; Lidoderm® [US/Can]; L-M-X™ 4 [US-OTC]; L-M-X™ 5 [US-OTC]; Premjact® [US-OTC]; Solarcaine® Aloe Extra Burn Relief [US-OTC]; Topicaine® [US-OTC]; Xylocaine® [US/Can]; Xylocaine® MPF [US]; Xylocaine® Viscous [US]; Xylocard® [Can]; Zilactin® [Can]; Zilactin-L® [US-OTC]

Therapeutic Category Analgesic, Topical; Antiarrhythmic Agent, Class I-B; Local Anesthetic

Use Local anesthetic and acute treatment of ventricular arrhythmias from myocardial infarction, cardiac manipulation, digitalis intoxication; drug of choice for ventricular ectopy, ventricular tachycardia (VT), ventricular fibrillation (VF); for pulseless VT or VF preferably administer **after** defibrillation and epinephrine; control of premature ventricular contractions, wide-complex paroxysmal supraventricular tachycardia (PSVT); control of hemodynamically compromising PVCs; hemodynamically stable VT

Rectal: Temporary relief of pain and itching due to anorectal disorders

Topical: Local anesthetic for use in laser, cosmetic, and outpatient surgeries; minor burns, cuts, and abrasions of the skin

Orphan drug: Lidoderm® Patch: Relief of allodynia (painful hypersensitivity) and chronic pain in postherpetic neuralgia

Usual Dosage

Antiarrhythmic:

I.V.: 1-1.5 mg/kg bolus over 2-3 minutes; may repeat doses of 0.5-0.75 mg/kg in 5-10 minutes up to a total of 3 mg/kg; continuous infusion: 1-4 mg/minute

Infusion rates: 2 g/250 mL D_5W (infusion pump should be used):

1 mg/minute: 7.5 mL/hour
2 mg/minute: 15 mL/hour
3 mg/minute: 22.5 mL/hour
4 mg/minute: 30 mL/hour

Ventricular fibrillation (after defibrillation and epinephrine): Initial: 1-1.5 mg/kg. Repeat 0.5-0.75 mg/kg bolus may be given 3-5 minutes after initial dose. Total dose should not exceed 200-300 mg during a 1-hour period or 3 mg/kg total dose. Follow with continuous infusion after return of perfusion.

Endotracheal: 2-2.5 times the I.V. dose (2-4 mg/kg diluted with NS to a total volume of 10 mL)

Decrease dose in patients with CHF, shock, or hepatic disease.

Anesthesia, topical:

Cream:

LidaMantle®: Skin irritation: Children and Adults: Apply to affected area 2-3 times/day as needed

L-M-X™ 4: Children ≥2 years and Adults: Apply 1/4 inch thick layer to intact skin. Leave on until adequate anesthetic effect is obtained. Remove cream and cleanse area before beginning procedure.

L-M-X™ 5: Relief of anorectal pain and itching: Children ≥12 years and Adults: Rectal: Apply topically to clean, dry area **or** using applicator, insert rectally, up to 6 times/day

Gel, ointment, solution: Adults: Apply to affected area ≤3 times/day as needed (maximum dose: 4.5 mg/kg, not to exceed 300 mg)

Jelly:

Children ≥10 years: Dose varies with age and weight (maximum dose: 4.5 mg/kg)

Adults (maximum dose: 600 mg in any 12-hour period): Anesthesia of male urethra: 5-30 mL Anesthesia of female urethra: 3-5 mL Lubrication of endotracheal tube: Apply a moderate amount to external surface only

Liquid: Cold sores and fever blisters: Children ≥5 years and Adults: Apply to affected area every 6 hours as needed

Patch: Postherpetic neuralgia: Adults: Apply patch to most painful area. Up to 3 patches may be applied in a single application. Patch may remain in place for up to 12 hours in any 24-hour period.

Anesthetic, local injectable: Children and Adults: Varies with procedure, degree of anesthesia needed, vascularity of tissue, duration of anesthesia required, and physical condition of patient; maximum: 4.5 mg/kg/dose; do not repeat within 2 hours.

Dosage Forms [DSC] = Discontinued product

Cream, rectal (L-M-X™ 5): 5% (30 g) [contains benzyl alcohol; previously named ELA-Max® 5]

Cream, topical (L-M-X™ 4): 4% (5 g, 30 g) [contains benzyl alcohol; previously named ELA-Max®]

Cream, topical, as hydrochloride (LidaMantle®): 3% (30 g, 85 g)

Gel, topical:

Burn-O-Jel: 0.5% (90 g)

Topicaine®: 4% (1 g, 10 g, 30 g, 113 g) [contains benzyl alcohol, aloe vera, and jojoba]

Gel, topical, as hydrochloride: 2% (30 g)

Burn Jel: 2% (3.5 g, 120 g)

Solarcaine® Aloe Extra Burn Relief: 0.5% (226 g) [contains aloe vera gel and tartrazine]

Infusion, as hydrochloride [premixed in D_5W]: 0.4% [4 mg/mL] (250 mL, 500 mL); 0.8% [8 mg/mL] (250 mL, 500 mL)

Injection, solution, as hydrochloride: 0.5% [5 mg/mL] (50 mL); 1% [10 mg/mL] (5 mL, 20 mL, 30 mL, 50 mL); 1.5% [15 mg/mL] (20 mL); 2% [20 mg/mL] (2 mL, 5 mL, 20 mL, 30 mL, 50 mL)

Xylocaine®: 0.5% [5 mg/mL] (50 mL); 1% [10 mg/mL] (10 mL, 20 mL, 50 mL); 2% [20 mg/mL] (1.8 mL, 10 mL, 20 mL, 50 mL); 4% [40 mg/mL] (5 mL)

Injection, solution, as hydrochloride [preservative free]: 0.5% [5 mg/mL] (50 mL); 1% [10 mg/mL] (2 mL, 5 mL, 30 mL); 1.5% [15 mg/mL] (20 mL); 2% [20 mg/mL] (5 mL, 10 mL); 4% [40 mg/mL] (5 mL); 10% [100 mg/mL] (10 mL); 20% [200 mg/mL] (10 mL)

Xylocaine® MPF: 0.5% [5 mg/mL] (50 mL); 1% [10 mg/mL] (2 mL, 5 mL, 10 mL, 20 mL, 30 mL); 1.5% [15 mg/mL] (10 mL, 20 mL); 2% [2 mg/mL] (2 mL, 5 mL, 10 mL); 4% [40 mg/mL] (5 mL)

Injection, solution, as hydrochloride [premixed in $D_{7.5}W$, preservative free]: 5% (2 mL)

Xylocaine®-MPF: 1.5% (2 mL)

Jelly, topical, as hydrochloride:

Anestacon®: 2% (15 mL, 240 mL) [contains benzalkonium chloride]

Xylocaine®: 2% (5 mL, 10 mL [DSC], 20 mL [DSC], 30 mL)

Liquid, topical (Zilactin®-L): 2.5% (7.5 mL)

Ointment, topical: 5% (37 g)

Xylocaine®: 2.5% (35 g) [OTC]; 5% (3.5 g, 35 g) [mint or unflavored]

Patch, transdermal (Lidoderm®): 5% (30s)

Solution, topical, as hydrochloride: 2% [20 mg/mL] (15 mL, 240 mL); 4% [40 mg/mL] (50 mL)

Band-Aid® Hurt-Free™ Antiseptic Wash: 2% (180 mL)

Xylocaine®: 4% [40 mg/mL] (50 mL)

Solution, viscous, as hydrochloride: 2% [20 mg/mL] (20 mL, 100 mL)

Xylocaine® Viscous: 2% [20 mg/mL] (20 mL, 100 mL, 450 mL)

Spray, topical:

Burnamycin: 0.5% (60 mL) [contains aloe vera gel]

Premjact®: 9.6% (13 mL)

Solarcaine® Aloe Extra Burn Relief: 0.5% (127 g) [contains aloe vera]

lidocaine and epinephrine (LYE doe kane & ep i NEF rin)

Synonyms epinephrine and lidocaine

U.S./Canadian Brand Names LidoSite™ [US]; Xylocaine® MPF With Epinephrine [US]; Xylocaine® With Epinephrine [Can]

Therapeutic Category Local Anesthetic

Use Local infiltration anesthesia; AVS for nerve block; topical local analgesia for superficial dermatologic procedures

Usual Dosage Children (dosage varies with the anesthetic procedure): Use lidocaine concentrations of 0.5% or 1% (or even more dilute) to decrease possibility of toxicity; lidocaine dose should not exceed 4.5 mg/kg/dose; do not repeat within 2 hours

Dosage Forms

Injection, solution, as hydrochloride, with epinephrine 1:50,000 (Xylocaine® with Epinephrine): Lidocaine 2% [20 mg/mL] (1.8 mL) [contains sodium metabisulfite]

Injection, solution, as hydrochloride, with epinephrine 1:100,000: Lidocaine 1% [10 mg/mL] (20 mL, 30 mL, 50 mL); Lidocaine 2% (20 mL, 30 mL, 50 mL)

Xylocaine® with Epinephrine: Lidocaine 1% [10 mg/mL] (10 mL 20 mL, 50 mL); Lidocaine 2% (1.8 mL, 10 mL, 20 mL, 50 mL) [contains sodium metabisulfite]

Injection, solution, as hydrochloride, with epinephrine 1:200,000: Lidocaine 0.5% [5 mg/mL] (50 mL)

Xylocaine® with Epinephrine: Lidocaine 0.5% [5 mg/mL] (50 mL) [contains sodium metabisulfite]

Injection, solution, as hydrochloride, with epinephrine 1:200,000 [methylparaben free]: Lidocaine 1% [10 mg/mL] (30 mL); Lidocaine 1.5% (5 mL, 30 mL); Lidocaine 2% (20 mL) [contains sodium metabisulfite]

Xylocaine® MPF with Epinephrine: Lidocaine 1% [10 mg/mL] (5 mL, 10 mL, 30 mL); 1.5% [15 mg/mL] (5 mL, 10 mL, 30 mL); Lidocaine 2% [20 mg/mL] (5 mL, 10 mL, 20 mL) [contains sodium metabisulfite]

Transdermal system (LidoSite™): Lidocaine 10%, epinephrine 0.1% (25s) [contains sodium metabisulfite; for use only with LidoSite™ controller]

lidocaine and hydrocortisone (LYE doe kane & hye droe KOR ti sone)

Synonyms hydrocortisone and lidocaine

U.S./Canadian Brand Names AnaMantle® HC [US]; LidaMantle® HC [US]

Therapeutic Category Anesthetic/Corticosteroid

Use Topical antiinflammatory and anesthetic for skin disorders; rectal for the treatment of hemorrhoids, anal fissures, pruritus ani, or similar conditions

Usual Dosage Adults:

Topical: Apply 2-3 times/day

Rectal: One applicatorful twice daily

Dosage Forms

Cream, rectal (AnaMantle® HC): Lidocaine hydrochloride 3% and hydrocortisone acetate 0.5% (7 g) [kit contains 14 single-use tubes (7 g each) and 14 applicators]

Cream, topical (LidaMantle® HC): Lidocaine hydrochloride 3% and hydrocortisone acetate 0.5% (30 g, 85 g)

lidocaine and prilocaine (LYE doe kane & PRIL oh kane)

Synonyms prilocaine and lidocaine

U.S./Canadian Brand Names EMLA® [US/Can]

Therapeutic Category Analgesic, Topical

Use Topical anesthetic for use on normal intact skin to provide local analgesia for minor procedures such as I.V. cannulation or venipuncture; has also been used for painful procedures such as lumbar puncture and skin graft harvesting; for superficial minor surgery of genital mucous membranes and as an adjunct for local infiltration anesthesia in genital mucous membranes.

Usual Dosage Although the incidence of systemic adverse effects with EMLA® is very low, caution should be exercised, particularly when applying over large areas and leaving on for >2 hours

Children (intact skin): EMLA® should **not** be used in neonates with a gestation age <37 weeks nor in infants <12 months of age who are receiving treatment with methemoglobin-inducing agents

Dosing is based on child's age and weight:

Age 0-3 months or <5 kg: Apply a maximum of 1 g over no more than 10 cm^2 of skin; leave on for no longer than 1 hour

Age 3 months to 12 months and >5 kg: Apply no more than a maximum 2 g total over no more than 20 cm^2 of skin; leave on for no longer than 4 hours

Age 1-6 years and >10 kg: Apply no more than a maximum of 10 g total over no more than 100 cm^2 of skin; leave on for no longer than 4 hours.

Age 7-12 years and >20 kg: Apply no more than a maximum 20 g total over no more than 200 cm^2 of skin; leave on for no longer than 4 hours.

Note: If a patient greater than 3 months old does not meet the minimum weight requirement, the maximum total dose should be restricted to the corresponding maximum based on patient weight.

Adults (intact skin):

EMLA® cream and EMLA® anesthetic disc: A thick layer of EMLA® cream is applied to intact skin and covered with an occlusive dressing, or alternatively, an EMLA® anesthetic disc is applied to intact skin

Minor dermal procedures (eg, I.V. cannulation or venipuncture): Apply 2.5 g of cream (1/2 of the 5 g tube) over 20-25 cm of skin surface area, or 1 anesthetic disc (1 g over 10 cm^2) for at least 1 hour. **Note:** In clinical trials, 2 sites were usually prepared in case there was a technical problem with cannulation or venipuncture at the first site.

Major dermal procedures (eg, more painful dermatological procedures involving a larger skin area such as split thickness skin graft harvesting): Apply 2 g of cream per 10 cm^2 of skin and allow to remain in contact with the skin for at least 2 hours.

Adult male genital skin (eg, pretreatment prior to local anesthetic infiltration): Apply a thick layer of cream (1 g/10 cm^2) to the skin surface for 15 minutes. Local anesthetic infiltration should be performed immediately after removal of EMLA® cream.

Note: Dermal analgesia can be expected to increase for up to 3 hours under occlusive dressing and persist for 1-2 hours after removal of the cream

Adult females: Genital mucous membranes: Minor procedures (eg, removal of condylomata acuminata, pretreatment for local anesthetic infiltration): Apply 5-10 g (thick layer) of cream for 5-10 minutes

Dosage Forms

Cream, topical: Lidocaine 2.5% and prilocaine 2.5% (30 g)

EMLA®: Lidocaine 2.5% and prilocaine 2.5% (5 g, 30 g) [each 5 g tube is packaged with two Tegaderm® dressings]

Disc, topical: 1 g (2s, 10s) [contains lidocaine 2.5% and prilocaine 2.5% per 10 cm^2 disc]

lidocaine hydrochloride *see* lidocaine *on page 518*

Lidodan™ [Can] *see* lidocaine *on page 518*

Lidoderm® [US/Can] *see* lidocaine *on page 518*

LidoPen® I.M. Injection Auto-Injector *(Discontinued)* *see page 1042*

LidoSite™ [US] *see* lidocaine and epinephrine *on previous page*

LID-Pack® [Can] *see* bacitracin and polymyxin B *on page 97*

lignocaine hydrochloride *see* lidocaine *on page 518*

Lilly CT-3231 *see* vindesine *on page 912*

Limbitrol® [US/Can] *see* amitriptyline and chlordiazepoxide *on page 48*

Limbitrol® DS [US] *see* amitriptyline and chlordiazepoxide *on page 48*

Lin-Amox [Can] *see* amoxicillin *on page 51*

Lin-Buspirone [Can] *see* buspirone *on page 137*

Lincorex® *(Discontinued)* *see page 1042*

lindane (LIN dane)

Synonyms benzene hexachloride; gamma benzene hexachloride; hexachlorocyclohexane

U.S./Canadian Brand Names Hexit™ [Can]; PMS-Lindane [Can]

Therapeutic Category Scabicides/Pediculicides

Use Treatment of *Sarcoptes scabiei* (scabies), *Pediculus capitis* (head lice), and *Pthirus pubis* (crab lice); FDA recommends reserving lindane as a second-line agent or with inadequate response to other therapies

Usual Dosage Children and Adults: Topical:

Scabies: Apply a thin layer of lotion and massage it on skin from the neck to the toes; after 8-12 hours, bathe and remove the drug

Head lice, crab lice: Apply shampoo to dry hair and massage into hair for 4 minutes; add small quantities of water to hair until lather forms, then rinse hair thoroughly and comb with a fine tooth comb to remove nits. Amount of shampoo needed is based on length and density of hair; most patients will require 30 mL (maximum: 60 mL).

Dosage Forms

Lotion, topical: 1% (60 mL, 473 mL)

Shampoo, topical: 1% (60 mL, 473 mL)

linezolid (li NE zoh lid)

Sound-Alike/Look-Alike Issues

Zyvox™ may be confused with Vioxx®, Zosyn®

U.S./Canadian Brand Names Zyvox™ [US]; Zyvoxam® [Can]

Therapeutic Category Antibiotic, Oxazolidinone

Use Treatment of vancomycin-resistant *Enterococcus faecium* (VRE) infections, nosocomial pneumonia caused by *Staphylococcus aureus* including MRSA or *Streptococcus pneumoniae* (including multidrug-resistant strains [MDRSP]), complicated and uncomplicated skin and skin structure infections (including diabetic foot infections without concomitant osteomyelitis), and community-acquired pneumonia caused by susceptible gram-positive organisms

Usual Dosage

VRE infections: Oral, I.V.:

Preterm neonates (<34 weeks gestational age): 10 mg/kg every 12 hours; neonates with a suboptimal clinical response can be advanced to 10 mg/kg every 8 hours. By day 7 of life, all neonates should receive 10 mg/kg every 8 hours.

Infants (excluding preterm neonates <1 week) and Children ≤11 years: 10 mg/kg every 8 hours for 14-28 days

Children ≥12 years and Adults: 600 mg every 12 hours for 14-28 days

Nosocomial pneumonia, complicated skin and skin structure infections, community acquired pneumonia including concurrent bacteremia: Oral, I.V.:

Infants (excluding preterm neonates <1 week) and Children ≤11 years: 10 mg/kg every 8 hours for 10-14 days

Children ≥12 years and Adults: 600 mg every 12 hours for 10-14 days

Uncomplicated skin and skin structure infections: Oral:

Infants (excluding preterm neonates <1 week) and Children <5 years: 10 mg/kg every 8 hours for 10-14 days

Children 5-11 years: 10 mg/kg every 12 hours for 10-14 days

Children ≥12-18 years: 600 mg every 12 hours for 10-14 days

Adults: 400 mg every 12 hours for 10-14 days

Dosage Forms

Infusion [premixed]: 200 mg (100 mL) [contains sodium 1.7 mEq]; 400 mg (200 mL) [contains sodium 3.3 mEq]; 600 mg (300 mL) [contains sodium 5 mEq]

Powder for oral suspension: 20 mg/mL (150 mL) [contains phenylalanine 20 mg/5 mL, sodium benzoate, and sodium 0.4 mEq/5 mL; orange flavor]

Tablet: 400 mg, 600 mg [each strength contains sodium 0.1 mEq/tablet]

Lin-Megestrol [Can] *see* megestrol acetate *on page 549*

Lin-Pravastatin [Can] *see* pravastatin *on page 721*

Lin-Sotalol [Can] *see* sotalol *on page 819*

Lioresal® [US/Can] *see* baclofen *on page 98*

Liotec [Can] *see* baclofen *on page 98*

liothyronine (lye oh THYE roe neen)

Sound-Alike/Look-Alike Issues

liothyronine may be confused with levothyroxine

Synonyms liothyronine sodium; sodium *L*-triiodothyronine; T_3 sodium

U.S./Canadian Brand Names Cytomel® [US/Can]; Triostat® [US]

Therapeutic Category Thyroid Product

Use

Oral: Replacement or supplemental therapy in hypothyroidism; management of nontoxic goiter; a diagnostic aid

I.V.: Treatment of myxedema coma/precoma

Usual Dosage Doses should be adjusted based on clinical response and laboratory parameters.

Children: Congenital hypothyroidism: Oral: 5 mcg/day increase by 5 mcg every 3-4 days until the desired response is achieved. Usual maintenance dose: 20 mcg/day for infants, 50 mcg/day for children 1-3 years of age, and adult dose for children >3 years.

Adults:

Hypothyroidism: Oral: 25 mcg/day increase by increments of 12.5-25 mcg/day every 1-2 weeks to a maximum of 100 mcg/day; usual maintenance dose: 25-75 mcg/day.

T_3 suppression test: Oral: 75-100 mcg/day for 7 days

Myxedema: Oral: Initial: 5 mcg/day; increase in increments of 5-10 mcg/day every 1-2 weeks. When 25 mcg/day is reached, dosage may be increased at intervals of 5-25 mcg/day every 1-2 weeks. Usual maintenance dose: 50-100 mcg/day.

Myxedema coma: I.V.: 25-50 mcg

Patients with known or suspected cardiovascular disease: 10-20 mcg

Note: Normally, at least 4 hours should be allowed between doses to adequately assess therapeutic response and no more than 12 hours should elapse between doses to avoid fluctuations in hormone levels. Oral therapy should be resumed as soon as the clinical situation has been stabilized and the patient is able to take oral medication. If levothyroxine rather than liothyronine sodium is used in initiating oral therapy, the physician should bear in mind that there is a delay of several days in the onset of levothyroxine activity and that I.V. therapy should be discontinued gradually.

Simple (nontoxic) goiter: Oral: Initial: 5 mcg/day; increase by 5-10 mcg every 1-2 weeks; after 25 mcg/day is reached, may increase dose by 12.5-25 mcg. Usual maintenance dose: 75 mcg/day

Dosage Forms

Injection, solution, as sodium (Triostat®): 10 mcg/mL (1 mL) [contains alcohol 6.8%]

Tablet, as sodium (Cytomel®): 5 mcg, 25 mcg, 50 mcg

liothyronine sodium *see* liothyronine *on this page*

liotrix (LYE oh triks)

Sound-Alike/Look-Alike Issues

Liotrix may be confused with Klotrix®

Thyrolar® may be confused with Theolair™, Thyrogen®, Thytropar®

Synonyms T_3/T_4 liotrix

U.S./Canadian Brand Names Thyrolar® [US/Can]

Therapeutic Category Thyroid Product

Use Replacement or supplemental therapy in hypothyroidism (uniform mixture of T_4:T_3 in 4:1 ratio by weight); little advantage to this product exists and cost is not justified

Usual Dosage Oral:

Congenital hypothyroidism:

Children (dose of T_4 or levothyroxine/day):

0-6 months: 8-10 mcg/kg or 25-50 mcg/day

(Continued)

liotrix *(Continued)*

6-12 months: 6-8 mcg/kg or 50-75 mcg/day
1-5 years: 5-6 mcg/kg or 75-100 mcg/day
6-12 years: 4-5 mcg/kg or 100-150 mcg/day
>12 years: 2-3 mcg/kg or >150 mcg/day

Hypothyroidism (dose of thyroid equivalent): Adults: 30 mg/day (15 mg/day if cardiovascular impairment), increasing by increments of 15 mg/day at 2- to 3-week intervals to a maximum of 180 mg/day (usual maintenance dose: 60-120 mg/day)

Dosage Forms Tablet:
$^{1}/_{4}$ [levothyroxine sodium 12.5 mcg and liothyronine sodium 3.1 mcg]
$^{1}/_{2}$ [levothyroxine sodium 25 mcg and liothyronine sodium 6.25 mcg]
1 [levothyroxine sodium 50 mcg and liothyronine sodium 12.5 mcg]
2 [levothyroxine sodium 100 mcg and liothyronine sodium 25 mcg]
3 [levothyroxine sodium 150 mcg and liothyronine sodium 37.5 mcg]

lipancreatin *see* pancrelipase *on page 663*
Lipidil Micro® [Can] *see* fenofibrate *on page 360*
Lipidil Supra® [Can] *see* fenofibrate *on page 360*
Lipitor® [US/Can] *see* atorvastatin *on page 86*
Liposyn® III [US] *see* fat emulsion *on page 358*
Lipram 4500 [US] *see* pancrelipase *on page 663*
Lipram-CR [US] *see* pancrelipase *on page 663*
Lipram-PN [US] *see* pancrelipase *on page 663*
Lipram-UL [US] *see* pancrelipase *on page 663*
Liquaemin® *(Discontinued)* *see page 1042*
Liquibid® *(Discontinued)* *see page 1042*
Liquibid® 1200 *(Discontinued)* *see page 1042*
Liquibid-D [US] *see* guaifenesin and phenylephrine *on page 418*
Liquibid-PD [US] *see* guaifenesin and phenylephrine *on page 418*
Liqui-Char® *(Discontinued)* *see page 1042*
liquid antidote *see* charcoal *on page 180*
Liquid Barosperse® [US] *see* radiological/contrast media (ionic) *on page 759*
Liquid Pred® *(Discontinued)* *see page 1042*
Liquifilm® Forte Solution *(Discontinued)* *see page 1042*
Liquifilm® Tears Solution *(Discontinued)* *see page 1042*
Liquifilm® Tears [US-OTC] *see* artificial tears *on page 78*
Liquipake® [US] *see* radiological/contrast media (ionic) *on page 759*

lisinopril (lyse IN oh pril)

Sound-Alike/Look-Alike Issues
lisinopril may be confused with fosinopril, Lioresal®, Risperdal®
Prinivil® may be confused with Pravachol®, Plendil®, Prevacid®, Prilosec®, Proventil®
Zestril® may be confused with Desyrel®, Restoril®, Vistaril®, Zetia™, Zostrix®

U.S./Canadian Brand Names Apo-Lisinopril® [Can]; Prinivil® [US/Can]; Zestril® [US/Can]

Therapeutic Category Angiotensin-Converting Enzyme (ACE) Inhibitor

Use Treatment of hypertension, either alone or in combination with other antihypertensive agents; adjunctive therapy in treatment of CHF (afterload reduction); treatment of acute myocardial infarction within 24 hours in hemodynamically-stable patients to improve survival; treatment of left ventricular dysfunction after myocardial infarction

Usual Dosage Oral:

Hypertension:

Children ≥6 years: Initial: 0.07 mg/kg once daily (up to 5 mg); increase dose at 1- to 2-week intervals; doses >0.61 mg/kg or >40 mg have not been evaluated.

Adults: Initial: 10 mg/day; increase doses 5-10 mg/day at 1- to 2-week intervals; maximum daily dose: 40 mg

Patients taking diuretics should have them discontinued 2-3 days prior to initiating lisinopril if possible. Restart diuretic after blood pressure is stable if needed. If diuretic cannot be discontinued prior to therapy, begin with 5 mg with close supervision until stable blood pressure. In patients with hyponatremia (<130 mEq/L), start dose at 2.5 mg/day,

Congestive heart failure: Adults: Initial: 5 mg; then increase by no more than 10 mg increments at intervals no less than 2 weeks to a maximum daily dose of 40 mg. Usual maintenance: 5-40 mg/day as a single dose. Patients should start/continue standard therapy, including diuretics, beta-blockers, and digoxin, as indicated.

Acute myocardial infarction (within 24 hours in hemodynamically stable patients): Oral: 5 mg immediately, then 5 mg at 24 hours, 10 mg at 48 hours, and 10 mg every day thereafter for 6 weeks. Patients should continue to receive standard treatments such as thrombolytics, aspirin, and beta-blockers.

Dosage Forms [DSC] = Discontinued product

Tablet: 2.5 mg, 5 mg, 10 mg, 20 mg, 30 mg, 40 mg

Prinivil®: 2.5 mg [DSC], 5 mg, 10 mg, 20 mg, 30 mg, 40 mg

Zestril®: 2.5 mg, 5 mg, 10 mg, 20 mg, 30 mg, 40 mg

lisinopril and hydrochlorothiazide

(lyse IN oh pril & hye droe klor oh THYE a zide)

Synonyms hydrochlorothiazide and lisinopril

U.S./Canadian Brand Names Prinzide® [US/Can]; Zestoretic® [US/Can]

Therapeutic Category Antihypertensive Agent, Combination

Use Treatment of hypertension

Usual Dosage Adults: Oral: Dosage is individualized; see each component for appropriate dosing suggestions; doses >80 mg/day lisinopril or >50 mg/day hydrochlorothiazide are not recommended.

Dosage Forms Tablet:

Lisinopril 10 mg and hydrochlorothiazide 12.5 mg

Lisinopril 20 mg and hydrochlorothiazide 12.5 mg

Lisinopril 20 mg and hydrochlorothiazide 25 mg

lispro, insulin *see* insulin preparations *on page 474*

Listerex® Scrub *(Discontinued)* *see page 1042*

Listermint® With Fluoride *(Discontinued)* *see page 1042*

Lithane™ [Can] *see* lithium *on this page*

Lithane® *(Discontinued)* *see page 1042*

lithium (LITH ee um)

Sound-Alike/Look-Alike Issues

Eskalith® may be confused with Estratest®

Lithobid® may be confused with Levbid®, Lithostat®

Synonyms lithium carbonate; lithium citrate

U.S./Canadian Brand Names Apo-Lithium® [Can]; Carbolith™ [Can]; Duralith® [Can]; Eskalith® [US]; Eskalith CR® [US]; Lithane™ [Can]; Lithobid® [US]; PMS-Lithium Carbonate [Can]; PMS-Lithium Citrate [Can]

Therapeutic Category Antimanic Agent

Use Management of bipolar disorders; treatment of mania in individuals with bipolar disorder (maintenance treatment prevents or diminishes intensity of subsequent episodes)

(Continued)

lithium *(Continued)*

Usual Dosage Oral: Monitor serum concentrations and clinical response (efficacy and toxicity) to determine proper dose

Children 6-12 years: Bipolar disorder: 15-60 mg/kg/day in 3-4 divided doses; dose not to exceed usual adult dosage

Adults: Bipolar disorder: 900-2400 mg/day in 3-4 divided doses or 900-1800 mg/day (sustained release) in 2 divided doses

Dosage Forms

Capsule, as carbonate: 150 mg, 300 mg, 600 mg

Eskalith®: 300 mg [contains benzyl alcohol]

Syrup, as citrate: 300 mg/5 mL (5 mL, 10 mL, 480 mL) [contains alcohol]

Tablet, as carbonate: 300 mg

Tablet, controlled release, as carbonate (Eskalith CR®): 450 mg

Tablet, slow release, as carbonate (Lithobid®): 300 mg

lithium carbonate *see* lithium *on previous page*

lithium citrate *see* lithium *on previous page*

Lithobid® [US] *see* lithium *on previous page*

Lithonate® ***(Discontinued)*** *see page 1042*

Lithostat® [US/Can] *see* acetohydroxamic acid *on page 15*

Lithotabs® ***(Discontinued)*** *see page 1042*

Livostin® [US/Can] *see* levocabastine *on page 512*

l-lysine (el-LYE seen)

Synonyms L-lysine hydrochloride

U.S./Canadian Brand Names Lysinyl® [US-OTC]

Therapeutic Category Dietary Supplement

Use Improves utilization of vegetable proteins

Usual Dosage Adults: Oral: 334-1500 mg/day

Dosage Forms

Capsule (Lysinyl): 500 mg

Tablet: 500 mg, 1000 mg

L-lysine hydrochloride *see* l-lysine *on this page*

LMD® [US] *see* dextran *on page 258*

L-M-X™ 4 [US-OTC] *see* lidocaine *on page 518*

L-M-X™ 5 [US-OTC] *see* lidocaine *on page 518*

LNg 20 *see* levonorgestrel *on page 515*

Locacorten® Vioform® [Can] *see* clioquinol and flumethasone *(Canada only) on page 211*

LoCHOLEST® ***(Discontinued)*** *see page 1042*

LoCHOLEST® Light ***(Discontinued)*** *see page 1042*

Locoid® [US/Can] *see* hydrocortisone (topical) *on page 451*

Lodine® [US/Can] *see* etodolac *on page 350*

Lodine® XL [US] *see* etodolac *on page 350*

Lodosyn® [US] *see* carbidopa *on page 157*

lodoxamide tromethamine (loe DOKS a mide troe METH a meen)

U.S./Canadian Brand Names Alomide® [US/Can]

Therapeutic Category Mast Cell Stabilizer

Use Treatment of vernal keratoconjunctivitis, vernal conjunctivitis, and vernal keratitis

Usual Dosage Ophthalmic: Instill 1-2 drops in eye(s) 4 times/day for up to 3 months

Dosage Forms Solution, ophthalmic: 0.1% (10 mL) [contains benzalkonium chloride]

Lodrane® [US] *see* brompheniramine and pseudoephedrine *on page 129*

Lodrane® 12D [US] *see* brompheniramine and pseudoephedrine *on page 129*

Lodrane® LD [US] *see* brompheniramine and pseudoephedrine *on page 129*

Loestrin® [US/Can] *see* ethinyl estradiol and norethindrone *on page 342*

Loestrin® 1.5.30 [Can] *see* ethinyl estradiol and norethindrone *on page 342*

Loestrin® Fe [US] *see* ethinyl estradiol and norethindrone *on page 342*

Lofibra™ [US] *see* fenofibrate *on page 360*

Logen® *(Discontinued)* *see page 1042*

L-OHP *see* oxaliplatin *on page 652*

LoKara™ [US] *see* desonide *on page 253*

Lomanate® *(Discontinued)* *see page 1042*

lomefloxacin (loe me FLOKS a sin)

Synonyms lomefloxacin hydrochloride

U.S./Canadian Brand Names Maxaquin® [US]

Therapeutic Category Quinolone

Use Lower respiratory infections, acute bacterial exacerbation of chronic bronchitis, and urinary tract infections caused by *E. coli, K. pneumoniae, P. mirabilis, P. aeruginosa*; also has gram-positive activity including *S. pneumoniae* and some staphylococci; surgical prophylaxis (transrectal prostate biopsy or transurethral procedures)

Usual Dosage Oral: Adults:

Lower respiratory and urinary tract infections (UTI): 400 mg once daily for 10-14 days

Urinary tract infection (UTI) due to susceptible organisms:

Females:

Uncomplicated cystitis caused by *Escherichia coli*: 400 mg once daily for 3 successive days

Uncomplicated cystitis caused by *Klebsiella pneumoniae, Proteus mirabilis*, or *Staphylococcus saprophyticus*: 400 mg once daily for 10 successive days

Complicated UTI caused by *Escherichia coli, Klebsiella pneumoniae, Proteus mirabilis*, or *Pseudomonas aeruginosa*: 400 mg once daily for 14 successive days

Surgical prophylaxis: 400 mg 2-6 hours before surgery

Dosage Forms Tablet: 400 mg

lomefloxacin hydrochloride *see* lomefloxacin *on this page*

Lomine [Can] *see* dicyclomine *on page 267*

Lomotil® [US/Can] *see* diphenoxylate and atropine *on page 279*

lomustine (loe MUS teen)

Synonyms CCNU

U.S./Canadian Brand Names CeeNU® [US/Can]

Therapeutic Category Antineoplastic Agent

Use Treatment of brain tumors and Hodgkin disease, non-Hodgkin lymphoma, melanoma, renal carcinoma, lung cancer, colon cancer

Usual Dosage Refer to individual protocols. Oral:

Children: 75-150 mg/m^2 as a single dose every 6 weeks; subsequent doses are readjusted after initial treatment according to platelet and leukocyte counts

Adults: 100-130 mg/m^2 as a single dose every 6 weeks; readjust after initial treatment according to platelet and leukocyte counts

With compromised marrow function: Initial dose: 100 mg/m^2 as a single dose every 6 weeks

Repeat courses should only be administered after adequate recovery: WBC >4000 and platelet counts >100,000

(Continued)

lomustine *(Continued)*

Subsequent dosing adjustment based on nadir:

Leukocytes 2000-2900/mm^3, platelets 25,000-74,999/mm^3: Administer 70% of prior dose

Leukocytes <2000/mm^3, platelets <25,000/mm^3: Administer 50% of prior dose

Dosage Forms

Capsule: 10 mg, 40 mg, 100 mg

Capsule [dose pack]: 10 mg (2s); 40 mg (2s); 100 mg (2s)

Loniten® [US] *see* minoxidil *on page 584*

Lonox® [US] *see* diphenoxylate and atropine *on page 279*

Lo/Ovral® [US] *see* ethinyl estradiol and norgestrel *on page 347*

loperamide (loe PER a mide)

Sound-Alike/Look-Alike Issues

Imodium® A-D may be confused with Indocin®, Ionamin®

Synonyms loperamide hydrochloride

U.S./Canadian Brand Names Apo-Loperamide® [Can]; Diarr-Eze [Can]; Imodium® [Can]; Imodium® A-D [US-OTC]; Lopercap [Can]; Novo-Loperamide [Can]; PMS-Loperamine [Can]; Rho®-Loperamine [Can]; Riva-Loperamine [Can]

Therapeutic Category Antidiarrheal

Use Treatment of acute diarrhea and chronic diarrhea associated with inflammatory bowel disease; chronic functional diarrhea (idiopathic), chronic diarrhea caused by bowel resection or organic lesions; to decrease the volume of ileostomy discharge

Usual Dosage Oral:

Children:

Acute diarrhea: Initial doses (in first 24 hours):

2-6 years: 1 mg 3 times/day

6-8 years: 2 mg twice daily

8-12 years: 2 mg 3 times/day

Maintenance: After initial dosing, 0.1 mg/kg doses after each loose stool, but not exceeding initial dosage

Chronic diarrhea: 0.08-0.24 mg/kg/day divided 2-3 times/day, maximum: 2 mg/dose

Adults:

Acute diarrhea: Initial: 4 mg (2 capsules), followed by 2 mg after each loose stool, up to 16 mg/day (8 capsules)

Chronic diarrhea: Initial: Follow acute diarrhea; maintenance dose should be slowly titrated downward to minimum required to control symptoms (typically, 4-8 mg/day in divided doses)

Traveler's diarrhea: Treat for no more than 2 days

6-8 years: 1 mg after first loose stool followed by 1 mg after each subsequent stool; maximum dose: 4 mg/day

9-11 years: 2 mg after first loose stool followed by 1 mg after each subsequent stool; maximum dose: 6 mg/day

12 years to Adults: 4 mg after first loose stool followed by 2 mg after each subsequent stool; maximum dose: 8 mg/day

Dosage Forms

Caplet, as hydrochloride (Imodium® A-D): 2 mg

Capsule, as hydrochloride: 2 mg

Liquid, oral, as hydrochloride: 1 mg/5 mL (5 mL, 10 mL, 120 mL)

Imodium® A-D: 1 mg/5 mL (60 mL, 120 mL) [contains sodium benzoate, benzoic acid; cherry mint flavor]

Tablet, as hydrochloride: 2 mg

loperamide hydrochloride *see* loperamide *on this page*

Lopercap [Can] *see* loperamide *on this page*

Lopid® [US/Can] *see* gemfibrozil *on page 400*

lopinavir and ritonavir (loe PIN a veer & rye TON a veer)

Synonyms ritonavir and lopinavir

U.S./Canadian Brand Names Kaletra™ [US/Can]

Therapeutic Category Antiretroviral Agent, Non-nucleoside Reverse Transcriptase Inhibitor (NNRTI)

Use Treatment of HIV infection in combination with other antiretroviral agents

Usual Dosage Oral (take with food):

Children 6 months to 12 years: Dosage based on weight, presented based on mg of lopinavir (maximum dose: Lopinavir 400 mg/ritonavir 100 mg)

7-<15 kg: 12 mg/kg twice daily

15-40 kg: 10 mg/kg twice daily

>40 kg: Refer to adult dosing

Children >12 years and Adults: Lopinavir 400 mg/ritonavir 100 mg twice daily

Dosage adjustment when taken with amprenavir, efavirenz, nelfinavir, or nevirapine:

Children 6 months to 12 years:

7-<15 kg: 13 mg/kg twice daily

15-45 kg: 11 mg/kg twice daily

>45 kg: Refer to adult dosing

Note: In the USHHS guidelines, the cutoff for adult dosing is 50 kg. (Pediatric Guidelines - December 14, 2001, are available at http://www.aidsinfo.nih.gov, last accessed January 22, 2003.)

Children >12 years and Adults: Lopinavir 533 mg/ritonavir 133 mg twice daily

Dosage Forms

Capsule: Lopinavir 133.3 mg and ritonavir 33.3 mg

Solution, oral: Lopinavir 80 mg and ritonavir 20 mg per mL (160 mL) [contains alcohol 42.4%]

lopremone *see* protirelin *on page 744*

Lopressor® [US/Can] *see* metoprolol *on page 575*

Loprox® [US/Can] *see* ciclopirox *on page 198*

Lorabid® [US/Can] *see* loracarbef *on this page*

loracarbef (lor a KAR bef)

Sound-Alike/Look-Alike Issues

Lorabid® may be confused with Levbid®, Lopid®, Lortab®, Slo-bid™

U.S./Canadian Brand Names Lorabid® [US/Can]

Therapeutic Category Antibiotic, Carbacephem

Use Infections caused by susceptible organisms involving the respiratory tract, acute otitis media, sinusitis, skin and skin structure, bone and joint, and urinary tract and gynecologic

Usual Dosage Oral:

Children:

Acute otitis media: 15 mg/kg twice daily for 10 days

Pharyngitis and impetigo: 7.5-15 mg/kg twice daily for 10 days

Adults:

Uncomplicated urinary tract infections: 200 mg once daily for 7 days

Skin and soft tissue: 200-400 mg every 12-24 hours

Uncomplicated pyelonephritis: 400 mg every 12 hours for 14 days

Upper/lower respiratory tract infection: 200-400 mg every 12-24 hours for 7-14 days

Dosage Forms

Capsule: 200 mg, 400 mg

Powder for oral suspension: 100 mg/5 mL (100 mL); 200 mg/5 mL (100 mL) [strawberry bubblegum flavor]

loratadine (lor AT a deen)

Sound-Alike/Look-Alike Issues

Dimetapp® may be confused with Dermatop®, Dimetabs®, Dimetane®

U.S./Canadian Brand Names Alavert™ [US-OTC]; Apo-Loratadine® [Can]; Claritin® Hives Relief [US-OTC]; Claritin® Kids [Can]; Claritin® [US-OTC/Can]; Dimetapp® Children's ND [US-OTC]; Tavist® ND [US-OTC]

Therapeutic Category Antihistamine

Use Relief of nasal and non-nasal symptoms of seasonal allergic rhinitis; treatment of chronic idiopathic urticaria

Usual Dosage Oral: Seasonal allergic rhinitis, chronic idiopathic urticaria:

Children 2-5 years: 5 mg once daily

Children ≥6 years and Adults: 10 mg once daily

Dosage Forms

Syrup (Claritin®): 1 mg/mL (120 mL) [contains sodium benzoate; fruit flavor]

Tablet (Alavert™, Claritin®, Claritin® Hives Relief; Tavist® ND): 10 mg

Tablet, rapidly-disintegrating: 10 mg

Alavert™: 10 mg [contains phenylalanine 8.4 mg/tablet]

Claritin® RediTabs®: 10 mg [mint flavor]

Dimetapp® Children's ND: 10 mg [contains phenylalanine 8.4 mg/tablet]

loratadine and pseudoephedrine (lor AT a deen & soo doe e FED rin)

Synonyms pseudoephedrine and loratadine

U.S./Canadian Brand Names Alavert™ Allergy and Sinus [US-OTC]; Chlor-Tripolon ND® [Can]; Claritin-D® 12-Hour [US-OTC]; Claritin-D® 24-Hour [US-OTC]; Claritin® Extra [Can]; Claritin® Liberator [Can]

Therapeutic Category Antihistamine/Decongestant Combination

Use Temporary relief of symptoms of seasonal allergic rhinitis, other upper respiratory allergies, or the common cold

Usual Dosage Children ≥12 years and Adults: Oral:

Claritin-D® 12-Hour: 1 tablet every 12 hours

Alavert™ Allergy and Sinus, Claritin-D® 24-Hour: 1 tablet daily

Dosage Forms

Tablet, extended release: Loratadine 10 mg and pseudoephedrine sulfate 240 mg

Alavert™ Allergy and Sinus, Claritin-D® 12-hour: Loratadine 5 mg and pseudoephedrine sulfate 120 mg

Claritin-D® 24-hour: Loratadine 10 mg and pseudoephedrine sulfate 240 mg

lorazepam (lor A ze pam)

Sound-Alike/Look-Alike Issues

lorazepam may be confused with alprazolam, clonazepam, diazepam, temazepam

Ativan® may be confused with Atarax®, Atgam®, Avitene®

U.S./Canadian Brand Names Apo-Lorazepam® [Can]; Ativan® [US/Can]; Lorazepam Intensol® [US]; Novo-Lorazem® [Can]; Nu-Loraz [Can]; PMS-Lorazepam [Can]; Riva-Lorazepam [Can]

Therapeutic Category Benzodiazepine

Controlled Substance C-IV

Use

Oral: Management of anxiety disorders or short-term relief of the symptoms of anxiety or anxiety associated with depressive symptoms

I.V.: Status epilepticus, preanesthesia for desired amnesia, antiemetic adjunct

Usual Dosage

Antiemetic:

Children 2-15 years: I.V.: 0.05 mg/kg (up to 2 mg/dose) prior to chemotherapy

Adults: Oral, I.V. (**Note:** May be administered sublingually; not a labeled route): 0.5-2 mg every 4-6 hours as needed

Anxiety and sedation:
Infants and Children: Oral, I.M., I.V.: Usual: 0.05 mg/kg/dose (range: 0.02-0.09 mg/kg) every 4-8 hours
I.V.: May use smaller doses (eg, 0.01-0.03 mg/kg) and repeat every 20 minutes, as needed to titrate to effect
Adults: Oral: 1-10 mg/day in 2-3 divided doses; usual dose: 2-6 mg/day in divided doses
Insomnia: Adults: Oral: 2-4 mg at bedtime
Preoperative: Adults:
I.M.: 0.05 mg/kg administered 2 hours before surgery (maximum: 4 mg/dose)
I.V.: 0.044 mg/kg 15-20 minutes before surgery (usual maximum: 2 mg/dose)
Operative amnesia: Adults: I.V.: Up to 0.05 mg/kg (maximum: 4 mg/dose)
Sedation (preprocedure): Infants and Children:
Oral, I.M., I.V.: Usual: 0.05 mg/kg (range: 0.02-0.09 mg/kg);
I.V.: May use smaller doses (eg, 0.01-0.03 mg/kg) and repeat every 20 minutes, as needed to titrate to effect
Status epilepticus: I.V.:
Infants and Children: 0.1 mg/kg slow I.V. over 2-5 minutes; do not exceed 4 mg/single dose; may repeat second dose of 0.05 mg/kg slow I.V. in 10-15 minutes if needed
Adolescents: 0.07 mg/kg slow I.V. over 2-5 minutes; maximum: 4 mg/dose; may repeat in 10-15 minutes
Adults: 4 mg/dose slow I.V. over 2-5 minutes; may repeat in 10-15 minutes; usual maximum dose: 8 mg
Rapid tranquilization of agitated patient (administer every 30-60 minutes):
Oral: 1-2 mg
I.M.: 0.5-1 mg
Average total dose for tranquilization: Oral, I.M.: 4-8 mg

Dosage Forms
Injection, solution (Ativan®): 2 mg/mL (1 mL, 10 mL); 4 mg/mL (1 mL, 10 mL) [contains benzyl alcohol]
Solution, oral concentrate (Lorazepam Intensol®): 2 mg/mL (30 mL) [alcohol free, dye free]
Tablet (Ativan®): 0.5 mg, 1 mg, 2 mg

Lorazepam Intensol® [US] *see* lorazepam *on previous page*

Lorcet® ***(Discontinued)*** *see page 1042*

Lorcet® 10/650 [US] *see* hydrocodone and acetaminophen *on page 443*

Lorcet®-HD [US] *see* hydrocodone and acetaminophen *on page 443*

Lorcet® Plus [US] *see* hydrocodone and acetaminophen *on page 443*

Lorelco® ***(Discontinued)*** *see page 1042*

Loroxide® [US-OTC] *see* benzoyl peroxide *on page 109*

Lorsin® ***(Discontinued)*** *see page 1042*

Lortab® [US] *see* hydrocodone and acetaminophen *on page 443*

Lortab® ASA ***(Discontinued)*** *see page 1042*

losartan (loe SAR tan)

Sound-Alike/Look-Alike Issues
losartan may be confused with valsartan
Cozaar® may be confused with Hyzaar®, Zocor®

Synonyms DuP 753; losartan potassium; MK594

U.S./Canadian Brand Names Cozaar® [US/Can]

Therapeutic Category Angiotensin II Receptor Antagonist

Use Treatment of hypertension (HTN); treatment of diabetic nephropathy in patients with type 2 diabetes mellitus (noninsulin dependent, NIDDM) and a history of hypertension; stroke risk reduction in patients with HTN and left ventricular hypertrophy (LVH)
(Continued)

losartan *(Continued)*

Usual Dosage Oral:

Hypertension:

Children 6-16 years: 0.7 mg/kg once daily (maximum: 50 mg/day); adjust dose based on response; doses >1.4 mg/kg (maximum: 100 mg) have not been studied

Adults: Usual starting dose: 50 mg once daily; can be administered once or twice daily with total daily doses ranging from 25-100 mg

Patients receiving diuretics or with intravascular volume depletion: Usual initial dose: 25 mg

Nephropathy in patients with type 2 diabetes and hypertension: Adults: Initial: 50 mg once daily; can be increased to 100 mg once daily based on blood pressure response

Stroke reduction (HTN with LVH): Adults: 50 mg once daily (maximum daily dose: 100 mg); may be used in combination with a thiazide diuretic

Dosage Forms Tablet [film coated], as potassium: 25 mg, 50 mg, 100 mg

losartan and hydrochlorothiazide

(loe SAR tan & hye droe klor oh THYE a zide)

Sound-Alike/Look-Alike Issues

Hyzaar® may be confused with Cozaar®

Synonyms hydrochlorothiazide and losartan

U.S./Canadian Brand Names Hyzaar® [US/Can]; Hyzaar® DS [Can]

Therapeutic Category Antihypertensive Agent, Combination

Use Treatment of hypertension

Usual Dosage Oral (dosage must be individualized): Adults: 1 tablet daily

Dosage Forms Tablet [film coated]:

50-12.5: Losartan potassium 50 mg and hydrochlorothiazide 12.5 mg

100-25: Losartan potassium 100 mg and hydrochlorothiazide 25 mg

losartan potassium *see* losartan *on previous page*

Losec® [Can] *see* omeprazole *on page 644*

Losopan® *(Discontinued)* *see page 1042*

Lotemax® [US/Can] *see* loteprednol *on this page*

Lotensin® [US/Can] *see* benazepril *on page 105*

Lotensin® HCT [US] *see* benazepril and hydrochlorothiazide *on page 105*

loteprednol (loe te PRED nol)

Synonyms loteprednol etabonate

U.S./Canadian Brand Names Alrex® [US/Can]; Lotemax® [US/Can]

Therapeutic Category Corticosteroid, Ophthalmic

Use

Suspension, 0.2% (Alrex™): Temporary relief of signs and symptoms of seasonal allergic conjunctivitis

Suspension, 0.5% (Lotemax™): Inflammatory conditions (treatment of steroid-responsive inflammatory conditions of the palpebral and bulbar conjunctiva, cornea, and anterior segment of the globe such as allergic conjunctivitis, acne rosacea, superficial punctate keratitis, herpes zoster keratitis, iritis, cyclitis, selected infective conjunctivitis, when the inherent hazard of steroid use is accepted to obtain an advisable diminution in edema and inflammation) and treatment of postoperative inflammation following ocular surgery

Usual Dosage Adults: Ophthalmic:

Suspension, 0.2% (Alrex™): Instill 1 drop into affected eye(s) 4 times/day

Suspension, 0.5% (Lotemax™):

Inflammatory conditions: Apply 1-2 drops into the conjunctival sac of the affected eye(s) 4 times/day. During the initial treatment within the first week, the dosing may be increased up to 1 drop every hour. Advise patients not to discontinue therapy prematurely. If signs and symptoms fail to improve after 2 days, reevaluate the patient.

Postoperative inflammation: Apply 1-2 drops into the conjunctival sac of the operated eye(s) 4 times/day beginning 24 hours after surgery and continuing throughout the first 2 weeks of the postoperative period

Dosage Forms Suspension, ophthalmic, as etabonate:

Alrex®: 0.2% (5 mL, 10 mL) [contains benzalkonium chloride]

Lotemax®: 0.5% (2.5 mL, 5 mL, 10 mL, 15 mL) [contains benzalkonium chloride]

loteprednol etabonate *see* loteprednol *on previous page*

Lotrel® [US] *see* amlodipine and benazepril *on page 49*

Lotriderm® [Can] *see* betamethasone and clotrimazole *on page 115*

Lotrimin® AF Athlete's Foot Cream [US-OTC] *see* clotrimazole *on page 218*

Lotrimin® AF Athlete's Foot Solution [US-OTC] *see* clotrimazole *on page 218*

Lotrimin® AF Cream *(Discontinued)* *see page 1042*

Lotrimin® AF Jock Itch Cream [US-OTC] *see* clotrimazole *on page 218*

Lotrimin® AF Lotion *(Discontinued)* *see page 1042*

Lotrimin® AF Powder/Spray [US-OTC] *see* miconazole *on page 578*

Lotrimin® AF Solution *(Discontinued)* *see page 1042*

Lotrimin® Ultra™ [US-OTC] *see* butenafine *on page 139*

Lotrisone® [US] *see* betamethasone and clotrimazole *on page 115*

Lotronex® [US] *see* alosetron *on page 34*

lovastatin (LOE va sta tin)

Sound-Alike/Look-Alike Issues

lovastatin may be confused with Leustatin™, Livostin®, Lotensin®

Mevacor® may be confused with Mivacron®

Synonyms mevinolin; monacolin K

U.S./Canadian Brand Names Altoprev™ [US]; Apo-Lovastatin® [Can]; Gen-Lovastatin [Can]; Mevacor® [US/Can]; Novo-Lovastatin [Can]; Nu-Lovastatin [Can]; PMS-Lovastatin [Can]; ratio-Lovastatin [Can]

Therapeutic Category HMG-CoA Reductase Inhibitor

Use

Adjunct to dietary therapy to decrease elevated serum total and LDL-cholesterol concentrations in primary hypercholesterolemia

Primary prevention of coronary artery disease (patients without symptomatic disease with average to moderately elevated total and LDL-cholesterol and below average HDL-cholesterol); slow progression of coronary atherosclerosis in patients with coronary heart disease

Adjunct to dietary therapy in adolescent patients (10-17 years of age, females >1 year postmenarche) with heterozygous familial hypercholesterolemia having LDL >189 mg/dL, **or** LDL >160 mg/dL with positive family history of premature cardiovascular disease (CVD), **or** LDL >160 mg/dL with the presence of at least two other CVD risk factors

Usual Dosage Oral:

Adolescents 10-17 years: Immediate release tablet:

LDL reduction <20%: Initial: 10 mg/day with evening meal

LDL reduction ≥20%: Initial: 20 mg/day with evening meal

Usual range: 10-40 mg with evening meal, then adjust dose at 4-week intervals

Adults: Initial: 20 mg with evening meal, then adjust at 4-week intervals; maximum dose: 80 mg/day immediate release tablet **or** 60 mg/day extended release tablet

Dosage modification/limits based on concurrent therapy:

Cyclosporine and other immunosuppressant drugs: Initial dose: 10 mg/day with a maximum recommended dose of 20 mg/day

(Continued)

lovastatin *(Continued)*

Concurrent therapy with fibrates and/or lipid-lowering doses of niacin (>1 g/day): Maximum recommended dose: 20 mg/day. Concurrent use with fibrates should be avoided unless risk to benefit favors use.

Concurrent therapy with amiodarone or verapamil: Maximum recommended dose: 40 mg/day of regular release or 20 mg/day with extended release.

Dosage Forms

Tablet: 10 mg, 20 mg, 40 mg

Mevacor®: 10 mg [DSC], 20 mg, 40 mg

Tablet, extended release (Altocor™ [DSC], Altoprev™): 10 mg, 20 mg, 40 mg, 60 mg

lovastatin and niacin *see* niacin and lovastatin *on page 617*

Lovenox® [US/Can] *see* enoxaparin *on page 310*

Lovenox® HP [Can] *see* enoxaparin *on page 310*

Low-Ogestrel® [US] *see* ethinyl estradiol and norgestrel *on page 347*

loxapine (LOKS a peen)

Sound-Alike/Look-Alike Issues

Loxitane® may be confused with Soriatane®

Synonyms loxapine hydrochloride; loxapine succinate; oxilapine succinate

U.S./Canadian Brand Names Apo-Loxapine® [Can]; Loxitane® [US]; Loxitane® C [US]; Nu-Loxapine [Can]; PMS-Loxapine [Can]

Therapeutic Category Antipsychotic Agent, Dibenzoxazepine

Use Management of psychotic disorders

Usual Dosage Oral: Adults: 10 mg twice daily, increase dose until psychotic symptoms are controlled; usual dose range: 20-100 mg/day in divided doses 2-4 times/day; dosages >250 mg/day are not recommended

Dosage Forms

Capsule, as succinate (Loxitane®): 5 mg, 10 mg, 25 mg, 50 mg

Solution, oral concentrate, as hydrochloride (Loxitane® C): 25 mg/mL [120 mL dropper bottle]

loxapine hydrochloride *see* loxapine *on this page*

loxapine succinate *see* loxapine *on this page*

Loxitane® [US] *see* loxapine *on this page*

Loxitane® C [US] *see* loxapine *on this page*

Loxitane® I.M. *(Discontinued)* *see page 1042*

Lozide® [Can] *see* indapamide *on page 470*

Lozi-Flur™ [US] *see* fluoride *on page 376*

Lozi-Tab® *(Discontinued)* *see page 1042*

Lozol® [US/Can] *see* indapamide *on page 470*

L-PAM *see* melphalan *on page 550*

LRH *see* gonadorelin *on page 412*

L-sarcolysin *see* melphalan *on page 550*

LTG *see* lamotrigine *on page 503*

***L*-thyroxine sodium** *see* levothyroxine *on page 516*

Lu-26-054 *see* escitalopram *on page 322*

Lubriderm® Fragrance Free [US-OTC] *see* lanolin, cetyl alcohol, glycerin, petrolatum, and mineral oil *on page 505*

Lubriderm® [US-OTC] *see* lanolin, cetyl alcohol, glycerin, petrolatum, and mineral oil *on page 505*

LubriTears® Solution *(Discontinued)* *see page 1042*

Ludiomil® ***(Discontinued)*** *see page 1042*

Lufyllin® [US/Can] *see* dyphylline *on page 301*

Lugol's solution *see* potassium iodide *on page 715*

Lumigan® [US/Can] *see* bimatoprost *on page 119*

Luminal® Sodium [US] *see* phenobarbital *on page 686*

Lumitene™ [US] *see* beta-carotene *on page 113*

Lunelle™ [US] *see* estradiol cypionate and medroxyprogesterone acetate *on page 328*

LupiCare™ Dandruff [US-OTC] *see* salicylic acid *on page 789*

LupiCare™ II Psoriasis [US-OTC] *see* salicylic acid *on page 789*

LupiCare™ Psoriasis [US-OTC] *see* salicylic acid *on page 789*

Lupron® [US/Can] *see* leuprolide acetate *on page 509*

Lupron Depot® [US/Can] *see* leuprolide acetate *on page 509*

Lupron Depot-Ped® [US] *see* leuprolide acetate *on page 509*

Luride® [US] *see* fluoride *on page 376*

Luride® Lozi-Tab® [US] *see* fluoride *on page 376*

Luride®-SF ***(Discontinued)*** *see page 1042*

Lustra® [US/Can] *see* hydroquinone *on page 454*

Lustra-AF™ [US] *see* hydroquinone *on page 454*

luteinizing hormone releasing hormone *see* gonadorelin *on page 412*

Lutrepulse™ [Can] *see* gonadorelin *on page 412*

Luvox® [Can] *see* fluvoxamine *on page 385*

Luvox® ***(Discontinued)*** *see page 1042*

Luxiq® [US] *see* betamethasone (topical) *on page 116*

LY139603 *see* atomoxetine *on page 86*

LY146032 *see* daptomycin *on page 245*

LY170053 *see* olanzapine *on page 641*

LY231514 *see* pemetrexed *on page 673*

Lycolan® Elixir ***(Discontinued)*** *see page 1042*

Lyderm® [Can] *see* fluocinonide *on page 375*

Lydonide [Can] *see* fluocinonide *on page 375*

LYMErix™ ***(Discontinued)*** *see page 1042*

Lymphazurin® [US/Can] *see* radiological/contrast media (ionic) *on page 759*

lymphocyte mitogenic factor *see* aldesleukin *on page 28*

Lyphocin® Injection ***(Discontinued)*** *see page 1042*

Lysinyl® [US-OTC] *see* l-lysine *on page 526*

Lysodren® [US/Can] *see* mitotane *on page 585*

Lyteprep™ [Can] *see* polyethylene glycol-electrolyte solution *on page 706*

Maalox® Anti-Gas ***(Discontinued)*** *see page 1042*

Maalox® Anti-Gas Extra Strength ***(Discontinued)*** *see page 1042*

Maalox® Extra Strength ***(Discontinued)*** *see page 1042*

Maalox® Max [US-OTC] *see* aluminum hydroxide, magnesium hydroxide, and simethicone *on page 40*

Maalox® Plus ***(Discontinued)*** *see page 1042*

Maalox® TC (Therapeutic Concentrate) ***(Discontinued)*** *see page 1042*

Maalox® [US-OTC] *see* aluminum hydroxide, magnesium hydroxide, and simethicone *on page 40*

Macrobid® [US/Can] *see* nitrofurantoin *on page 622*

Macrodantin® [US/Can] *see* nitrofurantoin *on page 622*

Macrodex® *(Discontinued)* *see page 1042*

mafenide (MA fe nide)

Synonyms mafenide acetate

U.S./Canadian Brand Names Sulfamylon® [US]

Therapeutic Category Antibacterial, Topical

Use Adjunct in the treatment of second- and third-degree burns to prevent septicemia caused by susceptible organisms such as *Pseudomonas aeruginosa*

Orphan drug: Prevention of graft loss of meshed autografts on excised burn wounds

Usual Dosage Children and Adults: Topical: Apply once or twice daily with a sterile gloved hand; apply to a thickness of approximately 16 mm; the burned area should be covered with cream at all times

Dosage Forms

Cream, topical, as acetate: 85 mg/g (60 g, 120 g, 454 g) [contains sodium metabisulfite]

Powder, for topical solution: 5% (5s) [50 g/packet]

mafenide acetate *see* mafenide *on this page*

magaldrate and simethicone (MAG al drate & sye METH i kone)

Sound-Alike/Look-Alike Issues

Riopan Plus® may be confused with Repan®

Synonyms simethicone and magaldrate

Therapeutic Category Antacid; Antiflatulent

Use Relief of hyperacidity associated with peptic ulcer, gastritis, peptic esophagitis and hiatal hernia which are accompanied by symptoms of gas

Usual Dosage Adults: Oral: 540-1080 mg magaldrate between meals and at bedtime

Dosage Forms Suspension, oral:

Riopan Plus®: Magaldrate 540 mg and simethicone 20 mg per 5 mL (360 mL)

Riopan Plus® Double Strength: Magaldrate 1080 mg and simethicone 40 mg per 5 mL (360 mL)

Magalox Plus® *(Discontinued)* *see page 1042*

Magan® *(Discontinued)* *see page 1042*

Mag Delay® [US-OTC] *see* magnesium chloride *on this page*

Mag G® [US-OTC] *see* magnesium gluconate *on next page*

Maginex™ DS [US-OTC] *see* magnesium L-aspartate hydrochloride *on page 539*

Maginex™ [US-OTC] *see* magnesium L-aspartate hydrochloride *on page 539*

magnesia magma *see* magnesium hydroxide *on next page*

magnesium carbonate and aluminum hydroxide *see* aluminum hydroxide and magnesium carbonate *on page 39*

magnesium chloride (mag NEE zhum KLOR ide)

U.S./Canadian Brand Names Chloromag® [US]; Mag Delay® [US-OTC]; Mag-SR® [US-OTC]; Slow-Mag® [US-OTC]

Therapeutic Category Electrolyte Supplement, Oral

Use Correction or prevention of hypomagnesemia

Usual Dosage Dietary supplement:

Oral: Adults: 54-483 mg/day in divided doses; refer to product labeling. The recommended dietary allowance (RDA) of magnesium is 4.5 mg/kg which is a total daily allowance of 350-400 mg for adult men and 280-300 mg for adult women. During pregnancy the RDA is 300 mg and during lactation the RDA is 355 mg.

I.V. in TPN:

Children: 2-10 mEq/day

The usual recommended pediatric maintenance intake of magnesium ranges from 0.2-0.6 mEq/kg/day. The dose of magnesium may also be based on the caloric intake; on that basis, 3-10 mEq/day of magnesium are needed; maximum maintenance dose: 8-16 mEq/day

Adults: 8-24 mEq/day

Dosage Forms

Injection, solution (Chloromag®): 200 mg/mL [1.97 mEq/mL] (50 mL)

Tablet [enteric coated] (Slo-Mag®): Elemental magnesium 64 mg [contains elemental calcium 106 mg]

Tablet, extended release (Mag Delay®, Mag-SR®): Magnesium chloride hexahydrate 535 mg [equivalent to elemental magnesium 64 mg]

magnesium citrate (mag NEE zhum SIT rate)

Synonyms citrate of magnesia

U.S./Canadian Brand Names Citro-Mag® [Can]

Therapeutic Category Laxative

Use Evacuation of bowel prior to certain surgical and diagnostic procedures or overdose situations

Usual Dosage Cathartic: Oral:

Children:

<6 years: 0.5 mL/kg up to a maximum of 200 mL repeated every 4-6 hours until stools are clear

6-12 years: 100-150 mL

Children ≥12 years and Adults: 1/2 to 1 full bottle (120-300 mL)

Dosage Forms

Solution, oral: 290 mg/5 mL (300 mL) [cherry and lemon flavors]

Tablets: 100 mg [as elemental magnesium]

magnesium gluconate (mag NEE zhum GLOO koe nate)

U.S./Canadian Brand Names Almora® [US-OTC]; Mag G® [US-OTC]; Magonate® Sport [US-OTC]; Magonate® [US-OTC]; Magtrate® [US-OTC]

Therapeutic Category Electrolyte Supplement, Oral

Use Dietary supplement for treatment of magnesium deficiencies

Usual Dosage The recommended dietary allowance (RDA) of magnesium is 4.5 mg/kg which is a total daily allowance of 350-400 mg for adult men and 280-300 mg for adult women. During pregnancy the RDA is 300 mg and during lactation the RDA is 355 mg.

Dietary supplement: Oral:

Children: 3-6 mg/kg/day in divided doses 3-4 times/day; maximum: 400 mg/day

Adults: 54-483 mg/day in divided doses; refer to product labeling

Dosage Forms

Solution:

Magonate®: 1000 mg/5 mL (480 mL) [magnesium 4.8 mEq/5 mL; equivalent to elemental magnesium 54 mg/5 mL; contains sodium benzoate]

Magonate® Sport: 1000 mg/5 mL (30 mL) [magnesium 4.8 mEq/5 mL; equivalent to elemental magnesium 54 mg/5 mL; contains sodium benzoate; fruit flavor]

Tablet (Almora®, Mag G®, Magonate®, Magtrate®): 500 mg [magnesium 2.4 mEq; equivalent to elemental magnesium 27 mg]

magnesium hydroxide (mag NEE zhum hye DROKS ide)

Synonyms magnesia magma; milk of magnesia; MOM

U.S./Canadian Brand Names Dulcolax® Milk of Magnesia [US-OTC]; Phillips'® Milk of Magnesia [US-OTC]

Therapeutic Category Antacid; Electrolyte Supplement, Oral; Laxative

(Continued)

magnesium hydroxide *(Continued)*

Use Short-term treatment of occasional constipation and symptoms of hyperacidity, magnesium replacement therapy

Usual Dosage Oral:

Average daily intakes of dietary magnesium have declined in recent years due to processing of food; the latest estimate of the average American dietary intake was 349 mg/day

Laxative:

Liquid:

Children <2 years: 0.5 mL/kg/dose 2-5 years: 5-15 mL/day (2.5-7.5 mL/day of liquid concentrate) or in divided doses 6-12 years: 15-30 mL/day (7.5-15 mL/day of liquid concentrate) or in divided doses

Children ≥12 years and Adults: 30-60 mL/day (15-30 mL/day of liquid concentrate) or in divided doses

Tablet:

Children: 2-5 years: 1-2 tablets before bedtime 6-11 years: 3-4 tablets before bedtime

Children ≥12 years and Adults: 6-8 tablets before bedtime

Antacid:

Liquid:

Children: 2.5-5 mL as needed up to 4 times/day

Adults: 5-15 mL (2.5-7.5 mL of liquid concentrate) as needed up to 4 times/day

Tablet:

Children 7-14 years: 1 tablet up to 4 times/day

Adults: 2-4 tablets up to 4 times/day

Dosage Forms

Liquid, oral: 400 mg/5 mL (360 mL, 480 mL, 960 mL, 3780 mL)

Dulcolax® Milk of Magnesia: 400 mg/5 mL (360 mL, 780 mL) [regular and mint flavors]

Phillips'® Milk of Magnesia: 400 mg/5 mL (120 mL, 360 mL, 780 mL) [original, French vanilla, cherry, and mint flavors]

Liquid, oral concentrate: 800 mg/5 mL (100 mL, 400 mL)

Phillips'® Milk of Magnesia [concentrate]: 800 mg/5 mL (240 mL) [strawberry créme flavor]

Tablet, chewable (Phillips'® Milk of Magnesia): 311 mg [mint flavor]

magnesium hydroxide, aluminum hydroxide, and simethicone *see* aluminum hydroxide, magnesium hydroxide, and simethicone *on page 40*

magnesium hydroxide and aluminum hydroxide *see* aluminum hydroxide and magnesium hydroxide *on page 40*

magnesium hydroxide and calcium carbonate *see* calcium carbonate and magnesium hydroxide *on page 146*

magnesium hydroxide and mineral oil emulsion

(mag NEE zhum hye DROKS ide & MIN er al oyl e MUL shun)

Synonyms Haley's M-O; MOM/mineral oil emulsion

U.S./Canadian Brand Names Phillips' M-O® [US-OTC]

Therapeutic Category Laxative

Use Short-term treatment of occasional constipation

Usual Dosage

Children 6-11 years: 5-15 mL at bedtime or upon rising

Children ≥12 years and Adults: 30-60 mL at bedtime or upon rising

Dosage Forms Suspension, oral: Magnesium hydroxide 300 mg and mineral oil 1.25 mL per 5 mL (360 mL, 780 mL) [original and mint flavors]

magnesium hydroxide, famotidine, and calcium carbonate *see* famotidine, calcium carbonate, and magnesium hydroxide *on page 357*

magnesium L-aspartate hydrochloride

(mag NEE zhum el-as PAR tate hye droe KLOR ide)

Synonyms MAH™

U.S./Canadian Brand Names Maginex™ [US-OTC]; Maginex™ DS [US-OTC]

Therapeutic Category Electrolyte Supplement, Oral

Use Dietary supplement

Usual Dosage Adults:

Recommended dietary allowance (RDA) of magnesium:

Male: 400-420 mg

Female: 310-320 mg

During pregnancy: 360 mg

During lactation: 320 mg

Dietary supplement: Oral: Magnesium-L-aspartate 1230 mg (magnesium 122 mg) up to 3 times/day

Dosage Forms

Granules (Maginex™ DS): 1230 mg [magnesium 10 mEq; equivalent to magnesium 122 mg; lemon flavor]

Tablet (Maginex™): 615 mg [magnesium 5 mEq; equivalent to magnesium 61 mg]

magnesium oxide (mag NEE zhum OKS ide)

U.S./Canadian Brand Names Mag-Ox® 400 [US-OTC]; Uro-Mag® [US-OTC]

Therapeutic Category Antacid; Electrolyte Supplement, Oral; Laxative

Use Electrolyte replacement

Usual Dosage The recommended dietary allowance (RDA) of magnesium is 4.5 mg/kg which is a total daily allowance of 350-400 mg for adult men and 280-300 mg for adult women. During pregnancy the RDA is 300 mg and during lactation the RDA is 355 mg.

Adults: Oral: Dietary supplement: 20-40 mEq (1-2 tablets) 2-3 times

Product labeling:

Mag-Ox 400®: 1-2 tablets daily with food

Uro-Mag®: 1-2 tablets 3 times/day with food

Note: Oral magnesium is not generally adequate for repletion in patients with serum magnesium concentrations <1.5 mEq/L

Dosage Forms

Capsule (Uro-Mag®): 140 mg [magnesium 7 mEq; equivalent to elemental magnesium 84 mg]

Tablet (Mag-Ox 400®): 400 mg [magnesium 20 mEq; equivalent to elemental magnesium 242 mg]

magnesium salicylate (mag NEE zhum sa LIS i late)

Sound-Alike/Look-Alike Issues

Mobidin® may be confused with Moban®, molindone

U.S./Canadian Brand Names Doan's® Extra Strength [US-OTC]; Doan's® [US-OTC]; Momentum® [US-OTC]

Therapeutic Category Nonsteroidal Antiinflammatory Drug (NSAID)

Use Mild to moderate pain, fever, various inflammatory conditions

Usual Dosage Oral: Adults: 650 mg 4 times daily or 1090 mg 3 times daily; may increase to 3.6-4.8 mg/day in 3 or 4 divided doses

Dosage Forms [DSC] = Discontinued product

Caplet, as anhydrous magnesium salicylate: 467 mg

Doan's®: 304 mg

Doan's® Extra Strength: 467 mg

Mobidin® [DSC]: 600 mg

Momentum®: 467 mg

magnesium sulfate (mag NEE zhum SUL fate)

Sound-Alike/Look-Alike Issues

magnesium sulfate may be confused with manganese sulfate

(Continued)

magnesium sulfate *(Continued)*

Synonyms epsom salts

Therapeutic Category Anticonvulsant; Electrolyte Supplement, Oral; Laxative

Use Treatment and prevention of hypomagnesemia; seizure prevention in severe pre-eclampsia or eclampsia, pediatric acute nephritis; short-term treatment torsade de pointes; treatment of cardiac arrhythmias (VT/VF) caused by hypomagnesemia; short-term treatment of constipation or soaking aid

Usual Dosage The recommended dietary allowance (RDA) of magnesium is 4.5 mg/kg which is a total daily allowance of 350-400 mg for adult men and 280-300 mg for adult women. During pregnancy the RDA is 300 mg and during lactation the RDA is 355 mg. Average daily intakes of dietary magnesium have declined in recent years due to processing of food. The latest estimate of the average American dietary intake was 349 mg/day. Dose represented as magnesium sulfate unless stated otherwise.

Note: Serum magnesium is poor reflection of repletional status as the majority of magnesium is intracellular; serum levels may be transiently normal for a few hours after a dose is given, therefore, aim for consistently high normal serum levels in patients with normal renal function for most efficient repletion

Hypomagnesemia:

Children: I.M., I.V.: 25-50 mg/kg/dose (0.2-0.4 mEq/kg/dose) every 4-6 hours for 3-4 doses, maximum single dose: 2000 mg (16 mEq), may repeat if hypomagnesemia persists (higher dosage up to 100 mg/kg/dose magnesium sulfate I.V. has been used); maintenance: I.V.: 30-60 mg/kg/day (0.25-0.5 mEq/kg/day)

Adults:

Oral: 3 g every 6 hours for 4 doses as needed

I.M., I.V.: 1 g every 6 hours for 4 doses; for severe hypomagnesemia: 8-12 g magnesium sulfate/day in divided doses has been used

Management of seizures and hypertension: Children: I.M., I.V.: 20-100 mg/kg/dose every 4-6 hours as needed; in severe cases doses as high as 200 mg/kg/dose have been used

Eclampsia, preeclampsia: Adults:

I.M.: 1-4 g every 4 hours

I.V.: Initial: 4 g, then switch to I.M. or 1-4 g/hour by continuous infusion

Note: Maximum dose not to exceed 30-40 g/day; maximum rate of infusion: 1-2 g/hour

Life-threatening arrhythmia: I.V.: 1-2 g (8-16 mEq) in 100 mL D_5W, administered over 5-60 minutes followed by an infusion of 0.5-1 g/hour, **or**

1-6 g administered over several minutes, followed by (in some cases) I.V. infusion of 3-20 mg/minute for 5-48 hours (depending on patient response and serum magnesium levels)

Maintenance electrolyte requirements:

Daily requirements: 0.2-0.5 mEq/kg/24 hours or 3-10 mEq/1000 kcal/24 hours

Maximum: 8-16 mEq/24 hours

Cathartic: Oral:

Children:

2-5 years: 2.5-5 g/kg/day in a single or divided doses

6-11 years: 5-10 g/day in a single or divided doses

Children ≥12 years and Adults: 10-30 g/day in a single or divided doses

Soaking aid: Topical: Adults: Dissolve 2 capfuls of powder per gallon of warm water

Dosage Forms

Infusion [premixed in D_5W]: 10 mg/mL (100 mL); 20 mg/mL (500 mL, 1000 mL)

Infusion [premixed in water for injection]: 40 mg/mL (100 mL, 500 mL, 1000 mL); 80 mg/mL (50 mL)

Injection, solution: 125 mg/mL (8 mL); 500 mg/mL (2 mL, 5 mL, 10 mL, 20 mL, 50 mL)

Powder: Magnesium sulfate USP (480 g, 1810 g, 1920 g)

Magnevist® [US/Can] *see* radiological/contrast media (ionic) *on page 759*

Magonate® Sport [US-OTC] *see* magnesium gluconate *on page 537*

Magonate® [US-OTC] *see* magnesium gluconate *on page 537*

Mag-Ox® 400 [US-OTC] *see* magnesium oxide *on page 539*

Magsal® *(Discontinued)* *see page 1042*

Mag-SR® [US-OTC] *see* magnesium chloride *on page 536*

Magtrate® [US-OTC] *see* magnesium gluconate *on page 537*

MAH™ *see* magnesium L-aspartate hydrochloride *on page 539*

Malarone™ [US/Can] *see* atovaquone and proguanil *on page 87*

Malatal® *(Discontinued)* *see page 1042*

malathion (mal a THYE on)

U.S./Canadian Brand Names Ovide® [US]

Therapeutic Category Scabicides/Pediculicides

Use Treatment of head lice and their ova

Usual Dosage Sprinkle Ovide™ lotion on dry hair and rub gently until the scalp is thoroughly moistened; pay special attention to the back of the head and neck. Allow to dry naturally - use no heat and leave uncovered. After 8-12 hours, the hair should be washed with a nonmedicated shampoo; rinse and use a fine-toothed comb to remove dead lice and eggs. If required, repeat with second application in 7-9 days. Further treatment is generally not necessary. Other family members should be evaluated to determine if infested and if so, receive treatment.

Dosage Forms Lotion: 0.5% (59 mL)

Mallisol® *(Discontinued)* *see page 1042*

Malotuss® Syrup *(Discontinued)* *see page 1042*

maltodextrin (mal toe DEK strin)

U.S./Canadian Brand Names Gelclair™ [US]; Multidex® [US-OTC]; OraRinse™ [US-OTC]

Therapeutic Category Skin and Mucous Membrane Agent

Use Topical: Treatment of infected or noninfected wounds

Usual Dosage Adults:

Oral: Management of pain due to oral lesions:

Gelclair™: Using contents of 1 reconstituted packet, rinse around mouth for ~1 minute, 3 times/day or more if needed; gargle and expectorate. May be used undiluted or with less dilution if adequate pain relief is not achieved.

OraRinse™: 1 tablespoonful, swish or gargle for ~1 minute, 4 times/day or more if needed

Topical: Wound dressing: Multidex®: After debridement and irrigation of wound, apply and cover with a nonadherent, nonocclusive dressing. May be applied to moist or dry, infected or noninfected wounds.

Dosage Forms

Gel, oral [concentrate] (Gelclair™): 15 mL/packet (21s) [contains benzalkonium chloride and sodium benzoate]

Gel, topical dressing (Multidex®): (4 mL, 7 mL, 14 mL, 85 mL)

Powder, for oral suspension (OraRinse™): (19 g) [contains phenylalanine; also contains aloe vera, fructose, and sodium benzoate; vanilla flavor]

Powder, topical dressing (Multidex®): (6 g, 12 g, 25 g, 45 g)

malt soup extract (malt soop EKS trakt)

U.S./Canadian Brand Names Maltsupex® [US-OTC]

Therapeutic Category Laxative

Use Short-term treatment of constipation

Usual Dosage Oral:

Infants >1 month:

Breast-fed:

Liquid: 1-2 teaspoonfuls in 2-4 oz of water or fruit juice 1-2 times/day for 3-4 days

Powder: 4 g in 2-4 oz of water or fruit juice daily for 3-4 days

(Continued)

malt soup extract *(Continued)*

Bottle-fed:

Liquid: $1/2$ to 2 tablespoonfuls/day in formula for 3-4 days, then 1-2 teaspoonfuls/day

Powder: 8-16 g/day in formula for 3-4 days, then 4-8 g/day

Children:

2-6 years:

Liquid: 7.5 mL 1-2 times/day for 3-4 days

Powder: 8 g twice daily for 3-4 days

6-12 years:

Liquid: 15-30 mL 1-2 times/day for 3-4 days

Powder: Up to 16 g/day for 3-4 days

Children ≥12 years and Adults:

Liquid: 30 mL twice daily for 3-4 days, then 15-30 mL at bedtime

Powder: Up to 32 g twice daily for 3-4 days, then 16-32 g at bedtime

Tablet: 4 tablets 4 times/day (maximum dose: 64 g/day)

Dosage Forms

Liquid: Nondiastatic barley malt extract 16 g/15 mL (240 mL, 480 mL)

Powder: Nondiastatic barley malt extract 8 g/tablespoonful (240 g, 480 g)

Tablet: Nondiastatic barley malt extract 750 mg

Maltsupex® [US-OTC] *see* malt soup extract *on previous page*

Mandelamine® [US/Can] *see* methenamine *on page 563*

Mandol® (all products) ***(Discontinued)*** *see page 1042*

mandrake *see* podophyllum resin *on page 705*

Manerix® [Can] *see* moclobemide *(Canada only)* *on page 587*

manganese *see* trace metals *on page 874*

mannitol (MAN i tole)

Sound-Alike/Look-Alike Issues

Osmitrol® may be confused with esmolol

Synonyms *D*-mannitol

U.S./Canadian Brand Names Osmitrol® [US/Can]; Resectisol® [US]

Therapeutic Category Diuretic, Osmotic

Use Reduction of increased intracranial pressure associated with cerebral edema; promotion of diuresis in the prevention and/or treatment of oliguria or anuria due to acute renal failure; reduction of increased intraocular pressure; promoting urinary excretion of toxic substances; genitourinary irrigant in transurethral prostatic resection or other transurethral surgical procedures

Usual Dosage I.V.:

Children:

Test dose (to assess adequate renal function): 200 mg/kg over 3-5 minutes to produce a urine flow of at least 1 mL/kg for 1-3 hours

Initial: 0.5-1 g/kg

Maintenance: 0.25-0.5 g/kg given every 4-6 hours

Adults:

Test dose (to assess adequate renal function): 12.5 g (200 mg/kg) over 3-5 minutes to produce a urine flow of at least 30-50 mL of urine per hour over the next 2-3 hours

Initial: 0.5-1 g/kg

Maintenance: 0.25-0.5 g/kg every 4-6 hours; usual adult dose: 20-200 g/24 hours

Intracranial pressure: Cerebral edema: 1.5-2 g/kg/dose I.V. as a 15% to 20% solution over ≥30 minutes; maintain serum osmolality 310-320 mOsm/kg

Preoperative for neurosurgery: 1.5-2 g/kg administered 1-1.5 hours prior to surgery

Transurethral irrigation: Use urogenital solution as required for irrigation

Dosage Forms

Injection, solution: 5% [50 mg/mL] (1000 mL); 10% [100 mg/mL] (500 mL, 1000 mL); 15% [150 mg/mL] (500 mL); 20% [200 mg/mL] (150 mL, 250 mL, 500 mL); 25% [250 mg/mL] (50 mL)

Osmitrol®: 5% [50 mg/mL] (1000 mL); 10% [100 mg/mL] (500 mL, 1000 mL); 15% [150 mg/mL] (500 mL); 20% [200 mg/mL] (250 mL, 500 mL)

Solution, urogenital (Resectisol®): 5% [50 mg/mL] (2000 mL, 4000 mL)

Mantadil® Cream ***(Discontinued)*** *see page 1042*

Mantoux *see* tuberculin tests *on page 893*

Maolate® ***(Discontinued)*** *see page 1042*

Maox® ***(Discontinued)*** *see page 1042*

Mapap® Arthritis [US-OTC] *see* acetaminophen *on page 5*

Mapap® Children's [US-OTC] *see* acetaminophen *on page 5*

Mapap® Extra Strength [US-OTC] *see* acetaminophen *on page 5*

Mapap® Infants [US-OTC] *see* acetaminophen *on page 5*

Mapap® Sinus Maximum Strength [US-OTC] *see* acetaminophen and pseudoephedrine *on page 9*

Mapap® [US-OTC] *see* acetaminophen *on page 5*

maprotiline (ma PROE ti leen)

Synonyms maprotiline hydrochloride

U.S./Canadian Brand Names Novo-Maprotiline [Can]

Therapeutic Category Antidepressant, Tetracyclic

Use Treatment of depression and anxiety associated with depression

Usual Dosage Oral:

Children 6-14 years: Depression/anxiety: 10 mg/day; increase to a maximum daily dose of 75 mg

Adults: Depression/anxiety: 75 mg/day to start, increase by 25 mg every 2 weeks up to 150-225 mg/day; given in 3 divided doses or in a single daily dose

Dosage Forms Tablet, as hydrochloride: 25 mg, 50 mg, 75 mg

maprotiline hydrochloride *see* maprotiline *on this page*

Marax® ***(Discontinued)*** *see page 1042*

Marcaine® [US/Can] *see* bupivacaine *on page 133*

Marcaine® Spinal [US] *see* bupivacaine *on page 133*

Margesic® H [US] *see* hydrocodone and acetaminophen *on page 443*

Marinol® [US/Can] *see* dronabinol *on page 297*

Marmine® Injection ***(Discontinued)*** *see page 1042*

Marmine® Oral ***(Discontinued)*** *see page 1042*

Marplan® [US] *see* isocarboxazid *on page 486*

Marthritic® ***(Discontinued)*** *see page 1042*

Marvelon® [Can] *see* ethinyl estradiol and desogestrel *on page 335*

Matulane® [US/Can] *see* procarbazine *on page 731*

3M™ Avagard™ ***(Discontinued)*** *see page 1042*

Mavik® [US/Can] *see* trandolapril *on page 875*

Maxair™ Autohaler™ [US] *see* pirbuterol *on page 698*

Maxalt® [US/Can] *see* rizatriptan *on page 781*

Maxalt-MLT® [US] *see* rizatriptan *on page 781*

Maxalt RPD™ [Can] *see* rizatriptan *on page 781*

Maxaquin® [US] *see* lomefloxacin *on page 527*

Max-Caro® *(Discontinued)* *see page 1042*

Maxidex® [US/Can] *see* dexamethasone (ophthalmic) *on page 254*

Maxidex® Ophthalmic Ointment *(Discontinued)* *see page 1042*

Maxidone™ [US] *see* hydrocodone and acetaminophen *on page 443*

Maxifed® [US] *see* guaifenesin and pseudoephedrine *on page 419*

Maxifed® DM [US] *see* guaifenesin, pseudoephedrine, and dextromethorphan *on page 422*

Maxifed-G® [US] *see* guaifenesin and pseudoephedrine *on page 419*

Maxiflor® *(Discontinued)* *see page 1042*

Maximum Strength Desenex® Antifungal Cream *(Discontinued)* *see page 1042*

Maximum Strength Dex-A-Diet® *(Discontinued)* *see page 1042*

Maximum Strength Dexatrim® *(Discontinued)* *see page 1042*

Maxipime® [US/Can] *see* cefepime *on page 167*

Maxitrol® [US/Can] *see* neomycin, polymyxin B, and dexamethasone *on page 611*

Maxivate® [US] *see* betamethasone (topical) *on page 116*

Maxolon® *(Discontinued)* *see page 1042*

Maxzide® [US] *see* hydrochlorothiazide and triamterene *on page 443*

Maxzide®-25 [US] *see* hydrochlorothiazide and triamterene *on page 443*

may apple *see* podophyllum resin *on page 705*

Mazanor® *(Discontinued)* *see page 1042*

3M™ Cavilon™ Skin Cleanser [US-OTC] *see* benzalkonium chloride *on page 107*

MCH *see* collagen hemostat *on page 225*

m-cresyl acetate (em-KREE sil AS e tate)

U.S./Canadian Brand Names Cresylate® [US]

Therapeutic Category Otic Agent, Antiinfective

Use Provides an acid medium; for external otitis infections caused by susceptible bacteria or fungus

Usual Dosage Otic: Instill 2-4 drops as required

Dosage Forms Solution, otic: 25% (15 mL) [with isopropanol 25%, chlorobutanol 1%, benzyl alcohol 1%, and castor oil 5% in propylene glycol]

MCT Oil® [US-OTC/Can] *see* medium chain triglycerides *on page 547*

MD-Gastroview® [US] *see* radiological/contrast media (ionic) *on page 759*

MDL 73,147EF *see* dolasetron *on page 287*

MDL-71754 *see* vigabatrin *(Canada only) on page 911*

ME-500® [US] *see* methionine *on page 564*

measles, mumps, and rubella vaccines, combined

(MEE zels, mumpz, & roo BEL a vak SEENS, kom BINED)

Synonyms MMR; mumps, measles and rubella vaccines, combined; rubella, measles and mumps vaccines, combined

U.S./Canadian Brand Names M-M-R® II [US/Can]; Priorix™ [Can]

Therapeutic Category Vaccine, Live Virus

Use Measles, mumps, and rubella prophylaxis

Usual Dosage SubQ:

Infants <12 months: If there is risk of exposure to measles, single-antigen measles vaccine should be administered at 6-11 months of age with a second dose (of MMR) at >12 months of age.

Children ≥12 months: 0.5 mL at 12 months and then repeated at 4-6 years of age. If the second dose was not received, the schedule should be completed by the 11- to 12-year old visit. Administer in outer aspect of the upper arm. Recommended age of primary immunization is 12-15 months; revaccination is recommended prior to elementary school.

Dosage Forms Injection, powder for reconstitution [preservative free]: Measles virus 1000 $TCID_{50}$, rubella virus 1000 $TCID_{50}$, and mumps virus 20,000 $TCID_{50}$ [contains neomycin 25 mcg, gelatin, human albumin, and bovine serum; produced in chick embryo cell culture]

measles virus vaccine (live) (MEE zels VYE rus vak SEEN live)

Sound-Alike/Look-Alike Issues

Attenuvax® may be confused with Meruvax®

Synonyms more attenuated enders strain; rubeola vaccine

U.S./Canadian Brand Names Attenuvax® [US]

Therapeutic Category Vaccine, Live Virus

Use Adults born before 1957 are generally considered to be immune. All those born in or after 1957 without documentation of live vaccine on or after first birthday, physician-diagnosed measles, or laboratory evidence of immunity should be vaccinated, ideally with two doses of vaccine separated by no less than 1 month. For those previously vaccinated with one dose of measles vaccine, revaccination is recommended for students entering colleges and other institutions of higher education, for healthcare workers at the time of employment, and for international travelers who visit endemic areas.

MMR is the vaccine of choice if recipients are likely to be susceptible to rubella and/or mumps as well as to measles. Persons vaccinated between 1963 and 1967 with a killed measles vaccine, followed by live vaccine within 3 months, or with a vaccine of unknown type should be revaccinated with live measles virus vaccine.

Usual Dosage Children ≥15 months and Adults: SubQ: 0.5 mL in outer aspect of the upper arm, no routine boosters

Dosage Forms Injection, powder for reconstitution [preservative free]: 1000 $TCID_{50}$ [contains human albumin, bovine serum, and neomycin; produced in chick embryo cell culture]

Measurin® *(Discontinued)* *see page 1042*

Mebaral® [US/Can] *see* mephobarbital *on page 553*

mebendazole (me BEN da zole)

U.S./Canadian Brand Names Vermox® [US/Can]

Therapeutic Category Anthelmintic

Use Treatment of pinworms (*Enterobius vermicularis*), whipworms (*Trichuris trichiura*), roundworms (*Ascaris lumbricoides*), and hookworms (*Ancylostoma duodenale*)

Usual Dosage Children and Adults: Oral:

Pinworms: 100 mg as a single dose; may need to repeat after 2 weeks; treatment should include family members in close contact with patient

Whipworms, roundworms, hookworms: One tablet twice daily, morning and evening on 3 consecutive days; if patient is not cured within 3-4 weeks, a second course of treatment may be administered

Capillariasis: 200 mg twice daily for 20 days

Dosage Forms Tablet, chewable: 100 mg

mecamylamine (mek a MIL a meen)

Sound-Alike/Look-Alike Issues
mecamylamine may be confused with mesalamine

Synonyms mecamylamine hydrochloride

U.S./Canadian Brand Names Inversine® [US/Can]

Therapeutic Category Ganglionic Blocking Agent

Use Treatment of moderately severe to severe hypertension and in uncomplicated malignant hypertension

Usual Dosage Adults: Oral: 2.5 mg twice daily after meals for 2 days; increased by increments of 2.5 mg at intervals ≥2 days until desired blood pressure response is achieved; average daily dose: 25 mg (usually in 3 divided doses)

Note: Reduce dosage of other antihypertensives when combined with mecamylamine with exception of thiazide diuretics which may be maintained at usual dose while decreasing mecamylamine by 50%

Dosage Forms Tablet, as hydrochloride: 2.5 mg

mecamylamine hydrochloride *see* mecamylamine *on this page*

mechlorethamine (me klor ETH a meen)

Synonyms chlorethazine; chlorethazine mustard; HN_2; mechlorethamine hydrochloride; mustine; nitrogen mustard; NSC-762

U.S./Canadian Brand Names Mustargen® [US/Can]

Therapeutic Category Antineoplastic Agent

Use Combination therapy of Hodgkin disease and malignant lymphomas; non-Hodgkin lymphoma; may be used by intracavitary injection for treatment of metastatic tumors; pleural and other malignant effusions; topical treatment of mycosis fungoides

Usual Dosage Refer to individual protocols.

Children and Adults: I.V.: 6 mg/m^2 on days 1 and 8 of a 28-day cycle (MOPP regimen)

Adults:

I.V.: 0.4 mg/kg **or** 12-16 mg/m^2 for one dose **or** divided into 0.1 mg/kg/day for 4 days, repeated at 4- to 6-week intervals

Intracavitary: 0.2-0.4 mg/kg (10-20 mg) as a single dose; may be repeated if fluid continues to accumulate.

Intrapericardially: 0.2-0.4 mg/kg as a single dose; may be repeated if fluid continues to accumulate.

Topical: 0.01% to 0.02% solution, lotion, or ointment

Dosage Forms Injection, powder for reconstitution, as hydrochloride: 10 mg

mechlorethamine hydrochloride *see* mechlorethamine *on this page*

Meclan® Topical *(Discontinued)* *see page 1042*

meclizine (MEK li zeen)

Synonyms meclizine hydrochloride; meclozine hydrochloride

U.S./Canadian Brand Names Antivert® [US/Can]; Bonamine™ [Can]; Bonine® [US-OTC/Can]; Dramamine® Less Drowsy Formula [US-OTC]

Therapeutic Category Antihistamine

Use Prevention and treatment of symptoms of motion sickness; management of vertigo with diseases affecting the vestibular system

Usual Dosage Children >12 years and Adults: Oral:

Motion sickness: 12.5-25 mg 1 hour before travel, repeat dose every 12-24 hours if needed; doses up to 50 mg may be needed

Vertigo: 25-100 mg/day in divided doses

Dosage Forms

Tablet, as hydrochloride: 12.5 mg, 25 mg

- Antivert®: 12.5 mg, 25 mg, 50 mg
- Dramamine® Less Drowsy Formula: 25 mg

Tablet, chewable, as hydrochloride (Bonine®): 25 mg

meclizine hydrochloride *see* meclizine *on previous page*

meclofenamate (me kloe fen AM ate)

Synonyms meclofenamate sodium

U.S./Canadian Brand Names Meclomen® [Can]

Therapeutic Category Analgesic, Nonnarcotic; Nonsteroidal Antiinflammatory Drug (NSAID)

Use Treatment of inflammatory disorders, arthritis, mild to moderate pain, dysmenorrhea

Usual Dosage Children >14 years and Adults: Oral:

Mild to moderate pain: 50 mg every 4-6 hours; increases to 100 mg may be required; maximum dose: 400 mg

Rheumatoid arthritis and osteoarthritis: 50 mg every 4-6 hours; increase, over weeks, to 200-400 mg/day in 3-4 divided doses; do not exceed 400 mg/day; maximal benefit for any dose may not be seen for 2-3 weeks

Dosage Forms Capsule, as sodium: 50 mg, 100 mg

meclofenamate sodium *see* meclofenamate *on this page*

Meclomen® [Can] *see* meclofenamate *on this page*

Meclomen® ***(Discontinued)*** *see page 1042*

meclozine hydrochloride *see* meclizine *on previous page*

Med-Diltiazem [Can] *see* diltiazem *on page 273*

medicinal carbon *see* charcoal *on page 180*

medicinal charcoal *see* charcoal *on page 180*

Medicone® [US-OTC] *see* phenylephrine *on page 689*

Medidin® Liquid ***(Discontinued)*** *see page 1042*

Medihaler-Epi® ***(Discontinued)*** *see page 1042*

Medihaler Ergotamine® ***(Discontinued)*** *see page 1042*

Medihaler-Iso® ***(Discontinued)*** *see page 1042*

Medipain 5® ***(Discontinued)*** *see page 1042*

Mediplast® [US-OTC] *see* salicylic acid *on page 789*

Medipren® ***(Discontinued)*** *see page 1042*

Medi-Quick® Topical Ointment ***(Discontinued)*** *see page 1042*

Medispaz® ***(Discontinued)*** *see page 1042*

Medi-Synal [US-OTC] *see* acetaminophen and pseudoephedrine *on page 9*

Medi-Tuss® ***(Discontinued)*** *see page 1042*

medium chain triglycerides (mee DEE um chane trye GLIS er ides)

Synonyms triglycerides, medium chain

U.S./Canadian Brand Names MCT Oil® [US-OTC/Can]

Therapeutic Category Nutritional Supplement

Use Dietary supplement for those who cannot digest long chain fats; malabsorption associated with disorders such as pancreatic insufficiency, bile salt deficiency, and bacterial overgrowth of the small bowel; induce ketosis as a prevention for seizures (akinetic, clonic, and petit mal)

Usual Dosage Oral:

Infants: Initial: 0.5 mL every other feeding, then advance to every feeding, then increase in increments of 0.25-0.5 mL/feeding at intervals of 2-3 days as tolerated

Seizures: About 39 mL with each meal or 50% to 70% (800-1120 kcal) of total calories (1600 kcal) as the oil will induce ketosis necessary for seizure control

Cystic fibrosis: 3 tablespoons/day is tolerated without adverse symptoms by most children

Adults: 15 mL 3-4 times/day

Dosage Forms Oil: 14 g/15 mL (960 mL)

Medralone® Injection *(Discontinued)* *see page 1042*

Medrapred® *(Discontinued)* *see page 1042*

Medrol® [US/Can] *see* methylprednisolone *on page 572*

Medrol® Acetate Topical *(Discontinued)* *see page 1042*

medroxyprogesterone acetate (me DROKS ee proe JES te rone AS e tate)

Sound-Alike/Look-Alike Issues

medroxyprogesterone may be confused with hydroxyprogesterone, methylprednisolone, methyltestosterone

Provera® may be confused with Covera®, Parlodel®, Premarin®

Synonyms acetoxymethylprogesterone; methylacetoxyprogesterone

Tall-Man medroxy**PROGESTER**one acetate

U.S./Canadian Brand Names Alti-MPA [Can]; Apo-Medroxy® [Can]; Depo-Provera® [US/Can]; Depo-Provera® Contraceptive [US]; Gen-Medroxy [Can]; Novo-Medrone [Can]; Provera® [US/Can]

Therapeutic Category Contraceptive, Progestin Only; Progestin

Use Endometrial carcinoma or renal carcinoma as well as secondary amenorrhea or abnormal uterine bleeding due to hormonal imbalance; reduction of endometrial hyperplasia in postmenopausal women receiving 0.625 mg conjugated estrogens for 12-14 consecutive days per month; Depo-Provera® injection is used for the prevention of pregnancy

Usual Dosage

Adolescents and Adults: Oral:

- Amenorrhea: 5-10 mg/day for 5-10 days or 2.5 mg/day
- Abnormal uterine bleeding: 5-10 mg for 5-10 days starting on day 16 or 21 of cycle
- Accompanying cyclic estrogen therapy, postmenopausal: 2.5-10 mg the last 10-13 days of estrogen dosing each month

Adults: I.M.:

- Endometrial or renal carcinoma: 400-1000 mg/week
- Contraception: 150 mg every 3 months

Dosage Forms

Injection, suspension, as acetate:

- Depo-Provera®: 400 mg/mL (2.5 mL, 10 mL)
- Depo-Provera® Contraceptive: 150 mg/mL (1 mL) [prefilled syringe or vial]

Tablet, as acetate (Provera®): 2.5 mg, 5 mg, 10 mg

medroxyprogesterone acetate and estradiol cypionate *see* estradiol cypionate and medroxyprogesterone acetate *on page 328*

medroxyprogesterone and estrogens (conjugated) *see* estrogens (conjugated/equine) and medroxyprogesterone *on page 330*

medrysone (ME dri sone)

U.S./Canadian Brand Names HMS Liquifilm® [US]

Therapeutic Category Adrenal Corticosteroid

Use Treatment of allergic conjunctivitis, vernal conjunctivitis, episcleritis, ophthalmic epinephrine sensitivity reaction

Usual Dosage Children ≥3 years and Adults: Ophthalmic: Instill 1 drop in conjunctival sac 2-4 times/day up to every 4 hours; may use every 1-2 hours during first 1-2 days

Dosage Forms Solution, ophthalmic: 1% (5 mL, 10 mL) [contains benzalkonium chloride]

mefenamic acid (me fe NAM ik AS id)

Sound-Alike/Look-Alike Issues

Ponstel® may be confused with Pronestyl®

U.S./Canadian Brand Names Apo-Mefenamic® [Can]; Nu-Mefenamic [Can]; PMS-Mefenamic Acid [Can]; Ponstan® [Can]; Ponstel® [US/Can]

Therapeutic Category Analgesic, Nonnarcotic; Nonsteroidal Antiinflammatory Drug (NSAID)

Use Short-term relief of mild to moderate pain including primary dysmenorrhea

Usual Dosage Children >14 years and Adults: Oral: 500 mg to start then 250 mg every 4 hours as needed; maximum therapy: 1 week

Dosage Forms Capsule: 250 mg

mefloquine (ME floe kwin)

Synonyms mefloquine hydrochloride

U.S./Canadian Brand Names Apo-Mefloquine® [Can]; Lariam® [US/Can]

Therapeutic Category Antimalarial Agent

Use Treatment of acute malarial infections and prevention of malaria

Usual Dosage Oral (dose expressed as mg of mefloquine hydrochloride):

Children ≥6 months and >5 kg:

Malaria treatment: 20-25 mg/kg in 2 divided doses, taken 6-8 hours apart (maximum: 1250 mg) Take with food and an ample amount of water. If clinical improvement is not seen within 48-72 hours, an alternative therapy should be used for retreatment.

Malaria prophylaxis: 5 mg/kg/once weekly (maximum dose: 250 mg) starting 1 week before, arrival in endemic area, continuing weekly during travel and for 4 weeks after leaving endemic area. Take with food and an ample amount of water.

Adults:

Malaria treatment (mild to moderate infection): 5 tablets (1250 mg) as a single dose. Take with food and at least 8 oz of water. If clinical improvement is not seen within 48-72 hours, an alternative therapy should be used for retreatment.

Malaria prophylaxis: 1 tablet (250 mg) weekly starting 1 week before, arrival in endemic area, continuing weekly during travel and for 4 weeks after leaving endemic area. Take with food and at least 8 oz of water.

Dosage Forms Tablet, as hydrochloride: 250 mg [equivalent to 228 mg base]

mefloquine hydrochloride *see* mefloquine *on this page*

Mefoxin® [US/Can] *see* cefoxitin *on page 169*

Megace® [US/Can] *see* megestrol acetate *on this page*

Megace® OS [US] *see* megestrol acetate *on this page*

Megadophilus® [US-OTC] *see* Lactobacillus *on page 501*

megestrol acetate (me JES trole AS e tate)

Sound-Alike/Look-Alike Issues

Megace® may be confused with Reglan®

Synonyms 5071-1DL(6); NSC-10363

U.S./Canadian Brand Names Apo-Megestrol® [Can]; Lin-Megestrol [Can]; Megace® [US/Can]; Megace® OS [US]; Nu-Megestrol [Can]

Therapeutic Category Antineoplastic Agent; Progestin

Use Palliative treatment of breast and endometrial carcinoma

Orphan drug: Treatment of anorexia, cachexia, or significant weight loss (≥10% baseline body weight) and confirmed diagnosis of AIDS

Usual Dosage Refer to individual protocols. Adults: Oral:

Female:

Breast carcinoma: 40 mg 4 times/day

Endometrial carcinoma: 40-320 mg/day in divided doses; use for 2 months to determine efficacy; maximum doses used have been up to 800 mg/day

Male/Female: HIV-related cachexia: Initial dose: 800 mg/day; daily doses of 400 and 800 mg/day were found to be clinically effective

Dosage Forms

Suspension, oral, as acetate: 40 mg/mL (240 mL) [contains alcohol 0.06% and sodium benzoate; lemon-lime flavor]

Tablet, as acetate: 20 mg, 40 mg

Melanex® [US] *see* hydroquinone *on page 454*

Melfiat® [US] *see* phendimetrazine *on page 685*

Mellaril® (all products) *(Discontinued)* *see page 1042*

Mellaril-S® *(Discontinued)* *see page 1042*

meloxicam (mel OX ee cam)

U.S./Canadian Brand Names Mobic® [US/Can]; Mobicox® [Can]

Therapeutic Category Nonsteroidal Antiinflammatory Drug (NSAID)

Use Relief of signs and symptoms of osteoarthritis and rheumatoid arthritis

Usual Dosage Adults: Oral: Initial: 7.5 mg once daily; some patients may receive additional benefit from an increased dose of 15 mg once daily; maximum dose: 15 mg/day

Dosage Forms

Suspension: 7.5 mg/5 mL (100 mL) [contains sodium benzoate; raspberry flavor]

Tablet: 7.5 mg, 15 mg

Melpaque HP® [US] *see* hydroquinone *on page 454*

melphalan (MEL fa lan)

Sound-Alike/Look-Alike Issues

melphalan may be confused with Mephyton®, Myleran®

Alkeran® may be confused with Alferon®, Leukeran®

Synonyms L-PAM; L-sarcolysin; phenylalanine mustard

U.S./Canadian Brand Names Alkeran® [US/Can]

Therapeutic Category Antineoplastic Agent

Use Palliative treatment of multiple myeloma and nonresectable epithelial ovarian carcinoma; neuroblastoma, rhabdomyosarcoma, breast cancer

Usual Dosage Refer to individual protocols.

Oral: Dose should always be adjusted to patient response and weekly blood counts:

Children: 4-20 mg/m^2/day for 1-21 days

Adults:

Multiple myeloma: 6 mg/day initially adjusted as indicated **or** 0.15 mg/kg/day for 7 days **or** 0.25 mg/kg/day for 4 days; repeat at 4- to 6-week intervals.

Ovarian carcinoma: 0.2 mg/kg/day for 5 days, repeat every 4-5 weeks.

I.V.:

Children:

Pediatric rhabdomyosarcoma: 10-35 mg/m^2/dose every 21-28 days

High-dose melphalan with bone marrow transplantation for neuroblastoma: I.V.: 100-220 mg/m^2 as a single dose or divided into 2-5 daily doses. Infuse over 20-60 minutes.

Adults: Multiple myeloma: 16 mg/m^2 administered at 2-week intervals for 4 doses, then repeat monthly as per protocol for multiple myeloma.

Dosage Forms

Injection, powder for reconstitution, as hydrochloride: 50 mg [diluent contains ethanol]

Tablet: 2 mg

Melquin-3® [US] *see* hydroquinone *on page 454*

Melquin HP® [US] *see* hydroquinone *on page 454*

memantine (me MAN teen)

Synonyms memantine hydrochloride

U.S./Canadian Brand Names Namenda™ [US]

Therapeutic Category N-Methyl-D-Aspartate Receptor Antagonist

Use Treatment of moderate to severe dementia of the Alzheimer type

Usual Dosage Oral: Adults: Alzheimer's disease: Initial: 5 mg/day; increase dose by 5 mg/day to a target dose of 20 mg/day; wait at least 1 week between dosage changes. Doses >5 mg/day should be given in 2 divided doses.

Suggested titration: 5 mg/day for ≥1 week; 5 mg twice daily for ≥1 week; 15 mg/day given in 5 mg and 10 mg separated doses for ≥1 week; then 10 mg twice daily

Dosage Forms

Tablet, as hydrochloride (Namenda™): 5 mg, 10 mg

Combination package (Namenda™) [titration pack contains 2 separate tablet formulations]: Memantine hydrochloride 5 mg (28s) and memantine hydrochloride 10 mg (21s)

memantine hydrochloride *see* memantine *on previous page*

Menadol® [US-OTC] *see* ibuprofen *on page 462*

Menest® [US/Can] *see* estrogens (esterified) *on page 331*

Meni-D® *(Discontinued)* *see page 1042*

meningococcal polysaccharide vaccine (groups A, C, Y and W-135)

(me NIN joe kok al pol i SAK a ride vak SEEN groops aye, see, why, & dubl yoo-won thur tee fyve)

U.S./Canadian Brand Names Menomune®-A/C/Y/W-135 [US]

Therapeutic Category Vaccine, Live Bacteria

Use Provide active immunity to meningococcal serogroups contained in the vaccine; prevention and control of outbreaks of serogroup C meningococcal disease; recommended for use in:

Immunization of persons ≥2 years of age in epidemic or endemic areas as might be determined in a population delineated by neighborhood, school, dormitory, or other reasonable boundary. The prevalent serogroup in such a situation should match a serogroup in the vaccine. Individuals at particular high-risk include persons with terminal component complement deficiencies and those with anatomic or functional asplenia.

Travelers visiting areas of a country that are recognized as having hyperendemic or epidemic meningococcal disease

Vaccinations should be considered for household or institutional contacts of persons with meningococcal disease as an adjunct to appropriate antibiotic chemoprophylaxis as well as medical and laboratory personnel at risk of exposure to meningococcal disease

Usual Dosage SubQ: Children ≥2 years and Adults: 0.5 mL; the need for booster is unknown, but may be considered in high-risk individuals, particularly children first vaccinated at <4 years of age. **Note:** Individuals who are sensitive to thimerosal should receive single-dose pack (reconstituted with 0.78 mL vial without preservative).

Dosage Forms Injection, powder for reconstitution: 50 mcg each of polysaccharide antigen groups A, C, Y, and W-135 [contains lactose; packaged with 1 mL preservative free diluent or 6 mL diluent containing thimerosal; vial stoppers contain dry, natural latex rubber]

Menomune®-A/C/Y/W-135 [US] *see* meningococcal polysaccharide vaccine (groups A, C, Y and W-135) *on this page*

Menostar™ [US] *see* estradiol *on page 324*

menotropins (men oh TROE pins)

Sound-Alike/Look-Alike Issues

Repronex® may be confused with Regranex®

U.S./Canadian Brand Names Pergonal® [US/Can]; Repronex® [US/Can]

Therapeutic Category Gonadotropin

Use Sequentially with hCG to induce ovulation and pregnancy in the infertile woman with functional anovulation or in patients who have previously received pituitary suppression;

(Continued)

menotropins *(Continued)*

stimulation of multiple follicle development in ovulatory patients as part of an *in vitro* fertilization program; used with hCG in men to stimulate spermatogenesis in those with primary hypogonadotropic hypogonadism

Usual Dosage Adults: I.M.:

Spermatogenesis (Male): Following pretreatment with hCG, 1 ampul 3 times/week and hCG 2000 units twice weekly until sperm is detected in the ejaculate (4-6 months) then may be increased to 2 ampuls of menotropins (150 units FSH/150 units LH) 3 times/week

Induction of ovulation (Female): 1 ampul/day (75 units of FSH and LH) for 9-12 days followed by 10,000 units hCG 1 day after the last dose; repeated at least twice at same level before increasing dosage to 2 ampuls (150 units FSH/150 units LH)

Repronex®: I.M., SubQ:

Infertile patients with oligo-anovulation: Initial: 150 int. units daily for the first 5 days of treatment. Adjustments should not be made more frequently than once every 2 days and should not exceed 75-150 int. units per adjustment. Maximum daily dose should not exceed 450 int. units and dosing beyond 12 days is not recommended. If patient's response to Repronex® is appropriate, hCG 5000-10,000 units should be given one day following the last dose of Repronex®. Hold dose if serum estradiol is >2000 pg/mL, if the ovaries are abnormally enlarged, or if abdominal pain occurs; the patient should also be advised to refrain from intercourse.

Assisted reproductive technologies: Initial (in patients who have received GnRH agonist or antagonist pituitary suppression): 225 int. units; adjustments in dose should not be made more frequently than once every 2 days and should not exceed more than 75-50 int. units per adjustment. The maximum daily doses of Repronex® given should not exceed 450 int. units and dosing beyond 12 days is not recommended. Once adequate follicular development is evident, hCG (5000-10,000 units) should be administered to induce final follicular maturation in preparation for oocyte retrieval. Withhold treatment when ovaries are abnormally enlarged on last day of therapy (to reduce chance of developing OHSS).

Dosage Forms Injection, powder for reconstitution:

Pergonal®: Follicle stimulating hormone activity 75 int. units and luteinizing hormone activity 75 int. units [packaged with diluent]

Repronex®:

Follicle stimulating hormone activity 75 int. units and luteinizing hormone activity 75 int. units [packaged with diluent]

Follicle stimulating hormone activity 150 int. units and luteinizing hormone activity 150 int. units [packaged with diluent]

Mentax® [US] *see* butenafine *on page 139*

292 MEP® [Can] *see* aspirin and meprobamate *on page 83*

mepenzolate (me PEN zoe late)

Sound-Alike/Look-Alike Issues

Cantil® may be confused with Bentyl®

Synonyms mepenzolate bromide

U.S./Canadian Brand Names Cantil® [US/Can]

Therapeutic Category Anticholinergic Agent

Use Adjunctive treatment of peptic ulcer disease

Usual Dosage Adults: Oral: 25-50 mg 4 times/day with meals and at bedtime

Dosage Forms Tablet, as bromide: 25 mg [contains tartrazine]

mepenzolate bromide *see* mepenzolate *on this page*

mepergan *see* meperidine and promethazine *on next page*

meperidine (me PER i deen)

Sound-Alike/Look-Alike Issues

meperidine may be confused with meprobamate

Demerol® may be confused with Demulen®, Desyrel®, Detrol®, dicumarol, Dilaudid®, Dymelor®, Pamelor®

Synonyms isonipecaine hydrochloride; meperidine hydrochloride; pethidine hydrochloride

U.S./Canadian Brand Names Demerol® [US/Can]; Meperitab® [US]

Therapeutic Category Analgesic, Narcotic

Controlled Substance C-II

Use Management of moderate to severe pain; adjunct to anesthesia and preoperative sedation

Usual Dosage **Note:** Doses should be titrated to necessary analgesic effect. When changing route of administration, note that oral doses are about half as effective as parenteral dose. Oral route not recommended for chronic pain. These are guidelines and do not represent the maximum doses that may be required in all patients.

Children: Pain: Oral, I.M., I.V., SubQ: 1-1.5 mg/kg/dose every 3-4 hours as needed; 1-2 mg/kg as a single dose preoperative medication may be used; maximum 100 mg/dose

Adults: Pain:

Oral: Initial: Opiate-naive: 50 mg every 3-4 hours as needed; usual dosage range: 50-150 mg every 2-4 hours as needed

I.M., SubQ: Initial: Opiate-naive: 50-75 mg every 3-4 hours as needed; patients with prior opiate exposure may require higher initial doses; usual dosage range: 50-150 mg every 2-4 hours as needed

Preoperatively: 50-100 mg given 30-90 minutes before the beginning of anesthesia

Slow I.V.: Initial: 5-10 mg every 5 minutes as needed

Patient-controlled analgesia (PCA): Usual concentration: 10 mg/mL

Initial dose: 10 mg

Demand dose: 1-5 mg (manufacturer recommendations); range 5-25 mg (American Pain Society, 1999).

Lockout interval: 5-10 minutes

Dosage Forms

Injection, solution, as hydrochloride [ampul]: 50 mg/mL (1.5 mL, 2 mL)

Injection, solution, as hydrochloride [prefilled syringe]: 25 mg/mL (1 mL); 50 mg/mL (1 mL); 75 mg/mL (1 mL); 100 mg/mL (1 mL)

Injection, solution, as hydrochloride [prefilled syringe for PCA pump]: 10 mg/mL (50 mL)

Injection, solution, as hydrochloride [vial]: 50 mg/mL (1 mL, 30 mL); 100 mg/mL (20 mL) [may contain sodium metabisulfite]

Syrup, as hydrochloride: 50 mg/5 mL (5 mL, 500 mL) [contains sodium benzoate]

Demerol®: 50 mg/5 mL (480 mL) [contains benzoic acid; banana flavor]

Tablet, as hydrochloride (Demerol®, Meperitab®): 50 mg, 100 mg

meperidine and promethazine (me PER i deen & proe METH a zeen)

Synonyms mepergan; promethazine and meperidine

Therapeutic Category Analgesic, Narcotic

Controlled Substance C-II

Use Management of moderate to severe pain

Usual Dosage Adults: Oral: One (1) capsule every 4-6 hours as needed

Dosage Forms Capsule: Meperidine hydrochloride 50 mg and promethazine hydrochloride 25 mg

meperidine hydrochloride *see* meperidine *on this page*

Meperitab® [US] *see* meperidine *on this page*

mephobarbital (me foe BAR bi tal)

Sound-Alike/Look-Alike Issues

mephobarbital may be confused with methocarbamol

(Continued)

mephobarbital *(Continued)*

Mebaral® may be confused with Medrol®, Mellaril®, Tegretol®

Synonyms methylphenobarbital

U.S./Canadian Brand Names Mebaral® [US/Can]

Therapeutic Category Barbiturate

Controlled Substance C-IV

Use Sedative; treatment of grand mal and petit mal epilepsy

Usual Dosage Oral:

Epilepsy:

Children: 6-12 mg/kg/day in 2-4 divided doses

Adults: 200-600 mg/day in 2-4 divided doses

Sedation:

Children:

<5 years: 16-32 mg 3-4 times/day

>5 years: 32-64 mg 3-4 times/day

Adults: 32-100 mg 3-4 times/day

Dosage Forms Tablet: 32 mg, 50 mg, 100 mg

Mephyton® [US/Can] *see* phytonadione *on page 693*

mepivacaine (me PIV a kane)

Sound-Alike/Look-Alike Issues

mepivacaine may be confused with bupivacaine

Polocaine® may be confused with prilocaine

Synonyms mepivacaine hydrochloride

U.S./Canadian Brand Names Carbocaine® [Can]; Polocaine® [US/Can]; Polocaine® MPF [US]

Therapeutic Category Local Anesthetic

Use Local anesthesia by nerve block; **not** for use in spinal anesthesia

Usual Dosage Children and Adults: Injectable local anesthetic: Varies with procedure, degree of anesthesia needed, vascularity of tissue, duration of anesthesia required, and physical condition of patient

Dosage Forms [DSC] = Discontinued product

Injection, solution, as hydrochloride:

Carbocaine® [DSC]: 1% (30 mL, 50 mL); 2% (20 mL, 50 mL)

Polocaine®: 1% (50 mL); 2% (50 mL)

Polocaine® MPF: 1% (30 mL); 1.5% (30 mL); 3% (20 mL)

mepivacaine hydrochloride *see* mepivacaine *on this page*

meprobamate (me proe BA mate)

Sound-Alike/Look-Alike Issues

meprobamate may be confused with Mepergan®, meperidine

U.S./Canadian Brand Names Miltown® [US]; Novo-Mepro [Can]

Therapeutic Category Antianxiety Agent, Miscellaneous

Controlled Substance C-IV

Use Management of anxiety disorders

Usual Dosage Oral:

Children 6-12 years: Anxiety: 100-200 mg 2-3 times/day

Adults: Anxiety: 400 mg 3-4 times/day, up to 2400 mg/day

Dosage Forms Tablet: 200 mg, 400 mg

meprobamate and aspirin *see* aspirin and meprobamate *on page 83*

Mepron® [US/Can] *see* atovaquone *on page 87*

Meprospan® ***(Discontinued)*** *see page 1042*

mequinol and tretinoin (ME kwi nol & TRET i noyn)

Synonyms tretinoin and mequinol

U.S./Canadian Brand Names Solagé™ [US/Can]

Therapeutic Category Retinoic Acid Derivative; Vitamin A Derivative; Vitamin, Topical

Use Treatment of solar lentigines; the efficacy of using Solagé™ daily for >24 weeks has not been established. The local cutaneous safety of Solagé™ in non-Caucasians has not been adequately established.

Usual Dosage Solar lentigines: Topical: Apply twice daily to solar lentigines using the applicator tip while avoiding application to the surrounding skin. Separate application by at least 8 hours or as directed by physician.

Dosage Forms Liquid, topical: Mequinol 2% and tretinoin 0.01% (30 mL) [contains alcohol 78%]

merbromin (mer BROE min)

U.S./Canadian Brand Names Mercurochrome® [US]

Therapeutic Category Topical Skin Product

Use Topical antiseptic

Usual Dosage Apply freely, until injury has healed

Dosage Forms Solution, topical: 2% (30 mL)

mercaptopurine (mer kap toe PYOOR een)

Synonyms 6-mercaptopurine; 6-MP; NSC-755

U.S./Canadian Brand Names Purinethol® [US/Can]

Therapeutic Category Antineoplastic Agent

Use Treatment (maintenance and induction) of acute lymphoblastic leukemia (ALL)

Usual Dosage Refer to individual protocols. Oral:

Children:

Induction: 2.5-5 mg/kg/day **or** 70-100 mg/m^2/day given once daily

Maintenance: 1.5-2.5 mg/kg/day **or** 50-75 mg/m^2/day given once daily

Adults:

Induction: 2.5-5 mg/kg/day (100-200 mg)

Maintenance: 1.5-2.5 mg/kg/day **or** 80-100 mg/m^2/day given once daily

Dosage adjustment with concurrent allopurinol: Reduce mercaptopurine dosage to $^1/_3$ to $^1/_2$ the usual dose.

Dosage adjustment in TPMT-deficiency: Not established; substantial reductions are generally required only in homozygous deficiency.

Note: In ALL, administration in the evening (vs morning administration) may lower the risk of relapse.

Dosage Forms Tablet [scored]: 50 mg

6-mercaptopurine *see* mercaptopurine *on this page*

mercapturic acid *see* acetylcysteine *on page 16*

mercuric oxide (mer KYOOR ik OKS ide)

Synonyms yellow mercuric oxide

Therapeutic Category Antibiotic, Ophthalmic

Use Treatment of irritation and minor infections of the eyelids

Usual Dosage Apply small amount to inner surface of lower eyelid once or twice daily

Dosage Forms Ointment, ophthalmic: 1%, 2% [OTC]

Mercurochrome® [US] *see* merbromin *on this page*

Meridia® [US/Can] *see* sibutramine *on page 803*

meropenem (mer oh PEN em)

U.S./Canadian Brand Names Merrem® I.V. [US/Can]

Therapeutic Category Carbapenem (Antibiotic)

(Continued)

meropenem *(Continued)*

Use Intra-abdominal infections (complicated appendicitis and peritonitis) caused by viridans group streptococci, *E. coli*, *K. pneumoniae*, *P. aeruginosa*, *B. fragilis*, *B. thetaiotaomicron*, and *Peptostreptococcus* sp; also indicated for bacterial meningitis in pediatric patients >3 months of age caused by *S. pneumoniae*, *H. influenzae*, and *N. meningitidis*; meropenem has also been used to treat soft tissue infections, febrile neutropenia, and urinary tract infections

Usual Dosage I.V.:

Neonates:

Preterm: 20 mg/kg/dose every 12 hours (may be increased to 40 mg/kg/dose if treating a highly resistant organism such as *Pseudomonas aeruginosa*)

Full-term (<3 months of age): 20 mg/kg/dose every 8 hours (may be increased to 40 mg/kg/dose if treating a highly resistant organism such as *Pseudomonas aeruginosa*)

Children >3 months (<50 kg):

Intra-abdominal infections: 20 mg/kg every 8 hours (maximum dose: 1 g every 8 hours)

Meningitis: 40 mg/kg every 8 hours (maximum dose: 2 g every 8 hours)

Children >50 kg:

Intra-abdominal infections: 1 g every 8 hours

Meningitis: 2 g every 8 hours

Adults: 1 g every 8 hours

Dosage Forms Injection, powder for reconstitution: 500 mg, 1 g

Merrem® I.V. [US/Can] *see* meropenem *on previous page*

Mersol® [US-OTC] *see* thimerosal *on page 857*

Merthiolate® [US-OTC] *see* thimerosal *on page 857*

Meruvax® II [US] *see* rubella virus vaccine (live) *on page 788*

mesalamine (me SAL a meen)

Sound-Alike/Look-Alike Issues

mesalamine may be confused with mecamylamine

Asacol® may be confused with Ansaid®, Os-Cal®

Synonyms 5-aminosalicylic acid; 5-ASA; fisalamine; mesalazine

U.S./Canadian Brand Names Asacol® [US/Can]; Canasa™ [US]; Mesasal® [Can]; Novo-5 ASA [Can]; Pentasa® [US/Can]; Quintasa® [Can]; Rowasa® [US/Can]; Salofalk® [Can]

Therapeutic Category 5-Aminosalicylic Acid Derivative

Use

Oral: Treatment and maintenance of remission of mildly to moderately active ulcerative colitis

Rectal: Treatment of active mild to moderate distal ulcerative colitis, proctosigmoiditis, or proctitis

Usual Dosage Adults (usual course of therapy is 3-8 weeks):

Oral:

Treatment of ulcerative colitis: Capsule: 1 g 4 times/day Tablet: Initial: 800 mg (2 tablets) 3 times/day for 6 weeks

Maintenance of remission of ulcerative colitis: Capsule: 1 g 4 times/day Tablet: 1.6 g/day in divided doses

Rectal:

Retention enema: 60 mL (4 g) at bedtime, retained overnight, approximately 8 hours

Rectal suppository: Insert 1 suppository in rectum twice daily; retain suppositories for at least 1-3 hours to achieve maximum benefit Canasa™: May increase to 3 times/day if inadequate response is seen after 2 weeks.

Note: Some patients may require rectal and oral therapy concurrently.

Dosage Forms

Capsule, controlled release (Pentasa®): 250 mg

Suppository, rectal (Canasa™): 500 mg

Suspension, rectal (Rowasa®): 4 g/60 mL (7s) [contains potassium metabisulfite and sodium benzoate]

Tablet, delayed release [enteric coated] (Asacol®): 400 mg

mesalazine *see* mesalamine *on previous page*

Mesantoin® *(Discontinued)* *see page 1042*

Mesasal® [Can] *see* mesalamine *on previous page*

M-Eslon® [Can] *see* morphine sulfate *on page 591*

mesna (MES na)

Synonyms sodium 2-mercaptoethane sulfonate

U.S./Canadian Brand Names Mesnex™ [US/Can]; Uromitexan™ [Can]

Therapeutic Category Antidote

Use **Orphan drug:** Prevention of hemorrhagic cystitis induced by ifosfamide

Usual Dosage Refer to individual protocols. Children and Adults:

I.V.: Recommended dose is 60% of the ifosfamide dose given in 3 divided doses (0, 4, and 8 hours after the start of ifosfamide)

Alternative I.V. regimens include 80% of the ifosfamide dose given in 4 divided doses (0, 3, 6, and 9 hours after the start of ifosfamide) and continuous infusions

Oral: 20% of the ifosfamide dose hour 0, followed by 40% of the ifosfamide dose given 4 and 8 hours (or 3, 6, and 9 hours) after start of ifosfamide

Dosage Forms

Injection, solution: 100 mg/mL (10 mL) [contains benzyl alcohol]

Tablet: 400 mg

Mesnex™ [US/Can] *see* mesna *on this page*

mesoridazine (mez oh RID a zeen)

Sound-Alike/Look-Alike Issues

Serentil® may be confused with selegiline, Serevent®, Seroquel®, sertraline, Serzone®, Sinequan®, Surgicel®

Synonyms mesoridazine besylate

U.S./Canadian Brand Names Serentil® [Can]

Therapeutic Category Phenothiazine Derivative

Use Management of schizophrenic patients who fail to respond adequately to treatment with other antipsychotic drugs, either because of insufficient effectiveness or the inability to achieve an effective dose due to intolerable adverse effects from these drugs

Usual Dosage Concentrate may be diluted just prior to administration with distilled water, acidified tap water, orange or grape juice; do not prepare and store bulk dilutions

Adults: Schizophrenia/psychoses:

Oral: 25-50 mg 3 times/day; maximum: 100-400 mg/day

I.M.: Initial: 25 mg, repeat in 30-60 minutes as needed; optimal dosage range: 25-200 mg/day

Dosage Forms [DSC] = Discontinued product

Injection, solution, as besylate [DSC]: 25 mg/mL (1 mL)

Liquid, oral, as besylate [DSC]: 25 mg/mL (118 mL) [contains alcohol 0.61%]

Tablet, as besylate [DSC]: 10 mg, 25 mg, 50 mg, 100 mg

mesoridazine besylate *see* mesoridazine *on this page*

Mestinon® [US/Can] *see* pyridostigmine *on page 751*

Mestinon® Injection *(Discontinued)* *see page 1042*

Mestinon®-SR [Can] *see* pyridostigmine *on page 751*

Mestinon® Timespan® [US] *see* pyridostigmine *on page 751*

mestranol and norethindrone (MES tra nole & nor eth IN drone)

Sound-Alike/Look-Alike Issues
Norinyl® may be confused with Nardil®

Synonyms norethindrone and mestranol

U.S./Canadian Brand Names Necon® 1/50 [US]; Norinyl® 1+50 [US]; Ortho-Novum® 1/50 [US/Can]

Therapeutic Category Contraceptive, Oral

Use Prevention of pregnancy

Usual Dosage Oral: Adults: Female: Contraception:

Schedule 1 (Sunday starter): Dose begins on first Sunday after onset of menstruation; if the menstrual period starts on Sunday, take first tablet that very same day. **With a Sunday start, an additional method of contraception should be used until after the first 7 days of consecutive administration.**

For 21-tablet package: Dosage is 1 tablet daily for 21 consecutive days, followed by 7 days off of the medication; a new course begins on the 8th day after the last tablet is taken.

For 28-tablet package: Dosage is 1 tablet daily without interruption.

Schedule 2 (Day 1 starter): Dose starts on first day of menstrual cycle taking 1 tablet daily.

For 21-tablet package: Dosage is 1 tablet daily for 21 consecutive days, followed by 7 days off of the medication; a new course begins on the 8th day after the last tablet is taken.

For 28-tablet package: Dosage is 1 tablet daily without interruption.

If all doses have been taken on schedule and one menstrual period is missed, continue dosing cycle. If two consecutive menstrual periods are missed, pregnancy test is required before new dosing cycle is started.

Missed doses **monophasic formulations** (refer to package insert for complete information):

One dose missed: Take as soon as remembered or take 2 tablets next day

Two consecutive doses missed in the first 2 weeks: Take 2 tablets as soon as remembered or 2 tablets next 2 days. **An additional method of contraception should be used for 7 days after missed dose.**

Two consecutive doses missed in week 3 or three consecutive doses missed at any time: **An additional method of contraception must be used for 7 days after a missed dose:**

Schedule 1 (Sunday starter): Continue dose of 1 tablet daily until Sunday, then discard the rest of the pack, and a new pack should be started that same day.

Schedule 2 (Day 1 starter): Current pack should be discarded, and a new pack should be started that same day.

Dosage Forms Tablet, monophasic formulations:

Necon® 1/50-21: Norethindrone 1 mg and mestranol 0.05 mg [light blue tablets] (21s)

Necon® 1/50-28: Norethindrone 1 mg and mestranol 0.05 mg [21 light blue tablets and 7 white inactive tablets] (28s)

Norinyl® 1+50: Norethindrone 1 mg and mestranol 0.05 mg [21 white tablets and 7 orange inactive tablets] (28s)

Ortho-Novum® 1/50: Norethindrone 1 mg and mestranol 0.05 mg [21 yellow tablets and 7 green inactive tablets] (28s)

metacortandralone *see* prednisolone (systemic) *on page 724*

Metadate® CD [US] *see* methylphenidate *on page 571*

Metadate™ ER [US] *see* methylphenidate *on page 571*

Metadol™ [Can] *see* methadone *on page 562*

Metaglip™ [US] *see* glipizide and metformin *on page 406*

Metahydrin® [Can] *see* trichlormethiazide *on page 883*

Metahydrin® *(Discontinued)* *see page 1042*

Metamucil® [Can] *see* psyllium *on page 749*

Metamucil® Smooth Texture [US-OTC] *see* psyllium *on page 749*

Metamucil® [US-OTC] *see* psyllium *on page 749*

Metaprel® Aerosol *(Discontinued)* *see page 1042*

Metaprel® Inhalation Solution *(Discontinued)* *see page 1042*

Metaprel® Syrup *(Discontinued)* *see page 1042*

Metaprel® Tablet *(Discontinued)* *see page 1042*

metaproterenol (met a proe TER e nol)

Sound-Alike/Look-Alike Issues

metaproterenol may be confused with metipranolol, metoprolol
Alupent® may be confused with Atrovent®

Synonyms metaproterenol sulfate; orciprenaline sulfate

U.S./Canadian Brand Names Alupent® [US]

Therapeutic Category Adrenergic Agonist Agent

Use Bronchodilator in reversible airway obstruction due to asthma or COPD; because of its delayed onset of action (1 hour) and prolonged effect (4 or more hours), this may not be the drug of choice for assessing response to a bronchodilator

Usual Dosage

Oral:

- Children:
  - <2 years: 0.4 mg/kg/dose given 3-4 times/day; in infants, the dose can be given every 8-12 hours
  - 2-6 years: 1-2.6 mg/kg/day divided every 6 hours
  - 6-9 years: 10 mg/dose 3-4 times/day
- Children >9 years and Adults: 20 mg 3-4 times/day

Inhalation: Children >12 years and Adults: 2-3 inhalations every 3-4 hours, up to 12 inhalations in 24 hours

Nebulizer:

- Infants and Children: 0.01-0.02 mL/kg of 5% solution; minimum dose: 0.1 mL; maximum dose: 0.3 mL diluted in 2-3 mL normal saline every 4-6 hours (may be given more frequently according to need)
- Adolescents and Adults: 5-20 breaths of full strength 5% metaproterenol **or** 0.2 to 0.3 mL 5% metaproterenol in 2.5-3 mL normal saline until nebulized every 4-6 hours (can be given more frequently according to need)

Dosage Forms

Aerosol for oral inhalation, as sulfate (Alupent®): 0.65 mg/inhalation (14 g) [200 doses]
Solution for oral inhalation, as sulfate [preservative free]: 0.4% [4 mg/mL] (2.5 mL); 0.6% [6 mg/mL] (2.5 mL); 5% [50 mg/mL] (10 mL, 30 mL)
Syrup, as sulfate: 10 mg/5 mL (480 mL) [may contain sodium benzoate]
Tablet, as sulfate: 10 mg, 20 mg

metaproterenol sulfate *see* metaproterenol *on this page*

metaraminol (met a RAM i nole)

Sound-Alike/Look-Alike Issues

Aramine® may be confused with Artane®

Synonyms metaraminol bitartrate

U.S./Canadian Brand Names Aramine® [Can]

Therapeutic Category Adrenergic Agonist Agent

Use Acute hypotensive crisis in the treatment of shock

Usual Dosage

Children:

- I.M.: 0.01 mg/kg as a single dose
- I.V.: 0.01 mg/kg as a single dose or intravenous infusion of 5 mcg/kg/minute

Adults:

- Prevention of hypotension: I.M., SubQ: 2-10 mg

(Continued)

metaraminol *(Continued)*

Adjunctive treatment of hypotension: I.V.: 15-100 mg in 250-500 mL NS or 5% dextrose in water

Severe shock: I.V.: 0.5-5 mg direct I.V. injection followed by intravenous infusion of 15-100 mg in 250-500 mL NS or D_5W; may also be administered endotracheally

Dosage Forms [DSC] = Discontinued product

Injection, solution, as bitartrate [DSC]: 10 mg/mL (10 mL) [contains sodium bisulfite]

metaraminol bitartrate *see* metaraminol *on previous page*

Metasep® *(Discontinued)* *see page 1042*

Metastron® [US/Can] *see* strontium-89 *on page 825*

Metatensin® [Can] *see* trichlormethiazide *on page 883*

metaxalone (me TAKS a lone)

Sound-Alike/Look-Alike Issues

metaxalone may be confused with metolazone

U.S./Canadian Brand Names Skelaxin® [US/Can]

Therapeutic Category Skeletal Muscle Relaxant

Use Relief of discomfort associated with acute, painful musculoskeletal conditions

Usual Dosage Children >12 years and Adults: Oral: 800 mg 3-4 times/day

Dosage Forms Tablet: 400 mg, 800 mg

metformin (met FOR min)

Sound-Alike/Look-Alike Issues

Glucophage® may be confused with Glucotrol®, Glutofac®

Synonyms metformin hydrochloride

U.S./Canadian Brand Names Alti-Metformin [Can]; Apo-Metformin® [Can]; Fortamet™ [US]; Gen-Metformin [Can]; Glucophage® [US/Can]; Glucophage® XR [US]; Glycon [Can]; Novo-Metformin [Can]; Nu-Metformin [Can]; PMS-Metformin [Can]; Rho®-Metformin [Can]; Rhoxal-metformin FC [Can]

Therapeutic Category Antidiabetic Agent, Oral

Use Management of type 2 diabetes mellitus (noninsulin dependent, NIDDM) as monotherapy when hyperglycemia cannot be managed on diet alone. May be used concomitantly with a sulfonylurea or insulin to improve glycemic control.

Usual Dosage Note: Allow 1-2 weeks between dose titrations: Generally, clinically significant responses are not seen at doses <1500 mg daily; however, a lower recommended starting dose and gradual increased dosage is recommended to minimize gastrointestinal symptoms

Children 10-16 years: Management of type 2 diabetes mellitus: Oral (500 mg tablet or oral solution): Initial: 500 mg twice daily (given with the morning and evening meals); increases in daily dosage should be made in increments of 500 mg at weekly intervals, given in divided doses, up to a maximum of 2000 mg/day

Adults ≥17 years: Management of type 2 diabetes mellitus: Oral:

Immediate release tablet or oral solution: Initial: 500 mg twice daily (give with the morning and evening meals) **or** 850 mg once daily; increase dosage incrementally.

Incremental dosing recommendations based on dosage form: 500 mg tablet: One tablet/day at weekly intervals 850 mg tablet: One tablet/day every other week Oral solution: 500 mg twice daily every other week

Doses of up to 2000 mg/day may be given twice daily. If a dose > 2000 mg/day is required, it may be better tolerated in three divided doses. Maximum recommended dose 2550 mg/day.

Extended release tablet: Initial: 500 mg once daily (with the evening meal); dosage may be increased by 500 mg weekly; maximum dose: 2000 mg once daily. If glycemic control is not achieved at maximum dose, may divide dose to 1000 mg twice daily. If doses >2000 mg/day are needed, switch to regular release tablets and titrate to maximum dose of 2550 mg/day.

Transfer from other antidiabetic agents: No transition period is generally necessary except when transferring from chlorpropamide. When transferring from chlorpropamide, care should be exercised during the first 2 weeks because of the prolonged retention of chlorpropamide in the body, leading to overlapping drug effects and possible hypoglycemia.

Concomitant metformin and oral sulfonylurea therapy: If patients have not responded to 4 weeks of the maximum dose of metformin monotherapy, consider a gradual addition of an oral sulfonylurea, even if prior primary or secondary failure to a sulfonylurea has occurred. Continue metformin at the maximum dose.

Failed sulfonylurea therapy: Patients with prior failure on glyburide may be treated by gradual addition of metformin. Initiate with glyburide 20 mg and metformin 500 mg daily. Metformin dosage may be increased by 500 mg/day at weekly intervals, up to a maximum of 2500 mg/day (dosage of glyburide maintained at 20 mg/day).

Concomitant metformin and insulin therapy: Initial: 500 mg metformin once daily, continue current insulin dose; increase by 500 mg metformin weekly until adequate glycemic control is achieved

Maximum dose: 2500 mg metformin; 2000 mg metformin extended release

Decrease insulin dose 10% to 25% when FPG <120 mg/dL; monitor and make further adjustments as needed

Dosage Forms

Solution, oral, as hydrochloride (Riomet™): 100 mg/mL (118 mL, 473 mL) [contains saccharin; cherry flavor]

Tablet, as hydrochloride (Glucophage®): 500 mg, 850 mg, 1000 mg

Tablet, extended release, as hydrochloride: 500 mg

Fortamet™: 500 mg, 1000 mg

Glucophage® XR: 500 mg, 750 mg

metformin and glipizide *see* glipizide and metformin *on page 406*

metformin and glyburide *see* glyburide and metformin *on page 409*

metformin and rosiglitazone *see* rosiglitazone and metformin *on page 786*

metformin hydrochloride *see* metformin *on previous page*

metformin hydrochloride and rosiglitazone maleate *see* rosiglitazone and metformin *on page 786*

methacholine (meth a KOLE leen)

Synonyms methacholine chloride

U.S./Canadian Brand Names Provocholine® [US/Can]

Therapeutic Category Diagnostic Agent

Use Diagnosis of bronchial airway hyperactivity

Usual Dosage The table is a suggested schedule for administration of methacholine challenge. Calculate cumulative units by multiplying number of breaths by concentration given. Total cumulative units is the sum of cumulative units for each concentration given.

Vial	Serial Concentration (mg/mL)	No. of Breaths	Cumulative Units per Concentration	Total Cumulative Units
E	0.025	5	0.125	0.125
D	0.25	5	1.25	1.375
C	2.5	5	12.5	13.88
B	10	5	50	63.88
A	25	5	125	188.88

Dosage Forms Powder for oral inhalation, as chloride: 100 mg

methacholine chloride *see* methacholine *on this page*

methadone (METH a done)

Sound-Alike/Look-Alike Issues

methadone may be confused with Mephyton®, methylphenidate

Synonyms methadone hydrochloride

U.S./Canadian Brand Names Dolophine® [US/Can]; Metadol™ [Can]; Methadone Intensol™ [US]; Methadose® [US/Can]

Therapeutic Category Analgesic, Narcotic

Controlled Substance C-II

Use Management of severe pain; detoxification and maintenance treatment of narcotic addiction (if used for detoxification and maintenance treatment of narcotic addiction, it must be part of an FDA-approved program)

Usual Dosage Note: These are guidelines and do not represent the maximum doses that may be required in all patients. Methadone accumulates with repeated doses and dosage may need reduction after 3-5 days to prevent CNS depressant effects. Some patients may benefit from every 8-12 hour dosing interval for chronic pain management. Doses should be titrated to appropriate effects.

Adults:

Pain (analgesia):

Oral: Initial: 5-10 mg; dosing interval may range from 4-12 hours during initial therapy; decrease in dose or frequency may be required (~days 2-5) due to accumulation with repeated doses

Manufacturer's labeling: 2.5-10 mg every 3-4 hours as needed

I.V.: Manufacturers labeling: Initial: 2.5-10 mg every 8-12 hours in opioid-naive patients; titrate slowly to effect; may also be administered by SubQ or I.M. injection

Conversion from oral to parenteral dose: Initial dose: Oral: parenteral: 2:1 ratio

Detoxification: Oral: 15-40 mg/day

Maintenance treatment of opiate dependence: Oral: 20-120 mg/day

Dosage Forms

Injection, solution, as hydrochloride: 10 mg/mL (20 mL)

Solution, oral, as hydrochloride: 5 mg/5 mL (500 mL); 10 mg/5 mL (500 mL) [contains alcohol 8%; citrus flavor]

Solution, oral concentrate, as hydrochloride: 10 mg/mL (30 mL)

Methadone Intensol™: 10 mg/mL (30 mL)

Methadose®: 10 mg/mL (30 mL) [cherry flavor]

Tablet, as hydrochloride (Dolophine®, Methadose®): 5 mg, 10 mg

Tablet, dispersible, as hydrochloride:

Methadose®: 40 mg

Methadone Diskets®: 40 mg [orange-pineapple flavor]

methadone hydrochloride *see* methadone *on this page*

Methadone Intensol™ [US] *see* methadone *on this page*

Methadose® [US/Can] *see* methadone *on this page*

methaminodiazepoxide hydrochloride *see* chlordiazepoxide *on page 183*

methamphetamine (meth am FET a meen)

Sound-Alike/Look-Alike Issues

Desoxyn® may be confused with digoxin

Synonyms desoxyephedrine hydrochloride; methamphetamine hydrochloride

U.S./Canadian Brand Names Desoxyn® [US/Can]

Therapeutic Category Amphetamine

Controlled Substance C-II

Use Treatment of attention-deficit/hyperactivity disorder (ADHD); exogenous obesity (short-term adjunct)

Usual Dosage Oral:

Children >6 years and Adults: ADHD: 2.5-5 mg 1-2 times/day; may increase by 5 mg increments at weekly intervals until optimum response is achieved, usually 20-25 mg/day

Children >12 years and Adults: Exogenous obesity: 5 mg 30 minutes before each meal; treatment duration should not exceed a few weeks

Dosage Forms Tablet, as hydrochloride: 5 mg

methamphetamine hydrochloride *see* methamphetamine *on previous page*

methazolamide (meth a ZOE la mide)

Sound-Alike/Look-Alike Issues

methazolamide may be confused with methenamine, metolazone

Neptazane® may be confused with Nesacaine®

U.S./Canadian Brand Names Apo-Methazolamide® [Can]

Therapeutic Category Carbonic Anhydrase Inhibitor

Use Adjunctive treatment of open-angle or secondary glaucoma; short-term therapy of narrow-angle glaucoma when delay of surgery is desired

Usual Dosage Adults: Oral: 50-100 mg 2-3 times/day

Dosage Forms Tablet: 25 mg, 50 mg

methenamine (meth EN a meen)

Sound-Alike/Look-Alike Issues

methenamine may be confused with methazolamide, methionine

Urex® may be confused with Eurax®, Serax®

Synonyms hexamethylenetetramine; methenamine hippurate; methenamine mandelate

U.S./Canadian Brand Names Dehydral® [Can]; Hiprex® [US/Can]; Mandelamine® [US/Can]; Urasal® [Can]; Urex® [US/Can]

Therapeutic Category Antibiotic, Miscellaneous

Use Prophylaxis or suppression of recurrent urinary tract infections; urinary tract discomfort secondary to hypermotility

Usual Dosage Oral:

Children:

>2-6 years: *Mandelate:* 50-75 mg/kg/day in 3-4 doses or 0.25 g/30 lb 4 times/day

6-12 years:

Hippurate: 0.5-1 g twice daily

Mandelate: 50-75 mg/kg/day in 3-4 doses or 0.5 g 4 times/day

>12 years and Adults:

Hippurate: 0.5-1 g twice daily

Mandelate: 1 g 4 times/day after meals and at bedtime

Dosage Forms

Tablet, as hippurate (Hiprex®, Urex®): 1 g [Hiprex® contains tartrazine dye]

Tablet, enteric coated, as mandelate (Mandelamine®): 500 mg, 1 g

methenamine hippurate *see* methenamine *on this page*

methenamine mandelate *see* methenamine *on this page*

methenamine, phenyl salicylate, atropine, hyoscyamine, benzoic acid, and methylene blue

(meth EN a meen, fen nil sa LIS i late, A troe peen, hye oh SYE a meen, ben ZOE ik AS id, & METH i leen bloo)

Therapeutic Category Antibiotic, Urinary Antiinfective; Urinary Tract Product

Use Urinary tract infections

Usual Dosage Adults: Oral: Two tablets 4 times/day

Dosage Forms Tablet: Methenamine 40.8 mg, phenyl salicylate 18.1 mg, atropine sulfate 0.03 mg, hyoscyamine sulfate 0.03 mg, benzoic acid 4.5 mg, and methylene blue 5.4 mg

Methergine® [US/Can] *see* methylergonovine *on page 570*

methicillin *(Discontinued)* *see page 1042*

methimazole (meth IM a zole)

Synonyms thiamazole

U.S./Canadian Brand Names Tapazole® [US/Can]

Therapeutic Category Antithyroid Agent

Use Palliative treatment of hyperthyroidism, return the hyperthyroid patient to a normal metabolic state prior to thyroidectomy, and to control thyrotoxic crisis that may accompany thyroidectomy. The use of antithyroid thioamides is as effective in elderly as they are in younger adults; however, the expense, potential adverse effects, and inconvenience (compliance, monitoring) make them undesirable. The use of radioiodine due to ease of administration and less concern for long-term side effects and reproduction problems (some older males) makes it a more appropriate therapy.

Usual Dosage Oral: Administer in 3 equally divided doses at approximately 8-hour intervals

Children: Initial: 0.4 mg/kg/day in 3 divided doses; maintenance: 0.2 mg/kg/day in 3 divided doses up to 30 mg/24 hours maximum

Alternatively: Initial: 0.5-0.7 mg/kg/day **or** 15-20 mg/m^2/day in 3 divided doses

Maintenance: $^1/_3$ to $^2/_3$ of the initial dose beginning when the patient is euthyroid

Maximum: 30 mg/24 hours

Adults: Initial: 15 mg/day for mild hyperthyroidism; 30-40 mg/day in moderately severe hyperthyroidism; 60 mg/day in severe hyperthyroidism; maintenance: 5-15 mg/day

Adjust dosage as required to achieve and maintain serum T_3, T_4, and TSH levels in the normal range. An elevated T_3 may be the sole indicator of inadequate treatment. An elevated TSH indicates excessive antithyroid treatment.

Dosage Forms Tablet: 5 mg, 10 mg

methionine (me THYE oh neen)

Sound-Alike/Look-Alike Issues

methionine may be confused with methenamine

U.S./Canadian Brand Names ME-500® [US]; Pedameth® [US]

Therapeutic Category Dietary Supplement

Use Treatment of diaper rash and control of odor, dermatitis and ulceration caused by ammoniacal urine

Usual Dosage Oral:

Children: Control of diaper rash: 75 mg in formula or other liquid 3-4 times/day for 3-5 days

Adults:

Control of odor in incontinent adults: 200-400 mg 3-4 times/day

Dietary supplement: 500 mg/day

Dosage Forms

Capsule (ME-500®): 500 mg

Liquid (Pedameth®): 75 mg/5 mL (480 mL)

Tablet: 500 mg

Methitest® [US] *see* methyltestosterone *on page 573*

methocarbamol (meth oh KAR ba mole)

Sound-Alike/Look-Alike Issues

methocarbamol may be confused with mephobarbital

Robaxin® may be confused with Rubex®

U.S./Canadian Brand Names Robaxin® [US/Can]

Therapeutic Category Skeletal Muscle Relaxant

Use Treatment of muscle spasm associated with acute painful musculoskeletal conditions; supportive therapy in tetanus

Usual Dosage

Tetanus: I.V.:

Children: Recommended **only** for use in tetanus: 15 mg/kg/dose or 500 mg/m^2/dose, may repeat every 6 hours if needed; maximum dose: 1.8 g/m^2/day for 3 days only

Adults: Initial dose: 1-3 g; may repeat dose every 6 hours until oral dosing is possible; injection should not be used for more than 3 consecutive days

Muscle spasm: Children ≥16 years and Adults:

Oral: 1.5 g 4 times/day for 2-3 days (up to 8 g/day may be given in severe conditions), then decrease to 4-4.5 g/day in 3-6 divided doses

I.M., I.V.: 1 g every 8 hours if oral not possible; injection should not be used for more than 3 consecutive days. If condition persists, may repeat course of therapy after a drug-free interval of 48 hours.

Dosage Forms

Injection, solution: 100 mg/mL (10 mL) [in polyethylene glycol; vial stopper contains latex]

Tablet: 500 mg, 750 mg

methocarbamol and aspirin (meth oh KAR ba mole & AS pir in)

Synonyms aspirin and methocarbamol

Therapeutic Category Skeletal Muscle Relaxant

Use Adjunct to rest, physical therapy, and other measures for the relief of discomfort associated with acute, painful musculoskeletal disorders

Usual Dosage Children >12 years and Adults: Oral: 2 tablets 4 times/day

Dosage Forms Tablet: Methocarbamol 400 mg and aspirin 325 mg

methohexital (meth oh HEKS i tal)

Sound-Alike/Look-Alike Issues

Brevital® may be confused with Brevibloc®

Synonyms methohexital sodium

U.S./Canadian Brand Names Brevital® Sodium [US/Can]

Therapeutic Category Barbiturate

Controlled Substance C-IV

Use Induction and maintenance of general anesthesia for short procedures

Can be used in pediatric patients ≥1 month of age as follows: For rectal or intramuscular induction of anesthesia prior to the use of other general anesthetic agents, as an adjunct to subpotent inhalational anesthetic agents for short surgical procedures, or for short surgical, diagnostic, or therapeutic procedures associated with minimal painful stimuli

Usual Dosage Doses must be titrated to effect

Manufacturer's recommendations:

Infants <1 month: Safety and efficacy not established

Infants ≥1 month and Children:

I.M.: Induction: 6.6-10 mg/kg of a 5% solution

Rectal: Induction: Usual: 25 mg/kg of a 1% solution

Alternative pediatric dosing:

Children 3-12 years:

I.M.: Preoperative: 5-10 mg/kg/dose

I.V.: Induction: 1-2 mg/kg/dose

Rectal: Preoperative/induction: 20-35 mg/kg/dose; usual: 25 mg/kg/dose; maximum dose: 500 mg/dose; give as 10% aqueous solution

Adults: I.V.:

Induction: 50-120 mg to start; 20-40 mg every 4-7 minutes

Dosage Forms Injection, powder for reconstitution, as sodium: 500 mg, 2.5 g, 5 g

methohexital sodium *see* methohexital *on this page*

methotrexate (meth oh TREKS ate)

Sound-Alike/Look-Alike Issues

methotrexate may be confused with metolazone

Synonyms amethopterin; methotrexate sodium; MTX; NSC-740

U.S./Canadian Brand Names Apo-Methotrexate® [Can]; ratio-Methotrexate [Can]; Rheumatrex® [US]; Trexall™ [US]

(Continued)

methotrexate *(Continued)*

Therapeutic Category Antineoplastic Agent

Use Treatment of trophoblastic neoplasms; leukemias; psoriasis; rheumatoid arthritis (RA), including polyarticular-course juvenile rheumatoid arthritis (JRA); breast, head and neck, and lung carcinomas; osteosarcoma; soft-tissue sarcomas; carcinoma of gastrointestinal tract, esophagus, testes; lymphomas

Dosage Forms

Injection, powder for reconstitution [preservative free]: 20 mg, 1 g

Injection, solution, as sodium: 25 mg/mL (2 mL, 10 mL) [contains benzyl alcohol]

Injection, solution, as sodium [preservative free]: 25 mg/mL (2 mL, 4 mL, 8 mL, 10 mL)

Tablet, as sodium: 2.5 mg

Rheumatrex®: 2.5 mg

Trexall™: 5 mg, 7.5 mg, 10 mg, 15 mg

Tablet, as sodium [dose pack] (Rheumatrex® Dose Pack): 2.5 mg (4 cards with 2, 3, 4, 5, or 6 tablets each)

methotrexate sodium *see* methotrexate *on previous page*

methotrimeprazine *(Canada only)* (meth oh trye MEP ra zeen)

Synonyms levomepromazine; methotrimeprazine hydrochloride

U.S./Canadian Brand Names Apo-Methoprazine® [Can]; Novo-Meprazine [Can]; Nozinan® [Can]

Therapeutic Category Neuroleptic Agent

Use Treatment of schizophrenia or psychosis; management of pain, including pain caused by neuralgia or cancer; adjunct to general anesthesia; management of nausea and vomiting; sedation

Usual Dosage

Children >2 years:

Oral: 0.25 mg/kg/day in 2-3 divided doses; may increase gradually based on response. Maximum dose: 40 mg/day in children <12 years

I.M.: 0.06-0.125 mg/kg/day in 1-3 divided doses

Adults:

Oral:

Anxiety, mild-moderate pain: 6-25 mg/day in 3 divided doses

Psychoses, severe pain: 50-75 mg/day in 2-3 divided doses; titrate to effect (doses up to 1000 mg/day or greater have been used in treatment of some patients with psychoses). If higher dosages are used to initiate therapy (100-200 mg/day), patients should be restricted to bed for the first few days of therapy.

Sedative: 10-25 mg at bedtime

I.M.:

Psychoses, severe pain: 75-100 mg (administered in 3-4 deep I.M. injections)

Analgesia (postoperative): 10-25 mg every 8 hours (2.5-7.5 mg every 4-6 hours is suggested postoperatively if residual effects of anesthetic may be present)

Premedication: 10-25 mg every 8 hours (final preoperative dose may be 25-50 mg administered ~1 hour prior to surgery)

I.V.: During surgical procedures/labor: 20-50 mcg/minute (some patients may require up to 100 mcg/minute)

SubQ (continuous infusion): Palliative care: : 25-200 mcg/day (via syringe driver)

Dosage Forms

Injection, solution, as hydrochloride: 25 mg/mL (1 mL)

Solution, oral: 5 mg/mL (500 mL) [contains ethanol 2%]

Solution, oral drops: 40 mg/mL (100 mL) [contains ethanol 16.5%]

Tablet, as maleate: 2 mg, 5 mg, 25 mg, 50 mg

methotrimeprazine hydrochloride *see* methotrimeprazine *(Canada only)* *on this page*

methoxsalen (meth OKS a len)

Synonyms methoxypsoralen; 8-methoxypsoralen

U.S./Canadian Brand Names 8-MOP® [US/Can]; Oxsoralen® [US/Can]; Oxsoralen-Ultra® [US/Can]; Ultramop™ [Can]; Uvadex® [US/Can]

Therapeutic Category Psoralen

Use

Oral: Symptomatic control of severe, recalcitrant disabling psoriasis; repigmentation of idiopathic vitiligo; palliative treatment of skin manifestations of cutaneous T-cell lymphoma (CTCL)

Topical: Repigmentation of idiopathic vitiligo

Extracorporeal: Palliative treatment of skin manifestations of CTCL

Usual Dosage Note: Refer to treatment protocols for UVA exposure guidelines.

Children >12 years and Adults: Vitiligo: Topical: Apply lotion 1-2 hours before exposure to UVA light, no more than once weekly

Adults:

Psoriasis: Oral: 10-70 mg 11/2-2 hours before exposure to UVA light; dose may be repeated 2-3 times per week, based on UVA exposure; doses must be given at least 48 hours apart; dosage is based upon patient's body weight and skin type:

<30 kg: 10 mg
30-50 kg: 20 mg
51-65 kg: 30 mg
66-80 kg: 40 mg
81-90 kg: 50 mg
91-115 kg: 60 mg
>115 kg: 70 mg

Vitiligo: (8-MOP®): Oral: 20 mg 2-4 hours before exposure to UVA light; dose may be repeated based on erythema and tenderness of skin; do not give on 2 consecutive days

CTCL: Extracorporeal (Uvadex®): 200 mcg injected into the photoactivation bag during the collection cycle using the UVAR® photopheresis system (consult user's guide). Treatment schedule: Two consecutive days every 4 weeks for a minimum of 7 treatment cycles

Dosage Forms

Capsule:

8-MOP®: 10 mg [hard-gelatin capsule]

Oxsoralen-Ultra®: 10 mg [soft-gelatin capsule]

Lotion (Oxsoralen®): 1% (30 mL) [contains alcohol 71%]

Solution, for extracorporeal administration (Uvadex®): 20 mcg/mL (10 mL) **[not for injection]**

methoxycinnamate and oxybenzone

(meth OKS ee SIN a mate & oks i BEN zone)

Synonyms sunscreen (paba-free)

Therapeutic Category Sunscreen

Use Reduce the chance of premature aging of the skin and skin cancer from overexposure to the sun

Usual Dosage Adults: Topical: Apply liberally to all exposed areas at least 30 minutes prior to sun exposure

Dosage Forms Lotion:

SPF 15: 120 mL
SPF 29: 120 mL

methoxypsoralen *see* methoxsalen *on this page*

8-methoxypsoralen *see* methoxsalen *on this page*

methscopolamine (meth skoe POL a meen)

Synonyms methscopolamine bromide

U.S./Canadian Brand Names Pamine® [US/Can]; Pamine® Forte [US]

(Continued)

methscopolamine *(Continued)*

Therapeutic Category Anticholinergic Agent

Use Adjunctive therapy in the treatment of peptic ulcer

Usual Dosage Adults: Oral: 2.5 mg 30 minutes before meals or food and 2.5-5 mg at bedtime; may increase dose to 5 mg twice daily

Dosage Forms Tablet, as bromide:

Pamine®: 2.5 mg

Pamine® Forte: 5 mg

methscopolamine bromide *see* methscopolamine *on previous page*

methscopolamine, chlorpheniramine, and phenylephrine *see* chlorpheniramine, phenylephrine, and methscopolamine *on page 192*

methsuximide (meth SUKS i mide)

Sound-Alike/Look-Alike Issues

methsuximide may be confused with ethosuximide

U.S./Canadian Brand Names Celontin® [US/Can]

Therapeutic Category Anticonvulsant

Use Control of absence (petit mal) seizures that are refractory to other drugs

Usual Dosage Oral:

Children: Anticonvulsant: Initial: 10-15 mg/kg/day in 3-4 divided doses; increase weekly up to maximum of 30 mg/kg/day

Adults: Anticonvulsant: 300 mg/day for the first week; may increase by 300 mg/day at weekly intervals up to 1.2 g/day in 2-4 divided doses/day

Dosage Forms Capsule: 150 mg, 300 mg

methyclothiazide (meth i kloe THYE a zide)

Sound-Alike/Look-Alike Issues

Enduron® may be confused with Empirin®, Imuran®, Inderal®

U.S./Canadian Brand Names Aquatensen® [US/Can]; Enduron® [US/Can]

Therapeutic Category Diuretic, Thiazide

Use Management of mild to moderate hypertension; treatment of edema in congestive heart failure and nephrotic syndrome

Usual Dosage Adults: Oral:

Edema: 2.5-10 mg/day

Hypertension: 2.5-5 mg/day; may add another antihypertensive if 5 mg is not adequate after a trial of 8-12 weeks of therapy

Dosage Forms Tablet: 5 mg

methyclothiazide and deserpidine

(meth i kloe THYE a zide & de SER pi deen)

Sound-Alike/Look-Alike Issues

Enduronyl® may be confused with Inderal®

Enduronyl® Forte may be confused with Inderal® 40

Synonyms deserpidine and methyclothiazide

U.S./Canadian Brand Names Enduronyl® Forte [US/Can]; Enduronyl® [US/Can]

Therapeutic Category Antihypertensive Agent, Combination

Use Management of mild to moderately severe hypertension

Usual Dosage Oral: Individualized, normally 1-4 tablets/day

Dosage Forms Tablet:

Enduronyl®: Methyclothiazide 5 mg and deserpidine 0.25 mg

Enduronyl® Forte: Methyclothiazide 5 mg and deserpidine 0.5 mg

methylacetoxyprogesterone *see* medroxyprogesterone acetate *on page 548*

methylcellulose (meth il SEL yoo lose)

Sound-Alike/Look-Alike Issues

Citrucel® may be confused with Citracal®

U.S./Canadian Brand Names Citrucel® [US-OTC]; FiberEase™ [US-OTC]

Therapeutic Category Laxative

Use Adjunct in treatment of constipation

Usual Dosage Oral:

Children 6-12 years:

Citrucel® caplet: 1 caplet up to 6 times/day; follow each dose with 8 oz of water

Citrucel® powder: Half the adult dose in 4 oz of cold water, 1-3 times/day

Children ≥12 years and Adults:

Citrucel® caplet: 2-4 caplets 1-3 times/day; follow each dose with 8 oz of water

Citrucel® powder: 1 heaping tablespoon (19 g) in 8 oz of cold water, 1-3 times/day

FiberEase™: 2 tablespoonsful mixed in 7 oz of water, 1-3 times/day

Dosage Forms

Caplet (Citrucel®): 500 mg

Liquid (FiberEase™): 4 g/30 mL (414 mL) [available in regular or dietetic formulations; orange and apple-raspberry flavors]

Powder:

Citrucel® [clear mix formulation]: 2 g/level scoop (275 g, 539 g)

Citrucel® [regular formulation]: 2 g/level scoop (448 g, 840 g); 2 g/packet (20s) [orange flavor]

Citrucel® [sugar free formulation]: 2 g/level scoop (241 g, 473 g) [contains phenylalanine 52 mg/level scoop; orange flavor]; 2 g/packet (20s) [contains phenylalanine 52 mg/packet; orange flavor]

methylcellulose, gelatin, and pectin *see* gelatin, pectin, and methylcellulose *on page 399*

methyldopa (meth il DOE pa)

Sound-Alike/Look-Alike Issues

methyldopa may be confused with l-dopa, levodopa

Synonyms methyldopate hydrochloride

U.S./Canadian Brand Names Apo-Methyldopa® [Can]; Nu-Medopa [Can]

Therapeutic Category Alpha-Adrenergic Blocking Agent

Use Management of moderate to severe hypertension

Usual Dosage

Children:

Oral: Initial: 10 mg/kg/day in 2-4 divided doses; increase every 2 days as needed to maximum dose of 65 mg/kg/day; do not exceed 3 g/day.

I.V.: 5-10 mg/kg/dose every 6-8 hours up to a total dose of 65 mg/kg/24 hours or 3 g/24 hours

Adults:

Oral: Initial: 250 mg 2-3 times/day; increase every 2 days as needed (maximum dose: 3 g/day): usual dose range (JNC 7): 250-1000 mg/day in 2 divided doses

I.V.: 250-500 mg every 6-8 hours; maximum dose: 1 g every 6 hours

Dosage Forms

Injection, solution, as methyldopate hydrochloride: 50 mg/mL (5 mL) [contains sodium bisulfite]

Tablet: 250 mg, 500 mg

methyldopa and hydrochlorothiazide

(meth il DOE pa & hye droe klor oh THYE a zide)

Sound-Alike/Look-Alike Issues

Aldoril® may be confused with Aldoclor®, Aldomet®, Elavil®

Synonyms hydrochlorothiazide and methyldopa

U.S./Canadian Brand Names Aldoril® [US]; Aldoril® D [US]; Apo-Methazide® [Can]

Therapeutic Category Antihypertensive Agent, Combination

(Continued)

methyldopa and hydrochlorothiazide *(Continued)*

Use Management of moderate to severe hypertension

Usual Dosage Oral: Dosage titrated on individual components, then switch to combination product; no more than methyldopa 3 g/day and/or hydrochlorothiazide 50 mg/day; maintain initial dose for first 48 hours, then decrease or increase at intervals of not less than 2 days until an adequate response is achieved

Methyldopa 250 mg and hydrochlorothiazide 15 mg: 2-3 times/day

Methyldopa 250 mg and hydrochlorothiazide 25 mg: Twice daily

Methyldopa 500 mg and hydrochlorothiazide 30 mg: Once daily

Dosage Forms Tablet: Methyldopa 250 mg and hydrochlorothiazide 15 mg; methyldopa 250 mg and hydrochlorothiazide 25 mg

Aldoril® 15: Methyldopa 250 mg and hydrochlorothiazide 15 mg

Aldoril® 25: Methyldopa 250 mg and hydrochlorothiazide 25 mg

Aldoril® D30: Methyldopa 500 mg and hydrochlorothiazide 30 mg

methyldopate hydrochloride *see* methyldopa *on previous page*

methylene blue (METH i leen bloo)

U.S./Canadian Brand Names Urolene Blue® [US]

Therapeutic Category Antidote

Use Antidote for cyanide poisoning and drug-induced methemoglobinemia, indicator dye

Usual Dosage

Children: NADPH-methemoglobin reductase deficiency: Oral: 1-1.5 mg/kg/day (maximum: 300 mg/day) given with 5-8 mg/kg/day of ascorbic acid

Children and Adults: Methemoglobinemia: I.V.: 1-2 mg/kg or 25-50 mg/m^2 over several minutes; may be repeated in 1 hour if necessary

Adults: Genitourinary antiseptic: Oral: 65-130 mg 3 times/day with a full glass of water (maximum: 390 mg/day)

Dosage Forms

Injection, solution: 10 mg/mL (1 mL, 10 mL)

Tablet (Urolene Blue®): 65 mg

methylergometrine maleate *see* methylergonovine *on this page*

methylergonovine (meth il er goe NOE veen)

Synonyms methylergometrine maleate; methylergonovine maleate

U.S./Canadian Brand Names Methergine® [US/Can]

Therapeutic Category Ergot Alkaloid and Derivative

Use Prevention and treatment of postpartum and postabortion hemorrhage caused by uterine atony or subinvolution

Usual Dosage Adults:

Oral: 0.2 mg 3-4 times/day for 2-7 days

I.M.: 0.2 mg after delivery of anterior shoulder, after delivery of placenta, or during puerperium; may be repeated as required at intervals of 2-4 hours

I.V.: Same dose as I.M., but should not be routinely administered I.V. because of possibility of inducing sudden hypertension and cerebrovascular accident

Dosage Forms

Injection, solution, as maleate: 0.2 mg/mL (1 mL)

Tablet, as maleate: 0.2 mg

methylergonovine maleate *see* methylergonovine *on this page*

Methylin™ [US] *see* methylphenidate *on next page*

Methylin™ ER [US] *see* methylphenidate *on next page*

methylmorphine *see* codeine *on page 221*

methylphenidate (meth il FEN i date)

Sound-Alike/Look-Alike Issues

methylphenidate may be confused with methadone

Ritalin® may be confused with Ismelin®, Rifadin®

Synonyms methylphenidate hydrochloride

U.S./Canadian Brand Names Concerta® [US/Can]; Metadate® CD [US]; Metadate™ ER [US]; Methylin™ [US]; Methylin™ ER [US]; PMS-Methylphenidate [Can]; Ritalin® [US/Can]; Ritalin® LA [US]; Ritalin-SR® [US/Can]

Therapeutic Category Central Nervous System Stimulant, Nonamphetamine

Controlled Substance C-II

Use Treatment of attention-deficit/hyperactivity disorder (ADHD); symptomatic management of narcolepsy

Usual Dosage Oral (discontinue periodically to re-evaluate or if no improvement occurs within 1 month):

Children ≥6 years: ADHD: Initial: 0.3 mg/kg/dose or 2.5-5 mg/dose given before breakfast and lunch; increase by 0.1 mg/kg/dose or by 5-10 mg/day at weekly intervals; usual dose: 0.5-1 mg/kg/day; maximum dose: 2 mg/kg/day or 90 mg/day

Extended release products:

Metadate™ ER, Methylin™ ER, Ritalin® SR: Duration of action is 8 hours. May be given in place of regular tablets, once the daily dose is titrated using the regular tablets and the titrated 8-hour dosage corresponds to sustained release tablet size.

Metadate® CD, Ritalin® LA: Initial: 20 mg once daily; may be adjusted in 10-20 mg increments at weekly intervals; maximum: 60 mg/day

Concerta®: Duration of action is 12 hours:

Children not currently taking methylphenidate: Initial: 18 mg once daily in the morning Adjustment: May increase to maximum of 54 mg/day in increments of 18 mg/day; dose may be adjusted at weekly intervals

Children currently taking methylphenidate: **Note:** Dosing based on current regimen and clinical judgment; suggested dosing listed below: Patients taking methylphenidate 5 mg 2-3 times/day or 20 mg/day sustained release formulation: Initial dose: 18 mg once every morning (maximum: 54 mg/day). Patients taking methylphenidate 10 mg 2-3 times/day or 40 mg/day sustained release formulation: Initial dose: 36 mg once every morning (maximum: 54 mg/day) Patients taking methylphenidate 15 mg 2-3 times/day or 60 mg/day sustained release formulation: Initial dose: 54 mg once every morning (maximum: 54 mg/day)

Note: A 27 mg dosage strength is available for situations in which a dosage between 18 mg and 36 mg is desired.

Adults: Narcolepsy: 10 mg 2-3 times/day, up to 60 mg/day

Dosage Forms

Capsule, extended release, as hydrochloride:

Metadate® CD: 10 mg, 20 mg, 30 mg

Ritalin® LA: 10 mg, 20 mg, 30 mg, 40 mg

Tablet, as hydrochloride (Methylin™, Ritalin®): 5 mg, 10 mg, 20 mg

Tablet, extended release, as hydrochloride: 20 mg

Concerta®: 18 mg, 27 mg, 36 mg, 54 mg [osmotic controlled release]

Metadate™ ER, Methylin™ ER: 10 mg, 20 mg

Tablet, sustained release, as hydrochloride (Ritalin-SR®): 20 mg

methylphenidate hydrochloride *see* methylphenidate *on this page*

methylphenobarbital *see* mephobarbital *on page 553*

methylphenoxy-benzene propanamine *see* atomoxetine *on page 86*

methylphenyl isoxazolyl penicillin *see* oxacillin *on page 651*

methylphytyl napthoquinone *see* phytonadione *on page 693*

methylprednisolone (meth il pred NIS oh lone)

Sound-Alike/Look-Alike Issues

methylprednisolone may be confused with medroxyprogesterone, prednisone
Depo-Medrol® may be confused with Solu-Medrol®
Medrol® may be confused with Mebaral®
Solu-Medrol® may be confused with Depo-Medrol®

Synonyms 6-α-methylprednisolone; methylprednisolone acetate; methylprednisolone sodium succinate

Tall-Man methyl**PREDNIS**olone

U.S./Canadian Brand Names A-methapred® [US]; Depo-Medrol® [US/Can]; Medrol® [US/Can]; Solu-Medrol® [US/Can]

Therapeutic Category Adrenal Corticosteroid

Use Primarily as an antiinflammatory or immunosuppressant agent in the treatment of a variety of diseases including those of hematologic, allergic, inflammatory, neoplastic, and autoimmune origin. Prevention and treatment of graft-versus-host disease following allogeneic bone marrow transplantation.

Usual Dosage Dosing should be based on the lesser of ideal body weight or actual body weight

Only sodium succinate may be given I.V.; methylprednisolone sodium succinate is highly soluble and has a rapid effect by I.M. and I.V. routes. Methylprednisolone acetate has a low solubility and has a sustained I.M. effect.

Children:

Antiinflammatory or immunosuppressive: Oral, I.M., I.V. (sodium succinate): 0.5-1.7 mg/kg/day **or** 5-25 mg/m²/day in divided doses every 6-12 hours; "Pulse" therapy: 15-30 mg/kg/dose over ≥30 minutes given once daily for 3 days

Status asthmaticus: I.V. (sodium succinate): Loading dose: 2 mg/kg/dose, then 0.5-1 mg/kg/dose every 6 hours for up to 5 days

Acute spinal cord injury: I.V. (sodium succinate): 30 mg/kg over 15 minutes, followed in 45 minutes by a continuous infusion of 5.4 mg/kg/hour for 23 hours

Lupus nephritis: I.V. (sodium succinate): 30 mg/kg over ≥30 minutes every other day for 6 doses

Adults: **Only sodium succinate may be given I.V.;** methylprednisolone sodium succinate is highly soluble and has a rapid effect by I.M. and I.V. routes. Methylprednisolone acetate has a low solubility and has a sustained I.M. effect.

Acute spinal cord injury: I.V. (sodium succinate): 30 mg/kg over 15 minutes, followed in 45 minutes by a continuous infusion of 5.4 mg/kg/hour for 23 hours

Antiinflammatory or immunosuppressive:

Oral: 2-60 mg/day in 1-4 divided doses to start, followed by gradual reduction in dosage to the lowest possible level consistent with maintaining an adequate clinical response.

I.M. (sodium succinate): 10-80 mg/day once daily

I.M. (acetate): 10-80 mg every 1-2 weeks

I.V. (sodium succinate): 10-40 mg over a period of several minutes and repeated I.V. or I.M. at intervals depending on clinical response; when high dosages are needed, give 30 mg/kg over a period ≥30 minutes and may be repeated every 4-6 hours for 48 hours.

Status asthmaticus: I.V. (sodium succinate): Loading dose: 2 mg/kg/dose, then 0.5-1 mg/kg/dose every 6 hours for up to 5 days

High-dose therapy for acute spinal cord injury: I.V. bolus: 30 mg/kg over 15 minutes, followed 45 minutes later by an infusion of 5.4 mg/kg/hour for 23 hours

Lupus nephritis: High-dose "pulse" therapy: I.V. (sodium succinate): 1 g/day for 3 days

Aplastic anemia: I.V. (sodium succinate): 1 mg/kg/day or 40 mg/day (whichever dose is higher), for 4 days. After 4 days, change to oral and continue until day 10 or until symptoms of serum sickness resolve, then rapidly reduce over approximately 2 weeks.

Pneumocystis pneumonia in AIDs patients: I.V.: 40-60 mg every 6 hours for 7-10 days

Intra-articular (acetate): Administer every 1-5 weeks.

Large joints: 20-80 mg

Small joints: 4-10 mg

Intralesional (acetate): 20-60 mg every 1-5 weeks

Dosage Forms

Injection, powder for reconstitution, as sodium succinate: 40 mg, 125 mg, 500 mg
A-Methapred®: 40 mg, 125 mg, 500 mg, 1000 mg [diluent contains benzyl alcohol]
Solu-Medrol®: 40 mg, 125 mg, 500 mg, 1 g, 2 g [packaged with diluent; diluent contains benzyl alcohol]
Solu-Medrol®: 500 mg, 1 g
Injection, suspension, as acetate (Depo-Medrol®): 20 mg/mL (5 mL); 40 mg/mL (5 mL); 80 mg/mL (5 mL) [contains benzyl alcohol]
Injection, suspension, as acetate [single-dose vial] (Depo-Medrol®): 40 mg/mL (1 mL); 80 mg/mL (1 mL)
Tablet: 4 mg
Medrol®: 2 mg, 4 mg, 8 mg, 16 mg, 32 mg
Tablet, dose-pack: 4 mg (21s)

6-α-methylprednisolone *see* methylprednisolone *on previous page*

methylprednisolone acetate *see* methylprednisolone *on previous page*

methylprednisolone sodium succinate *see* methylprednisolone *on previous page*

4-methylpyrazole *see* fomepizole *on page 387*

methyltestosterone (meth il tes TOS te rone)

Sound-Alike/Look-Alike Issues

methyltestosterone may be confused with medroxyprogesterone
Virilon® may be confused with Verelan®

Tall-Man methyl**TESTOSTER**one

U.S./Canadian Brand Names Android® [US]; Methitest® [US]; Testred® [US]; Virilon® [US]

Therapeutic Category Androgen

Use

Male: Hypogonadism; delayed puberty; impotence and climacteric symptoms
Female: Palliative treatment of metastatic breast cancer

Usual Dosage Adults (buccal absorption produces twice the androgenic activity of oral tablets):

Male:
- Hypogonadism, male climacteric and impotence: Oral: 10-40 mg/day
- Androgen deficiency:
  - Oral: 10-50 mg/day
  - Buccal: 5-25 mg/day
- Postpubertal cryptorchidism: Oral: 30 mg/day

Female:
- Breast pain/engorgement:
  - Oral: 80 mg/day for 3-5 days
  - Buccal: 40 mg/day for 3-5 days
- Breast cancer:
  - Oral: 50-200 mg/day
  - Buccal: 25-100 mg/day

Dosage Forms

Capsule (Android®, Testred®, Virilon®): 10 mg
Tablet (Methitest®): 10 mg

Meticorten® ***(Discontinued)*** *see page 1042*

metipranolol (met i PRAN oh lol)

Sound-Alike/Look-Alike Issues

metipranolol may be confused with metaproterenol

Synonyms metipranolol hydrochloride

U.S./Canadian Brand Names OptiPranolol® [US/Can]

(Continued)

metipranolol *(Continued)*

Therapeutic Category Beta-Adrenergic Blocker

Use Agent for lowering intraocular pressure in patients with chronic open-angle glaucoma

Usual Dosage Ophthalmic: Adults: Instill 1 drop in the affected eye(s) twice daily

Dosage Forms Solution, ophthalmic: 0.3% (5 mL, 10 mL) [contains benzalkonium chloride]

metipranolol hydrochloride *see* metipranolol *on previous page*

Metizol® Tablet *(Discontinued)* *see page 1042*

metoclopramide (met oh kloe PRA mide)

Sound-Alike/Look-Alike Issues

metoclopramide may be confused with metolazone

Reglan® may be confused with Megace®, Regonol®, Renagel®

U.S./Canadian Brand Names Apo-Metoclop® [Can]; Nu-Metoclopramide [Can]; Reglan® [US]

Therapeutic Category Gastrointestinal Agent, Prokinetic

Use Symptomatic treatment of diabetic gastric stasis; gastroesophageal reflux

Usual Dosage

Children:

Gastroesophageal reflux: Oral: 0.1-0.2 mg/kg/dose up to 4 times/day; efficacy of continuing metoclopramide beyond 12 weeks in reflux has not been determined; total daily dose should not exceed 0.5 mg/kg/day

Gastrointestinal hypomotility (gastroparesis): Oral, I.M., I.V.: 0.1 mg/kg/dose up to 4 times/day, not to exceed 0.5 mg/kg/day

Adults:

Gastroesophageal reflux: Oral: 10-15 mg/dose up to 4 times/day 30 minutes before meals or food and at bedtime; single doses of 20 mg are occasionally needed for provoking situations

Gastrointestinal hypomotility (gastroparesis):

Oral: 10 mg 30 minutes before each meal and at bedtime for 2-8 weeks

I.V. (for severe symptoms): 10 mg over 1-2 minutes; 10 days of I.V. therapy may be necessary for best response

Elderly:

Gastroesophageal reflux: Oral: 5 mg 4 times/day (30 minutes before meals and at bedtime); increase dose to 10 mg 4 times/day if no response at lower dose

Gastrointestinal hypomotility:

Oral: Initial: 5 mg 30 minutes before meals and at bedtime for 2-8 weeks; increase if necessary to 10 mg doses

I.V.: Initiate at 5 mg over 1-2 minutes; increase to 10 mg if necessary

Dosage Forms

Injection, solution, as hydrochloride (Reglan®): 5 mg/mL (2 mL, 10 mL, 30 mL)

Syrup, as hydrochloride: 5 mg/5 mL (10 mL, 480 mL) [some products contain sodium benzoate; sugar free]

Tablet, as hydrochloride (Reglan®): 5 mg, 10 mg

metolazone (me TOLE a zone)

Sound-Alike/Look-Alike Issues

metolazone may be confused with metaxalone, methazolamide, methotrexate, metoclopramide, metoprolol, minoxidil

Zaroxolyn® may be confused with Zarontin®

U.S./Canadian Brand Names Mykrox® [Can]; Zaroxolyn® [US/Can]

Therapeutic Category Diuretic, Miscellaneous

Use Management of mild to moderate hypertension; treatment of edema in congestive heart failure and nephrotic syndrome, impaired renal function

Usual Dosage Adults: Oral:

Edema: 5-20 mg/dose every 24 hours

Hypertension (Zaroxolyn®): 2.5-5 mg/dose every 24 hours
Hypertension (Mykrox®): 0.5 mg/day; if response is not adequate, increase dose to maximum of 1 mg/day
Dialysis: Not dialyzable (0% to 5%) via hemo- or peritoneal dialysis; supplemental dose is not necessary

Dosage Forms [DSC] = Discontinued product
Tablet, rapid acting (Mykrox®): 0.5 mg [DSC]
Tablet, slow acting: 2.5 mg
Zaroxolyn®: 2.5 mg, 5 mg, 10 mg

Metopirone® [US] *see* metyrapone *on page 577*

metoprolol (me toe PROE lole)

Sound-Alike/Look-Alike Issues
metoprolol may be confused with metaproterenol, metolazone, misoprostol

Synonyms metoprolol succinate; metoprolol tartrate

U.S./Canadian Brand Names Apo-Metoprolol® [Can]; Betaloc® [Can]; Betaloc® Durules®; Lopressor® [US/Can]; Novo-Metoprolol [Can]; Nu-Metop [Can]; PMS-Metoprolol [Can]; Toprol-XL® [US/Can]

Therapeutic Category Beta-Adrenergic Blocker

Use Treatment of hypertension and angina pectoris; prevention of myocardial infarction, atrial fibrillation, flutter, symptomatic treatment of hypertrophic subaortic stenosis; to reduce mortality/hospitalization in patients with congestive heart failure (stable NYHA Class II or III) in patients already receiving ACE inhibitors, diuretics, and/or digoxin (sustained-release only)

Usual Dosage
Children: Oral: 1-5 mg/kg/24 hours divided twice daily; allow 3 days between dose adjustments
Adults:
Hypertension: Oral: 100-450 mg/day in 2-3 divided doses, begin with 50 mg twice daily and increase doses at weekly intervals to desired effect; usual dosage range (JNC 7): 50-100 mg/day
Extended release: Same daily dose administered as a single dose
Angina, SVT, MI prophylaxis: Oral: 100-450 mg/day in 2-3 divided doses, begin with 50 mg twice daily and increase doses at weekly intervals to desired effect
Extended release: Same daily dose administered as a single dose
Hypertension/ventricular rate control: I.V. (in patients having nonfunctioning GI tract): Initial: 1.25-5 mg every 6-12 hours; titrate initial dose to response. Initially, low doses may be appropriate to establish response; however, up to 15 mg every 3-6 hours has been employed.
Congestive heart failure: Oral (extended release): Initial: 25 mg once daily (reduce to 12.5 mg once daily in NYHA class higher than class II); may double dosage every 2 weeks as tolerated, up to 200 mg/day
Myocardial infarction (acute): I.V.: 5 mg every 2 minutes for 3 doses in early treatment of myocardial infarction; thereafter give 50 mg orally every 6 hours 15 minutes after last I.V. dose and continue for 48 hours; then administer a maintenance dose of 100 mg twice daily.
Extended release: 25-50 mg/day initially as a single dose; increase at 1- to 2-week intervals.

Dosage Forms
Injection, solution, as tartrate (Lopressor®): 1 mg/mL (5 mL)
Tablet, as tartrate 25 mg, 50 mg, 100 mg
Lopressor®: 50 mg, 100 mg
Tablet, extended release, as succinate (Toprol-XL®): 25 mg, 50 mg, 100 mg, 200 mg [expressed as mg equivalent to tartrate]

metoprolol succinate *see* metoprolol *on this page*

metoprolol tartrate *see* metoprolol *on this page*

Metra® *(Discontinued)* *see page 1042*

Metreton® *(Discontinued)* *see page 1042*

metrizamide *see* radiological/contrast media (nonionic) *on page 761*

MetroCream® [US/Can] *see* metronidazole *on this page*

Metrodin® *(Discontinued)* *see page 1042*

MetroGel® [US/Can] *see* metronidazole *on this page*

MetroGel-Vaginal® [US] *see* metronidazole *on this page*

Metro I.V.® Injection *(Discontinued)* *see page 1042*

MetroLotion® [US] *see* metronidazole *on this page*

metronidazole (me troe NI da zole)

Synonyms metronidazole hydrochloride

U.S./Canadian Brand Names Apo-Metronidazole® [Can]; Flagyl® [US/Can]; Flagyl ER® [US]; Florazole ER® [Can]; MetroCream® [US/Can]; MetroGel® [US/Can]; MetroGel-Vaginal® [US]; MetroLotion® [US]; Nidagel™ [Can]; Noritate® [US/Can]; Novo-Nidazol [Can]; Rozex™ [US]; Trikacide® [Can]

Therapeutic Category Amebicide; Antibiotic, Topical; Antibiotic, Miscellaneous; Antiprotozoal

Use Treatment of susceptible anaerobic bacterial and protozoal infections in the following conditions: Amebiasis, symptomatic and asymptomatic trichomoniasis; skin and skin structure infections; CNS infections; intra-abdominal infections (as part of combination regimen); systemic anaerobic infections; treatment of antibiotic-associated pseudomembranous colitis (AAPC), bacterial vaginosis; as part of a multidrug regimen for *H. pylori* eradication to reduce the risk of duodenal ulcer recurrence

Topical: Treatment of inflammatory lesions and erythema of rosacea

Usual Dosage

Infants and Children:

Amebiasis: Oral: 35-50 mg/kg/day in divided doses every 8 hours for 10 days

Trichomoniasis: Oral: 15-30 mg/kg/day in divided doses every 8 hours for 7 days

Anaerobic infections:

Oral: 15-35 mg/kg/day in divided doses every 8 hours

I.V.: 30 mg/kg/day in divided doses every 6 hours

Clostridium difficile (antibiotic-associated colitis): Oral: 20 mg/kg/day divided every 6 hours

Maximum dose: 2 g/day

Adults:

Amebiasis: Oral: 500-750 mg every 8 hours for 5-10 days

Trichomoniasis: Oral: 250 mg every 8 hours for 7 days **or** 375 mg twice daily for 7 days **or** 2 g as a single dose

Anaerobic infections: Oral, I.V.: 500 mg every 6-8 hours, not to exceed 4 g/day

Antibiotic-associated pseudomembranous colitis: Oral: 250-500 mg 3-4 times/day for 10-14 days

Helicobacter pylori eradication: Oral: 250-500 mg with meals and at bedtime for 14 days; requires combination therapy with at least one other antibiotic and an acid-suppressing agent (proton pump inhibitor or H_2 blocker)

Bacterial vaginosis:

Oral: 750 mg (extended release tablet) once daily for 7 days

Vaginal: 1 applicatorful (~37.5 mg metronidazole) intravaginally once or twice daily for 5 days; apply once in morning and evening if using twice daily, if daily, use at bedtime

Acne rosacea: Topical:

0.75%: Apply and rub a thin film twice daily, morning and evening, to entire affected areas after washing. Significant therapeutic results should be noticed within 3 weeks. Clinical studies have demonstrated continuing improvement through 9 weeks of therapy.

1%: Apply thin film to affected area once daily

Dosage Forms [DSC] = Discontinued product

Capsule (Flagyl®): 375 mg
Cream, topical: 0.75% (45 g)
MetroCream®: 0.75% (45 g) [contains benzyl alcohol]
Noritate®: 1% (60 g)
Emulsion, topical (Rozex™): 0.75% (60 g) [contains benzyl alcohol]
Gel, topical (MetroGel®): 0.75% [7.5 mg/mL] (45 g)
Gel, vaginal (MetroGel-Vaginal®): 0.75% (70 g)
Infusion [premixed iso-osmotic sodium chloride solution]: 500 mg (100 mL)
Injection, powder for reconstitution, as hydrochloride (Flagyl®): 500 mg [DSC]
Lotion, topical (MetroLotion®): 0.75% (60 mL) [contains benzyl alcohol]
Tablet (Flagyl®): 250 mg, 500 mg
Tablet, extended release (Flagyl® ER): 750 mg

metronidazole, bismuth subsalicylate, and tetracycline *see* bismuth subsalicylate, metronidazole, and tetracycline *on page 121*

metronidazole hydrochloride *see* metronidazole *on previous page*

metronidazole, tetracycline, and bismuth subsalicylate *see* bismuth subsalicylate, metronidazole, and tetracycline *on page 121*

Metubine® Iodide *(Discontinued)* *see page 1042*

metyrapone (me TEER a pone)

Sound-Alike/Look-Alike Issues
metyrapone may be confused with metyrosine

U.S./Canadian Brand Names Metopirone® [US]

Therapeutic Category Diagnostic Agent

Use Diagnostic test for hypothalamic-pituitary ACTH function

Usual Dosage Oral:
Children: 15 mg/kg every 4 hours for 6 doses; minimum dose: 250 mg
Adults: 750 mg every 4 hours for 6 doses

Dosage Forms Capsule: 250 mg

metyrosine (me TYE roe seen)

Sound-Alike/Look-Alike Issues
metyrosine may be confused with metyrapone

Synonyms AMPT; OGMT

U.S./Canadian Brand Names Demser® [US/Can]

Therapeutic Category Tyrosine Hydroxylase Inhibitor

Use Short-term management of pheochromocytoma before surgery, long-term management when surgery is contraindicated or when chronic malignant pheochromocytoma exists

Usual Dosage Children >12 years and Adults: Oral: Initial: 250 mg 4 times/day, increased by 250-500 mg/day up to 4 g/day; maintenance: 2-3 g/day in 4 divided doses; for preoperative preparation, administer optimum effective dosage for 5-7 days

Dosage Forms Capsule: 250 mg

Mevacor® [US/Can] *see* lovastatin *on page 533*

mevinolin *see* lovastatin *on page 533*

mexiletine (MEKS i le teen)

U.S./Canadian Brand Names Mexitil® [US]; Novo-Mexiletine [Can]

Therapeutic Category Antiarrhythmic Agent, Class I-B

Use Management of serious ventricular arrhythmias; suppression of PVCs

Usual Dosage Adults: Oral: Initial: 200 mg every 8 hours (may load with 400 mg if necessary); adjust dose every 2-3 days; usual dose: 200-300 mg every 8 hours; maximum dose: 1.2 g/day (some patients respond to every 12-hour dosing). When switching from another antiarrhythmic, initiate a 200 mg dose 6-12 hours after stopping former agents, 3-6 hours after stopping procainamide.

Dosage Forms Capsule, as hydrochloride: 150 mg, 200 mg, 250 mg

Mexitil® [US] *see* mexiletine *on previous page*

Mezlin® *(Discontinued)* *see page 1042*

MG217® Medicated Tar [US-OTC] *see* coal tar *on page 219*

MG217 Sal-Acid® [US-OTC] *see* salicylic acid *on page 789*

MG217® [US-OTC] *see* coal tar *on page 219*

Miacalcin® [US] *see* calcitonin *on page 143*

Miacalcin® NS [Can] *see* calcitonin *on page 143*

Micaderm® [US-OTC] *see* miconazole *on this page*

Micanol® [Can] *see* anthralin *on page 60*

Micardis® [US/Can] *see* telmisartan *on page 842*

Micardis® HCT [US] *see* telmisartan and hydrochlorothiazide *on page 843*

Micardis® Plus [Can] *see* telmisartan and hydrochlorothiazide *on page 843*

Micatin® [US-OTC/Can] *see* miconazole *on this page*

miconazole (mi KON a zole)

Sound-Alike/Look-Alike Issues

miconazole may be confused with Micronase®, Micronor®
Lotrimin® may be confused with Lotrisone®, Otrivin®
Micatin® may be confused with Miacalcin®

Synonyms miconazole nitrate

U.S./Canadian Brand Names Aloe Vesta® 2-n-1 Antifungal [US-OTC]; Baza® Antifungal [US-OTC]; Carrington Antifungal [US-OTC]; Dermazole [Can]; Femizol-M™ [US-OTC]; Fungoid® Tincture [US-OTC]; Lotrimin® AF Powder/Spray [US-OTC]; Micaderm® [US-OTC]; Micatin® [US-OTC/Can]; Micozole [Can]; Micro-Guard® [US-OTC]; Mitrazol™ [US-OTC]; Monistat® [Can]; Monistat® 1 Combination Pack [US-OTC]; Monistat® 3 [US-OTC]; Monistat® 7 [US-OTC]; Monistat-Derm® [US]; Triple Care® Antifungal [OTC]; Zeasorb®-AF [US-OTC]

Therapeutic Category Antifungal Agent

Use Treatment of vulvovaginal candidiasis and a variety of skin and mucous membrane fungal infections

Usual Dosage

Topical: Children and Adults: **Note:** Not for OTC use in children <2 years:
Tinea pedis and tinea corporis: Apply twice daily for 4 weeks
Tinea cruris: Apply twice daily for 2 weeks

Vaginal: Adults: Vulvovaginal candidiasis:
Cream, 2%: Insert 1 applicatorful at bedtime for 7 days
Cream, 4%: Insert 1 applicatorful at bedtime for 3 days
Suppository, 100 mg: Insert 1 suppository at bedtime for 7 days
Suppository, 200 mg: Insert 1 suppository at bedtime for 3 days
Suppository, 1200 mg: Insert 1 suppository (a one-time dose); may be used at bedtime or during the day

Note: Many products are available as a combination pack, with a suppository for vaginal instillation and cream to relieve external symptoms. External cream may be used twice daily, as needed, for up to 7 days.

Dosage Forms

Combination products: Miconazole nitrate vaginal suppository 200 mg (3s) and miconazole nitrate external cream 2%; Miconazole nitrate vaginal suppository 100 mg (7s) and miconazole nitrate external cream 2%

Monistat® 1 Combination Pack: Miconazole nitrate vaginal insert 1200 mg (1) and miconazole external cream 2% (5 g) [Note: Do not confuse with 1-Day™ (formerly Monistat® 1) which contains tioconazole]

Monistat® 3 Combination Pack: Miconazole nitrate vaginal suppository 200 mg (3s) and miconazole nitrate external cream 2%
Monistat® 3 Cream Combination Pack: Miconazole nitrate vaginal cream 4% and miconazole nitrate external cream 2%
Monistat® 7 Combination Pack:
Miconazole nitrate vaginal suppository 100 mg (7s) and miconazole nitrate external cream 2%
Miconazole nitrate vaginal cream 2% (7 prefilled applicators) and miconazole nitrate external cream 2%
Cream, topical, as nitrate: 2% (15 g, 30 g, 45 g)
Baza® Antifungal: 2% (4 g, 57 g, 142 g) [zinc oxide based formula]
Carrington Antifungal: 2% (150 g)
Micaderm®: 2% (30 g)
Micatin®: 2% (15 g)
Micro-Guard®, Mitrazol™: 2% (60 g)
Monistat-Derm®: 2% (15 g, 30 g, 85 g)
Triple Care® Antifungal: 2% (60 g, 98 g)
Cream, vaginal, as nitrate [prefilled or with single refillable applicator]: 2% (45 g)
Femizol-M™: 2% (47 g)
Monistat® 3: 4% (15 g, 25 g)
Monistat® 7: 2% (45 g)
Liquid, spray, as nitrate (Micatin®): 2% (90 mL, 105 mL)
Lotion, powder, as nitrate (Zeasorb®-AF): 2% (56 g) [contains alcohol 70%]
Ointment, topical, as nitrate: (Aloe Vesta® 2-n-1 Antifungal): 2% (60 g, 150 g)
Powder, topical, as nitrate:
Lotrimin® AF, Micatin®, Micro-Guard®: 2% (90 g)
Mitrazol™: 2% (30 g)
Zeasorb®-AF: 2% (70 g)
Powder spray, topical, as nitrate (Lotrimin® AF): 2% (100 g)
Suppository, vaginal, as nitrate: 100 mg (7s); 200 mg (3s)
Monistat® 3: 200 mg (3s)
Monistat® 7: 100 mg (7s)
Tincture, topical, as nitrate (Fungoid®): 2% (30 mL, 473 mL) [contains isopropyl alcohol 30%]

miconazole nitrate *see* miconazole *on previous page*

Micozole [Can] *see* miconazole *on previous page*

MICRhoGAM® [US] *see* Rh_0(D) immune globulin *on page 771*

Microgestin™ Fe [US] *see* ethinyl estradiol and norethindrone *on page 342*

Micro-Guard® [US-OTC] *see* miconazole *on previous page*

Micro-K® 10 Extencaps® [US] *see* potassium chloride *on page 713*

Micro-K® Extencaps [US-OTC/Can] *see* potassium chloride *on page 713*

Micro-K® LS *(Discontinued)* *see page 1042*

Micronase® [US] *see* glyburide *on page 409*

microNefrin® *(Discontinued)* *see page 1042*

Micronor® [US/Can] *see* norethindrone *on page 627*

Microzide™ [US] *see* hydrochlorothiazide *on page 441*

Midamor® [Can] *see* amiloride *on page 44*

Midamor® *(Discontinued)* *see page 1042*

midazolam (MID aye zoe lam)

Synonyms midazolam hydrochloride
U.S./Canadian Brand Names Apo-Midazolam® [Can]
Therapeutic Category Benzodiazepine
Controlled Substance C-IV
(Continued)

midazolam *(Continued)*

Use Preoperative sedation and provides conscious sedation prior to diagnostic or radiographic procedures; ICU sedation (continuous infusion); intravenous anesthesia (induction); intravenous anesthesia (maintenance)

Usual Dosage The dose of midazolam needs to be individualized based on the patient's age, underlying diseases, and concurrent medications. Decrease dose (by ~30%) if narcotics or other CNS depressants are administered concomitantly. **Personnel and equipment needed for standard respiratory resuscitation should be immediately available during midazolam administration.**

Children <6 years may require higher doses and closer monitoring than older children; calculate dose on ideal body weight

Conscious sedation for procedures or preoperative sedation:

Oral: 0.25-0.5 mg/kg as a single dose preprocedure, up to a maximum of 20 mg; administer 30-45 minutes prior to procedure. Children <6 years or less cooperative patients may require as much as 1 mg/kg as a single dose; 0.25 mg/kg may suffice for children 6-16 years of age.

Intranasal (not an approved route): 0.2 mg/kg (up to 0.4 mg/kg in some studies), to a maximum of 15 mg; may be administered 30-45 minutes prior to procedure

I.M.: 0.1-0.15 mg/kg 30-60 minutes before surgery or procedure; range 0.05-0.15 mg/kg; doses up to 0.5 mg/kg have been used in more anxious patients; maximum total dose: 10 mg

I.V.:

Infants <6 months: Limited information is available in nonintubated infants; dosing recommendations not clear; infants <6 months are at higher risk for airway obstruction and hypoventilation; titrate dose in small increments to desired effect; monitor carefully

Infants 6 months to Children 5 years: Initial: 0.05-0.1 mg/kg; titrate dose carefully; total dose of 0.6 mg/kg may be required; usual maximum total dose: 6 mg

Children 6-12 years: Initial: 0.025-0.05 mg/kg; titrate dose carefully; total doses of 0.4 mg/kg may be required; usual maximum total dose: 10 mg

Children 12-16 years: Dose as adults; usual maximum total dose: 10 mg

Conscious sedation during mechanical ventilation: Children: Loading dose: 0.05-0.2 mg/kg, followed by initial continuous infusion: 0.06-0.12 mg/kg/hour (1-2 mcg/kg/minute); titrate to the desired effect; usual range: 0.4-6 mcg/kg/minute

Adults:

Preoperative sedation:

I.M.: 0.07-0.08 mg/kg 30-60 minutes prior to surgery/procedure; usual dose: 5 mg; **Note:** Reduce dose in patients with COPD, high-risk patients, patients ≥60 years of age, and patients receiving other narcotics or CNS depressants

I.V.: 0.02-0.04 mg/kg; repeat every 5 minutes as needed to desired effect or up to 0.1-0.2 mg/kg

Intranasal (not an approved route): 0.2 mg/kg (up to 0.4 mg/kg in some studies); administer 30-45 minutes prior to surgery/procedure

Conscious sedation: I.V.: Initial: 0.5-2 mg slow I.V. over at least 2 minutes; slowly titrate to effect by repeating doses every 2-3 minutes if needed; usual total dose: 2.5-5 mg; use decreased doses in elderly

Healthy Adults <60 years: Some patients respond to doses as low as 1 mg; no more than 2.5 mg should be administered over a period of 2 minutes. Additional doses of midazolam may be administered after a 2-minute waiting period and evaluation of sedation after each dose increment. A total dose >5 mg is generally not needed. If narcotics or other CNS depressants are administered concomitantly, the midazolam dose should be reduced by 30%.

Anesthesia: I.V.:

Induction: Unpremedicated patients: 0.3-0.35 mg/kg (up to 0.6 mg/kg in resistant cases) Premedicated patients: 0.15-0.35 mg/kg

Maintenance: 0.05-0.3 mg/kg as needed, or continuous infusion 0.25-1.5 mcg/kg/minute

Sedation in mechanically-ventilated patients: I.V. continuous infusion: 100 mg in 250 mL D_5W or NS (if patient is fluid-restricted, may concentrate up to a maximum of 0.5 mg/mL); initial dose: 0.02-0.08 mg/kg (~1 mg to 5 mg in 70 kg adult) initially and either repeated at 5-15 minute intervals until adequate sedation is achieved or continuous infusion rates of 0.04-0.2 mg/kg/hour and titrate to reach desired level of sedation

Elderly: I.V.: Conscious sedation: Initial: 0.5 mg slow I.V.; give no more than 1.5 mg in a 2-minute period; if additional titration is needed, give no more than 1 mg over 2 minutes, waiting another 2 or more minutes to evaluate sedative effect; a total dose of >3.5 mg is rarely necessary

Dosage Forms [DSC] = Discontinued product

Injection, solution, as hydrochloride (Versed® [DSC]): 1 mg/mL (2 mL, 5 mL, 10 mL); 5 mg/mL (1 mL, 2 mL, 5 mL, 10 mL) [contains benzyl alcohol 1%]

Injection, solution, as hydrochloride [preservative free]: 1 mg/mL (2 mL, 5 mL); 5 mg/mL (1 mL, 2 mL)

Syrup, as hydrochloride (Versed® [DSC]): 2 mg/mL (118 mL) [contains sodium benzoate; cherry flavor]

midazolam hydrochloride *see* midazolam *on page 579*

midodrine (MI doe dreen)

Sound-Alike/Look-Alike Issues

ProAmatine® may be confused with protamine

Synonyms midodrine hydrochloride

U.S./Canadian Brand Names Amatine® [Can]; ProAmatine® [US]

Therapeutic Category Alpha-Adrenergic Agonist

Use Orphan drug: Treatment of symptomatic orthostatic hypotension

Usual Dosage Adults: Oral: 10 mg 3 times/day during daytime hours (every 3-4 hours) when patient is upright (maximum: 40 mg/day)

Dosage Forms Tablet, as hydrochloride: 2.5 mg, 5 mg, 10 mg

midodrine hydrochloride *see* midodrine *on this page*

Midol® Maximum Strength Cramp Formula [US-OTC] *see* ibuprofen *on page 462*

Midrin® [US] *see* acetaminophen, isometheptene, and dichloralphenazone *on page 13*

Mifeprex® [US] *see* mifepristone *on this page*

mifepristone (mi fe PRIS tone)

Sound-Alike/Look-Alike Issues

Mifeprex® may be confused with Mirapex®

Synonyms RU-486; RU-38486

U.S./Canadian Brand Names Mifeprex® [US]

Therapeutic Category Abortifacient; Antineoplastic Agent, Hormone Antagonist; Antiprogestin

Use Medical termination of intrauterine pregnancy, through day 49 of pregnancy. Patients may need treatment with misoprostol and possibly surgery to complete therapy

Usual Dosage Oral:

Adults: Termination of pregnancy: Treatment consists of three office visits by the patient; the patient must read medication guide and sign patient agreement prior to treatment:

Day 1: 600 mg (three 200 mg tablets) taken as a single dose under physician supervision

Day 3: Patient must return to the healthcare provider 2 days following administration of mifepristone; if termination of pregnancy cannot be confirmed using ultrasound or clinical examination: 400 mcg (two 200 mcg tablets) of misoprostol; patient may need treatment for cramps or gastrointestinal symptoms at this time

(Continued)

mifepristone *(Continued)*

Day 14: Patient must return to the healthcare provider ~14 days after administration of mifepristone; confirm complete termination of pregnancy by ultrasound or clinical exam. Surgical termination is recommended to manage treatment failures.

Dosage Forms Tablet: 200 mg

Miflex® Tablet ***(Discontinued)*** *see page 1042*

miglitol (MIG li tol)

U.S./Canadian Brand Names Glyset® [US/Can]

Therapeutic Category Antidiabetic Agent, Oral

Use Type 2 diabetes mellitus (noninsulin-dependent, NIDDM):

Monotherapy adjunct to diet to improve glycemic control in patients with type 2 diabetes mellitus (noninsulin-dependent, NIDDM) whose hyperglycemia cannot be managed with diet alone

Combination therapy with a sulfonylurea when diet plus either miglitol or a sulfonylurea alone do not result in adequate glycemic control. The effect of miglitol to enhance glycemic control is additive to that of sulfonylureas when used in combination.

Usual Dosage Adults: Oral: 25 mg 3 times/day with the first bite of food at each meal; the dose may be increased to 50 mg 3 times/day after 4-8 weeks; maximum recommended dose: 100 mg 3 times/day

Dosage Forms Tablet: 25 mg, 50 mg, 100 mg

miglustat (MIG loo stat)

Synonyms OGT-918

U.S./Canadian Brand Names Zavesca® [US]

Therapeutic Category Enzyme Inhibitor

Use Treatment of mild-to-moderate type 1 Gaucher disease when enzyme replacement therapy is not a therapeutic option

Usual Dosage Oral: Adults: Type 1 Gaucher disease: 100 mg 3 times/day; dose may be reduced to 100 mg 1-2 times/day in patients with adverse effects (ie, tremor, GI distress)

Dosage Forms Capsule: 100 mg

Migranal® [US/Can] *see* dihydroergotamine *on page 271*

Migrapap® ***(Discontinued)*** *see page 1042*

Migratine® ***(Discontinued)*** *see page 1042*

Migrin-A [US] *see* acetaminophen, isometheptene, and dichloralphenazone *on page 13*

Milkinol® ***(Discontinued)*** *see page 1042*

milk of magnesia *see* magnesium hydroxide *on page 537*

Milontin® ***(Discontinued)*** *see page 1042*

Milophene® [Can] *see* clomiphene *on page 214*

Milophene® ***(Discontinued)*** *see page 1042*

Milprem® ***(Discontinued)*** *see page 1042*

milrinone (MIL ri none)

Sound-Alike/Look-Alike Issues

Primacor® may be confused with Primaxin®

Synonyms milrinone lactate

U.S./Canadian Brand Names Primacor® [US/Can]

Therapeutic Category Cardiovascular Agent, Other

Use Short-term I.V. therapy of congestive heart failure; calcium antagonist intoxication

Usual Dosage Adults: I.V.: Loading dose: 50 mcg/kg administered over 10 minutes, then 0.375-0.75 mcg/kg/min as a continuous infusion for a total daily dose of 0.59-1.13 mg/kg

Dosage Forms

Infusion, as lactate [premixed in D_5W] (Primacor®): 200 mcg/mL (100 mL, 200 mL)

Injection, solution, as lactate: 1 mg/mL (10 mL, 20 mL, 50 mL)

Primacor®: 1 mg/mL (5 mL, 10 mL, 20 mL, 50 mL)

milrinone lactate *see* milrinone *on previous page*

Miltown® [US] *see* meprobamate *on page 554*

mineral oil, petrolatum, lanolin, cetyl alcohol, and glycerin *see* lanolin, cetyl alcohol, glycerin, petrolatum, and mineral oil *on page 505*

Minestrin™ 1/20 [Can] *see* ethinyl estradiol and norethindrone *on page 342*

Minidyne® [US-OTC] *see* povidone-iodine *on page 718*

Mini-Gamulin® Rh *(Discontinued)* *see page 1042*

Minim's Atropine Solution [Can] *see* atropine *on page 88*

Minim's Gentamicin 0.3% [Can] *see* gentamicin *on page 403*

Minipress® [US/Can] *see* prazosin *on page 722*

Minirin® [Can] *see* desmopressin acetate *on page 252*

Minitran™ [US/Can] *see* nitroglycerin *on page 623*

Minizide® [US] *see* prazosin and polythiazide *on page 722*

Minocin® [US/Can] *see* minocycline *on this page*

Minocin® Tablet *(Discontinued)* *see page 1042*

minocycline (mi noe SYE kleen)

Sound-Alike/Look-Alike Issues

Dynacin® may be confused with Dyazide®, Dynabac®, DynaCirc®, Dynapen®

Minocin® may be confused with Indocin®, Lincocin®, Minizide®, Mithracin®, niacin

Synonyms minocycline hydrochloride

U.S./Canadian Brand Names Alti-Minocycline [Can]; Apo-Minocycline® [Can]; Dynacin® [US]; Gen-Minocycline [Can]; Minocin® [US/Can]; Novo-Minocycline [Can]; PMS-Minocycline [Can]; Rhoxal-minocycline [Can]

Therapeutic Category Tetracycline Derivative

Use Treatment of susceptible bacterial infections of both gram-negative and gram-positive organisms; treatment of anthrax (inhalational, cutaneous, and gastrointestinal); acne; meningococcal carrier state; Rickettsial diseases (including Rocky Mountain spotted fever, Q fever); nongonococcal urethritis, gonorrhea; acute intestinal amebiasis

Usual Dosage

Children >8 years: Oral, I.V.: Initial: 4 mg/kg followed by 2 mg/kg/dose every 12 hours

Adults:

Infection: Oral, I.V.: 200 mg stat, 100 mg every 12 hours not to exceed 400 mg/24 hours

Acne: Oral: 50 mg 1-3 times/day

Dosage Forms

Capsule, as hydrochloride: 50 mg, 75 mg, 100 mg

Dynacin®: 50 mg, 75 mg, 100 mg

Capsule, pellet-filled, as hydrochloride (Minocin®): 50 mg, 100 mg

Injection, powder for reconstitution, as hydrochloride (Minocin®): 100 mg

Tablet, as hydrochloride (Dynacin®): 50 mg, 75 mg, 100 mg

minocycline hydrochloride *see* minocycline *on this page*

Min-Ovral® [Can] *see* ethinyl estradiol and levonorgestrel *on page 339*

Minox [Can] *see* minoxidil *on next page*

minoxidil (mi NOKS i dil)

Sound-Alike/Look-Alike Issues

minoxidil may be confused with metolazone, Monopril®

Loniten® may be confused with clonidine, Lioresal®, Lotensin®

U.S./Canadian Brand Names Apo-Gain® [Can]; Loniten® [US]; Minox [Can]; Rogaine® [Can]; Rogaine® Extra Strength for Men [US-OTC]; Rogaine® for Men [US-OTC]; Rogaine® for Women [US-OTC]

Therapeutic Category Topical Skin Product; Vasodilator

Use Management of severe hypertension (usually in combination with a diuretic and beta-blocker); treatment (topical formulation) of alopecia androgenetica in males and females

Usual Dosage

Children <12 years: Hypertension: Oral: Initial: 0.1-0.2 mg/kg once daily; maximum: 5 mg/day; increase gradually every 3 days; usual dosage: 0.25-1 mg/kg/day in 1-2 divided doses; maximum: 50 mg/day

Children >12 years and Adults: Hypertension: Oral: Initial: 5 mg once daily, increase gradually every 3 days (maximum: 100 mg/day); usual dose range (JNC 7): 2.5-80 mg/day in 1-2 divided doses

Adults: Alopecia: Topical: Apply twice daily; 4 months of therapy may be necessary for hair growth.

Dosage Forms

Solution, topical: 2% [20 mg/metered dose] (60 mL); 5% [50 mg/metered dose] (60 mL)
 Rogaine® for Men, Rogaine® for Women: 2% [20 mg/metered dose] (60 mL)
 Rogaine® Extra Strength for Men: 5% [50 mg/metered dose] (60 mL)

Tablet (Loniten®): 2.5 mg, 10 mg

Mintezol® [US] *see* thiabendazole *on page 856*

Minute-Gel® ***(Discontinued)*** *see page 1042*

Miochol® ***(Discontinued)*** *see page 1042*

Miochol-E® [US/Can] *see* acetylcholine *on page 16*

Miostat® [US/Can] *see* carbachol *on page 154*

MiraLax™ [US] *see* polyethylene glycol-electrolyte solution *on page 706*

Mirapex® [US/Can] *see* pramipexole *on page 720*

Miraphen PSE [US] *see* guaifenesin and pseudoephedrine *on page 419*

Mircette® [US] *see* ethinyl estradiol and desogestrel *on page 335*

Mirena® [US] *see* levonorgestrel *on page 515*

mirtazapine (mir TAZ a peen)

Sound-Alike/Look-Alike Issues

Remeron® may be confused with Premarin®, Zemuron®

U.S./Canadian Brand Names Remeron® [US/Can]; Remeron® SolTab® [US]

Therapeutic Category Antidepressant, Alpha-2 Antagonist

Use Treatment of depression

Usual Dosage

Children: Safety and efficacy in children have not been established

Treatment of depression: Adults: Oral: Initial: 15 mg nightly, titrate up to 15-45 mg/day with dose increases made no more frequently than every 1-2 weeks; there is an inverse relationship between dose and sedation

Dosage Forms

Tablet (Remeron®): 15 mg, 30 mg, 45 mg

Tablet, orally-disintegrating: 15 mg, 30 mg
 Remeron SolTab®:
  15 mg [contains phenylalanine 2.6 mg/tablet; orange flavor]
  30 mg [contains phenylalanine 5.2 mg/tablet; orange flavor]
  45 mg [contains phenylalanine 7.8 mg/tablet; orange flavor]

misoprostol (mye soe PROST ole)

Sound-Alike/Look-Alike Issues

misoprostol may be confused with metoprolol

Cytotec® may be confused with Cytoxan®, Sytobex®

U.S./Canadian Brand Names Apo-Misoprostil® [Can]; Cytotec® [US/Can]; Novo-Misoprostol [Can]

Therapeutic Category Prostaglandin

Use Prevention of NSAID-induced gastric ulcers; medical termination of pregnancy of ≤49 days (in conjunction with mifepristone)

Usual Dosage Oral: Adults:

Prevention of NSAID-induced gastric ulcers: 200 mcg 4 times/day with food; if not tolerated, may decrease dose to 100 mcg 4 times/day with food or 200 mcg twice daily with food; last dose of the day should be taken at bedtime

Medical termination of pregnancy: Refer to Mifepristone monograph.

Dosage Forms Tablet: 100 mcg, 200 mcg

misoprostol and diclofenac *see* diclofenac and misoprostol *on page 267*

Mithracin® ***(Discontinued)*** *see page 1042*

Mito-Carn® ***(Discontinued)*** *see page 1042*

mitomycin (mye toe MYE sin)

Sound-Alike/Look-Alike Issues

mitomycin may be confused with mithramycin, mitotane, mitoxantrone, Mutamycin®

Mutamycin® may be confused with mitomycin

Synonyms mitomycin-C; mitomycin-X; MTC; NSC-26980

U.S./Canadian Brand Names Mutamycin® [US/Can]

Therapeutic Category Antineoplastic Agent

Use Treatment of adenocarcinoma of stomach or pancreas, bladder cancer, breast cancer, or colorectal cancer

Usual Dosage Refer to individual protocols. Children and Adults:

Single agent therapy: I.V.: 20 mg/m^2 every 6-8 weeks

Combination therapy: I.V.: 10 mg/m^2 every 6-8 weeks

Bladder carcinoma: Intravesicular instillation (unapproved route): 20-40 mg/dose instilled into the bladder for 3 hours repeated up to 3 times/week for up to 20 procedures per course

Dosage Forms Injection, powder for reconstitution (Mutamycin®): 5 mg, 20 mg, 40 mg

mitomycin-C *see* mitomycin *on this page*

mitomycin-X *see* mitomycin *on this page*

mitotane (MYE toe tane)

Sound-Alike/Look-Alike Issues

mitotane may be confused with mitomycin

Synonyms NSC-38721; o,p′-DDD

U.S./Canadian Brand Names Lysodren® [US/Can]

Therapeutic Category Antineoplastic Agent

Use Treatment of adrenocortical carcinoma

Usual Dosage Oral:

Children: 0.1-0.5 mg/kg or 1-2 g/day in divided doses increasing gradually to a maximum of 5-7 g/day

Adults: Start at 1-6 g/day in divided doses, then increase incrementally to 8-10 g/day in 3-4 divided doses (maximum daily dose: 18 g)

Dosage Forms Tablet [scored]: 500 mg

mitoxantrone (mye toe ZAN trone)

Sound-Alike/Look-Alike Issues

mitoxantrone may be confused with mitomycin

Synonyms DAD; DHAD; DHAQ; dihydroxyanthracenedione dihydrochloride; mitoxantrone hydrochloride CL-232315; mitozantrone; NSC-301739

U.S./Canadian Brand Names Novantrone® [US/Can]

Therapeutic Category Antineoplastic Agent

Use Treatment of acute leukemias, lymphoma, breast cancer, pediatric sarcoma, progressive or relapsing-remitting multiple sclerosis, prostate cancer

Usual Dosage Refer to individual protocols. I.V. (dilute in D_5W or NS):

Acute leukemias:

Children ≤2 years: 0.4 mg/kg/day once daily for 3-5 days

Children >2 years and Adults: 8-12 mg/m²/day once daily for 4-5 days

Solid tumors:

Children: 18-20 mg/m² every 3-4 weeks **or** 5-8 mg/m² every week

Adults: 12-14 mg/m² every 3-4 weeks **or** 2-4 mg/m²/day for 5 days every 4 weeks

Hormone-refractory prostate cancer: Adults: 12-14 mg/m²

Multiple sclerosis: Adults: 12 mg/m²

Dosage Forms Injection, solution, as hydrochloride: 2 mg base/mL (10 mL, 12.5 mL, 15 mL)

mitoxantrone hydrochloride CL-232315 *see* mitoxantrone *on this page*

mitozantrone *see* mitoxantrone *on this page*

Mitran® Oral *(Discontinued)* *see page 1042*

Mitrazol™ [US-OTC] *see* miconazole *on page 578*

Mivacron® [US/Can] *see* mivacurium *on this page*

mivacurium (mye va KYOO ree um)

Sound-Alike/Look-Alike Issues

Mivacron® may be confused with Mevacor®

Synonyms mivacurium chloride

U.S./Canadian Brand Names Mivacron® [US/Can]

Therapeutic Category Skeletal Muscle Relaxant

Use Adjunct to general anesthesia to facilitate endotracheal intubation and to relax skeletal muscles during surgery; to facilitate mechanical ventilation in ICU patients; does not relieve pain or produce sedation

Usual Dosage Continuous infusion requires an infusion pump; dose to effect; doses will vary due to interpatient variability; use ideal body weight for obese patients

Children 2-12 years (duration of action is shorter and dosage requirements are higher): 0.2 mg/kg I.V. followed by average infusion rate of 14 mcg/kg/minute (range: 5-31 mcg/kg/minute) upon evidence of spontaneous recovery from initial dose

Adults: Initial: I.V.: 0.15-0.25 mg/kg bolus followed by maintenance doses of 0.1 mg/kg at approximately 15-minute intervals; for prolonged neuromuscular block, initial infusion of 9-10 mcg/kg/minute is used upon evidence of spontaneous recovery from initial dose, usual infusion rate of 6-7 mcg/kg/minute (1-15 mcg/kg/minute) under balanced anesthesia; initial dose after succinylcholine for intubation (balanced anesthesia): Adults: 0.1 mg/kg

Pretreatment/priming: 10% of intubating dose given 3-5 minutes before initial dose

Dosage Forms

Injection, solution, as chloride: 2 mg/mL (20 mL, 50 mL) [with benzyl alcohol]

Injection, solution, as chloride [preservative free]: 2 mg/mL (5 mL, 10 mL)

mivacurium chloride *see* mivacurium *on this page*

MK383 *see* tirofiban *on page 866*

MK462 *see* rizatriptan *on page 781*

MK594 *see* losartan *on page 531*

MK0826 *see* ertapenem *on page 319*

MK 869 *see* aprepitant *on page 74*

MLN341 *see* bortezomib *on page 124*

MMF *see* mycophenolate *on page 596*

MMR *see* measles, mumps, and rubella vaccines, combined *on page 544*

M-M-R® II [US/Can] *see* measles, mumps, and rubella vaccines, combined *on page 544*

Moban® [US/Can] *see* molindone *on next page*

Mobic® [US/Can] *see* meloxicam *on page 550*

Mobicox® [Can] *see* meloxicam *on page 550*

Mobidin® *(Discontinued)* *see page 1042*

Mobisyl® [US-OTC] *see* triethanolamine salicylate *on page 884*

moclobemide *(Canada only)* (moe KLOE be mide)

Synonyms Ro 11-1163

U.S./Canadian Brand Names Alti-Moclobemide [Can]; Apo-Moclobemide® [Can]; Manerix® [Can]; Novo-Moclobemide [Can]; Nu-Moclobemide [Can]; PMS-Moclobemide [Can]

Therapeutic Category Antidepressant, Monoamine Oxidase Inhibitor

Use Symptomatic relief of depressive illness

Usual Dosage Oral: Adults: Initial: 300 mg/day in 2 divided doses; increase gradually to maximum of 600 mg/day; **Note:** Individual patient response may allow a reduction in daily dose in long-term therapy.

Dosage Forms Tablet: 150 mg, 300 mg

Moctanin® *(Discontinued)* *see page 1042*

modafinil (moe DAF i nil)

U.S./Canadian Brand Names Alertec® [Can]; Provigil® [US/Can]

Therapeutic Category Central Nervous System Stimulant, Nonamphetamine

Controlled Substance C-IV

Use Improve wakefulness in patients with excessive daytime sleepiness associated with narcolepsy and shift work sleep disorder (SWSD); adjunctive therapy for obstructive sleep apnea/hypopnea syndrome (OSAHS)

Usual Dosage Oral: Adults:

Narcolepsy, OSAHS: Initial: 200 mg as a single daily dose in the morning

SWSD: Initial: 200 mg as a single dose taken ~1 hour prior to start of work shift

Note: Doses of 400 mg/day, given as a single dose, have been well tolerated, but there is no consistent evidence that this dose confers additional benefit

Dosage Forms Tablet: 100 mg, 200 mg

Modane® Bulk [US-OTC] *see* psyllium *on page 749*

Modane® Soft *(Discontinued)* *see page 1042*

Modane Tablets® [US-OTC] *see* bisacodyl *on page 120*

Modecate® [Can] *see* fluphenazine *on page 380*

Modicon® [US] *see* ethinyl estradiol and norethindrone *on page 342*

modified Dakin's solution *see* sodium hypochlorite solution *on page 813*

Moditen® Enanthate [Can] *see* fluphenazine *on page 380*

Moditen® HCl [Can] *see* fluphenazine *on page 380*

Moducal® [US-OTC] *see* glucose polymers *on page 408*

Modulon® [Can] *see* trimebutine *(Canada only) on page 886*

Moduret® [Can] *see* amiloride and hydrochlorothiazide *on page 45*

Moduretic® [Can] *see* amiloride and hydrochlorothiazide *on page 45*

Moduretic® ***(Discontinued)*** *see page 1042*

moexipril (mo EKS i pril)

Sound-Alike/Look-Alike Issues
moexipril may be confused with Monopril®

Synonyms moexipril hydrochloride

U.S./Canadian Brand Names Univasc® [US]

Therapeutic Category Angiotensin-Converting Enzyme (ACE) Inhibitor

Use Treatment of hypertension, alone or in combination with thiazide diuretics; treatment of left ventricular dysfunction after myocardial infarction

Usual Dosage Adults: Oral: Initial: 7.5 mg once daily (in patients **not** receiving diuretics), 1 hour prior to a meal **or** 3.75 mg once daily (when combined with thiazide diuretics); maintenance dose: 7.5-30 mg/day in 1 or 2 divided doses 1 hour before meals

Dosage Forms Tablet, as hydrochloride [film coated, scored]: 7.5 mg, 15 mg

moexipril and hydrochlorothiazide

(mo EKS i pril & hye droe klor oh THYE a zide)

Synonyms hydrochlorothiazide and moexipril

U.S./Canadian Brand Names Uniretic® [US/Can]

Therapeutic Category Angiotensin-Converting Enzyme (ACE) Inhibitor; Diuretic, Thiazide

Use Combination therapy for hypertension, however, not indicated for initial treatment of hypertension; replacement therapy in patients receiving separate dosage forms (for patient convenience); when monotherapy with one component fails to achieve desired antihypertensive effect, or when dose-limiting adverse effects limit upward titration of monotherapy

Usual Dosage Adults: Oral: 7.5-30 mg of moexipril, taken either in a single or divided dose one hour before meals; hydrochlorothiazide dose should be ≤50 mg/day

Dosage Forms Tablet [film coated, scored]:
7.5/12.5: Moexipril hydrochloride 7.5 mg and hydrochlorothiazide 12.5 mg
15/12.5: Moexipril hydrochloride 15 mg and hydrochlorothiazide 12.5 mg
15/25: Moexipril hydrochloride 15 mg and hydrochlorothiazide 25 mg

moexipril hydrochloride *see* moexipril *on this page*

Moi-Stir® [US-OTC] *see* saliva substitute *on page 792*

Moisture® Eyes PM [US-OTC] *see* artificial tears *on page 78*

Moisture® Eyes [US-OTC] *see* artificial tears *on page 78*

Moisturel® Lotion ***(Discontinued)*** *see page 1042*

molindone (moe LIN done)

Sound-Alike/Look-Alike Issues
molindone may be confused with Mobidin®
Moban® may be confused with Mobidin®, Modane®

Synonyms molindone hydrochloride

U.S./Canadian Brand Names Moban® [US/Can]

Therapeutic Category Antipsychotic Agent, Dihydroindoline

Use Management of schizophrenia

Usual Dosage Oral:
Children: Schizophrenia/psychoses:
3-5 years: 1-2.5 mg/day in 4 divided doses
5-12 years: 0.5-1 mg/kg/day in 4 divided doses
Adults: Schizophrenia/psychoses: 50-75 mg/day increase at 3- to 4-day intervals up to 225 mg/day

Dosage Forms

Solution, oral concentrate, as hydrochloride: 20 mg/mL (120 mL) [contains alcohol and sodium metabisulfite; cherry flavor]

Tablet, as hydrochloride: 5 mg, 10 mg, 25 mg, 50 mg, 100 mg

molindone hydrochloride *see* molindone *on previous page*

molybdenum *see* trace metals *on page 874*

Molypen® [US] *see* trace metals *on page 874*

MOM *see* magnesium hydroxide *on page 537*

Momentum® [US-OTC] *see* magnesium salicylate *on page 539*

mometasone furoate (moe MET a sone FYOOR oh ate)

U.S./Canadian Brand Names Elocom® [Can]; Elocon® [US]; Nasonex® [US/Can]

Therapeutic Category Corticosteroid, Intranasal; Corticosteroid, Topical

Use Relief of the inflammatory and pruritic manifestations of corticosteroid-responsive dermatoses (medium potency topical corticosteroid); treatment of nasal symptoms of seasonal and perennial allergic rhinitis in adults and children ≥2 years of age; prevention of nasal symptoms associated with seasonal allergic rhinitis in children ≥12 years of age and adults

Usual Dosage

Nasal spray:

Children 2-11 years: 1 spray (50 mcg) in each nostril daily

Children ≥12 years and Adults: 2 sprays (100 mcg) in each nostril daily; when used for the prevention of allergic rhinitis, treatment should begin 2-4 weeks prior to pollen season

Topical: Apply sparingly, do not use occlusive dressings. Therapy should be discontinued when control is achieved; if no improvement is seen in 2 weeks, reassessment of diagnosis may be necessary.

Cream, ointment: Children ≥2 years and Adults: Apply a thin film to affected area once daily; do not use in pediatric patients for longer than 3 weeks

Lotion: Children ≥12 years and Adults: Apply a few drops to affected area once daily

Dosage Forms

Cream, topical (Elocon®): 0.1% (15 g, 45 g)

Lotion, topical (Elocon®): 0.1% (30 mL, 60 mL) [contains isopropyl alcohol 40%]

Ointment, topical (Elocon®): 0.1% (15 g, 45 g)

Suspension, intranasal spray (Nasonex®): 50 mcg/spray (17 g) [delivers 120 sprays; contains benzalkonium chloride]

MOM/mineral oil emulsion *see* magnesium hydroxide and mineral oil emulsion *on page 538*

monacolin K *see* lovastatin *on page 533*

Monafed® *(Discontinued)* *see page 1042*

Monafed® DM *(Discontinued)* *see page 1042*

Monarc® M [US] *see* antihemophilic factor (human) *on page 62*

***Monilia* skin test** *see Candida albicans (Monilia)* *on page 152*

Monistat® [Can] *see* miconazole *on page 578*

Monistat® 1 Combination Pack [US-OTC] *see* miconazole *on page 578*

Monistat® 3 [US-OTC] *see* miconazole *on page 578*

Monistat® 7 [US-OTC] *see* miconazole *on page 578*

Monistat-Derm® [US] *see* miconazole *on page 578*

Monistat i.v.™ Injection *(Discontinued)* *see page 1042*

Monitan® [Can] *see* acebutolol *on page 4*

monobenzone (mon oh BEN zone)

U.S./Canadian Brand Names Benoquin® [US]

Therapeutic Category Topical Skin Product

Use Final depigmentation in extensive vitiligo

Usual Dosage Children ≥12 years and Adults: Topical: Apply 2-3 times daily; once desired degree of pigmentation is obtained, may apply as needed (usually 2 times/ week)

Dosage Forms Cream, topical: 20% (35 g)

Monocete® Topical Liquid *(Discontinued)* *see page 1042*

Monocid® *(Discontinued)* *see page 1042*

Monoclate-P® [US] *see* antihemophilic factor (human) *on page 62*

monoclonal antibody *see* muromonab-CD3 *on page 595*

monoclonal antibody purified *see* factor IX *on page 354*

Monocor® [Can] *see* bisoprolol *on page 122*

Monodox® [US] *see* doxycycline *on page 294*

monoethanolamine *see* ethanolamine oleate *on page 335*

Mono-Gesic® [US] *see* salsalate *on page 793*

Monoket® [US] *see* isosorbide mononitrate *on page 489*

MonoNessa™ [US] *see* ethinyl estradiol and norgestimate *on page 346*

Mononine® [US/Can] *see* factor IX *on page 354*

Monopril® [US/Can] *see* fosinopril *on page 390*

Monopril-HCT® [US/Can] *see* fosinopril and hydrochlorothiazide *on page 391*

montelukast (mon te LOO kast)

Sound-Alike/Look-Alike Issues

Singulair® may be confused with Sinequan®

Synonyms montelukast sodium

U.S./Canadian Brand Names Singulair® [US/Can]

Therapeutic Category Leukotriene Receptor Antagonist

Use Prophylaxis and chronic treatment of asthma in adults and children ≥1 year of age; relief of symptoms of seasonal allergic rhinitis in adults and children ≥2 years of age

Usual Dosage Oral:

Children:

<1 year: Safety and efficacy have not been established

12-23 months: Asthma: 4 mg (oral granules) once daily, taken in the evening

2-5 years: Asthma or seasonal allergic rhinitis: 4 mg (chewable tablet or oral granules) once daily, taken in the evening

6-14 years: Asthma or seasonal allergic rhinitis: Chew one 5 mg chewable tablet/day, taken in the evening

Children ≥15 years and Adults: Asthma or seasonal allergic rhinitis: 10 mg/day, taken in the evening

Dosage Forms

Granules: 4 mg/packet

Tablet: 10 mg

Tablet, chewable: 4 mg [contains phenylalanine 0.674 mg; cherry flavor]; 5 mg [contains phenylalanine 0.842 mg; cherry flavor]

montelukast sodium *see* montelukast *on this page*

Monurol™ [US/Can] *see* fosfomycin *on page 390*

8-MOP® [US/Can] *see* methoxsalen *on page 567*

more attenuated enders strain *see* measles virus vaccine (live) *on page 545*

MoreDophilus® [US-OTC] *see* Lactobacillus *on page 501*

moricizine (mor EYE siz een)

Sound-Alike/Look-Alike Issues

Ethmozine® may be confused with Erythrocin®, erythromycin

Synonyms noricizine hydrochloride

U.S./Canadian Brand Names Ethmozine® [US/Can]

Therapeutic Category Antiarrhythmic Agent, Class I

Use Treatment of ventricular tachycardia and life-threatening ventricular arrhythmias

Usual Dosage Adults: Oral: 200-300 mg every 8 hours, adjust dosage at 150 mg/day at 3-day intervals

Dosage Forms Tablet, as hydrochloride: 200 mg, 250 mg, 300 mg

morning after pill *see* ethinyl estradiol and norgestrel *on page 347*

Morphine HP® [Can] *see* morphine sulfate *on this page*

Morphine LP® Epidural [Can] *see* morphine sulfate *on this page*

morphine sulfate (MOR feen SUL fate)

Sound-Alike/Look-Alike Issues

morphine may be confused with hydromorphone

Avinza™ may be confused with Evista®

Roxanol® may be confused with Roxicet®

Synonyms MS

U.S./Canadian Brand Names Astramorph/PF™ [US]; Avinza™ [US]; DepoDur™ [US]; Duramorph® [US]; Infumorph® [US]; Kadian® [US/Can]; M-Eslon® [Can]; Morphine HP® [Can]; Morphine LP® Epidural [Can]; M.O.S.-Sulfate® [Can]; MS Contin® [US/Can]; MSIR® [US/Can]; Oramorph SR® [US]; PMS-Morphine Sulfate SR [Can]; ratio-Morphine SR [Can]; RMS® [US]; Roxanol® [US]; Roxanol 100® [US]; Roxanol®-T [US]; Statex® [Can]

Therapeutic Category Analgesic, Narcotic

Controlled Substance C-II

Use Relief of moderate to severe acute and chronic pain; relief of pain of myocardial infarction; relief of dyspnea of acute left ventricular failure and pulmonary edema; preanesthetic medication

DepoDur™: Epidural (lumbar) single-dose management of surgical pain

Orphan drug: Infumorph™: Used in microinfusion devices for intraspinal administration in treatment of intractable chronic pain

Usual Dosage Note: These are guidelines and do not represent the maximum doses that may be required in all patients. Doses should be titrated to pain relief/prevention.

Children >6 months and <50 kg: Acute pain (moderate-to-severe):

Oral (prompt release): 0.15-0.3 mg/kg every 3-4 hours as needed

I.M.: 0.1 mg/kg every 3-4 hours as needed

I.V.: 0.05-0.1 mg/kg every 3-4 hours as needed

I.V. infusion: Range: 10-30 mcg/kg/hour

Adolescents >12 years: Sedation/analgesia for procedures: I.V.: 3-4 mg and repeat in 5 minutes if necessary

Adults: Acute pain (moderate-to-severe):

Oral: Prompt release formulations: Opiate-naive: Initial: 10 mg every 3-4 hours as needed; patients with prior opiate exposure may require higher initial doses: usual dosage range: 10-30 mg every 3-4 hours as needed

Oral: Controlled-, extended-, or sustained-release formulations: **Note:** A patient's morphine requirement should be established using prompt-release formulations. Conversion to long-acting products may be considered when chronic, continuous treatment is required. Higher dosages should be reserved for use only in opioid-tolerant patients.

Capsules, extended release (Avinza™): Daily dose administered once daily (for best results, administer at same time each day)

Capsules, sustained release (Kadian®): Daily dose administered once daily or in 2 divided doses daily (every 12 hours)

(Continued)

morphine sulfate *(Continued)*

Tablets, controlled release (MS Contin®), sustained release (Oramorph SR®), or extended release: Daily dose divided and administered every 8 or every 12 hours

I.V.: Initial: Opiate-naive: 2.5-5 mg every 3-4 hours; patients with prior opiate exposure may require higher initial doses. **Note:** Repeated doses (up to every 5 minutes if needed) in small increments (eg, 1-4 mg) may be preferred to larger and less frequent doses.

I.V., SubQ continuous infusion: 0.8-10 mg/hour; may increase depending on pain relief/adverse effects: usual range: up to 80 mg/hour although higher doses may be required

Mechanically-ventilated patients (based on 70 kg patient): 0.7-10 mg every 1-2 hours as needed; infusion: 5-35 mg/hour

Patient-controlled analgesia (PCA): (Opiate-naive: Consider lower end of dosing range): Usual concentration: 1 mg/mL Demand dose: Usual: 1 mg; range: 0.5-2.5 mg Lockout interval: 5-10 minutes

Epidural: **Note:** Administer with extreme caution and in reduced dosage to geriatric or debilitated patients.

Infusion: Bolus dose: 1-6 mg Infusion rate: 0.1-1 mg/hour Maximum dose: 10 mg/24 hours

Single-dose (extended release, Depo-Dur™): Cesarean section: 10 mg Lower abdominal/pelvic surgery: 10-15 mg **Note:** Some patients may benefit from a 20 mg dose, however, the incidence of adverse effects may be increased.

Intrathecal (I.T.): One-tenth of epidural dose; **Note:** Administer with extreme caution and in reduced dosage to geriatric or debilitated patients.

Opiate-naive: 0.2-1 mg/dose (may provide adequate relief for 24 hours); repeat doses **not** recommended except to establish initial IT dose.

I.M., SubQ: **Note:** Repeated SubQ administration causes local tissue irritation, pain, and induration.

Initial: Opiate-naive: 5-10 mg every 3-4 hours as needed; patients with prior opiate exposure may require higher initial doses; usual dosage range: 5-20 mg every 3-4 hours as needed

Rectal: 10-20 mg every 3-4 hours

Chronic pain: Patients taking opioids chronically may become tolerant and require doses higher than the usual dosage range to maintain the desired effect. Tolerance can be managed by appropriate dose titration. There is no optimal or maximal dose for morphine in chronic pain. The appropriate dose is one that relieves pain throughout its dosing interval without causing unmanageable side effects.

Dosage Forms

Capsule (MSIR®): 15 mg, 30 mg

Capsule, extended release (Avinza™): 30 mg, 60 mg, 90 mg, 120 mg

Capsule, sustained release (Kadian®): 20 mg, 30 mg, 50 mg, 60 mg, 100 mg

Infusion [premixed in D_5W]: 0.2 mg/mL (250 mL, 500 mL); 1 mg/mL (100 mL, 250 mL, 500 mL)

Injection, extended release liposomal suspension [lumbar epidural injection, preservative free] (DepoDur™): 10 mg/mL (1 mL, 1.5 mL, 2 mL)

Injection, solution: 2 mg/mL (1 mL); 4 mg/mL (1 mL); 5 mg/mL (1 mL); 8 mg/mL (1 mL); 10 mg/mL (1 mL, 2 mL, 10 mL); 15 mg/mL (1 mL, 20 mL); 25 mg/mL (4 mL, 10 mL, 20 mL, 40 mL) [some preparations contain sodium metabisulfite]

Injection, solution [epidural, intrathecal, or I.V. infusion; preservative free]:

Astramorph/PF™: 0.5 mg/mL (2 mL, 10 mL); 1 mg/mL (2 mL, 10 mL)

Duramorph®: 0.5 mg/mL (10 mL); 1 mg/mL (10 mL)

Injection, solution [epidural or intrathecal infusion via microinfusion device; preservative free] (Infumorph®): 10 mg/mL (20 mL); 25 mg/mL (20 mL)

Injection, solution [I.V. infusion via PCA pump]: 1 mg/mL (50 mL); 5 mg/mL (50 mL)

Injection, solution [preservative free]: 0.5 mg/mL (10 mL); 1 mg/mL (10 mL, 30 mL); 10 mg/mL (10 mL); 15 mg/mL (20 mL); 25 mg/mL (4 mL, 10 mL, 20 mL); 50 mg/mL (10 mL, 20 mL, 50 mL)

Solution, oral: 10 mg/5 mL (5 mL, 10 mL, 100 mL, 500 mL); 20 mg/5 mL (100 mL, 500 mL); 20 mg/mL (30 mL, 120 mL, 240 mL)
MSIR®: 10 mg/5 mL (120 mL); 20 mg/5 mL (120 mL); 20 mg/mL (30 mL, 120 mL) [contains sodium benzoate]
Roxanol™: 20 mg/mL (30 mL, 120 mL)
Roxanol 100™: 100 mg/5 mL (240 mL) [with calibrated spoon]
Roxanol T™: 20 mg/mL (30 mL, 120 mL) [tinted, flavored]
Suppository, rectal (RMS®): 5 mg (12s), 10 mg (12s), 20 mg (12s), 30 mg (12s)
Tablet (MSIR®): 15 mg, 30 mg
Tablet, controlled release (MS Contin®): 15 mg, 30 mg, 60 mg, 100 mg, 200 mg
Tablet, extended release: 15 mg, 30 mg, 60 mg, 100 mg, 200 mg
Tablet, sustained release (Oramorph SR®): 15 mg, 30 mg, 60 mg, 100 mg

morrhuate sodium (MOR yoo ate SOW dee um)

U.S./Canadian Brand Names Scleromate™ [US]
Therapeutic Category Sclerosing Agent
Use Treatment of small, uncomplicated varicose veins of the lower extremities
Usual Dosage Adults: I.V.: 50-250 mg, repeated at 5- to 7-day intervals (50-100 mg for small veins, 150-250 mg for large veins)
Dosage Forms Injection, solution: 50 mg/mL (30 mL)

Mosco® Corn and Callus Remover [US-OTC] *see* salicylic acid *on page 789*

M.O.S.-Sulfate® [Can] *see* morphine sulfate *on page 591*

Motilium® [Can] *see* domperidone *(Canada only) on page 288*

Motofen® [US] *see* difenoxin and atropine *on page 269*

Motrin® [US/Can] *see* ibuprofen *on page 462*

Motrin® Children's [US-OTC/Can] *see* ibuprofen *on page 462*

Motrin® Cold and Sinus [US-OTC] *see* pseudoephedrine and ibuprofen *on page 747*

Motrin® Cold, Children's [US-OTC] *see* pseudoephedrine and ibuprofen *on page 747*

Motrin® IB Sinus *(Discontinued)* *see page 1042*

Motrin® IB [US-OTC/Can] *see* ibuprofen *on page 462*

Motrin® Infants' [US-OTC] *see* ibuprofen *on page 462*

Motrin® Junior Strength [US-OTC] *see* ibuprofen *on page 462*

Motrin® Migraine Pain [US-OTC] *see* ibuprofen *on page 462*

MouthKote® [US-OTC] *see* saliva substitute *on page 792*

Moxam® Injection *(Discontinued)* *see page 1042*

moxifloxacin (mox i FLOX a sin)

Sound-Alike/Look-Alike Issues
Avelox® may be confused with Avonex®
Synonyms moxifloxacin hydrochloride
U.S./Canadian Brand Names Avelox® [US/Can]; Avelox® I.V. [US]; Vigamox™ [US]
Therapeutic Category Antibiotic, Quinolone
Use Treatment of mild-to-moderate community-acquired pneumonia, including multidrug-resistant *Streptococcus pneumoniae* (MDRSP); acute bacterial exacerbation of chronic bronchitis; acute bacterial sinusitis; uncomplicated skin infections; bacterial conjunctivitis (ophthalmic formulation)
Usual Dosage
Oral, I.V.: Adults:
Acute bacterial sinusitis: 400 mg every 24 hours for 10 days
Chronic bronchitis, acute bacterial exacerbation: 400 mg every 24 hours for 5 days
(Continued)

moxifloxacin *(Continued)*

Note: Avelox® ABC Pack™ (Avelox® Bronchitis Course) contains five tablets of 400 mg each.

Community-acquired pneumonia (including MDRSP): 400 mg every 24 hours for 7-14 days

Uncomplicated skin infections: 400 mg every 24 hours for 7 days

Ophthalmic: Children ≥1 year and Adults: Instill 1 drop into affected eye(s) 3 times/day for 7 days

Dosage Forms

Infusion, as hydrochloride [premixed in sodium chloride 0.8%] (Avelox® I.V.): 400 mg (250 mL)

Solution, ophthalmic, as hydrochloride (Vigamox™): 0.5% (3 mL)

Tablet [film coated], as hydrochloride:

Avelox®: 400 mg

Avelox® ABC Pack [unit-dose pack]: 400 mg (5s)

moxifloxacin hydrochloride *see* moxifloxacin *on previous page*

Moxilin® [US] *see* amoxicillin *on page 51*

4-MP *see* fomepizole *on page 387*

6-MP *see* mercaptopurine *on page 555*

MPA *see* mycophenolate *on page 596*

MPA and estrogens (conjugated) *see* estrogens (conjugated/equine) and medroxyprogesterone *on page 330*

M-Prednisol® Injection *(Discontinued)* *see page 1042*

M-R-VAX® II *(Discontinued)* *see page 1042*

MS *see* morphine sulfate *on page 591*

MS Contin® [US/Can] *see* morphine sulfate *on page 591*

MSIR® [US/Can] *see* morphine sulfate *on page 591*

MSTA® Mumps *(Discontinued)* *see page 1042*

MTA *see* pemetrexed *on page 673*

MTC *see* mitomycin *on page 585*

M.T.E.-4® [US] *see* trace metals *on page 874*

M.T.E.-5® [US] *see* trace metals *on page 874*

M.T.E.-6® [US] *see* trace metals *on page 874*

M.T.E.-7® [US] *see* trace metals *on page 874*

MTX *see* methotrexate *on page 565*

Mucinex®-D [US] *see* guaifenesin and pseudoephedrine *on page 419*

Mucinex® [US-OTC] *see* guaifenesin *on page 415*

Mucomyst® [US/Can] *see* acetylcysteine *on page 16*

Mucosil™ *(Discontinued)* *see page 1042*

Multidex® [US-OTC] *see* maltodextrin *on page 541*

multiple vitamins *see* vitamins (multiple/oral) *on page 927*

multitargeted antifolate *see* pemetrexed *on page 673*

Multitest CMI® *(Discontinued)* *see page 1042*

Multitrace™-4 [US] *see* trace metals *on page 874*

Multitrace™-4 Neonatal [US] *see* trace metals *on page 874*

Multitrace™-4 Pediatric [US] *see* trace metals *on page 874*

Multitrace™-5 [US] *see* trace metals *on page 874*

multivitamins/fluoride *see* vitamins (multiple/pediatric) *on page 927*

mumps, measles and rubella vaccines, combined *see* measles, mumps, and rubella vaccines, combined *on page 544*

Mumpsvax® [US/Can] *see* mumps virus vaccine, live, attenuated *on this page*

mumps virus vaccine, live, attenuated

(mumpz VYE rus vak SEEN, live, a ten YOO ate ed)

U.S./Canadian Brand Names Mumpsvax® [US/Can]

Therapeutic Category Vaccine, Live Virus

Use Mumps prophylaxis by promoting active immunity

Note: Trivalent measles-mumps-rubella (MMR) vaccine is the preferred agent for most children and many adults; persons born prior to 1957 are generally considered immune and need not be vaccinated

Usual Dosage Children ≥15 months and Adults: 0.5 mL SubQ in outer aspect of the upper arm, no booster

Dosage Forms Injection, powder for reconstitution [preservative free]: 20,000 $TCID_{50}$ [contains human albumin, neomycin; packaged with diluent]

mupirocin (myoo PEER oh sin)

Sound-Alike/Look-Alike Issues

Bactroban® may be confused with bacitracin, baclofen

Synonyms mupirocin calcium; pseudomonic acid A

U.S./Canadian Brand Names Bactroban® Nasal [US]; Bactroban® [US/Can]

Therapeutic Category Antibiotic, Topical

Use

Intranasal: Eradication of nasal colonization with MRSA in adult patients and healthcare workers

Topical treatment of impetigo due to *Staphylococcus aureus*, beta-hemolytic *Streptococcus*, and *S. pyogenes*

Usual Dosage

Children ≥3 months and Adults: Topical: Apply small amount to affected area 2-5 times/day for 5-14 days

Children ≥12 years and Adults: Intranasal: Approximately one-half of the ointment from the single-use tube should be applied into one nostril and the other half into the other nostril twice daily for 5 days

Dosage Forms

Cream, topical, as calcium (Bactroban®): 2% (15 g, 30 g) [contains benzyl alcohol]

Ointment, intranasal, topical, as calcium (Bactroban® Nasal): 2% (1 g) [single-use tube]

Ointment, topical (Bactroban®): 2% (22 g)

mupirocin calcium *see* mupirocin *on this page*

Murine® Ear [US-OTC] *see* carbamide peroxide *on page 155*

Murine® Tears Plus [US-OTC] *see* tetrahydrozoline *on page 852*

Murine® Tears [US-OTC] *see* artificial tears *on page 78*

Muro 128® [US-OTC] *see* sodium chloride *on page 810*

Murocel® [US-OTC] *see* artificial tears *on page 78*

Murocoll-2® [US] *see* phenylephrine and scopolamine *on page 690*

muromonab-CD3 (myoo roe MOE nab-see dee three)

Synonyms monoclonal antibody; OKT3

U.S./Canadian Brand Names Orthoclone OKT® 3 [US/Can]

Therapeutic Category Immunosuppressant Agent

Use Treatment of acute allograft rejection in renal transplant patients; treatment of acute hepatic, kidney, and pancreas rejection episodes resistant to conventional treatment.

(Continued)

muromonab-CD3 *(Continued)*

Acute graft-versus-host disease following bone marrow transplantation resistant to conventional treatment.

Usual Dosage Refer to individual protocols. I.V.:

Children <30 kg: 2.5 mg/day once daily for 7-14 days
Children >30 kg: 5 mg/day once daily for 7-14 days
OR
Children <12 years: 0.1 mg/kg/day once daily for 10-14 days
Children ≥12 years and Adults: 5 mg/day once daily for 10-14 days

Dosage Forms Injection, solution: 1 mg/mL (5 mL)

Muroptic-5® ***(Discontinued)*** *see page 1042*

Muse® [Can] *see* alprostadil *on page 35*

Muse® Pellet [US] *see* alprostadil *on page 35*

Mus-Lax® ***(Discontinued)*** *see page 1042*

Mustargen® [US/Can] *see* mechlorethamine *on page 546*

mustine *see* mechlorethamine *on page 546*

Mutamycin® [US/Can] *see* mitomycin *on page 585*

M.V.I.®-12 [US] *see* vitamins (multiple/injectable) *on page 919*

M.V.I.-Adult® [US] *see* vitamins (multiple/injectable) *on page 919*

M.V.I.-Pediatric® [US] *see* vitamins (multiple/injectable) *on page 919*

Myambutol® [US] *see* ethambutol *on page 334*

Mycelex® [US] *see* clotrimazole *on page 218*

Mycelex®-3 [US-OTC] *see* butoconazole *on page 139*

Mycelex®-7 [US-OTC] *see* clotrimazole *on page 218*

Mycelex®-G ***(Discontinued)*** *see page 1042*

Mycelex® Twin Pack [US-OTC] *see* clotrimazole *on page 218*

Mycifradin® Sulfate ***(Discontinued)*** *see page 1042*

Myciguent [US-OTC] *see* neomycin *on page 609*

Mycinettes® [US-OTC] *see* benzocaine *on page 107*

Mycobutin® [US/Can] *see* rifabutin *on page 775*

Mycolog®-II ***(Discontinued)*** *see page 1042*

Myco-Nail [US-OTC] *see* triacetin *on page 879*

Myconel® Topical ***(Discontinued)*** *see page 1042*

mycophenolate (mye koe FEN oh late)

Synonyms MMF; MPA; mycophenolate mofetil; mycophenolate sodium; mycophenolic acid

U.S./Canadian Brand Names CellCept® [US/Can]; Myfortic® [US]

Therapeutic Category Immunosuppressant Agent

Use Prophylaxis of organ rejection concomitantly with cyclosporine and corticosteroids in patients receiving allogenic renal (CellCept®, Myfortic®), cardiac (CellCept®), or hepatic (CellCept®) transplants

Usual Dosage

Children: Renal transplant: Oral:

CellCept® suspension: 600 mg/m^2/dose twice daily; maximum dose: 1 g twice daily
Alternatively, may use solid dosage forms according to BSA as follows:
BSA 1.25-1.5 m^2: 750 mg capsule twice daily
BSA >1.5 m^2: 1 g capsule or tablet twice daily

Myfortic®:
BSA <1.19 m^2: Use of this formulation is not recommended

BSA 1.19-1.58 m^2: 400 mg/m^2 twice daily (maximum: 1080 mg/day)
BSA >1.58 m^2: 400 mg/m^2 twice daily (maximum: 1440 mg/day)

Adults: The initial dose should be given as soon as possible following transplantation; intravenous solution may be given until the oral medication can be tolerated (up to 14 days)

Renal transplant:

CellCept®: Oral: 1 g twice daily. Although a dose of 1.5 g twice daily was used in clinical trials and shown to be effective, no efficacy advantage was established. Patients receiving 2 g/day demonstrated an overall better safety profile than patients receiving 3 g/day. Doses >2 g/day are not recommended in these patients because of the possibility for enhanced immunosuppression as well as toxicities. I.V.: 1 g twice daily

Myfortic®: Oral: 720 mg twice daily (1440 mg/day)

Cardiac transplantation:

Oral (CellCept®): 1.5 g twice daily
I.V. (CellCept®): 1.5 g twice daily

Hepatic transplantation:

Oral (CellCept®): 1.5 g twice daily
I.V. (CellCept®): 1 g twice daily

Dosage Forms

Capsule, as mofetil (CellCept®): 250 mg

Injection, powder for reconstitution, as mofetil hydrochloride (CellCept®): 500 mg [contains polysorbate 80]

Powder for oral suspension, as mofetil (CellCept®): 200 mg/mL (225 mL) [contains phenylalanine 0.56 mg/mL; mixed fruit flavor]

Tablet, as mofetil [film coated] (CellCept®): 500 mg [may contain ethyl alcohol]

Tablet, delayed release, as mycophenolic acid [film coated] (Myfortic®): 180 mg, 360 mg [formulated as a sodium salt]

mycophenolate mofetil *see* mycophenolate *on previous page*

mycophenolate sodium *see* mycophenolate *on previous page*

mycophenolic acid *see* mycophenolate *on previous page*

Mycostatin® [US/Can] *see* nystatin *on page 637*

Mydfrin® [US/Can] *see* phenylephrine *on page 689*

Mydriacyl® [US/Can] *see* tropicamide *on page 892*

My First Flintstones® [US-OTC] *see* vitamins (multiple/pediatric) *on page 927*

Myfortic® [US] *see* mycophenolate *on previous page*

Mykrox® [Can] *see* metolazone *on page 574*

Mykrox® ***(Discontinued)*** *see page 1042*

Mylanta® [Can] *see* aluminum hydroxide and magnesium hydroxide *on page 40*

Mylanta AR® ***(Discontinued)*** *see page 1042*

Mylanta® Children's [US-OTC] *see* calcium carbonate *on page 144*

Mylanta® Double Strength [Can] *see* aluminum hydroxide, magnesium hydroxide, and simethicone *on page 40*

Mylanta® Extra Strength [Can] *see* aluminum hydroxide, magnesium hydroxide, and simethicone *on page 40*

Mylanta® Gas Maximum Strength [US-OTC] *see* simethicone *on page 804*

Mylanta® Gas [US-OTC] *see* simethicone *on page 804*

Mylanta® Gelcaps® [US-OTC] *see* calcium carbonate and magnesium hydroxide *on page 146*

Mylanta®-II ***(Discontinued)*** *see page 1042*

Mylanta® Liquid [US-OTC] *see* aluminum hydroxide, magnesium hydroxide, and simethicone *on page 40*

Mylanta® Maximum Strength Liquid [US-OTC] *see* aluminum hydroxide, magnesium hydroxide, and simethicone *on page 40*

Mylanta® Regular Strength [Can] *see* aluminum hydroxide, magnesium hydroxide, and simethicone *on page 40*

Mylanta® Supreme [US-OTC] *see* calcium carbonate and magnesium hydroxide *on page 146*

Mylanta® Ultra [US-OTC] *see* calcium carbonate and magnesium hydroxide *on page 146*

Mylaxen® Injection *(Discontinued)* *see page 1042*

Myleran® [US/Can] *see* busulfan *on page 137*

Mylicon® Infants [US-OTC] *see* simethicone *on page 804*

Mylocel™ [US] *see* hydroxyurea *on page 457*

Mylotarg® [US/Can] *see* gemtuzumab ozogamicin *on page 400*

Myminic® Expectorant *(Discontinued)* *see page 1042*

Myobloc® [US] *see* botulinum toxin type B *on page 125*

Myochrysine® [Can] *see* gold sodium thiomalate *on page 412*

Myochrysine® *(Discontinued)* *see page 1042*

Myoflex® [US-OTC/Can] *see* triethanolamine salicylate *on page 884*

Myotonachol® [Can] *see* bethanechol *on page 117*

Myotonachol™ *(Discontinued)* *see page 1042*

Myphetane DC® *(Discontinued)* *see page 1042*

Mysoline® [US/Can] *see* primidone *on page 728*

Mytelase® [US/Can] *see* ambenonium *on page 42*

Mytussin® AC [US] *see* guaifenesin and codeine *on page 416*

Mytussin® DAC [US] *see* guaifenesin, pseudoephedrine, and codeine *on page 422*

Mytussin® DM [US-OTC] *see* guaifenesin and dextromethorphan *on page 416*

Nabi-HB® [US] *see* hepatitis B immune globulin *on page 433*

nabumetone (na BYOO me tone)

U.S./Canadian Brand Names Apo-Nabumetone® [Can]; Gen-Nabumetone [Can]; Relafen® [US/Can]; Rhoxal-nabumetone [Can]

Therapeutic Category Analgesic, Nonnarcotic; Nonsteroidal Antiinflammatory Drug (NSAID)

Use Management of osteoarthritis and rheumatoid arthritis

Usual Dosage Adults: Oral: 1000 mg/day; an additional 500-1000 mg may be needed in some patients to obtain more symptomatic relief; may be administered once or twice daily

Dosage Forms Tablet: 500 mg, 750 mg

NAC *see* acetylcysteine *on page 16*

***n*-acetylcysteine** *see* acetylcysteine *on page 16*

***n*-acetyl-L-cysteine** *see* acetylcysteine *on page 16*

n-acetyl-p-aminophenol *see* acetaminophen *on page 5*

NaCl *see* sodium chloride *on page 810*

nadolol (nay DOE lole)

Sound-Alike/Look-Alike Issues

nadolol may be confused with Mandol®

Corgard® may be confused with Cognex®

U.S./Canadian Brand Names Alti-Nadolol [Can]; Apo-Nadol® [Can]; Corgard® [US/Can]; Novo-Nadolol [Can]

Therapeutic Category Beta-Adrenergic Blocker

Use Treatment of hypertension and angina pectoris; prophylaxis of migraine headaches

Usual Dosage Oral:

Adults: Initial: 40 mg/day, increase dosage gradually by 40-80 mg increments at 3- to 7-day intervals until optimum clinical response is obtained with profound slowing of heart rate; doses up to 160-240 mg/day in angina and 240-320 mg/day in hypertension may be necessary.

Hypertension: Usual dosage range (JNC 7): 40-120 mg once daily

Dosage Forms Tablet: 20 mg, 40 mg, 80 mg, 120 mg, 160 mg

Nadopen-V® [Can] *see* penicillin V potassium *on page 677*

nadroparin calcium *see* nadroparin *(Canada only)* *on this page*

nadroparin *(Canada only)* (nad roe PA rin)

Synonyms nadroparin calcium

U.S./Canadian Brand Names Fraxiparine™ [Can]; Fraxiparine™ Forte [Can]

Therapeutic Category Low Molecular Weight Heparin

Use Prophylaxis of thromboembolic disorders (particularly deep venous thrombosis and pulmonary embolism) in general and orthopedic surgery; treatment of deep venous thrombosis; prevention of clotting during hemodialysis

Usual Dosage SubQ: Adults:

Prophylaxis of thromboembolic disorders in general surgery: 2850 anti-Xa int. units once daily; begin 2-4 hours before surgery and continue for 7 days

Prophylaxis of thromboembolic disorders in hip replacement: 38 anti-Xa int. units/kg 12 hours before and 12 hours after surgery, **followed by** 38 anti-Xa int. units/kg/day up to and including day 3, **then** 57 anti-Xa int. units/kg/day for up to 10 days total therapy

Treatment of thromboembolic disorders: 171 anti-Xa int. units/kg/day to a maximum of 17,100 int. units; plasma anti-Xa levels should be 1.2-1.8 anti-Xa int. units/mL 3-4 hours postinjection

Patients at increased risk of bleeding: 86 anti-Xa int. units/kg twice daily; plasma anti-Xa levels should be 0.5-1.1 anti-Xa int. units/mL 3-4 hours postinjection

Prevention of clotting during hemodialysis: Single dose of 65 anti-Xa int. units/kg into arterial line at start of each dialysis session; may give additional dose if session lasts longer than 4 hours

Patients at risk of hemorrhage: Administer 50% of dose

Dosage Forms Injection, solution, as calcium:

Fraxiparine™:

9500 anti-Xa int. units/mL (0.2 mL, 0.3 mL, 0.4 mL) [ungraduated prefilled syringe]

9500 anti-Xa int. units/mL (0.6 mL, 0.8 mL, 1 mL) [graduated prefilled syringe]

Fraxiparine™ Forte: 19,000 anti-Xa int. units/mL (0.6 mL, 0.8 mL, 1 mL) [graduated prefilled syringe]

nafarelin (NAF a re lin)

Sound-Alike/Look-Alike Issues

nafarelin may be confused with Anafranil®, enalapril

Synonyms nafarelin acetate

U.S./Canadian Brand Names Synarel® [US/Can]

Therapeutic Category Hormone, Posterior Pituitary

Use Treatment of endometriosis, including pain and reduction of lesions; treatment of central precocious puberty (gonadotropin-dependent precocious puberty) in children of both sexes

(Continued)

nafarelin *(Continued)*

Usual Dosage

Endometriosis: Adults: Female: 1 spray (200 mcg) in 1 nostril each morning and the other nostril each evening starting on days 2-4 of menstrual cycle for 6 months

Central precocious puberty: Children: Males/Females: 2 sprays (400 mcg) into each nostril in the morning 2 sprays (400 mcg) into each nostril in the evening. If inadequate suppression, may increase dose to 3 sprays (600 mcg) into alternating nostrils 3 times/day.

Dosage Forms Solution, intranasal spray, as acetate: 2 mg/mL (8 mL) [200 mcg/spray: 60 metered doses]

nafarelin acetate *see* nafarelin *on previous page*

Nafazair® Ophthalmic *(Discontinued)* *see page 1042*

Nafcil™ *(Discontinued)* *see page 1042*

nafcillin (naf SIL in)

Synonyms ethoxynaphthamido penicillin sodium; nafcillin sodium; sodium nafcillin

U.S./Canadian Brand Names Nallpen® [Can]; Unipen® [Can]

Therapeutic Category Penicillin

Use Treatment of infections such as osteomyelitis, septicemia, endocarditis, and CNS infections caused by susceptible strains of staphylococci species

Usual Dosage

Neonates:

<2000 g, <7 days: 50 mg/kg/day divided every 12 hours

<2000 g, >7 days: 75 mg/kg/day divided every 8 hours

>2000 g, <7 days: 50 mg/kg/day divided every 8 hours

>2000 g, >7 days: 75 mg/kg/day divided every 6 hours

Children:

I.M.: 25 mg/kg twice daily

I.V.:

Mild to moderate infections: 50-100 mg/kg/day in divided doses every 6 hours

Severe infections: 100-200 mg/kg/day in divided doses every 4-6 hours

Maximum dose: 12 g/day

Adults:

I.M.: 500 mg every 4-6 hours

I.V.: 500-2000 mg every 4-6 hours

Dosage Forms

Infusion [premixed iso-osmotic dextrose solution]: 1 g (50 mL); 2 g (100 mL)

Injection, powder for reconstitution, as sodium: 1 g, 2 g, 10 g

nafcillin sodium *see* nafcillin *on this page*

naftifine (NAF ti feen)

Synonyms naftifine hydrochloride

U.S./Canadian Brand Names Naftin® [US]

Therapeutic Category Antifungal Agent

Use Topical treatment of tinea cruris (jock itch), tinea corporis (ringworm), and tinea pedis (athlete's foot)

Usual Dosage Adults: Topical: Apply cream once daily and gel twice daily (morning and evening) for up to 4 weeks

Dosage Forms

Cream, as hydrochloride: 1% (15 g, 30 g, 60 g) [contains alcohol]

Gel, as hydrochloride: 1% (20 g, 40 g, 60 g) [contains alcohol]

naftifine hydrochloride *see* naftifine *on this page*

Naftin® [US] *see* naftifine *on this page*

$NaHCO_3$ *see* sodium bicarbonate *on page 809*

nalbuphine (NAL byoo feen)

Sound-Alike/Look-Alike Issues
Nubain® may be confused with Navane®, Nebcin®

Synonyms nalbuphine hydrochloride

U.S./Canadian Brand Names Nubain® [US/Can]

Therapeutic Category Analgesic, Narcotic

Use Relief of moderate to severe pain; preoperative analgesia, postoperative and surgical anesthesia, and obstetrical analgesia during labor and delivery

Usual Dosage I.M., I.V., SubQ:
Children 10 months to 14 years: Premedication: 0.2 mg/kg; maximum: 20 mg/dose
Adults: 10 mg/70 kg every 3-6 hours; maximum single dose: 20 mg; maximum daily dose: 160 mg

Dosage Forms Injection, solution, as hydrochloride: 10 mg/mL (1 mL, 10 mL); 20 mg/mL (1 mL, 10 mL)

nalbuphine hydrochloride *see* nalbuphine *on this page*

Nalcrom® [Can] *see* cromolyn sodium *on page 230*

Naldecon® *(Discontinued)* *see page 1042*

Naldecon® DX Adult Liquid *(Discontinued)* *see page 1042*

Naldecon-EX® Children's Syrup *(Discontinued)* *see page 1042*

Naldecon Senior EX® [US-OTC] *see* guaifenesin *on page 415*

Naldelate® *(Discontinued)* *see page 1042*

Nalex®-A [US] *see* chlorpheniramine, phenylephrine, and phenyltoloxamine *on page 193*

Nalfon® [US/Can] *see* fenoprofen *on page 361*

Nalgest® *(Discontinued)* *see page 1042*

nalidixic acid (nal i DIKS ik AS id)

Synonyms nalidixinic acid

U.S./Canadian Brand Names NegGram® [US/Can]

Therapeutic Category Quinolone

Use Treatment of urinary tract infections

Usual Dosage Oral:
Children 3 months to 12 years: 55 mg/kg/day divided every 6 hours; suppressive therapy is 33 mg/kg/day divided every 6 hours
Adults: 1 g 4 times/day for 2 weeks; then suppressive therapy of 500 mg 4 times/day

Dosage Forms [DSC] = Discontinued product
Suspension, oral: 250 mg/5 mL (473 mL) [raspberry flavor]
Tablet: 250 mg [DSC], 500 mg, 1 g [DSC]

nalidixinic acid *see* nalidixic acid *on this page*

Nallpen® [Can] *see* nafcillin *on previous page*

Nallpen® *(Discontinued)* *see page 1042*

***N*-allylnoroxymorphine hydrochloride** *see* naloxone *on next page*

nalmefene (NAL me feen)

Sound-Alike/Look-Alike Issues
Revex® may be confused with Nimbex®, ReVia®

Synonyms nalmefene hydrochloride

U.S./Canadian Brand Names Revex® [US]

Therapeutic Category Antidote

Use Complete or partial reversal of opioid drug effects, including respiratory depression induced by natural or synthetic opioids; reversal of postoperative opioid depression; management of known or suspected opioid overdose

(Continued)

nalmefene *(Continued)*

Usual Dosage

Reversal of postoperative opioid depression: Blue labeled product (100 mcg/mL): Titrate to reverse the undesired effects of opioids; initial dose for nonopioid dependent patients: 0.25 mcg/kg followed by 0.25 mcg/kg incremental doses at 2- to 5-minute intervals; after a total dose >1 mcg/kg, further therapeutic response is unlikely

Management of known/suspected opioid overdose: Green labeled product (1000 mcg/mL): Initial dose: 0.5 mg/70 kg; may repeat with 1 mg/70 kg in 2-5 minutes; further increase beyond a total dose of 1.5 mg/70 kg will not likely result in improved response and may result in cardiovascular stress and precipitated withdrawal syndrome. (If opioid dependency is suspected, administer a challenge dose of 0.1 mg/70 kg; if no withdrawal symptoms are observed in 2 minutes, the recommended doses can be administered.)

Note: If recurrence of respiratory depression is noted, dose may again be titrated to clinical effect using incremental doses.

Note: If I.V. access is lost or not readily obtainable, a single SubQ or I.M. dose of 1 mg may be effective in 5-15 minutes.

Dosing adjustment in renal or hepatic impairment: Not necessary with single uses, however, slow administration (over 60 seconds) of incremental doses is recommended to minimize hypertension and dizziness

Dosage Forms Injection, solution, as hydrochloride: 100 mcg/mL [blue label] (1 mL); 1000 mcg/mL [green label] (2 mL)

nalmefene hydrochloride *see* nalmefene *on previous page*

naloxone (nal OKS one)

Sound-Alike/Look-Alike Issues

naloxone may be confused with naltrexone

Narcan® may be confused with Marcaine®, Norcuron®

Synonyms *N*-allylnoroxymorphine hydrochloride; naloxone hydrochloride

U.S./Canadian Brand Names Narcan® [US/Can]

Therapeutic Category Antidote

Use

Complete or partial reversal of opioid depression, including respiratory depression, induced by natural and synthetic opioids, including propoxyphene, methadone, and certain mixed agonist-antagonist analgesics: nalbuphine, pentazocine, and butorphanol

Diagnosis of suspected opioid tolerance or acute opioid overdose

Adjunctive agent to increase blood pressure in the management of septic shock

Usual Dosage I.M., I.V. (preferred), intratracheal, SubQ:

Postanesthesia narcotic reversal: Infants and Children: 0.01 mg/kg; may repeat every 2-3 minutes, as needed based on response

Opiate intoxication:

Children:

Birth (including premature infants) to 5 years or <20 kg: 0.1 mg/kg; repeat every 2-3 minutes if needed; may need to repeat doses every 20-60 minutes

>5 years or ≥20 kg: 2 mg/dose; if no response, repeat every 2-3 minutes; may need to repeat doses every 20-60 minutes

Children and Adults: Continuous infusion: I.V.: If continuous infusion is required, calculate dosage/hour based on effective intermittent dose used and duration of adequate response seen, titrate dose 0.04-0.16 mg/kg/hour for 2-5 days in children, adult dose typically 0.25-6.25 mg/hour (short-term infusions as high as 2.4 mg/kg/hour have been tolerated in adults during treatment for septic shock); alternatively, continuous infusion utilizes $^2/_3$ of the initial naloxone bolus on an hourly basis; add 10 times this dose to each liter of D_5W and infuse at a rate of 100 mL/hour; $^1/_2$ of the initial bolus dose should be readministered 15 minutes after initiation of the continuous infusion to prevent a drop in naloxone levels; increase infusion rate as needed to assure adequate ventilation

Narcotic overdose: Adults: I.V.: 0.4-2 mg every 2-3 minutes as needed; may need to repeat doses every 20-60 minutes, if no response is observed after 10 mg, question the diagnosis. **Note:** Use 0.1-0.2 mg increments in patients who are opioid dependent and in postoperative patients to avoid large cardiovascular changes.

Dosage Forms

Injection, neonatal solution, as hydrochloride: 0.02 mg/mL (2 mL)

Injection, solution, as hydrochloride: 0.4 mg/mL (1 mL, 10 mL); 1 mg/mL (2 mL, 10 mL)

naloxone and buprenorphine *see* buprenorphine and naloxone *on page 135*

naloxone hydrochloride *see* naloxone *on previous page*

naloxone hydrochloride and pentazocine hydrochloride *see* pentazocine *on page 678*

naloxone hydrochloride dihydrate and buprenorphine hydrochloride *see* buprenorphine and naloxone *on page 135*

Nalspan® *(Discontinued)* *see page 1042*

naltrexone (nal TREKS one)

Sound-Alike/Look-Alike Issues

naltrexone may be confused with naloxone

ReVia® may be confused with Revex®

Synonyms naltrexone hydrochloride

U.S./Canadian Brand Names ReVia® [US/Can]

Therapeutic Category Antidote

Use Treatment of ethanol dependence; blockade of the effects of exogenously administered opioids

Usual Dosage Do not give until patient is opioid-free for 7-10 days as determined by urine analysis

Adults: Oral: 25 mg; if no withdrawal signs within 1 hour give another 25 mg; maintenance regimen is flexible, variable and individualized (50 mg/day to 100-150 mg 3 times/week for 12 weeks); up to 800 mg/day has been tolerated in adults without an adverse effect

Dosage Forms Tablet, as hydrochloride: 50 mg

naltrexone hydrochloride *see* naltrexone *on this page*

Namenda™ [US] *see* memantine *on page 550*

Nandrobolic® Injection *(Discontinued)* *see page 1042*

nandrolone (NAN droe lone)

Synonyms nandrolone decanoate; nandrolone phenpropionate

U.S./Canadian Brand Names Deca-Durabolin® [Can]; Durabolin® [Can]

Therapeutic Category Androgen

Controlled Substance C-III

Use Control of metastatic breast cancer; management of anemia of renal insufficiency

Usual Dosage Deep I.M. (into gluteal muscle):

Children 2-13 years (decanoate): 25-50 mg every 3-4 weeks

Adults:

- Male:
  - Breast cancer (phenpropionate): 50-100 mg/week
  - Anemia of renal insufficiency (decanoate): 100-200 mg/week
- Female: 50-100 mg/week
  - Breast cancer (phenpropionate): 50-100 mg/week
  - Anemia of renal insufficiency (decanoate): 50-100 mg/week

Dosage Forms Injection, solution, as decanoate [in sesame oil]: 100 mg/mL (2 mL); 200 mg/mL (1 mL) [contains benzyl alcohol]

nandrolone decanoate *see* nandrolone *on this page*

nandrolone phenpropionate *see* nandrolone *on previous page*

naphazoline (naf AZ oh leen)

Synonyms naphazoline hydrochloride

U.S./Canadian Brand Names AK-Con™ [US]; Albalon® [US]; Allersol® [US]; Clear Eyes® ACR [US-OTC]; Clear Eyes® [US-OTC]; Naphcon Forte® [Can]; Naphcon® [US-OTC]; Privine® [US-OTC]; VasoClear® [US-OTC]; Vasocon® [Can]

Therapeutic Category Adrenergic Agonist Agent

Use Topical ocular vasoconstrictor; will temporarily relieve congestion, itching, and minor irritation, and to control hyperemia in patients with superficial corneal vascularity; treatment of nasal congestion; adjunct for sinusitis

Usual Dosage

Nasal:

Children:

<6 years: Not recommended (especially infants) due to CNS depression

6-12 years: 1 spray of 0.05% into each nostril every 6 hours if necessary; therapy should not exceed 3-5 days

Children >12 years and Adults: 0.05%, instill 1-2 drops or sprays every 6 hours if needed; therapy should not exceed 3-5 days

Ophthalmic:

Children <6 years: Not recommended for use due to CNS depression (especially in infants)

Children >6 years and Adults: Instill 1-2 drops into conjunctival sac of affected eye(s) every 3-4 hours; therapy generally should not exceed 3-4 days

Dosage Forms

Solution, intranasal drops, as hydrochloride (Privine®): 0.05% (25 mL)

Solution, intranasal spray, as hydrochloride (Privine®): 0.05% (20 mL, 480 mL)

Solution, ophthalmic, as hydrochloride: 0.1% (15 mL)

AK-Con™, Albalon®, Allersol®: 0.1% (15 mL) [contains benzalkonium chloride]

Clear Eyes®: 0.012% (6 mL, 15 mL, 30 mL) [contains glycerin 0.2% and benzalkonium chloride]

Clear Eyes® ACR: 0.012% (15 mL, 30 mL) [contains glycerin 0.2%, zinc sulfate 0.25%, and benzalkonium chloride]

Naphcon®: 0.012% (15 mL) [contains benzalkonium chloride]

VasoClear®: 0.02% (15 mL) [contains benzalkonium chloride]

naphazoline and antazoline (naf AZ oh leen & an TAZ oh leen)

Synonyms antazoline and naphazoline

U.S./Canadian Brand Names Albalon®-A Liquifilm [Can]; Vasocon-A® [US-OTC/Can]

Therapeutic Category Antihistamine/Decongestant Combination

Use Topical ocular congestion, irritation and itching

Usual Dosage Ophthalmic: 1-2 drops every 3-4 hours

Dosage Forms Solution, ophthalmic: Naphazoline hydrochloride 0.05% and antazoline phosphate 0.5% (15 mL) [contains benzalkonium chloride]

naphazoline and pheniramine (naf AZ oh leen & fen NIR a meen)

Sound-Alike/Look-Alike Issues

Visine® may be confused with Visken®

Synonyms pheniramine and naphazoline

U.S./Canadian Brand Names Naphcon-A® [US-OTC/Can]; Opcon-A® [US-OTC]; Visine-A™ [US-OTC]

Therapeutic Category Antihistamine/Decongestant Combination

Use Treatment of ocular congestion, irritation, and itching

Usual Dosage Ophthalmic: Children ≥6 years and Adults: 1-2 drops up to 4 times/day

Dosage Forms Solution, ophthalmic: Naphazoline hydrochloride 0.025% and pheniramine 0.3% (15 mL) [contains benzalkonium chloride]

naphazoline hydrochloride *see* naphazoline *on this page*

Naphcon-A® [US-OTC/Can] *see* naphazoline and pheniramine *on previous page*

Naphcon Forte® [Can] *see* naphazoline *on previous page*

Naphcon Forte® Ophthalmic *(Discontinued)* *see page 1042*

Naphcon® [US-OTC] *see* naphazoline *on previous page*

NapraPAC™ *see* lansoprazole and naproxen *on page 506*

Naprelan® [US] *see* naproxen *on this page*

Naprosyn® [US/Can] *see* naproxen *on this page*

naproxen (na PROKS en)

Sound-Alike/Look-Alike Issues

naproxen may be confused with Naprosyn®
Aleve® may be confused with Alesse®
Anaprox® may be confused with Anaspaz®, Avapro®
Naprelan® may be confused with Naprosyn®
Naprosyn® may be confused with Naprelan®, naproxen, Natacyn®, Nebcin®

Synonyms naproxen sodium

U.S./Canadian Brand Names Aleve® [US-OTC]; Anaprox® [US/Can]; Anaprox® DS [US/Can]; Apo-Napro-Na® [Can]; Apo-Napro-Na DS® [Can]; Apo-Naproxen® [Can]; Apo-Naproxen SR® [Can]; EC-Naprosyn® [US]; Gen-Naproxen EC [Can]; Naprelan® [US]; Naprosyn® [US/Can]; Naxen® [Can]; Novo-Naproc EC [Can]; Novo-Naprox [Can]; Novo-Naprox Sodium [Can]; Novo-Naprox Sodium DS [Can]; Novo-Naprox SR [Can]; Nu-Naprox [Can]; Pamprin® Maximum Strength All Day Relief [US-OTC]; Riva-Naproxen [Can]

Therapeutic Category Analgesic, Nonnarcotic; Antipyretic; Nonsteroidal Antiinflammatory Drug (NSAID)

Use Management of inflammatory disease and rheumatoid disorders (including juvenile rheumatoid arthritis); acute gout; mild to moderate pain; dysmenorrhea; fever, migraine headache

Usual Dosage Oral:

Children >2 years:
- Fever: 2.5-10 mg/kg/dose; maximum: 10 mg/kg/day
- Juvenile arthritis: 10 mg/kg/day in 2 divided doses

Adults:
- Rheumatoid arthritis, osteoarthritis, and ankylosing spondylitis: 500-1000 mg/day in 2 divided doses; may increase to 1.5 g/day of naproxen base for limited time period
- Mild to moderate pain or dysmenorrhea: Initial: 500 mg, then 250 mg every 6-8 hours; maximum: 1250 mg/day naproxen base

OTC labeling: Pain/fever:
- Children ≥12 years and Adults ≤65 years: 200 mg naproxen base every 8-12 hours; if needed, may take 400 mg naproxen base for the initial dose; maximum: 600 mg naproxen base/24 hours
- Adults >65 years: 200 mg naproxen base every 12 hours

Dosage Forms

Caplet, as sodium (Aleve®, Pamprin® Maximum Strength All Day Relief): 220 mg [equivalent to naproxen 200 mg and sodium 20 mg]

Gelcap, as sodium (Aleve®): 220 mg [equivalent to naproxen 200 mg and sodium 20 mg]

Suspension, oral (Naprosyn®): 125 mg/5 mL (480 mL) [contains sodium 0.3 mEq/mL; orange-pineapple flavor]

Tablet (Naprosyn®): 250 mg, 375 mg, 500 mg

Tablet, as sodium: 220 mg [equivalent to naproxen 200 mg and sodium 20 mg]; 275 mg [equivalent to naproxen 250 mg and sodium 25 mg]; 550 mg [equivalent to naproxen 500 mg and sodium 50 mg]
- Aleve®: 220 mg [equivalent to naproxen 200 mg and sodium 20 mg]
- Anaprox®: 275 mg [equivalent to naproxen 250 mg and sodium 25 mg]
- Anaprox® DS: 550 mg [equivalent to naproxen 500 mg and sodium 50 mg]

(Continued)

naproxen *(Continued)*

Tablet, controlled release, as sodium: 550 mg [equivalent to naproxen 500 mg and sodium 50 mg]

Naprelan®: 421.5 mg [equivalent to naproxen 375 mg and sodium 37.5 mg]; 550 mg [equivalent to naproxen 500 mg and sodium 50 mg]

Tablet, delayed release (EC-Naprosyn®): 375 mg, 500 mg

naproxen and lansoprazole *see* lansoprazole and naproxen *on page 506*

naproxen sodium *see* naproxen *on previous page*

Naqua® [US/Can] *see* trichlormethiazide *on page 883*

naratriptan (NAR a trip tan)

Sound-Alike/Look-Alike Issues

Amerge® may be confused with Altace®, Amaryl®

Synonyms naratriptan hydrochloride

U.S./Canadian Brand Names Amerge® [US/Can]

Therapeutic Category Antimigraine Agent; Serotonin Agonist

Use Treatment of acute migraine headache with or without aura

Usual Dosage Adults: Oral: 1-2.5 mg at the onset of headache; it is recommended to use the lowest possible dose to minimize adverse effects. If headache returns or does not fully resolve, the dose may be repeated after 4 hours; do not exceed 5 mg in 24 hours.

Dosage Forms Tablet: 1 mg, 2.5 mg

naratriptan hydrochloride *see* naratriptan *on this page*

Narcan® [US/Can] *see* naloxone *on page 602*

Nardil® [US/Can] *see* phenelzine *on page 685*

Naropin® [US/Can] *see* ropivacaine *on page 785*

Nasacort® [HFA] [US] *see* triamcinolone (inhalation, nasal) *on page 880*

Nasacort® *(Discontinued)* *see page 1042*

Nasacort® AQ [US/Can] *see* triamcinolone (inhalation, nasal) *on page 880*

Nasahist B® *(Discontinued)* *see page 1042*

NasalCrom® [US-OTC] *see* cromolyn sodium *on page 230*

Nasalide® [Can] *see* flunisolide *on page 373*

Nasal Moist® [US-OTC] *see* sodium chloride *on page 810*

NaSal™ [US-OTC] *see* sodium chloride *on page 810*

Nasarel® [US] *see* flunisolide *on page 373*

Nasatab® LA [US] *see* guaifenesin and pseudoephedrine *on page 419*

Nascobal® [US] *see* cyanocobalamin *on page 232*

Nasonex® [US/Can] *see* mometasone furoate *on page 589*

Natabec® *(Discontinued)* *see page 1042*

Natabec® FA *(Discontinued)* *see page 1042*

Natabec® Rx *(Discontinued)* *see page 1042*

NataChew™ [US] *see* vitamins (multiple/prenatal) *on page 927*

Natacyn® [US/Can] *see* natamycin *on next page*

NataFort® [US] *see* vitamins (multiple/prenatal) *on page 927*

NatalCare® CFe 60 [US] *see* vitamins (multiple/prenatal) *on page 927*

NatalCare® GlossTabs™ [US] *see* vitamins (multiple/prenatal) *on page 927*

NatalCare® PIC [US] *see* vitamins (multiple/prenatal) *on page 927*

NatalCare® PIC Forte [US] *see* vitamins (multiple/prenatal) *on page 927*

NatalCare® Plus [US] *see* vitamins (multiple/prenatal) *on page 927*

NatalCare® Rx [US] *see* vitamins (multiple/prenatal) *on page 927*

NatalCare® Three [US] *see* vitamins (multiple/prenatal) *on page 927*

Natalins® Rx *(Discontinued)* *see page 1042*

natamycin (na ta MYE sin)

Sound-Alike/Look-Alike Issues

Natacyn® may be confused with Naprosyn®

Synonyms pimaricin

U.S./Canadian Brand Names Natacyn® [US/Can]

Therapeutic Category Antifungal Agent

Use Treatment of blepharitis, conjunctivitis, and keratitis caused by susceptible fungi (*Aspergillus, Candida*), *Cephalosporium, Curvularia, Fusarium, Penicillium, Microsporum, Epidermophyton, Blastomyces dermatitidis, Coccidioides immitis, Cryptococcus neoformans, Histoplasma capsulatum, Sporothrix schenckii*, and *Trichomonas vaginalis*

Usual Dosage Adults: Ophthalmic: Instill 1 drop in conjunctival sac every 1-2 hours, after 3-4 days reduce to one drop 6-8 times/day; usual course of therapy is 2-3 weeks.

Dosage Forms Suspension, ophthalmic: 5% (15 mL) [contains benzalkonium chloride]

NataTab™ CFe [US] *see* vitamins (multiple/prenatal) *on page 927*

NataTab™ FA [US] *see* vitamins (multiple/prenatal) *on page 927*

NataTab™ Rx [US] *see* vitamins (multiple/prenatal) *on page 927*

nateglinide (na TEG li nide)

U.S./Canadian Brand Names Starlix® [US/Can]

Therapeutic Category Antidiabetic Agent

Use Management of type 2 diabetes mellitus (noninsulin dependent, NIDDM) as monotherapy when hyperglycemia cannot be managed by diet and exercise alone; in combination with metformin or a thiazolidinedione to lower blood glucose in patients whose hyperglycemia cannot be controlled by exercise, diet, or a single agent alone

Usual Dosage

Children: Safety and efficacy have not been established

Adults: Management of type 2 diabetes mellitus: Oral: Initial and maintenance dose: 120 mg 3 times/day, 1-30 minutes before meals; may be given alone or in combination with metformin or a thiazolidinedione; patients close to Hb A_{1c} goal may be started at 60 mg 3 times/day

Dosage Forms Tablet: 60 mg, 120 mg

Natrecor® [US] *see* nesiritide *on page 614*

natriuretic peptide *see* nesiritide *on page 614*

Natulan® [Can] *see* procarbazine *on page 731*

natural lung surfactant *see* beractant *on page 113*

Nature's Tears® [US-OTC] *see* artificial tears *on page 78*

Nature-Throid® NT [US] *see* thyroid *on page 860*

Naturetin® *(Discontinued)* *see page 1042*

Naus-A-Way® *(Discontinued)* *see page 1042*

Nausea Relief [US-OTC] *see* fructose, dextrose, and phosphoric acid *on page 392*

Nausetrol® [US-OTC] *see* fructose, dextrose, and phosphoric acid *on page 392*

Navane® [US/Can] *see* thiothixene *on page 859*

Navelbine® [US/Can] *see* vinorelbine *on page 912*

Naxen® [Can] *see* naproxen *on page 605*

Na-Zone® [US-OTC] *see* sodium chloride *on page 810*
N-B-P® Ointment *(Discontinued)* *see page 1042*
***n*-docosanol** *see* docosanol *on page 285*
Nebcin® [Can] *see* tobramycin *on page 866*
Nebcin® *(Discontinued)* *see page 1042*
NebuPent® [US] *see* pentamidine *on page 678*
Necon® 0.5/35 [US] *see* ethinyl estradiol and norethindrone *on page 342*
Necon® 1/35 [US] *see* ethinyl estradiol and norethindrone *on page 342*
Necon® 1/50 [US] *see* mestranol and norethindrone *on page 558*
Necon® 7/7/7 [US] *see* ethinyl estradiol and norethindrone *on page 342*
Necon® 10/11 [US] *see* ethinyl estradiol and norethindrone *on page 342*

nedocromil (inhalation) (ne doe KROE mil in hil LA shun)

U.S./Canadian Brand Names Tilade® [US/Can]
Therapeutic Category Mast Cell Stabilizer
Use Maintenance therapy in patients with mild to moderate bronchial asthma
Usual Dosage Adults: Inhalation: 2 inhalations 4 times/day
Dosage Forms Aerosol, as sodium: 1.75 mg/activation (16.2 g)

nedocromil (ophthalmic) (ne doe KROE mil op THAL mik)

U.S./Canadian Brand Names Alocril™ [US/Can]
Therapeutic Category Mast Cell Stabilizer
Use Treatment of itching associated with allergic conjunctivitis
Usual Dosage Adults: Ophthalmic: 1-2 drops in eye(s) twice daily
Dosage Forms Solution, ophthalmic, as sodium: 2% (5 mL)

nefazodone (nef AY zoe done)

Synonyms nefazodone hydrochloride
U.S./Canadian Brand Names Apo-Nefazodone® [Can]
Therapeutic Category Antidepressant, Miscellaneous
Use Treatment of depression
Usual Dosage Oral: Depression:
Children and Adolescents: Target dose: 300-400 mg/day (mean: 3.4 mg/kg)
Adults: 200 mg/day, administered in 2 divided doses initially, with a range of 300-600 mg/day in 2 divided doses thereafter
Dosage Forms Tablet, as hydrochloride: 100 mg, 150 mg, 200 mg, 250 mg
Serzone® [DSC]: 50 mg, 100 mg, 150 mg, 200 mg, 250 mg

nefazodone hydrochloride *see* nefazodone *on this page*
NegGram® [US/Can] *see* nalidixic acid *on page 601*

nelfinavir (nel FIN a veer)

Sound-Alike/Look-Alike Issues
nelfinavir may be confused with nevirapine
Viracept® may be confused with Viramune®
Synonyms NFV
U.S./Canadian Brand Names Viracept® [US/Can]
Therapeutic Category Antiviral Agent
Use In combination with other antiretroviral therapy in the treatment of HIV infection
Usual Dosage Oral:
Children 2-13 years: 45-55 mg/kg twice daily **or** 25-35 mg/kg 3 times/day (maximum: 2500 mg/day); all doses should be taken with a meal. If tablets are unable to be taken, use oral powder in small amount of water, milk, formula, or dietary supplements; do not use acidic food/juice or store for >6 hours.

Adults: 750 mg 3 times/day with meals or 1250 mg twice daily with meals in combination with other antiretroviral therapies

Note: Dosage adjustments for nelfinavir when administered in combination with ritonavir: Nelfinavir 500-750 mg twice daily plus ritonavir 400 mg twice daily

Dosage Forms

Powder, oral: 50 mg/g (144 g) [contains phenylalanine 11.2 mg/g]
Tablet [film coated]: 250 mg, 625 mg

Nelova™ 0.5/35E *(Discontinued)* *see page 1042*

Nelova™ 1/35E *(Discontinued)* *see page 1042*

Nelova™ 1/50M *(Discontinued)* *see page 1042*

Nelova™ 10/11 *(Discontinued)* *see page 1042*

Nembutal® [US] *see* pentobarbital *on page 679*

Nembutal® Sodium [Can] *see* pentobarbital *on page 679*

Neo-Calglucon® *(Discontinued)* *see page 1042*

Neo-Castaderm® *(Discontinued)* *see page 1042*

NeoCeuticals™ Acne Spot Treatment [US-OTC] *see* salicylic acid *on page 789*

Neo-Cortef® *(Discontinued)* *see page 1042*

NeoDecadron® [US] *see* neomycin and dexamethasone *on next page*

NeoDecadron® Topical *(Discontinued)* *see page 1042*

Neo-Dexameth® Ophthalmic *(Discontinued)* *see page 1042*

Neo-Durabolic® *(Discontinued)* *see page 1042*

Neofed® *(Discontinued)* *see page 1042*

Neo-Fradin™ [US] *see* neomycin *on this page*

Neo-Medrol® Acetate Topical *(Discontinued)* *see page 1042*

Neomixin® Topical *(Discontinued)* *see page 1042*

neomycin (nee oh MYE sin)

Sound-Alike/Look-Alike Issues

Myciguent may be confused with Mycitracin®

Synonyms neomycin sulfate

U.S./Canadian Brand Names Myciguent [US-OTC]; Neo-Fradin™ [US]; Neo-Rx [US]

Therapeutic Category Aminoglycoside (Antibiotic); Antibiotic, Topical

Use Orally to prepare GI tract for surgery; topically to treat minor skin infections; treatment of diarrhea caused by *E. coli*; adjunct in the treatment of hepatic encephalopathy; bladder irrigation; ocular infections

Usual Dosage

Children: Oral:

Preoperative intestinal antisepsis: 90 mg/kg/day divided every 4 hours for 2 days; or 25 mg/kg at 1 PM, 2 PM, and 11 PM on the day preceding surgery as an adjunct to mechanical cleansing of the intestine and in combination with erythromycin base

Hepatic encephalopathy: 50-100 mg/kg/day in divided doses every 6-8 hours or 2.5-7 g/m^2/day divided every 4-6 hours for 5-6 days not to exceed 12 g/day

Adults: Oral:

Preoperative intestinal antisepsis: 1 g each hour for 4 doses then 1 g every 4 hours for 5 doses; or 1 g at 1 PM, 2 PM, and 11 PM on day preceding surgery as an adjunct to mechanical cleansing of the bowel and oral erythromycin; or 6 g/day divided every 4 hours for 2-3 days

Hepatic encephalopathy: 500-2000 mg every 6-8 hours or 4-12 g/day divided every 4-6 hours for 5-6 days

Chronic hepatic insufficiency: 4 g/day for an indefinite period

(Continued)

neomycin *(Continued)*

Children and Adults: Topical: Apply ointment 1-4 times/day; topical solutions containing 0.1% to 1% neomycin have been used for irrigation

Dosage Forms

Ointment, topical, as sulfate (Myciguent): 3.5 mg/g (15 g, 30 g)

Powder, micronized, as sulfate [for prescription compounding] (Neo-Rx): (10 g, 100 g)

Solution, oral, as sulfate (Neo-Fradin™): 125 mg/5 mL (480 mL) [contains benzoic acid; cherry flavor]

Tablet, as sulfate: 500 mg

neomycin and dexamethasone (nee oh MYE sin & deks a METH a sone)

Synonyms dexamethasone and neomycin

U.S./Canadian Brand Names NeoDecadron® [US]

Therapeutic Category Antibiotic/Corticosteroid, Ophthalmic; Antibiotic/Corticosteroid, Topical

Use Treatment of steroid responsive inflammatory conditions of the palpebral and bulbar conjunctiva, lid, cornea, and anterior segment of the globe

Usual Dosage Ophthalmic: Instill 1-2 drops in eye(s) every 3-4 hours

Dosage Forms Solution, ophthalmic: Neomycin sulfate 0.35% [3.5 mg/mL] and dexamethasone sodium phosphate 0.1% [1 mg/mL] (5 mL) [contains benzalkonium chloride and sodium bisulfite]

neomycin and polymyxin B (nee oh MYE sin & pol i MIKS in bee)

Synonyms polymyxin B and neomycin

U.S./Canadian Brand Names Neosporin® G.U. Irrigant [US]; Neosporin® Irrigating Solution [Can]

Therapeutic Category Antibiotic, Topical; Genitourinary Irrigant

Use Short-term as a continuous irrigant or rinse in the urinary bladder to prevent bacteriuria and gram-negative rod septicemia associated with the use of indwelling catheters; to help prevent infection in minor cuts, scrapes, and burns

Usual Dosage Children and Adults: Bladder irrigation: **Not for injection**; add 1 mL irrigant to 1 liter isotonic saline solution and connect container to the inflow of lumen of 3-way catheter. Continuous irrigant or rinse in the urinary bladder for up to a maximum of 10 days with administration rate adjusted to patient's urine output; usually no more than 1 L of irrigant is used per day.

Dosage Forms Solution, irrigant: Neomycin sulfate 40 mg and polymyxin B sulfate 200,000 units per mL (1 mL, 20 mL)

neomycin, bacitracin, and polymyxin B *see* bacitracin, neomycin, and polymyxin B *on page 97*

neomycin, bacitracin, polymyxin B, and hydrocortisone *see* bacitracin, neomycin, polymyxin B, and hydrocortisone *on page 98*

neomycin, colistin, hydrocortisone, and thonzonium
(nee oh MYE sin, koe LIS tin, hye droe KOR ti sone, & thon ZOE nee um)

Synonyms colistin, neomycin, hydrocortisone, and thonzonium; hydrocortisone, neomycin, colistin, and thonzonium; thonzonium, neomycin, colistin, and hydrocortisone

U.S./Canadian Brand Names Coly-Mycin® S [US]; Cortisporin®-TC [US]

Therapeutic Category Antibiotic/Corticosteroid, Otic

Use Treatment of superficial and susceptible bacterial infections of the external auditory canal; for treatment of susceptible bacterial infections of mastoidectomy and fenestration cavities

Usual Dosage Otic:

Calibrated dropper:

Children: 4 drops in affected ear 3-4 times/day

Adults: 5 drops in affected ear 3-4 times/day

Dropper bottle:
Children: 3 drops in affected ear 3-4 times/day
Adults: 4 drops in affected ear 3-4 times/day
Note: Alternatively, a cotton wick may be inserted in the ear canal and saturated with suspension every 4 hours; wick should be replaced at least every 24 hours

Dosage Forms
Suspension, otic [drops]:
Coly-Mycin® S: Colistin sulfate 0.3%, neomycin sulfate 0.33%, and hydrocortisone acetate 1% (5 mL) [contains thonzonium bromide 0.05% and thimerosal; packaged with dropper]
Cortisporin®-TC: Colistin sulfate 0.3%, neomycin sulfate 0.33%, and hydrocortisone acetate 1% (10 mL) [contains thonzonium bromide 0.05% and thimerosal; packaged with dropper]

neomycin, polymyxin B, and dexamethasone

(nee oh MYE sin, pol i MIKS in bee, & deks a METH a sone)

Sound-Alike/Look-Alike Issues
AK-Trol® may be confused with AKTob®

Synonyms dexamethasone, neomycin, and polymyxin B; polymyxin B, neomycin, and dexamethasone

U.S./Canadian Brand Names AK-Trol® [US]; Dexacidin® [US]; Dexacine™ [US]; Dioptrol® [Can]; Maxitrol® [US/Can]

Therapeutic Category Antibiotic/Corticosteroid, Ophthalmic

Use Steroid-responsive inflammatory ocular conditions in which a corticosteroid is indicated and where bacterial infection or a risk of bacterial infection exists

Usual Dosage Children and Adults: Ophthalmic:
Ointment: Place a small amount (~½") in the affected eye 3-4 times/day or apply at bedtime as an adjunct with drops
Suspension: Instill 1-2 drops into affected eye(s) every 3-4 hours; in severe disease, drops may be used hourly and tapered to discontinuation

Dosage Forms
Ointment, ophthalmic (Dexacine™, Maxitrol®): Neomycin sulfate 3.5 mg, polymyxin B sulfate 10,000 units, and dexamethasone 0.1% per g (3.5 g)
Suspension, ophthalmic (AK-Trol®, Dexacidin®, Maxitrol®): Neomycin sulfate 3.5 mg, polymyxin B sulfate 10,000 units, and dexamethasone 0.1% per mL (5 mL) [contains benzalkonium chloride]

neomycin, polymyxin B, and gramicidin

(nee oh MYE sin, pol i MIKS in bee, & gram i SYE din)

Synonyms gramicidin, neomycin, and polymyxin B; polymyxin B, neomycin, and gramicidin

U.S./Canadian Brand Names Neosporin® Ophthalmic Solution [US/Can]; Optimyxin Plus® [Can]

Therapeutic Category Antibiotic, Ophthalmic

Use Treatment of superficial ocular infection

Usual Dosage Children and Adults: Ophthalmic: Instill 1-2 drops 4-6 times/day or more frequently as required for severe infections

Dosage Forms Solution, ophthalmic: Neomycin 1.75 mg, polymyxin B 10,000 units, and gramicidin 0.025 mg per mL (10 mL) [contains alcohol 0.5% and thimerosal]

neomycin, polymyxin B, and hydrocortisone

(nee oh MYE sin, pol i MIKS in bee, & hye droe KOR ti sone)

Synonyms hydrocortisone, neomycin, and polymyxin B; polymyxin B, neomycin, and hydrocortisone

U.S./Canadian Brand Names AntibiOtic® Ear [US]; Cortimyxin® [Can]; Cortisporin® Cream [US]; Cortisporin® Ophthalmic [US]; Cortisporin® Otic [US/Can]; PediOtic® [US]

Therapeutic Category Antibiotic/Corticosteroid, Ophthalmic; Antibiotic/Corticosteroid, Otic; Antibiotic/Corticosteroid, Topical

(Continued)

neomycin, polymyxin B, and hydrocortisone *(Continued)*

Use Steroid-responsive inflammatory condition for which a corticosteroid is indicated and where bacterial infection or a risk of bacterial infection exists

Usual Dosage Duration of use should be limited to 10 days unless otherwise directed by the physician

Otic solution is used **only** for swimmer's ear (infections of external auditory canal)

Otic:

Children: Instill 3 drops into affected ear 3-4 times/day

Adults: Instill 4 drops 3-4 times/day; otic suspension is the preferred otic preparation

Children and Adults:

Ophthalmic: Drops: Instill 1-2 drops 2-4 times/day, or more frequently as required for severe infections; in acute infections, instill 1-2 drops every 15-30 minutes gradually reducing the frequency of administration as the infection is controlled

Topical: Apply a thin layer 1-4 times/day. Therapy should be discontinued when control is achieved; if no improvement is seen, reassessment of diagnosis may be necessary.

Dosage Forms

Cream, topical (Cortisporin®): Neomycin sulfate 5 mg [equivalent to 3.5 mg base], polymyxin B sulfate 10,000 units, and hydrocortisone 5 mg per g (7.5 g)

Solution, otic (AntibiOtic® Ear; Cortisporin®): Neomycin sulfate 5 mg [equivalent to 3.5 mg base], polymyxin B sulfate 10,000 units, and hydrocortisone 10 mg per mL (10 mL) [contains potassium metabisulfite]

Suspension, ophthalmic (Cortisporin®): Neomycin sulfate 5 mg [equivalent to 3.5 mg base], polymyxin B sulfate 10,000 units, and hydrocortisone 10 mg per mL (7.5 mL) [contains thimerosal]

Suspension, otic: Neomycin sulfate 5 mg [equivalent to 3.5 mg base], polymyxin B sulfate 10,000 units, and hydrocortisone 10 mg per mL (10 mL)

AntibiOtic® Ear, Cortisporin®: Neomycin sulfate 5 mg [equivalent to 3.5 mg base], polymyxin B sulfate 10,000 units, and hydrocortisone 10 mg per mL (10 mL)

PediOtic®: Neomycin sulfate 5 mg [equivalent to 3.5 mg base], polymyxin B sulfate 10,000 units, and hydrocortisone 10 mg per mL (7.5 mL)

neomycin, polymyxin B, and prednisolone

(nee oh MYE sin, pol i MIKS in bee, & pred NIS oh lone)

Synonyms polymyxin B, neomycin, and prednisolone; prednisolone, neomycin, and polymyxin B

U.S./Canadian Brand Names Poly-Pred® [US]

Therapeutic Category Antibiotic/Corticosteroid, Ophthalmic

Use Steroid-responsive inflammatory ocular condition in which bacterial infection or a risk of bacterial ocular infection exists

Usual Dosage Children and Adults: Ophthalmic: Instill 1-2 drops every 3-4 hours; acute infections may require every 30-minute instillation initially with frequency of administration reduced as the infection is brought under control. To treat the lids: Instill 1-2 drops every 3-4 hours, close the eye and rub the excess on the lids and lid margins.

Dosage Forms Suspension, ophthalmic: Neomycin sulfate 0.35%, polymyxin B sulfate 10,000 units, and prednisolone acetate 0.5% per mL (5 mL, 10 mL)

neomycin sulfate *see* neomycin *on page 609*

neonatal trace metals *see* trace metals *on page 874*

Neoquess® Injection *(Discontinued)* *see page 1042*

Neoquess® Tablet *(Discontinued)* *see page 1042*

Neoral® [US/Can] *see* cyclosporine *on page 235*

Neo-Rx [US] *see* neomycin *on page 609*

Neosporin® G.U. Irrigant [US] *see* neomycin and polymyxin B *on page 610*

Neosporin® Irrigating Solution [Can] *see* neomycin and polymyxin B *on page 610*

Neosporin® Neo To Go® [US-OTC] *see* bacitracin, neomycin, and polymyxin B *on page 97*

Neosporin® Ophthalmic Ointment [US/Can] *see* bacitracin, neomycin, and polymyxin B *on page 97*

Neosporin® Ophthalmic Solution [US/Can] *see* neomycin, polymyxin B, and gramicidin *on page 611*

Neosporin® Topical [US-OTC] *see* bacitracin, neomycin, and polymyxin B *on page 97*

neostigmine (nee oh STIG meen)

Sound-Alike/Look-Alike Issues

Prostigmin® may be confused with physostigmine

Synonyms neostigmine bromide; neostigmine methylsulfate

U.S./Canadian Brand Names Prostigmin® [US/Can]

Therapeutic Category Cholinergic Agent

Use Diagnosis and treatment of myasthenia gravis; prevention and treatment of postoperative bladder distention and urinary retention; reversal of the effects of nondepolarizing neuromuscular-blocking agents after surgery

Usual Dosage

Myasthenia gravis: Diagnosis: I.M.:
- Children: 0.04 mg/kg as a single dose
- Adults: 0.02 mg/kg as a single dose

Myasthenia gravis: Treatment:
- Children:
  - Oral: 2 mg/kg/day divided every 3-4 hours
  - I.M., I.V., SubQ: 0.01-0.04 mg/kg every 2-4 hours
- Adults:
  - Oral: 15 mg/dose every 3-4 hours up to 375 mg/day maximum; interval between doses must be individualized to maximal response
  - I.M., I.V., SubQ: 0.5-2.5 mg every 1-3 hours up to 10 mg/24 hours maximum

Reversal of nondepolarizing neuromuscular blockade after surgery in conjunction with atropine (must administer atropine several minutes prior to neostigmine): I.V.:
- Infants: 0.025-0.1 mg/kg/dose
- Children: 0.025-0.08 mg/kg/dose
- Adults: 0.5-2.5 mg; total dose not to exceed 5 mg

Bladder atony: Adults: I.M., SubQ:
- Prevention: 0.25 mg every 4-6 hours for 2-3 days
- Treatment: 0.5-1 mg every 3 hours for 5 doses after bladder has emptied

Dosage Forms

Injection, solution, as methylsulfate: 0.5 mg/mL (1 mL, 10 mL); 1 mg/mL (10 mL)

Tablet, as bromide: 15 mg

neostigmine bromide *see* neostigmine *on this page*

neostigmine methylsulfate *see* neostigmine *on this page*

NeoStrata® AHA [US-OTC] *see* hydroquinone *on page 454*

NeoStrata® HQ [Can] *see* hydroquinone *on page 454*

Neo-Synalar® Topical *(Discontinued)* *see page 1042*

Neo-Synephrine® 12 Hour Extra Moisturizing [US-OTC] *see* oxymetazoline *on page 658*

Neo-Synephrine® 12 Hour [US-OTC] *see* oxymetazoline *on page 658*

Neo-Synephrine® Extra Strength [US-OTC] *see* phenylephrine *on page 689*

Neo-Synephrine® Mild [US-OTC] *see* phenylephrine *on page 689*

Neo-Synephrine® Ophthalmic [US] *see* phenylephrine *on page 689*

Neo-Synephrine® Regular Strength [US-OTC] *see* phenylephrine *on page 689*

Neo-Tabs® *(Discontinued)* *see page 1042*

Neotopic® [Can] *see* bacitracin, neomycin, and polymyxin B *on page 97*

Neotrace-4® [US] *see* trace metals *on page 874*

NeoVadrin® *(Discontinued)* *see page 1042*

NephPlex® Rx [US] *see* vitamin B complex combinations *on page 915*

Nephro-Calci® [US-OTC] *see* calcium carbonate *on page 144*

Nephrocaps® [US] *see* vitamin B complex combinations *on page 915*

Nephro-Fer® [US-OTC] *see* ferrous fumarate *on page 363*

Nephron FA® [US] *see* vitamin B complex combinations *on page 915*

Nephro-Vite® [US] *see* vitamin B complex combinations *on page 915*

Nephro-Vite® Rx [US] *see* vitamin B complex combinations *on page 915*

Nephrox Suspension *(Discontinued)* *see page 1042*

Neptazane® *(Discontinued)* *see page 1042*

Nervocaine® Injection *(Discontinued)* *see page 1042*

Nesacaine® [US] *see* chloroprocaine *on page 185*

Nesacaine®-CE [Can] *see* chloroprocaine *on page 185*

Nesacaine®-MPF [US] *see* chloroprocaine *on page 185*

nesiritide (ni SIR i tide)

Synonyms B-type natriuretic peptide (human); hBNP; natriuretic peptide

U.S./Canadian Brand Names Natrecor® [US]

Therapeutic Category Natriuretic Peptide, B-type, Human; Vasodilator

Use Treatment of acutely decompensated congestive heart failure (CHF) in patients with dyspnea at rest or with minimal activity

Usual Dosage Adults: I.V.: Initial: 2 mcg/kg (bolus); followed by continuous infusion at 0.01 mcg/kg/minute; **Note:** Should not be initiated at a dosage higher than initial recommended dose. At intervals of ≥3 hours, the dosage may be increased by 0.005 mcg/kg/minute (preceded by a bolus of 1 mcg/kg), up to a maximum of 0.03 mcg/kg/minute. Increases beyond the initial infusion rate should be limited to selected patients and accompanied by hemodynamic monitoring.

Patients experiencing hypotension during the infusion: Infusion should be interrupted. May attempt to restart at a lower dose (reduce initial infusion dose by 30% and omit bolus).

Dosage Forms Injection, powder for reconstitution: 1.5 mg

Nestabs® CBF [US] *see* vitamins (multiple/prenatal) *on page 927*

Nestabs® FA [US] *see* vitamins (multiple/prenatal) *on page 927*

Nestabs® RX [US] *see* vitamins (multiple/prenatal) *on page 927*

Nestrex® *(Discontinued)* *see page 1042*

Netromycin® *(Discontinued)* *see page 1042*

Neucalm-50® Injection *(Discontinued)* *see page 1042*

Neulasta™ [US] *see* pegfilgrastim *on page 671*

Neumega® [US] *see* oprelvekin *on page 647*

Neupogen® [US/Can] *see* filgrastim *on page 368*

Neuramate® *(Discontinued)* *see page 1042*

Neurontin® [US/Can] *see* gabapentin *on page 395*

Neut® [US] *see* sodium bicarbonate *on page 809*

NeutraCare® [US] *see* fluoride *on page 376*

NeutraGard® [US-OTC] *see* fluoride *on page 376*

Neutra-Phos® Capsule ***(Discontinued)*** *see page 1042*

Neutra-Phos®-K [US-OTC] *see* potassium phosphate *on page 716*

Neutra-Phos® [US-OTC] *see* potassium phosphate and sodium phosphate *on page 717*

NeuTrexin® [US] *see* trimetrexate glucuronate *on page 888*

Neutrogena® Acne Mask [US-OTC] *see* benzoyl peroxide *on page 109*

Neutrogena® Acne Wash [US-OTC] *see* salicylic acid *on page 789*

Neutrogena® Body Clear™ [US-OTC] *see* salicylic acid *on page 789*

Neutrogena® Clear Pore Shine Control [US-OTC] *see* salicylic acid *on page 789*

Neutrogena® Clear Pore [US-OTC] *see* salicylic acid *on page 789*

Neutrogena® Healthy Scalp [US-OTC] *see* salicylic acid *on page 789*

Neutrogena® Maximum Strength T/Sal® [US-OTC] *see* salicylic acid *on page 789*

Neutrogena® On The Spot® Acne Patch [US-OTC] *see* salicylic acid *on page 789*

Neutrogena® On The Spot® Acne Treatment [US-OTC] *see* benzoyl peroxide *on page 109*

Neutrogena® T/Gel Extra Strength [US-OTC] *see* coal tar *on page 219*

Neutrogena® T/Gel [US-OTC] *see* coal tar *on page 219*

nevirapine (ne VYE ra peen)

Sound-Alike/Look-Alike Issues

nevirapine may be confused with nelfinavir

Viramune® may be confused with Viracept®

Synonyms NVP

U.S./Canadian Brand Names Viramune® [US/Can]

Therapeutic Category Antiviral Agent

Use In combination therapy with other antiretroviral agents for the treatment of HIV-1

Usual Dosage Oral:

Children 2 months to <8 years: Initial: 4 mg/kg/dose once daily for 14 days; increase dose to 7 mg/kg/dose every 12 hours if no rash or other adverse effects occur; maximum dose: 200 mg/dose every 12 hours

Children ≥8 years: Initial: 4 mg/kg/dose once daily for 14 days; increase dose to 4 mg/kg/dose every 12 hours if no rash or other adverse effects occur; maximum dose: 200 mg/dose every 12 hours

Adults: Initial: 200 mg once daily for 14 days; maintenance: 200 mg twice daily (in combination with an additional antiretroviral agent)

Note: If patient experiences a rash during the 14-day lead-in period, dose should not be increased until the rash has resolved. Discontinue if severe rash, or rash with constitutional symptoms, is noted. If therapy is interrupted for >7 days, restart with initial dose for 14 days

Dosage Forms

Suspension, oral: 50 mg/5 mL (240 mL)

Tablet: 200 mg

New Decongestant® ***(Discontinued)*** *see page 1042*

Nexium® [US/Can] *see* esomeprazole *on page 323*

NFV *see* nelfinavir *on page 608*

N.G.A.® Topical ***(Discontinued)*** *see page 1042*

Niac® ***(Discontinued)*** *see page 1042*

Niacels™ ***(Discontinued)*** *see page 1042*

niacin (NYE a sin)

Sound-Alike/Look-Alike Issues

niacin may be confused with Minocin®, Niaspan®, Nispan®

Niaspan® may be confused with niacin

Synonyms nicotinic acid; vitamin B_3

U.S./Canadian Brand Names Niacor® [US]; Niaspan® [US/Can]; Nicotinex [US-OTC]; Slo-Niacin® [US-OTC]

Therapeutic Category Vitamin, Water Soluble

Use Adjunctive treatment of dyslipidemias (alone or with lovastatin or bile acid sequestrant); peripheral vascular disease and circulatory disorders; treatment of pellagra; dietary supplement

Usual Dosage Oral:

Children:

Pellagra: 50-100 mg/dose 3 times/day

Recommended daily allowances:

0-0.5 years: 5 mg/day

0.5-1 year: 6 mg/day

1-3 years: 9 mg/day

4-6 years: 12 mg/day

7-10 years: 13 mg/day

Children and Adolescents: Recommended daily allowances:

Male:

11-14 years: 17 mg/day

15-18 years: 20 mg/day

19-24 years: 19 mg/day

Female: 11-24 years: 15 mg/day

Adults:

Recommended daily allowances:

Male: 25-50 years: 19 mg/day; >51 years: 15 mg/day

Female: 25-50 years: 15 mg/day; >51 years: 13 mg/day

Hyperlipidemia: Usual target dose: 1.5-6 g/day in 3 divided doses with or after meals using a dosage titration schedule; extended release: 375 mg to 2 g once daily at bedtime

Regular release formulation (Niacor®): Initial: 250 mg once daily (with evening meal); increase frequency and/or dose every 4-7 days to desired response or first-level therapeutic dose (1.5-2 g/day in 2-3 divided doses); after 2 months, may increase at 2- to 4-week intervals to 3 g/day in 3 divided doses

Extended release formulation (Niaspan®): 500 mg at bedtime for 4 weeks, then 1 g at bedtime for 4 weeks; adjust dose to response and tolerance; can increase to a maximum of 2 g/day, but only at 500 mg/day at 4-week intervals

With lovastatin: Maximum lovastatin dose: 40 mg/day

Pellagra: 50-100 mg 3-4 times/day, maximum: 500 mg/day

Niacin deficiency: 10-20 mg/day, maximum: 100 mg/day

Dosage Forms

Capsule, extended release: 125 mg, 250 mg, 400 mg, 500 mg

Capsule, timed release: 250 mg

Elixir (Nicotinex): 50 mg/5 mL (473 mL) [contains alcohol 10% (sherry wine)]

Tablet: 50 mg, 100 mg, 250 mg, 500 mg

Niacor®: 500 mg

Tablet, controlled release (Slo-Niacin®): 250 mg, 500 mg, 750 mg

Tablet, extended release (Niaspan®): 500 mg, 750 mg, 1000 mg

Tablet, timed release: 250 mg, 500 mg, 750 mg, 1000 mg

niacinamide (nye a SIN a mide)

Sound-Alike/Look-Alike Issues

niacinamide may be confused with nicardipine

Synonyms nicotinamide; vitamin B_3

Therapeutic Category Vitamin, Water Soluble

Use Prophylaxis and treatment of pellagra

Usual Dosage Oral:

Children: Pellagra: 100-300 mg/day in divided doses

Adults: 50 mg 3-10 times/day

Pellagra: 300-500 mg/day

Recommended daily allowance: 13-19 mg/day

Dosage Forms Tablet: 100 mg, 250 mg, 500 mg

niacin and lovastatin (NYE a sin & LOE va sta tin)

Sound-Alike/Look-Alike Issues

Advicor™ may be confused with Advair Diskus®, Altocor™

Synonyms lovastatin and niacin

U.S./Canadian Brand Names Advicor™ [US]

Therapeutic Category HMG-CoA Reductase Inhibitor; Vitamin, Water Soluble

Use Treatment of primary hypercholesterolemia (heterozygous familial and nonfamilial) and mixed dyslipidemia (Fredrickson types IIa and IIb) in patients previously treated with either agent alone (patients who require further lowering of triglycerides (TG) or increase in HDL-cholesterol (HDL-C) from addition of niacin or further lowering of LDL-cholesterol (LDL-C) from addition of lovastatin). Combination product; not intended for initial treatment.

Usual Dosage Dosage forms are a fixed combination of niacin and lovastatin.

Oral: Adults: Lowest dose: Niacin 500 mg/lovastatin 20 mg; may increase by not more than 500 mg (niacin) at 4-week intervals (maximum dose: Niacin 2000 mg/lovastatin 40 mg daily); should be taken at bedtime with a low-fat snack

Not for use as initial therapy of dyslipidemias. May be substituted for equivalent dose of Niaspan®, however, manufacturer does not recommend direct substitution with other niacin products.

Dosage Forms [DSC] = Discontinued product

Tablet, variable release:

500/20: Niacin 500 mg [extended release] and lovastatin 20 mg [immediate release]

750/20: Niacin 750 mg [extended release] and lovastatin 20 mg [immediate release] [DSC]

1000/20: Niacin 1000 mg [extended release] and lovastatin 20 mg [immediate release]

Niacor® [US] *see* niacin *on previous page*

Niaspan® [US/Can] *see* niacin *on previous page*

Niastase® [Can] *see* factor VIIa (recombinant) *on page 354*

nicardipine (nye KAR de peen)

Sound-Alike/Look-Alike Issues

nicardipine may be confused with niacinamide, nifedipine, nimodipine

Cardene® may be confused with Cardizem®, Cardura®, codeine

Synonyms nicardipine hydrochloride

Tall-Man ni**CAR**dipine

U.S./Canadian Brand Names Cardene® I.V. [US]; Cardene® SR [US]; Cardene® [US]

Therapeutic Category Calcium Channel Blocker

Use Chronic stable angina (immediate-release product only); management of essential hypertension (immediate- and sustained-release; parenteral only for short time that oral treatment is not feasible)

Usual Dosage Adults:

Oral:

Immediate release: Initial: 20 mg 3 times/day; usual: 20-40 mg 3 times/day (allow 3 days between dose increases)

Sustained release: Initial: 30 mg twice daily, titrate up to 60 mg twice daily

Note: The total daily dose of immediate-release product may not automatically be equivalent to the daily sustained-release dose; use caution in converting.

(Continued)

nicardipine *(Continued)*

I.V. (dilute to 0.1 mg/mL):

Acute hypertension: Initial: 5 mg/hour increased by 2.5 mg/hour every 15 minutes to a maximum of 15 mg/hour; consider reduction to 3 mg/hour after response is achieved. Monitor and titrate to lowest dose necessary to maintain stable blood pressure.

Substitution for oral therapy (approximate equivalents):

20 mg every 8 hours oral, equivalent to 0.5 mg/hour I.V. infusion
30 mg every 8 hours oral, equivalent to 1.2 mg/hour I.V. infusion
40 mg every 8 hours oral, equivalent to 2.2 mg/hour I.V. infusion

Dosage Forms

Capsule (Cardene®): 20 mg, 30 mg
Capsule, sustained-release (Cardene® SR): 30 mg, 45 mg, 60 mg
Injection, solution (Cardene® IV): 2.5 mg/mL (10 mL)

nicardipine hydrochloride *see* nicardipine *on previous page*

N'ice® *(Discontinued)* *see page 1042*

Niclocide® *(Discontinued)* *see page 1042*

Nicobid® *(Discontinued)* *see page 1042*

NicoDerm® [Can] *see* nicotine *on this page*

NicoDerm® CQ® [US-OTC] *see* nicotine *on this page*

Nicolar® *(Discontinued)* *see page 1042*

Nicorette® Plus [Can] *see* nicotine *on this page*

Nicorette® [US-OTC/Can] *see* nicotine *on this page*

nicotinamide *see* niacinamide *on page 616*

nicotine (nik oh TEEN)

Sound-Alike/Look-Alike Issues

NicoDerm® may be confused with Nitroderm®
Nicorette® may be confused with Nordette®

U.S./Canadian Brand Names Commit™ [US-OTC]; Habitrol® [Can]; NicoDerm® [Can]; NicoDerm® CQ® [US-OTC]; Nicorette® Plus [Can]; Nicorette® [US-OTC/Can]; Nicotrol® [Can]; Nicotrol® Inhaler [US]; Nicotrol® NS [US]; Nicotrol® Patch [US-OTC/Can]

Therapeutic Category Smoking Deterrent

Use Treatment to aid smoking cessation for the relief of nicotine withdrawal symptoms (including nicotine craving)

Usual Dosage Adults:

Smoking deterrent: Patients should be advised to completely stop smoking upon initiation of therapy.

Gum: Chew 1 piece of gum when urge to smoke, up to 30 pieces/day; most patients require 10-12 pieces of gum/day

Inhaler: Usually 6 to 16 cartridges per day; best effect was achieved by frequent continuous puffing (20 minutes); recommended duration of treatment is 3 months, after which patients may be weaned from the inhaler by gradual reduction of the daily dose over 6-12 weeks

Lozenge: Patients who smoke their first cigarette within 30 minutes of waking should use the 4 mg strength; otherwise the 2 mg strength is recommended.

Weeks 1-6: One lozenge every 1-2 hours
Weeks 7-9: One lozenge every 2-4 hours
Weeks 10-12: One lozenge every 4-8 hours

Note: Use at least 9 lozenges/day during first 6 weeks to improve chances of quitting; do not use more than one lozenge at a time (maximum: 5 lozenges every 6 hours, 20 lozenges/day)

Transdermal patch: Apply new patch every 24 hours to nonhairy, clean, dry skin on the upper body or upper outer arm; each patch should be applied to a different site.

Note: Adjustment may be required during initial treatment (move to higher dose if experiencing withdrawal symptoms; lower dose if side effects are experienced).

Habitrol®, NicoDerm CQ®: Patients smoking ≥10 cigarettes/day: Begin with **step 1** (21 mg/day) for 4-6 weeks, followed by **step 2** (14 mg/day) for 2 weeks; finish with **step 3** (7 mg/day) for 2 weeks Patients smoking <10 cigarettes/day: Begin with **step 2** (14 mg/day) for 6 weeks, followed by **step 3** (7 mg/day) for 2 weeks **Note:** Initial starting dose for patients <100 pounds, history of cardiovascular disease: 14 mg/day for 4-6 weeks, followed by 7 mg/day for 2-4 weeks **Note:** Patients receiving >600 mg/day of cimetidine: Decrease to the next lower patch size

Nicotrol®: One patch daily for 6 weeks

Note: Benefits of use of nicotine transdermal patches beyond 3 months have not been demonstrated.

Spray: 1-2 sprays/hour; do not exceed more than 5 doses (10 sprays) per hour; each dose (2 sprays) contains 1 mg of nicotine. **Warning:** A dose of 40 mg can cause fatalities.

Dosage Forms

Gum, chewing, as polacrilex (Nicorette®): 2 mg/square (48s, 108s, 168s); 4 mg/square (48s, 108s, 168s) [mint, orange, and original flavors]

Lozenge, as polacrilex (Commit™): 2 mg, 4 mg [contains phenylalanine 3.4 mg/lozenge; mint flavor]

Oral inhalation system (Nicotrol® Inhaler): 10 mg cartridge [delivering 4 mg nicotine] (42s) [each unit consists of 1 mouthpiece, 7 storage trays each containing 6 cartridges, and 1 storage case]

Patch, transdermal: 7 mg/24 (7s, 30s); 14 mg/24 hours (7s, 14s, 30s); 21 mg/24 hours (7s, 14s, 30s)

Kit: Step 1: 21 mg/24 hours (28s); Step 2: 14 mg/24 hours (14s); Step 3: 7 mg/24 hours (14s) [kit also contains support material]

NicoDerm® CQ® [clear patch]: 7 mg/24 hours (14s); 14 mg/24 hours (14s); 21 mg/24 hours (14s)

NicoDerm® CQ® [tan patch]: 7 mg/24 hours (14s); 14 mg/24 hours (14s); 21 mg/24 hours (7s, 14s)

Nicotrol®: 15 mg/16 hours (7s)

Solution, intranasal spray (Nicotrol® NS): 10 mg/mL (10 mL) [delivers 0.5 mg/spray; 200 sprays]

Nicotinex [US-OTC] *see* niacin *on page 616*

nicotinic acid *see* niacin *on page 616*

Nicotrol® [Can] *see* nicotine *on previous page*

Nicotrol® Inhaler [US] *see* nicotine *on previous page*

Nicotrol® NS [US] *see* nicotine *on previous page*

Nicotrol® Patch [US-OTC/Can] *see* nicotine *on previous page*

Nico-Vert® ***(Discontinued)*** *see page 1042*

Nidagel™ [Can] *see* metronidazole *on page 576*

Nidryl® ***(Discontinued)*** *see page 1042*

Nifedical™ XL [US] *see* nifedipine *on this page*

nifedipine (nye FED i peen)

Sound-Alike/Look-Alike Issues

nifedipine may be confused with nicardipine, nimodipine, nisoldipine

Procardia XL® may be confused with Cartia® XT

Tall-Man NIFEdipine

U.S./Canadian Brand Names Adalat® CC [US]; Adalat® XL® [Can]; Apo-Nifed® [Can]; Apo-Nifed PA® [Can]; Nifedical™ XL [US]; Novo-Nifedin [Can]; Nu-Nifed [Can]; Procardia® [US/Can]; Procardia XL® [US]

Therapeutic Category Calcium Channel Blocker

Use Angina and hypertension (sustained release only), pulmonary hypertension

(Continued)

nifedipine *(Continued)*

Usual Dosage Oral:

Children: Hypertrophic cardiomyopathy: 0.6-0.9 mg/kg/24 hours in 3-4 divided doses

Adolescents and Adults: (**Note:** When switching from immediate release to sustained release formulations, total daily dose will start the same)

Initial: 30 mg once daily as sustained release formulation, or if indicated, 10 mg 3 times/day as capsules

Usual dose: 10-30 mg 3 times/day as capsules or 30-60 mg once daily as sustained release

Maximum dose: 120-180 mg/day

Increase sustained release at 7- to 14-day intervals

Dosage Forms

Capsule, liquid-filled (Procardia®): 10 mg, 20 mg

Tablet, extended release: 30 mg, 60 mg, 90 mg

Adalat® CC, Procardia XL®: 30 mg, 60 mg, 90 mg

Nifedical™ XL: 30 mg, 60 mg

Niferex® 150 [US-OTC] *see* polysaccharide-iron complex *on page 709*

Niferex Forte® ***(Discontinued)*** *see page 1042*

Niferex®-PN [US] *see* vitamins (multiple/prenatal) *on page 927*

Niferex®-PN Forte [US] *see* vitamins (multiple/prenatal) *on page 927*

Niferex® [US-OTC] *see* polysaccharide-iron complex *on page 709*

niftolid *see* flutamide *on page 382*

Nilandron® [US] *see* nilutamide *on this page*

Niloric® ***(Discontinued)*** *see page 1042*

Nilstat® [Can] *see* nystatin *on page 637*

Nilstat® ***(Discontinued)*** *see page 1042*

nilutamide (ni LU ta mide)

Synonyms RU-23908

U.S./Canadian Brand Names Anandron® [Can]; Nilandron® [US]

Therapeutic Category Antineoplastic Agent

Use Treatment of metastatic prostate cancer

Usual Dosage Refer to individual protocols.

Adults: Oral: 300 mg daily for 30 days starting the same day or day after surgical castration, then 150 mg/day

Dosage Forms Tablet: 150 mg

Nimbex® [US/Can] *see* cisatracurium *on page 204*

nimodipine (nye MOE di peen)

Sound-Alike/Look-Alike Issues

nimodipine may be confused with nicardipine, nifedipine

U.S./Canadian Brand Names Nimotop® [US/Can]

Therapeutic Category Calcium Channel Blocker

Use Spasm following subarachnoid hemorrhage from ruptured intracranial aneurysms regardless of the patients neurological condition postictus (Hunt and Hess grades I-V)

Usual Dosage Adults: Oral: 60 mg every 4 hours for 21 days, start therapy within 96 hours after subarachnoid hemorrhage.

Dosage Forms Capsule, liquid filled: 30 mg

Nimotop® [US/Can] *see* nimodipine *on this page*

Nipent® [US/Can] *see* pentostatin *on page 680*

Nipride® [Can] *see* nitroprusside *on page 624*

Nipride® Injection *(Discontinued)* *see page 1042*

Nisaval® *(Discontinued)* *see page 1042*

nisoldipine (NYE sole di peen)

Sound-Alike/Look-Alike Issues

nisoldipine may be confused with nifedipine

U.S./Canadian Brand Names Sular® [US]

Therapeutic Category Calcium Channel Blocker

Use Management of hypertension, alone or in combination with other antihypertensive agents

Usual Dosage Adults: Oral: Initial: 20 mg once daily, then increase by 10 mg/week (or longer intervals) to attain adequate control of blood pressure; usual dose range (JNC 7): 10-40 mg once daily; doses >60 mg once daily are not recommended. A starting dose not exceeding 10 mg/day is recommended for the elderly and those with hepatic impairment.

Dosage Forms Tablet, extended release: 10 mg, 20 mg, 30 mg, 40 mg

nitalapram *see* citalopram *on page 205*

nitazoxanide (nye ta ZOX a nide)

Synonyms NTZ

U.S./Canadian Brand Names Alinia® [US]

Therapeutic Category Antiprotozoal

Use Treatment of diarrhea caused by *Cryptosporidium parvum* or *Giardia lamblia*

Usual Dosage Oral:

Diarrhea caused by *Cryptosporidium parvum*:

Children 12-47 months: 100 mg every 12 hours for 3 days

Children 4-11 years: 200 mg every 12 hours for 3 days

Diarrhea caused by *Giardia lamblia:*

Children 12-47 months: 100 mg every 12 hours for 3 days

Children 4-11 years: 200 mg every 12 hours for 3 days

Children ≥12 years and Adults: 500 mg every 12 hours for 3 days

Dosage Forms

Powder for oral suspension: 100 mg/5 mL (60 mL) [contains sucrose 1.48 g/5 mL, sodium benzoate; strawberry flavor]

Tablet: 500 mg

nitisinone (ni TIS i known)

U.S./Canadian Brand Names Orfadin® [US]

Therapeutic Category 4-Hydroxyphenylpyruvate Dioxygenase Inhibitor

Use Treatment of hereditary tyrosinemia type 1 (HT-1); to be used with dietary restriction of tyrosine and phenylalanine

Usual Dosage Oral: **Note:** Must be used in conjunction with a low protein diet restricted in tyrosine and phenylalanine.

Infants: See dosing for Children and Adults; infants may require maximal dose once liver function has improved

Children and Adults: Initial: 1 mg/kg/day in divided doses, given in the morning and evening, 1 hour before meals; doses do not need to be divided evenly

Dosage Forms Capsule: 2 mg, 5 mg, 10 mg

nitrazepam *(Canada only)* (nye TRA ze pam)

Synonyms nitrozepamum

Therapeutic Category Benzodiazepine

Use Short-term management of insomnia; treatment of infantile spasm and seizures

(Continued)

nitrazepam *(Canada only)* *(Continued)*

Usual Dosage Oral:
Insomnia:
Children:
1-6 years: 2.5 mg
≥7 years: 5 mg
Adults: 5-10 mg at night
Epilepsy: Children and Adults: 1-6 mg/day; dosage should be decreased in elderly, hypothyroid patients, and cirrhosis
Children maximum dose: 60 mg
Adult maximum dose: 20 mg

Dosage Forms Tablet: 5 mg, 10 mg

Nitrek® [US] *see* nitroglycerin *on next page*

nitric oxide (NYE trik OKS ide)

U.S./Canadian Brand Names INOmax® [US/Can]

Therapeutic Category Vasodilator, Pulmonary

Use Treatment of term and near-term (>34 weeks) neonates with hypoxic respiratory failure associated with pulmonary hypertension; used concurrently with ventilatory support and other agents

Usual Dosage Inhalation: Neonates (up to 14 days old): 20 ppm. Treatment should be maintained up to 14 days or until the underlying oxygen desaturation has resolved and the neonate is ready to be weaned from therapy. In the CINRGI trial, patients whose oxygenation improved had their dose reduced to 5 ppm at the end of 4 hours of treatment. Doses above 20 ppm should not be used because of the risk of methemoglobinemia and elevated NO_2.

Dosage Forms Gas, for inhalation:
100 ppm [nitric oxide 0.01% and nitrogen 99.9%] (353 L) [delivers 344 L], (1963 L) [delivers 1918 L]
800 ppm [nitric oxide 0.08% and nitrogen 99.92%] (353 L) [delivers 344 L], (1963 L) [delivers 1918 L]

4′-nitro-3′-trifluoromethylisobutyrantide *see* flutamide *on page 382*

Nitro-Bid® [US] *see* nitroglycerin *on next page*

Nitro-Bid® I.V. Injection *(Discontinued)* *see page 1042*

Nitro-Bid® Oral *(Discontinued)* *see page 1042*

Nitrocine® Oral *(Discontinued)* *see page 1042*

Nitrodisc® Patch *(Discontinued)* *see page 1042*

Nitro-Dur® [US/Can] *see* nitroglycerin *on next page*

nitrofural *see* nitrofurazone *on next page*

nitrofurantoin (nye troe fyoor AN toyn)

U.S./Canadian Brand Names Apo-Nitrofurantoin® [Can]; Furadantin® [US]; Macrobid® [US/Can]; Macrodantin® [US/Can]; Novo-Furantoin [Can]

Therapeutic Category Antibiotic, Miscellaneous

Use Prevention and treatment of urinary tract infections caused by susceptible gram-negative and some gram-positive organisms; *Pseudomonas*, *Serratia*, and most species of *Proteus* are generally resistant to nitrofurantoin

Usual Dosage Oral:
Children >1 month: 5-7 mg/kg/day in divided doses every 6 hours; maximum: 400 mg/day
UTI prophylaxis (chronic): 1-2 mg/kg/day in divided doses every 12-24 hours; maximum: 100 mg/day
Adults: 50-100 mg/dose every 6 hours
Macrocrystal/monohydrate: 100 mg twice daily

UTI prophylaxis (chronic): 50-100 mg/dose at bedtime

Dosage Forms

Capsule, macrocrystal: 50 mg, 100 mg

Macrodantin®: 25 mg, 50 mg, 100 mg

Capsule, macrocrystal/monohydrate (Macrobid®): 100 mg

Suspension, oral (Furadantin®): 25 mg/5 mL (470 mL)

nitrofurazone (nye troe FYOOR a zone)

Synonyms nitrofural

Therapeutic Category Antibacterial, Topical

Use Antibacterial agent used in second- and third-degree burns and skin grafting

Usual Dosage Children and Adults: Topical: Apply once daily or every few days to lesion or place on gauze

Dosage Forms

Cream: 0.2% (28 g)

Ointment, soluble dressing: 0.2% (28 g, 56 g, 454 g, 480 g)

Solution, topical: 0.2% (480 mL)

Nitrogard® [US] *see* nitroglycerin *on this page*

nitrogen mustard *see* mechlorethamine *on page 546*

nitroglycerin (nye troe GLI ser in)

Sound-Alike/Look-Alike Issues

nitroglycerin may be confused with nitroprusside

Nitro-Bid® may be confused with Nicobid®

Nitrol® may be confused with Nizoral®

Nitrostat® may be confused with Hyperstat®, Nilstat®, nystatin

Synonyms glyceryl trinitrate; nitroglycerol; NTG

U.S./Canadian Brand Names Gen-Nitro [Can]; Minitran™ [US/Can]; Nitrek® [US]; Nitro-Bid® [US]; Nitro-Dur® [US/Can]; Nitrogard® [US]; Nitrol® [Can]; Nitrolingual® [US]; NitroQuick® [US]; Nitrostat® [US/Can]; Nitro-Tab® [US]; NitroTime® [US]; Rho®-Nitro [Can]; Transderm-Nitro® [Can]

Therapeutic Category Vasodilator

Use Treatment of angina pectoris; I.V. for congestive heart failure (especially when associated with acute myocardial infarction); pulmonary hypertension; hypertensive emergencies occurring perioperatively (especially during cardiovascular surgery)

Usual Dosage Note: Hemodynamic and antianginal tolerance often develop within 24-48 hours of continuous nitrate administration. Nitrate-free interval (10-12 hours/day) is recommended to avoid tolerance development; gradually decrease dose in patients receiving NTG for prolonged period to avoid withdrawal reaction.

Children: Pulmonary hypertension: Continuous infusion: Start 0.25-0.5 mcg/kg/minute and titrate by 1 mcg/kg/minute at 20- to 60-minute intervals to desired effect; usual dose: 1-3 mcg/kg/minute; maximum: 5 mcg/kg/minute

Adults:

Buccal: Initial: 1 mg every 3-5 hours while awake (3 times/day); titrate dosage upward if angina occurs with tablet in place

Oral: 2.5-9 mg 2-4 times/day (up to 26 mg 4 times/day)

I.V.: 5 mcg/minute, increase by 5 mcg/minute every 3-5 minutes to 20 mcg/minute; if no response at 20 mcg/minute increase by 10 mcg/minute every 3-5 minutes, up to 200 mcg/minute

Ointment: 1/2" upon rising and 1/2" 6 hours later; the dose may be doubled and even doubled again as needed

Patch, transdermal: Initial: 0.2-0.4 mg/hour, titrate to doses of 0.4-0.8 mg/hour; tolerance is minimized by using a patch-on period of 12-14 hours and patch-off period of 10-12 hours

Sublingual: 0.2-0.6 mg every 5 minutes for maximum of 3 doses in 15 minutes; may also use prophylactically 5-10 minutes prior to activities which may provoke an attack

(Continued)

nitroglycerin *(Continued)*

Translingual: 1-2 sprays into mouth under tongue every 3-5 minutes for maximum of 3 doses in 15 minutes, may also be used 5-10 minutes prior to activities which may provoke an attack prophylactically

Dosage Forms [DSC] = Discontinued product

Aerosol, translingual spray (Nitrolingual®): 0.4 mg/metered spray (12 g) [contains alcohol 20%; 200 metered sprays]
Capsule, extended release (Nitro-Time®): 2.5 mg, 6.5 mg, 9 mg
Infusion [premixed in D_5W]: 0.1 mg/mL (250 mL, 500 mL); 0.2 mg/mL (250 mL); 0.4 mg/mL (250 mL, 500 mL)
Injection, solution: 5 mg/mL (5 mL, 10 mL) [contains alcohol and propylene glycol]
Ointment, topical:
Nitro-Bid®: 2% [20 mg/g] (30 g, 60 g)
Nitrol® [DSC]: 2% [20 mg/g] (3 g, 60 g)
Tablet, buccal, extended release (Nitrogard®): 2 mg, 3 mg
Tablet, sublingual (NitroQuick®, Nitrostat®, Nitro-Tab®): 0.3 mg, 0.4 mg, 0.6 mg
Transdermal system [once daily patch]: 0.1 mg/hour (30s); 0.2 mg/hour (30s); 0.4 mg/hour (30s); 0.6 mg/hour (30s)
Minitran™: 0.1 mg/hour (30s); 0.2 mg/hour (30s); 0.4 mg/hour (30s); 0.6 mg/hour (30s)
Nitrek®: 0.2 mg/hour (30s); 0.4 mg/hour (30s); 0.6 mg/hour (30s)
Nitro-Dur®: 0.1 mg/hour (30s); 0.2 mg/hour (30s); 0.3 mg/hour (30s); 0.4 mg/hour (30s); 0.6 mg/hour (30s); 0.8 mg/hour (30s)

nitroglycerol *see* nitroglycerin *on previous page*

Nitrol® [Can] *see* nitroglycerin *on previous page*

Nitrol® *(Discontinued)* *see page 1042*

Nitrolingual® [US] *see* nitroglycerin *on previous page*

Nitrong® Oral Tablet *(Discontinued)* *see page 1042*

Nitropress® [US] *see* nitroprusside *on this page*

nitroprusside (nye troe PRUS ide)

Sound-Alike/Look-Alike Issues

nitroprusside may be confused with nitroglycerin

Synonyms nitroprusside sodium; sodium nitroferricyanide; sodium nitroprusside

U.S./Canadian Brand Names Nipride® [Can]; Nitropress® [US]

Therapeutic Category Vasodilator

Use Management of hypertensive crises; congestive heart failure; used for controlled hypotension to reduce bleeding during surgery

Usual Dosage Administration requires the use of an infusion pump. Average dose: 5 mcg/kg/minute.

Children: Pulmonary hypertension: I.V.: Initial: 1 mcg/kg/minute by continuous I.V. infusion; increase in increments of 1 mcg/kg/minute at intervals of 20-60 minutes; titrating to the desired response; usual dose: 3 mcg/kg/minute, rarely need >4 mcg/kg/minute; maximum: 5 mcg/kg/minute.

Adults: I.V. Initial: 0.3-0.5 mcg/kg/minute; increase in increments of 0.5 mcg/kg/minute, titrating to the desired hemodynamic effect or the appearance of headache or nausea; usual dose: 3 mcg/kg/minute; rarely need >4 mcg/kg/minute; maximum: 10 mcg/kg/minute. When administered by prolonged infusion faster than 2 mcg/kg/minute, cyanide is generated faster than an unaided patient can handle.

Dosage Forms [DSC] = Discontinued product

Injection, powder for reconstitution, as sodium: 50 mg [DSC]
Injection, solution, as sodium: 25 mg/mL (2 mL)

nitroprusside sodium *see* nitroprusside *on this page*

NitroQuick® [US] *see* nitroglycerin *on previous page*

Nitrostat® [US/Can] *see* nitroglycerin *on previous page*

Nitrostat® 0.15 mg Tablet *(Discontinued)* *see page 1042*

Nitro-Tab® [US] *see* nitroglycerin *on page 623*

NitroTime® [US] *see* nitroglycerin *on page 623*

nitrous oxide (NYE trus OKS ide)

Therapeutic Category Anesthetic, Gas

Use Produces sedation and analgesia; principal adjunct to inhalation and intravenous general anesthesia

Usual Dosage Children and Adults:

Surgical: For sedation and analgesia: Concentrations of 25% to 50% nitrous oxide with oxygen. For general anesthesia, concentrations of 40% to 70% via mask or endotracheal tube. Minimal alveolar concentration (MAC), which can be considered the ED_{50} of inhalational anesthetics, is 105%; therefore delivery in a hyperbaric chamber is necessary to use as a complete anesthetic. When administered at 70%, reduces the MAC of other anesthetics by half.

Dental: For sedation and analgesia: Concentrations of 25% to 50% nitrous oxide with oxygen

Dosage Forms Supplied in blue cylinders

nitrozepamum *see* nitrazepam *(Canada only) on page 621*

Nix® [US/Can] *see* permethrin *on page 683*

nizatidine (ni ZA ti deen)

Sound-Alike/Look-Alike Issues

Axid® may be confused with Ansaid®

U.S./Canadian Brand Names Apo-Nizatidine® [Can]; Axid® [US/Can]; Axid® AR [US-OTC]; Gen-Nizatidine [Can]; Novo-Nizatidine [Can]; Nu-Nizatidine [Can]; PMS-Nizatidine [Can]

Therapeutic Category Histamine H_2 Antagonist

Use Treatment and maintenance of duodenal ulcer; treatment of benign gastric ulcer; treatment of gastroesophageal reflux disease (GERD); OTC tablet used for the prevention of meal-induced heartburn, acid indigestion, and sour stomach

Usual Dosage Oral:

Children:

GERD: Refer to Adults dosing

Meal-induced heartburn, acid indigestion and sour stomach: Refer to Adults dosing

Adults:

Duodenal ulcer:

Treatment of active ulcer: 300 mg at bedtime or 150 mg twice daily

Maintenance of healed ulcer: 150 mg/day at bedtime

Gastric ulcer: 150 mg twice daily or 300 mg at bedtime

GERD: 150 mg twice daily

Meal-induced heartburn, acid indigestion, and sour stomach: 75 mg tablet [OTC] twice daily, 30 to 60 minutes prior to consuming food or beverages

Dosage Forms

Capsule (Axid®): 150 mg, 300 mg

Solution, oral (Axid®): 15 mg/mL (480 mL) [bubblegum flavor]

Tablet (Axid® AR): 75 mg

Nizoral® [US/Can] *see* ketoconazole *on page 495*

Nizoral® A-D [US-OTC] *see* ketoconazole *on page 495*

N-methylhydrazine *see* procarbazine *on page 731*

Nocosyn™ [US] *see* sulfur and sulfacetamide *on page 834*

Noctec® *(Discontinued)* *see page 1042*

Nolahist® [US-OTC/Can] *see* phenindamine *on page 686*

Nolamine® *(Discontinued)* *see page 1042*

Nolex® LA *(Discontinued)* *see page 1042*

Noludar® *(Discontinued)* *see page 1042*

Nolvadex® [US/Can] *see* tamoxifen *on page 839*

Nolvadex®-D [Can] *see* tamoxifen *on page 839*

nonoxynol 9 (non OKS i nole nine)

Sound-Alike/Look-Alike Issues

Delfen® may be confused with Delsym®

U.S./Canadian Brand Names Advantage 24™ [Can]; Advantage-S™ [US-OTC]; Aqua Lube Plus [US-OTC]; Conceptrol® [US-OTC]; Delfen® [US-OTC]; Emko® [US-OTC]; Encare® [US-OTC]; Gynol II® [US-OTC]; Semicid® [US-OTC]; Shur-Seal® [US-OTC]; VCF™ [US-OTC]

Therapeutic Category Spermicide

Use Spermatocide in contraception

Usual Dosage Insert into vagina at least 10 minutes before intercourse (but not longer than 1 hour); refer to specific product labeling

Dosage Forms

Film, vaginal (VCF™): 28% (3s, 6s,12s)

Foam, vaginal:

Delfen®: 12.5% (17 g)

Emko®: 8% (40 g, 90 g)

VCF™: 12.5% (40 g)

Gel, vaginal:

Advantage-S™: 3.5% (1.5 g) [packaged in 3s or 6s with reusable applicator]; (30g) [packaged with reusable applicator]

Aqua Lube Plus: 1% (60 g, 120 g)

Conceptrol®: 4% (2.7 g) [packaged in 10s with applicator]

Gynol II: 2% (85 g, 114 g)

Shur-Seal®: 2% (6 g) [packaged in 24s]

Suppository, vaginal:

Encare®: 100 mg (12s, 18s)

Semicid®: 100 mg (9s, 18s)

No Pain-HP® *(Discontinued)* *see page 1042*

Nora-BE™ [US] *see* norethindrone *on next page*

noradrenaline *see* norepinephrine *on next page*

noradrenaline acid tartrate *see* norepinephrine *on next page*

Norcet® *(Discontinued)* *see page 1042*

Norco® [US] *see* hydrocodone and acetaminophen *on page 443*

Norcuron® [Can] *see* vecuronium *on page 907*

Norcuron® *(Discontinued)* *see page 1042*

nordeoxyguanosine *see* ganciclovir *on page 396*

Nordette® [US] *see* ethinyl estradiol and levonorgestrel *on page 339*

Norditropin® [US/Can] *see* human growth hormone *on page 437*

Norditropin® Cartridges [US] *see* human growth hormone *on page 437*

Nordryl® Injection *(Discontinued)* *see page 1042*

Nordryl® Oral *(Discontinued)* *see page 1042*

norelgestromin and ethinyl estradiol *see* ethinyl estradiol and norelgestromin *on page 342*

norepinephrine (nor ep i NEF rin)

Synonyms levarterenol bitartrate; noradrenaline; noradrenaline acid tartrate; norepinephrine bitartrate

U.S./Canadian Brand Names Levophed® [US/Can]

Therapeutic Category Adrenergic Agonist Agent

Use Treatment of shock which persists after adequate fluid volume replacement

Usual Dosage **Administration requires the use of an infusion pump!**

Note: Norepinephrine dosage is stated in terms of norepinephrine base and intravenous formulation is norepinephrine bitartrate

Norepinephrine bitartrate 2 mg = Norepinephrine base 1 mg

Continuous I.V. infusion:

Children: Initial: 0.05-0.1 mcg/kg/minute; titrate to desired effect; maximum dose: 1-2 mcg/kg/minute

Adults: Initial: 0.5-1 mcg/minute and titrate to desired response; 8-30 mcg/minute is usual range; range used in clinical trials: 0.01-3 mcg/kg/minute; ACLS dosage range: 0.5-30 mcg/minute

Dosage Forms Injection, solution, as bitartrate: 1 mg/mL (4 mL) [contains sodium metabisulfite]

norepinephrine bitartrate *see* norepinephrine *on this page*

Norethin™ 1/35E *(Discontinued)* *see page 1042*

norethindrone (nor eth IN drone)

Sound-Alike/Look-Alike Issues

Micronor® may be confused with miconazole, Micronase®

Synonyms norethindrone acetate; norethisterone

U.S./Canadian Brand Names Aygestin® [US]; Camila™ [US]; Errin™ [US]; Jolivette™ [US]; Micronor® [US/Can]; Nora-BE™ [US]; Norlutate® [Can]; Nor-QD® [US]

Therapeutic Category Contraceptive, Progestin Only; Progestin

Use Treatment of amenorrhea; abnormal uterine bleeding; endometriosis, oral contraceptive; **higher rate of failure with progestin only contraceptives**

Usual Dosage Oral: Adolescents and Adults: Female:

Contraception: Progesterone only: Norethindrone 0.35 mg every day of the year starting on first day of menstruation; if one dose is missed, discontinue and use an alternative method of contraception

Amenorrhea and abnormal uterine bleeding:

Norethindrone: 5-20 mg/day for 5-10 days during the second half of the menstrual cycle

Acetate salt: 2.5-10 mg/day for 5-10 days during the second half of the menstrual cycle

Endometriosis:

Norethindrone: 10 mg/day for 2 weeks; increase at increments of 5 mg/day every 2 weeks until 30 mg/day; continue for 6-9 months or until breakthrough bleeding demands temporary termination

Acetate salt: 5 mg/day for 14 days; increase at increments of 2.5 mg/day every 2 weeks up to 15 mg/day; continue for 6-9 months or until breakthrough bleeding demands temporary termination

Dosage Forms

Tablet (Camila™, Errin™, Jolivette™, Micronor®, Nora-BE™, Nor-QD®): 0.35 mg

Tablet, as acetate (Aygestin®): 5 mg

norethindrone acetate *see* norethindrone *on this page*

norethindrone acetate and ethinyl estradiol *see* ethinyl estradiol and norethindrone *on page 342*

norethindrone and estradiol *see* estradiol and norethindrone *on page 327*

norethindrone and mestranol *see* mestranol and norethindrone *on page 558*

norethisterone *see* norethindrone *on this page*

Norflex™ [US/Can] *see* orphenadrine *on page 649*

norfloxacin (nor FLOKS a sin)

Sound-Alike/Look-Alike Issues

norfloxacin may be confused with Norflex®, Noroxin®

Noroxin® may be confused with Neurontin®, Norflex®, norfloxacin

U.S./Canadian Brand Names Apo-Norflox® [Can]; Norfloxacine® [Can]; Noroxin® [US]; Novo-Norfloxacin [Can]; PMS-Norfloxacin [Can]; Riva-Norfloxacin [Can]

Therapeutic Category Quinolone

Use Uncomplicated urinary tract infections and cystitis caused by susceptible gram-negative and gram-positive bacteria; sexually-transmitted disease (eg, uncomplicated urethral and cervical gonorrhea) caused by *N. gonorrhoeae*; prostatitis due to *E. coli*

Usual Dosage Oral: Adults:

Urinary tract infections: 400 mg twice daily for 3-21 days depending on severity of infection or organism sensitivity; maximum: 800 mg/day

Uncomplicated gonorrhea: 800 mg as a single dose (CDC recommends as an alternative regimen to ciprofloxacin or ofloxacin)

Prostatitis: 400 mg every 12 hours for 4 weeks

Dosage Forms Tablet: 400 mg

Norfloxacine® [Can] *see* norfloxacin *on this page*

Norgesic™ [US/Can] *see* orphenadrine, aspirin, and caffeine *on page 649*

Norgesic™ Forte [US/Can] *see* orphenadrine, aspirin, and caffeine *on page 649*

norgestimate and estradiol *see* estradiol and norgestimate *on page 328*

norgestimate and ethinyl estradiol *see* ethinyl estradiol and norgestimate *on page 346*

norgestrel (nor JES trel)

U.S./Canadian Brand Names Ovrette® [US/Can]

Therapeutic Category Contraceptive, Progestin Only

Use Prevention of pregnancy; **progestin only products have higher risk of failure in contraceptive use**

Usual Dosage Oral: Administer daily, starting the first day of menstruation, take 1 tablet at the same time each day, every day of the year. If one dose is missed, take as soon as remembered, then next tablet at regular time; if two doses are missed, take 1 tablet as soon as it is remembered, followed by an additional dose that same day at the usual time. When one or two doses are missed, additional contraceptive measures should be used until 14 consecutive tablets have been taken. If three doses are missed, discontinue norgestrel and use an additional form of birth control until menses or pregnancy is ruled out.

Dosage Forms Tablet: 0.075 mg [contains tartrazine]

norgestrel and ethinyl estradiol *see* ethinyl estradiol and norgestrel *on page 347*

noricizine hydrochloride *see* moricizine *on page 591*

Norinyl® 1+35 [US] *see* ethinyl estradiol and norethindrone *on page 342*

Norinyl® 1+50 [US] *see* mestranol and norethindrone *on page 558*

Noritate® [US/Can] *see* metronidazole *on page 576*

Norlutate® [Can] *see* norethindrone *on previous page*

Norlutate® ***(Discontinued)*** *see page 1042*

Norlutin® ***(Discontinued)*** *see page 1042*

normal human serum albumin *see* albumin *on page 25*

normal saline *see* sodium chloride *on page 810*

normal serum albumin (human) *see* albumin *on page 25*

Normiflo® ***(Discontinued)*** *see page 1042*

Normodyne® [US/Can] *see* labetalol *on page 499*

Noroxin® [US] *see* norfloxacin *on previous page*

Norpace® [US/Can] *see* disopyramide *on page 283*

Norpace® CR [US] *see* disopyramide *on page 283*

Norplant® Implant [Can] *see* levonorgestrel *on page 515*

Norplant® Implant ***(Discontinued)*** *see page 1042*

Norpramin® [US/Can] *see* desipramine *on page 251*

Nor-QD® [US] *see* norethindrone *on page 627*

North American coral snake antivenin *see* antivenin *(Micrurus fulvius) on page 67*

North and South American antisnake-bite serum *see* antivenin *(Crotalidae)* polyvalent *on page 67*

Nortrel™ [US] *see* ethinyl estradiol and norethindrone *on page 342*

Nortrel™ 7/7/7 [US] *see* ethinyl estradiol and norethindrone *on page 342*

nortriptyline (nor TRIP ti leen)

Sound-Alike/Look-Alike Issues

nortriptyline may be confused with amitriptyline, desipramine, Norpramin®

Aventyl® HCl may be confused with Bentyl®

Pamelor® may be confused with Demerol®, Dymelor®

Synonyms nortriptyline hydrochloride

U.S./Canadian Brand Names Alti-Nortriptyline [Can]; Apo-Nortriptyline® [Can]; Aventyl® [Can]; Aventyl® HCl [US]; Gen-Nortriptyline [Can]; Norventyl [Can]; Novo-Nortriptyline [Can]; Nu-Nortriptyline [Can]; Pamelor® [US]; PMS-Nortriptyline [Can]

Therapeutic Category Antidepressant, Tricyclic (Secondary Amine)

Use Treatment of symptoms of depression

Usual Dosage Oral:

Nocturnal enuresis:

Children:

6-7 years (20-25 kg): 10 mg/day

8-11 years (25-35 kg): 10-20 mg/day

>11 years (35-54 kg): 25-35 mg/day

Depression:

Adults: 25 mg 3-4 times/day up to 150 mg/day

Elderly (**Note:** Nortriptyline is one of the best tolerated TCAs in the elderly)

Initial: 10-25 mg at bedtime

Dosage can be increased by 25 mg every 3 days for inpatients and weekly for outpatients if tolerated

Usual maintenance dose: 75 mg as a single bedtime dose or 2 divided doses; however, lower or higher doses may be required to stay within the therapeutic window

Dosage Forms

Capsule, as hydrochloride: 10 mg, 25 mg, 50 mg, 75 mg

Aventyl® HCl: 10 mg, 25 mg

Pamelor®: 10 mg, 25 mg, 50 mg, 75 mg [may contain benzyl alcohol; 50 mg may also contain sodium bisulfite]

Solution, as hydrochloride (Aventyl® HCl, Pamelor®): 10 mg/5 mL (473 mL) [contains alcohol 4% and benzoic acid]

nortriptyline hydrochloride *see* nortriptyline *on this page*

Norvasc® [US/Can] *see* amlodipine *on page 49*

Norventyl [Can] *see* nortriptyline *on this page*

Norvir® [US/Can] *see* ritonavir *on page 780*

Novo-Clobazam [Can] *see* clobazam *(Canada only) on page 212*
Novo-Clobetasol [Can] *see* clobetasol *on page 212*
Novo-Clonazepam [Can] *see* clonazepam *on page 215*
Novo-Clonidine [Can] *see* clonidine *on page 215*
Novo-Clopate [Can] *see* clorazepate *on page 217*
Novo-Clopramine [Can] *see* clomipramine *on page 214*
Novo-Cloxin [Can] *see* cloxacillin *on page 218*
Novo-Cycloprine [Can] *see* cyclobenzaprine *on page 233*
Novo-Desipramine [Can] *see* desipramine *on page 251*
Novo-Difenac® [Can] *see* diclofenac *on page 266*
Novo-Difenac-K [Can] *see* diclofenac *on page 266*
Novo-Difenac® SR [Can] *see* diclofenac *on page 266*
Novo-Diflunisal [Can] *see* diflunisal *on page 270*
Novo-Digoxin [Can] *see* digoxin *on page 270*
Novo-Diltazem [Can] *see* diltiazem *on page 273*
Novo-Diltazem SR [Can] *see* diltiazem *on page 273*
Novo-Diltiazem-CD [Can] *see* diltiazem *on page 273*
Novo-Dimenate [Can] *see* dimenhydrinate *on page 274*
Novo-Dipiradol [Can] *see* dipyridamole *on page 282*
Novo-Divalproex [Can] *see* valproic acid and derivatives *on page 901*
Novo-Docusate Calcium [Can] *see* docusate *on page 285*
Novo-Docusate Sodium [Can] *see* docusate *on page 285*
Novo-Domperidone [Can] *see* domperidone *(Canada only) on page 288*
Novo-Doxazosin [Can] *see* doxazosin *on page 291*
Novo-Doxepin [Can] *see* doxepin *on page 292*
Novo-Doxylin [Can] *see* doxycycline *on page 294*
Novo-Famotidine [Can] *see* famotidine *on page 356*
Novo-Fenofibrate [Can] *see* fenofibrate *on page 360*
Novo-Ferrogluc [Can] *see* ferrous gluconate *on page 364*
Novo-Fluconazole [Can] *see* fluconazole *on page 371*
Novo-Fluoxetine [Can] *see* fluoxetine *on page 379*
Novo-Flurprofen [Can] *see* flurbiprofen *on page 381*
Novo-Flutamide [Can] *see* flutamide *on page 382*
Novo-Fluvoxamine [Can] *see* fluvoxamine *on page 385*
Novo-Furantoin [Can] *see* nitrofurantoin *on page 622*
Novo-Gabapentin [Can] *see* gabapentin *on page 395*
Novo-Gemfibrozil [Can] *see* gemfibrozil *on page 400*
Novo-Gliclazide [Can] *see* gliclazide *(Canada only) on page 405*
Novo-Glyburide [Can] *see* glyburide *on page 409*
Novo-Hydrazide [Can] *see* hydrochlorothiazide *on page 441*
Novo-Hydroxyzin [Can] *see* hydroxyzine *on page 458*
Novo-Hylazin [Can] *see* hydralazine *on page 440*
Novo-Indapamide [Can] *see* indapamide *on page 470*
Novo-Ipramide [Can] *see* ipratropium *on page 482*

Novo-Peridol [Can] *see* haloperidol *on page 428*
Novo-Pheniram® [Can] *see* chlorpheniramine *on page 187*
Novo-Pindol [Can] *see* pindolol *on page 696*
Novo-Pirocam® [Can] *see* piroxicam *on page 698*
Novo-Pravastatin [Can] *see* pravastatin *on page 721*
Novo-Prazin [Can] *see* prazosin *on page 722*
Novo-Prednisolone [Can] *see* prednisolone (ophthalmic) *on page 723*
Novo-Profen® [Can] *see* ibuprofen *on page 462*
Novo-Propamide [Can] *see* chlorpropamide *on page 195*
Novo-Quinidin [Can] *see* quinidine *on page 756*
Novo-Ranidine [Can] *see* ranitidine hydrochloride *on page 763*
NovoRapid® [Can] *see* insulin preparations *on page 474*
Novo-Selegiline [Can] *see* selegiline *on page 798*
Novo-Sertraline [Can] *see* sertraline *on page 801*
NovoSeven® [US] *see* factor VIIa (recombinant) *on page 354*
Novo-Sorbide [Can] *see* isosorbide dinitrate *on page 488*
Novo-Sotalol [Can] *see* sotalol *on page 819*
Novo-Soxazole® [Can] *see* sulfisoxazole *on page 833*
Novo-Spiroton [Can] *see* spironolactone *on page 821*
Novo-Spirozine [Can] *see* hydrochlorothiazide and spironolactone *on page 443*
Novo-Sucralate [Can] *see* sucralfate *on page 827*
Novo-Sundac [Can] *see* sulindac *on page 835*
Novo-Tamoxifen [Can] *see* tamoxifen *on page 839*
Novo-Temazepam [Can] *see* temazepam *on page 843*
Novo-Terazosin [Can] *see* terazosin *on page 845*
Novo-Tetra [Can] *see* tetracycline *on page 851*
Novo-Theophyl SR [Can] *see* theophylline *on page 854*
Novothyrox [US] *see* levothyroxine *on page 516*
Novo-Tiaprofenic [Can] *see* tiaprofenic acid *(Canada only) on page 861*
Novo-Ticlopidine [Can] *see* ticlopidine *on page 862*
Novo-Trazodone [Can] *see* trazodone *on page 877*
Novo-Triamzide [Can] *see* hydrochlorothiazide and triamterene *on page 443*
Novo-Trifluzine [Can] *see* trifluoperazine *on page 885*
Novo-Trimel [Can] *see* sulfamethoxazole and trimethoprim *on page 831*
Novo-Trimel D.S. [Can] *see* sulfamethoxazole and trimethoprim *on page 831*
Novo-Tripramine [Can] *see* trimipramine *on page 888*
Novo-Veramil [Can] *see* verapamil *on page 908*
Novo-Veramil SR [Can] *see* verapamil *on page 908*
Novoxapram® [Can] *see* oxazepam *on page 653*
Nozinan® [Can] *see* methotrimeprazine *(Canada only) on page 566*
NP-27® *(Discontinued)* *see page 1042*
NPH Iletin® II [US] *see* insulin preparations *on page 474*
NPH Iletin® I Insulin *(Discontinued)* *see page 1042*
NPH, insulin *see* insulin preparations *on page 474*

NSC-740 *see* methotrexate *on page 565*
NSC-752 *see* thioguanine *on page 857*
NSC-755 *see* mercaptopurine *on page 555*
NSC-762 *see* mechlorethamine *on page 546*
NSC-3053 *see* dactinomycin *on page 241*
NSC-3088 *see* chlorambucil *on page 182*
NSC-10363 *see* megestrol acetate *on page 549*
NSC-13875 *see* altretamine *on page 38*
NSC-26271 *see* cyclophosphamide *on page 234*
NSC-26980 *see* mitomycin *on page 585*
NSC-27640 *see* floxuridine *on page 371*
NSC-38721 *see* mitotane *on page 585*
NSC-49842 *see* vinblastine *on page 911*
NSC-63878 *see* cytarabine *on page 239*
NSC-67574 *see* vincristine *on page 912*
NSC-77213 *see* procarbazine *on page 731*
NSC-82151 *see* daunorubicin hydrochloride *on page 246*
NSC-85998 *see* streptozocin *on page 825*
NSC-89199 *see* estramustine *on page 329*
NSC-102816 *see* azacitidine *on page 92*
NSC-106977 (*Erwinia*) *see* asparaginase *on page 80*
NSC-109229 (*E. coli*) *see* asparaginase *on page 80*
NSC-109724 *see* ifosfamide *on page 464*
NSC-123127 *see* doxorubicin *on page 293*
NSC-125066 *see* bleomycin *on page 123*
NSC-125973 *see* paclitaxel *on page 660*
NSC-147834 *see* flutamide *on page 382*
NSC-180973 *see* tamoxifen *on page 839*
NSC-218321 *see* pentostatin *on page 680*
NSC-245467 *see* vindesine *on page 912*
NSC-256439 *see* idarubicin *on page 464*
NSC-266046 *see* oxaliplatin *on page 652*
NSC-301739 *see* mitoxantrone *on page 586*
NSC-352122 *see* trimetrexate glucuronate *on page 888*
NSC-362856 *see* temozolomide *on page 843*
NSC-373364 *see* aldesleukin *on page 28*
NSC-377526 *see* leuprolide acetate *on page 509*
NSC-409962 *see* carmustine *on page 162*
NSC-606864 *see* goserelin *on page 413*
NSC-609699 *see* topotecan *on page 872*
NSC-616348 *see* irinotecan *on page 484*
NSC-628503 *see* docetaxel *on page 284*
NSC-639186 *see* raltitrexed *(Canada only) on page 762*
NSC-644954 *see* pegaspargase *on page 670*

Nuprin® ***(Discontinued)*** *see page 1042*
Nu-Prochlor [Can] *see* prochlorperazine *on page 731*
Nu-Propranolol [Can] *see* propranolol *on page 741*
Nuquin HP® Cream [US] *see* hydroquinone *on page 454*
Nu-Ranit [Can] *see* ranitidine hydrochloride *on page 763*
Nuromax® [US/Can] *see* doxacurium *on page 290*
Nursoy® ***(Discontinued)*** *see page 1042*
Nu-Selegiline [Can] *see* selegiline *on page 798*
Nu-Sertraline [Can] *see* sertraline *on page 801*
Nu-Sotalol [Can] *see* sotalol *on page 819*
Nu-Sucralate [Can] *see* sucralfate *on page 827*
Nu-Sulfinpyrazone [Can] *see* sulfinpyrazone *on page 833*
Nu-Sundac [Can] *see* sulindac *on page 835*
Nu-Tears® II [US-OTC] *see* artificial tears *on page 78*
Nu-Tears® [US-OTC] *see* artificial tears *on page 78*
Nu-Temazepam [Can] *see* temazepam *on page 843*
Nu-Terazosin [Can] *see* terazosin *on page 845*
Nu-Tetra [Can] *see* tetracycline *on page 851*
Nu-Tiaprofenic [Can] *see* tiaprofenic acid *(Canada only) on page 861*
Nu-Ticlopidine [Can] *see* ticlopidine *on page 862*
Nu-Timolol [Can] *see* timolol *on page 863*
Nutracort® [US] *see* hydrocortisone (topical) *on page 451*
Nutraplus® [US-OTC] *see* urea *on page 897*
Nu-Trazodone [Can] *see* trazodone *on page 877*
Nu-Triazide [Can] *see* hydrochlorothiazide and triamterene *on page 443*
Nu-Trimipramine [Can] *see* trimipramine *on page 888*
NutriNate® [US] *see* vitamins (multiple/prenatal) *on page 927*
Nutropin® [US] *see* human growth hormone *on page 437*
Nutropin AQ® [US/Can] *see* human growth hormone *on page 437*
Nutropin Depot® ***(Discontinued)*** *see page 1042*
Nutropine® [Can] *see* human growth hormone *on page 437*
NuvaRing® [US] *see* ethinyl estradiol and etonogestrel *on page 338*
Nu-Zopiclone [Can] *see* zopiclone *(Canada only) on page 944*
NVB *see* vinorelbine *on page 912*
NVP *see* nevirapine *on page 615*
Nyaderm [Can] *see* nystatin *on this page*
Nydrazid® ***(Discontinued)*** *see page 1042*

nystatin (nye STAT in)

Sound-Alike/Look-Alike Issues
nystatin may be confused with Nitrostat®

U.S./Canadian Brand Names Bio-Statin® [US]; Candistatin® [Can]; Mycostatin® [US/Can]; Nilstat® [Can]; Nyaderm [Can]; Nystat-Rx® [US]; Nystop® [US]; Pedi-Dri® [US]; PMS-Nystatin [Can]

Therapeutic Category Antifungal Agent

Use Treatment of susceptible cutaneous, mucocutaneous, and oral cavity fungal infections normally caused by the *Candida* species

(Continued)

nystatin *(Continued)*

Usual Dosage

Oral candidiasis:

Suspension (swish and swallow orally):

Premature infants: 100,000 units 4 times/day

Infants: 200,000 units 4 times/day or 100,000 units to each side of mouth 4 times/day

Children and Adults: 400,000-600,000 units 4 times/day

Troche: Children and Adults: 200,000-400,000 units 4-5 times/day

Powder for compounding: Children and Adults: $^1/_8$ teaspoon (500,000 units) to equal approximately $^1/_2$ cup of water; give 4 times/day

Mucocutaneous infections: Children and Adults: Topical: Apply 2-3 times/day to affected areas; very moist topical lesions are treated best with powder

Intestinal infections: Adults: Oral: 500,000-1,000,000 units every 8 hours

Vaginal infections: Adults: Vaginal tablets: Insert 1 tablet/day at bedtime for 2 weeks

Dosage Forms [DSC] = Discontinued product

Capsule (Bio-Statin®): 500,000 units, 1 million units

Cream: 100,000 units/g (15 g, 30 g)

Mycostatin®: 100,000 units/g (30 g)

Lozenge (Mycostatin®): 200,000 units [DSC]

Ointment, topical: 100,000 units/g (15 g, 30 g)

Powder, for prescription compounding: 50 million units (10 g); 150 million units (30 g); 500 million units (100 g); 2 billion units (400 g)

Nystat-Rx®: 50 million units (10 g); 150 million units (30 g); 500 million units (100 g); 1 billion units (190 g); 2 billion units (350 g)

Powder, topical:

Mycostatin®: 100,000 units/g (15 g)

Nystop®: 100,000 units/g (15 g, 30 g, 60 g)

Pedi-Dri®: 100,000 units/g (56.7 g)

Suspension, oral: 100,000 units/mL (5 mL, 60 mL, 480 mL)

Mycostatin® [DSC]: 100,000 units/mL (60 mL, 480 mL) [contains alcohol ≤1%; cherry-mint flavor]

Tablet: 500,000 units

Tablet, vaginal: 100,000 units (15s) [packaged with applicator]

nystatin and triamcinolone (nye STAT in & trye am SIN oh lone)

Synonyms triamcinolone and nystatin

Therapeutic Category Antifungal/Corticosteroid

Use Treatment of cutaneous candidiasis

Usual Dosage Children and Adults: Topical: Apply sparingly 2-4 times/day. Therapy should be discontinued when control is achieved; if no improvement is seen, reassessment of diagnosis may be necessary.

Dosage Forms [DSC] = Discontinued product

Cream (Mycolog®-II [DSC]): Nystatin 100,000 units and triamcinolone acetonide 0.1% (15 g, 30 g, 60 g)

Ointment: Nystatin 100,000 units and triamcinolone acetonide 0.1% (15 g, 30 g, 60 g)

Mycolog®-II: Nystatin 100,000 units and triamcinolone acetonide 0.1% (15 g, 30 g, 60 g) [DSC]

Nystat-Rx® [US] *see* nystatin *on previous page*

Nystex® *(Discontinued)* *see page 1042*

Nystop® [US] *see* nystatin *on previous page*

Nytol® Extra Strength [Can] *see* diphenhydramine *on page 277*

Nytol® Maximum Strength [US-OTC] *see* diphenhydramine *on page 277*

Nytol® [US-OTC/Can] *see* diphenhydramine *on page 277*

OB-20 [US] *see* vitamins (multiple/prenatal) *on page 927*

Obegyn™ [US] *see* vitamins (multiple/prenatal) *on page 927*

Obezine® [US] *see* phendimetrazine *on page 685*

OCBZ *see* oxcarbazepine *on page 653*

Occlusal™ [Can] *see* salicylic acid *on page 789*

Occlusal®-HP [US/Can] *see* salicylic acid *on page 789*

Ocean® [US-OTC] *see* sodium chloride *on page 810*

OCL® *(Discontinued)* *see page 1042*

Octagam® [US] *see* immune globulin (intravenous) *on page 468*

Octamide® *(Discontinued)* *see page 1042*

Octicair® Otic *(Discontinued)* *see page 1042*

Octocaine® *(Discontinued)* *see page 1042*

Octostim® [Can] *see* desmopressin acetate *on page 252*

octreotide (ok TREE oh tide)

Sound-Alike/Look-Alike Issues

Sandostatin® may be confused with Sandimmune®

Synonyms octreotide acetate

U.S./Canadian Brand Names Sandostatin LAR® [US/Can]; Sandostatin® [US/Can]

Therapeutic Category Somatostatin Analog

Use Control of symptoms in patients with metastatic carcinoid and vasoactive intestinal peptide-secreting tumors (VIPomas); pancreatic tumors, gastrinoma, secretory diarrhea, acromegaly

Usual Dosage

Infants and Children:

Diarrhea: I.V., SubQ: Doses of 1-10 mcg/kg every 12 hours have been used in children beginning at the low end of the range and increasing by 0.3 mcg/kg/dose at 3-day intervals. Suppression of growth hormone (animal data) is of concern when used as long-term therapy.

Adults: SubQ: Initial: 50 mcg 1-2 times/day and titrate dose based on patient tolerance and response

Carcinoid: 100-600 mcg/day in 2-4 divided doses

VIPomas: 200-300 mcg/day in 2-4 divided doses

Diarrhea: Initial: I.V.: 50-100 mcg every 8 hours; increase by 100 mcg/dose at 48-hour intervals; maximum dose: 500 mcg every 8 hours

Esophageal varices bleeding: I.V. bolus: 25-50 mcg followed by continuous I.V. infusion of 25-50 mcg/hour

Acromegaly: Initial: SubQ: 50 mcg 3 times/day; titrate to achieve growth hormone levels <5 ng/mL or IGF-I (somatomedin C) levels <1.9 U/mL in males and <2.2 U/mL in females; usual effective dose 100 mcg 3 times/day; range 300-1500 mcg/day

Note: Should be withdrawn yearly for a 4-week interval in patients who have received irradiation. Resume if levels increase and signs/symptoms recur.

Acromegaly, carcinoid tumors, and VIPomas (depot injection): Patients must be stabilized on subcutaneous octreotide for at least 2 weeks before switching to the long-acting depot: Upon switch: 20 mg I.M. intragluteally every 4 weeks for 2-3 months, then the dose may be modified based upon response

Dosage adjustment for acromegaly: After 3 months of depot injections the dosage may be continued or modified as follows:

GH ≤2.5 ng/mL, IGF-1 is normal, symptoms controlled: Maintain octreotide LAR® at 20 mg I.M. every 4 weeks

GH >2.5 ng/mL, IGF-1 is elevated, and/or symptoms uncontrolled: Increase octreotide LAR® to 30 mg I.M. every 4 weeks

GH ≤1 ng/mL, IGF-1 is normal, symptoms controlled: Reduce octreotide LAR® to 10 mg I.M. every 4 weeks

Dosages >40 mg are not recommended

(Continued)

octreotide *(Continued)*

Dosage adjustment for carcinoid tumors and VIPomas: After 2 months of depot injections the dosage may be continued or modified as follows:

Increase to 30 mg I.M. every 4 weeks if symptoms are inadequately controlled

Decrease to 10 mg I.M. every 4 weeks, for a trial period, if initially responsive to 20 mg dose

Dosage >30 mg is not recommended

Dosage Forms

Injection, microspheres for suspension, as acetate [depot formulation] (Sandostatin LAR®): 10 mg, 20 mg, 30 mg [with diluent and syringe]

Injection, solution, as acetate (Sandostatin®): 0.05 mg/mL (1 mL); 0.1 mg/mL (1 mL); 0.2 mg/mL (5 mL); 0.5 mg/mL (1 mL); 1 mg/mL (5 mL)

octreotide acetate *see* octreotide *on previous page*

OcuClear® ***(Discontinued)*** *see page 1042*

OcuCoat® PF [US-OTC] *see* artificial tears *on page 78*

OcuCoat® [US-OTC] *see* artificial tears *on page 78*

Ocufen® [US/Can] *see* flurbiprofen *on page 381*

Ocuflox® [US/Can] *see* ofloxacin *on this page*

Ocupress® ***(Discontinued)*** *see page 1042*

Ocupress® Ophthalmic [Can] *see* carteolol *on page 163*

Ocusert Pilo-20® ***(Discontinued)*** *see page 1042*

Ocusert Pilo-40® ***(Discontinued)*** *see page 1042*

Ocu-Sul® ***(Discontinued)*** *see page 1042*

Ocusulf-10 [US] *see* sulfacetamide *on page 829*

Ocutricin® Topical Ointment ***(Discontinued)*** *see page 1042*

Oesclim® [Can] *see* estradiol *on page 324*

ofloxacin (oh FLOKS a sin)

Sound-Alike/Look-Alike Issues

Floxin® may be confused with Flexeril®

Ocuflox® may be confused with Ocufen®

Synonyms floxin otic singles

U.S./Canadian Brand Names Apo-Oflox® [Can]; Floxin® [US/Can]; Ocuflox® [US/Can]

Therapeutic Category Antibiotic, Ophthalmic; Antibiotic, Otic; Quinolone

Use Quinolone antibiotic for the treatment of acute exacerbations of chronic bronchitis, community-acquired pneumonia, skin and skin structure infections (uncomplicated), urethral and cervical gonorrhea (acute, uncomplicated), urethritis and cervicitis (nongonococcal), mixed infections of the urethra and cervix, pelvic inflammatory disease (acute), cystitis (uncomplicated), urinary tract infections (complicated), prostatitis

Ophthalmic: Treatment of superficial ocular infections involving the conjunctiva or cornea due to strains of susceptible organisms

Otic: Otitis externa, chronic suppurative otitis media, acute otitis media

Usual Dosage

Oral: Adults:

Chronic bronchitis (acute exacerbation), community-acquired pneumonia, skin and skin structure infections (uncomplicated): 400 mg every 12 hours for 10 days

Urethral and cervical gonorrhea (acute, uncomplicated): 400 mg as a single dose

Cervicitis/urethritis (nongonococcal) due to *C. trachomatis*, mixed infection of urethra and cervix due to *C. trachomatis* and *N. gonorrhoeae*: 300 mg every 12 hours for 7 days

Pelvic inflammatory disease (acute): 400 mg every 12 hours for 10-14 days

Cystitis (uncomplicated):
Due to *E. coli* or *K. pneumoniae*: 200 mg every 12 hours for 3 days
Due to other organisms: 200 mg every 12 hours for 7 days
UTI (complicated): 200 mg every 12 hours for 10 days
Prostatitis: 200 mg every 12 hours for 6 weeks
Ophthalmic: Children >1 year and Adults:
Conjunctivitis: Instill 1-2 drops in affected eye(s) every 2-4 hours for the first 2 days, then use 4 times/day for an additional 5 days
Corneal ulcer: Instill 1-2 drops every 30 minutes while awake and every 4-6 hours after retiring for the first 2 days; beginning on day 3, instill 1-2 drops every hour while awake for 4-6 additional days; thereafter, 1-2 drops 4 times/day until clinical cure.
Otic:
Acute otitis media with tympanostomy tubes: Children 1-12 years: Instill 5 drops (or the contents of 1 single-dose container) into affected ear(s) twice daily for 10 days
Chronic suppurative otitis media with perforated tympanic membranes: Children >12 years and Adults: Instill 10 drops (or the contents of 2 single-dose containers) into affected ear twice daily for 14 days
Otitis externa:
Children 6 months to 13 years: Instill 5 drops (or the contents of 1 single-dose container) into affected ear(s) once daily for 7 days
Children ≥13 years and Adults: Instill 10 drops (or the contents of 2 single-dose containers) into affected ear(s) once daily for 7 days

Dosage Forms
Solution, ophthalmic (Ocuflox®): 0.3% (5 mL, 10 mL) [contains benzalkonium chloride]
Solution, otic:
Floxin®: 0.3% (5 mL, 10 mL) [contains benzalkonium chloride]
Floxin® Otic Singles™: 0.3% (0.25 mL) [contains benzalkonium chloride; packaged as 2 single-dose containers per pouch, 10 pouches per carton, total net volume 5 mL]
Tablet (Floxin®): 200 mg, 300 mg, 400 mg

Ogen® [US/Can] *see* estropipate *on page 332*

Ogestrel® *see* ethinyl estradiol and norgestrel *on page 347*

OGMT *see* metyrosine *on page 577*

OGT-918 *see* miglustat *on page 582*

OKT3 *see* muromonab-CD3 *on page 595*

olanzapine (oh LAN za peen)

Sound-Alike/Look-Alike Issues
olanzapine may be confused with olsalazine
Zyprexa® may be confused with Celexa®, Zyrtec®

Synonyms LY170053

U.S./Canadian Brand Names Zyprexa® [US/Can]; Zyprexa® Zydis® [US/Can]

Therapeutic Category Antipsychotic Agent

Use Treatment of the manifestations of schizophrenia; treatment of acute mania episodes associated with bipolar disorder (as monotherapy or in combination with lithium or valproate); maintenance treatment of bipolar disorder; acute agitation (patients with schizophrenia or bipolar mania)

Usual Dosage
Children: Schizophrenia/bipolar disorder: Oral: Initial: 2.5 mg/day; titrate as necessary to 20 mg/day (0.12-0.29 mg/kg/day)
Adults:
Schizophrenia: Oral: Usual starting dose: 5-10 mg once daily; increase to 10 mg once daily within 5-7 days, thereafter adjust by 5-10 mg/day at 1-week intervals, up to a maximum of 20 mg/day; doses of 30-50 mg/day have been used; typical dosage range: 10-30 mg/day
(Continued)

olanzapine *(Continued)*

Bipolar mania: Oral:

Monotherapy: Usual starting dose: 10-15 mg once daily; increase by 5 mg/day at intervals of not less than 24 hours; maintenance: 5-20 mg/day; maximum dose: 20 mg/day

Combination therapy (olanzapine in combination with lithium or valproate): Initial: 10 mg once daily; dosing range: 5-20 mg/day

Agitation (acute, associated with bipolar disorder or schizophrenia): I.M.: Initial dose: 5-10 mg (a lower dose of 2.5 mg may be considered when clinical factors warrant); additional doses (2.5-10 mg) may be considered; however, 2-4 hours should be allowed between doses to evaluate response (maximum total daily dose: 30 mg, per manufacturer's recommendation)

Dosage Forms

Injection, powder for reconstitution (Zyprexa® IntraMuscular): 10 mg [contains lactose 50 mg]

Tablet (Zyprexa®): 2.5 mg, 5 mg, 7.5 mg, 10 mg, 15 mg, 20 mg

Tablet, orally-disintegrating (Zyprexa® Zydis®): 5 mg [contains phenylalanine 0.34 mg/tablet], 10 mg [contains phenylalanine 0.45 mg/tablet], 15 mg [contains phenylalanine 0.67 mg/tablet], 20 mg [contains phenylalanine 0.9 mg/tablet]

olanzapine and fluoxetine (oh LAN za peen & floo OKS e teen)

Synonyms fluoxetine and olanzapine; olanzapine and fluoxetine hydrochloride

U.S./Canadian Brand Names Symbyax™ [US]

Therapeutic Category Antidepressant, Selective Serotonin Reuptake Inhibitor; Antipsychotic Agent, Thienobenzodiaepine

Use Treatment of depressive episodes associated with bipolar disorder

Usual Dosage Oral: Adults: Depression associated with bipolar disorder: Initial: Olanzapine 6 mg/fluoxetine 25 mg once daily in the evening. Dosing range: Olanzapine 6-12 mg/fluoxetine 25-50 mg. Use caution adjusting dose in patients predisposed to hypotension, in females, and in nonsmokers (metabolism may be decreased). Safety of daily doses of olanzapine >18 mg/fluoxetine >75 mg have not been evaluated.

Dosage Forms Capsule (Symbyax™):

6/25: Olanzapine 6 mg and fluoxetine 25 mg

6/50: Olanzapine 6 mg and fluoxetine 50 mg

12/25: Olanzapine 12 mg and fluoxetine 25 mg

12/50: Olanzapine 12 mg and fluoxetine 50 mg

olanzapine and fluoxetine hydrochloride *see* olanzapine and fluoxetine *on this page*

oleovitamin A *see* vitamin A *on page 914*

oleum ricini *see* castor oil *on page 165*

olmesartan (ole me SAR tan)

Synonyms olmesartan medoxomil

U.S./Canadian Brand Names Benicar™ [US]

Therapeutic Category Angiotensin II Receptor Antagonist

Use Treatment of hypertension with or without concurrent use of other antihypertensive agents

Usual Dosage Oral: Adults: Initial: Usual starting dose is 20 mg once daily; if initial response is inadequate, may be increased to 40 mg once daily after 2 weeks. May administer with other antihypertensive agents if blood pressure inadequately controlled with olmesartan. Consider lower starting dose in patients with possible depletion of intravascular volume (eg, patients receiving diuretics).

Dosage Forms Tablet [film coated], as medoxomil: 5 mg, 20 mg, 40 mg

olmesartan and hydrochlorothiazide

(ole me SAR tan & hye droe klor oh THYE a zide)

Synonyms hydrochlorothiazide and olmesartan medoxomil; olmesartan medoxomil and hydrochlorothiazide

U.S./Canadian Brand Names Benicar HCT™ [US]

Therapeutic Category Angiotensin II Receptor Antagonist; Diuretic, Thiazide

Use Treatment of hypertension (not recommended for initial treatment)

Usual Dosage Oral: Adults: One tablet daily; dosage must be individualized (see below). May be titrated at 2- to 4-week intervals.

Replacement therapy: May be substituted for previously titrated dosages of the individual components.

Patients not controlled with single-agent therapy: Initiate by adding the lowest available dose of the alternative component (hydrochlorothiazide 12.5 mg or olmesartan 20 mg). Titrate to effect (maximum daily hydrochlorothiazide dose: 25 mg; maximum daily olmesartan dose: 40 mg).

Dosage Forms Tablet:

20/125: Olmesartan medoxomil 20 mg and hydrochlorothiazide 12.5 mg
40/12.5: Olmesartan medoxomil 40 mg and hydrochlorothiazide 12.5 mg
40/25: Olmesartan medoxomil 40 mg and hydrochlorothiazide 25 mg

olmesartan medoxomil *see* olmesartan *on previous page*

olmesartan medoxomil and hydrochlorothiazide *see* olmesartan and hydrochlorothiazide *on this page*

olopatadine (oh LOP ah tah deen)

Sound-Alike/Look-Alike Issues

Patanol® may be confused with Platinol®

U.S./Canadian Brand Names Patanol® [US/Can]

Therapeutic Category Antihistamine

Use Treatment of the signs and symptoms of allergic conjunctivitis

Usual Dosage Adults: Ophthalmic: 1 to 2 drops in affected eye(s) twice daily every 6 to 8 hours; results from an environmental study demonstrated that olopatadine was effective when dosed twice daily for up to 6 weeks

Dosage Forms Solution, ophthalmic: 0.1% (5 mL) [contains benzalkonium chloride]

olsalazine (ole SAL a zeen)

Sound-Alike/Look-Alike Issues

olsalazine may be confused with olanzapine
Dipentum® may be confused with Dilantin®

Synonyms olsalazine sodium

U.S./Canadian Brand Names Dipentum® [US/Can]

Therapeutic Category 5-Aminosalicylic Acid Derivative

Use Maintenance of remission of ulcerative colitis in patients intolerant to sulfasalazine

Usual Dosage Adults: Oral: 1 g/day in 2 divided doses

Dosage Forms Capsule, as sodium: 250 mg

olsalazine sodium *see* olsalazine *on this page*

Olux® [US] *see* clobetasol *on page 212*

omalizumab (oh mah lye ZOO mab)

Synonyms rhuMAb-E25

U.S./Canadian Brand Names Xolair® [US]

Therapeutic Category Monoclonal Antibody

Use Treatment of moderate-to-severe, persistent allergic asthma not adequately controlled with inhaled corticosteroids

Usual Dosage SubQ: Children ≥12 years and Adults: Asthma: Dose is based on pretreatment IgE serum levels and body weight. Dosing should not be adjusted based

(Continued)

omalizumab *(Continued)*

on IgE levels taken during treatment or <1 year following therapy; doses should be adjusted during treatment for significant changes in body weight

IgE ≥30-100 int. units/mL:
- 30-90 kg: 150 mg every 4 weeks
- >90-150 kg: 300 mg every 4 weeks

IgE >100-200 int. units/mL:
- 30-90 kg: 300 mg every 4 weeks
- >90-150 kg: 225 mg every 2 weeks

IgE >200-300 int. units/mL:
- 30-60 kg: 300 mg every 4 weeks
- >60-90 kg: 225 mg every 2 weeks
- >90-150 kg: 300 mg every 2 weeks

IgE >300-400 int. units/mL:
- 30-70 kg: 225 mg every 2 weeks
- >70-90 kg: 300 mg every 2 weeks
- >90 kg: Do not administer dose

IgE >400-500 int. units/mL:
- 30-70 kg: 300 mg every 2 weeks
- >70-90 kg: 375 mg every 2 weeks
- >90 kg: Do not administer dose

IgE >500-600 int. units/mL:
- 30-60 kg: 300 mg every 2 weeks
- >60-70 kg: 375 mg every 2 weeks
- >70 kg: Do not administer dose

IgE >600-700 int. units/mL:
- 30-60 kg: 375 mg every 2 weeks
- >60 kg: Do not administer dose

Dosage Forms Injection, powder for reconstitution [preservative free]: 150 mg

omeprazole (oh ME pray zol)

Sound-Alike/Look-Alike Issues

Prilosec® may be confused with Plendil®, Prevacid®, prednisone, prilocaine, Prinivil®, Proventil®, Prozac®

U.S./Canadian Brand Names Losec® [Can]; Prilosec® [US]; Prilosec OTC™ [US-OTC]; Zegerid™ [US]

Therapeutic Category Gastric Acid Secretion Inhibitor

Use Short-term (4-8 weeks) treatment of active duodenal ulcer disease or active benign gastric ulcer; treatment of heartburn and other symptoms associated with gastroesophageal reflux disease (GERD); short-term (4-8 weeks) treatment of endoscopically-diagnosed erosive esophagitis; maintenance healing of erosive esophagitis; long-term treatment of pathological hypersecretory conditions; as part of a multidrug regimen for *H. pylori* eradication to reduce the risk of duodenal ulcer recurrence

OTC labeling: Short-term treatment of frequent, uncomplicated heartburn occurring ≥2 days/week

Usual Dosage Oral:

Children ≥2 years: GERD or other acid-related disorders:
- <20 kg: 10 mg once daily
- ≥20 kg: 20 mg once daily

Adults:
- Active duodenal ulcer: 20 mg/day for 4-8 weeks
- Gastric ulcers: 40 mg/day for 4-8 weeks
- Symptomatic GERD: 20 mg/day for up to 4 weeks
- Erosive esophagitis: 20 mg/day for 4-8 weeks
- *Helicobacter pylori* eradication: Dose varies with regimen: 20 mg once daily **or** 40 mg/day as single dose or in 2 divided doses; requires combination therapy with antibiotics
- Pathological hypersecretory conditions: Initial: 60 mg once daily; doses up to 120 mg 3 times/day have been administered; administer daily doses >80 mg in divided doses

Frequent heartburn (OTC labeling): 20 mg/day for 14 days; treatment may be repeated after 4 months if needed

Dosage Forms

Capsule, delayed release: 10 mg, 20 mg

Prilosec®: 10 mg, 20 mg, 40 mg

Prilosec OTC™: 20 mg

Powder for oral suspension (Zegerid™): 20 mEq/packet (30s) [contains sodium bicarbonate 1680 mg, equivalent to sodium 460 mg]

Omnicef® [US/Can] *see* cefdinir *on page 167*

OmniHIB™ *(Discontinued)* *see page 1042*

Omnipaque® [US] *see* radiological/contrast media (nonionic) *on page 761*

Omnipen® *(Discontinued)* *see page 1042*

Omnipen®-N *(Discontinued)* *see page 1042*

Oncaspar® [US] *see* pegaspargase *on page 670*

Oncet® *(Discontinued)* *see page 1042*

Oncotice™ [Can] *see* BCG vaccine *on page 101*

Oncovin® *(Discontinued)* *see page 1042*

Oncovin® [Can] *see* vincristine *on page 912*

ondansetron (on DAN se tron)

Sound-Alike/Look-Alike Issues

Zofran® may be confused with Zantac®, Zosyn®

Synonyms GR38032R; ondansetron hydrochloride

U.S./Canadian Brand Names Zofran® ODT [US/Can]; Zofran® [US/Can]

Therapeutic Category Selective 5-HT_3 Receptor Antagonist

Use Prevention of nausea and vomiting associated with moderately- to highly-emetogenic cancer chemotherapy; radiotherapy in patients receiving total body irradiation or fractions to the abdomen; prevention and treatment of postoperative nausea and vomiting

Generally **not** recommended for treatment of existing chemotherapy-induced emesis (CIE) or for prophylaxis of nausea from agents with a low emetogenic potential.

Usual Dosage

Children:

I.V.:

Chemotherapy-induced emesis: 4-18 years: 0.15 mg/kg/dose administered 30 minutes prior to chemotherapy, 4 and 8 hours after the first dose **or** 0.45 mg/kg/day as a single dose

Postoperative nausea and vomiting: 2-12 years: ≤40 kg: 0.1 mg/kg >40 kg: 4 mg

Oral: Chemotherapy-induced emesis:

4-11 years: 4 mg 30 minutes before chemotherapy; repeat 4 and 8 hours after initial dose, then 4 mg every 8 hours for 1-2 days after chemotherapy completed

≥12 years: Refer to adult dosing.

Adults:

I.V.: Chemotherapy-induced emesis:

0.15 mg/kg 3 times/day beginning 30 minutes prior to chemotherapy **or**

0.45 mg/kg once daily **or**

8-10 mg 1-2 times/day **or**

24 mg or 32 mg once daily

I.M., I.V.: Postoperative nausea and vomiting: 4 mg as a single dose approximately 30 minutes before the end of anesthesia, or as treatment if vomiting occurs after surgery

Oral:

Chemotherapy-induced emesis: Highly-emetogenic agents/single-day therapy: 24 mg given 30 minutes prior to the start of therapy Moderately-emetogenic agents: 8 mg

(Continued)

ondansetron *(Continued)*

every 12 hours beginning 30 minutes before chemotherapy, continuously for 1-2 days after chemotherapy completed

Total body irradiation: 8 mg 1-2 hours before daily each fraction of radiotherapy

Single high-dose fraction radiotherapy to abdomen: 8 mg 1-2 hours before irradiation, then 8 mg every 8 hours after first dose for 1-2 days after completion of radiotherapy

Daily fractionated radiotherapy to abdomen: 8 mg 1-2 hours before irradiation, then 8 mg 8 hours after first dose for each day of radiotherapy

Postoperative nausea and vomiting: 16 mg given 1 hour prior to induction of anesthesia

Dosage Forms

Infusion, as hydrochloride [premixed in D_5W] (Zofran®): 32 mg (50 mL)

Injection, solution, as hydrochloride (Zofran®): 2 mg/mL (2 mL, 20 mL)

Solution, as hydrochloride (Zofran®): 4 mg/5 mL (50 mL) [contains sodium benzoate; strawberry flavor]

Tablet, as hydrochloride (Zofran®): 4 mg, 8 mg, 24 mg

Tablet, orally-disintegrating (Zofran® ODT): 4 mg, 8 mg [each strength contains phenylalanine <0.03 mg/tablet; strawberry flavor]

ondansetron hydrochloride *see* ondansetron *on previous page*

One-A-Day® 50 Plus Formula [US-OTC] *see* vitamins (multiple/oral) *on page 927*

One-A-Day® Active Formula [US-OTC] *see* vitamins (multiple/oral) *on page 927*

One-A -Day® Essential Formula [US-OTC] *see* vitamins (multiple/oral) *on page 927*

One-A-Day® Kids Bugs Bunny and Friends Complete [US-OTC] *see* vitamins (multiple/pediatric) *on page 927*

One-A-Day® Kids Bugs Bunny and Friends Plus Extra C [US-OTC] *see* vitamins (multiple/pediatric) *on page 927*

One-A-Day® Kids Extreme Sports [US-OTC] *see* vitamins (multiple/pediatric) *on page 927*

One-A-Day® Kids Scooby-Doo! Complete [US-OTC] *see* vitamins (multiple/pediatric) *on page 927*

One-A-Day® Kids Scooby Doo! Plus Calcium [US-OTC] *see* vitamins (multiple/pediatric) *on page 927*

One-A-Day® Maximum Formula [US-OTC] *see* vitamins (multiple/oral) *on page 927*

One-A-Day® Men's Formula [US-OTC] *see* vitamins (multiple/oral) *on page 927*

One-A-Day® Today [US-OTC] *see* vitamins (multiple/oral) *on page 927*

One-A-Day® Women's Formula [US-OTC] *see* vitamins (multiple/oral) *on page 927*

ONTAK® [US] *see* denileukin diftitox *on page 249*

Onxol™ [US] *see* paclitaxel *on page 660*

Ony-Clear *(Discontinued)* *see page 1042*

OPC-13013 *see* cilostazol *on page 199*

OPC-14597 *see* aripiprazole *on page 77*

OP-CCK *see* sincalide *on page 806*

Opcon-A® [US-OTC] *see* naphazoline and pheniramine *on page 604*

Opcon® Ophthalmic *(Discontinued)* *see page 1042*

o,p′-DDD *see* mitotane *on page 585*

Operand® Chlorhexidine Gluconate [US-OTC] *see* chlorhexidine gluconate *on page 183*

Operand® [US-OTC] *see* povidone-iodine *on page 718*

Ophthaine® ***(Discontinued)*** *see page 1042*

Ophthalgan® Ophthalmic ***(Discontinued)*** *see page 1042*

Ophthetic® [US] *see* proparacaine *on page 738*

Ophthifluor® ***(Discontinued)*** *see page 1042*

Ophthochlor® Ophthalmic ***(Discontinued)*** *see page 1042*

Ophthocort® ***(Discontinued)*** *see page 1042*

Ophtho-Dipivefrin™ [Can] *see* dipivefrin *on page 281*

opium and belladonna *see* belladonna and opium *on page 103*

opium tincture (OH pee um TINGK chur)

Sound-Alike/Look-Alike Issues

opium tincture may be confused with paregoric

Synonyms DTO; opium tincture, deodorized

Therapeutic Category Analgesic, Narcotic

Controlled Substance C-II

Use Treatment of diarrhea or relief of pain

Usual Dosage Oral:

Children:

Diarrhea: 0.005-0.01 mL/kg/dose every 3-4 hours for a maximum of 6 doses/24 hours

Analgesia: 0.01-0.02 mL/kg/dose every 3-4 hours

Adults:

Diarrhea: 0.3-1 mL/dose every 2-6 hours to maximum of 6 mL/24 hours

Analgesia: 0.6-1.5 mL/dose every 3-4 hours

Dosage Forms Liquid: 10% (120 mL, 480 mL) [0.6 mL equivalent to morphine 6 mg; contains alcohol 19%]

opium tincture, deodorized *see* opium tincture *on this page*

oprelvekin (oh PREL ve kin)

Sound-Alike/Look-Alike Issues

oprelvekin may be confused with aldesleukin, Proleukin®

Neumega® may be confused with Neupogen®

Synonyms IL-11; interleukin-11; recombinant human interleukin-11; recombinant interleukin-11; rhIL-11; rIL-11

U.S./Canadian Brand Names Neumega® [US]

Therapeutic Category Platelet Growth Factor

Use Prevention of severe thrombocytopenia and the reduction of the need for platelet transfusions following myelosuppressive chemotherapy

Usual Dosage SubQ: **Note:** First dose should not be administered until 24-36 hours after the end of chemotherapy. Discontinue the drug at least 48 hours before beginning the next cycle of chemotherapy.

Children: 75-100 mcg/kg once daily for 10-21 days (until postnadir platelet count ≥50,000 cells/µL)

Note: The manufacturer states that, until efficacy/toxicity parameters are established, the use of oprelvekin in pediatric patients (particularly those <12 years of age) should be restricted to use in controlled clinical trials.

Adults: 50 mcg/kg once daily for 10-21 days (until postnadir platelet count ≥50,000 cells/µL)

Dosage Forms Injection, powder for reconstitution: 5 mg

Optho-Bunolol® [Can] *see* levobunolol *on page 511*

Opticaine® [US] *see* tetracaine *on page 851*

Opticrom® [US/Can] *see* cromolyn sodium *on page 230*
Opticyl® [US] *see* tropicamide *on page 892*
Optigene® 3 [US-OTC] *see* tetrahydrozoline *on page 852*
Optimine® ***(Discontinued)*** *see page 1042*
Optimoist® Solution ***(Discontinued)*** *see page 1042*
Optimyxin® [Can] *see* bacitracin and polymyxin B *on page 97*
Optimyxin Plus® [Can] *see* neomycin, polymyxin B, and gramicidin *on page 611*
OptiPranolol® [US/Can] *see* metipranolol *on page 573*
Optiray® [US] *see* radiological/contrast media (nonionic) *on page 761*
Optivar® [US] *see* azelastine *on page 93*
Orabase®-B [US-OTC] *see* benzocaine *on page 107*
Orabase®-O ***(Discontinued)*** *see page 1042*
Oracort [Can] *see* triamcinolone (topical) *on page 882*
Oradex-C® ***(Discontinued)*** *see page 1042*
Oragrafin® Calcium [US] *see* radiological/contrast media (ionic) *on page 759*
Oragrafin® Sodium [US] *see* radiological/contrast media (ionic) *on page 759*
Orajel® Baby Nighttime [US-OTC] *see* benzocaine *on page 107*
Orajel® Baby [US-OTC] *see* benzocaine *on page 107*
Orajel® Brace-Aid Oral Anesthetic ***(Discontinued)*** *see page 1042*
Orajel® Maximum Strength [US-OTC] *see* benzocaine *on page 107*
Orajel® Perioseptic® Spot Treatment [US-OTC] *see* carbamide peroxide *on page 155*
Orajel® [US-OTC] *see* benzocaine *on page 107*
Oramorph SR® [US] *see* morphine sulfate *on page 591*
Oranyl [US-OTC] *see* pseudoephedrine *on page 745*
Orap™ [US/Can] *see* pimozide *on page 695*
Orapred™ [US] *see* prednisolone (systemic) *on page 724*
OraRinse™ [US-OTC] *see* maltodextrin *on page 541*
Orasol® [US-OTC] *see* benzocaine *on page 107*
Orasone® ***(Discontinued)*** *see page 1042*
Oratect® ***(Discontinued)*** *see page 1042*
Orazinc® [US-OTC] *see* zinc sulfate *on page 941*
orciprenaline sulfate *see* metaproterenol *on page 559*
Ordrine AT® Extended Release Capsule ***(Discontinued)*** *see page 1042*
Oretic® [US] *see* hydrochlorothiazide *on page 441*
Oreticyl® ***(Discontinued)*** *see page 1042*
Oreton® Methyl ***(Discontinued)*** *see page 1042*
Orfadin® [US] *see* nitisinone *on page 621*
ORG 946 *see* rocuronium *on page 783*
Orgalutran® [Can] *see* ganirelix *on page 397*
Organ-1 NR [US] *see* guaifenesin *on page 415*
Organidin® ***(Discontinued)*** *see page 1042*
Organidin® NR [US] *see* guaifenesin *on page 415*
Orgaran® [Can] *see* danaparoid *on page 243*

Orgaran® *(Discontinued)* *see page 1042*

ORG NC 45 *see* vecuronium *on page 907*

Orimune® *(Discontinued)* *see page 1042*

Orinase Diagnostic® *(Discontinued)* *see page 1042*

Orinase® Oral *(Discontinued)* *see page 1042*

ORLAAM® *(Discontinued)* *see page 1042*

orlistat (OR li stat)

U.S./Canadian Brand Names Xenical® [US/Can]

Therapeutic Category Lipase Inhibitor

Use Management of obesity, including weight loss and weight management when used in conjunction with a reduced-calorie diet; reduce the risk of weight regain after prior weight loss; indicated for obese patients with an initial body mass index (BMI) ≥30 kg/m^2 or ≥27 kg/m^2 in the presence of other risk factors

Usual Dosage Oral: Children ≥12 years and Adults: 120 mg 3 times/day with each main meal containing fat (during or up to 1 hour after the meal); omit dose if meal is occasionally missed or contains no fat.

Dosage Forms Capsule: 120 mg

Ormazine® *(Discontinued)* *see page 1042*

Ornade® Spansule® Capsules *(Discontinued)* *see page 1042*

Ornex® Maximum Strength [US-OTC] *see* acetaminophen and pseudoephedrine *on page 9*

Ornex® [US-OTC] *see* acetaminophen and pseudoephedrine *on page 9*

Ornidyl® Injection *(Discontinued)* *see page 1042*

ORO-Clense [Can] *see* chlorhexidine gluconate *on page 183*

Orphenace® [Can] *see* orphenadrine *on this page*

orphenadrine (or FEN a dreen)

Sound-Alike/Look-Alike Issues

Norflex™ may be confused with norfloxacin, Noroxin®

Synonyms orphenadrine citrate

U.S./Canadian Brand Names Norflex™ [US/Can]; Orphenace® [Can]; Rhoxal-orphendrine [Can]

Therapeutic Category Skeletal Muscle Relaxant

Use Treatment of muscle spasm associated with acute painful musculoskeletal conditions; supportive therapy in tetanus

Usual Dosage Adults:

Oral: 100 mg twice daily

I.M., I.V.: 60 mg every 12 hours

Dosage Forms

Injection, solution, as citrate: 30 mg/mL (2 mL) [contains sodium bisulfite]

Tablet, extended release, as citrate: 100 mg

orphenadrine, aspirin, and caffeine

(or FEN a dreen, AS pir in, & KAF een)

Sound-Alike/Look-Alike Issues

Norgesic™ Forte may be confused with Norgesic® 40

Synonyms aspirin, orphenadrine, and caffeine; caffeine, orphenadrine, and aspirin

U.S./Canadian Brand Names Norgesic™ Forte [US/Can]; Norgesic™ [US/Can]; Orphengesic Forte [US]; Orphengesic [US]

Therapeutic Category Analgesic, Nonnarcotic; Skeletal Muscle Relaxant

Use Relief of discomfort associated with skeletal muscular conditions

Usual Dosage Oral: 1-2 tablets 3-4 times/day

(Continued)

orphenadrine, aspirin, and caffeine *(Continued)*

Dosage Forms

Tablet: Orphenadrine citrate 25 mg, aspirin 385 mg, and caffeine 30 mg; orphenadrine citrate 50 mg, aspirin 770 mg, and caffeine 60 mg

Norgesic™, Orphengesic: Orphenadrine citrate 25 mg, aspirin 385 mg, and caffeine 30 mg

Norgesic™ Forte, Orphengesic Forte: Orphenadrine citrate 50 mg, aspirin 770 mg, and caffeine 60 mg

orphenadrine citrate *see* orphenadrine *on previous page*

Orphengesic [US] *see* orphenadrine, aspirin, and caffeine *on previous page*

Orphengesic Forte [US] *see* orphenadrine, aspirin, and caffeine *on previous page*

Ortho® 0.5/35 [Can] *see* ethinyl estradiol and norethindrone *on page 342*

Ortho® 1/35 [Can] *see* ethinyl estradiol and norethindrone *on page 342*

Ortho® 7/7/7 [Can] *see* ethinyl estradiol and norethindrone *on page 342*

Ortho-Cept® [US/Can] *see* ethinyl estradiol and desogestrel *on page 335*

Orthoclone OKT® 3 [US/Can] *see* muromonab-CD3 *on page 595*

Ortho-Cyclen® [US] *see* ethinyl estradiol and norgestimate *on page 346*

ortho est *see* estropipate *on page 332*

Ortho-Est® [US] *see* estropipate *on page 332*

Ortho Evra™ [US] *see* ethinyl estradiol and norelgestromin *on page 342*

Ortho-Novum® [US] *see* ethinyl estradiol and norethindrone *on page 342*

Ortho-Novum® 1/50 [US/Can] *see* mestranol and norethindrone *on page 558*

ortho prefest *see* estradiol and norgestimate *on page 328*

Ortho Tri-Cyclen® [US] *see* ethinyl estradiol and norgestimate *on page 346*

Ortho-Tri-Cyclen® Lo [US] *see* ethinyl estradiol and norgestimate *on page 346*

Or-Tyl® Injection *(Discontinued)* *see page 1042*

Orudis® *(Discontinued)* *see page 1042*

Orudis® KT [US-OTC] *see* ketoprofen *on page 495*

Orudis® SR [Can] *see* ketoprofen *on page 495*

Oruvail® [US/Can] *see* ketoprofen *on page 495*

Os-Cal® [Can] *see* calcium carbonate *on page 144*

Os-Cal® 500 [US-OTC] *see* calcium carbonate *on page 144*

oseltamivir (o sel TAM e veer)

Sound-Alike/Look-Alike Issues

Tamiflu® may be confused with Thera-Flu®

U.S./Canadian Brand Names Tamiflu™ [US/Can]

Therapeutic Category Antiviral Agent, Oral

Controlled Substance [FS100]influenza

Use Treatment of uncomplicated acute illness due to influenza (A or B) infection in adults and children >1 year of age who have been symptomatic for no more than 2 days; prophylaxis against influenza (A or B) infection in adults and adolescents ≥13 years of age

Usual Dosage Oral:

Treatment: Initiate treatment within 2 days of onset of symptoms; duration of treatment: 5 days:

Children: 1-12 years:

≤15 kg: 30 mg twice daily

>15 kg - ≤23 kg: 45 mg twice daily

>23 kg - ≤40 kg: 60 mg twice daily

>40 kg: 75 mg twice daily
Adolescents ≥13 years and Adults: 75 mg twice daily
Prophylaxis: Adolescents ≥13 years and Adults: 75 mg once daily for at least 7 days; treatment should begin within 2 days of contact with an infected individual. During community outbreaks, dosing is 75 mg once daily. May be used for up to 6 weeks; duration of protection lasts for length of dosing period

Dosage Forms
Capsule, as phosphate: 75 mg
Powder for oral suspension: 12 mg/mL (25 mL) [contains sodium benzoate; tutti-frutti flavor]

Osmitrol® [US/Can] *see* mannitol *on page 542*

Osmoglyn® [US] *see* glycerin *on page 410*

Ostac® [Can] *see* clodronate disodium *(Canada only) on page 213*

Osteocalcin® ***(Discontinued)*** *see page 1042*

Osteocit® [Can] *see* calcium citrate *on page 147*

Ostoforte® [Can] *see* ergocalciferol *on page 317*

Otic-Care® Otic ***(Discontinued)*** *see page 1042*

Otic Domeboro® ***(Discontinued)*** *see page 1042*

Otic Tridesilon® ***(Discontinued)*** *see page 1042*

Otobiotic® ***(Discontinued)*** *see page 1042*

Otocort® Otic ***(Discontinued)*** *see page 1042*

Otosporin® Otic ***(Discontinued)*** *see page 1042*

Otrivin® ***(Discontinued)*** *see page 1042*

Otrivin® Pediatric ***(Discontinued)*** *see page 1042*

Ovace™ [US] *see* sulfacetamide *on page 829*

Ovcon® [US] *see* ethinyl estradiol and norethindrone *on page 342*

Ovide® [US] *see* malathion *on page 541*

Ovidrel® [US] *see* chorionic gonadotropin (recombinant) *on page 197*

Ovol® [Can] *see* simethicone *on page 804*

Ovral® ***(Discontinued)*** *see page 1042*

Ovral® [Can] *see* ethinyl estradiol and norgestrel *on page 347*

Ovrette® [US/Can] *see* norgestrel *on page 628*

O-V Staticin® ***(Discontinued)*** *see page 1042*

oxacillin (oks a SIL in)

Synonyms methylphenyl isoxazolyl penicillin; oxacillin sodium
Therapeutic Category Penicillin
Use Treatment of infections such as osteomyelitis, septicemia, endocarditis, and CNS infections caused by susceptible strains of *Staphylococcus*
Usual Dosage I.M., I.V.:
Neonates:
Postnatal age <7 days:
<2000 g: 25 mg/kg/dose every 12 hours
>2000 g: 25 mg/kg/dose every 8 hours
Postnatal age >7 days:
<1200 g: 25 mg/kg/dose every 12 hours
1200-2000 g: 30 mg/kg/dose every 8 hours
>2000 g: 37.5 mg/kg/dose every 6 hours
Infants and Children: 150-200 mg/kg/day in divided doses every 6 hours; maximum dose: 12 g/day
(Continued)

oxacillin *(Continued)*

Adults: 250 mg to 2 g/dose every 4-6 hours

Dosage Forms

Infusion [premixed iso-osmotic dextrose solution]: 1 g (50 mL); 2 g (50 mL)

Injection, powder for reconstitution, as sodium: 1 g, 2 g, 10 g

oxacillin sodium *see* oxacillin *on previous page*

oxaliplatin (ox AL i pla tin)

Synonyms diaminocyclohexane oxalatoplatinum; L-OHP; NSC-266046

U.S./Canadian Brand Names Eloxatin™ [US]

Therapeutic Category Antineoplastic Agent, Alkylating Agent

Use Treatment of advanced colon or rectal carcinoma

Usual Dosage I.V.: Colorectal cancer (labeled dosing): Refer to individual protocols.

Adults:

85 mg/m^2 every 2 weeks **or**

20-25 mg/m^2 days 1-5 every 3 weeks **or**

100-130 mg/m^2 every 2-3 weeks

Dosage Forms Injection, powder for reconstitution: 50 mg, 100 mg [contains lactose]

Oxandrin® [US] *see* oxandrolone *on this page*

oxandrolone (oks AN droe lone)

U.S./Canadian Brand Names Oxandrin® [US]

Therapeutic Category Androgen

Controlled Substance C-III

Use Adjunctive therapy to promote weight gain after weight loss following extensive surgery, chronic infections, or severe trauma, and in some patients who, without definite pathophysiologic reasons, fail to gain or to maintain normal weight; to offset protein catabolism with prolonged corticosteroid administration; relief of bone pain associated with osteoporosis

Usual Dosage Oral:

Children: Total daily dose: ≤0.1 mg/kg **or** ≤0.045 mg/lb

Adults: 2.5-20 mg in divided doses 2-4 times/day based on individual response; a course of therapy of 2-4 weeks is usually adequate. This may be repeated intermittently as needed.

Dosage Forms Tablet: 2.5 mg, 10 mg

oxaprozin (oks a PROE zin)

Sound-Alike/Look-Alike Issues

oxaprozin may be confused with oxazepam

Daypro® may be confused with Diupres®

U.S./Canadian Brand Names Apo-Oxaprozin® [Can]; Daypro® [US/Can]; Rhoxal-oxaprozin [Can]

Therapeutic Category Analgesic, Nonnarcotic; Nonsteroidal Antiinflammatory Drug (NSAID)

Use Acute and long-term use in the management of signs and symptoms of osteoarthritis and rheumatoid arthritis; juvenile rheumatoid arthritis

Usual Dosage Oral (individualize dosage to lowest effective dose to minimize adverse effects):

Children 6-16 years: Juvenile rheumatoid arthritis:

22-31 kg: 600 mg once daily

32-54 kg: 900 mg once daily

≥55 kg: 1200 mg once daily

Adults:

Osteoarthritis: 600-1200 mg once daily; patients should be titrated to lowest dose possible; patients with low body weight should start with 600 mg daily

Rheumatoid arthritis: 1200 mg once daily; a one-time loading dose of up to 1800 mg/day or 26 mg/kg (whichever is lower) may be given

Maximum daily dose: 1800 mg or 26 mg/kg (whichever is lower) in divided doses

Dosage Forms Tablet: 600 mg

oxazepam (oks A ze pam)

Sound-Alike/Look-Alike Issues

oxazepam may be confused with oxaprozin, quazepam

Serax® may be confused with Eurax®, Urex®, Zyrtec®

U.S./Canadian Brand Names Apo-Oxazepam® [Can]; Novoxapram® [Can]; Oxpram® [Can]; PMS-Oxazepam [Can]; Serax® [US]

Therapeutic Category Anticonvulsant; Benzodiazepine

Controlled Substance C-IV

Use Treatment of anxiety; management of ethanol withdrawal

Usual Dosage Oral:

Children: Anxiety: 1 mg/kg/day has been administered

Adults:

Anxiety: 10-30 mg 3-4 times/day

Ethanol withdrawal: 15-30 mg 3-4 times/day

Hypnotic: 15-30 mg

Dosage Forms

Capsule: 10 mg, 15 mg, 30 mg

Tablet: 15 mg

oxcarbazepine (ox car BAZ e peen)

Synonyms GP 47680; OCBZ

U.S./Canadian Brand Names Trileptal® [US/Can]

Therapeutic Category Anticonvulsant, Miscellaneous

Use Monotherapy or adjunctive therapy in the treatment of partial seizures in adults and children (4-16 years of age) with epilepsy

Usual Dosage Oral:

Children 4-16 years:

Adjunctive therapy: 8-10 mg/kg/day, not to exceed 600 mg/day, given in 2 divided daily doses. Maintenance dose should be achieved over 2 weeks, and is dependent upon patient weight, according to the following:

20-29 kg: 900 mg/day in 2 divided doses

29.1-39 kg: 1200 mg/day in 2 divided doses

>39 kg: 1800 mg/day in 2 divided doses

Conversion to monotherapy: Oxcarbazepine 8-10 mg/kg/day in twice daily divided doses, while simultaneously initiating the reduction of the dose of the concomitant antiepileptic drug; the concomitant drug should be withdrawn over 3-6 weeks. Oxcarbazepine dose may be increased by a maximum of 10 mg/kg/day at weekly intervals. See below for recommended total daily dose by weight.

Initiation of monotherapy: Oxcarbazepine should be initiated at 8-10 mg/kg/day in twice daily divided doses; doses may be titrated by 5 mg/kg/day every third day. See below for recommended total daily dose by weight.

Range of maintenance doses by weight during monotherapy:

20 kg: 600-900 mg/day

25-30 kg: 900-1200 mg/day

35-40 kg: 900-1500 mg/day

45 kg: 1200-1500 mg/day

50-55 kg: 1200-1800 mg/day

60-65 kg: 1200-2100 mg/day

70 kg: 1500-2100 mg/day

Adults:

Adjunctive therapy: Initial: 300 mg twice daily; dose may be increased by as much as 600 mg/day at weekly intervals; recommended daily dose: 1200 mg/day in 2 divided

(Continued)

oxcarbazepine *(Continued)*

doses. Although daily doses >1200 mg/day demonstrated greater efficacy, most patients were unable to tolerate 2400 mg/day (due to CNS effects).

Conversion to monotherapy: Oxcarbazepine 600 mg/day in twice daily divided doses while simultaneously initiating the reduction of the dose of the concomitant antiepileptic drug. The concomitant dosage should be withdrawn over 3-6 weeks, while the maximum dose of oxcarbazepine should be reached in about 2-4 weeks. Recommended daily dose: 2400 mg/day.

Initiation of monotherapy: Oxcarbazepine should be initiated at a dose of 600 mg/day in twice daily divided doses; doses may be titrated upward by 300 mg/day every third day to a final dose of 1200 mg/day given in 2 daily divided doses

Dosage Forms

Suspension, oral: 300 mg/5 mL (250 mL) [contains ethanol]

Tablet [film coated]: 150 mg, 300 mg, 600 mg

Oxeze® Turbuhaler® [Can] *see* formoterol *on page 388*

oxiconazole (oks i KON a zole)

Synonyms oxiconazole nitrate

U.S./Canadian Brand Names Oxistat® [US/Can]; Oxizole® [Can]

Therapeutic Category Antifungal Agent

Use Treatment of tinea pedis (athlete's foot), tinea cruris (jock itch), and tinea corporis (ringworm)

Usual Dosage Topical:

Children and Adults:

Tinea corporis/tinea cruris: Cream, lotion: Apply to affected areas 1-2 times daily for 2 weeks

Tinea pedis: Cream, lotion: Apply to affected areas 1-2 times daily for 1 month

Adults: Tinea versicolor: Cream: Apply to affected areas once daily for 2 weeks

Dosage Forms

Cream, as nitrate: 1% (15 g, 30 g, 60 g)

Lotion, as nitrate: 1% (30 mL)

oxiconazole nitrate *see* oxiconazole *on this page*

oxidized regenerated cellulose *see* cellulose, oxidized regenerated *on page 174*

oxilapine succinate *see* loxapine *on page 534*

Oxipor® VHC [US-OTC] *see* coal tar *on page 219*

Oxistat® [US/Can] *see* oxiconazole *on this page*

Oxizole® [Can] *see* oxiconazole *on this page*

oxpentifylline *see* pentoxifylline *on page 680*

Oxpram® [Can] *see* oxazepam *on previous page*

oxprenolol *(Canada only)* (ox PREN oh lole)

Synonyms oxprenolol hydrochloride

U.S./Canadian Brand Names Slow-Trasicor® [Can]; Trasicor® [Can]

Therapeutic Category Beta-Adrenergic Blocker

Use Treatment of mild or moderate hypertension

Usual Dosage Oral: Adults:

Initial: 20 mg 3 times/day (regular-release formulation); increase by 60 mg/day (in 3 divided doses) at 1-2 week intervals until adequate control is obtained

Maintenance: 120-320 mg/day; do not exceed 480 mg; may switch to slow-release formulation once-daily dosing at this time

Dosage Forms

Tablet (Trasicor®): 40 mg, 80 mg

Tablet, slow release (Slow-Trasicor®): 80 mg, 160 mg

oxprenolol hydrochloride *see* oxprenolol *(Canada only) on previous page*

Oxsoralen® [US/Can] *see* methoxsalen *on page 567*

Oxsoralen® Oral *(Discontinued)* *see page 1042*

Oxsoralen-Ultra® [US/Can] *see* methoxsalen *on page 567*

Oxy-5® *(Discontinued)* *see page 1042*

Oxy 10® Balanced Medicated Face Wash [US-OTC] *see* benzoyl peroxide *on page 109*

Oxy 10® Balance Spot Treatment [US-OTC] *see* benzoyl peroxide *on page 109*

Oxy® Balance Deep Pore [US-OTC] *see* salicylic acid *on page 789*

Oxy® Balance [US-OTC] *see* salicylic acid *on page 789*

oxybutynin (oks i BYOO ti nin)

Sound-Alike/Look-Alike Issues

oxybutynin may be confused with OxyContin®

Ditropan® may be confused with Detrol®, diazepam, Diprivan®, dithranol

Synonyms oxybutynin chloride

U.S./Canadian Brand Names Ditropan® [US/Can]; Ditropan® XL [US/Can]; Gen-Oxybutynin [Can]; Novo-Oxybutynin [Can]; Nu-Oxybutyn [Can]; Oxytrol™ [US]; PMS-Oxybutynin [Can]

Therapeutic Category Antispasmodic Agent, Urinary

Use Antispasmodic for neurogenic bladder (urgency, frequency, urge incontinence) and uninhibited bladder

Usual Dosage

Oral:

Children:

>5 years: 5 mg twice daily, up to 5 mg 3 times/day maximum

>6 years: Extended release: 5 mg once daily; maximum dose: 20 mg/day

Adults: 5 mg 2-3 times/day up to 5 mg 4 times/day maximum

Extended release: Initial: 5-10 mg once daily, may increase in 5-10 mg increments; maximum: 30 mg daily

Transdermal: Adults: Apply one 3.9 mg/day patch twice weekly (every 3-4 days)

Note: Should be discontinued periodically to determine whether the patient can manage without the drug and to minimize resistance to the drug

Dosage Forms

Syrup, as chloride (Ditropan®): 5 mg/5 mL (473 mL)

Tablet, as chloride (Ditropan®): 5 mg

Tablet, extended release, as chloride (Ditropan® XL): 5 mg, 10 mg, 15 mg

Transdermal system (Oxytrol™): 3.9 mg/day (8s, 24s) [39 cm^2; total oxybutynin 36 mg]

oxybutynin chloride *see* oxybutynin *on this page*

oxychlorosene (oks i KLOR oh seen)

Synonyms oxychlorosene sodium

U.S./Canadian Brand Names Clorpactin® WCS-90 [US-OTC]

Therapeutic Category Antibiotic, Topical

Use Treatment of localized infections

Usual Dosage Topical (0.1% to 0.5% solutions): Apply by irrigation, instillation, spray, soaks, or wet compresses

Dosage Forms Powder for solution, as sodium: 2 g

oxychlorosene sodium *see* oxychlorosene *on this page*

Oxycocet® [Can] *see* oxycodone and acetaminophen *on next page*

Oxycodan® [Can] *see* oxycodone and aspirin *on page 657*

oxycodone (oks i KOE done)

Sound-Alike/Look-Alike Issues

oxycodone may be confused with OxyContin®

OxyContin® may be confused with oxybutynin, oxycodone

Synonyms dihydrohydroxycodeinone; oxycodone hydrochloride

U.S./Canadian Brand Names OxyContin® [US/Can]; Oxydose™ [US]; OxyFast® [US]; OxyIR® [US/Can]; Roxicodone™ Intensol™ [US]; Roxicodone™ [US]; Supeudol® [Can]

Therapeutic Category Analgesic, Narcotic

Controlled Substance C-II

Use Management of moderate to severe pain, normally used in combination with non-narcotic analgesics

OxyContin® is indicated for around-the-clock management of moderate to severe pain when an analgesic is needed for an extended period of time. **Note:** OxyContin® is not intended for use as an "as needed" analgesic or for immediately-postoperative pain management (should be used postoperatively only if the patient has received it prior to surgery or if severe, persistent pain is anticipated).

Usual Dosage Oral:

Immediate release:

Children:

6-12 years: 1.25 mg every 6 hours as needed

>12 years: 2.5 mg every 6 hours as needed

Adults: 5 mg every 6 hours as needed

Controlled release: Adults:

Opioid naive (not currently on opioid): 10 mg every 12 hours

Currently on opioid/ASA or acetaminophen or NSAID combination:

1-5 tablets: 10-20 mg every 12 hours

6-9 tablets: 20-30 mg every 12 hours

10-12 tablets: 30-40 mg every 12 hours

May continue the nonopioid as a separate drug.

Currently on opioids: Use standard conversion chart to convert daily dose to oxycodone equivalent. Divide daily dose in 2 (for every 12-hour dosing) and round down to nearest dosage form.

Note: 80 mg or 160 mg tablets are for use **only** in opioid-tolerant patients. Special safety considerations must be addressed when converting to OxyContin® doses ≥160 mg every 12 hours. Dietary caution must be taken when patients are initially titrated to 160 mg tablets.

Dosage Forms

Capsule, immediate release, as hydrochloride (OxyIR®): 5 mg

Solution, oral, as hydrochloride: 5 mg/5 mL (500 mL)

Roxicodone™: 5 mg/5 mL (5 mL, 500 mL) [contains alcohol]

Solution, oral concentrate, as hydrochloride: 20 mg/mL (30 mL)

Oxydose™: 20 mg/mL (30 mL) [contains sodium benzoate; berry flavor]

OxyFast®, Roxicodone™ Intensol™: 20 mg/mL (30 mL) [contains sodium benzoate]

Tablet, as hydrochloride: 5 mg

Roxicodone™: 5 mg, 15 mg, 30 mg

Tablet, controlled release, as hydrochloride (OxyContin®): 10 mg, 20 mg, 40 mg, 80 mg, 160 mg

Tablet, extended release, as hydrochloride: 80 mg

oxycodone and acetaminophen (oks i KOE done & a seet a MIN oh fen)

Sound-Alike/Look-Alike Issues

Percocet® may be confused with Percodan®

Roxicet™ may be confused with Roxanol®

Tylox® may be confused with Trimox®, Tylenol®, Wymox®, Xanax®

Synonyms acetaminophen and oxycodone

U.S./Canadian Brand Names Endocet® [US/Can]; Oxycocet® [Can]; Percocet® [US/Can]; Percocet®-Demi [Can]; PMS-Oxycodone-Acetaminophen [Can]; Roxicet™ [US]; Roxicet® 5/500 [US]; Tylox® [US]

Therapeutic Category Analgesic, Narcotic

Controlled Substance C-II

Use Management of moderate to severe pain

Usual Dosage Oral: Doses should be given every 4-6 hours as needed and titrated to appropriate analgesic effects. **Note:** Initial dose is based on the **oxycodone** content; however, the maximum daily dose is based on the **acetaminophen** content.

Children: Maximum acetaminophen dose: Children <45 kg: 90 mg/kg/day; children >45 kg: 4 g/day

Mild to moderate pain: Initial dose, **based on oxycodone content:** 0.05-0.1 mg/kg/dose

Severe pain: Initial dose, **based on oxycodone content:** 0.3 mg/kg/dose

Adults:

Mild to moderate pain: Initial dose, **based on oxycodone content:** 5 mg

Severe pain: Initial dose, **based on oxycodone content:** 15-30 mg. Do not exceed acetaminophen 4 g/day.

Dosage Forms

Caplet (Roxicet™ 5/500): Oxycodone hydrochloride 5 mg and acetaminophen 500 mg

Capsule: Oxycodone hydrochloride 5 mg and acetaminophen 500 mg

Tylox®: Oxycodone hydrochloride 5 mg and acetaminophen 500 mg [contains sodium benzoate and sodium metabisulfite]

Solution, oral (Roxicet™): Oxycodone hydrochloride 5 mg and acetaminophen 325 mg per 5 mL (5 mL, 500 mL) [contains alcohol <0.5%]

Tablet: Oxycodone hydrochloride 5 mg and acetaminophen 325 mg; oxycodone hydrochloride 7.5 mg and acetaminophen 325 mg; oxycodone hydrochloride 7.5 mg and acetaminophen 500 mg; oxycodone hydrochloride 10 mg and acetaminophen 325 mg; oxycodone hydrochloride 10 mg and acetaminophen 650 mg

Endocet® 5/325 [scored]: Oxycodone hydrochloride 5 mg and acetaminophen 325 mg

Endocet® 7.5/325: Oxycodone hydrochloride 7.5 mg and acetaminophen 325 mg

Endocet® 7.5/500: Oxycodone hydrochloride 7.5 mg and acetaminophen 500 mg

Endocet® 10/325: Oxycodone hydrochloride 10 mg and acetaminophen 325 mg

Endocet® 10/650: Oxycodone hydrochloride 10 mg and acetaminophen 650 mg

Percocet® 2.5/325: Oxycodone hydrochloride 2.5 mg and acetaminophen 325 mg

Percocet® 5/325 [scored]: Oxycodone hydrochloride 5 mg and acetaminophen 325 mg

Percocet® 7.5/325: Oxycodone hydrochloride 7.5 mg and acetaminophen 325 mg

Percocet® 7.5/500: Oxycodone hydrochloride 7.5 mg and acetaminophen 500 mg

Percocet® 10/325: Oxycodone hydrochloride 10 mg and acetaminophen 325 mg

Percocet® 10/650: Oxycodone hydrochloride 10 mg and acetaminophen 650 mg

Roxicet™ [scored]: Oxycodone hydrochloride 5 mg and acetaminophen 325 mg

oxycodone and aspirin (oks i KOE done & AS pir in)

Sound-Alike/Look-Alike Issues

Percodan® may be confused with Decadron®, Percocet®, Percogesic®, Periactin®

Synonyms aspirin and oxycodone

U.S./Canadian Brand Names Endodan® [US/Can]; Oxycodan® [Can]; Percodan® [US/Can]

Therapeutic Category Analgesic, Narcotic

Controlled Substance C-II

Use Management of moderate to severe pain

Usual Dosage Oral (based on oxycodone combined salts):

Children: Maximum oxycodone: 5 mg/dose; maximum aspirin dose should not exceed 4 g/day. Doses should be given every 6 hours as needed.

Mild-to-moderate pain: Initial dose, **based on oxycodone content:**: 0.05-0.1 mg/kg/dose

Severe pain: Initial dose, **based on oxycodone content**: 0.3 mg/kg/dose

Adults: Percodan®: 1 tablet every 6 hours as needed for pain; maximum aspirin dose should not exceed 4 g/day.

(Continued)

oxycodone and aspirin *(Continued)*

Dosage Forms

Tablet: Oxycodone hydrochloride 4.5 mg, oxycodone terephthalate 0.38 mg, and aspirin 325 mg

Endodan®, Percodan®: Oxycodone hydrochloride 4.5 mg, oxycodone terephthalate 0.38 mg, and aspirin 325 mg

oxycodone hydrochloride *see* oxycodone *on page 656*

OxyContin® [US/Can] *see* oxycodone *on page 656*

Oxyderm™ [Can] *see* benzoyl peroxide *on page 109*

Oxydose™ [US] *see* oxycodone *on page 656*

OxyFast® [US] *see* oxycodone *on page 656*

OxyIR® [US/Can] *see* oxycodone *on page 656*

oxymetazoline (oks i met AZ oh leen)

Sound-Alike/Look-Alike Issues

oxymetazoline may be confused with oxymetholone

Afrin® may be confused with aspirin

Visine® may be confused with Visken®

Synonyms oxymetazoline hydrochloride

U.S./Canadian Brand Names Afrin® Extra Moisturizing [US-OTC]; Afrin® Original [US-OTC]; Afrin® Severe Congestion [US-OTC]; Afrin® Sinus [US-OTC]; Afrin® [US-OTC]; Claritin® Allergic Decongestant [Can]; Dristan® Long Lasting Nasal [Can]; Drixoral® Nasal [Can]; Duramist® Plus [US-OTC]; Duration® [US-OTC]; Genasal [US-OTC]; Neo-Synephrine® 12 Hour Extra Moisturizing [US-OTC]; Neo-Synephrine® 12 Hour [US-OTC]; Nōstrilla® [US-OTC]; Twice-A-Day® [US-OTC]; Vicks® Sinex® 12 Hour Ultrafine Mist [US-OTC]; Visine® L.R. [US-OTC]; 4-Way® Long Acting [US-OTC]

Therapeutic Category Adrenergic Agonist Agent

Use Adjunctive therapy of middle ear infections, associated with acute or chronic rhinitis, the common cold, sinusitis, hay fever, or other allergies

Ophthalmic: Relief of redness of eye due to minor eye irritations

Usual Dosage

Intranasal (therapy should not exceed 3-5 days):

Children 2-5 years: 0.025% solution: Instill 2-3 drops in each nostril twice daily

Children ≥6 years and Adults: 0.05% solution: Instill 2-3 drops or 2-3 sprays into each nostril twice daily

Ophthalmic: Children >6 years and Adults: 0.025% solution: Instill 1-2 drops in affected eye(s) every 6 hours as needed or as directed by healthcare provider

Dosage Forms [DSC] = Discontinued product

Solution, intranasal spray, as hydrochloride: 0.05% (15 mL, 30 mL)

Afrin®, Afrin® Extra Moisturizing, Afrin® Sinus: 0.05% (15 mL) [contains benzyl alcohol; no drip formula]

Afrin® Original: 0.05% (15 mL, 30 mL, 45 mL)

Afrin® Severe Congestion: 0.05% (15 mL) [contains benzyl alcohol and menthol; no drip formula]

Duramist® Plus, Neo-Synephrine® 12 Hour, Nōstrilla®, Vicks® Sinex® 12 Hour Ultrafine Mist, 4-Way® Long Acting Nasal: 0.05% (15 mL)

Duration®: 0.05% (30 mL)

Genasal: 0.05% (15 mL, 30 mL)

Neo-Synephrine® 12 Hour Extra Moisturizing: 0.05% (15 mL) [contains glycerin]

Solution, ophthalmic, as hydrochloride (OcuClear® [DSC], Visine® L.R.): 0.025% (15 mL, 30 mL) [contains benzalkonium chloride]

oxymetazoline hydrochloride *see* oxymetazoline *on this page*

oxymetholone (oks i METH oh lone)

Sound-Alike/Look-Alike Issues
oxymetholone may be confused with oxymetazoline, oxymorphone
U.S./Canadian Brand Names Anadrol® [US]
Therapeutic Category Anabolic Steroid
Controlled Substance C-III
Use Treatment of anemias caused by deficient red cell production
Usual Dosage Children and Adults: Erythropoietic effects: Oral: 1-5 mg/kg/day in one daily dose; usual effective dose: 1-2 mg/kg/day; give for a minimum trial of 3-6 months because response may be delayed
Dosage Forms Tablet: 50 mg

oxymorphone (oks i MOR fone)

Sound-Alike/Look-Alike Issues
oxymorphone may be confused with oxymetholone
Synonyms oxymorphone hydrochloride
U.S./Canadian Brand Names Numorphan® [US/Can]
Therapeutic Category Analgesic, Narcotic
Controlled Substance C-II
Use Management of moderate to severe pain and preoperatively as a sedative and a supplement to anesthesia
Usual Dosage Adults: **Note:** More frequent dosing may be required.
I.M., SubQ: 0.5 mg initially, 1-1.5 mg every 4-6 hours as needed
I.V.: 0.5 mg initially
Rectal: 5 mg every 4-6 hours
Dosage Forms
Injection, solution, as hydrochloride: 1 mg (1 mL); 1.5 mg/mL (10 mL)
Suppository, rectal, as hydrochloride: 5 mg

oxymorphone hydrochloride *see* oxymorphone *on this page*
oxyphenbutazone *(Discontinued)* *see page 1042*

oxytetracycline (oks i tet ra SYE kleen)

Sound-Alike/Look-Alike Issues
Terramycin® may be confused with Garamycin®
Synonyms oxytetracycline hydrochloride
U.S./Canadian Brand Names Terramycin® [Can]; Terramycin® I.M. [US]
Therapeutic Category Tetracycline Derivative
Use Treatment of susceptible bacterial infections; both gram-positive and gram-negative, as well as, *Rickettsia* and *Mycoplasma* organisms
Usual Dosage I.M.:
Children >8 years: 15-25 mg/kg/day (maximum: 250 mg/dose) in divided doses every 8-12 hours
Adults: 250 mg every 24 hours or 300 mg/day divided every 8-12 hours
Dosage Forms Injection, solution: 5% [50 mg/mL] (10 mL) [contains lidocaine hydrochloride 2%]

oxytetracycline and polymyxin B

(oks i tet ra SYE kleen & pol i MIKS in bee)
Synonyms polymyxin B and oxytetracycline
U.S./Canadian Brand Names Terramycin® w/Polymyxin B Ophthalmic [US]
Therapeutic Category Antibiotic, Ophthalmic
Use Treatment of superficial ocular infections involving the conjunctiva and/or cornea
Usual Dosage Topical: Apply 1/2" of ointment onto the lower lid of affected eye 2-4 times/day
Dosage Forms Ointment, ophthalmic: Oxytetracycline hydrochloride 5 mg and polymyxin B 10,000 units per g (3.5 g)

oxytetracycline hydrochloride *see* oxytetracycline *on previous page*

oxytocin (oks i TOE sin)

Sound-Alike/Look-Alike Issues
Pitocin® may be confused with Pitressin®

Synonyms pit

U.S./Canadian Brand Names Pitocin® [US/Can]; Syntocinon® [Can]

Therapeutic Category Oxytocic Agent

Use Induction of labor at term; control of postpartum bleeding; adjunctive therapy in management of abortion

Usual Dosage I.V. administration requires the use of an infusion pump. Adults:

Induction of labor: I.V.: 0.5-1 milliunits/minute; gradually increase dose in increments of 1-2 milliunits/minute until desired contraction pattern is established; dose may be decreased after desired frequency of contractions is reached and labor has progressed to 5-6 cm dilation. Infusion rates of 6 milliunits/minute provide oxytocin levels similar to those at spontaneous labor; rates of >9-10 milliunits/minute are rarely required.

Postpartum bleeding:
I.M.: Total dose of 10 units after delivery
I.V.: 10-40 units by I.V. infusion in 1000 mL of intravenous fluid at a rate sufficient to control uterine atony

Adjunctive treatment of abortion: I.V.: 10-20 milliunits/minute; maximum total dose: 30 units/12 hours

Dosage Forms Injection, solution: 10 units/mL (1 mL, 10 mL)
Pitocin®: 10 units/mL (1 mL)

Oxytrol™ [US] *see* oxybutynin *on page 655*

Oysco 500 [US-OTC] *see* calcium carbonate *on page 144*

Oyst-Cal 500 [US-OTC] *see* calcium carbonate *on page 144*

P-071 *see* cetirizine *on page 178*

Pacerone® [US] *see* amiodarone *on page 47*

Pacis™ [Can] *see* BCG vaccine *on page 101*

paclitaxel (PAK li taks el)

Sound-Alike/Look-Alike Issues
paclitaxel may be confused with docetaxel, paroxetine, Paxil®
Taxol® may be confused with Paxil®, Taxotere®

Synonyms NSC-125973

U.S./Canadian Brand Names Onxol™ [US]; Taxol® [US/Can]

Therapeutic Category Antineoplastic Agent

Use Treatment of breast, lung (small cell and nonsmall cell), and ovarian cancers

Usual Dosage Premedication with dexamethasone (20 mg orally or I.V. at 12 and 6 hours **or** 14 and 7 hours before the dose), diphenhydramine (50 mg I.V. 30-60 minutes prior to the dose), and cimetidine, famotidine or ranitidine (I.V. 30-60 minutes prior to the dose) is recommended

Adults: I.V.: Refer to individual protocols.
Ovarian carcinoma: 135-175 mg/m^2 over 3 hours every 3 weeks **or**
50-80 mg/m^2 over 1-3 hours weekly **or**
1.4-4 mg/m^2/day continuous infusion for 14 days every 4 weeks
Metastatic breast cancer: 175-250 mg/m^2 over 3 hours every 3 weeks **or**
50-80 mg/m^2 weekly **or**
1.4-4 mg/m^2/day continuous infusion for 14 days every 4 weeks
Nonsmall-cell lung carcinoma: 135 mg/m^2 over 24 hours every 3 weeks
AIDS-related Kaposi sarcoma: 135 mg/m^2 over 3 hours every 3 weeks **or**
100 mg/m^2 over 3 hours every 2 weeks

Dosage modification for toxicity (solid tumors, including ovary, breast, and lung carcinoma): Courses of paclitaxel should not be repeated until the neutrophil count is

≥1500 cells/mm^3 and the platelet count is ≥100,000 cells/mm^3; reduce dosage by 20% for patients experiencing severe peripheral neuropathy or severe neutropenia (neutrophil <500 cells/mm^3 for a week or longer)

Dosage modification for immunosuppression in advanced HIV disease: Paclitaxel should not be given to patients with HIV if the baseline or subsequent neutrophil count is <1000 cells/mm^3. Additional modifications include: Reduce dosage of dexamethasone in premedication to 10 mg orally; reduce dosage by 20% in patients experiencing severe peripheral neuropathy or severe neutropenia (neutrophil <500 cells/mm^3 for a week or longer); initiate concurrent hematopoietic growth factor (G-CSF) as clinically indicated

Dosage Forms Injection, solution: 6 mg/mL (5 mL, 16.7 mL, 50 mL) [contains alcohol and purified Cremophor® EL (polyoxyethylated castor oil)]

Onxol™: 6 mg/mL (5 mL, 25 mL, 50 mL) [contains alcohol] [contains alcohol and purified Cremophor® EL (polyoxyethylated castor oil)]

Taxol®: 6 mg/mL (5 mL, 16.7 mL, 50 mL) [contains alcohol and purified Cremophor® EL (polyoxyethylated castor oil)]

Pain-A-Lay® [US-OTC] *see* phenol *on page 687*

Pain-Off [US-OTC] *see* acetaminophen, aspirin, and caffeine *on page 10*

Palafer® [Can] *see* ferrous fumarate *on page 363*

Palgic®-D [US] *see* carbinoxamine and pseudoephedrine *on page 157*

Palgic®-DS [US] *see* carbinoxamine and pseudoephedrine *on page 157*

palivizumab (pah li VIZ u mab)

Sound-Alike/Look-Alike Issues

Synagis® may be confused with Synalgos®-DC, Synvisc®

U.S./Canadian Brand Names Synagis® [US/Can]

Therapeutic Category Monoclonal Antibody

Use Prevention of serious lower respiratory tract disease caused by respiratory syncytial virus (RSV) in infants and children <2 years of age at high risk of RSV disease

Usual Dosage I.M.: Infants and Children: 15 mg/kg of body weight, monthly throughout RSV season (First dose administered prior to commencement of RSV season)

Dosage Forms Injection, powder for reconstitution: 50 mg, 100 mg

Palmer's® Skin Success Acne Cleanser [US-OTC] *see* salicylic acid *on page 789*

Palmer's® Skin Success Acne [US-OTC] *see* benzoyl peroxide *on page 109*

Palmer's® Skin Success Fade Cream™ [US-OTC] *see* hydroquinone *on page 454*

Palmitate-A® [US-OTC] *see* vitamin A *on page 914*

palonosetron (pal oh NOE se tron)

Synonyms palonosetron hydrochloride; RS-25259; RS-25259-197

U.S./Canadian Brand Names Aloxi™ [US]

Therapeutic Category Antiemetic; Selective 5-HT_3 Receptor Antagonist

Use Prevention of acute (within 24 hours) and delayed (2-5 days) chemotherapy-induced nausea and vomiting

Usual Dosage I.V.: Adults: Chemotherapy-induced nausea and vomiting: 0.25 mg 30 minutes prior to chemotherapy administration, day 1 of each cycle (doses should not be given more than once weekly)

Dosage Forms Injection, solution, as hydrochloride: 0.05 mg/mL (5 mL)

palonosetron hydrochloride *see* palonosetron *on this page*

2-PAM *see* pralidoxime *on page 719*

Pamelor® [US] *see* nortriptyline *on page 629*

pamidronate (pa mi DROE nate)

Sound-Alike/Look-Alike Issues

Aredia® may be confused with Adriamycin®

Synonyms pamidronate disodium

U.S./Canadian Brand Names Aredia® [US/Can]

Therapeutic Category Bisphosphonate Derivative

Use Treatment of hypercalcemia associated with malignancy; treatment of osteolytic bone lesions associated with multiple myeloma or metastatic breast cancer; moderate to severe Paget disease of bone

Usual Dosage Drug must be diluted properly before administration and infused intravenously slowly. Due to risk of nephrotoxicity, doses should not exceed 90 mg. I.V.:

Adults:

Hypercalcemia of malignancy:

Moderate cancer-related hypercalcemia (corrected serum calcium: 12-13.5 mg/dL): 60-90 mg, as a single dose, given as a slow infusion over 2-24 hours; dose should be diluted in 1000 mL 0.45% NaCl, 0.9% NaCl, or D_5W

Severe cancer-related hypercalcemia (corrected serum calcium: >13.5 mg/dL): 90 mg, as a single dose, as a slow infusion over 2-24 hours; dose should be diluted in 1000 mL 0.45% NaCl, 0.9% NaCl, or D_5W

A period of 7 days should elapse before the use of second course; repeat infusions every 2-3 weeks have been suggested, however, could be administered every 2-3 months according to the degree and of severity of hypercalcemia and/or the type of malignancy.

Note: Some investigators have suggested a lack of a dose-response relationship. Courses of pamidronate for hypercalcemia may be repeated at varying intervals, depending on the duration of normocalcemia (median 2-3 weeks), but the manufacturer recommends a minimum interval between courses of 7 days. Oral etidronate at a dose of 20 mg/kg/day has been used to maintain the calcium lowering effect following I.V. bisphosphonates, although it is of limited effectiveness.

Osteolytic bone lesions with multiple myeloma: 90 mg in 500 mL D_5W, 0.45% NaCl or 0.9% NaCl administered over 4 hours on a monthly basis

Osteolytic bone lesions with metastatic breast cancer: 90 mg in 250 mL D_5W, 0.45% NaCl or 0.9% NaCl administered over 2 hours, repeated every 3-4 weeks

Paget disease: 30 mg in 500 mL 0.45% NaCl, 0.9% NaCl or D_5W administered over 4 hours for 3 consecutive days

Dosage Forms

Injection, powder for reconstitution, as disodium (Aredia®): 30 mg, 90 mg

Injection, solution: 3 mg/mL (10 mL); 6 mg/mL (10 mL); 9 mg/mL (10 mL)

pamidronate disodium *see* pamidronate *on this page*

Pamine® [US/Can] *see* methscopolamine *on page 567*

Pamine® Forte [US] *see* methscopolamine *on page 567*

p-aminoclonidine *see* apraclonidine *on page 74*

Pamprin IB® *(Discontinued)* *see page 1042*

Pamprin® Maximum Strength All Day Relief [US-OTC] *see* naproxen *on page 605*

Panadol® *(Discontinued)* *see page 1042*

Panasal® 5/500 *(Discontinued)* *see page 1042*

pan-B antibody *see* rituximab *on page 780*

Pancof®-XP [US] *see* hydrocodone, pseudoephedrine, and guaifenesin *on page 447*

Pancrease® [US/Can] *see* pancrelipase *on next page*

Pancrease® MT [US/Can] *see* pancrelipase *on next page*

Pancrecarb MS® [US] *see* pancrelipase *on next page*

pancrelipase (pan kre LI pase)

Synonyms lipancreatin

U.S./Canadian Brand Names Cotazym® [Can]; Creon® [US]; Creon® 5 [Can]; Creon® 10 [Can]; Creon® 20 [Can]; Creon® 25 [Can]; Ku-Zyme® HP [US]; Lipram 4500 [US]; Lipram-CR [US]; Lipram-PN [US]; Lipram-UL [US]; Pancrease® [US/Can]; Pancrease® MT [US/Can]; Pancrecarb MS® [US]; Pangestyme™ CN; Pangestyme™ EC; Pangestyme™ MT; Pangestyme™ UL; Ultrase® MT [US/Can]; Viokase® [US/Can]

Therapeutic Category Enzyme

Use Replacement therapy in symptomatic treatment of malabsorption syndrome caused by pancreatic insufficiency

Usual Dosage Oral:

Powder: Actual dose depends on the condition being treated and the digestive requirements of the patient

Children <1 year: Start with 1/8 teaspoonful with feedings

Adults: 0.7 g (1/4 teaspoonful) with meals

Capsules/tablets: The following dosage recommendations are only an approximation for initial dosages. The actual dosage will depend on the condition being treated and the digestive requirements of the individual patient. Adjust dose based on body weight and stool fat content. Total daily dose reflects ~3 meals/day and 2-3 snacks/day, with half the mealtime dose given with a snack. Older patients may need less units/kg due to increased weight, but decreased ingestion of fat/kg. Maximum dose: 2500 units of lipase/kg/meal (10,000 units of lipase/kg/day)

Children:

<1 year: 2000 units of lipase with meals

1-6 years: 4000-8000 units of lipase with meals and 4000 units with snacks

7-12 years: 4000-12,000 units of lipase with meals and snacks

Adults: 4000-48,000 units of lipase with meals and with snacks

Occluded feeding tubes: One tablet of Viokase® crushed with one 325 mg tablet of sodium bicarbonate (to activate the Viokase®) in 5 mL of water can be instilled into the nasogastric tube and clamped for 5 minutes; then, flushed with 50 mL of tap water

Dosage Forms

Capsule (Ku-Zyme® HP): Lipase 8000 units, protease 30,000 units, amylase 30,000 units

Capsule, delayed release:

Pangestyme™ CN-10: Lipase 10,000 units, protease 37,500 units, amylase 33,200 units

Pangestyme™ CN-20: Lipase 20,000 units, protease 75,000 units, amylase 66,400 units

Capsule, delayed release, enteric coated microspheres:

Creon® 5: Lipase 5000 units, protease 18,750 units, amylase 16,600 units

Creon® 10: Lipase 10,000 units, protease 37,500 units, amylase 33,200 units

Creon® 20: Lipase 20,000 units, protease 75,000 units, amylase 66,400 units

Lipram 4500: Lipase 4500 units, protease 25,000 units, amylase 20,000 units

Lipram-CR10: Lipase 10,000 units, protease 37,500 units, amylase 33,200 units

Lipram-CR20: Lipase 20,000 units, protease 75,000 units, amylase 66,400 units

Lipram-PN10: Lipase 10,000 units, protease 30,000 units, amylase 30,000 units

Lipram-PN16: Lipase 16,000 units, protease 48,000 units, amylase 48,000 units

Lipram-UL12: Lipase 12,000 units, protease 39,000 units, amylase 39,000 units

Lipram-UL18: Lipase 18,000 units, protease 58,500 units, amylase 58,500 units

Lipram-UL20: Lipase 20,000 units, protease 65,000 units, amylase 65,000 units

Pancrecarb MS-4®: Lipase 4000 units, protease 25,000 units, amylase 25,000 units [buffered]

Pancrecarb MS-8®: Lipase 8000 units, protease 45,000 units, amylase 40,000 units [buffered]

Capsule, enteric coated microspheres (Pancrease®, Pangestyme™ EC, Ultrase®): Lipase 4500 units, protease 25,000 units, amylase 20,000 units

Capsule, enteric coated microtablets:

Pancrease® MT 4: Lipase 4000 units, protease 12,000 units, amylase 12,000 units

(Continued)

pancrelipase *(Continued)*

Pancrease® MT 10: Lipase 10,000 units, protease 30,000 units, amylase 30,000 units
Pancrease® MT 16, Pangestyme™ MT 16: Lipase 16,000 units, protease 48,000 units, amylase 48,000 units
Pancrease® MT 20: Lipase 20,000 units, protease 44,000 units, amylase 56,000 units
Pangestyme™ UL 12: Lipase 12,000 units, protease 39,000 units, amylase 39,000 units
Pangestyme™ UL 18: Lipase 18,000 units, protease 58,500 units, amylase 58,500 units
Pangestyme™ UL 20: Lipase 20,000 units, protease 65,000 units, amylase 65,000 units

Capsule, enteric coated minitablets:
Ultrase® MT12: Lipase 12,000 units, protease 39,000 units, amylase 39,000 units
Ultrase® MT18: Lipase 18,000 units, protease 58,500 units, amylase 58,500 units
Ultrase® MT20: Lipase 20,000 units, protease 65,000 units, amylase 65,000 units

Powder (Viokase®): Lipase 16,800 units, protease 70,000 units, amylase 70,000 units per 0.7 g (227 g)

Tablet:
Viokase® 8: Lipase 8000 units, protease 30,000 units, amylase 30,000 units
Viokase® 16: Lipase 16,000 units, protease 60,000 units, amylase 60,000 units

pancuronium (pan kyoo ROE nee um)

Sound-Alike/Look-Alike Issues
pancuronium may be confused with pipecuronium

Synonyms pancuronium bromide

Therapeutic Category Skeletal Muscle Relaxant

Use Adjunct to general anesthesia to facilitate endotracheal intubation and to relax skeletal muscles during surgery; to facilitate mechanical ventilation in ICU patients; does not relieve pain or produce sedation

Drug of choice for neuromuscular blockade except in patients with renal failure, hepatic failure, or cardiovascular instability or in situations not suited for pancuronium's long duration of action

Usual Dosage Administer I.V.; dose to effect; doses will vary due to interpatient variability; use ideal body weight for obese patients

Surgery:
Neonates <1 month:
Test dose: 0.02 mg/kg to measure responsiveness
Initial: 0.03 mg/kg/dose repeated twice at 5- to 10-minute intervals as needed; maintenance: 0.03-0.09 mg/kg/dose every 30 minutes to 4 hours as needed
Infants >1 month, Children, and Adults: Initial: 0.06-0.1 mg/kg or 0.05 mg/kg after initial dose of succinylcholine for intubation; maintenance dose: 0.01 mg/kg 60-100 minutes after initial dose and then 0.01 mg/kg every 25-60 minutes
Pretreatment/priming: 10% of intubating dose given 3-5 minutes before initial dose
ICU: 0.05-0.1 mg/kg bolus followed by 0.8-1.7 mcg/kg/minute once initial recovery from bolus observed or 0.1-0.2 mg/kg every 1-3 hours

Dosage Forms Injection, solution, as bromide: 1 mg/mL (10 mL); 2 mg/mL (2 mL, 5 mL) [may contain benzyl alcohol]

pancuronium bromide *see* pancuronium *on this page*

Pandel® [US] *see* hydrocortisone (topical) *on page 451*

Pangestyme™ CN *see* pancrelipase *on previous page*

Pangestyme™ EC *see* pancrelipase *on previous page*

Pangestyme™ MT *see* pancrelipase *on previous page*

Pangestyme™ UL *see* pancrelipase *on previous page*

Panglobulin® [US] *see* immune globulin (intravenous) *on page 468*

Panhematin® [US] *see* hemin *on page 430*

Panixine DisperDose™ [US] *see* cephalexin *on page 176*

PanMist®-DM [US] *see* guaifenesin, pseudoephedrine, and dextromethorphan *on page 422*

PanMist® Jr. [US] *see* guaifenesin and pseudoephedrine *on page 419*

PanMist® LA [US] *see* guaifenesin and pseudoephedrine *on page 419*

PanMist® S [US] *see* guaifenesin and pseudoephedrine *on page 419*

PanOxyl® [US/Can] *see* benzoyl peroxide *on page 109*

PanOxyl®-AQ [US/Can] *see* benzoyl peroxide *on page 109*

PanOxyl® Aqua Gel [US] *see* benzoyl peroxide *on page 109*

PanOxyl® Bar [US-OTC] *see* benzoyl peroxide *on page 109*

Panretin® [US/Can] *see* alitretinoin *on page 32*

Panscol® Lotion *(Discontinued)* *see page 1042*

Panscol® Ointment *(Discontinued)* *see page 1042*

Panthoderm® [US-OTC] *see* dexpanthenol *on page 257*

Panto™ IV [Can] *see* pantoprazole *on this page*

Pantoloc™ [Can] *see* pantoprazole *on this page*

Pantopon® *(Discontinued)* *see page 1042*

pantoprazole (pan TOE pra zole)

Sound-Alike/Look-Alike Issues

Protonix® may be confused with Lotronex®

U.S./Canadian Brand Names Panto™ IV [Can]; Pantoloc™ [Can]; Protonix® [US/Can]

Therapeutic Category Proton Pump Inhibitor

Use

Oral: Treatment and maintenance of healing of erosive esophagitis associated with GERD; reduction in relapse rates of daytime and nighttime heartburn symptoms in GERD; hypersecretory disorders associated with Zollinger-Ellison syndrome or other neoplastic disorders

I.V.: As an alternative to oral therapy in patients unable to continue oral pantoprazole; hypersecretory disorders associated with Zollinger-Ellison syndrome or other neoplastic disorders

Usual Dosage Adults:

Oral:

Erosive esophagitis associated with GERD:

Treatment: 40 mg once daily for up to 8 weeks; an additional 8 weeks may be used in patients who have not healed after an 8-week course

Maintenance of healing: 40 mg once daily

Note: Lower doses (20 mg once daily) have been used successfully in mild GERD treatment and maintenance of healing

Hypersecretory disorders (including Zollinger-Ellison): Initial: 40 mg twice daily; adjust dose based on patient needs; doses up to 240 mg/day have been administered

I.V.:

Erosive esophagitis associated with GERD: 40 mg once daily for 7-10 days

Hypersecretory disorders: 80 mg twice daily; adjust dose based on acid output measurements; 160-240 mg/day in divided doses has been used for a limited period (up to 7 days)

Dosage Forms

Injection, powder for reconstitution, as sodium: 40 mg [original formulation]

Injection, powder for reconstitution, as sodium: 40 mg [contains edetate sodium 1 mg]

Tablet, delayed release, as sodium: 20 mg, 40 mg

pantothenic acid (pan toe THEN ik AS id)

Synonyms calcium pantothenate; vitamin B_5
Therapeutic Category Vitamin, Water Soluble
Use Pantothenic acid deficiency
Usual Dosage Adults: Oral: Recommended daily dose 4-7 mg/day
Dosage Forms Tablet: 100 mg, 200 mg, 250 mg, 500 mg

pantothenyl alcohol *see* dexpanthenol *on page 257*

Panwarfarin® *(Discontinued)* *see page 1042*

papain and urea (pa PAY in & yoor EE a)

Therapeutic Category Enzyme, Topical Debridement; Topical Skin Product
Use Enzymatic debriding ointment for treatment of chronic and acute wounds
Usual Dosage Cleanse wound with cleanser or saline (not hydrogen peroxide); apply directly to the wound, cover with appropriate dressing, secure into place and reapply 1-2 times/day. Irrigate wound at each dressing.
Dosage Forms Ointment, topical: Papain 1.1×10^4 int. units and urea 10% in hydrophilic ointment (30 g)

papaverine (pa PAV er een)

Synonyms papaverine hydrochloride
U.S./Canadian Brand Names Para-Time S.R.® [US]
Therapeutic Category Vasodilator
Use Oral: Relief of peripheral and cerebral ischemia associated with arterial spasm and myocardial ischemia complicated by arrhythmias
Usual Dosage
I.M., I.V.:
Children: 6 mg/kg/day in 4 divided doses
Adults: 30-65 mg (rarely up to 120 mg); may repeat every 3 hours
Oral, sustained release: Adults: 150-300 mg every 12 hours; in difficult cases: 150 mg every 8 hours
Dosage Forms
Capsule, sustained release, as hydrochloride (Para-Time SR®): 150 mg
Injection, solution, as hydrochloride: 30 mg/mL (2 mL, 10 mL)

papaverine hydrochloride *see* papaverine *on this page*

Paplex® *(Discontinued)* *see page 1042*

parabromdylamine *see* brompheniramine *on page 128*

paracetamol *see* acetaminophen *on page 5*

Paradione® *(Discontinued)* *see page 1042*

Paraflex® *(Discontinued)* *see page 1042*

Parafon Forte® [Can] *see* chlorzoxazone *on page 196*

Parafon Forte® DSC [US] *see* chlorzoxazone *on page 196*

Para-Hist AT® *(Discontinued)* *see page 1042*

paraldehyde *(Discontinued)* *see page 1042*

Paraplatin® [US] *see* carboplatin *on page 160*

Paraplatin-AQ [Can] *see* carboplatin *on page 160*

parathyroid hormone (1-34) *see* teriparatide *on page 847*

Para-Time S.R.® [US] *see* papaverine *on this page*

Par Decon® *(Discontinued)* *see page 1042*

Paredrine® *(Discontinued)* *see page 1042*

paregoric (par e GOR ik)

Sound-Alike/Look-Alike Issues

paregoric may be confused with opium tincture, Percogesic®

Synonyms camphorated tincture of opium

Therapeutic Category Analgesic, Narcotic

Controlled Substance C-III

Use Treatment of diarrhea or relief of pain; neonatal opiate withdrawal

Usual Dosage Oral:

Neonatal opiate withdrawal: 3-6 drops every 3-6 hours as needed, or initially 0.2 mL every 3 hours; increase dosage by approximately 0.05 mL every 3 hours until withdrawal symptoms are controlled; it is rare to exceed 0.7 mL/dose. Stabilize withdrawal symptoms for 3-5 days, then gradually decrease dosage over a 2- to 4-week period.

Children: 0.25-0.5 mL/kg 1-4 times/day

Adults: 5-10 mL 1-4 times/day

Dosage Forms Liquid: 2 mg morphine equivalent/5 mL (473 mL) [equivalent to 20 mg opium powder; contains alcohol 45% and benzoic acid; licorice flavor]

Paremyd® Ophthalmic *(Discontinued)* *see page 1042*

Parepectolin® *(Discontinued)* *see page 1042*

Pargen Fortified® *(Discontinued)* *see page 1042*

Par Glycerol® *(Discontinued)* *see page 1042*

paricalcitol (par eh CAL ci tol)

U.S./Canadian Brand Names Zemplar™ [US/Can]

Therapeutic Category Vitamin D Analog

Use Prevention and treatment of secondary hyperparathyroidism associated with chronic renal failure. Has been evaluated only in hemodialysis patients.

Usual Dosage Children >5 years and Adults: I.V.: 0.04-0.1 mcg/kg (2.8-7 mcg) given as a bolus dose no more frequently than every other day at any time during dialysis; doses as high as 0.24 mcg/kg (16.8 mcg) have been administered safely; usually start with 0.04 mcg/kg 3 times/week by I.V. bolus, increased by 0.04 mcg/kg every 2 weeks; the dose of paricalcitol should be adjusted based on serum PTH levels, as follows:

Same or increasing serum PTH level: Increase paricalcitol dose

Serum PTH level decreased by <30%: Increase paricalcitol dose

Serum PTH level decreased by >30% and <60%: Maintain paricalcitol dose

Serum PTH level decrease by >60%: Decrease paricalcitol dose

Serum PTH level 1.5-3 times upper limit of normal: Maintain paricalcitol dose

Dosage Forms Injection, solution: 5 mcg/mL (1 mL, 2 mL) [contains alcohol]

Pariet® [Can] *see* rabeprazole *on page 758*

pariprazole *see* rabeprazole *on page 758*

Parlodel® [US/Can] *see* bromocriptine *on page 128*

Parnate® [US/Can] *see* tranylcypromine *on page 877*

paromomycin (par oh moe MYE sin)

Synonyms paromomycin sulfate

U.S./Canadian Brand Names Humatin® [US/Can]

Therapeutic Category Amebicide

Use Treatment of acute and chronic intestinal amebiasis; hepatic coma

Usual Dosage Oral:

Intestinal amebiasis: Children and Adults: 25-35 mg/kg/day in 3 divided doses for 5-10 days

Dientamoeba fragilis: Children and Adults: 25-30 mg/kg/day in 3 divided doses for 7 days

Tapeworm (fish, dog, bovine, porcine):

Children: 11 mg/kg every 15 minutes for 4 doses

(Continued)

paromomycin *(Continued)*

Adults: 1 g every 15 minutes for 4 doses
Hepatic coma: Adults: 4 g/day in 2-4 divided doses for 5-6 days
Dwarf tapeworm: Children and Adults: 45 mg/kg/dose every day for 5-7 days

Dosage Forms Capsule, as sulfate: 250 mg

paromomycin sulfate *see* paromomycin *on previous page*

paroxetine (pa ROKS e teen)

Sound-Alike/Look-Alike Issues
paroxetine may be confused with paclitaxel, pyridoxine
Paxil® may be confused with Doxil®, paclitaxel, Plavix®, Taxol®

Synonyms paroxetine hydrochloride; paroxetine mesylate

U.S./Canadian Brand Names Paxil® [US/Can]; Paxil® CR™ [US/Can]; Pexeva™ [US]

Therapeutic Category Antidepressant, Selective Serotonin Reuptake Inhibitor

Use Treatment of depression in adults; treatment of panic disorder with or without agoraphobia; obsessive-compulsive disorder (OCD) in adults; social anxiety disorder (social phobia); generalized anxiety disorder (GAD); post-traumatic stress disorder (PTSD)

Paxil CR™: Treatment of depression; panic disorder; premenstrual dysphoric disorder (PMDD); social anxiety disorder (social phobia)

Usual Dosage Oral:
Adults:
Depression:
Paxil®, Pexeva™: Initial: 20 mg once daily, preferably in the morning; increase if needed by 10 mg/day increments at intervals of at least 1 week; maximum dose: 50 mg/day
Paxil CR™: Initial: 25 mg once daily; increase if needed by 12.5 mg/day increments at intervals of at least 1 week; maximum dose: 62.5 mg/day
GAD (Paxil®): Initial: 20 mg once daily, preferably in the morning; doses of 20-50 mg/day were used in clinical trials, however, no greater benefit was seen with doses >20 mg. If dose is increased, adjust in increments of 10 mg/day at 1-week intervals.
OCD (Paxil®, Pexeva™): Initial: 20 mg once daily, preferably in the morning; increase if needed by 10 mg/day increments at intervals of at least 1 week; recommended dose: 40 mg/day; range: 20-60 mg/day; maximum dose: 60 mg/day
Panic disorder:
Paxil®, Pexeva™: Initial: 10 mg once daily, preferably in the morning; increase if needed by 10 mg/day increments at intervals of at least 1 week; recommended dose: 40 mg/day; range: 10-60 mg/day; maximum dose: 60 mg/day
Paxil CR™: Initial: 12.5 mg once daily; increase if needed by 12.5 mg/day at intervals of at least 1 week; maximum dose: 75 mg/day
PMDD (Paxil CR™): Initial: 12.5 mg once daily in the morning; may be increased to 25 mg/day; dosing changes should occur at intervals of at least 1 week. May be given daily throughout the menstrual cycle or limited to the luteal phase.
PTSD (Paxil®): Initial: 20 mg once daily, preferably in the morning; increase if needed by 10 mg/day increments at intervals of at least 1 week; range: 20-50 mg
Social anxiety disorder:
Paxil®: Initial: 20 mg once daily, preferably in the morning; recommended dose: 20 mg/day; range: 20-60 mg/day; doses >20 mg may not have additional benefit
Paxil CR™: Initial: 12.5 mg once daily, preferably in the morning; may be increased by 12.5 mg/day at intervals of at least 1 week; maximum dose: 37.5 mg/day

Dosage Forms Note: Available as paroxetine hydrochloride or mesylate; mg strength refers to paroxetine
Suspension, oral, as hydrochloride (Paxil®): 10 mg/5 mL (250 mL) [orange flavor]
Tablet, as hydrochloride (Paxil®): 10 mg, 20 mg, 30 mg, 40 mg
Tablet, as mesylate (Pexeva™): 10 mg, 20 mg, 30 mg, 40 mg
Tablet, controlled release, as hydrochloride (Paxil CR™): 12.5 mg, 25 mg, 37.5 mg

paroxetine hydrochloride *see* paroxetine *on previous page*

paroxetine mesylate *see* paroxetine *on previous page*

Parsidol® *(Discontinued)* *see page 1042*

Partuss® LA *(Discontinued)* *see page 1042*

Parvolex® [Can] *see* acetylcysteine *on page 16*

PAS *see* aminosalicylate sodium *on page 46*

Patanol® [US/Can] *see* olopatadine *on page 643*

Pathilon® *(Discontinued)* *see page 1042*

Pathocil® [Can] *see* dicloxacillin *on page 267*

Pathocil® *(Discontinued)* *see page 1042*

Pavabid® (all products) *(Discontinued)* *see page 1042*

Pavasule® *(Discontinued)* *see page 1042*

Pavatine® *(Discontinued)* *see page 1042*

Pavatym® *(Discontinued)* *see page 1042*

Pavesed® *(Discontinued)* *see page 1042*

Pavulon® *(Discontinued)* *see page 1042*

Paxene® *(Discontinued)* *see page 1042*

Paxil® [US/Can] *see* paroxetine *on previous page*

Paxil® CR™ [US/Can] *see* paroxetine *on previous page*

Paxipam® *(Discontinued)* *see page 1042*

PBZ® (all products) *(Discontinued)* *see page 1042*

PCA *see* procainamide *on page 730*

PCE® [US/Can] *see* erythromycin *on page 320*

PCEC *see* rabies virus vaccine *on page 759*

PCM [US] *see* chlorpheniramine, phenylephrine, and methscopolamine *on page 192*

PCM Allergy [US] *see* chlorpheniramine, phenylephrine, and methscopolamine *on page 192*

PCV7 *see* pneumococcal conjugate vaccine (7-valent) *on page 703*

pectin and kaolin *see* kaolin and pectin *on page 493*

pectin, gelatin, and methylcellulose *see* gelatin, pectin, and methylcellulose *on page 399*

Pedameth® [US] *see* methionine *on page 564*

PediaCare® Cold and Allergy [US-OTC] *see* chlorpheniramine and pseudoephedrine *on page 189*

PediaCare® Decongestant Infants [US-OTC] *see* pseudoephedrine *on page 745*

Pediacare® Decongestant Plus Cough [US-OTC] *see* pseudoephedrine and dextromethorphan *on page 746*

PediaCare® Infants' Long-Acting Cough [US-OTC] *see* dextromethorphan *on page 261*

Pediacare® Long Acting Cough Plus Cold [US-OTC] *see* pseudoephedrine and dextromethorphan *on page 746*

Pediacof® [US] *see* chlorpheniramine, phenylephrine, codeine, and potassium iodide *on page 193*

Pediaflor® [US] *see* fluoride *on page 376*

Pediamist® [US-OTC] *see* sodium chloride *on page 810*

PediaPatch Transdermal Patch *(Discontinued)* *see page 1042*

Pediapred® [US/Can] *see* prednisolone (systemic) *on page 724*

Pedia-Profen™ *(Discontinued)* *see page 1042*

Pediatex™-D [US] *see* carbinoxamine and pseudoephedrine *on page 157*

Pediatex™-DM [US] *see* carbinoxamine, pseudoephedrine, and dextromethorphan *on page 159*

Pediatric Triban® *(Discontinued)* *see page 1042*

Pediatrix [Can] *see* acetaminophen *on page 5*

Pediazole® [US/Can] *see* erythromycin and sulfisoxazole *on page 321*

Pedi-Boro® [US-OTC] *see* aluminum sulfate and calcium acetate *on page 41*

Pedi-Dri® [US] *see* nystatin *on page 637*

PediOtic® [US] *see* neomycin, polymyxin B, and hydrocortisone *on page 611*

Pedisilk® [US-OTC] *see* salicylic acid *on page 789*

Pedtrace-4® [US] *see* trace metals *on page 874*

PedvaxHIB® [US/Can] *see* *Haemophilus* B conjugate vaccine *on page 426*

pegademase (bovine) (peg A de mase BOE vine)

U.S./Canadian Brand Names Adagen™ [US/Can]

Therapeutic Category Enzyme

Use **Orphan drug:** Enzyme replacement therapy for adenosine deaminase (ADA) deficiency in patients with severe combined immunodeficiency disease (SCID) who can not benefit from bone marrow transplant; not a cure for SCID, unlike bone marrow transplants, injections must be used the rest of the child's life, therefore is not really an alternative

Usual Dosage Children: I.M.: Dose given every 7 days, 10 units/kg the first dose, 15 units/kg the second dose, and 20 units/kg the third dose; maintenance dose: 20 units/kg/week is recommended depending on patient's ADA level; maximum single dose: 30 units/kg

Dosage Forms Injection, solution: 250 units/mL (1.5 mL)

Peganone® [US/Can] *see* ethotoin *on page 349*

pegaspargase (peg AS par jase)

Sound-Alike/Look-Alike Issues

pegaspargase may be confused with asparaginase

Synonyms NSC-644954; PEG-L-asparaginase

U.S./Canadian Brand Names Oncaspar® [US]

Therapeutic Category Antineoplastic Agent

Use Treatment of acute lymphocytic leukemia, blast crisis of chronic lymphocytic leukemia (CLL), salvage therapy of non-Hodgkin lymphoma; may be used in some patients who have had hypersensitivity reactions to *E. coli* asparaginase

Usual Dosage Refer to individual protocols.

I.M. administration is **preferred** over I.V. administration; I.M. administration may decrease the incidence of hepatotoxicity, coagulopathy, and GI and renal disorders

Children: I.M., I.V.:

Body surface area <0.6 m^2: 82.5 int. units/kg every 14 days

Body surface area ≥0.6 m^2: 2500 int. units/m^2 every 14 days

Adults: I.M., I.V.: 2500 int. units/m^2 every 14 days

Dosage Forms Injection, solution [preservative free]: 750 units/mL (5 mL)

Pegasys® [US/Can] *see* peginterferon alfa-2a *on next page*

pegfilgrastim (peg fil GRA stim)

Synonyms G-CSF (PEG conjugate); granulocyte colony stimulating factor (PEG conjugate)

U.S./Canadian Brand Names Neulasta™ [US]

Therapeutic Category Colony-Stimulating Factor

Use Decrease the incidence of infection, by stimulation of granulocyte production, in patients with nonmyeloid malignancies receiving myelosuppressive therapy associated with a significant risk of febrile neutropenia

Usual Dosage SubQ: Adolescents >45 kg and Adults: 6 mg once per chemotherapy cycle; do not administer in the period between 14 days before and 24 hours after administration of cytotoxic chemotherapy; do not use in patients, infants, children, and smaller adolescents weighing <45 kg

Dosage Forms Injection, solution [preservative free]: 10 mg/mL (0.6 mL) [prefilled syringe]

peginterferon alfa-2a (peg in ter FEER on AL fa-too aye)

Synonyms interferon alfa-2a (PEG conjugate); pegylated interferon alfa-2a

U.S./Canadian Brand Names Pegasys® [US/Can]

Therapeutic Category Interferon

Use Treatment of chronic hepatitis C, alone or in combination with ribavirin, in patients with compensated liver disease

Usual Dosage SubQ: Adults: Chronic hepatitis C:

Monotherapy: 180 mcg once weekly for 48 weeks

Combination therapy with ribavirin: Recommended dosage: 180 mcg once/week with ribavirin (Copegus™)

Note: Duration of therapy based on genotype:

Genotype 1,4: Treat for 48 weeks

Genotype 2,3: Treat for 24 weeks

Dose modification:

For moderate to severe adverse reactions: Initial: 135 mcg/week; may need decreased to 90 mcg/week in some cases

Based on hematologic parameters:

ANC <750/mm^3: 135 mcg/week

ANC <500/mm^3: Suspend therapy until >1000/mm^3, then restart at 90 mcg/week and monitor

Platelet count <50,000/mm^3: 90 mcg/week

Platelet count <25,000/mm^3: Discontinue therapy

Depression (severity based on DSM-IV criteria):

Mild depression: No dosage adjustment required; evaluate once weekly by visit/phone call. If depression remains stable, continue weekly visits. If depression improves, resume normal visit schedule

Moderate depression: Decrease interferon dose to 90-135 mcg once/week; evaluate once weekly with an office visit at least every other week. If depression remains stable, consider psychiatric evaluation and continue with reduced dosing. If symptoms improve and remain stable for 4 weeks, resume normal visit schedule; continue reduced dosing or return to normal dose.

Severe depression: Discontinue interferon permanently. Obtain immediate psychiatric consultation. Discontinue ribavirin if using concurrently.

Dosage Forms

Injection, solution: 180 mcg/mL (1.2 mL) [contains benzyl alcohol]

Injection, solution [prefilled syringe]: 180 mcg/mL (0.5 mL) [contains benzyl alcohol; packaged with needles and alcohol swabs]

peginterferon alfa-2b (peg in ter FEER on AL fa-too bee)

Synonyms interferon alfa-2b (PEG conjugate); pegylated interferon alfa-2b

U.S./Canadian Brand Names PEG-Intron™ [US/Can]

Therapeutic Category Interferon

(Continued)

peginterferon alfa-2b *(Continued)*

Use Treatment of chronic hepatitis C (as monotherapy or in combination with ribavirin) in adult patients who have never received interferon alpha and have compensated liver disease

Usual Dosage SubQ:

Children: Safety and efficacy have not been established

Adults: Chronic hepatitis C: Administer dose once weekly; **Note:** Usual duration is for 1 year; after 24 weeks of treatment, if serum HCV RNA is not below the limit of detection of the assay, consider discontinuation:

Monotherapy: Initial:
- ≤45 kg: 40 mcg
- 46-56 kg: 50 mcg
- 57-72 kg: 64 mcg
- 73-88 kg: 80 mcg
- 89-106 kg: 96 mcg
- 107-136 kg: 120 mcg
- 137-160 kg: 150 mcg

Combination therapy with ribavirin (400 mg twice daily): Initial: 1.5 mcg/kg/week
- <40 kg: 50 mcg
- 40-50 kg: 64 mcg
- 51-60 kg: 80 mcg
- 61-75 kg: 96 mcg
- 76-85 kg: 120 mcg
- >85 kg: 150 mcg

Dosage adjustment if serious adverse event occurs: Depression (severity based upon DSM-IV criteria):

Mild depression: No dosage adjustment required; evaluate once weekly by visit/phone call. If depression remains stable, continue weekly visits. If depression improves, resume normal visit schedule.

Moderate depression: Decrease interferon dose by 50%; evaluate once weekly with an office visit at least every other week. If depression remains stable, consider psychiatric evaluation and continue with reduced dosing. If symptoms improve and remain stable for 4 weeks, resume normal visit schedule; continue reduced dosing or return to normal dose.

Severe depression: Discontinue interferon and ribavirin permanently. Obtain immediate psychiatric consultation.

Dosage Forms

Injection, powder for reconstitution [prefilled syringe] (Redipen™): 50 mcg, 80 mcg, 120 mcg, 150 mcg [packaged with alcohol swabs and needle for injection]

Injection, powder for reconstitution [vial]: 50 mcg, 80 mcg, 120 mcg, 150 mcg [packaged with SWFI, alcohol swabs, and syringes]

PEG-Intron™ [US/Can] *see* peginterferon alfa-2b *on previous page*

PEG-L-asparaginase *see* pegaspargase *on page 670*

PegLyte® [Can] *see* polyethylene glycol-electrolyte solution *on page 706*

pegvisomant (peg VI soe mant)

Synonyms B2036-PEG

U.S./Canadian Brand Names Somavert® [US]

Therapeutic Category Growth Hormone Receptor Antagonist

Use Treatment of acromegaly in patients resistant to or unable to tolerate other therapies

Usual Dosage SubQ: Adults: Initial loading dose: 40 mg; maintenance dose: 10 mg once daily; doses may be adjusted by 5 mg in 4- to 6-week intervals based on IGF-I concentrations (maximum dose: 30 mg/day)

Dosage Forms Injection, powder for reconstitution [preservative free]: 10 mg, 15 mg, 20 mg [vial stopper contains latex; packaged with SWFI]

pegylated interferon alfa-2a *see* peginterferon alfa-2a *on page 671*

pegylated interferon alfa-2b *see* peginterferon alfa-2b *on page 671*

PemADD® [US] *see* pemoline *on this page*

PemADD® CT [US] *see* pemoline *on this page*

pemetrexed (pem e TREKS ed)

Synonyms LY231514; MTA; multitargeted antifolate; NSC-698037; pemetrexed disodium

U.S./Canadian Brand Names Alimta® [US]

Therapeutic Category Antineoplastic Agent, Antimetabolite; Antineoplastic Agent, Antimetabolite (Antifolate)

Use Treatment of malignant pleural mesothelioma in combination with cisplatin; treatment of nonsmall-cell lung cancer

Usual Dosage I.V.: Adults:

Nonsmall-cell lung cancer: 500 mg/m^2 on day 1 of each 21-day cycle

Malignant pleural mesothelioma: 500-600 mg/m^2 on day 1 of each 21-day cycle in combination with cisplatin

Note: Start vitamin supplements 1 week before initial dose of pemetrexed. Folic acid 350-1000 mcg/day orally (continuing for 21 days after last dose of pemetrexed) and vitamin B_{12} 1000 mcg I.M. every 9 weeks. Dexamethasone 4 mg twice daily can be started the day before therapy, and continued the day of and the day after to minimize cutaneous reactions.

Dosage Forms Injection, powder for reconstitution: 500 mg

pemetrexed disodium *see* pemetrexed *on this page*

pemirolast (pe MIR oh last)

U.S./Canadian Brand Names Alamast™ [US/Can]

Therapeutic Category Mast Cell Stabilizer; Ophthalmic Agent, Miscellaneous

Use Prevention of itching of the eye due to allergic conjunctivitis

Usual Dosage Children >3 years and Adults: 1-2 drops instilled in affected eye(s) 4 times/day

Dosage Forms Solution, ophthalmic, as potassium: 0.1% (10 mL)

pemoline (PEM oh leen)

Synonyms phenylisohydantoin; PIO

U.S./Canadian Brand Names Cylert® [US]; PemADD® [US]; PemADD® CT [US]

Therapeutic Category Central Nervous System Stimulant, Nonamphetamine

Controlled Substance C-IV

Use Treatment of attention-deficit/hyperactivity disorder (ADHD) (not first-line)

Usual Dosage Children ≥6 years: Oral: Initial: 37.5 mg given once daily in the morning, increase by 18.75 mg/day at weekly intervals; usual effective dose range: 56.25-75 mg/day; maximum: 112.5 mg/day; dosage range: 0.5-3 mg/kg/24 hours; significant benefit may not be evident until third or fourth week of administration

Dosage Forms

Tablet (Cylert®, PemADD®): 18.75 mg, 37.5 mg, 75 mg

Tablet, chewable (Cylert®, PemADD® CT): 37.5 mg

penbutolol (pen BYOO toe lole)

Sound-Alike/Look-Alike Issues

Levatol® may be confused with Lipitor®

Synonyms penbutolol sulfate

U.S./Canadian Brand Names Levatol® [US/Can]

Therapeutic Category Beta-Adrenergic Blocker

Use Treatment of mild to moderate arterial hypertension

(Continued)

penbutolol *(Continued)*

Usual Dosage Adults: Oral: Initial: 20 mg once daily, full effect of a 20 or 40 mg dose is seen by the end of a 2-week period, doses of 40-80 mg have been tolerated but have shown little additional antihypertensive effects; usual dose range (JNC 7): 10-40 mg once daily

Dosage Forms Tablet, as sulfate: 20 mg

penbutolol sulfate *see* penbutolol *on previous page*

penciclovir (pen SYE kloe veer)

Sound-Alike/Look-Alike Issues

Denavir® may be confused with indinavir

U.S./Canadian Brand Names Denavir™ [US]

Therapeutic Category Antiviral Agent

Use Topical treatment of herpes simplex labialis (cold sores)

Usual Dosage Children ≥12 years and Adults: Topical: Apply cream at the first sign or symptom of cold sore (eg, tingling, swelling); apply every 2 hours during waking hours for 4 days

Dosage Forms Cream: 1% (1.5 g)

Penetrex® ***(Discontinued)*** *see page 1042*

penicillamine (pen i SIL a meen)

Sound-Alike/Look-Alike Issues

penicillamine may be confused with penicillin

Depen® may be confused with Endal®

Synonyms D-3-mercaptovaline; β,β-dimethylcysteine; D-penicillamine

U.S./Canadian Brand Names Cuprimine® [US/Can]; Depen® [US/Can]

Therapeutic Category Chelating Agent

Use Treatment of Wilson's disease, cystinuria, adjunct in the treatment of rheumatoid arthritis

Usual Dosage Oral:

Rheumatoid arthritis:

Children: Initial: 3 mg/kg/day (≤250 mg/day) for 3 months, then 6 mg/kg/day (≤500 mg/day) in divided doses twice daily for 3 months to a maximum of 10 mg/kg/day in 3-4 divided doses

Adults: 125-250 mg/day, may increase dose at 1- to 3-month intervals up to 1-1.5 g/day (maximum in older adults: 750 mg/day)

Wilson's disease (doses titrated to maintain urinary copper excretion >1 mg/day)

Infants <6 months: 250 mg/dose once daily

Children <12 years: 250 mg/dose 2-3 times/day

Adults: 250 mg 4 times/day (maximum in older adults: 750 mg/day)

Cystinuria:

Children: 30 mg/kg/day in 4 divided doses

Adults: 1-4 g/day in divided doses every 6 hours lead level is <15 mcg/dL; may also be used in other heavy metal poisoning:

Children: 25-35 mg/kg/day, administered in 3-4 divided doses; initiating treatment at 25% of this dose and gradually increasing to the full dose over 2-3 weeks may minimize adverse reactions

Adults: 250-500 mg/dose every 8-12 hours

Primary biliary cirrhosis: 250 mg/day to start, increase by 250 mg every 2 weeks up to a maintenance dose of 1 g/day, usually given 250 mg 4 times/day

Arsenic poisoning: Children: 100 mg/kg/day in divided doses every 6 hours for 5 days; maximum: 1 g/day

Dosage Forms

Capsule (Cuprimine®): 125 mg, 250 mg

Tablet (Depen®): 250 mg

penicillin G benzathine (pen i SIL in jee BENZ a theen)

Sound-Alike/Look-Alike Issues
Bicillin® may be confused with Wycillin®

Synonyms benzathine benzylpenicillin; benzathine penicillin G; benzylpenicillin benzathine

U.S./Canadian Brand Names Bicillin® L-A [US]; Permapen® Isoject® [US]

Therapeutic Category Penicillin

Use Active against some gram-positive organisms, few gram-negative organisms such as *Neisseria gonorrhoeae*, and some anaerobes and spirochetes; used in the treatment of syphilis; used only for the treatment of mild to moderately severe infections caused by organisms susceptible to low concentrations of penicillin G or for prophylaxis of infections caused by these organisms

Usual Dosage I.M.: Administer undiluted injection; higher doses result in more sustained rather than higher levels. Use a penicillin G benzathine-penicillin G procaine combination to achieve early peak levels in acute infections.

Infants and Children:
- Group A streptococcal upper respiratory infection: 25,000-50,000 units/kg as a single dose; maximum: 1.2 million units
- Prophylaxis of recurrent rheumatic fever: 25,000-50,000 units/kg every 3-4 weeks; maximum: 1.2 million units/dose
- Early syphilis: 50,000 units/kg as a single injection; maximum: 2.4 million units
- Syphilis of more than 1-year duration: 50,000 units/kg every week for 3 doses; maximum: 2.4 million units/dose

Adults:
- Group A streptococcal upper respiratory infection: 1.2 million units as a single dose
- Prophylaxis of recurrent rheumatic fever: 1.2 million units every 3-4 weeks or 600,000 units twice monthly
- Early syphilis: 2.4 million units as a single dose in 2 injection sites
- Syphilis of more than 1-year duration: 2.4 million units in 2 injection sites once weekly for 3 doses
- Not indicated as single drug therapy for neurosyphilis, but may be given 1 time/week for 3 weeks following I.V. treatment; refer to Penicillin G Parenteral/Aqueous monograph for dosing

Dosage Forms Injection, suspension [prefilled syringe]:
Bicillin® L-A: 600,000 units/mL (1 mL, 2 mL, 4 mL)
Permapen® Isoject®: 600,000 units/mL (2 mL)

penicillin G benzathine and penicillin G procaine

(pen i SIL in jee BENZ a theen & pen i SIL in jee PROE kane)

Sound-Alike/Look-Alike Issues
Bicillin® may be confused with Wycillin®

Synonyms penicillin G procaine and benzathine combined

U.S./Canadian Brand Names Bicillin® C-R 900/300 [US]; Bicillin® C-R [US]

Therapeutic Category Penicillin

Use May be used in specific situations in the treatment of streptococcal infections

Usual Dosage I.M.:

Children:
- <30 lb: 600,000 units in a single dose
- 30-60 lb: 900,000 units to 1.2 million units in a single dose

Children >60 lb and Adults: 2.4 million units in a single dose

Dosage Forms Injection, suspension [prefilled syringe]:
Bicillin® C-R:
- 600,000 units: Penicillin G benzathine 300,000 units and penicillin G procaine 300,000 units per 1 mL (1 mL)
- 1,200,000 units: Penicillin G benzathine 600,000 units and penicillin G procaine 600,000 units per 2 mL (2 mL)

(Continued)

penicillin G benzathine and penicillin G procaine *(Continued)*

2,400,000 units: Penicillin G benzathine 1,200,000 units and penicillin G procaine 1,200,000 units per 4 mL (4 mL)

Bicillin® C-R 900/300: 1,200,000 units: Penicillin G benzathine 900,000 units and penicillin G procaine 300,000 units per 2 mL (2 mL)

penicillin G (parenteral/aqueous)

(pen i SIL in jee pa REN ter al/AYE kwee us)

Sound-Alike/Look-Alike Issues

Penicillin may be confused with penicillamine

Synonyms benzylpenicillin potassium; benzylpenicillin sodium; crystalline penicillin; penicillin G potassium; penicillin G sodium

U.S./Canadian Brand Names Pfizerpen® [US/Can]

Therapeutic Category Penicillin

Use Active against some gram-positive organisms, generally not *Staphylococcus aureus*; some gram-negative organisms such as *Neisseria gonorrhoeae*, and some anaerobes and spirochetes

Usual Dosage I.M., I.V.:

Infants:

<7 days, <2000 g: 50,000 units/kg/day in divided doses every 12 hours

<7 days, >2000 g: 50,000 units/kg/day in divided doses every 8 hours

>7 days, <2000 g: 75,000 units/kg/day in divided doses every 8 hours

>7 days, >2000 g: 100,000 units/kg/day in divided doses every 6 hours

Infants and Children (sodium salt is preferred in children): 100,000-250,000 units/kg/day in divided doses every 4 hours

Severe infections: Up to 400,000 units/kg/day in divided doses every 4 hours; maximum dose: 24 million units/day

Congenital syphilis:

Newborns: 50,000 units/kg/day I.V. every 8-12 hours for 10-14 days

Infants: 50,000 units/kg every 4-6 hours for 10-14 days

Disseminated gonococcal infections or gonococcus ophthalmia (if organism proven sensitive): 100,000 units/kg/day in 2 equal doses (4 equal doses/day for infants >1 week)

Gonococcal meningitis: 150,000 units/kg in 2 equal doses (4 doses/day for infants >1 week)

Adults: 2-24 million units/day in divided doses every 4 hours depending on sensitivity of the organism and severity of the infection

Neurosyphilis: 18-24 million units/day in divided doses every 3-4 hours for 10-14 days

Dosage Forms

Infusion, as potassium [premixed iso-osmotic dextrose solution, frozen]: 1 million units (50 mL), 2 million units (50 mL), 3 million units (50 mL)

Injection, powder for reconstitution, as potassium (Pfizerpen®): 5 million units, 20 million units

Injection, powder for reconstitution, as sodium: 5 million units

penicillin G potassium *see* penicillin G (parenteral/aqueous) *on this page*

penicillin G procaine (pen i SIL in jee PROE kane)

Sound-Alike/Look-Alike Issues

Penicillin G procaine may be confused with penicillin V potassium

Wycillin® may be confused with Bicillin®

Synonyms APPG; aqueous procaine penicillin G; procaine benzylpenicillin; procaine penicillin G

U.S./Canadian Brand Names Pfizerpen-AS® [Can]; Wycillin® [Can]

Therapeutic Category Penicillin

Use Moderately severe infections due to *Treponema pallidum* and other penicillin G-sensitive microorganisms that are susceptible to low, but prolonged serum penicillin concentrations; anthrax due to *Bacillus anthracis* (postexposure) to reduce the incidence or progression of disease following exposure to aerolized *Bacillus anthracis*

Usual Dosage I.M.:

Children: 25,000-50,000 units/kg/day in divided doses 1-2 times/day; not to exceed 4.8 million units/24 hours

Anthrax, inhalational (postexposure prophylaxis): 25,000 units/kg every 12 hours (maximum: 1,200,000 units every 12 hours); see "Note" in Adults dosing

Congenital syphilis: 50,000 units/kg/day for 10-14 days

Adults: 0.6-4.8 million units/day in divided doses every 12-24 hours

Anthrax:

Inhalational (postexposure prophylaxis): 1,200,000 units every 12 hours

Note: Overall treatment duration should be 60 days. Available safety data suggest continued administration of penicillin G procaine for longer than 2 weeks may incur additional risk for adverse reactions. Clinicians may consider switching to effective alternative treatment for completion of therapy beyond 2 weeks.

Cutaneous (treatment): 600,000-1,200,000 units/day; alternative therapy is recommended in severe cutaneous or other forms of anthrax infection

Endocarditis caused by susceptible viridans *Streptococcus* (when used in conjunction with an aminoglycoside): 1.2 million units every 6 hours for 2-4 weeks

Neurosyphilis: I.M.: 2-4 million units/day with 500 mg probenecid by mouth 4 times/day for 10-14 days; **penicillin G aqueous I.V. is the preferred agent**

Dosage Forms Injection, suspension: 600,000 units/mL (1 mL, 2 mL)

penicillin G procaine and benzathine combined *see* penicillin G benzathine and penicillin G procaine *on page 675*

penicillin G sodium *see* penicillin G (parenteral/aqueous) *on previous page*

penicillin V potassium (pen i SIL in vee poe TASS ee um)

Sound-Alike/Look-Alike Issues

penicillin V procaine may be confused with penicillin G potassium

Synonyms pen VK; phenoxymethyl penicillin

U.S./Canadian Brand Names Apo-Pen VK® [Can]; Nadopen-V® [Can]; Novo-Pen-VK® [Can]; Nu-Pen-VK® [Can]; PVF® K [Can]; Veetids® [US]

Therapeutic Category Penicillin

Use Treatment of infections caused by susceptible organisms involving the respiratory tract, otitis media, sinusitis, skin, and urinary tract; prophylaxis in rheumatic fever

Usual Dosage Oral:

Systemic infections:

Children <12 years: 25-50 mg/kg/day in divided doses every 6-8 hours; maximum dose: 3 g/day

Children ≥12 years and Adults: 125-500 mg every 6-8 hours

Prophylaxis of pneumococcal infections:

Children <5 years: 125 mg twice daily

Children ≥5 years and Adults: 250 mg twice daily

Prophylaxis of recurrent rheumatic fever:

Children <5 years: 125 mg twice daily

Children ≥5 years and Adults: 250 mg twice daily

Dosage Forms Note: 250 mg = 400,000 units

Powder for oral solution: 125 mg/5 mL (100 mL, 200 mL); 250 mg/5 mL (100 mL, 200 mL)

Tablet: 250 mg, 500 mg

penicilloyl-polylysine *see* benzylpenicilloyl-polylysine *on page 112*

Penlac™ [US/Can] *see* ciclopirox *on page 198*

Pennsaid® [Can] *see* diclofenac *on page 266*

Pentacarinat® [Can] *see* pentamidine *on next page*

Pentacarinat® Injection *(Discontinued)* *see page 1042*

pentahydrate *see* sodium thiosulfate *on page 817*

Pentam-300® [US] *see* pentamidine *on this page*

pentamidine (pen TAM i deen)

Synonyms pentamidine isethionate

U.S./Canadian Brand Names NebuPent® [US]; Pentacarinat® [Can]; Pentam-300® [US]

Therapeutic Category Antiprotozoal

Use Treatment and prevention of pneumonia caused by *Pneumocystis carinii* (PCP)

Usual Dosage

Children:

Treatment of PCP pneumonia: I.M., I.V. (I.V. preferred): 4 mg/kg/day once daily for 10-14 days

Prevention of PCP pneumonia:

I.M., I.V.: 4 mg/kg monthly or every 2 weeks

Inhalation (aerosolized pentamidine in children ≥5 years): 300 mg/dose given every 3-4 weeks via Respirgard® II inhaler (8 mg/kg dose has also been used in children <5 years)

Adults:

Treatment: I.M., I.V. (I.V. preferred): 4 mg/kg/day once daily for 14-21 days

Prevention: Inhalation: 300 mg every 4 weeks via Respirgard® II nebulizer

Dialysis: Not removed by hemo or peritoneal dialysis or continuous arteriovenous or venovenous hemofiltration; supplemental dosage is not necessary

Dosage Forms

Injection, powder for reconstitution, as isethionate (Pentam® 300): 300 mg

Powder for nebulization, as isethionate (NebuPent®): 300 mg

pentamidine isethionate *see* pentamidine *on this page*

Pentamycetin® [Can] *see* chloramphenicol *on page 182*

Pentasa® [US/Can] *see* mesalamine *on page 556*

Pentaspan® [US/Can] *see* pentastarch *on this page*

pentastarch (PEN ta starch)

U.S./Canadian Brand Names Pentaspan® [US/Can]

Therapeutic Category Blood Modifiers

Use Orphan drug: Adjunct in leukapheresis to improve harvesting and increase yield of leukocytes by centrifugal means

Usual Dosage 250-700 mL to which citrate anticoagulant has been added is administered by adding to the input line of the centrifugation apparatus at a ratio of 1:8-1:13 to venous whole blood

Dosage Forms Infusion [premixed in NS]: 10% (500 mL)

Penta-Triamterene HCTZ [Can] *see* hydrochlorothiazide and triamterene *on page 443*

pentazocine (pen TAZ oh seen)

Synonyms naloxone hydrochloride and pentazocine hydrochloride; pentazocine hydrochloride; pentazocine hydrochloride and naloxone hydrochloride; pentazocine lactate

U.S./Canadian Brand Names Talwin® NX [US]; Talwin® [US/Can]

Therapeutic Category Analgesic, Narcotic

Controlled Substance C-IV

Use Relief of moderate to severe pain; has also been used as a sedative prior to surgery and as a supplement to surgical anesthesia

Usual Dosage

Preoperative/pre-anesthetic: Children 1-16 years: I.M.: 0.5 mg/kg

Analgesia:
Children: I.M.:
5-8 years: 15 mg
8-14 years: 30 mg
Children >12 years and Adults: Oral: 50 mg every 3-4 hours; may increase to 100 mg/dose if needed, but should not exceed 600 mg/day
Adults:
I.M., SubQ: 30-60 mg every 3-4 hours, not to exceed total daily dose of 360 mg
I.V.: 30 mg every 3-4 hours (maximum: 360 mg/day)

Dosage Forms
Injection, solution, as lactate (Talwin®): 30 mg/mL (1 mL, 2 mL, 10 mL) [multidose vial and prefilled syringe contain sodium bisulfite]
Tablet (Talwin® NX): Pentazocine hydrochloride 50 mg and naloxone hydrochloride 0.5 mg

pentazocine and acetaminophen (pen TAZ oh seen & a seet a MIN oh fen)

Therapeutic Category Analgesic, Narcotic
Use Relief of moderate to severe pain; has also been used as a sedative prior to surgery and as a supplement to surgical anesthesia
Usual Dosage Adults: Oral: 2 tablets 3-4 times/day
Dosage Forms Tablet:
Talacen®: Pentazocine hydrochloride 25 mg and acetaminophen 650 mg
Talwin® Compound: Pentazocine hydrochloride 12.5 mg and aspirin 325 mg

pentazocine hydrochloride *see* pentazocine *on previous page*

pentazocine hydrochloride and naloxone hydrochloride *see* pentazocine *on previous page*

pentazocine lactate *see* pentazocine *on previous page*

Penthrane® *(Discontinued)* *see page 1042*

Pentids® *(Discontinued)* *see page 1042*

pentobarbital (pen toe BAR bi tal)

Sound-Alike/Look-Alike Issues
pentobarbital may be confused with phenobarbital
Nembutal® may be confused with Myambutol®
Synonyms pentobarbital sodium
U.S./Canadian Brand Names Nembutal® [US]; Nembutal® Sodium [Can]
Therapeutic Category Barbiturate
Controlled Substance C-II
Use Sedative/hypnotic; preanesthetic; high-dose barbiturate coma for treatment of increased intracranial pressure or status epilepticus unresponsive to other therapy
Usual Dosage
Children:
Hypnotic: I.M.: 2-6 mg/kg; maximum: 100 mg/dose
Preoperative/preprocedure sedation: ≥6 months:
Note: Limited information is available for infants <6 months of age.
I.M.: 2-6 mg/kg; maximum: 100 mg/dose
I.V.: 1-3 mg/kg to a maximum of 100 mg until asleep
Conscious sedation prior to a procedure: Children 5-12 years: I.V.: 2 mg/kg 5-10 minutes before procedures, may repeat one time
Adolescents: Conscious sedation: I.V.: 100 mg prior to a procedure
Children and Adults: Barbiturate coma in head injury patients: I.V.: Loading dose: 5-10 mg/kg given slowly over 1-2 hours; monitor blood pressure and respiratory rate; Maintenance infusion: Initial: 1 mg/kg/hour; may increase to 2-3 mg/kg/hour; maintain burst suppression on EEG
Status epilepticus: I.V.: **Note**: Intubation required; monitor hemodynamics
(Continued)

pentobarbital *(Continued)*

Children: Loading dose: 5-15 mg/kg given slowly over 1-2 hours; maintenance infusion: 0.5-5 mg/kg/hour

Adults: Loading dose: 2-15 mg/kg given slowly over 1-2 hours; maintenance infusion: 0.5-3 mg/kg/hour

Adults:

Hypnotic:

I.M.: 150-200 mg

I.V.: Initial: 100 mg, may repeat every 1-3 minutes up to 200-500 mg total dose

Preoperative sedation: I.M.: 150-200 mg

Dosage Forms Injection, solution, as sodium: 50 mg/mL (20 mL, 50 mL) [contains alcohol 10%]

pentobarbital sodium *see* pentobarbital *on previous page*

pentosan polysulfate sodium (PEN toe san pol i SUL fate SOW dee um)

Sound-Alike/Look-Alike Issues

pentosan may be confused with pentostatin

Elmiron® may be confused with Imuran®

Synonyms PPS

U.S./Canadian Brand Names Elmiron® [US/Can]

Therapeutic Category Analgesic, Urinary

Use **Orphan drug:** Relief of bladder pain or discomfort due to interstitial cystitis

Usual Dosage Adults: Oral: 100 mg 3 times/day taken with water 1 hour before or 2 hours after meals

Patients should be evaluated at 3 months and may be continued an additional 3 months if there has been no improvement and if there are no therapy-limiting side effects. **The risks and benefits of continued use beyond 6 months in patients who have not responded is not yet known.**

Dosage Forms Capsule: 100 mg

pentostatin (PEN toe stat in)

Sound-Alike/Look-Alike Issues

pentostatin may be confused with pentosan

Synonyms CL-825; co-vidarabine; dCF; deoxycoformycin; 2′-deoxycoformycin; NSC-218321

U.S./Canadian Brand Names Nipent® [US/Can]

Therapeutic Category Antineoplastic Agent

Use Treatment of hairy cell leukemia; non-Hodgkin lymphoma, cutaneous T-cell lymphoma

Usual Dosage Refractory hairy cell leukemia: Adults (refer to individual protocols):

4 mg/m^2 every other week **or**

4 mg/m^2 weekly for 3 weeks, then every 2 weeks **or**

5 mg/m^2 daily for 3 days every 3 weeks

Dosage Forms Injection, powder for reconstitution: 10 mg

Pentothal® [US/Can] *see* thiopental *on page 857*

Pentothal® Sodium Rectal Suspension *(Discontinued)* *see page 1042*

pentoxifylline (pen toks I fi leen)

Sound-Alike/Look-Alike Issues

pentoxifylline may be confused with tamoxifen

Trental® may be confused with Bentyl®, Tegretol®, Trandate®

Synonyms oxpentifylline

U.S./Canadian Brand Names Albert® Pentoxifylline [Can]; Apo-Pentoxifylline SR® [Can]; Nu-Pentoxifylline SR [Can]; Pentoxil® [US]; ratio-Pentoxifylline [Can]; Trental® [US/Can]

Therapeutic Category Blood Viscosity Reducer Agent

Use Treatment of intermittent claudication on the basis of chronic occlusive arterial disease of the limbs; may improve function and symptoms, but not intended to replace more definitive therapy

Usual Dosage Adults: Oral: 400 mg 3 times/day with meals; may reduce to 400 mg twice daily if GI or CNS side effects occur

Dosage Forms

Tablet, controlled release (Trental®): 400 mg

Tablet, extended release (Pentoxil®): 400 mg

Pentoxil® [US] *see* pentoxifylline *on previous page*

Pentrax® [US-OTC] *see* coal tar *on page 219*

Pen.Vee® K ***(Discontinued)*** *see page 1042*

pen VK *see* penicillin V potassium *on page 677*

Pepcid® [US/Can] *see* famotidine *on page 356*

Pepcid® AC [US-OTC/Can] *see* famotidine *on page 356*

Pepcid® Complete [US-OTC/Can] *see* famotidine, calcium carbonate, and magnesium hydroxide *on page 357*

Pepcid® I.V. [Can] *see* famotidine *on page 356*

Pepcid RPD™ ***(Discontinued)*** *see page 1042*

Peptavlon® ***(Discontinued)*** *see page 1042*

Pepto-Bismol® Maximum Strength [US-OTC] *see* bismuth *on page 120*

Pepto-Bismol® [US-OTC] *see* bismuth *on page 120*

Pepto® Diarrhea Control ***(Discontinued)*** *see page 1042*

Perchloracap® [US] *see* radiological/contrast media (ionic) *on page 759*

Percocet® [US/Can] *see* oxycodone and acetaminophen *on page 656*

Percocet®-Demi [Can] *see* oxycodone and acetaminophen *on page 656*

Percodan® [US/Can] *see* oxycodone and aspirin *on page 657*

Percodan®-Demi ***(Discontinued)*** *see page 1042*

Percogesic® Extra Strength [US-OTC] *see* acetaminophen and diphenhydramine *on page 7*

Percogesic® [US-OTC] *see* acetaminophen and phenyltoloxamine *on page 8*

Percolone® ***(Discontinued)*** *see page 1042*

Perdiem® Fiber Therapy [US-OTC] *see* psyllium *on page 749*

Perfectoderm® Gel ***(Discontinued)*** *see page 1042*

perflutren lipid microspheres (per FLOO tren LIP id MIKE roe sfeers)

U.S./Canadian Brand Names Definity® [US/Can]

Therapeutic Category Diagnostic Agent

Use Opacification of left ventricular chamber and improvement of delineation of the left ventricular endocardial border in patients with suboptimal echocardiograms

Usual Dosage Adults: Dose should be given following baseline noncontrast echocardiography. Imaging should begin immediately following dose and compared to noncontrast image. Mechanical index for the ultrasound device should be set at ≤0.8.

I.V. bolus: 10 μL/kg of activated product, followed by 10 mL saline flush. May repeat in 30 minutes if needed (maximum dose: 2 bolus infusions).

I.V. infusion: Initial: 4 mL/minute of prepared infusion; titrate to achieve optimal image; maximum rate: 10 mL/minute (maximum dose: 1 intravenous infusion).

Dosage Forms Injection, solution [preservative free]: OFP 6.52 mg/mL and lipid blend 0.75 mg/mL (2 mL) [following activation, forms a suspension containing perflutren lipid microspheres 1.2 x 10^{10}/mL and OFP 1.1 mg/mL]

pergolide (PER go lide)

Sound-Alike/Look-Alike Issues

Permax® may be confused with Bumex®, Pentrax®, Pernox®

Synonyms pergolide mesylate

U.S./Canadian Brand Names Permax® [US/Can]

Therapeutic Category Anti-Parkinson Agent; Dopaminergic Agent (Anti-Parkinson); Ergot Alkaloid and Derivative

Use Adjunctive treatment to levodopa/carbidopa in the management of Parkinson disease

Usual Dosage When adding pergolide to levodopa/carbidopa, the dose of the latter can usually and should be decreased. Patients no longer responsive to bromocriptine may benefit by being switched to pergolide. Oral:

Adults: Parkinson disease: Start with 0.05 mg/day for 2 days, then increase dosage by 0.1 or 0.15 mg/day every 3 days over next 12 days, increase dose by 0.25 mg/day every 3 days until optimal therapeutic dose is achieved, up to 5 mg/day maximum; usual dosage range: 2-3 mg/day in 3 divided doses

Dosage Forms Tablet, as mesylate: 0.05 mg, 0.25 mg, 1 mg

pergolide mesylate *see* pergolide *on this page*

Pergonal® [US/Can] *see* menotropins *on page 551*

Periactin® [Can] *see* cyproheptadine *on page 237*

Periactin® *(Discontinued)* *see page 1042*

Peri-Colace® *(Discontinued)* *see page 1042*

Peri-Colace® *(reformulation)* [US-OTC] *see* docusate and senna *on page 286*

pericyazine *(Canada only)* (per ee CYE ah zeen)

Therapeutic Category Phenothiazine Derivative

Use As adjunctive medication in some psychotic patients, for the control of residual prevailing hostility, impulsiveness and aggressiveness

Usual Dosage Oral:

Children and adolescents (5 years of age and over): 2.5-10 mg in the morning and 5-30 mg in the evening. These dosages approximate a daily dosage range of 1-3 mg/year of age.

Adults: 5-20 mg in the morning and 10-40 mg in the evening. For maintenance therapy, the dosage should be reduced to the minimum effective dose. Lower doses of 2.5-15 mg in the morning, and 5-30 mg in the evening have been suggested. For elderly patients the initial total daily dosage should be in the order of 5 mg and increased gradually as tolerated, until an adequate response is obtained. A daily dosage of more than 30 mg will rarely be needed. Children and adolescents (5 years of age and over): 2.5-10 mg in the morning and 5-30 mg in the evening. These dosages approximate a daily dosage range of 1-3 mg/year of age.

Dosage Forms

Capsule: 5 mg, 10 mg, 20 mg

Drops, oral: 10 mg/mL (100 mL)

Peridex® [US] *see* chlorhexidine gluconate *on page 183*

Peridol [Can] *see* haloperidol *on page 428*

perindopril and indapamide *(Canada only)*

(per IN doe pril & in DAP a mide)

Therapeutic Category Miscellaneous Product

Use Hypertension

Dosage Forms Tablet: Perindopril 2 mg and indapamide 0.625 mg

perindopril erbumine (per IN doe pril er BYOO meen)

U.S./Canadian Brand Names Aceon® [US]; Coversyl® [Can]

Therapeutic Category Miscellaneous Product

Use Treatment of stage I or II hypertension and congestive heart failure; treatment of left ventricular dysfunction after myocardial infarction

Usual Dosage Adults: Oral:

Congestive heart failure: 4 mg once daily; increase at 1- to 2-week intervals (maximum 16 mg/day)

Hypertension: Initial: 4 mg/day but may be titrated to response; usual range: 4-8 mg/day; increase at 1- to 2-week intervals; maximum: 16 mg/day

Dosage Forms Tablet: 2 mg, 4 mg, 8 mg

Periochip® [US] *see* chlorhexidine gluconate *on page 183*

PerioGard® [US] *see* chlorhexidine gluconate *on page 183*

Periostat® [US] *see* doxycycline *on page 294*

Peritrate® *(Discontinued)* *see page 1042*

Peritrate® SA *(Discontinued)* *see page 1042*

Permapen® Isoject® [US] *see* penicillin G benzathine *on page 675*

Permax® [US/Can] *see* pergolide *on previous page*

permethrin (per METH rin)

U.S./Canadian Brand Names A200® Lice [US-OTC]; Acticin® [US]; Elimite® [US]; Kwellada-P™ [Can]; Nix® [US/Can]; Rid® Spray [US-OTC]

Therapeutic Category Scabicides/Pediculicides

Use Single-application treatment of infestation with *Pediculus humanus capitis* (head louse) and its nits or *Sarcoptes scabiei* (scabies); indicated for prophylactic use during epidemics of lice

Usual Dosage Topical:

Head lice: Children >2 months and Adults: After hair has been washed with shampoo, rinsed with water, and towel dried, apply a sufficient volume of topical liquid (lotion or cream rinse) to saturate the hair and scalp. Leave on hair for 10 minutes before rinsing off with water; remove remaining nits; may repeat in 1 week if lice or nits still present.

Scabies: Apply cream from head to toe; leave on for 8-14 hours before washing off with water; for infants, also apply on the hairline, neck, scalp, temple, and forehead; may reapply in 1 week if live mites appear

Permethrin 5% cream was shown to be safe and effective when applied to an infant <1 month of age with neonatal scabies; time of application was limited to 6 hours before rinsing with soap and water

Dosage Forms

Cream, topical (Acticin®, Elimite®): 5% (60 g) [contains coconut oil]

Liquid, topical [creme rinse formulation] (Nix®): 1% (60 mL) [contains isopropyl alcohol 20%]

Lotion, topical: 1% (59 mL)

Solution, spray [for bedding and furniture]:

A200® Lice: 0.5% (180 mL)

Nix®: 0.25% (148 mL)

Rid®: 0.5% (150 mL)

Permitil® Oral *(Discontinued)* *see page 1042*

Peroxin A5® *(Discontinued)* *see page 1042*

Peroxin A10® *(Discontinued)* *see page 1042*

perphenazine (per FEN a zeen)

Sound-Alike/Look-Alike Issues

Trilafon® may be confused with Tri-Levlen®

(Continued)

perphenazine *(Continued)*

U.S./Canadian Brand Names Apo-Perphenazine® [Can]; Trilafon® [Can]

Therapeutic Category Phenothiazine Derivative

Use Treatment of schizophrenia; nausea and vomiting

Usual Dosage Oral:

Children:

Schizophrenia/psychoses:

1-6 years: 4-6 mg/day in divided doses

6-12 years: 6 mg/day in divided doses

>12 years: 4-16 mg 2-4 times/day

Adults:

Schizophrenia/psychoses: 4-16 mg 2-4 times/day not to exceed 64 mg/day

Nausea/vomiting: 8-16 mg/day in divided doses up to 24 mg/day

Dosage Forms Tablet: 2 mg, 4 mg, 8 mg, 16 mg

perphenazine and amitriptyline *see* amitriptyline and perphenazine *on page 48*

Persa-Gel® ***(Discontinued)*** *see page 1042*

Persantine® [US/Can] *see* dipyridamole *on page 282*

Pertussin® CS ***(Discontinued)*** *see page 1042*

Pertussin® ES ***(Discontinued)*** *see page 1042*

pethidine hydrochloride *see* meperidine *on page 553*

Pexeva™ [US] *see* paroxetine *on page 668*

Pexicam® [Can] *see* piroxicam *on page 698*

PFA *see* foscarnet *on page 390*

Pfizerpen® [US/Can] *see* penicillin G (parenteral/aqueous) *on page 676*

Pfizerpen-AS® ***(Discontinued)*** *see page 1042*

Pfizerpen-AS® [Can] *see* penicillin G procaine *on page 676*

PGE_1 *see* alprostadil *on page 35*

PGE_2 *see* dinoprostone *on page 275*

PGI_2 *see* epoprostenol *on page 316*

PGX *see* epoprostenol *on page 316*

Phanasin® Diabetic Choice [US-OTC] *see* guaifenesin *on page 415*

Phanasin [US-OTC] *see* guaifenesin *on page 415*

Pharmaflur® [US] *see* fluoride *on page 376*

Pharmaflur® 1.1 [US] *see* fluoride *on page 376*

Pharmorubicin® [Can] *see* epirubicin *on page 313*

Phazyme® ***(Discontinued)*** *see page 1042*

Phazyme™ [Can] *see* simethicone *on page 804*

Phazyme® Quick Dissolve [US-OTC] *see* simethicone *on page 804*

Phazyme® Ultra Strength [US-OTC] *see* simethicone *on page 804*

Phenadex® Senior ***(Discontinued)*** *see page 1042*

Phenadoz™ [US] *see* promethazine *on page 734*

Phenahist-TR® ***(Discontinued)*** *see page 1042*

Phenameth® DM ***(Discontinued)*** *see page 1042*

Phenaphen® ***(Discontinued)*** *see page 1042*

Phenaphen®/Codeine #4 ***(Discontinued)*** *see page 1042*

Phenaseptic® ***(Discontinued)*** *see page 1042*

PhenaVent™ [US] *see* guaifenesin and phenylephrine *on page 418*

PhenaVent™ D [US] *see* guaifenesin and phenylephrine *on page 418*

PhenaVent™ Ped [US] *see* guaifenesin and phenylephrine *on page 418*

Phenazine® Injection *(Discontinued)* *see page 1042*

Phenazo™ [Can] *see* phenazopyridine *on this page*

phenazopyridine (fen az oh PEER i deen)

Sound-Alike/Look-Alike Issues
Pyridium® may be confused with Dyrenium®, Perdiem®, pyridoxine, pyrithione

Synonyms phenazopyridine hydrochloride; phenylazo diamino pyridine hydrochloride

U.S./Canadian Brand Names Azo-Gesic® [US-OTC]; Azo-Standard® [US-OTC]; Phenazo™ [Can]; Prodium® [US-OTC]; Pyridium® [US/Can]; ReAzo [US-OTC]; Uristat® [US-OTC]; UTI Relief® [US-OTC]

Therapeutic Category Analgesic, Urinary

Use Symptomatic relief of urinary burning, itching, frequency and urgency in association with urinary tract infection or following urologic procedures

Usual Dosage Oral:
Children: 12 mg/kg/day in 3 divided doses administered after meals for 2 days
Adults: 100-200 mg 3 times/day after meals for 2 days when used concomitantly with an antibacterial agent

Dosage Forms Tablet, as hydrochloride: 100 mg, 200 mg
Azo-Gesic®, Azo-Standard®, Prodium®, Uristat®: 95 mg
ReAzo: 97 mg
Pyridium®: 100 mg, 200 mg [contains sodium benzoate]
UTI Relief®: 97.2 mg

phenazopyridine hydrochloride *see* phenazopyridine *on this page*

Phencen-50® *(Discontinued)* *see page 1042*

Phenclor® S.H.A. *(Discontinued)* *see page 1042*

phendimetrazine (fen dye ME tra zeen)

Sound-Alike/Look-Alike Issues
Bontril PDM® may be confused with Bentyl®

Synonyms phendimetrazine tartrate

U.S./Canadian Brand Names Bontril® [Can]; Bontril PDM® [US]; Bontril® Slow-Release [US]; Melfiat® [US]; Obezine® [US]; Plegine® [Can]; Prelu-2® [US]; Statobex® [Can]

Therapeutic Category Anorexiant

Controlled Substance C-III

Use Appetite suppressant during the first few weeks of dieting to help establish new eating habits; its effectiveness lasts only for short periods (3-12 weeks)

Usual Dosage Adults: Oral:
Tablet: 35 mg 2 or 3 times daily, 1 hour before meals
Capsule, timed release: 105 mg once daily in the morning before breakfast

Dosage Forms
Capsule, timed release, as tartrate (Bontril® Slow Release, Melfiat®, Prelu-2®): 105 mg
Tablet, as tartrate (Bontril PDM®, Obenzine®): 35 mg

phendimetrazine tartrate *see* phendimetrazine *on this page*

Phendry® Oral *(Discontinued)* *see page 1042*

phenelzine (FEN el zeen)

Sound-Alike/Look-Alike Issues
phenelzine may be confused with phenytoin
Nardil® may be confused with Norinyl®

Synonyms phenelzine sulfate

U.S./Canadian Brand Names Nardil® [US/Can]
(Continued)

phenelzine *(Continued)*

Therapeutic Category Antidepressant, Monoamine Oxidase Inhibitor

Use Symptomatic treatment of atypical, nonendogenous, or neurotic depression

Usual Dosage Oral: Adults: Depression: 15 mg 3 times/day; may increase to 60-90 mg/day during early phase of treatment, then reduce dose for maintenance therapy slowly after maximum benefit is obtained; takes 2-4 weeks for a significant response to occur

Dosage Forms Tablet, as sulfate: 15 mg

phenelzine sulfate *see* phenelzine *on previous page*

Phenerbel-S® *(Discontinued)* *see page 1042*

Phenergan® [US/Can] *see* promethazine *on page 734*

Phenergan® VC With Codeine *(Discontinued)* *see page 1042*

Phenergan® With Codeine [US] *see* promethazine and codeine *on page 735*

Phenergan® With Dextromethorphan *(Discontinued)* *see page 1042*

Phenetron® *(Discontinued)* *see page 1042*

phenindamine (fen IN dah meen)

Synonyms phenindamine tartrate

U.S./Canadian Brand Names Nolahist® [US-OTC/Can]

Therapeutic Category Antihistamine

Use Treatment of perennial and seasonal allergic rhinitis and chronic urticaria

Usual Dosage Oral:

Children <6 years: As directed by physician

Children 6 to <12 years: 12.5 mg every 4-6 hours, up to 75 mg/24 hours

Adults: 25 mg every 4-6 hours, up to 150 mg/24 hours

Dosage Forms Tablet, as tartrate: 25 mg

phenindamine tartrate *see* phenindamine *on this page*

pheniramine and naphazoline *see* naphazoline and pheniramine *on page 604*

phenobarbital (fee noe BAR bi tal)

Sound-Alike/Look-Alike Issues

phenobarbital may be confused with pentobarbital

Luminal® may be confused with Tuinal®

Synonyms phenobarbital sodium; phenobarbitone; phenylethylmalonylurea

U.S./Canadian Brand Names Luminal® Sodium [US]; PMS-Phenobarbital [Can]

Therapeutic Category Anticonvulsant; Barbiturate

Controlled Substance C-IV

Use Management of generalized tonic-clonic (grand mal) and partial seizures; sedative

Usual Dosage

Children:

Sedation: Oral: 2 mg/kg 3 times/day

Hypnotic: I.M., I.V., SubQ: 3-5 mg/kg at bedtime

Preoperative sedation: Oral, I.M., I.V.: 1-3 mg/kg 1-1.5 hours before procedure

Adults:

Sedation: Oral, I.M.: 30-120 mg/day in 2-3 divided doses

Hypnotic: Oral, I.M., I.V., SubQ: 100-320 mg at bedtime

Preoperative sedation: I.M.: 100-200 mg 1-1.5 hours before procedure

Anticonvulsant: Status epilepticus: **Loading dose:** I.V.:

Infants and Children: 10-20 mg/kg in a single or divided dose; in select patients may administer additional 5 mg/kg/dose every 15-30 minutes until seizure is controlled or a total dose of 40 mg/kg is reached

Adults: 300-800 mg initially followed by 120-240 mg/dose at 20-minute intervals until seizures are controlled or a total dose of 1-2 g

Anticonvulsant maintenance dose: Oral, I.V.:
Infants: 5-8 mg/kg/day in 1-2 divided doses
Children:
1-5 years: 6-8 mg/kg/day in 1-2 divided doses
5-12 years: 4-6 mg/kg/day in 1-2 divided doses
Children >12 years and Adults: 1-3 mg/kg/day in divided doses or 50-100 mg 2-3 times/day

Dosage Forms

Elixir: 20 mg/5 mL (5 mL, 7.5 mL, 15 mL, 473 mL, 946 mL, 4000 mL) [contains alcohol]
Injection, solution, as sodium: 60 mg/mL (1 mL); 130 mg/mL (1 mL) [contains alcohol]
Luminal® Sodium: 60 mg/mL (1 mL); 130 mg/mL (1 mL) [contains alcohol 10%]
Tablet: 15 mg, 30 mg, 32 mg, 60 mg, 65 mg, 100 mg

phenobarbital, belladonna, and ergotamine tartrate *see* belladonna, phenobarbital, and ergotamine tartrate *on page 104*

phenobarbital, hyoscyamine, atropine, and scopolamine *see* hyoscyamine, atropine, scopolamine, and phenobarbital *on page 460*

phenobarbital sodium *see* phenobarbital *on previous page*

phenobarbitone *see* phenobarbital *on previous page*

phenol (FEE nol)

Sound-Alike/Look-Alike Issues

Cēpastat® may be confused with Capastat®

Synonyms carbolic acid

U.S./Canadian Brand Names Cēpastat® Extra Strength [US-OTC]; Cēpastat® [US-OTC]; Chloraseptic® Gargle [US-OTC]; Chloraseptic® Mouth Pain Spray [US-OTC]; Chloraseptic® Rinse [US-OTC]; Chloraseptic® Spray for Kids [US-OTC]; Chloraseptic® Spray [US-OTC]; Pain-A-Lay® [US-OTC]; P & S™ Liquid Phenol [Can]; Ulcerease® [US-OTC]

Therapeutic Category Pharmaceutical Aid

Use Relief of sore throat pain, mouth, gum, and throat irritations; neurologic pain, rectal prolapse, hemorrhoids, hydrocele

Usual Dosage

Allow to dissolve slowly in mouth; may be repeated every 2 hours as needed
For each neurolysis procedure: 0.5-2 mL (up to 7.5 mL may be needed)

Dosage Forms

Liquid, oral (Ulcerease®): 0.6% (180 mL) [contains glycerin; sugar free]
Lozenge:
Cēpastat®: 14.5 mg (18s) [contains eucalyptus oil and menthol; sugar free; cherry flavor]
Cēpastat® Extra Strength: 29 mg (18s) [contains eucalyptus oil and menthol; sugar free; eucalyptus flavor]
Solution, oral:
Chloraseptic® [gargle]: 1.4% (296 mL) [cool mint flavor]
Chloraseptic® [rinse]: 1.4% (240 mL) [cinnamon flavor]
Pain-A-Lay®: 1.4% (240 mL) [gargle; contains tartrazine]
Solution, oral spray: 1.4% (180 mL)
Chloraseptic®: 1.4% (180 mL) [cherry flavor]
Chloraseptic® for Kids: 0.5% (177 mL) [grape flavor]
Chloraseptic® Mouth Pain Spray: 1.4% (30 mL) [cherry blast or cool mint flavor]
Pain-A-Lay®: 1.4% (180 mL) [contains tartrazine]

phenol and camphor *see* camphor and phenol *on page 151*

phenolsulfonphthalein *(Discontinued)* *see page 1042*

Phenoptic® [US] *see* phenylephrine *on page 689*

Phenoxine® *(Discontinued)* *see page 1042*

phenoxybenzamine (fen oks ee BEN za meen)

Synonyms phenoxybenzamine hydrochloride

U.S./Canadian Brand Names Dibenzyline® [US/Can]

Therapeutic Category Alpha-Adrenergic Blocking Agent

Use Symptomatic management of pheochromocytoma; treatment of hypertensive crisis caused by sympathomimetic amines

Usual Dosage Oral:

Children: Initial: 0.2 mg/kg (maximum: 10 mg) once daily, increase by 0.2 mg/kg increments; usual maintenance dose: 0.4-1.2 mg/kg/day every 6-8 hours, higher doses may be necessary

Adults: Initial: 10 mg twice daily, increase by 10 mg every other day until optimum dose is achieved; usual range: 20-40 mg 2-3 times/day

Dosage Forms Capsule, as hydrochloride: 10 mg [contains benzyl alcohol]

phenoxybenzamine hydrochloride *see* phenoxybenzamine *on this page*

phenoxymethyl penicillin *see* penicillin V potassium *on page 677*

phentermine (FEN ter meen)

Sound-Alike/Look-Alike Issues

phentermine may be confused with phentolamine, phenytoin

Ionamin® may be confused with Imodium®

Synonyms phentermine hydrochloride

U.S./Canadian Brand Names Adipex-P® [US]; Ionamin® [US/Can]

Therapeutic Category Anorexiant

Controlled Substance C-IV

Use Short-term adjunct in a regimen of weight reduction based on exercise, behavioral modification, and caloric reduction in the management of exogenous obesity for patients with an initial body mass index ≥30 kg/m^2 or ≥27 kg/m^2 in the presence of other risk factors (diabetes, hypertension)

Usual Dosage Oral: Adults: Obesity: 8 mg 3 times/day 30 minutes before meals or food or 15-37.5 mg/day before breakfast or 10-14 hours before retiring

Dosage Forms

Capsule, as hydrochloride: 15 mg, 30 mg

Adipex-P®: 37.5 mg

Capsule, resin complex (Ionamin®): 15 mg, 30 mg

Tablet, as hydrochloride: 37.5 mg

Adipex-P®: 37.5 mg

phentermine hydrochloride *see* phentermine *on this page*

phentolamine (fen TOLE a meen)

Sound-Alike/Look-Alike Issues

phentolamine may be confused with phentermine, Ventolin®

Synonyms phentolamine mesylate

U.S./Canadian Brand Names Regitine® [Can]; Rogitine® [Can]

Therapeutic Category Alpha-Adrenergic Blocking Agent; Diagnostic Agent

Use Diagnosis of pheochromocytoma and treatment of hypertension associated with pheochromocytoma or other forms of hypertension caused by excess sympathomimetic amines; as treatment of dermal necrosis after extravasation of drugs with alpha-adrenergic effects (norepinephrine, dopamine, epinephrine)

Usual Dosage

Treatment of alpha-adrenergic drug extravasation: SubQ:

Children: 0.1-0.2 mg/kg diluted in 10 mL 0.9% sodium chloride infiltrated into area of extravasation within 12 hours

Adults: Infiltrate area with small amount of solution made by diluting 5-10 mg in 10 mL 0.9% sodium chloride within 12 hours of extravasation; do not exceed 0.1-0.2 mg/kg or 5 mg total

If dose is effective, normal skin color should return to the blanched area within 1 hour
Diagnosis of pheochromocytoma: I.M., I.V.:
Children: 0.05-0.1 mg/kg/dose, maximum single dose: 5 mg
Adults: 5 mg
Surgery for pheochromocytoma: Hypertension: I.M., I.V.:
Children: 0.05-0.1 mg/kg/dose given 1-2 hours before procedure; repeat as needed every 2-4 hours until hypertension is controlled; maximum single dose: 5 mg
Adults: 5 mg given 1-2 hours before procedure and repeated as needed every 2-4 hours
Hypertensive crisis: Adults: 5-20 mg

Dosage Forms Injection, powder for reconstitution, as mesylate: 5 mg

phentolamine mesylate *see* phentolamine *on previous page*

Phenurone® *(Discontinued)* *see page 1042*

phenylalanine mustard *see* melphalan *on page 550*

phenylazo diamino pyridine hydrochloride *see* phenazopyridine *on page 685*

Phenyldrine® *(Discontinued)* *see page 1042*

phenylephrine (fen il EF rin)

Sound-Alike/Look-Alike Issues
Mydfrin® may be confused with Midrin®

Synonyms phenylephrine hydrochloride

U.S./Canadian Brand Names AK-Dilate® [US]; AK-Nefrin® [US]; Dionephrine® [Can]; Formulation R™ [US-OTC]; Medicone® [US-OTC]; Mydfrin® [US/Can]; Neo-Synephrine® Extra Strength [US-OTC]; Neo-Synephrine® Mild [US-OTC]; Neo-Synephrine® Ophthalmic [US]; Neo-Synephrine® Regular Strength [US-OTC]; Nostril® [US-OTC]; Phenoptic® [US]; Relief® [US-OTC]; Vicks® Sinex® Nasal [US-OTC]; Vicks® Sinex® UltraFine Mist [US-OTC]

Therapeutic Category Adrenergic Agonist Agent

Use Treatment of hypotension, vascular failure in shock; as a vasoconstrictor in regional analgesia; as a mydriatic in ophthalmic procedures and treatment of wide-angle glaucoma; supraventricular tachycardia

For OTC use as symptomatic relief of nasal and nasopharyngeal mucosal congestion, treatment of hemorrhoids, relief of redness of the eye due to irritation

Usual Dosage
Ocular procedures:
Infants <1 year: Instill 1 drop of 2.5% 15-30 minutes before procedures
Children and Adults: Instill 1 drop of 2.5% or 10% solution, may repeat in 10-60 minutes as needed
Ophthalmic irritation (OTC formulation for relief of eye redness): Adults: Instill 1-2 drops 0.12% solution into affected eye, up to 4 times/day; do not use for >72 hours
Nasal decongestant (therapy should not exceed 3 continuous days):
Children:
2-6 years: Instill 1 drop every 2-4 hours of 0.125% solution as needed
6-12 years: Instill 1-2 sprays or instill 1-2 drops every 4 hours of 0.25% solution as needed
Children >12 years and Adults: Instill 1-2 sprays or instill 1-2 drops every 4 hours of 0.25% to 0.5% solution as needed; 1% solution may be used in adult in cases of extreme nasal congestion; do not use nasal solutions more than 3 days
Hypotension/shock:
Children:
I.M., SubQ: 0.1 mg/kg/dose every 1-2 hours as needed (maximum: 5 mg)
I.V. bolus: 5-20 mcg/kg/dose every 10-15 minutes as needed
I.V. infusion: 0.1-0.5 mcg/kg/minute

(Continued)

phenylephrine *(Continued)*

Adults:

I.M., SubQ: 2-5 mg/dose every 1-2 hours as needed (initial dose should not exceed 5 mg)

I.V. bolus: 0.1-0.5 mg/dose every 10-15 minutes as needed (initial dose should not exceed 0.5 mg)

I.V. infusion: 10 mg in 250 mL D_5W or NS (1:25,000 dilution) (40 mcg/mL); start at 100-180 mcg/minute (2-5 mL/minute; 50-90 drops/minute) initially; when blood pressure is stabilized, maintenance rate: 40-60 mcg/minute (20-30 drops/minute); rates up to 360 mcg/minute have been reported; dosing range: 0.4-9.1 mcg/kg/minute **Note:** Concentrations up to 100-500 mg in 250 mL have been used.

Paroxysmal supraventricular tachycardia: I.V.:

Children: 5-10 mcg/kg/dose over 20-30 seconds

Adults: 0.25-0.5 mg/dose over 20-30 seconds

Hemorrhoids: Children ≥12 years and Adults: Rectal:

Cream/ointment: Apply to clean dry area, up to 4 times/day; may be used externally or inserted rectally using applicator.

Suppository: Insert 1 suppository rectally, up to 4 times/day

Dosage Forms [DSC] = Discontinued product

Cream, rectal (Formulation R™): 0.25% (30 g, 60 g) [contains sodium benzoate]

Injection, solution, as hydrochloride: 1% [10 mg/mL] (1 mL) [may contain sodium metabisulfite]

Ointment, rectal (Formulation R™): 0.25% (30 g, 60 g) [contains benzoic acid]

Solution, intranasal drops, as hydrochloride:

Neo-Synephrine® Extra Strength: 1% (15 mL)

Neo-Synephrine® Regular Strength: 0.5% (15 mL)

Solution, intranasal spray, as hydrochloride:

Neo-Synephrine® Extra Strength: 1% (15 mL)

Neo-Synephrine® Mild: 0.25% (15 mL)

Neo-Synephrine® Regular Strength: 0.5% (15 mL)

Nostril®: 0.25% (15 mL); 0.5% (15 mL)

Vicks® Sinex®, Vicks® Sinex® UltraFine Mist: 0.5% (15 mL)

Solution, ophthalmic, as hydrochloride: 2.5% (2 mL, 3 mL, 5 mL, 15 mL) [may contain sodium bisulfite]

AK-Dilate®: 2.5% (2 mL, 15 mL); 10% (5 mL)

AK-Nefrin®: 0.12% (15 mL)

Mydfrin®: 2.5% (3 mL, 5 mL) [contains sodium bisulfite]

Neo-Synephrine®: 2.5% (15 mL); 10% (5 mL)

Neo-Synephrine® Viscous: 10% (5 mL)

Phenoptic®: 2.5% (15 mL)

Prefrin™ [DSC], Relief®: 0.12% (15 mL)

Suppository, rectal: 0.25% (12s)

Medicone®: 0.25% (18s, 24s)

phenylephrine and chlorpheniramine *see* chlorpheniramine and phenylephrine *on page 188*

phenylephrine and cyclopentolate *see* cyclopentolate and phenylephrine *on page 234*

phenylephrine and promethazine *see* promethazine and phenylephrine *on page 736*

phenylephrine and scopolamine (fen il EF rin & skoe POL a meen)

Sound-Alike/Look-Alike Issues

Murocoll-2® may be confused with Murocel®

Synonyms scopolamine and phenylephrine

U.S./Canadian Brand Names Murocoll-2® [US]

Therapeutic Category Anticholinergic/Adrenergic Agonist

Use Mydriasis, cycloplegia, and to break posterior synechiae in iritis

Usual Dosage Ophthalmic: Instill 1-2 drops into eye(s); repeat in 5 minutes

Dosage Forms Solution, ophthalmic: Phenylephrine hydrochloride 10% and scopolamine hydrobromide 0.3% (5 mL)

phenylephrine and zinc sulfate (fen il EF rin & zingk SUL fate)

Synonyms zinc sulfate and phenylephrine

U.S./Canadian Brand Names Zincfrin® [US-OTC/Can]

Therapeutic Category Adrenergic Agonist Agent

Use Soothe, moisturize, and remove redness due to minor eye irritation

Usual Dosage Ophthalmic: Instill 1-2 drops in eye(s) 2-4 times/day as needed

Dosage Forms Solution, ophthalmic: Phenylephrine hydrochloride 0.12% and zinc sulfate 0.25% (15 mL)

phenylephrine, chlorpheniramine, and dextromethorphan *see* chlorpheniramine, phenylephrine, and dextromethorphan *on page 191*

phenylephrine, chlorpheniramine, and methscopolamine *see* chlorpheniramine, phenylephrine, and methscopolamine *on page 192*

phenylephrine, chlorpheniramine, and phenyltoloxamine *see* chlorpheniramine, phenylephrine, and phenyltoloxamine *on page 193*

phenylephrine, chlorpheniramine, codeine, and potassium iodide *see* chlorpheniramine, phenylephrine, codeine, and potassium iodide *on page 193*

phenylephrine, ephedrine, chlorpheniramine, and carbetapentane *see* chlorpheniramine, ephedrine, phenylephrine, and carbetapentane *on page 190*

phenylephrine hydrochloride *see* phenylephrine *on page 689*

phenylephrine hydrochloride and guaifenesin *see* guaifenesin and phenylephrine *on page 418*

phenylephrine, hydrocodone, chlorpheniramine, acetaminophen, and caffeine *see* hydrocodone, chlorpheniramine, phenylephrine, acetaminophen, and caffeine *on page 446*

phenylephrine, promethazine, and codeine *see* promethazine, phenylephrine, and codeine *on page 736*

phenylethylmalonylurea *see* phenobarbital *on page 686*

Phenylfenesin® L.A. *(Discontinued)* *see page 1042*

Phenylgesic® [US-OTC] *see* acetaminophen and phenyltoloxamine *on page 8*

phenylisohydantoin *see* pemoline *on page 673*

phenyltoloxamine and acetaminophen *see* acetaminophen and phenyltoloxamine *on page 8*

phenyltoloxamine, chlorpheniramine, and phenylephrine *see* chlorpheniramine, phenylephrine, and phenyltoloxamine *on page 193*

Phenytek™ [US] *see* phenytoin *on this page*

phenytoin (FEN i toyn)

Sound-Alike/Look-Alike Issues

phenytoin may be confused with phenelzine, phentermine

Dilantin® may be confused with Dilaudid®, diltiazem, Dipentum®

Synonyms diphenylhydantoin; DPH; phenytoin sodium; phenytoin sodium, extended; phenytoin sodium, prompt

U.S./Canadian Brand Names Dilantin® [US/Can]; Phenytek™ [US]

Therapeutic Category Antiarrhythmic Agent, Class I-B; Hydantoin

Use Management of generalized tonic-clonic (grand mal), complex partial seizures; prevention of seizures following head trauma/neurosurgery

(Continued)

phenytoin *(Continued)*

Usual Dosage

Status epilepticus: I.V.:

Infants and Children: Loading dose: 15-20 mg/kg in a single or divided dose; maintenance dose: Initial: 5 mg/kg/day in 2 divided doses; usual doses:

6 months to 3 years: 8-10 mg/kg/day

4-6 years: 7.5-9 mg/kg/day

7-9 years: 7-8 mg/kg/day

10-16 years: 6-7 mg/kg/day, some patients may require every 8 hours dosing

Adults: Loading dose: Manufacturer recommends 10-15 mg/kg, however, 15-25 mg/kg has been used clinically; maintenance dose: 300 mg/day or 5-6 mg/kg/day in 3 divided doses or 1-2 divided doses using extended release

Anticonvulsant: Children and Adults: Oral:

Loading dose: 15-20 mg/kg; based on phenytoin serum concentrations and recent dosing history; administer oral loading dose in 3 divided doses given every 2-4 hours to decrease GI adverse effects and to ensure complete oral absorption; maintenance dose: same as I.V.

Neurosurgery (prophylactic): 100-200 mg at approximately 4-hour intervals during surgery and during the immediate postoperative period

Dosage Forms

Capsule, extended release, as sodium:

Dilantin®: 30 mg [contains sodium benzoate], 100 mg

Phenytek™: 200 mg, 300 mg

Capsule, prompt release, as sodium: 100 mg

Injection, solution, as sodium: 50 mg/mL (2 mL, 5 mL) [contains alcohol]

Suspension, oral (Dilantin®): 125 mg/5 mL (240 mL) [contains alcohol <0.6%, sodium benzoate; orange-vanilla flavor]

Tablet, chewable (Dilantin®): 50 mg

phenytoin sodium *see* phenytoin *on previous page*

phenytoin sodium, extended *see* phenytoin *on previous page*

phenytoin sodium, prompt *see* phenytoin *on previous page*

Pherazine® VC With Codeine *(Discontinued)* *see page 1042*

Pherazine® With Codeine *(Discontinued)* *see page 1042*

Pherazine® With DM *(Discontinued)* *see page 1042*

Phillips'® Fibercaps [US-OTC] *see* polycarbophil *on page 706*

Phillips'® Milk of Magnesia [US-OTC] *see* magnesium hydroxide *on page 537*

Phillips' M-O® [US-OTC] *see* magnesium hydroxide and mineral oil emulsion *on page 538*

Phillips'® Stool Softener Laxative [US-OTC] *see* docusate *on page 285*

pHisoHex® [US/Can] *see* hexachlorophene *on page 435*

Phos-Ex® 62.5 *(Discontinued)* *see page 1042*

Phos-Ex® 125 *(Discontinued)* *see page 1042*

Phos-Ex® 167 *(Discontinued)* *see page 1042*

Phos-Ex® 250 *(Discontinued)* *see page 1042*

Phos-Flur® [US] *see* fluoride *on page 376*

Phos-Flur® Rinse [US-OTC] *see* fluoride *on page 376*

PhosLo® [US] *see* calcium acetate *on page 144*

pHos-pHaid® *(Discontinued)* *see page 1042*

Phosphaljel® *(Discontinued)* *see page 1042*

phosphate, potassium *see* potassium phosphate *on page 716*

Phospholine Iodide® [US] *see* echothiophate iodide *on page 301*

phosphonoformate *see* foscarnet *on page 390*

phosphonoformic acid *see* foscarnet *on page 390*

phosphorated carbohydrate solution *see* fructose, dextrose, and phosphoric acid *on page 392*

phosphoric acid, levulose and dextrose *see* fructose, dextrose, and phosphoric acid *on page 392*

Photofrin® [US/Can] *see* porfimer *on page 710*

Phoxal-timolol [Can] *see* timolol *on page 863*

Phrenilin® With Caffeine and Codeine [US] *see* butalbital, aspirin, caffeine, and codeine *on page 139*

***p*-hydroxyampicillin** *see* amoxicillin *on page 51*

Phyllocontin® [Can] *see* aminophylline *on page 46*

Phyllocontin®-350 [Can] *see* aminophylline *on page 46*

phylloquinone *see* phytonadione *on this page*

physostigmine (fye zoe STIG meen)

Sound-Alike/Look-Alike Issues

physostigmine may be confused with Prostigmin®, pyridostigmine

Synonyms eserine salicylate; physostigmine salicylate; physostigmine sulfate

U.S./Canadian Brand Names Eserine® [Can]; Isopto® Eserine [Can]

Therapeutic Category Cholinesterase Inhibitor

Use Reverse toxic CNS effects caused by anticholinergic drugs

Usual Dosage

Children: Anticholinergic drug overdose: Reserve for life-threatening situations only: I.V.: 0.01-0.03 mg/kg/dose (maximum: 0.5 mg/minute); may repeat after 5-10 minutes to a maximum total dose of 2 mg or until response occurs or adverse cholinergic effects occur

Adults: Anticholinergic drug overdose:

I.M., I.V., SubQ: 0.5-2 mg to start, repeat every 20 minutes until response occurs or adverse effect occurs

Repeat 1-4 mg every 30-60 minutes as life-threatening signs (arrhythmias, seizures, deep coma) recur; maximum I.V. rate: 1 mg/minute

Dosage Forms Injection, solution, as salicylate: 1 mg/mL (2 mL) [contains benzyl alcohol and sodium metabisulfite]

physostigmine salicylate *see* physostigmine *on this page*

physostigmine sulfate *see* physostigmine *on this page*

phytomenadione *see* phytonadione *on this page*

phytonadione (fye toe na DYE one)

Sound-Alike/Look-Alike Issues

Mephyton® may be confused with melphalan, methadone

Synonyms methylphytyl napthoquinone; phylloquinone; phytomenadione; vitamin K_1

U.S./Canadian Brand Names AquaMEPHYTON® [Can]; Konakion [Can]; Mephyton® [US/Can]

Therapeutic Category Vitamin, Fat Soluble

Use Prevention and treatment of hypoprothrombinemia caused by drug-induced or anticoagulant-induced vitamin K deficiency, hemorrhagic disease of the newborn; phytonadione is more effective and is preferred to other vitamin K preparations in the presence of impending hemorrhage; oral absorption depends on the presence of bile salts

Usual Dosage SubQ is the preferred (per manufacturer) parenteral route; I.V. route should be restricted for emergency use only

Minimum daily requirement: Not well established

Infants: 1-5 mcg/kg/day

(Continued)

phytonadione *(Continued)*

Adults: 0.03 mcg/kg/day
Hemorrhagic disease of the newborn:
Prophylaxis: I.M.: 0.5-1 mg within 1 hour of birth
Treatment: I.M., SubQ: 1-2 mg/dose/day
Oral anticoagulant overdose:
Infants and Children:
No bleeding, rapid reversal needed, patient **will require** further oral anticoagulant therapy: SubQ, I.V.: 0.5-2 mg
No bleeding, rapid reversal needed, patient **will not require** further oral anticoagulant therapy: SubQ, I.V.: 2-5 mg
Significant bleeding, not life-threatening: SubQ, I.V.: 0.5-2 mg
Significant bleeding, life-threatening: I.V.: 5 mg over 10-20 minutes
Adults: Oral, I.V., SubQ: 1-10 mg/dose depending on degree of INR elevation
Serious bleeding or major overdose: 10 mg I.V. (slow infusion); may repeat every 12 hours (have required doses up to 25 mg)
Vitamin K deficiency: Due to drugs, malabsorption, or decreased synthesis of vitamin K
Infants and Children:
Oral: 2.5-5 mg/24 hours
I.M., I.V., SubQ: 1-2 mg/dose as a single dose
Adults:
Oral: 5-25 mg/24 hours
I.M., I.V., SubQ: 10 mg

Dosage Forms [DSC] = Discontinued product
Injection, aqueous colloidal: 2 mg/mL (0.5 mL); 10 mg/mL (1 mL) [contains benzyl alcohol]
AquaMEPHYTON® [DSC]: 2 mg/mL (0.5 mL); 10 mg/mL (1 mL) [contains benzyl alcohol]
Tablet (Mephyton®): 5 mg

α_1-PI *see* alpha$_1$-proteinase inhibitor *on page 34*

pidorubicin *see* epirubicin *on page 313*

pidorubicin hydrochloride *see* epirubicin *on page 313*

Pilagan® Ophthalmic *(Discontinued)* *see page 1042*

Pilocar® [US] *see* pilocarpine *on this page*

pilocarpine (pye loe KAR peen)

Sound-Alike/Look-Alike Issues
Isopto® Carpine may be confused with Isopto® Carbachol
Salagen® may be confused with Salacid®

Synonyms pilocarpine hydrochloride

U.S./Canadian Brand Names Diocarpine [Can]; Isopto® Carpine [US/Can]; Pilocar® [US]; Pilopine HS® [US/Can]; Salagen® [US/Can]

Therapeutic Category Cholinergic Agent

Use
Ophthalmic: Management of chronic simple glaucoma, chronic and acute angle-closure glaucoma
Oral: Symptomatic treatment of xerostomia caused by salivary gland hypofunction resulting from radiotherapy for cancer of the head and neck or Sjögren syndrome

Usual Dosage Adults:
Ophthalmic: Glaucoma:
Solution: Instill 1-2 drops up to 6 times/day; adjust the concentration and frequency as required to control elevated intraocular pressure
Gel: Instill 0.5" ribbon into lower conjunctival sac once daily at bedtime

Oral: Xerostomia:

Following head and neck cancer: 5 mg 3 times/day, titration up to 10 mg 3 times/day may be considered for patients who have not responded adequately; do not exceed 2 tablets/dose

Sjögren syndrome: 5 mg 4 times/day

Dosage Forms

Gel, ophthalmic, as hydrochloride (Pilopine HS®): 4% (3.5 g) [contains benzalkonium chloride]

Solution, ophthalmic, as hydrochloride: 1% (15 mL); 2% (15 mL); 4% (15 mL); 6% (15 mL) [may contain benzalkonium chloride]

Isopto® Carpine: 1% (15 mL); 2% (15 mL, 30 mL); 4% (15 mL, 30 mL); 6% (15 mL); 8% (15 mL) [contains benzalkonium chloride]

Pilocar®: 0.5% (15 mL); 1% (1 mL, 15 mL); 2% (1 mL, 15 mL); 3% (15 mL); 4% (1 mL, 15 mL); 6% (15 mL) [contains benzalkonium chloride]

Tablet, as hydrochloride (Salagen®): 5 mg, 7.5 mg

pilocarpine and epinephrine (pye loe KAR peen & ep i NEF rin)

Synonyms epinephrine and pilocarpine

Therapeutic Category Cholinergic Agent

Use Treatment of glaucoma; counter effect of cycloplegics

Usual Dosage Ophthalmic: Instill 1-2 drops up to 6 times/day

Dosage Forms Solution, ophthalmic: Epinephrine bitartrate 1% and pilocarpine hydrochloride 6% (15 mL)

pilocarpine hydrochloride *see* pilocarpine *on previous page*

Pilopine HS® [US/Can] *see* pilocarpine *on previous page*

Pilostat® Ophthalmic *(Discontinued)* *see page 1042*

Pima® [US] *see* potassium iodide *on page 715*

pimaricin *see* natamycin *on page 607*

pimecrolimus (pim e KROE li mus)

U.S./Canadian Brand Names Elidel® [US/Can]

Therapeutic Category Immunosuppressant Agent; Topical Skin Product

Use Short-term and intermittent long-term treatment of mild to moderate atopic dermatitis in patients not responsive to conventional therapy or when conventional therapy is not appropriate

Usual Dosage Children ≥2 years and Adults: Topical: Apply thin layer to affected area twice daily; rub in gently and completely. **Note:** Continue as long as signs and symptoms persist; discontinue if resolution occurs; re-evaluate if symptoms persist >6 weeks.

Dosage Forms Cream, topical: 1% (15 g, 30 g, 60 g, 100 g)

pimozide (PI moe zide)

U.S./Canadian Brand Names Orap™ [US/Can]

Therapeutic Category Neuroleptic Agent

Use Suppression of severe motor and phonic tics in patients with Tourette disorder who have failed to respond satisfactorily to standard treatment

Usual Dosage Oral: **Note:** An ECG should be performed baseline and periodically thereafter, especially during dosage adjustment:

Children ≤12 years: Initial: 0.05 mg/kg preferably once at bedtime; may be increased every third day; usual range: 2-4 mg/day; do not exceed 10 mg/day (0.2 mg/kg/day)

Children >12 years and Adults: Initial: 1-2 mg/day in divided doses, then increase dosage as needed every other day; range is usually 7-16 mg/day, maximum dose: 10 mg/day or 0.2 mg/kg/day are not generally recommended

Note: Sudden unexpected deaths have occurred in patients taking doses >10 mg. Therefore, dosages exceeding 10 mg/day are generally not recommended.

Dosage Forms Tablet: 1 mg, 2 mg

pinaverium bromide *see* pinaverium *(Canada only) on this page*

pinaverium *(Canada only)* (pin ah VEER ee um)

Synonyms pinaverium bromide

U.S./Canadian Brand Names Dicetel® [Can]

Therapeutic Category Calcium Antagonist; Gastrointestinal Agent, Miscellaneous

Use Treatment and relief of symptoms associated with irritable bowel syndrome (IBS); treatment of symptoms related to functional disorders of the biliary tract

Usual Dosage Oral: Adults: 50 mg 3 times/day; in exceptional cases, the dosage may be increased up to 100 mg 3 times/day (maximum dose: 300 mg/day). Tablets should be taken with a full glass of water during a meal/snack.

Dosage Forms Tablet, as bromide: 50 mg, 100 mg

Pindac® ***(Discontinued)*** *see page 1042*

pindolol (PIN doe lole)

Sound-Alike/Look-Alike Issues

pindolol may be confused with Parlodel®, Plendil®

Visken® may be confused with Visine®

U.S./Canadian Brand Names Apo-Pindol® [Can]; Gen-Pindolol [Can]; Novo-Pindol [Can]; Nu-Pindol [Can]; PMS-Pindolol [Can]; Visken® [Can]

Therapeutic Category Beta-Adrenergic Blocker

Use Management of hypertension

Usual Dosage Oral: Adults:

Hypertension: Initial: 5 mg twice daily, increase as necessary by 10 mg/day every 3-4 weeks (maximum daily dose: 60 mg); usual dose range (JNC 7): 10-40 mg twice daily

Antidepressant augmentation: 2.5 mg 3 times/day

Dosage Forms Tablet: 5 mg, 10 mg

pink bismuth *see* bismuth *on page 120*

Pin-Rid® ***(Discontinued)*** *see page 1042*

Pin-X® [US-OTC] *see* pyrantel pamoate *on page 750*

PIO *see* pemoline *on page 673*

pioglitazone (pye oh GLI ta zone)

Sound-Alike/Look-Alike Issues

Actos® may be confused with Actidose®

U.S./Canadian Brand Names Actos® [US/Can]

Therapeutic Category Antidiabetic Agent; Thiazolidinedione Derivative

Use

Type 2 diabetes mellitus (noninsulin dependent, NIDDM), monotherapy: Adjunct to diet and exercise, to improve glycemic control

Type 2 diabetes mellitus (noninsulin dependent, NIDDM), combination therapy with sulfonylurea, metformin, or insulin: When diet, exercise, and a single agent alone does not result in adequate glycemic control

Usual Dosage Oral: Adults:

Monotherapy: Initial: 15-30 mg once daily; if response is inadequate, the dosage may be increased in increments up to 45 mg once daily; maximum recommended dose: 45 mg once daily

Combination therapy: Maximum recommended dose: 45 mg/day

With sulfonylureas: Initial: 15-30 mg once daily; dose of sulfonylurea should be reduced if the patient reports hypoglycemia

With metformin: Initial: 15-30 mg once daily; it is unlikely that the dose of metformin will need to be reduced due to hypoglycemia

With insulin: Initial: 15-30 mg once daily; dose of insulin should be reduced by 10% to 25% if the patient reports hypoglycemia or if the plasma glucose falls to <100 mg/dL.

Dosage adjustment in patients with CHF (NYHA Class II) in mono- or combination therapy: Initial: 15 mg once daily; may be increased after several months of treatment, with close attention to heart failure symptoms

Dosage Forms Tablet: 15 mg, 30 mg, 45 mg

piperacillin (pi PER a sil in)

Synonyms piperacillin sodium

Therapeutic Category Penicillin

Use Treatment of susceptible infections such as septicemia, acute and chronic respiratory tract infections, skin and soft tissue infections, and urinary tract infections due to susceptible strains of *Pseudomonas*, *Proteus*, and *Escherichia coli* and *Enterobacter*, active against some streptococci and some anaerobic bacteria; febrile neutropenia (as part of combination regimen)

Usual Dosage Safety and efficacy in children <12 years of age has not been established

I.M., I.V.:

Neonates:

≤7 days: 150 mg/kg/day divided every 8 hours

>7 days: 200 mg/kg/day divided every 6 hours

Infants and Children: 200-300 mg/kg/day in divided doses every 4-6 hours; maximum dose: 24 g/day

Higher doses have been used in cystic fibrosis: 350-500 mg/kg/day in divided doses every 4 hours

Adults: 2-4 g/dose every 4-8 hours; maximum dose: 24 g/day

Dosage Forms Injection, powder for reconstitution, as sodium: 2 g, 3 g, 4 g

piperacillin and tazobactam sodium

(pi PER a sil in & ta zoe BAK tam SOW dee um)

Sound-Alike/Look-Alike Issues

Zosyn® may be confused with Zofran®, Zyvox™

Synonyms piperacillin sodium and tazobactam sodium

U.S./Canadian Brand Names Tazocin® [Can]; Zosyn® [US]

Therapeutic Category Penicillin

Use Treatment of infections caused by susceptible organisms, including infections of the lower respiratory tract (community-acquired pneumonia, nosocomial pneumonia); urinary tract; skin and skin structures; gynecologic (endometritis, pelvic inflammatory disease); bone and joint infections; intra-abdominal infections (appendicitis with rupture/abscess, peritonitis); and septicemia. Tazobactam expands activity of piperacillin to include beta-lactamase producing strains of *S. aureus*, *H. influenzae*, *Bacteroides*, and other gram-negative bacteria.

Usual Dosage

Infants and Children ≥6 months: **Note:** Not FDA-approved for use in children <12 years of age:

I.V.: 240 mg of piperacillin component/kg/day in divided doses every 8 hours; higher doses have been used for serious pseudomonal infections: 300-400 mg of piperacillin component/kg/day in divided doses every 6 hours.

Children >12 years and Adults:

Nosocomial pneumonia: I.V.: Piperacillin/tazobactam 4/0.5 g every 6 hours for 7-14 days (when used empirically, combination with an aminoglycoside is recommended; consider discontinuation of aminoglycoside if *P. aeruginosa* is not isolated)

Severe infections: I.V.: Piperacillin/tazobactam 4/0.5 g every 8 hours or 3/0.375 g every 6 hours for 7-10 days

Moderate infections: I.M.: Piperacillin/tazobactam 2/0.25 g every 6-8 hours; treatment should be continued for ≥7-10 days depending on severity of disease (**Note:** I.M. route not FDA-approved)

Dosage Forms Note: 8:1 ratio of piperacillin sodium/tazobactam sodium:

Infusion [premixed iso-osmotic solution, frozen]:

Piperacillin sodium 2 g and tazobactam sodium 0.25 g (50 mL)

Piperacillin sodium 3 g and tazobactam sodium 0.375 g (50 mL)

(Continued)

piperacillin and tazobactam sodium *(Continued)*

Piperacillin sodium 4 g and tazobactam sodium 0.5 g (50 mL)
Injection, powder for reconstitution:
Piperacillin sodium 2 g and tazobactam sodium 0.25 g
Piperacillin sodium 3 g and tazobactam sodium 0.375 g
Piperacillin sodium 4 g and tazobactam sodium 0.5 g
Piperacillin sodium 36 g and tazobactam sodium 4.5 g [bulk pharmacy vial]

piperacillin sodium *see* piperacillin *on previous page*

piperacillin sodium and tazobactam sodium *see* piperacillin and tazobactam sodium *on previous page*

piperazine estrone sulfate *see* estropipate *on page 332*

piperonyl butoxide and pyrethrins *see* pyrethrins and piperonyl butoxide *on page 751*

Pipracil® *(Discontinued)* *see page 1042*

pirbuterol (peer BYOO ter ole)

Synonyms pirbuterol acetate
U.S./Canadian Brand Names Maxair™ Autohaler™ [US]
Therapeutic Category Adrenergic Agonist Agent
Use Prevention and treatment of reversible bronchospasm including asthma
Usual Dosage Children ≥12 years and Adults: 2 inhalations every 4-6 hours for prevention; two inhalations at an interval of at least 1-3 minutes, followed by a third inhalation in treatment of bronchospasm, not to exceed 12 inhalations/day
Dosage Forms Aerosol for oral inhalation, as acetate: Maxair™ Autohaler™: 0.2 mg/inhalation (2.8 g) [80 inhalations]; 14 g [400 inhalations]

pirbuterol acetate *see* pirbuterol *on this page*

piroxicam (peer OKS i kam)

U.S./Canadian Brand Names Apo-Piroxicam® [Can]; Feldene® [US/Can]; Gen-Piroxicam [Can]; Novo-Pirocam® [Can]; Nu-Pirox [Can]; Pexicam® [Can]
Therapeutic Category Analgesic, Nonnarcotic; Nonsteroidal Antiinflammatory Drug (NSAID)
Use Symptomatic treatment of acute and chronic rheumatoid arthritis and osteoarthritis
Usual Dosage Oral:
Children: 0.2-0.3 mg/kg/day once daily; maximum dose: 15 mg/day
Adults: 10-20 mg/day once daily; although associated with increase in GI adverse effects, doses >20 mg/day have been used (ie, 30-40 mg/day)
Dosage Forms Capsule: 10 mg, 20 mg

piroxicam and cyclodextrin *(Canada only)*

(peer OKS i kam & sye kloe DEKS trin)
Therapeutic Category Analgesic, Nonnarcotic; Nonsteroidal Antiinflammatory Drug (NSAID)
Use For the short-term relief of mild to moderately severe acute pain. Complexation with cyclodextrin allows faster absorption of piroxicam
Dosage Forms Tablet: Piroxicam-cyclodextrin 191.2 mg, equivalent to piroxicam 20 mg and beta-cyclodextrin 171.2 mg

***p*-isobutylhydratropic acid** *see* ibuprofen *on page 462*

pit *see* oxytocin *on page 660*

Pitocin® [US/Can] *see* oxytocin *on page 660*

Pitressin® [US] *see* vasopressin *on page 906*

Pitrex [Can] *see* tolnaftate *on page 870*

pit viper antivenin *see* antivenin *(Crotalidae)* polyvalent *on page 67*

pivampicillin *(Canada only)* (piv am pi SIL in)

Therapeutic Category Antibiotic, Penicillin

Use For the treatment of respiratory tract infections (including acute bronchitis, acute exacerbations of chronic bronchitis and pneumonia); ear, nose and throat infections; gynecological infections; urinary tract infections (including acute uncomplicated gonococcal urethritis) when caused by nonpenicillinase-producing susceptible strains of the following organisms: gram-positive organisms, ie, streptococci, pneumococci and staphylococci; gram-negative organisms, ie, *H. influenzae, N. gonorrhoeae, E. coli, P. mirabilis.*

Usual Dosage Oral:

Suspension:

Infants 3 to 12 months: 40-60 mg/kg body weight daily divided into 2 equal doses

Children:

1 to 3 years: 5 mL (175 mg) twice daily

4 to 6 years: 7.5 mL (262.5 mg) twice daily

7 to 10 years: 10 mL (350 mg) twice daily

Children ≤ 10 years: Dosage range: 25-35 mg/kg/day ; should not exceed the recommended adult dose of 500 mg twice daily

Children ≥10 years and Adults: 15 mL (525 mg) twice daily; for severe infections: Dosage may be doubled

Tablet: Children ≥ 10 years and Adults: 500 mg twice daily; for severe infections: Dosage may be doubled

In gonococcal urethritis: 1.5 g as a single dose with 1 g probenecid concurrently

Dosage Forms

Suspension, oral: 35 mg/5 mL (100 mL, 150 mL, 200 mL)

Tablet: 500 mg (equivalent to ampicillin 377 mg)

pix carbonis *see* coal tar *on page 219*

pizotifen *(Canada only)* (pi ZOE ti fen)

Synonyms pizotifen malate

U.S./Canadian Brand Names Sandomigran® [Can]; Sandomigran DS® [Can]

Therapeutic Category Antimigraine Agent

Use Migraine prophylaxis

Usual Dosage Oral: Children ≥12 years and Adults: Migraine prophylaxis: Initial: 0.5 mg at bedtime; increase gradually to 0.5 mg 3 times/day; usual dosage range: 1-6 mg/day

Note: Therapeutic response may require several weeks of therapy. Do not discontinue abruptly (reduce gradually over 2-week period).

Dosage Forms

Tablet (Sandomigran®): 0.5 mg [pizotifen malate 0.73 mg]

Tablet, double strength (Sandomigran® DS): 1 mg [pizotifen malate 1.46 mg]

pizotifen malate *see* pizotifen *(Canada only)* *on this page*

Placidyl® ***(Discontinued)*** *see page 1042*

plague vaccine (plaig vak SEEN)

Therapeutic Category Vaccine, Inactivated Bacteria

Use Selected travelers to countries reporting cases for whom avoidance of rodents and fleas is impossible; all laboratory and field personnel working with *Yersinia pestis* organisms possibly resistant to antimicrobials; those engaged in *Yersinia pestis* aerosol experiments or in field operations in areas with enzootic plague where regular exposure to potentially infected wild rodents, rabbits, or their fleas cannot be prevented. Prophylactic antibiotics may be indicated following definite exposure, whether or not the exposed persons have been vaccinated.

(Continued)

plague vaccine *(Continued)*

Usual Dosage Three I.M. doses: First dose 1 mL, second dose (0.2 mL) 1 month later, third dose (0.2 mL) 5 months after the second dose; booster doses (0.2 mL) at 1- to 2-year intervals if exposure continues

Dosage Forms Injection: 2 mL, 20 mL

Plan B® [US/Can] *see* levonorgestrel *on page 515*

plantago seed *see* psyllium *on page 749*

plantain seed *see* psyllium *on page 749*

Plaquase® ***(Discontinued)*** *see page 1042*

Plaquenil® [US/Can] *see* hydroxychloroquine *on page 455*

Plasbumin® [US] *see* albumin *on page 25*

Plasbumin®-5 [Can] *see* albumin *on page 25*

Plasbumin®-25 [Can] *see* albumin *on page 25*

Plasmanate® [US] *see* plasma protein fraction *on this page*

Plasma-Plex® ***(Discontinued)*** *see page 1042*

plasma protein fraction (PLAS mah PROE teen FRAK shun)

U.S./Canadian Brand Names Plasmanate® [US]

Therapeutic Category Blood Product Derivative

Use Plasma volume expansion and maintenance of cardiac output in the treatment of certain types of shock or impending shock

Usual Dosage I.V.: 250-1500 mL/day

Dosage Forms Injection, solution [human]: 5% (50 mL, 250 mL, 500 mL)

Plasmatein® ***(Discontinued)*** *see page 1042*

Platinol®-AQ [US] *see* cisplatin *on page 205*

Plavix® [US/Can] *see* clopidogrel *on page 217*

Plegine® ***(Discontinued)*** *see page 1042*

Plegine® [Can] *see* phendimetrazine *on page 685*

Plenaxis™ [US] *see* abarelix *on page 2*

Plendil® [US/Can] *see* felodipine *on page 359*

Pletal® [US/Can] *see* cilostazol *on page 199*

Plexion® [US] *see* sulfur and sulfacetamide *on page 834*

Plexion SCT™ [US] *see* sulfur and sulfacetamide *on page 834*

Plexion TS™ [US] *see* sulfur and sulfacetamide *on page 834*

PMPA *see* tenofovir *on page 845*

PMS-Amantadine [Can] *see* amantadine *on page 41*

PMS-Amitriptyline [Can] *see* amitriptyline *on page 47*

PMS-Amoxicillin [Can] *see* amoxicillin *on page 51*

PMS-Atenolol [Can] *see* atenolol *on page 85*

PMS-Baclofen [Can] *see* baclofen *on page 98*

PMS-Benzydamine [Can] *see* benzydamine *(Canada only) on page 112*

PMS-Bethanechol [Can] *see* bethanechol *on page 117*

PMS-Bezafibrate [Can] *see* bezafibrate *(Canada only) on page 118*

PMS-Brimonidine Tartrate [Can] *see* brimonidine *on page 127*

PMS-Bromocriptine [Can] *see* bromocriptine *on page 128*

PMS-Buspirone [Can] *see* buspirone *on page 137*

PMS-Butorphanol [Can] *see* butorphanol *on page 140*
PMS-Captopril [Can] *see* captopril *on page 153*
PMS-Carbamazepine [Can] *see* carbamazepine *on page 155*
PMS-Cefaclor [Can] *see* cefaclor *on page 165*
PMS-Chloral Hydrate [Can] *see* chloral hydrate *on page 181*
PMS-Cholestyramine [Can] *see* cholestyramine resin *on page 196*
PMS-Cimetidine [Can] *see* cimetidine *on page 199*
PMS-Clobazam [Can] *see* clobazam *(Canada only) on page 212*
PMS-Clonazepam [Can] *see* clonazepam *on page 215*
PMS-Deferoxamine [Can] *see* deferoxamine *on page 247*
PMS-Desipramine *see* desipramine *on page 251*
PMS-Desonide [Can] *see* desonide *on page 253*
PMS-Dexamethasone [Can] *see* dexamethasone (systemic) *on page 254*
PMS-Diclofenac [Can] *see* diclofenac *on page 266*
PMS-Diclofenac SR [Can] *see* diclofenac *on page 266*
PMS-Diphenhydramine [Can] *see* diphenhydramine *on page 277*
PMS-Dipivefrin [Can] *see* dipivefrin *on page 281*
PMS-Docusate Calcium [Can] *see* docusate *on page 285*
PMS-Docusate Sodium [Can] *see* docusate *on page 285*
PMS-Erythromycin [Can] *see* erythromycin *on page 320*
PMS-Fenofibrate Micro [Can] *see* fenofibrate *on page 360*
PMS-Fluorometholone [Can] *see* fluorometholone *on page 377*
PMS-Fluoxetine [Can] *see* fluoxetine *on page 379*
PMS-Fluphenazine Decanoate [Can] *see* fluphenazine *on page 380*
PMS-Flutamide [Can] *see* flutamide *on page 382*
PMS-Fluvoxamine [Can] *see* fluvoxamine *on page 385*
PMS-Gabapentin [Can] *see* gabapentin *on page 395*
PMS-Gemfibrozil [Can] *see* gemfibrozil *on page 400*
PMS-Glyburide [Can] *see* glyburide *on page 409*
PMS-Haloperidol LA [Can] *see* haloperidol *on page 428*
PMS-Hydromorphone [Can] *see* hydromorphone *on page 453*
PMS-Hydroxyzine [Can] *see* hydroxyzine *on page 458*
PMS-Indapamide [Can] *see* indapamide *on page 470*
PMS-Ipratropium [Can] *see* ipratropium *on page 482*
PMS-Isoniazid [Can] *see* isoniazid *on page 487*
PMS-Isosorbide [Can] *see* isosorbide dinitrate *on page 488*
PMS-Lactulose [Can] *see* lactulose *on page 502*
PMS-Lamotrigine [Can] *see* lamotrigine *on page 503*
PMS-Levobunolol [Can] *see* levobunolol *on page 511*
PMS-Lindane [Can] *see* lindane *on page 522*
PMS-Lithium Carbonate [Can] *see* lithium *on page 525*
PMS-Lithium Citrate [Can] *see* lithium *on page 525*
PMS-Loperamine [Can] *see* loperamide *on page 528*
PMS-Lorazepam [Can] *see* lorazepam *on page 530*

pneumococcal 7-valent conjugate vaccine *see* pneumococcal conjugate vaccine (7-valent) *on this page*

pneumococcal conjugate vaccine (7-valent)

(noo moe KOK al KON ju gate vak SEEN seven-vay lent)

Sound-Alike/Look-Alike Issues

Prevnar® may be confused with PREVEN®

Synonyms diphtheria CRM_{197} protein; PCV7; pneumococcal 7-valent conjugate vaccine

U.S./Canadian Brand Names Prevnar® [US/Can]

Therapeutic Category Vaccine

Use Immunization of infants and toddlers against *Streptococcus pneumoniae* infection caused by serotypes included in the vaccine

Advisory Committee on Immunization Practices (ACIP) guidelines also recommend PCV7 for use in:

Children ≥2-59 months with cochlear implants

All children ≥23 months

Children ages 24-59 months with: Sickle cell disease (including other sickle cell hemoglobinopathies, asplenia, splenic dysfunction), HIV infection, immunocompromising conditions (congenital immunodeficiencies, renal failure, nephrotic syndrome, diseases associated with immunosuppressive or radiation therapy, solid organ transplant), chronic illnesses (cardiac disease, cerebrospinal fluid leaks, diabetes mellitus, pulmonary disease excluding asthma unless on high dose corticosteroids)

Consider use in all children 24-59 months with priority given to:

Children 24-35 months

Children 24-59 months who are of Alaska native, American Indian, or African-American descent

Children 24-59 months who attend group day care centers

Usual Dosage I.M.:

Infants: 2-6 months: 0.5 mL at approximately 2-month intervals for 3 consecutive doses, followed by a fourth dose of 0.5 mL at 12-15 months of age; first dose may be given as young as 6 weeks of age, but is typically given at 2 months of age. In case of a moderate shortage of vaccine, defer the fourth dose until shortage is resolved; in case of a severe shortage of vaccine, defer third and fourth doses until shortage is resolved.

Previously Unvaccinated Infants and Children:

7-11 months: 0.5 mL for a total of 3 doses; 2 doses at least 4 weeks apart, followed by a third dose after the 1-year birthday (12-15 months), separated from the second dose by at least 2 months. In case of a severe shortage of vaccine, defer the third dose until shortage is resolved.

12-23 months: 0.5 mL for a total of 2 doses, separated by at least 2 months. In case of a severe shortage of vaccine, defer the second dose until shortage is resolved.

24-59 months:

Healthy Children: 0.5 mL as a single dose. In case of a severe shortage of vaccine, defer dosing until shortage is resolved.

Children with sickle cell disease, asplenia, HIV infection, chronic illness or immunocompromising conditions (not including bone marrow transplants - results pending; use PPV23 [pneumococcal polysaccharide vaccine, polyvalent] at 12- and 24-months until studies are complete): 0.5 mL for a total of 2 doses, separated by 2 months

Previously Vaccinated Children with a lapse in vaccine administration:

7-11 months: Previously received 1 or 2 doses PCV7: 0.5 mL dose at 7-11 months of age, followed by a second dose ≥2 months later at 12-15 months of age

12-23 months:

Previously received 1 dose before 12 months of age: 0.5 mL dose, followed by a second dose ≥2 months later

Previously received 2 doses before age 12 months: 0.5 mL dose ≥2 months after the most recent dose

24-59 months: Any incomplete schedule: 0.5 mL as a single dose; **Note:** Patients with chronic diseases or immunosuppressing conditions should receive 2 doses ≥2 months apart

(Continued)

pneumococcal conjugate vaccine (7-valent) *(Continued)*

Dosage Forms Injection, suspension: 2 mcg of each saccharide for serotypes 4, 9V, 14, 18C, 19F, and 23F, and 4 mcg of serotype 6B per 0.5 mL (0.5 mL) [contains 16 mcg total saccharide; also contains CRM197 carrier protein ~20 mcg/0.5 mL and aluminum 0.125 mg/0.5 mL (as aluminum phosphate adjuvant)]

pneumococcal polysaccharide vaccine (polyvalent)

(noo moe KOK al pol i SAK a ride vak SEEN, pol i VAY lent)

Synonyms PPV23; 23PS; 23-valent pneumococcal polysaccharide vaccine

U.S./Canadian Brand Names Pneumo 23™ [Can]; Pneumovax® 23 [US/Can]

Therapeutic Category Vaccine, Inactivated Bacteria

Use Children >2 years of age and adults who are at increased risk of pneumococcal disease and its complications because of underlying health conditions (including patients with cochlear implants); older adults, including all those ≥65 years of age

Current Advisory Committee on Immunization Practices (ACIP) guidelines recommend **pneumococcal 7-valent conjugate vaccine (PCV7)** be used for children 2-23 months of age and, in certain situations, children up to 59 months of age

Usual Dosage I.M., SubQ:

Children >2 years and Adults: 0.5 mL

Previously vaccinated with PCV7 vaccine: Children ≥2 years and Adults:

With sickle cell disease, asplenia, immunocompromised or HIV infection: 0.5 mL at ≥2 years of age and ≥2 months after last dose of PCV7; revaccination with PPV23 should be given ≥5 years for children >10 years of age and every 3-5 years for children ≤10 years of age; revaccination should not be administered <3 years after the previous PPV23 dose

With chronic illness: 0.5 mL at ≥2 years of age and ≥2 months after last dose of PCV7; revaccination with PPV23 is not recommended

Following bone marrow transplant (use of PCV7 under study): Administer one dose PPV23 at 12- and 24-months following BMT

Revaccination should be considered:

1. If ≥6 years since initial vaccination has elapsed, or
2. In patients who received 14-valent pneumococcal vaccine and are at highest risk (asplenic) for fatal infection or
3. At ≥6 years in patients with nephrotic syndrome, renal failure, or transplant recipients, or
4. 3-5 years in children with nephrotic syndrome, asplenia, or sickle cell disease

Dosage Forms

Injection, solution: 25 mcg each of 23 polysaccharide isolates/0.5 mL dose (0.5 mL) [prefilled syringe]

Injection, solution: 25 mcg each of 23 polysaccharide isolates/0.5 mL dose (0.5 mL, 2.5 mL) [vial]

Pneumomist® *(Discontinued)* *see page 1042*

Pneumotussin® [US] *see* hydrocodone and guaifenesin *on page 445*

Pneumovax® 23 [US/Can] *see* pneumococcal polysaccharide vaccine (polyvalent) *on this page*

Pnu-Imune® 23 *(Discontinued)* *see page 1042*

Pod-Ben-25® *(Discontinued)* *see page 1042*

Podocon-25™ [US] *see* podophyllum resin *on next page*

Podofilm® [Can] *see* podophyllum resin *on next page*

podofilox (po do FIL oks)

U.S./Canadian Brand Names Condyline™ [Can]; Condylox® [US]; Wartec® [Can]

Therapeutic Category Keratolytic Agent

Use Treatment of external genital warts

Usual Dosage Topical: Adults: Apply twice daily (morning and evening) for 3 consecutive days, then withhold use for 4 consecutive days; this cycle may be repeated up to 4 times until there is no visible wart tissue

Dosage Forms

Gel: 0.5% (3.5 g) [contains alcohol]

Solution, topical: 0.5% (3.5 mL) [contains alcohol]

Podofin® ***(Discontinued)*** *see page 1042*

podophyllin *see* podophyllum resin *on this page*

podophyllum resin (po DOF fil um REZ in)

Synonyms mandrake; may apple; podophyllin

U.S./Canadian Brand Names Podocon-25™ [US]; Podofilm® [Can]

Therapeutic Category Keratolytic Agent

Use Topical treatment of benign growths including external genital and perianal warts, papillomas, fibroids; compound benzoin tincture generally is used as the medium for topical application

Usual Dosage Children and Adults: Topical: 10% to 25% solution in compound benzoin tincture; use 1 drop at a time allowing drying between drops until area is covered; total volume should be limited to <0.5 mL to an area <10 cm^2 for genital or perianal warts or <2 cm^2 for vaginal warts per treatment session; therapy may be repeated once weekly for up to 4 applications for the treatment of genital or perianal warts; use 10% solution when applied to or near mucous membranes

Verrucae: 25% solution is applied directly to the wart; remove drug from area of application within 6 hours

Dosage Forms Liquid, topical: 25% (15 mL) [in benzoin tincture]

Point-Two® ***(Discontinued)*** *see page 1042*

Poladex® ***(Discontinued)*** *see page 1042*

Polaramine® ***(Discontinued)*** *see page 1042*

Polargen® ***(Discontinued)*** *see page 1042*

Poliovax® Injection ***(Discontinued)*** *see page 1042*

poliovirus vaccine (inactivated)

(POE lee oh VYE rus vak SEEN in ak ti VAY ted)

Synonyms enhanced-potency inactivated poliovirus vaccine; IPV; salk vaccine

U.S./Canadian Brand Names IPOL® [US/Can]

Therapeutic Category Vaccine, Live Virus and Inactivated Virus

Use

As the global eradication of poliomyelitis continues, the risk for importation of wild-type poliovirus into the United States decreases dramatically. To eliminate the risk for vaccine-associated paralytic poliomyelitis (VAPP), an all-IPV schedule is recommended for routine childhood vaccination in the United States. All children should receive four doses of IPV (at age 2 months, age 4 months, between ages 6-18 months, and between ages 4-6 years). Oral poliovirus vaccine (OPV), if available, may be used only for the following special circumstances:

- Mass vaccination campaigns to control outbreaks of paralytic polio
- Unvaccinated children who will be traveling within 4 weeks to areas where polio is endemic or epidemic
- Children of parents who do not accept the recommended number of vaccine injections; these children may receive OPV only for the third or fourth dose or both. In this situation, healthcare providers should administer OPV only after discussing the risk for VAPP with parents or caregivers.

OPV supplies are expected to be very limited in the United States after inventories are depleted. ACIP reaffirms its support for the global eradication initiative and use of OPV as the vaccine of choice to eradicate polio where it is endemic.

(Continued)

poliovirus vaccine (inactivated) *(Continued)*

Usual Dosage SubQ: **Enhanced-potency inactivated poliovirus vaccine (E-IPV) is preferred for primary vaccination of adults**, two doses SubQ 4-8 weeks apart, a third dose 6-12 months after the second. For adults with a completed primary series and for whom a booster is indicated, either OPV or E-IPV can be given (E-IPV preferred). If immediate protection is needed, either OPV or E-IPV is recommended.

Dosage Forms Injection, suspension: Type 1 poliovirus 40 D antigen units/0.5 mL, Type 2 poliovirus 8 D antigen units/0.5 mL, and Type 3 poliovirus 32 D antigen units/0.5 mL (0.5 mL, 5 mL) [contains calf serum protein, neomycin, streptomycin, and polymyxin B]

Polocaine® [US/Can] *see* mepivacaine *on page 554*

Polocaine® MPF [US] *see* mepivacaine *on page 554*

polycarbophil (pol i KAR boe fil)

U.S./Canadian Brand Names Equalactin® [US-OTC]; FiberCon® [US-OTC]; Fiber-Lax® [US-OTC]; FiberNorm™ [US-OTC]; Konsyl® Tablets [US-OTC]; Phillips'® Fibercaps [US-OTC]

Therapeutic Category Gastrointestinal Agent, Miscellaneous; Laxative

Use Treatment of constipation or diarrhea

Usual Dosage Oral: General dosing guidelines (OTC labeling):

Children 6-12 years: 625 mg 1-4 times/day

Children ≥12 years and Adults: 1250 mg 1-4 times/day

Dosage Forms

Caplet (FiberCon®, FiberNorm™, Phillips'® Fibercaps): 625 mg

Tablet (Fiber-Lax®, Konsyl®): 625 mg

Tablet, chewable (Equalactin®): 625 mg

Polycidin® Ophthalmic Ointment [Can] *see* bacitracin and polymyxin B *on page 97*

Polycillin-N® Injection *(Discontinued)* *see page 1042*

Polycillin® Oral *(Discontinued)* *see page 1042*

Polycillin-PRB® *(Discontinued)* *see page 1042*

Polycitra® [US] *see* citric acid, sodium citrate, and potassium citrate *on page 206*

Polycitra®-K [US] *see* potassium citrate and citric acid *on page 714*

Polycitra®-LC [US] *see* citric acid, sodium citrate, and potassium citrate *on page 206*

Polycose® [US-OTC] *see* glucose polymers *on page 408*

polyethylene glycol-electrolyte solution

(pol i ETH i leen GLY kol-EE lec tro e lyte soe LOO shun)

Sound-Alike/Look-Alike Issues

GoLYTELY® may be confused with NuLytely®

MiraLax™ may be confused with Mirapex®

NuLytely® may be confused with GoLYTELY®

Synonyms electrolyte lavage solution

U.S./Canadian Brand Names Colyte® [US/Can]; GlycoLax™ [US]; GoLYTELY® [US]; Klean-Prep® [Can]; Lyteprep™ [Can]; MiraLax™ [US]; NuLYTELY® [US]; PegLyte® [Can]; TriLyte™ [US]

Therapeutic Category Laxative

Use Bowel cleansing prior to GI examination or following toxic ingestion (electrolyte containing solutions only); treatment of occasional constipation (MiraLax™)

Usual Dosage

Oral:

Children ≥6 months: Bowel cleansing prior to GI exam (solutions with electrolytes only): 25-40 mL/kg/hour for 4-10 hours (until rectal effluent is clear). Ideally, patients should fast for ~3-4 hours prior to administration; absolutely no solid food for at least 2 hours before the solution is given. The solution may be given via nasogastric tube to patients who are unwilling or unable to drink the solution. Patients <2 years should be monitored closely.

Adults:

Bowel cleansing prior to GI exam (solutions with electrolytes only): 240 mL (8 oz) every 10 minutes, until 4 L are consumed or the rectal effluent is clear; rapid drinking of each portion is preferred to drinking small amounts continuously. Ideally, patients should fast for ~3-4 hours prior to administration; absolutely no solid food for at least 2 hours before the solution is given. The solution may be given via nasogastric tube to patients who are unwilling or unable to drink the solution.

Occasional constipation (MiraLax™): 17 g of powder (~1 heaping tablespoon) dissolved in 8 oz of water; once daily; do not use for >2 weeks.

Nasogastric tube:

Children ≥6 months: Bowel cleansing prior to GI exam (solutions with electrolytes only): 25 mL/kg/hour until rectal effluent is clear. Ideally, patients should fast for ~3-4 hours prior to administration; absolutely no solid food for at least 2 hours before the solution is given.

Adults: Bowel cleansing prior to GI exam (solutions with electrolytes only): 20-30 mL/minute (1.2-1.8 L/hour); the first bowel movement should occur ~1 hour after the start of administration. Ideally, patients should fast for ~3-4 hours prior to administration; absolutely no solid food for at least 2 hours before the solution is given.

Dosage Forms

Powder, for oral solution: PEG 3350 240 g, sodium sulfate 22.72 g, sodium bicarbonate 6.72 g, sodium chloride 5.84 g, and potassium chloride 2.98 g (4000 mL)

Colyte®:

PEG 3350 240 g, sodium sulfate 22.72 g, sodium bicarbonate 6.72 g, sodium chloride 5.84 g, and potassium chloride 2.98 g (4000 mL) [available with citrus berry, lemon lime, cherry, and pineapple flavor packets]

PEG 3350 227.1 g, sodium sulfate 21.5 g, sodium bicarbonate 6.36 g, sodium chloride 5.53 g, and potassium chloride 2.82 g (4000 mL) [regular and pineapple flavor]

GlycoLax™: PEG 3350 17 g/packet (14s); PEG 3350 255 g (16 oz); PEG 3350 527 g (24 oz)

GoLYTELY®:

Disposable jug: PEG 3350 236 g, sodium sulfate 22.74 g, sodium bicarbonate 6.74 g, sodium chloride 5.86 g, and potassium chloride 2.97 g (4000 mL) [regular and pineapple flavor]

Packets: PEG 3350 227.1 g, sodium sulfate 21.5 g, sodium bicarbonate 6.36 g, sodium chloride 5.53 g, and potassium chloride 2.82 g (4000 mL) [regular flavor]

MiraLax™: PEG 3350 17 g/packet (12s); PEG 3350 255 g (14 oz); PEG 3350 527 g (26 oz)

NuLYTELY®: PEG 3350 420 g, sodium bicarbonate 5.72 g, sodium chloride 11.2 g, and potassium chloride 1.48 (4000 mL) [cherry, lemon-lime, and orange flavors]

TriLyte™: PEG 3350 420 g, sodium bicarbonate 5.72 g, sodium chloride 11.2 g, and potassium chloride 1.48 (4000 mL) [supplied with flavor packets]

polyethylene glycol-electrolyte solution and bisacodyl

(pol i ETH i leen GLY kol-ee LEK troe lite soe LOO shun & bis a KOE dil)

U.S./Canadian Brand Names HalfLytely® and Bisacodyl [US]

Therapeutic Category Laxative, Bowel Evacuant; Laxative, Stimulant

Use Bowel cleansing prior to GI examination

Usual Dosage Oral: Adults: Bowel cleansing:

Bisacodyl: 4 tablets as a single dose. After bowel movement or 6 hours (whichever occurs first), initiate polyethylene glycol-electrolyte solution

Polyethylene glycol-electrolyte solution: 8 ounces every 10 minutes until 2 L are consumed

(Continued)

polyethylene glycol-electrolyte solution and bisacodyl *(Continued)*

Dosage Forms Kit (HalfLytely® and Bisacodyl) [each kit contains]:

Powder for oral solution (HalfLytely®):PEG 3350 210 g, sodium bicarbonate 2.86 g, sodium chloride 5.6 g, potassium chloride 0.74 g (2000 mL) [sulfate-free, regular, cherry, lemon-lime, orange flavor]

Tablet, delayed release: Bisacodyl: 5 mg (4s)

Polyflex® Tablet *(Discontinued)* *see page 1042*

Polygam® Injection *(Discontinued)* *see page 1042*

Polygam® S/D [US] *see* immune globulin (intravenous) *on page 468*

Poly-Histine CS® *(Discontinued)* *see page 1042*

Poly-Histine-D® Capsule *(Discontinued)* *see page 1042*

Polymox® *(Discontinued)* *see page 1042*

polymyxin B (pol i MIKS in bee)

Synonyms polymyxin B sulfate

U.S./Canadian Brand Names Poly-Rx [US]

Therapeutic Category Antibiotic, Irrigation; Antibiotic, Miscellaneous

Use Treatment of acute infections caused by susceptible strains of *Pseudomonas aeruginosa*; used occasionally for gut decontamination; parenteral use of polymyxin B has mainly been replaced by less toxic antibiotics, reserved for life-threatening infections caused by organisms resistant to the preferred drugs (eg, pseudomonal meningitis - intrathecal administration)

Usual Dosage

Otic (in combination with other drugs): 1-2 drops, 3-4 times/day; should be used sparingly to avoid accumulation of excess debris

Infants <2 years:

I.M.: Up to 40,000 units/kg/day divided every 6 hours (not routinely recommended due to pain at injection sites)

I.V.: Up to 40,000 units/kg/day divided every 12 hours

Intrathecal: 20,000 units/day for 3-4 days, then 25,000 units every other day for at least 2 weeks after CSF cultures are negative and CSF (glucose) has returned to within normal limits

Children ≥2 years and Adults:

I.M.: 25,000-30,000 units/kg/day divided every 4-6 hours (not routinely recommended due to pain at injection sites)

I.V.: 15,000-25,000 units/kg/day divided every 12 hours

Intrathecal: 50,000 units/day for 3-4 days, then every other day for at least 2 weeks after CSF cultures are negative and CSF (glucose) has returned to within normal limits

Total daily dose should not exceed 2,000,000 units/day

Bladder irrigation: Continuous irrigant or rinse in the urinary bladder for up to 10 days using 20 mg (equal to 200,000 units) added to 1 L of normal saline; usually no more than 1 L of irrigant is used per day unless urine flow rate is high; administration rate is adjusted to patient's urine output

Topical irrigation or topical solution: 500,000 units/L of normal saline; topical irrigation should not exceed 2 million units/day in adults

Gut sterilization: Oral: 15,000-25,000 units/kg/day in divided doses every 6 hours

Clostridium difficile enteritis: Oral: 25,000 units every 6 hours for 10 days

Ophthalmic: A concentration of 0.1% to 0.25% is administered as 1-3 drops every hour, then increasing the interval as response indicates to 1-2 drops 4-6 times/day

Dosage Forms

Injection, powder for reconstitution: 500,000 units

Powder [for prescription compounding] (Poly-Rx): 100 million units (13 g)

polymyxin B and bacitracin *see* bacitracin and polymyxin B *on page 97*

polymyxin B and neomycin *see* neomycin and polymyxin B *on page 610*

polymyxin B and oxytetracycline *see* oxytetracycline and polymyxin B *on page 659*

polymyxin B and trimethoprim *see* trimethoprim and polymyxin B *on page 888*

polymyxin B, bacitracin, and neomycin *see* bacitracin, neomycin, and polymyxin B *on page 97*

polymyxin B, bacitracin, neomycin, and hydrocortisone *see* bacitracin, neomycin, polymyxin B, and hydrocortisone *on page 98*

polymyxin B, neomycin, and dexamethasone *see* neomycin, polymyxin B, and dexamethasone *on page 611*

polymyxin B, neomycin, and gramicidin *see* neomycin, polymyxin B, and gramicidin *on page 611*

polymyxin B, neomycin, and hydrocortisone *see* neomycin, polymyxin B, and hydrocortisone *on page 611*

polymyxin B, neomycin, and prednisolone *see* neomycin, polymyxin B, and prednisolone *on page 612*

polymyxin B sulfate *see* polymyxin B *on previous page*

Poly-Pred® [US] *see* neomycin, polymyxin B, and prednisolone *on page 612*

Poly-Rx [US] *see* polymyxin B *on previous page*

polysaccharide-iron complex (pol i SAK a ride-EYE ern KOM pleks)

Sound-Alike/Look-Alike Issues
Niferex® may be confused with Nephrox®

Synonyms iron-polysaccharide complex

U.S./Canadian Brand Names Fe-Tinic™ 150 [US-OTC]; Hytinic® [US-OTC]; Niferex® 150 [US-OTC]; Niferex® [US-OTC]; Nu-Iron® 150 [US-OTC]

Therapeutic Category Electrolyte Supplement, Oral

Use Prevention and treatment of iron-deficiency anemias

Usual Dosage
Children ≥6 years: Tablets/elixir: 50-100 mg/day; may be given in divided doses
Adults:
Tablets/elixir: 50-100 mg twice daily
Capsules: 150-300 mg/day

Dosage Forms
Capsule (Fe-Tinic™ 150, Hytinic®, Niferex® 150, Nu-Iron® 150): Elemental iron 150 mg
Elixir (Niferex®): Elemental iron 100 mg/5 mL (240 mL) [contains alcohol 10%]
Tablet (Niferex®): Elemental iron 50 mg

Polysporin® Ophthalmic [US] *see* bacitracin and polymyxin B *on page 97*

Polysporin® Topical [US-OTC] *see* bacitracin and polymyxin B *on page 97*

Polytar® [US-OTC] *see* coal tar *on page 219*

polythiazide (pol i THYE a zide)

U.S./Canadian Brand Names Renese® [US]

Therapeutic Category Diuretic, Thiazide

Use Adjunctive therapy in treatment of edema and hypertension

Usual Dosage Adults: Oral:
Edema: 1-4 mg/day
Hypertension: 2-4 mg/day

Dosage Forms [DSC] = Discontinued product
Tablet: 1 mg [DSC], 2 mg

polythiazide and prazosin *see* prazosin and polythiazide *on page 722*

Polytrim® [US/Can] *see* trimethoprim and polymyxin B *on page 888*

Poly-Vi-Flor® [US] *see* vitamins (multiple/pediatric) *on page 927*

Poly-Vi-Flor® With Iron [US] *see* vitamins (multiple/pediatric) *on page 927*

polyvinyl alcohol *see* artificial tears *on page 78*

Poly-Vi-Sol® [US-OTC] *see* vitamins (multiple/pediatric) *on page 927*

Poly-Vi-Sol® with Iron [US-OTC] *see* vitamins (multiple/pediatric) *on page 927*

Pondimin® *(Discontinued)* *see page 1042*

Ponstan® [Can] *see* mefenamic acid *on page 548*

Ponstel® [US/Can] *see* mefenamic acid *on page 548*

Pontocaine® [US/Can] *see* tetracaine *on page 851*

Pontocaine® With Dextrose [US] *see* tetracaine and dextrose *on page 851*

poractant alfa (por AKT ant AL fa)

U.S./Canadian Brand Names Curosurf® [US/Can]

Therapeutic Category Lung Surfactant

Use **Orphan drug:** Treatment and prevention of respiratory distress syndrome (RDS) in premature infants

Usual Dosage Intratracheal use **only**: Premature infant with RDS: Initial dose is 2.5 mL/kg of birth weight. Up to 2 subsequent doses of 1.25 mL/kg birth weight can be administered at 12-hour intervals if needed in infants who continue to require mechanical ventilation and supplemental oxygen.

Dosage Forms Suspension for intratracheal instillation: 80 mg/mL (1.5 mL, 3 mL)

Porcelana® Sunscreen *(Discontinued)* *see page 1042*

porfimer (POR fi mer)

Synonyms CL-184116; dihematoporphyrin ether; porfimer sodium

U.S./Canadian Brand Names Photofrin® [US/Can]

Therapeutic Category Antineoplastic Agent

Use Adjunct to laser light therapy for obstructing esophageal cancer, obstructing endobronchial nonsmall-cell lung cancer (NSCLC), ablation of high-grade dysplasia in Barrett's esophagus

Usual Dosage Refer to individual protocols. I.V.:

Children: Safety and efficacy have not been established

Adults: 2 mg/kg, followed by exposure to the appropriate laser light

Dosage Forms Injection, powder for reconstitution, as sodium: 75 mg

porfimer sodium *see* porfimer *on this page*

Portia™ [US] *see* ethinyl estradiol and levonorgestrel *on page 339*

Posicor® *(Discontinued)* *see page 1042*

Post Peel Healing Balm [US] *see* hydrocortisone (topical) *on page 451*

Posture® [US-OTC] *see* calcium phosphate (tribasic) *on page 150*

Potasalan® *(Discontinued)* *see page 1042*

potassium acetate (poe TASS ee um AS e tate)

Therapeutic Category Electrolyte Supplement, Oral

Use Potassium deficiency; to avoid chloride when high concentration of potassium is needed, source of bicarbonate

Usual Dosage I.V. doses should be incorporated into the patient's maintenance I.V. fluids, intermittent I.V. potassium administration should be reserved for severe depletion situations and requires ECG monitoring; doses listed as mEq of potassium

Children:

Treatment of hypokalemia: I.V.: 2-5 mEq/kg/day

I.V. intermittent infusion (must be diluted prior to administration): 0.5-1 mEq/kg/dose (maximum: 30 mEq/dose) to infuse at 0.3-0.5 mEq/kg/hour (maximum: 1 mEq/kg/hour)

Note: Use caution in premature neonates; potassium acetate for injection contains aluminum.

Adults:

Treatment of hypokalemia: I.V.: 40-100 mEq/day

I.V. intermittent infusion (must be diluted prior to administration): 5-10 mEq/dose (maximum: 40 mEq/dose) to infuse over 2-3 hours (maximum: 40 mEq over 1 hour)

Note: Continuous cardiac monitor recommended for rates >0.5 mEq/hour

Potassium dosage/rate of infusion guidelines:

Serum potassium >2.5 mEq/L: Maximum infusion rate: 10 mEq/hour; maximum concentration: 40 mEq/L; maximum 24-hour dose: 200 mEq

Serum potassium <2.5 mEq/L: Maximum infusion rate: 40 mEq/hour; maximum concentration: 80 mEq/L; maximum 24-hour dose: 400 mEq

Dosage Forms Injection, solution: 2 mEq/mL (20 mL, 50 mL, 100 mL); 4 mEq/mL (50 mL) [contains aluminum ≤200 mcg/mL]

potassium acetate, potassium bicarbonate, and potassium citrate

(poe TASS ee um AS e tate, poe TASS ee um bye KAR bun ate, & poe TASS ee um SIT rate)

Synonyms potassium acetate, potassium citrate, and potassium bicarbonate; potassium bicarbonate, potassium acetate, and potassium citrate; potassium bicarbonate, potassium citrate, and potassium acetate; potassium citrate, potassium acetate, and potassium bicarbonate; potassium citrate, potassium bicarbonate, and potassium acetate

U.S./Canadian Brand Names Tri-K® [US]

Therapeutic Category Electrolyte Supplement, Oral

Use Treatment or prevention of hypokalemia

Usual Dosage Oral:

Children: 1-4 mEq/kg/24 hours in divided doses as required to maintain normal serum potassium

Adults:

Prevention: 16-24 mEq/day in 2-4 divided doses

Treatment: 40-100 mEq/day in 2-4 divided doses

Dosage Forms Solution, oral: Potassium 45 mEq/15 mL (480 mL) [from potassium acetate 1500 mg, potassium bicarbonate 1500 mg, and potassium citrate 1500 mg per 15 mL]

potassium acetate, potassium citrate, and potassium bicarbonate

see potassium acetate, potassium bicarbonate, and potassium citrate *on this page*

potassium acid phosphate

(poe TASS ee um AS id FOS fate)

U.S./Canadian Brand Names K-Phos® Original [US]

Therapeutic Category Urinary Acidifying Agent

Use Acidifies urine and lowers urinary calcium concentration; reduces odor and rash caused by ammoniacal urine; increases the antibacterial activity of methenamine

Usual Dosage Adults: Oral: 1000 mg dissolved in 6-8 oz of water 4 times/day with meals and at bedtime; for best results, soak tablets in water for 2-5 minutes, then stir and swallow

Dosage Forms Tablet [scored]: 500 mg [phosphorus 114 mg and potassium 144 mg (3.7 mEq) per tablet; sodium free]

potassium bicarbonate

(poe TASS ee um bye KAR bun ate)

U.S./Canadian Brand Names K+ Care® ET [US]

Therapeutic Category Electrolyte Supplement, Oral

Use Potassium deficiency, hypokalemia

(Continued)

potassium bicarbonate *(Continued)*

Usual Dosage Oral:

Children: 1-4 mEq/kg/day

Adults: 25 mEq 2-4 times/day

Dosage Forms Tablet for oral solution, effervescent: Potassium 25 mEq

potassium bicarbonate and potassium chloride, effervescent

(poe TASS ee um bye KAR bun ate & poe TASS ee um KLOR ide, ef er VES ent)

Synonyms potassium bicarbonate and potassium chloride (effervescent)

U.S./Canadian Brand Names K-Lyte/Cl® [US]; K-Lyte/Cl® 50 [US]

Therapeutic Category Electrolyte Supplement, Oral

Use Treatment or prevention of hypokalemia

Usual Dosage Oral:

Children: 1-4 mEq/kg/24 hours in divided doses as required to maintain normal serum potassium

Adults:

Prevention: 16-24 mEq/day in 2-4 divided doses

Treatment: 40-100 mEq/day in 2-4 divided doses

Dosage Forms Tablet for oral solution, effervescent:

K-Lyte/Cl®: Potassium chloride 25 mEq [potassium chloride 1.5 g and potassium bicarbonate 0.5 g; citrus or fruit punch flavor]

K-Lyte/Cl® 50: Potassium chloride 50 mEq [potassium chloride 2.24 g and potassium bicarbonate 2 g; citrus or fruit punch flavor]

potassium bicarbonate and potassium chloride (effervescent) *see* potassium bicarbonate and potassium chloride, effervescent *on this page*

potassium bicarbonate and potassium citrate, effervescent

(poe TASS ee um bye KAR bun ate & poe TASS ee um SIT rate, ef er VES ent)

Sound-Alike/Look-Alike Issues

Klor-Con® may be confused with Klaron®, K-Lor®

Synonyms potassium bicarbonate and potassium citrate (effervescent)

U.S./Canadian Brand Names Effer-K™ [US]; Klor-Con®/EF [US]; K-Lyte® [US/Can]; K-Lyte® DS [US]

Therapeutic Category Electrolyte Supplement, Oral

Use Treatment or prevention of hypokalemia

Usual Dosage Oral:

Children: 1-4 mEq/kg/24 hours in divided doses as required to maintain normal serum potassium

Adults:

Prevention: 16-24 mEq/day in 2-4 divided doses

Treatment: 40-100 mEq/day in 2-4 divided doses

Dosage Forms Tablet, effervescent: Potassium 25 mEq

Effer-K™: Potassium 25 mEq

Klor-Con®/EF: Potassium 25 mEq [orange flavor]

K-Lyte®: Potassium 25 mEq [lime or orange flavor]

K-Lyte® DS: Potassium 50 mEq [lime or orange flavor]

potassium bicarbonate and potassium citrate (effervescent) *see* potassium bicarbonate and potassium citrate, effervescent *on this page*

potassium bicarbonate, potassium acetate, and potassium citrate *see* potassium acetate, potassium bicarbonate, and potassium citrate *on previous page*

potassium bicarbonate, potassium citrate, and potassium acetate *see* potassium acetate, potassium bicarbonate, and potassium citrate *on previous page*

potassium chloride (poe TASS ee um KLOR ide)

Sound-Alike/Look-Alike Issues

Kaon-Cl®-10 may be confused with kaolin
K-Dur® may be confused with Cardura®, Imdur®
K-Lor™ may be confused with Kaochlor®, Klor-Con®
Klor-Con® may be confused with Klaron®, K-Lor®
Klotrix® may be confused with liotrix
Micro-K® may be confused with Micronase®

Synonyms KCl

U.S./Canadian Brand Names Apo-K® [Can]; K+8 [US]; K+10 [US]; Kaon-Cl®-10 [US]; Kaon-Cl® 20 [US]; Kay Ciel® [US]; K+ Care® [US]; K-Dur® [Can]; K-Dur® 10 [US]; K-Dur® 20 [US]; K-Lor™ [US/Can]; Klor-Con® [US]; Klor-Con® 8 [US]; Klor-Con® 10 [US]; Klor-Con®/25 [US]; Klor-Con® M [US]; Klotrix® [US]; K-Tab® [US]; Micro-K® 10 Extencaps® [US]; Micro-K® Extencaps [US-OTC/Can]; Roychlor® [Can]; Rum-K® [US]; Slow-K® [Can]

Therapeutic Category Electrolyte Supplement, Oral

Use Treatment or prevention of hypokalemia

Usual Dosage I.V. doses should be incorporated into the patient's maintenance I.V. fluids; intermittent I.V. potassium administration should be reserved for severe depletion situations in patients undergoing ECG monitoring.

Normal daily requirements: Oral, I.V.:
- Premature infants: 2-6 mEq/kg/24 hours
- Term infants 0-24 hours: 0-2 mEq/kg/24 hours
- Infants >24 hours: 1-2 mEq/kg/24 hours
- Children: 2-3 mEq/kg/day
- Adults: 40-80 mEq/day

Prevention during diuretic therapy: Oral:
- Children: 1-2 mEq/kg/day in 1-2 divided doses
- Adults: 20-40 mEq/day in 1-2 divided doses

Treatment of hypokalemia: Children:
- Oral: 1-2 mEq/kg initially, then as needed based on frequently obtained lab values. If deficits are severe or ongoing losses are great, I.V. route should be considered.
- I.V.: 1 mEq/kg over 1-2 hours initially, then repeated as needed based on frequently obtained lab values; severe depletion or ongoing losses may require >200% of normal limit needs
- I.V. intermittent infusion: Dose should not exceed 1 mEq/kg/hour, or 40 mEq/hour; if it exceeds 0.5 mEq/kg/hour, physician should be at bedside and patient should have continuous ECG monitoring; usual pediatric maximum: 3 mEq/kg/day or 40 mEq/m^2/day

Treatment of hypokalemia: Adults:
- I.V. intermittent infusion: 5-10 mEq/hour (continuous cardiac monitor recommended for rates >5 mEq/hour), not to exceed 40 mEq/hour; usual adult maximum per 24 hours: 400 mEq/day.
  - Potassium dosage/rate of infusion guidelines: Serum potassium >2.5 mEq/L: Maximum infusion rate: 10 mEq/hour; maximum concentration: 40 mEq/L; maximum 24-hour dose: 200 mEq Serum potassium <2.5 mEq/L: Maximum infusion rate: 40 mEq/hour; maximum concentration: 80 mEq/L; maximum 24-hour dose: 400 mEq
- Potassium >2.5 mEq/L:
  - Oral: 60-80 mEq/day plus additional amounts if needed
  - I.V.: 10 mEq over 1 hour with additional doses if needed
- Potassium <2.5 mEq/L:
  - Oral: Up to 40-60 mEq initial dose, followed by further doses based on lab values
  - I.V.: Up to 40 mEq over 1 hour, with doses based on frequent lab monitoring; deficits at a plasma level of 2 mEq/L may be as high as 400-800 mEq of potassium

Dosage Forms

Capsule, extended release: 10 mEq [800 mg]
- microK® [microencapsulated]: 8 mEq [600 mg]
- microK® 10 [microencapsulated]: 10 mEq [800 mg]

(Continued)

potassium chloride *(Continued)*

Infusion [premixed in D_5W]: 20 mEq (1000 mL); 30 mEq (1000 mL); 40 mEq (1000 mL)
Infusion [premixed in D_5W and LR]: 20 mEq (1000 mL); 30 mEq (1000 mL)
Infusion [premixed in D_5W and ¹/₄NS]: 10 mEq (500 mL, 1000 mL); 20 mEq (1000 mL); 30 mEq (1000 mL); 40 mEq (1000 mL)
Infusion [premixed in D_5W and ¹/₂NS]: 20 mEq (1000 mL); 40 mEq (1000 mL)
Infusion [premixed in D_5 and NS]: 20 mEq (1000 mL); 40 mEq (1000 mL)
Infusion [premixed in D_5W and sodium chloride 0.3%]: 10 mEq (500 mL); 20 mEq (1000 mL)
Infusion [premixed in NS]: 20 mEq (1000 mL); 40 mEq (1000 mL)
Infusion [premixed in SWFI]: 10 mEq (50 mL, 100 mL); 20 mEq (50 mL, 100 mL); 30 mEq (100 mL); 40 mEq (100 mL)
Injection, solution [concentrate]: 2 mEq/mL (5 mL, 10 mL, 15 mL, 20 mL, 250 mL)
Powder, for oral solution: 20 mEq/packet (30s, 100s, 1000s)
K+ Care®: 20 mEq/packet (30s) [fruit or orange flavor]
K-Lor®: 20 mEq/packet (30s, 100s)
Kay Ciel® 10%: 20 mEq/packet (30s, 100s) [sugar free]
Klor-Con®: 20 mEq/packet (30s, 100s) [sugar free]
Klor-Con®/25: 25 mEq/packet (30s, 100s) [sugar free]
Solution, oral: 20 mEq/15 mL (480 mL); 40 mEq/15 mL (480 mL)
Kaon-Cl® 20: 40 mEq/15 mL (480 mL) [sugar free; contains alcohol; cherry flavor]
Kay Ciel®: 10%: 20 mEq/15 mL (120 mL, 480 mL) [sugar free; contains alcohol]
Rum-K®: 20 mEq/10 mL (480 mL) [alcohol free, sugar free; butter/rum flavor]
Tablet, extended release: 8 mEq [600 mg]; 10 mEq [800 mg]; 20 mEq [1500 mg]
K+8: 8 mEq [600 mg]
K+10: 10 mEq [800 mg]
K-Dur® 10 [microencapsulated]: 10 mEq [800 mg]
K-Dur® 20 [microencapsulated]: 20 mEq [1500 mg; scored]
K-Tab®: 10 mEq [800 mg]
Kaon-Cl® 10 [film coated]: 10 mEq [800 mg
Klor-Con® 8: 8 mEq [600 mg; wax matrix]
Klor-Con® 10: 10 mEq [800 mg; wax matrix]
Klor-Con® M10 [microencapsulated]: 10 mEq [800 mg]
Klor-Con® M15 [microencapsulated]: 15 mEq [1125 mg]
Klor-Con® M20 [microencapsulated]: 20 mEq [1500 mg; scored]
Tablet, slow release [film coated] (Klotrix®): 10 mEq [800 mg; wax matrix]

potassium citrate (poe TASS ee um SIT rate)

Sound-Alike/Look-Alike Issues
Urocit®-K may be confused with Urised®
U.S./Canadian Brand Names K-Citra® [Can]; Urocit®-K [US]
Therapeutic Category Alkalinizing Agent
Use Prevention of uric acid nephrolithiasis; prevention of calcium renal stones in patients with hypocitraturia; urinary alkalinizer when sodium citrate is contraindicated
Usual Dosage Adults: Oral: 10-20 mEq 3 times/day with meals up to 100 mEq/day
Dosage Forms Tablet: 540 mg [5 mEq]; 1080 mg [10 mEq]

potassium citrate and citric acid

(poe TASS ee um SIT rate & SI trik AS id)
Synonyms citric acid and potassium citrate
U.S./Canadian Brand Names Cytra-K [US]; Polycitra®-K [US]
Therapeutic Category Alkalinizing Agent
Use Treatment of metabolic acidosis; alkalinizing agent in conditions where long-term maintenance of an alkaline urine is desirable
Usual Dosage Urine alkalizing agent:
Children: Solution: 5-15 mL after meals and at bedtime; adjust dose based on urinary pH

Adults:

Powder: One packet dissolved in water after meals and at bedtime; adjust dose to urinary pH

Solution: 15-30 mL after meals and at bedtime; adjust dose based on urinary pH

Dosage Forms Note: Equivalent to potassium 2 mEq/mL and bicarbonate 2 mEq/mL

Powder:

Cytra-K: Potassium citrate 3300 mg and citric acid 1002 mg per packet (100s) [sugar free; fruit flavor]

Polycitra®-K: Potassium citrate 3300 mg and citric acid 1002 mg per packet (100s) [sugar free]

Solution:

Cytra-K: Potassium citrate 1100 mg and citric acid monohydrate 334 mg per 5 mL (480 mL) [alcohol free, sugar free; contains sodium benzoate; cherry flavor]

Polycitra®-K: Potassium citrate 1100 mg and citric acid monohydrate 334 mg per 5 mL (480 mL) [alcohol free, sugar free]

potassium citrate, citric acid, and sodium citrate *see* citric acid, sodium citrate, and potassium citrate *on page 206*

potassium citrate, potassium acetate, and potassium bicarbonate *see* potassium acetate, potassium bicarbonate, and potassium citrate *on page 711*

potassium citrate, potassium bicarbonate, and potassium acetate *see* potassium acetate, potassium bicarbonate, and potassium citrate *on page 711*

potassium gluconate (poe TASS ee um GLOO coe nate)

U.S./Canadian Brand Names Glu-K® [US-OTC]; Kaon® [US]

Therapeutic Category Electrolyte Supplement, Oral

Use Treatment or prevention of hypokalemia

Usual Dosage Oral (doses listed as mEq of potassium):

Normal daily requirement:

Children: 2-3 mEq/kg/day

Adults: 40-80 mEq/day

Prevention of hypokalemia during diuretic therapy:

Children: 1-2 mEq/kg/day in 1-2 divided doses

Adults: 16-24 mEq/day in 1-2 divided doses

Treatment of hypokalemia:

Children: 2-5 mEq/kg/day in 2-4 divided doses

Adults: 40-100 mEq/day in 2-4 divided doses

Dosage Forms

Tablet: 500 mg, 610 mg

Glu-K®: 486 mg

Tablet, timed release: 595 mg

potassium iodide (poe TASS ee um EYE oh dide)

Synonyms KI; Lugol's solution; strong iodine solution

U.S./Canadian Brand Names Iosat™ [US-OTC]; Pima® [US]; SSKI® [US]

Therapeutic Category Antithyroid Agent; Expectorant

Use Expectorant for the symptomatic treatment of chronic pulmonary diseases complicated by mucous; reduce thyroid vascularity prior to thyroidectomy and management of thyrotoxic crisis; block thyroidal uptake of radioactive isotopes of iodine in a radiation emergency or other exposure to radioactive iodine

Usual Dosage Oral:

Adults: RDA: 150 mcg (iodide)

Expectorant:

Children (Pima®):

<3 years: 162 mg 3 times day

>3 years: 325 mg 3 times/day

(Continued)

potassium iodide *(Continued)*

Adults:
Pima®: 325-650 mg 3 times/day
SSKI®: 300-600 mg 3-4 times/day
Preoperative thyroidectomy: Children and Adults: 50-250 mg (1-5 drops SSKI®) 3 times/day **or** 0.1-0.3 mL (3-5 drops) of strong iodine (Lugol's solution) 3 times/day; administer for 10 days before surgery
Radiation protectant to radioactive isotopes of iodine (Pima®):
Children:
Infants up to 1 year: 65 mg once daily for 10 days; start 24 hours prior to exposure
>1 year: 130 mg once daily for 10 days; start 24 hours prior to exposure
Adults: 195 mg once daily for 10 days; start 24 hours prior to exposure
To reduce risk of thyroid cancer following nuclear accident (dosing should continue until risk of exposure has passed or other measures are implemented):
Children (see adult dose for children >68 kg):
Infants <1 month: 16 mg once daily
1 month to 3 years: 32 mg once daily
3-18 years: 65 mg once daily
Children >68 kg and Adults (including pregnant/lactating women): 130 mg once daily
Thyrotoxic crisis:
Infants <1 year: 150-250 mg (3-5 drops SSKI®) 3 times/day
Children and Adults: 300-500 mg (6-10 drops SSKI®) 3 times/day or 1 mL strong iodine (Lugol's solution) 3 times/day
Sporotrichosis (cutaneous, lymphocutaneous): Adults: Oral: Initial: 5 drops (SSKI®) 3 times/day; increase to 40-50 drops (SSKI®) 3 times/day as tolerated for 3-6 months

Dosage Forms
Solution, oral:
SSKI®: 1 g/mL (30 mL, 240 mL) [contains sodium thiosulfate]
Lugol's solution, strong iodine: Potassium iodide 100 mg/mL and iodine 50 mg/mL (15 mL, 480 mL)
Syrup (Pima®): 325 mg/5 mL [equivalent to iodide 249 mg/5 mL] (473 mL) [black raspberry flavor]
Tablet: 65 mg [equivalent to iodide 50 mg]
Iosat™: 130 mg

potassium iodide, chlorpheniramine, phenylephrine, and codeine *see* chlorpheniramine, phenylephrine, codeine, and potassium iodide *on page 193*

potassium perchlorate *see* radiological/contrast media (ionic) *on page 759*

potassium phosphate (poe TASS ee um FOS fate)

Sound-Alike/Look-Alike Issues
Neutra-Phos®-K may be confused with K-Phos Neutral®

Synonyms phosphate, potassium

U.S./Canadian Brand Names Neutra-Phos®-K [US-OTC]

Therapeutic Category Electrolyte Supplement, Oral

Use Treatment and prevention of hypophosphatemia or hypokalemia

Usual Dosage I.V. doses should be incorporated into the patient's maintenance I.V. fluids; intermittent I.V. infusion should be reserved for severe depletion situations in patients undergoing continuous ECG monitoring. It is difficult to determine total body phosphorus deficit; the following dosages are empiric guidelines:

Normal requirements elemental phosphorus: Oral:
0-6 months: 240 mg
6-12 months: 360 mg
1-10 years: 800 mg
>10 years: 1200 mg
Pregnancy lactation: Additional 400 mg/day
Adults: 800 mg

Treatment: It is difficult to provide concrete guidelines for the treatment of severe hypophosphatemia because the extent of total body deficits and response to therapy are difficult to predict. Aggressive doses of phosphate may result in a transient serum elevation followed by redistribution into intracellular compartments or bone tissue. It is recommended that repletion of severe hypophosphatemia (<1 mg/dL in adults) be done I.V. because large doses of oral phosphate may cause diarrhea and intestinal absorption may be unreliable

Pediatric I.V. phosphate repletion:

Children: 0.25-0.5 mmol/kg **administer over 4-6 hours and repeat if symptomatic hypophosphatemia persists**; to assess the need for further phosphate administration, obtain serum inorganic phosphate after administration of the first dose and base further doses on serum levels and clinical status

Adult I.V. phosphate repletion:

Initial dose: 0.08 mmol/kg if recent uncomplicated hypophosphatemia

Initial dose: 0.16 mmol/kg if prolonged hypophosphatemia with presumed total body deficits; increase dose by 25% to 50% if patient symptomatic with severe hypophosphatemia

Do not exceed 0.24 mmol/kg/dose; administer over 6-12 hours by I.V. infusion. Some investigators have used more rapid infusions.

With orders for I.V. phosphate, there is considerable confusion associated with the use of millimoles (mmol) versus milliequivalents (mEq) to express the phosphate requirement. Because inorganic phosphate exists as monobasic and dibasic anions, with the mixture of valences dependent on pH, ordering by mEq amounts is unreliable and may lead to large dosing errors. In addition, I.V. phosphate is available in the sodium and potassium salt; therefore, the content of these cations must be considered when ordering phosphate. The most reliable method of ordering I.V. phosphate is by millimoles, then specifying the potassium or sodium salt. For example, an order for 15 mmol of phosphate as potassium phosphate in one liter of normal saline. The dosing of phosphate should be 0.2-0.3 mmol/kg with a usual daily requirement of 30-60 mmol/day or 15 mmol of phosphate per liter of TPN or 15 mmol phosphate per 1000 calories of dextrose. Would also provide 22 mEq of potassium.

Maintenance:

I.V. solutions:

Children: 0.5-1.5 mmol/kg/24 hours I.V. or 2-3 mmol/kg/24 hours orally in divided doses

Adults: 15-30 mmol/24 hours I.V. or 50-150 mmol/24 hours orally in divided doses

Oral:

Children <4 years: 1 capsule (250 mg phosphorus/8 mmol) 4 times/day; dilute as instructed

Children >4 years and Adults: 1-2 capsules (250-500 mg phosphorus/8-16 mmol) 4 times/day; dilute as instructed

Dosage Forms

Injection, solution: Phosphate 3 mmol and potassium 4.4 mEq per mL (5 mL, 15 mL, 50 mL) [equivalent to phosphate 285 mg and potassium 170 mg per mL]

Powder for oral solution [packet] (Neutra-Phos®-K): Monobasic potassium phosphate and dibasic potassium phosphate/packet (100s) [equivalent to elemental phosphorus 250 mg and potassium 556 mg (14.2 mEq) per packet; sodium free]

potassium phosphate and sodium phosphate

(poe TASS ee um FOS fate & SOW dee um FOS fate)

Sound-Alike/Look-Alike Issues

K-Phos Neutral® may be confused with Neutra-Phos-K®

Synonyms sodium phosphate and potassium phosphate

U.S./Canadian Brand Names K-Phos® MF [US]; K-Phos® Neutral [US]; K-Phos® No. 2 [US]; Neutra-Phos® [US-OTC]; Uro-KP-Neutral® [US]

Therapeutic Category Electrolyte Supplement, Oral

Use Treatment of conditions associated with excessive renal phosphate loss or inadequate GI absorption of phosphate; to acidify the urine to lower calcium concentrations;

(Continued)

potassium phosphate and sodium phosphate *(Continued)*

to increase the antibacterial activity of methenamine; reduce odor and rash caused by ammonia in urine

Usual Dosage All dosage forms to be mixed in 6-8 oz of water prior to administration

Children ≥4 years: Elemental phosphorus 250 mg 4 times/day after meals and at bedtime

Adults: Elemental phosphorus 250-500 mg 4 times/day after meals and at bedtime

Dosage Forms

Powder, for oral suspension (Neutra-Phos®): Monobasic sodium, dibasic sodium, and potassium phosphate/packet (100s) [equivalent to elemental phosphorus 250 mg, sodium 164 mg (7.1 mEq), and potassium 278 mg (7.1 mEq) per packet]

Tablet:

K-Phos® MF: Potassium acid phosphate 155 mg and sodium acid phosphate 250 mg [equivalent to elemental phosphorus 125.6 mg, sodium 67 mg (2.9 mEq), and potassium 44.5 mg (1.1 mEq)]

K-Phos® Neutral: Dibasic sodium phosphate 852 mg, monobasic potassium phosphate 155 mg, and monobasic sodium phosphate 130 mg [equivalent to elemental phosphorus 250 mg, sodium 298 mg (13 mEq), and potassium 45 mg (1.1 mEq)]

K-Phos® No. 2: Potassium acid phosphate 305 mg and sodium acid phosphate 700 mg [equivalent to elemental phosphorus 250 mg, sodium 134 mg (5.8 mEq), and potassium 88 mg (2.3 mEq)]

Uro-KP-Neutral®: Sodium phosphate monobasic, dipotassium phosphate, and disodium phosphate [equivalent to elemental phosphorus 258 mg, phosphate 8 mmol, sodium 262.4 mg (10.8 mEq), and potassium 49.4 mg (1.3 mEq)]

povidone-iodine (POE vi done-EYE oh dyne)

Sound-Alike/Look-Alike Issues

Betadine® may be confused with Betagan®, betaine

U.S./Canadian Brand Names ACU-dyne® [US-OTC]; Betadine® Ophthalmic [US]; Betadine® [US-OTC/Can]; Minidyne® [US-OTC]; Operand® [US-OTC]; Proviodine [Can]; Summer's Eve® Medicated Douche [US-OTC]; Vagi-Gard® [US-OTC]

Therapeutic Category Antibacterial, Topical

Use External antiseptic with broad microbicidal spectrum against bacteria, fungi, viruses, protozoa, and yeasts

Usual Dosage

Shampoo: Apply 2 teaspoons to hair and scalp, lather and rinse; repeat application 2 times/week until improvement is noted, then shampoo weekly

Topical: Apply as needed for treatment and prevention of susceptible microbial infections

Dosage Forms

Gel, topical (Operand®): 10% (120 g)

Liquid, topical: 7.5% (120 mL)
- ACU-dyne®: 7.5% (60 mL, 240 mL, 480 mL, 960 mL, 3840 mL)
- Betadine®: 7.5% (120 mL)

Liquid, topical scrub: 7.5% (120 mL)
- Betadine®: 7.5% (120 mL, 480 mL, 960 mL, 3840 mL)
- Operand®: 7.5% (960 mL)

Ointment, topical: 10% (1 g, 3.5 g, 30 g)
- Betadine®: 10% (0.9 g, 3.7 g, 30 g)

Pad [prep pads]: 10% (200s)

Solution, ophthalmic (Betadine®): 5% (50 mL)

Solution, perineal (Betadine®, Operand®): 10% (240 mL)

Solution, topical: 10% (30 mL, 120 mL, 240 mL, 480 mL, 3840 mL)
- Betadine®: 10% (15 mL, 120 mL, 240 mL, 480 mL, 960 mL, 3840 mL)
- Minidyne®: 10% (15 mL)
- Operand®: 10% (60 mL, 120 mL, 240 mL, 480 mL, 960 mL, 3840 mL)

Solution, topical scrub: 7.5% (120 mL, 240 mL, 480 mL, 3840 mL)
- Operand®: 7.5% (60 mL, 120 mL, 240 mL, 480 mL, 960 mL, 3840 mL)

Solution, topical spray (Betadine®): 5% (90 mL)
Solution, vaginal douche: 10% (240 mL) [concentrate]
Betadine®: 10% (180 mL, 240 mL) [concentrate]
Operand®: 10% (240 mL) [concentrate]
Summer's Eve® Medicated Douche: 0.3% (135 mL)
Vagi-Gard®: 10% (240 mL) [concentrate]
Solution, whirlpool: 10% (3840 mL) [concentrate]
Operand®: 1% (3840 mL)
Swabsticks: 7.5% (25s, 50s); 10% (25s, 50s)
Betadine®: 10% (50s, 150s, 200s, 1000s)

PPD *see* tuberculin tests *on page 893*

PPI-149 *see* abarelix *on page 2*

PPL *see* benzylpenicilloyl-polylysine *on page 112*

PPS *see* pentosan polysulfate sodium *on page 680*

PPV23 *see* pneumococcal polysaccharide vaccine (polyvalent) *on page 704*

pralidoxime (pra li DOKS eem)

Sound-Alike/Look-Alike Issues
pralidoxime may be confused with pramoxine, pyridoxine
Protopam® may be confused with Proloprim®, protamine, Protropin®

Synonyms 2-PAM; pralidoxime chloride; 2-pyridine aldoxime methochloride

U.S./Canadian Brand Names Protopam® [US/Can]

Therapeutic Category Antidote

Use Reverse muscle paralysis caused by toxic exposure to organophosphate anticholinesterase pesticides and chemicals; control of overdose of anticholinesterase medications used to treat myasthenia gravis (ambenonium, neostigmine, pyridostigmine)

Usual Dosage
Organic phosphorus poisoning (use in conjunction with atropine; atropine effects should be established before pralidoxime is administered): I.V. (may be given I.M. or SubQ if I.V. is not feasible):
Children: 20-50 mg/kg/dose; repeat in 1-2 hours if muscle weakness has not been relieved, then at 8- to 12-hour intervals if cholinergic signs recur
Adults: 1-2 g; repeat in 1 hour if muscle weakness has not been relieved, then at 8- to 12-hour intervals if cholinergic signs recur. When the poison has been ingested, continued absorption from the lower bowel may require additional doses; patients should be titrated as long as signs of poisoning recur; dosing may need repeated every 3-8 hours.
Treatment of acetylcholinesterase inhibitor toxicity: Adults: I.V.: Initial: 1-2 g followed by increments of 250 mg every 5 minutes until response is observed
Infants and Children:
Prehospital ("in the field"): Mild-to-moderate symptoms: I.M.: 15 mg/kg; severe symptoms: 25 mg/kg
Hospital/emergency department: Mild-to-severe symptoms: I.V.: 15 mg/kg (up to 1 g)
Adults:
Prehospital ("in the field"): Mild-to-moderate symptoms: I.M.: 600 mg; severe symptoms: 1800 mg
Hospital/emergency department: Mild-to-severe symptoms: I.V.: 15 mg/kg (up to 1 g)
Frail patients, elderly:
Prehospital ("in the field"): Mild-to-moderate symptoms: I.M.: 10 mg/kg; severe symptoms: 25 mg/kg
Hospital/emergency department: Mild-to-severe symptoms: I.V.: 5-10 mg/kg

Dosage Forms Injection, powder for reconstitution, as chloride: 1 g

pralidoxime chloride *see* pralidoxime *on this page*

Pramet® FA *(Discontinued)* *see page 1042*

Pramilet® FA *(Discontinued)* *see page 1042*

pramipexole (pra mi PEX ole)

Sound-Alike/Look-Alike Issues
Mirapex® may be confused with Mifeprex®, MiraLax™

U.S./Canadian Brand Names Mirapex® [US/Can]

Therapeutic Category Dopaminergic Agent (Anti-Parkinson)

Use Treatment of the signs and symptoms of idiopathic Parkinson disease

Usual Dosage Adults: Oral: Initial: 0.375 mg/day given in 3 divided doses, increase gradually by 0.125 mg/dose every 5-7 days; range: 1.5-4.5 mg/day

Dosage Forms Tablet, as dihydrochloride monohydrate: 0.125 mg, 0.25 mg, 0.5 mg, 1 mg, 1.5 mg

Pramosone® [US] *see* pramoxine and hydrocortisone *on this page*

Pramox® HC [Can] *see* pramoxine and hydrocortisone *on this page*

pramoxine (pra MOKS een)

Sound-Alike/Look-Alike Issues
pramoxine may be confused with pralidoxime
Anusol® may be confused with Anusol-HC®, Aplisol®, Aquasol®
Tronolane® may be confused with Tronothane®

Synonyms pramoxine hydrochloride

U.S./Canadian Brand Names Anusol® Ointment [US-OTC]; Itch-X® [US-OTC]; Prax® [US-OTC]; ProctoFoam® NS [US-OTC]; Tronolane® [US-OTC]

Therapeutic Category Local Anesthetic

Use Temporary relief of pain and itching associated with anogenital pruritus or irritation; dermatosis, minor burns, or hemorrhoids

Usual Dosage Adults: Topical: Apply as directed, usually every 3-4 hours to affected area (maximum adult dose: 200 mg)

Dosage Forms
Aerosol, foam, as hydrochloride (ProctoFoam® NS): 1% (15 g)
Cream, as hydrochloride (Tronolane®): 1% (30 g, 60 g)
Gel, topical, as hydrochloride (Itch-X®): 1% (35.4 g) [contains benzyl alcohol]
Lotion, as hydrochloride (Prax®): 1% (15 mL, 120 mL, 240 mL)
Ointment, as hydrochloride (Anusol®): 1% (30 g) [contains zinc oxide 12.5%, benzyl alcohol, and mineral oil]
Solution, topical spray, as hydrochloride (Itch-X®): 1% (60 mL) [contains benzyl alcohol]
Suppositories, as hydrochloride (Tronolane®): 1% (10s, 20s)

pramoxine and hydrocortisone (pra MOKS een & hye droe KOR ti sone)

Sound-Alike/Look-Alike Issues
Pramosone® may be confused with predniSONE
Zone-A Forte® may be confused with Zonalon®

Synonyms hydrocortisone and pramoxine

U.S./Canadian Brand Names Analpram-HC® [US]; Enzone® [US]; Epifoam® [US]; Pramosone® [US]; Pramox® HC [Can]; ProctoFoam®-HC [US/Can]; Zone-A® [US]; Zone-A Forte® [US]

Therapeutic Category Anesthetic/Corticosteroid

Use Relief of inflammatory and pruritic manifestations of corticosteroid-responsive dermatoses

Usual Dosage Topical/rectal: Apply to affected areas 3-4 times/day

Dosage Forms
Cream, rectal (Analpram-HC®): Pramoxine hydrochloride 1% and hydrocortisone acetate 1% (30 g); pramoxine hydrochloride 1% and hydrocortisone acetate 2.5% (30 g)
Cream, topical:
Enzone®: Pramoxine hydrochloride 1% and hydrocortisone acetate 1% (30 g)
Pramosone®: Pramoxine hydrochloride 1% and hydrocortisone acetate 1% (30 g, 60 g); pramoxine hydrochloride 1% and hydrocortisone acetate 2.5% (30 g, 60 g)

Foam, rectal (ProctoFoam®-HC): Pramoxine hydrochloride 1% and hydrocortisone acetate 1% (10 g)
Foam, topical (Epifoam®): Pramoxine hydrochloride 1% and hydrocortisone acetate 1% (10 g)
Lotion, rectal (Analpram-HC®): Pramoxine hydrochloride 1% and hydrocortisone 2.5% (60 mL)
Lotion, topical:
Pramosone®: Pramoxine hydrochloride 1% and hydrocortisone 1% (60 mL, 120 mL, 240 mL); pramoxine hydrochloride 1% and hydrocortisone 2.5% (60 mL, 120 mL)
Zone-A®: Pramoxine hydrochloride 1% and hydrocortisone 1% (60 mL)
Zone-A Forte®: Pramoxine hydrochloride 1% and hydrocortisone 2.5% (60 mL)
Ointment, topical: Pramoxine hydrochloride 1% and hydrocortisone 1% (30 g); pramoxine hydrochloride 1% and hydrocortisone 2.5% (30 g)

pramoxine hydrochloride *see* pramoxine *on previous page*

Prandase® [Can] *see* acarbose *on page 4*

Prandin® [US/Can] *see* repaglinide *on page 768*

Pravachol® [US/Can] *see* pravastatin *on this page*

pravastatin (PRA va stat in)

Sound-Alike/Look-Alike Issues
Pravachol® may be confused with Prevacid®, Prinivil®, propranolol

Synonyms pravastatin sodium

U.S./Canadian Brand Names Apo-Pravastatin® [Can]; Lin-Pravastatin [Can]; Novo-Pravastatin [Can]; PMS-Pravastatin [Can]; Pravachol® [US/Can]; ratio-Pravastatin [Can]

Therapeutic Category HMG-CoA Reductase Inhibitor

Use Use with dietary therapy for the following:
Primary prevention of coronary events: In hypercholesterolemic patients without established coronary heart disease to reduce cardiovascular morbidity (myocardial infarction, coronary revascularization procedures) and mortality.
Secondary prevention of cardiovascular events in patients with established coronary heart disease: To slow the progression of coronary atherosclerosis; to reduce cardiovascular morbidity (myocardial infarction, coronary vascular procedures) and to reduce mortality; to reduce the risk of stroke and transient ischemic attacks
Hyperlipidemias: Reduce elevations in total cholesterol, LDL-C, apolipoprotein B, and triglycerides (elevations of 1 or more components are present in Fredrickson type IIa, IIb, III, and IV hyperlipidemias)
Heterozygous familial hypercholesterolemia (HeFH): In pediatric patients, 8-18 years of age, with HeFH having LDL-C ≥190 mg/dL **or** LDL ≥160 mg/dL with positive family history of premature cardiovascular disease (CVD) or 2 or more CVD risk factors in the pediatric patient

Usual Dosage Oral: **Note:** Doses should be individualized according to the baseline LDL-cholesterol levels, the recommended goal of therapy, and patient response; adjustments should be made at intervals of 4 weeks or more; doses may need adjusted based on concomitant medications
Children: HeFH:
8-13 years: 20 mg/day
14-18 years: 40 mg/day
Dosage adjustment for pravastatin based on concomitant immunosuppressants (ie, cyclosporine): Refer to Adults dosing section
Adults: Hyperlipidemias, primary prevention of coronary events, secondary prevention of cardiovascular events: Initial: 40 mg once daily; titrate dosage to response; usual range: 10-80 mg; (maximum dose: 80 mg once daily)
Dosage adjustment for pravastatin based on concomitant immunosuppressants (ie, cyclosporine): Initial: 10 mg/day, titrate with caution (maximum dose: 20 mg/day)

Dosage Forms Tablet, as sodium: 10 mg, 20 mg, 40 mg, 80 mg

pravastatin and aspirin *see* aspirin and pravastatin *on page 83*

pravastatin sodium *see* pravastatin *on previous page*

Pravigard™ PAC [US] *see* aspirin and pravastatin *on page 83*

Prax® [US-OTC] *see* pramoxine *on page 720*

praziquantel (pray zi KWON tel)

U.S./Canadian Brand Names Biltricide® [US/Can]

Therapeutic Category Anthelmintic

Use All stages of schistosomiasis caused by all *Schistosoma* species pathogenic to humans; clonorchiasis and opisthorchiasis

Usual Dosage Children >4 years and Adults: Oral:

Schistosomiasis: 20 mg/kg/dose 2-3 times/day for 1 day at 4- to 6-hour intervals

Clonorchiasis/opisthorchiasis: 3 doses of 25 mg/kg as a 1-day treatment

Dosage Forms Tablet [tri-scored]: 600 mg

prazosin (PRA zoe sin)

Sound-Alike/Look-Alike Issues

prazosin may be confused with prazepam, prednisone

Synonyms furazosin; prazosin hydrochloride

U.S./Canadian Brand Names Apo-Prazo® [Can]; Minipress® [US/Can]; Novo-Prazin [Can]; Nu-Prazo [Can]

Therapeutic Category Alpha-Adrenergic Blocking Agent

Use Treatment of hypertension

Usual Dosage Oral:

Children: Initial: 5 mcg/kg/dose (to assess hypotensive effects); usual dosing interval: every 6 hours; increase dosage gradually up to maximum of 25 mcg/kg/dose every 6 hours

Adults:

Hypertension: Initial: 1 mg/dose 2-3 times/day; usual maintenance dose: 3-15 mg/day in divided doses 2-4 times/day; maximum daily dose: 20 mg

Hypertensive urgency: 10-20 mg once, may repeat in 30 minutes

Dosage Forms Capsule, as hydrochloride: 1 mg, 2 mg, 5 mg

prazosin and polythiazide (PRA zoe sin & pol i THYE a zide)

Sound-Alike/Look-Alike Issues

Minizide® may be confused with Minocin®

Synonyms polythiazide and prazosin

U.S./Canadian Brand Names Minizide® [US]

Therapeutic Category Antihypertensive Agent, Combination

Use Management of mild to moderate hypertension

Usual Dosage Adults: Oral: 1 capsule 2-3 times/day

Dosage Forms Capsule:

Minizide® 1: Prazosin 1 mg and polythiazide 0.5 mg

Minizide® 2: Prazosin 2 mg and polythiazide 0.5 mg

Minizide® 5: Prazosin 5 mg and polythiazide 0.5 mg

prazosin hydrochloride *see* prazosin *on this page*

PreCare® [US] *see* vitamins (multiple/prenatal) *on page 927*

Precedex™ [US/Can] *see* dexmedetomidine *on page 256*

Precose® [US] *see* acarbose *on page 4*

Predair® ***(Discontinued)*** *see page 1042*

Predaject-50® ***(Discontinued)*** *see page 1042*

Predalone® ***(Discontinued)*** *see page 1042*

Predcor® ***(Discontinued)*** *see page 1042*

Predcor-TBA® ***(Discontinued)*** *see page 1042*

Pred Forte® [US/Can] *see* prednisolone (ophthalmic) *on this page*

Pred-G® [US] *see* prednisolone and gentamicin *on this page*

Predicort-50® ***(Discontinued)*** *see page 1042*

Pred Mild® [US/Can] *see* prednisolone (ophthalmic) *on this page*

prednicarbate (PRED ni kar bate)

Sound-Alike/Look-Alike Issues

Dermatop® may be confused with Dimetapp®

U.S./Canadian Brand Names Dermatop® [US/Can]

Therapeutic Category Corticosteroid, Topical

Use Relief of the inflammatory and pruritic manifestations of corticosteroid-responsive dermatoses (medium potency topical corticosteroid)

Usual Dosage Adults: Topical: Apply a thin film to affected area twice daily. Therapy should be discontinued when control is achieved; if no improvement is seen, reassessment of diagnosis may be necessary.

Dosage Forms

Cream: 0.1% (15 g, 60 g)

Ointment: 0.1% (15 g, 60 g)

Prednicen-M® ***(Discontinued)*** *see page 1042*

Prednicot® [US] *see* prednisone *on page 725*

prednisolone acetate *see* prednisolone (systemic) *on next page*

prednisolone acetate, ophthalmic *see* prednisolone (ophthalmic) *on this page*

prednisolone and gentamicin (pred NIS oh lone & jen ta MYE sin)

Synonyms gentamicin and prednisolone

U.S./Canadian Brand Names Pred-G® [US]

Therapeutic Category Antibiotic/Corticosteroid, Ophthalmic

Use Treatment of steroid responsive inflammatory conditions and superficial ocular infections due to microorganisms susceptible to gentamicin

Usual Dosage Ophthalmic: Children and Adults:

Ointment: Apply 1/2 inch ribbon in the conjunctival sac 1-3 times/day

Suspension: 1 drop 2-4 times/day; during the initial 24-48 hours, the dosing frequency may be increased if necessary up to 1 drop every hour

Dosage Forms

Ointment, ophthalmic: Prednisolone acetate 0.6% and gentamicin sulfate 0.3% (3.5 g)

Suspension, ophthalmic: Prednisolone acetate 1% and gentamicin sulfate 0.3% (2 mL, 5 mL, 10 mL) [contains benzalkonium chloride]

prednisolone and sulfacetamide *see* sulfacetamide and prednisolone *on page 829*

prednisolone, neomycin, and polymyxin B *see* neomycin, polymyxin B, and prednisolone *on page 612*

prednisolone (ophthalmic) (pred NIS oh lone op THAL mik)

Synonyms prednisolone acetate, ophthalmic; prednisolone sodium phosphate, ophthalmic

Tall-Man predniso**LONE** (ophthalmic)

U.S./Canadian Brand Names AK-Pred® [US]; Diopred® [Can]; Econopred® [US]; Econopred® Plus [US]; Hydeltra-T.B.A.® [Can]; Inflamase® Forte [US/Can]; Inflamase® Mild [US/Can]; Novo-Prednisolone [Can]; Pred Forte® [US/Can]; Pred Mild® [US/Can]; Sab-Prenase® [Can]

Therapeutic Category Adrenal Corticosteroid

(Continued)

prednisolone (ophthalmic) *(Continued)*

Use Treatment of palpebral and bulbar conjunctivitis; corneal injury from chemical, radiation, thermal burns, or foreign body penetration; endocrine disorders, rheumatic disorders, collagen diseases, dermatologic diseases, allergic states, ophthalmic diseases, respiratory diseases, hematologic disorders, neoplastic diseases, edematous states, and gastrointestinal diseases; useful in patients with inability to activate prednisone (liver disease)

Usual Dosage Ophthalmic suspension/solution: Children and Adults: Instill 1-2 drops into conjunctival sac every hour during day, every 2 hours at night until favorable response is obtained, then use 1 drop every 4 hours

Dosage Forms

Solution, ophthalmic, as sodium phosphate: 1% (5 mL, 10 mL, 15 mL) [contains benzalkonium chloride]

AK-Pred®: 1% (5 mL, 15 mL) [contains benzalkonium chloride]

Inflamase® Forte: 1% (5 mL, 10 mL, 15 mL) [contains benzalkonium chloride]

Inflamase® Mild: 0.125% (5 mL, 10 mL) [contains benzalkonium chloride]

Suspension, ophthalmic, as acetate: 1% (5 mL, 10 mL, 15 mL) [contains benzalkonium chloride]

Econopred®: 0.125% (5 mL, 10 mL) [contains benzalkonium chloride]

Econopred® Plus: 1% (5 mL, 10 mL) [contains benzalkonium chloride]

Pred Forte®: 1% (1 mL, 5 mL, 10 mL, 15 mL) [contains benzalkonium chloride and sodium bisulfite]

Pred Mild®: 0.12% (5 mL, 10 mL) [contains benzalkonium chloride and sodium bisulfite]

prednisolone sodium phosphate *see* prednisolone (systemic) *on this page*

prednisolone sodium phosphate, ophthalmic *see* prednisolone (ophthalmic) *on previous page*

prednisolone (systemic) (pred NIS oh lone sis TEM ik)

Sound-Alike/Look-Alike Issues

prednisolone may be confused with prednisone

Pediapred® may be confused with Pediazole®

Synonyms deltahydrocortisone; metacortandralone; prednisolone acetate; prednisolone sodium phosphate

Tall-Man predniso**LONE** (systemic)

U.S./Canadian Brand Names Orapred™ [US]; Pediapred® [US/Can]; Prednisol® TBA [US]; Prelone® [US]

Therapeutic Category Adrenal Corticosteroid

Use Treatment of palpebral and bulbar conjunctivitis; corneal injury from chemical, radiation, thermal burns, or foreign body penetration; endocrine disorders, rheumatic disorders, collagen diseases, dermatologic diseases, allergic states, ophthalmic diseases, respiratory diseases, hematologic disorders, neoplastic diseases, edematous states, and gastrointestinal diseases; useful in patients with inability to activate prednisone (liver disease)

Usual Dosage Dose depends upon condition being treated and response of patient; dosage for infants and children should be based on severity of the disease and response of the patient rather than on strict adherence to dosage indicated by age, weight, or body surface area. Consider alternate day therapy for long-term therapy. Discontinuation of long-term therapy requires gradual withdrawal by tapering the dose.

Children: Oral:

Acute asthma: 1-2 mg/kg/day in divided doses 1-2 times/day for 3-5 days

Antiinflammatory or immunosuppressive dose: 0.1-2 mg/kg/day in divided doses 1-4 times/day

Nephrotic syndrome:

Initial (first 3 episodes): 2 mg/kg/day **or** 60 mg/m²/day (maximum: 80 mg/day) in divided doses 3-4 times/day until urine is protein free for 3 consecutive days (maximum: 28 days); followed by 1-1.5 mg/kg/dose **or** 40 mg/m²/dose given every other day for 4 weeks

Maintenance (long-term maintenance dose for frequent relapses): 0.5-1 mg/kg/dose given every other day for 3-6 months

Adults: Oral:

Usual range: 5-60 mg/day

Multiple sclerosis: 200 mg/day for 1 week followed by 80 mg every other day for 1 month

Rheumatoid arthritis: Initial: 5-7.5 mg/day; adjust dose as necessary

Dosage Forms

Solution, oral, as sodium phosphate: Prednisolone base 5 mg/5 mL (120 mL)

Orapred®: 20 mg/5 mL (240 mL) [equivalent to prednisolone base 15 mg/5 mL; dye free; contains alcohol 2%, sodium benzoate; grape flavor]

Pediapred®: 6.7 mg/5 mL (120 mL) [equivalent to prednisolone base 5 mg/5 mL; dye free; raspberry flavor]

Syrup, as base: 5 mg/5 mL (120 mL); 15 mg/5 mL (240 mL, 480 mL)

Prelone®: 5 mg/5 mL (120 mL) [dye free, sugar free; contains alcohol ≤0.4%, benzoic acid; wild cherry flavor]; 15 mg/5 mL (240 mL, 480 mL) [contains alcohol 5%, benzoic acid; wild cherry flavor]

Tablet, as base: 5 mg [contains sodium benzoate]

Prednisol® TBA [US] *see* prednisolone (systemic) *on previous page*

prednisone (PRED ni sone)

Sound-Alike/Look-Alike Issues

prednisone may be confused with methylprednisolone, Pramosone®, prazosin, prednisolone, Prilosec®, primidone, promethazine

Synonyms deltacortisone; deltadehydrocortisone

Tall-Man predni**SONE**

U.S./Canadian Brand Names Apo-Prednisone® [Can]; Deltasone® [US]; Prednicot® [US]; Prednisone Intensol™ [US]; Sterapred® [US]; Sterapred® DS [US]; Winpred™ [Can]

Therapeutic Category Adrenal Corticosteroid

Use Treatment of a variety of diseases including adrenocortical insufficiency, hypercalcemia, rheumatic, and collagen disorders; dermatologic, ocular, respiratory, gastrointestinal, and neoplastic diseases; organ transplantation and a variety of diseases including those of hematologic, allergic, inflammatory, and autoimmune in origin; not available in injectable form, prednisolone must be used

Usual Dosage Oral: Dose depends upon condition being treated and response of patient; dosage for infants and children should be based on severity of the disease and response of the patient rather than on strict adherence to dosage indicated by age, weight, or body surface area. Consider alternate day therapy for long-term therapy. Discontinuation of long-term therapy requires gradual withdrawal by tapering the dose.

Children:

Antiinflammatory or immunosuppressive dose: 0.05-2 mg/kg/day divided 1-4 times/day

Acute asthma: 1-2 mg/kg/day in divided doses 1-2 times/day for 3-5 days

Alternatively (for 3- to 5-day "burst"):

<1 year: 10 mg every 12 hours

1-4 years: 20 mg every 12 hours

5-13 years: 30 mg every 12 hours

>13 years: 40 mg every 12 hours

Asthma long-term therapy (alternative dosing by age):

<1 year: 10 mg every other day

1-4 years: 20 mg every other day

5-13 years: 30 mg every other day

>13 years: 40 mg every other day

Nephrotic syndrome:

Initial (first 3 episodes): 2 mg/kg/day **or** 60 mg/m²/day (maximum: 80 mg/day) in divided doses 3-4 times/day until urine is protein free for 3 consecutive days

(Continued)

prednisone *(Continued)*

(maximum: 28 days); followed by 1-1.5 mg/kg/dose **or** 40 mg/m²/dose given every other day for 4 weeks

Maintenance dose (long-term maintenance dose for frequent relapses): 0.5-1 mg/kg/dose given every other day for 3-6 months

Children and Adults: Physiologic replacement: 4-5 mg/m²/day

Children ≥5 years and Adults: Asthma:

Moderate persistent: Inhaled corticosteroid (medium dose) or inhaled corticosteroid (low-medium dose) with a long-acting bronchodilator

Severe persistent: Inhaled corticosteroid (high dose) and corticosteroid tablets or syrup long term: 2 mg/kg/day, generally not to exceed 60 mg/day

Adults:

Immunosuppression/chemotherapy adjunct: Range: 5-60 mg/day in divided doses 1-4 times/day

Allergic reaction (contact dermatitis):

Day 1: 30 mg divided as 10 mg before breakfast, 5 mg at lunch, 5 mg at dinner, 10 mg at bedtime

Day 2: 5 mg at breakfast, 5 mg at lunch, 5 mg at dinner, 10 mg at bedtime

Day 3: 5 mg 4 times/day (with meals and at bedtime)

Day 4: 5 mg 3 times/day (breakfast, lunch, bedtime)

Day 5: 5 mg 2 times/day (breakfast, bedtime)

Day 6: 5 mg before breakfast

Pneumocystis carinii pneumonia (PCP):

40 mg twice daily for 5 days **followed by**

40 mg once daily for 5 days **followed by**

20 mg once daily for 11 days or until antimicrobial regimen is completed

Thyrotoxicosis: Oral: 60 mg/day

Chemotherapy (refer to individual protocols): Oral: Range: 20 mg/day to 100 mg/m²/day

Rheumatoid arthritis: Oral: Use lowest possible daily dose (often ≤7.5 mg/day)

Idiopathic thrombocytopenia purpura (ITP): Oral: 60 mg daily for 4-6 weeks, gradually tapered over several weeks

Systemic lupus erythematosus (SLE): Oral:

Acute: 1-2 mg/kg/day in 2-3 divided doses

Maintenance: Reduce to lowest possible dose, usually <1 mg/kg/day as single dose (morning)

Dosage Forms

Solution, oral: 1 mg/mL (5 mL, 120 mL, 500 mL) [contains alcohol 5%, sodium benzoate; vanilla flavor]

Solution, oral concentrate (Prednisone Intensol™): 5 mg/mL (30 mL) [contains alcohol 30%]

Tablet: 1 mg, 2.5 mg, 5 mg, 10 mg, 20 mg, 50 mg

Deltasone®: 2.5 mg, 10 mg, 20 mg, 50 mg

Sterapred®: 5 mg [supplied as 21 tablet 6-day unit-dose package or 48 tablet 12-day unit-dose package]

Sterapred® DS: 10 mg [supplied as 21 tablet 6-day unit-dose package or 48 tablet 12-day unit-dose package]

Prednisone Intensol™ [US] *see* prednisone *on previous page*

Prefest™ [US] *see* estradiol and norgestimate *on page 328*

Prefrin™ *(Discontinued)* *see page 1042*

pregnenedione *see* progesterone *on page 733*

Prelone® [US] *see* prednisolone (systemic) *on page 724*

Prelu-2® [US] *see* phendimetrazine *on page 685*

Preludin® *(Discontinued)* *see page 1042*

Premarin® [US/Can] *see* estrogens (conjugated/equine) *on page 329*

Premarin® With Methyltestosterone ***(Discontinued)*** *see page 1042*

Premjact® [US-OTC] *see* lidocaine *on page 518*

Premphase® [US/Can] *see* estrogens (conjugated/equine) and medroxyprogesterone *on page 330*

Premplus® [Can] *see* estrogens (conjugated/equine) and medroxyprogesterone *on page 330*

Prempro™ [US/Can] *see* estrogens (conjugated/equine) and medroxyprogesterone *on page 330*

Prenatal 1-A-Day [US] *see* vitamins (multiple/prenatal) *on page 927*

Prenatal AD [US] *see* vitamins (multiple/prenatal) *on page 927*

Prenatal H [US] *see* vitamins (multiple/prenatal) *on page 927*

Prenatal MR 90 Fe™ [US] *see* vitamins (multiple/prenatal) *on page 927*

Prenatal MTR with Selenium [US] *see* vitamins (multiple/prenatal) *on page 927*

Prenatal Plus [US] *see* vitamins (multiple/prenatal) *on page 927*

Prenatal Rx 1 [US] *see* vitamins (multiple/prenatal) *on page 927*

Prenatal U [US] *see* vitamins (multiple/prenatal) *on page 927*

prenatal vitamins *see* vitamins (multiple/prenatal) *on page 927*

Prenatal Z [US] *see* vitamins (multiple/prenatal) *on page 927*

Prenate Elite™ [US] *see* vitamins (multiple/prenatal) *on page 927*

Prenate GT™ [US] *see* vitamins (multiple/prenatal) *on page 927*

Preparation H® Cleansing Pads [Can] *see* witch hazel *on page 934*

Preparation H® Hydrocortisone [US] *see* hydrocortisone (rectal) *on page 448*

Prepcat® [US] *see* radiological/contrast media (ionic) *on page 759*

Pre-Pen® [US] *see* benzylpenicilloyl-polylysine *on page 112*

Prepidil® [US/Can] *see* dinoprostone *on page 275*

Prescription Strength Desenex® ***(Discontinued)*** *see page 1042*

Pressyn® [Can] *see* vasopressin *on page 906*

Pressyn® AR [Can] *see* vasopressin *on page 906*

Pretz-D® [US-OTC] *see* ephedrine *on page 311*

Pretz® Irrigation [US-OTC] *see* sodium chloride *on page 810*

Prevacid® [US/Can] *see* lansoprazole *on page 505*

Prevacid® NapraPAC™ [US] *see* lansoprazole and naproxen *on page 506*

Prevacid® SoluTab™ [US] *see* lansoprazole *on page 505*

Prevalite® [US] *see* cholestyramine resin *on page 196*

PREVEN® [US] *see* ethinyl estradiol and levonorgestrel *on page 339*

Prevex® B [Can] *see* betamethasone (topical) *on page 116*

PreviDent® [US] *see* fluoride *on page 376*

PreviDent® 5000 Plus™ [US] *see* fluoride *on page 376*

Previfem™ [US] *see* ethinyl estradiol and norgestimate *on page 346*

Prevnar® [US/Can] *see* pneumococcal conjugate vaccine (7-valent) *on page 703*

Prevpac® [US/Can] *see* lansoprazole, amoxicillin, and clarithromycin *on page 506*

Priftin® [US/Can] *see* rifapentine *on page 777*

prilocaine (PRIL oh kane)

Sound-Alike/Look-Alike Issues

prilocaine may be confused with Polocaine®, Prilosec®

U.S./Canadian Brand Names Citanest® Plain [US/Can]

Therapeutic Category Local Anesthetic

Use In dentistry for infiltration anesthesia and for nerve block anesthesia

Usual Dosage

Children <10 years: Doses >40 mg (1 mL) as a 4% solution per procedure rarely needed

Children >10 years and Adults: Dental anesthesia, infiltration, or conduction block: Initial: 40-80 mg (1-2 mL) as a 4% solution; up to a maximum of 400 mg (10 mL) as a 4% solution within a 2-hour period. Manufacturer's maximum recommended dose is not more than 600 mg to normal healthy adults. The effective anesthetic dose varies with procedure, intensity of anesthesia needed, duration of anesthesia required and physical condition of the patient. Always use the lowest effective dose along with careful aspiration.

The following numbers of dental carpules (1.8 mL) provide the indicated amounts of prilocaine hydrochloride 4%.

Note: Adult and children doses of prilocaine hydrochloride cited from USP Dispensing Information (USP DI), 17th ed, The United States Pharmacopeial Convention, Inc, Rockville, MD, 1997, 139.

Dosage Forms Injection, solution: 4% (1.8 mL) [prefilled cartridge]

prilocaine and lidocaine *see* lidocaine and prilocaine *on page 520*

Prilosec® [US] *see* omeprazole *on page 644*

Prilosec OTC™ [US-OTC] *see* omeprazole *on page 644*

primaclone *see* primidone *on this page*

Primacor® [US/Can] *see* milrinone *on page 582*

primaquine (PRIM a kween)

Synonyms primaquine phosphate; prymaccone

Therapeutic Category Aminoquinoline (Antimalarial)

Use Treatment of malaria

Usual Dosage Oral: Dosage expressed as mg of base (15 mg base = 26.3 mg primaquine phosphate)

Treatment of malaria (decrease risk of delayed primary attacks and prevent relapse):

Children: 0.3 mg base/kg/day once daily for 14 days (not to exceed 15 mg/day) or 0.9 mg base/kg once weekly for 8 weeks not to exceed 45 mg base/week

Adults: 15 mg/day (base) once daily for 14 days or 45 mg base once weekly for 8 weeks

CDC treatment recommendations: Begin therapy during last 2 weeks of, or following a course of, suppression with chloroquine or a comparable drug

Note: A second course (30 mg/day) for 14 days may be required in patients with relapse. Higher initial doses (30 mg/day) have also been used following exposure in S.E. Asia or Somalia.

Dosage Forms Tablet, as phosphate: 26.3 mg [15 mg base]

primaquine phosphate *see* primaquine *on this page*

Primatene® Mist [US-OTC] *see* epinephrine *on page 311*

Primaxin® [US/Can] *see* imipenem and cilastatin *on page 466*

primidone (PRI mi done)

Sound-Alike/Look-Alike Issues

primidone may be confused with prednisone

Synonyms desoxyphenobarbital; primaclone

U.S./Canadian Brand Names Apo-Primidone® [Can]; Mysoline® [US/Can]

Therapeutic Category Anticonvulsant; Barbiturate

Use Management of grand mal, psychomotor, and focal seizures

Usual Dosage Oral:

Children <8 years: Initial: 50-125 mg/day given at bedtime; increase by 50-125 mg/day increments every 3-7 days; usual dose: 10-25 mg/kg/day in divided doses 3-4 times/day

Children ≥8 years and Adults: Initial: 125-250 mg/day at bedtime; increase by 125-250 mg/day every 3-7 days; usual dose: 750-1500 mg/day in divided doses 3-4 times/day with maximum dosage of 2 g/day

Dosage Forms Tablet: 50 mg, 250 mg [generic tablet may contain sodium benzoate]

Primsol® [US] *see* trimethoprim *on page 887*

Principen® [US] *see* ampicillin *on page 56*

Prinivil® [US/Can] *see* lisinopril *on page 524*

Prinzide® [US/Can] *see* lisinopril and hydrochlorothiazide *on page 525*

Priorix™ [Can] *see* measles, mumps, and rubella vaccines, combined *on page 544*

Priscoline® *(Discontinued)* *see page 1042*

pristinamycin *see* quinupristin and dalfopristin *on page 758*

Privine® [US-OTC] *see* naphazoline *on page 604*

ProAmatine® [US] *see* midodrine *on page 581*

Proampacin® *(Discontinued)* *see page 1042*

Pro-Banthine® *(Discontinued)* *see page 1042*

probenecid (proe BEN e sid)

Sound-Alike/Look-Alike Issues

probenecid may be confused with Procanbid®

U.S./Canadian Brand Names Benuryl™ [Can]

Therapeutic Category Uricosuric Agent

Use Prevention of gouty arthritis; hyperuricemia; prolongation of beta-lactam effect (ie, serum levels)

Usual Dosage Oral:

Children:

<2 years: Not recommended

2-14 years: Prolong penicillin serum levels: 25 mg/kg starting dose, then 40 mg/kg/day given 4 times/day

Gonorrhea: <45 kg: 25 mg/kg x 1 (maximum: 1 g/dose) 30 minutes before penicillin, ampicillin or amoxicillin

Adults:

Hyperuricemia with gout: 250 mg twice daily for one week; increase to 250-500 mg/day; may increase by 500 mg/month, if needed, to maximum of 2-3 g/day (dosages may be increased by 500 mg every 6 months if serum urate concentrations are controlled)

Prolong penicillin serum levels: 500 mg 4 times/day

Gonorrhea: 1 g 30 minutes before penicillin, ampicillin, procaine, or amoxicillin

Pelvic inflammatory disease: Cefoxitin 2 g I.M. plus probenecid 1 g orally as a single dose

Neurosyphilis: Aqueous procaine penicillin 2.4 million units/day I.M. plus probenecid 500 mg 4 times/day for 10-14 days

Dosage Forms Tablet: 500 mg

probenecid and colchicine *see* colchicine and probenecid *on page 223*

Pro-Bionate® *(Discontinued)* *see page 1042*

Probiotica® [US-OTC] *see* Lactobacillus *on page 501*

procainamide (proe kane A mide)

Sound-Alike/Look-Alike Issues

Procanbid® may be confused with probenecid

Pronestyl® may be confused with Ponstel®

Synonyms PCA; procainamide hydrochloride; procaine amide hydrochloride

U.S./Canadian Brand Names Apo-Procainamide® [Can]; Procanbid® [US]; Procan™ SR [Can]; Pronestyl®-SR [Can]

Therapeutic Category Antiarrhythmic Agent, Class I-A

Use Treatment of ventricular tachycardia (VT), premature ventricular contractions, paroxysmal atrial tachycardia (PSVT), and atrial fibrillation (AF); prevent recurrence of ventricular tachycardia, paroxysmal supraventricular tachycardia, atrial fibrillation or flutter

Usual Dosage Must be titrated to patient's response

Children:

Oral: 15-50 mg/kg/24 hours divided every 3-6 hours

I.M.: 50 mg/kg/24 hours divided into doses of $1/8$ to $1/4$ every 3-6 hours in divided doses until oral therapy is possible

I.V. (infusion requires use of an infusion pump):

Load: 3-6 mg/kg/dose over 5 minutes not to exceed 100 mg/dose; may repeat every 5-10 minutes to maximum of 15 mg/kg/load

Maintenance as continuous I.V. infusion: 20-80 mcg/kg/minute; maximum: 2 g/24 hours

Adults:

Oral: 250-500 mg/dose every 3-6 hours or 500 mg to 1 g every 6 hours extended release; usual dose: 50 mg/kg/24 hours; maximum: 4 g/24 hours (**Note:** Twice daily dosing approved for Procanbid®)

I.M.: 0.5-1 g every 4-8 hours until oral therapy is possible

I.V. (infusion requires use of an infusion pump): Loading dose: 15-18 mg/kg administered as slow infusion over 25-30 minutes or 100-200 mg/dose repeated every 5 minutes as needed to a total dose of 1 g; maintenance dose: 1-4 mg/minute by continuous infusion

Infusion rate: **2 g/250 mL** D_5W/NS (I.V. infusion requires use of an infusion pump):

1 mg/minute: 7.5 mL/hour

2 mg/minute: 15 mL/hour

3 mg/minute: 22.5 mL/hour

4 mg/minute: 30 mL/hour

5 mg/minute: 37.5 mL/hour

6 mg/minute: 45 mL/hour

Intermittent/recurrent VF or pulseless VT:

Initial: 20-30 mg/minute (maximum: 50 mg/minute if necessary), up to a total of 17 mg/kg. ACLS guidelines: I.V.: Infuse 20 mg/minute until arrhythmia is controlled, hypotension occurs, QRS complex widens by 50% of its original width, or total of 17 mg/kg is given. **Note:** Reduce to 12 mg/kg in setting of cardiac or renal dysfunction

I.V. maintenance infusion: 1-4 mg/minute; monitor levels and do not exceed 3 mg/minute for >24 hours in adults with renal failure.

Dosage Forms [DSC] = Discontinued product

Capsule, as hydrochloride: 250 mg, 500 mg

Pronestyl®: 250 mg [DSC]

Injection, solution, as hydrochloride: 100 mg/mL (10 mL); 500 mg/mL (2 mL) [contains sodium metabisulfite]

Pronestyl®: 100 mg/mL (10 mL) [contains benzyl alcohol and sodium bisulfite] [DSC]

Tablet, as hydrochloride (Pronestyl®): 250 mg, 375 mg, 500 mg [contains tartrazine] [DSC]

Tablet, extended release, as hydrochloride: 500 mg, 750 mg, 1000 mg

Procanbid®: 500 mg, 1000 mg

Pronestyl-SR®: 500 mg [DSC]

procainamide hydrochloride *see* procainamide *on this page*

procaine (PROE kane)

Synonyms procaine hydrochloride

U.S./Canadian Brand Names Novocain® [US/Can]

Therapeutic Category Local Anesthetic

Use Produces spinal anesthesia and epidural and peripheral nerve block by injection and infiltration methods

Usual Dosage Dose varies with procedure, desired depth, and duration of anesthesia, desired muscle relaxation, vascularity of tissues, physical condition, and age of patient

Dosage Forms Injection, solution, as hydrochloride: 1% (30 mL); 2% (30 mL)

Novocain®: 1% [10 mg/mL] (2 mL, 6 mL, 30 mL); 2% [20 mg/mL] (30 mL); 10% (2 mL)

procaine amide hydrochloride *see* procainamide *on previous page*

procaine benzylpenicillin *see* penicillin G procaine *on page 676*

procaine hydrochloride *see* procaine *on this page*

procaine penicillin G *see* penicillin G procaine *on page 676*

Pro-Cal-Sof® *(Discontinued)* *see page 1042*

Procanbid® [US] *see* procainamide *on previous page*

Procan™ SR *(Discontinued)* *see page 1042*

Procan™ SR [Can] *see* procainamide *on previous page*

procarbazine (proe KAR ba zeen)

Sound-Alike/Look-Alike Issues

procarbazine may be confused with dacarbazine

Matulane® may be confused with Modane®

Synonyms benzmethyzin; N-methylhydrazine; NSC-77213; procarbazine hydrochloride

U.S./Canadian Brand Names Matulane® [US/Can]; Natulan® [Can]

Therapeutic Category Antineoplastic Agent

Use Treatment of Hodgkin disease

Usual Dosage Refer to individual protocols. Dose based on patient's ideal weight if the patient is obese or has abnormal fluid retention. Oral (may be given as a single daily dose or in 2-3 divided doses):

Children:

- BMT aplastic anemia conditioning regimen: 12.5 mg/kg/dose every other day for 4 doses
- Hodgkin disease: MOPP/IC-MOPP regimens: 100 mg/m^2/day for 14 days and repeated every 4 weeks
- Neuroblastoma and medulloblastoma: Doses as high as 100-200 mg/m^2/day once daily have been used

Adults: Initial: 2-4 mg/kg/day in single or divided doses for 7 days then increase dose to 4-6 mg/kg/day until response is obtained or leukocyte count decreased <4000/mm^3 or the platelet count decreased <100,000/mm^3; maintenance: 1-2 mg/kg/day

Dosage Forms Capsule, as hydrochloride: 50 mg

procarbazine hydrochloride *see* procarbazine *on this page*

Procardia® [US/Can] *see* nifedipine *on page 619*

Procardia XL® [US] *see* nifedipine *on page 619*

procetofene *see* fenofibrate *on page 360*

Prochieve™ [US] *see* progesterone *on page 733*

prochlorperazine (proe klor PER a zeen)

Sound-Alike/Look-Alike Issues

prochlorperazine may be confused with chlorpromazine

Compazine® may be confused with chlorpromazine, Copaxone®, Coumadin®

Synonyms chlormeprazine; prochlorperazine edisylate; prochlorperazine maleate

(Continued)

prochlorperazine *(Continued)*

U.S./Canadian Brand Names Apo-Prochlorperazine® [Can]; Compazine® [Can]; Compro™ [US]; Nu-Prochlor [Can]; Stemetil® [Can]

Therapeutic Category Phenothiazine Derivative

Use Management of nausea and vomiting; psychosis; anxiety

Usual Dosage

Antiemetic: Children (not recommended in children <10 kg or <2 years):

Oral, rectal: >10 kg: 0.4 mg/kg/24 hours in 3-4 divided doses; **or**

9-14 kg: 2.5 mg every 12-24 hours as needed; maximum: 7.5 mg/day

14-18 kg: 2.5 mg every 8-12 hours as needed; maximum: 10 mg/day

18-39 kg: 2.5 mg every 8 hours or 5 mg every 12 hours as needed; maximum: 15 mg/day

I.M.: 0.1-0.15 mg/kg/dose; usual: 0.13 mg/kg/dose; change to oral as soon as possible

Antiemetic: Adults:

Oral:

Tablet: 5-10 mg 3-4 times/day; usual maximum: 40 mg/day

Capsule, sustained action: 15 mg upon arising or 10 mg every 12 hours

I.M.: 5-10 mg every 3-4 hours; usual maximum: 40 mg/day

I.V.: 2.5-10 mg; maximum 10 mg/dose or 40 mg/day; may repeat dose every 3-4 hours as needed

Rectal: 25 mg twice daily

Surgical nausea/vomiting: Adults:

I.M.: 5-10 mg 1-2 hours before induction; may repeat once if necessary

I.V.: 5-10 mg 15-30 minutes before induction; may repeat once if necessary

Antipsychotic:

Children 2-12 years (not recommended in children <10 kg or <2 years):

Oral, rectal: 2.5 mg 2-3 times/day; increase dosage as needed to maximum daily dose of 20 mg for 2-5 years and 25 mg for 6-12 years

I.M.: 0.13 mg/kg/dose; change to oral as soon as possible

Adults:

Oral: 5-10 mg 3-4 times/day; doses up to 150 mg/day may be required in some patients for treatment of severe disturbances

I.M.: 10-20 mg every 4-6 hours may be required in some patients for treatment of severe disturbances; change to oral as soon as possible

Nonpsychotic anxiety: Oral: Adults: Usual dose: 15-20 mg/day in divided doses; do not give doses >20 mg/day or for longer than 12 weeks

Dosage Forms [DSC] = Discontinued product

Capsule, sustained release, as maleate (Compazine®) [DSC]: 10 mg, 15 mg

Injection, solution, as edisylate: 5 mg/mL (2 mL) [contains benzyl alcohol]

Compazine® [DSC]: 5 mg/mL (2 mL, 10 mL) [contains benzyl alcohol]

Suppository, rectal: 2.5 mg (12s), 5 mg (12s), 25 mg (12s) [may contain coconut and palm oil]

Compazine® [DSC]: 2.5 mg (12s), 5 mg (12s), 25 mg (12s) [contains coconut and palm oils]

Compro™: 25 mg (12s) [contains coconut and palm oils]

Syrup, as edisylate (Compazine® [DSC]): 5 mg/5 mL (120 mL) [contains sodium benzoate; fruit flavor]

Tablet, as maleate (Compazine® [DSC]): 5 mg, 10 mg

prochlorperazine edisylate *see* prochlorperazine *on previous page*

prochlorperazine maleate *see* prochlorperazine *on previous page*

Procrit® [US] *see* epoetin alfa *on page 314*

Proctocort™ Rectal [US] *see* hydrocortisone (rectal) *on page 448*

ProctoCream® HC [US] *see* hydrocortisone (rectal) *on page 448*

ProctoCream® HC Cream [US] *see* hydrocortisone (rectal) *on page 448*

proctofene *see* fenofibrate *on page 360*

ProctoFoam®-HC [US/Can] *see* pramoxine and hydrocortisone *on page 720*

ProctoFoam® NS [US-OTC] *see* pramoxine *on page 720*

Proctosol-HC® [US] *see* hydrocortisone (rectal) *on page 448*

Procyclid™ [Can] *see* procyclidine *on this page*

procyclidine (proe SYE kli deen)

Sound-Alike/Look-Alike Issues
Kemadrin® may be confused with Coumadin®

Synonyms procyclidine hydrochloride

U.S./Canadian Brand Names Kemadrin® [US]; PMS-Procyclidine [Can]; Procyclid™ [Can]

Therapeutic Category Anticholinergic Agent; Anti-Parkinson Agent

Use Relieves symptoms of parkinsonian syndrome and drug-induced extrapyramidal symptoms

Usual Dosage Adults: Oral: 2.5 mg 3 times/day after meals; if tolerated, gradually increase dose, maximum of 20 mg/day if necessary

Dosage Forms Tablet, as hydrochloride [scored]: 5 mg

procyclidine hydrochloride *see* procyclidine *on this page*

Procytox® [Can] *see* cyclophosphamide *on page 234*

Prodium® [US-OTC] *see* phenazopyridine *on page 685*

Profasi® *(Discontinued)* *see page 1042*

Profenal® *(Discontinued)* *see page 1042*

Profen Forte® [US] *see* guaifenesin and pseudoephedrine *on page 419*

Profen Forte® DM [US] *see* guaifenesin, pseudoephedrine, and dextromethorphan *on page 422*

Profen® II [US] *see* guaifenesin and pseudoephedrine *on page 419*

Profen II DM® [US] *see* guaifenesin, pseudoephedrine, and dextromethorphan *on page 422*

Profen LA® *(Discontinued)* *see page 1042*

Profilate-HP® *(Discontinued)* *see page 1042*

Profilnine® SD [US] *see* factor IX complex (human) *on page 355*

Proflavanol C™ [Can] *see* ascorbic acid *on page 79*

Progestaject® Injection *(Discontinued)* *see page 1042*

Progestasert® [US] *see* progesterone *on this page*

progesterone (proe JES ter one)

Synonyms pregnenedione; progestin

U.S./Canadian Brand Names Crinone® [US/Can]; Prochieve™ [US]; Progestasert® [US]; Prometrium® [US/Can]

Therapeutic Category Progestin

Use

Oral: Prevention of endometrial hyperplasia in nonhysterectomized, postmenopausal women who are receiving conjugated estrogen tablets; secondary amenorrhea

I.M.: Amenorrhea; abnormal uterine bleeding due to hormonal imbalance

Intrauterine device (IUD): Contraception in women who have had at least one child, are in a stable and mutually-monogamous relationship, and have no history of pelvic inflammatory disease; amenorrhea; functional uterine bleeding

Intravaginal gel: Part of assisted reproductive technology (ART) for infertile women with progesterone deficiency; secondary amenorrhea

Usual Dosage

I.M.: Adults: Female:

Amenorrhea: 5-10 mg/day for 6-8 consecutive days

(Continued)

progesterone *(Continued)*

Functional uterine bleeding: 5-10 mg/day for 6 doses

IUD: Adults: Female: Contraception: Insert a single system into the uterine cavity; contraceptive effectiveness is retained for 1 year and system must be replaced 1 year after insertion

Oral: Adults: Female:

Prevention of endometrial hyperplasia (in postmenopausal women with a uterus who are receiving daily conjugated estrogen tablets): 200 mg as a single daily dose every evening for 12 days sequentially per 28-day cycle

Amenorrhea: 400 mg every evening for 10 days

Intravaginal gel: Adults: Female:

ART in women who require progesterone supplementation: 90 mg (8% gel) once daily; if pregnancy occurs, may continue treatment for up to 10-12 weeks

ART in women with partial or complete ovarian failure: 90 mg (8% gel) intravaginally twice daily; if pregnancy occurs, may continue up to 10-12 weeks

Secondary amenorrhea: 45 mg (4% gel) intravaginally every other day for up to 6 doses; women who fail to respond may be increased to 90 mg (8% gel) every other day for up to 6 doses

Dosage Forms

Capsule (Prometrium®): 100 mg, 200 mg [contains peanut oil]

Gel, vaginal (Crinone®, Prochieve™): 4% (45 mg); 8% (90 mg) [contains palm oil; prefilled applicators]

Injection, oil: 50 mg/mL (10 mL) [contains benzyl alcohol 10%, sesame oil]

Intrauterine system (Progestasert®): 38 mg [delivers progesterone 65 mcg/day over 1 year; in silicone fluid]

progestin *see* progesterone *on previous page*

Proglycem® [US/Can] *see* diazoxide *on page 264*

Prograf® [US/Can] *see* tacrolimus *on page 837*

proguanil and atovaquone *see* atovaquone and proguanil *on page 87*

ProHance® [US] *see* radiological/contrast media (nonionic) *on page 761*

ProHIBiT® ***(Discontinued)*** *see page 1042*

Prokine™ Injection ***(Discontinued)*** *see page 1042*

Prolamine® ***(Discontinued)*** *see page 1042*

Prolastin® [US/Can] *see* alpha$_1$-proteinase inhibitor *on page 34*

Proleukin® [US/Can] *see* aldesleukin *on page 28*

Prolex™-D [US] *see* guaifenesin and phenylephrine *on page 418*

Prolixin® ***(Discontinued)*** *see page 1042*

Prolixin Decanoate® [US] *see* fluphenazine *on page 380*

Prolixin Enanthate® ***(Discontinued)*** *see page 1042*

Proloid® ***(Discontinued)*** *see page 1042*

Prolopa® [Can] *see* benserazide and levodopa *(Canada only) on page 106*

Proloprim® [US/Can] *see* trimethoprim *on page 887*

Promatussin® DM [Can] *see* promethazine and dextromethorphan *on page 736*

Prometa® ***(Discontinued)*** *see page 1042*

Prometh® ***(Discontinued)*** *see page 1042*

promethazine (proe METH a zeen)

Sound-Alike/Look-Alike Issues

promethazine may be confused with chlorpromazine, prednisone, promazine

Phenergan® may be confused with Phenaphen®, Phrenilin®, Theragran®

Synonyms promethazine hydrochloride

U.S./Canadian Brand Names Phenadoz™ [US]; Phenergan® [US/Can]

Therapeutic Category Antiemetic; Phenothiazine Derivative

Use Symptomatic treatment of various allergic conditions; antiemetic; motion sickness; sedative; postoperative pain (adjunctive therapy); anesthetic (adjunctive therapy); anaphylactic reactions (adjunctive therapy)

Usual Dosage

Children ≥2 years:

Allergic conditions: Oral, rectal: 0.1 mg/kg/dose (maximum: 12.5 mg) every 6 hours during the day and 0.5 mg/kg/dose (maximum: 25 mg) at bedtime as needed

Antiemetic: Oral, I.M., I.V., rectal: 0.25-1 mg/kg 4-6 times/day as needed (maximum: 25 mg/dose)

Motion sickness: Oral, rectal: 0.5 mg/kg/dose 30 minutes to 1 hour before departure, then every 12 hours as needed (maximum dose: 25 mg twice daily)

Sedation: Oral, I.M., I.V., rectal: 0.5-1 mg/kg/dose every 6 hours as needed (maximum: 50 mg/dose)

Adults:

Allergic conditions (including allergic reactions to blood or plasma):

Oral, rectal: 12.5 mg 3 times/day and 25 mg at bedtime

I.M., I.V.: 25 mg, may repeat in 2 hours when necessary; switch to oral route as soon as feasible

Antiemetic: Oral, I.M., I.V., rectal: 12.5-25 mg every 4-6 hours as needed

Motion sickness: Oral, rectal: 25 mg 30-60 minutes before departure, then every 12 hours as needed

Sedation: Oral, I.M., I.V., rectal: 12.5-50 mg/dose

Dosage Forms

Injection, solution, as hydrochloride: 25 mg/mL (1 mL); 50 mg/mL (1 mL)

Phenergan®: 25 mg/mL (1 mL); 50 mg/mL (1 mL) [contains sodium metabisulfite] [DSC]

Suppository, rectal, as hydrochloride: 12.5 mg, 25 mg, 50 mg

Phenadoz™: 12.5 mg, 25 mg

Phenergan®: 12.5 mg, 25 mg, 50 mg

Syrup, as hydrochloride: 6.25 mg/5 mL (120 mL, 480 mL) [contains alcohol]

Tablet, as hydrochloride: 12.5 mg, 25 mg, 50 mg

Phenergan®: 12.5 mg, 25 mg, 50 mg

promethazine and codeine (proe METH a zeen & KOE deen)

Synonyms codeine and promethazine

U.S./Canadian Brand Names Phenergan® With Codeine [US]

Therapeutic Category Antihistamine/Antitussive

Controlled Substance C-V

Use Temporary relief of coughs and upper respiratory symptoms associated with allergy or the common cold

Usual Dosage Oral (in terms of codeine):

Children: 1-1.5 mg/kg/day every 4 hours as needed; maximum: 30 mg/day **or**

2-6 years: 1.25-2.5 mL every 4-6 hours or 2.5-5 mg/dose every 4-6 hours as needed; maximum: 30 mg codeine/day

6-12 years: 2.5-5 mL every 4-6 hours as needed or 5-10 mg/dose every 4-6 hours as needed; maximum: 60 mg codeine/day

Adults: 10-20 mg/dose every 4-6 hours as needed; maximum: 120 mg codeine/day; or 5-10 mL every 4-6 hours as needed

Dosage Forms Syrup: Promethazine hydrochloride 6.25 mg and codeine phosphate 10 mg per 5 mL (120 mL, 473 mL, 3840 mL) [contains alcohol]

Phenergan® with Codeine: Promethazine hydrochloride 6.25 mg and codeine phosphate 10 mg per 5 mL (120 mL) [contains alcohol 7% and sodium benzoate]

promethazine and dextromethorphan

(proe METH a zeen & deks troe meth OR fan)

Synonyms dextromethorphan and promethazine

U.S./Canadian Brand Names Promatussin® DM [Can]

Therapeutic Category Antihistamine/Antitussive

Use Temporary relief of coughs and upper respiratory symptoms associated with allergy or the common cold

Usual Dosage Oral:

Children:

2-6 years: 1.25-2.5 mL every 4-6 hours up to 10 mL in 24 hours

6-12 years: 2.5-5 mL every 4-6 hours up to 20 mL in 24 hours

Adults: 5 mL every 4-6 hours up to 30 mL in 24 hours

Dosage Forms Syrup: Promethazine hydrochloride 6.25 mg and dextromethorphan hydrobromide 15 mg per 5 mL (120 mL, 480 mL, 4000 mL) [contains alcohol 7%]

promethazine and meperidine *see* meperidine and promethazine *on page 553*

promethazine and phenylephrine (proe METH a zeen & fen il EF rin)

Synonyms phenylephrine and promethazine

Therapeutic Category Antihistamine/Decongestant Combination

Use Temporary relief of upper respiratory symptoms associated with allergy or the common cold

Usual Dosage Oral:

Children:

2-6 years: 1.25 mL every 4-6 hours, not to exceed 7.5 mL in 24 hours

6-12 years: 2.5 mL every 4-6 hours, not to exceed 15 mL in 24 hours

Children >12 years and Adults: 5 mL every 4-6 hours, not to exceed 30 mL in 24 hours

Dosage Forms Syrup: Promethazine hydrochloride 6.25 mg and phenylephrine hydrochloride 5 mg per 5 mL (120 mL, 473 mL, 3840 mL) [contains alcohol]

promethazine hydrochloride *see* promethazine *on page 734*

promethazine, phenylephrine, and codeine

(proe METH a zeen, fen il EF rin, & KOE deen)

Synonyms codeine, promethazine, and phenylephrine; phenylephrine, promethazine, and codeine

Therapeutic Category Antihistamine/Decongestant/Antitussive

Controlled Substance C-V

Use Temporary relief of coughs and upper respiratory symptoms including nasal congestion

Usual Dosage Oral:

Children (expressed in terms of codeine dosage): 1-1.5 mg/kg/day every 4 hours, maximum: 30 mg/day **or**

<2 years: Not recommended

2-6 years:

Weight 25 lb: 1.25-2.5 mL every 4-6 hours, not to exceed 6 mL/24 hours

Weight 30 lb: 1.25-2.5 mL every 4-6 hours, not to exceed 7 mL/24 hours

Weight 35 lb: 1.25-2.5 mL every 4-6 hours, not to exceed 8 mL/24 hours

Weight 40 lb: 1.25-2.5 mL every 4-6 hours, not to exceed 9 mL/24 hours

6 to <12 years: 2.5-5 mL every 4-6 hours, not to exceed 15 mL/24 hours

Adults: 5 mL every 4-6 hours, not to exceed 30 mL/24 hours

Dosage Forms Syrup: Promethazine hydrochloride 6.25 mg, phenylephrine hydrochloride 5 mg, and codeine phosphate 10 mg per 5 mL with alcohol 7% (120 mL, 480 mL) [contains alcohol]

Promethist® With Codeine *(Discontinued)* *see page 1042*

Prometh® VC Plain Liquid *(Discontinued)* *see page 1042*

Prometh® VC With Codeine ***(Discontinued)*** *see page 1042*

Prometrium® [US/Can] *see* progesterone *on page 733*

Promit® [US] *see* dextran 1 *on page 258*

Pronap-100® [US] *see* propoxyphene and acetaminophen *on page 740*

Pronestyl® ***(Discontinued)*** *see page 1042*

Pronestyl®-SR ***(Discontinued)*** *see page 1042*

Pronestyl®-SR [Can] *see* procainamide *on page 730*

Pronto® Lice Control [Can] *see* pyrethrins and piperonyl butoxide *on page 751*

Pronto® [US-OTC] *see* pyrethrins and piperonyl butoxide *on page 751*

Propacet® ***(Discontinued)*** *see page 1042*

Propaderm® [Can] *see* beclomethasone *on page 102*

propafenone (proe pa FEEN one)

Synonyms propafenone hydrochloride

U.S./Canadian Brand Names Apo-Propafenone® [Can]; Gen-Propafenone [Can]; Rythmol® [US/Can]; Rythmol® SR [US]

Therapeutic Category Antiarrhythmic Agent, Class I-C

Use Treatment of life-threatening ventricular arrhythmias

Rythmol® SR: Maintenance of normal sinus rhythm in patients with symptomatic atrial fibrillation

Usual Dosage Oral: Adults: **Note:** Patients who exhibit significant widening of QRS complex or second- or third-degree AV block may need dose reduction.

Immediate release tablet: Initial: 150 mg every 8 hours, increase at 3- to 4-day intervals up to 300 mg every 8 hours.

Extended release capsule: Initial: 225 mg every 12 hours; dosage increase may be made at a minimum of 5-day intervals; may increase to 325 mg every 12 hours; if further increase is necessary, may increase to 425 mg every 12 hours

Dosage Forms

Capsule, extended release, as hydrochloride: 225 mg, 325 mg, 425 mg

Tablet, as hydrochloride: 150 mg, 225 mg, 300 mg

propafenone hydrochloride *see* propafenone *on this page*

Propagest® ***(Discontinued)*** *see page 1042*

Propanthel™ [Can] *see* propantheline *on this page*

propantheline (proe PAN the leen)

Synonyms propantheline bromide

U.S./Canadian Brand Names Propanthel™ [Can]

Therapeutic Category Anticholinergic Agent

Use Adjunctive treatment of peptic ulcer, irritable bowel syndrome, pancreatitis, ureteral and urinary bladder spasm; reduce duodenal motility during diagnostic radiologic procedures

Usual Dosage Oral:

Antisecretory:

Children: 1-2 mg/kg/day in 3-4 divided doses

Adults: 15 mg 3 times/day before meals or food and 30 mg at bedtime

Elderly: 7.5 mg 3 times/day before meals and at bedtime

Antispasmodic:

Children: 2-3 mg/kg/day in divided doses every 4-6 hours and at bedtime

Adults: 15 mg 3 times/day before meals or food and 30 mg at bedtime

Dosage Forms Tablet, as bromide: 15 mg

propantheline bromide *see* propantheline *on this page*

Propa pH [US-OTC] *see* salicylic acid *on page 789*

proparacaine (proe PAR a kane)

Sound-Alike/Look-Alike Issues

proparacaine may be confused with propoxyphene

Synonyms proparacaine hydrochloride; proxymetacaine

U.S./Canadian Brand Names Alcaine® [US/Can]; Diocaine® [Can]; Ophthetic® [US]

Therapeutic Category Local Anesthetic

Use Anesthesia for tonometry, gonioscopy; suture removal from cornea; removal of corneal foreign body; cataract extraction, glaucoma surgery; short operative procedure involving the cornea and conjunctiva

Usual Dosage Children and Adults:

Ophthalmic surgery: Instill 1 drop of 0.5% solution in eye every 5-10 minutes for 5-7 doses

Tonometry, gonioscopy, suture removal: Instill 1-2 drops of 0.5% solution in eye just prior to procedure

Dosage Forms Solution, ophthalmic, as hydrochloride: 0.5% (15 mL) [contains benzalkonium chloride]

proparacaine and fluorescein (proe PAR a kane & FLURE e seen)

Synonyms fluorescein and proparacaine

U.S./Canadian Brand Names Flucaine® [US]; Fluoracaine® [US]

Therapeutic Category Diagnostic Agent; Local Anesthetic

Use Anesthesia for tonometry, gonioscopy; suture removal from cornea; removal of corneal foreign body; cataract extraction, glaucoma surgery

Usual Dosage

Ophthalmic surgery: Children and Adults: Instill 1 drop in each eye every 5-10 minutes for 5-7 doses

Tonometry, gonioscopy, suture removal: Adults: Instill 1-2 drops in each eye just prior to procedure

Dosage Forms Solution, ophthalmic: Proparacaine hydrochloride 0.5% and fluorescein sodium 0.25% (5 mL)

proparacaine hydrochloride *see* proparacaine *on this page*

Propecia® [US/Can] *see* finasteride *on page 368*

Propine® [US/Can] *see* dipivefrin *on page 281*

Proplex® SX-T Injection *(Discontinued)* *see page 1042*

Proplex® T [US] *see* factor IX complex (human) *on page 355*

propofol (PROE po fole)

Sound-Alike/Look-Alike Issues

Diprivan® may be confused with Diflucan®, Ditropan®

U.S./Canadian Brand Names Diprivan® [US/Can]

Therapeutic Category General Anesthetic

Use Induction of anesthesia for inpatient or outpatient surgery in patients ≥3 years of age; maintenance of anesthesia for inpatient or outpatient surgery in patients >2 months of age; in adults, for the induction and maintenance of monitored anesthesia care sedation during diagnostic procedures; treatment of agitation in intubated, mechanically-ventilated ICU patients

Usual Dosage Dosage must be individualized based on total body weight and titrated to the desired clinical effect; wait at least 3-5 minutes between dosage adjustments to clinically assess drug effects; smaller doses are required when used with narcotics; the following are general dosing guidelines:

General anesthesia:

Induction: I.V.:

Children 3-16 years, ASA I or II: 2.5-3.5 mg/kg over 20-30 seconds; use a lower dose for children ASA III or IV

Adults, ASA I or II, <55 years: 2-2.5 mg/kg (~40 mg every 10 seconds until onset of induction)
Elderly, debilitated, hypovolemic, or ASA III or IV: 1-1.5 mg/kg (~20 mg every 10 seconds until onset of induction)
Cardiac anesthesia: 0.5-1.5 mg/kg (~20 mg every 10 seconds until onset of induction)
Neurosurgical patients: 1-2 mg/kg (~20 mg every 10 seconds until onset of induction)
Maintenance: I.V. infusion:
Children 2 months to 16 years, ASA I or II: Initial: 200-300 mcg/kg/minute; decrease dose after 30 minutes if clinical signs of light anesthesia are absent; usual infusion rate: 125-150 mcg/kg/minute (range: 125-300 mcg/kg/minute; 7.5-18 mg/kg/hour); children ≤5 years may require larger infusion rates compared to older children
Adults, ASA I or II, <55 years: Initial: 150-200 mcg/kg/minute for 10-15 minutes; decrease by 30% to 50% during first 30 minutes of maintenance; usual infusion rate: 100-200 mcg/kg/minute (6-12 mg/kg/hour)
Elderly, debilitated, hypovolemic, ASA III or IV: 50-100 mcg/kg/minute (3-6 mg/kg/hour)
Cardiac anesthesia:
Low-dose propofol with primary opioid: 50-100 mcg/kg/minute (see manufacturer's labeling)
Primary propofol with secondary opioid: 100-150 mcg/kg/minute
Neurosurgical patients: 100-200 mcg/kg/minute (6-12 mg/kg/hour)
Maintenance: I.V. intermittent bolus: Adults, ASA I or II, <55 years: 20-50 mg increments as needed

Monitored anesthesia care sedation:
Initiation:
Adults, ASA I or II, <55 years: Slow I.V. infusion: 100-150 mcg/kg/minute for 3-5 minutes **or** slow injection: 0.5 mg/kg over 3-5 minutes
Elderly, debilitated, neurosurgical, or ASA III or IV patients: Use similar doses to healthy adults; avoid rapid I.V. boluses
Maintenance:
Adults, ASA I or II, <55 years: I.V. infusion using variable rates (preferred over intermittent boluses): 25-75 mcg/kg/minute **or** incremental bolus doses: 10 mg or 20 mg
Elderly, debilitated, neurosurgical, or ASA III or IV patients: Use 80% of healthy adult dose; **do not** use rapid bolus doses (single or repeated)

ICU sedation in intubated mechanically-ventilated patients: Avoid rapid bolus injection; individualize dose and titrate to response Continuous infusion: Initial: 0.3 mg/kg/hour (5 mcg/kg/min); increase by 0.3-0.6 mg/kg/hour (5-10 mcg/kg/min) every 5-10 minutes until desired sedation level is achieved; usual maintenance: 0.3-4.8 mg/kg/hour (5-80 mcg/kg/min) or higher; reduce dose by 80% in elderly, debilitated, and ASA III or IV patients; reduce dose after adequate sedation established and adjust to response (ie, evaluate frequently to use minimum dose for sedation). Some clinicians recommend daily interruption of infusion to perform clinical evaluation.

Dosage Forms Injection, emulsion: 10 mg/mL (20 mL, 50 mL, 100 mL) [contains sodium metabisulfite, egg lecithin, and soybean oil]
Diprivan®: 10 mg/mL (20 mL, 50 mL, 100 mL) [contains egg lecithin, soybean oil, and disodium edetate]

Propoxacet-N® *(Discontinued)* *see page 1042*

propoxyphene (proe POKS i feen)

Sound-Alike/Look-Alike Issues
propoxyphene may be confused with proparacaine
Darvon® may be confused with Devrom®, Diovan®
Darvon-N® may be confused with Darvocet-N®

Synonyms dextropropoxyphene; propoxyphene hydrochloride; propoxyphene napsylate
U.S./Canadian Brand Names Darvon® [US]; Darvon-N® [US/Can]; 642® Tablet [Can]
Therapeutic Category Analgesic, Narcotic
Controlled Substance C-IV
(Continued)

propoxyphene *(Continued)*

Use Management of mild to moderate pain

Usual Dosage Oral:

Children: Doses for children are not well established; doses of the hydrochloride of 2-3 mg/kg/d divided every 6 hours have been used

Adults:

Hydrochloride: 65 mg every 3-4 hours as needed for pain; maximum: 390 mg/day

Napsylate: 100 mg every 4 hours as needed for pain; maximum: 600 mg/day

Dosage Forms

Capsule, as hydrochloride (Darvon®): 65 mg

Tablet, as napsylate (Darvon-N®): 100 mg

propoxyphene and acetaminophen

(proe POKS i feen & a seet a MIN oh fen)

Sound-Alike/Look-Alike Issues

Darvocet-N® may be confused with Darvon-N®

Synonyms propoxyphene hydrochloride and acetaminophen; propoxyphene napsylate and acetaminophen

U.S./Canadian Brand Names Darvocet A500™ [US]; Darvocet-N® 50 [US/Can]; Darvocet-N® 100 [US/Can]; Pronap-100® [US]

Therapeutic Category Analgesic, Narcotic

Controlled Substance C-IV

Use Management of mild to moderate pain

Usual Dosage Oral: Adults:

Darvocet A500™, Darvocet-N® 100: 1 tablet every 4 hours as needed; maximum: 600 mg propoxyphene napsylate/day

Darvocet-N® 50: 1-2 tablets every 4 hours as needed; maximum: 600 mg propoxyphene napsylate/day

Note: Dosage of acetaminophen should not exceed 4 g/day (6 tablets of Darvocet-N® 100); possibly less in patients with ethanol

Dosage Forms Tablet: Propoxyphene hydrochloride 65 mg and acetaminophen 650 mg, propoxyphene napsylate 100 mg, and acetaminophen 650 mg

Darvocet A500™: Propoxyphene napsylate 100 mg and acetaminophen 500 mg [contains lactose]

Darvocet-N® 50: Propoxyphene napsylate 50 mg and acetaminophen 325 mg

Darvocet-N® 100, Pronap-100®: Propoxyphene napsylate 100 mg and acetaminophen 650 mg

propoxyphene and aspirin (proe POKS i feen & AS pir in)

Synonyms aspirin and propoxyphene

Therapeutic Category Analgesic, Narcotic

Controlled Substance C-IV

Use Management of mild to moderate pain

Usual Dosage Oral: 1-2 capsules every 4 hours as needed

Dosage Forms Capsule: Propoxyphene hydrochloride 65 mg and aspirin 389 mg with caffeine 32.4 mg

propoxyphene hydrochloride *see* propoxyphene *on previous page*

propoxyphene hydrochloride and acetaminophen *see* propoxyphene and acetaminophen *on this page*

propoxyphene napsylate *see* propoxyphene *on previous page*

propoxyphene napsylate and acetaminophen *see* propoxyphene and acetaminophen *on this page*

propranolol (proe PRAN oh lole)

Sound-Alike/Look-Alike Issues

propranolol may be confused with Pravachol®, Propulsid®

Inderal® may be confused with Adderall®, Enduron®, Enduronyl®, Imdur®, Imuran®, Inderide®, Isordil®, Toradol®

Inderal® 40 may be confused with Enduronyl® Forte

Synonyms propranolol hydrochloride

U.S./Canadian Brand Names Apo-Propranolol® [Can]; Inderal® [US/Can]; Inderal® LA [US/Can]; InnoPran XL™ [US]; Nu-Propranolol [Can]; Propranolol Intensol™ [US]

Therapeutic Category Antiarrhythmic Agent, Class II; Beta-Adrenergic Blocker

Use Management of hypertension; angina pectoris; pheochromocytoma; essential tremor; tetralogy of Fallot cyanotic spells; arrhythmias (such as atrial fibrillation and flutter, AV nodal re-entrant tachycardias, and catecholamine-induced arrhythmias); prevention of myocardial infarction; migraine headache; symptomatic treatment of hypertrophic subaortic stenosis

Usual Dosage

Akathisia: Oral: Adults: 30-120 mg/day in 2-3 divided doses

Angina: Oral: Adults: 80-320 mg/day in doses divided 2-4 times/day

Long-acting formulation: Initial: 80 mg once daily; maximum dose: 320 mg once daily

Essential tremor: Oral: Adults: 20-40 mg twice daily initially; maintenance doses: usually 120-320 mg/day

Hypertension:

Oral:

Children: Initial: 0.5-1 mg/kg/day in divided doses every 6-12 hours; increase gradually every 5-7 days; maximum: 16 mg/kg/24 hours

Adults: Initial: 40 mg twice daily; increase dosage every 3-7 days; usual dose: ≤320 mg divided in 2-3 doses/day; maximum daily dose: 640 mg; usual dosage range (JNC 7): 40-160 mg/day in 2 divided doses Long-acting formulation: Initial: 80 mg once daily; usual maintenance: 120-160 mg once daily; maximum daily dose: 640 mg; usual dosage range (JNC 7): 60-180 mg/day once daily

I.V.: Children: 0.01-0.05 mg/kg over 1 hour; maximum dose: 10 mg

Hypertrophic subaortic stenosis: Oral: Adults: 20-40 mg 3-4 times/day

Long-acting formulation: 80-160 mg once daily

Migraine headache prophylaxis: Oral:

Children: Initial: 2-4 mg/kg/day **or**

≤35 kg: 10-20 mg 3 times/day

>35 kg: 20-40 mg 3 times/day

Adults: Initial: 80 mg/day divided every 6-8 hours; increase by 20-40 mg/dose every 3-4 weeks to a maximum of 160-240 mg/day given in divided doses every 6-8 hours; if satisfactory response not achieved within 6 weeks of starting therapy, drug should be withdrawn gradually over several weeks

Long-acting formulation: Initial: 80 mg once daily; effective dose range: 160-240 mg once daily

Myocardial infarction prophylaxis: Oral: Adults: 180-240 mg/day in 3-4 divided doses

Pheochromocytoma: Oral: Adults: 30-60 mg/day in divided doses

Tachyarrhythmias:

Oral:

Children: Initial: 0.5-1 mg/kg/day in divided doses every 6-8 hours; titrate dosage upward every 3-7 days; usual dose: 2-6 mg/kg/day; higher doses may be needed; do not exceed 16 mg/kg/day or 60 mg/day

Adults: 10-30 mg/dose every 6-8 hours

Elderly: Initial: 10 mg twice daily; increase dosage every 3-7 days; usual dosage range: 10-320 mg given in 2 divided doses

I.V.:

Children: 0.01-0.1 mg/kg/dose slow IVP over 10 minutes; maximum dose: 1 mg for infants; 3 mg for children

Adults (in patients having nonfunctional GI tract): 1 mg/dose slow IVP; repeat every 5 minutes up to a total of 5 mg; titrate initial dose to desired response

(Continued)

propranolol *(Continued)*

Tetralogy spells: Children:

Oral: Palliation: Initial: 1 mg/kg/day every 6 hours; if ineffective, may increase dose after 1 week by 1 mg/kg/day to a maximum of 5 mg/kg/day; if patient becomes refractory, may increase slowly to a maximum of 10-15 mg/kg/day. Allow 24 hours between dosing changes.

I.V.: 0.01-0.2 mg/kg/dose infused over 10 minutes; maximum initial dose: 1 mg

Thyrotoxicosis:

Oral:

Children: 2 mg/kg/day, divided every 6-8 hours, titrate to effective dose

Adolescents and Adults: Oral: 10-40 mg/dose every 6 hours

I.V.: Adults: 1-3 mg/dose slow IVP as a single dose

Dosage Forms

Capsule, extended release, as hydrochloride (InnoPran XL™): 80 mg, 120 mg

Capsule, sustained release, as hydrochloride (Inderal® LA): 60 mg, 80 mg, 120 mg, 160 mg

Injection, solution, as hydrochloride (Inderal®): 1 mg/mL (1 mL)

Solution, oral, as hydrochloride: 4 mg/mL (5 mL, 500 mL); 8 mg/mL (500 mL) [strawberry-mint flavor; contains alcohol 0.6%]

Solution, oral concentrate, as hydrochloride (Propranolol Intensol™): 80 mg/mL (30 mL)

Tablet, as hydrochloride (Inderal®): 10 mg, 20 mg, 40 mg, 60 mg, 80 mg

propranolol and hydrochlorothiazide

(proe PRAN oh lole & hye droe klor oh THYE a zide)

Sound-Alike/Look-Alike Issues

Inderide® may be confused with Inderal®

Synonyms hydrochlorothiazide and propranolol

U.S./Canadian Brand Names Inderide® [US]

Therapeutic Category Antihypertensive Agent, Combination

Use Management of hypertension

Usual Dosage Oral: Adults: Hypertension: Dose is individualized; typical dosages of **hydrochlorothiazide**: 12.5-50 mg/day; initial dose of **propranolol**: 80 mg/day

Daily dose of tablet form should be divided into 2 daily doses; may be used to maximum dosage of up to 160 mg of propranolol; higher dosages would result in higher than optimal thiazide dosages.

Dosage Forms Tablet (Inderide®):

40/25: Propranolol hydrochloride 40 mg and hydrochlorothiazide 25 mg

80/25: Propranolol hydrochloride 80 mg and hydrochlorothiazide 25 mg

propranolol hydrochloride *see* propranolol *on previous page*

Propranolol Intensol™ [US] *see* propranolol *on previous page*

Propulsid® [US] *see* cisapride *on page 204*

propylene glycol and salicylic acid *see* salicylic acid and propylene glycol *on page 792*

propylene glycol diacetate, acetic acid, and hydrocortisone *see* acetic acid, propylene glycol diacetate, and hydrocortisone *on page 15*

propylene glycol diacetate, hydrocortisone, and acetic acid *see* acetic acid, propylene glycol diacetate, and hydrocortisone *on page 15*

propylhexedrine (proe pil HEKS e dreen)

U.S./Canadian Brand Names Benzedrex® [US-OTC]

Therapeutic Category Adrenergic Agonist Agent

Use Topical nasal decongestant

Usual Dosage Nasal: Children 6-12 years and Adults: Two inhalations in each nostril, not more frequently than every 2 hours

Dosage Forms Inhaler, nasal: 250 mg/0.42 mL (0.42 mL)

propyliodone *see* radiological/contrast media (ionic) *on page 759*

2-propylpentanoic acid *see* valproic acid and derivatives *on page 901*

propylthiouracil (proe pil thye oh YOOR a sil)

Synonyms PTU

U.S./Canadian Brand Names Propyl-Thyracil® [Can]

Therapeutic Category Antithyroid Agent

Use Palliative treatment of hyperthyroidism as an adjunct to ameliorate hyperthyroidism in preparation for surgical treatment or radioactive iodine therapy; management of thyrotoxic crisis

Usual Dosage Oral: Administer in 3 equally divided doses at approximately 8-hour intervals. Adjust dosage to maintain T_3, T_4, and TSH levels in normal range; elevated T_3 may be sole indicator of inadequate treatment. Elevated TSH indicates excessive antithyroid treatment.

Children: Initial: 5-7 mg/kg/day **or** 150-200 mg/m^2/day in divided doses every 8 hours **or**

6-10 years: 50-150 mg/day

>10 years: 150-300 mg/day

Maintenance: Determined by patient response **or** 1/3 to 2/3 of the initial dose in divided doses every 8-12 hours. This usually begins after 2 months on an effective initial dose.

Adults: Initial: 300 mg/day in divided doses every 8 hours. In patients with severe hyperthyroidism, very large goiters, or both, the initial dosage is usually 450 mg/day; an occasional patient will require 600-900 mg/day; maintenance: 100-150 mg/day in divided doses every 8-12 hours

Withdrawal of therapy: Therapy should be withdrawn gradually with evaluation of the patient every 4-6 weeks for the first 3 months then every 3 months for the first year after discontinuation of therapy to detect any reoccurrence of a hyperthyroid state.

Dosage Forms Tablet: 50 mg

Propyl-Thyracil® [Can] *see* propylthiouracil *on this page*

2-propylvaleric acid *see* valproic acid and derivatives *on page 901*

Proscar® [US/Can] *see* finasteride *on page 368*

Pro-Sof® *(Discontinued)* *see page 1042*

Pro-Sof® Plus *(Discontinued)* *see page 1042*

ProSom™ [US] *see* estazolam *on page 324*

prostacyclin *see* epoprostenol *on page 316*

prostaglandin E_1 *see* alprostadil *on page 35*

prostaglandin E_2 *see* dinoprostone *on page 275*

Prostaphlin® *(Discontinued)* *see page 1042*

ProStep® Patch *(Discontinued)* *see page 1042*

Prostigmin® [US/Can] *see* neostigmine *on page 613*

Prostin E_2® [US/Can] *see* dinoprostone *on page 275*

Prostin F_2 Alpha® *(Discontinued)* *see page 1042*

Prostin® VR [Can] *see* alprostadil *on page 35*

Prostin VR Pediatric® [US] *see* alprostadil *on page 35*

protamine sulfate (PROE ta meen SUL fate)

Sound-Alike/Look-Alike Issues

protamine may be confused with ProAmatine®, Protopam®, Protropin®

Therapeutic Category Antidote

Use Treatment of heparin overdosage; neutralize heparin during surgery or dialysis procedures

(Continued)

protamine sulfate *(Continued)*

Usual Dosage Children and Adults: I.V.: 1 mg of protamine neutralizes 90 USP units of heparin (lung) and 115 USP units of heparin (intestinal); heparin neutralization occurs within 5 minutes following I.V. injection; administer 1 mg for each 100 units of heparin administered in preceding 3-4 hours up to a maximum dose of 50 mg

Note: Excessive protamine doses may worsen bleeding potential.

Dosage Forms Injection, solution, as sulfate [preservative free]: 10 mg/mL (5 mL, 25 mL)

protein C (activated), human, recombinant *see* drotrecogin alfa *on page 297*

Protenate® *(Discontinued)* *see page 1042*

Prothazine-DC® *(Discontinued)* *see page 1042*

prothrombin complex concentrate *see* factor IX complex (human) *on page 355*

Protilase® *(Discontinued)* *see page 1042*

protirelin (proe TYE re lin)

Synonyms lopremone; thyrotropin releasing hormone; TRH

U.S./Canadian Brand Names Relefact® TRH [Can]

Therapeutic Category Diagnostic Agent

Use Adjunct in the diagnostic assessment of thyroid function, and an adjunct to other diagnostic procedures in patients with pituitary or hypothalamic dysfunction; also causes release of prolactin from the pituitary and is used to detect defective control of prolactin secretion

Usual Dosage I.V.:

Infants and Children <6 years: Experience limited, but doses of 7 mcg/kg have been administered

Children 6-16 years: 7 mcg/kg to a maximum dose of 500 mcg

Adults: 500 mcg (range 200-500 mcg)

Dosage Forms Injection, solution: 500 mcg/mL (1 mL)

Protonix® [US/Can] *see* pantoprazole *on page 665*

Protopam® [US/Can] *see* pralidoxime *on page 719*

Protopam® Tablet *(Discontinued)* *see page 1042*

Protopic® [US/Can] *see* tacrolimus *on page 837*

Protostat® Oral *(Discontinued)* *see page 1042*

protriptyline (proe TRIP ti leen)

Synonyms protriptyline hydrochloride

U.S./Canadian Brand Names Vivactil® [US]

Therapeutic Category Antidepressant, Tricyclic (Secondary Amine)

Use Treatment of depression

Usual Dosage Oral:

Adolescents: 15-20 mg/day

Adults: 15-60 mg in 3-4 divided doses

Dosage Forms Tablet, as hydrochloride [film coated]: 5 mg, 10 mg

protriptyline hydrochloride *see* protriptyline *on this page*

Protropin® [US/Can] *see* human growth hormone *on page 437*

Protropine® [Can] *see* human growth hormone *on page 437*

Protuss®-DM *(Discontinued)* *see page 1042*

Provatene® *(Discontinued)* *see page 1042*

Proventil® [US] *see* albuterol *on page 25*

Proventil® HFA [US] *see* albuterol *on page 25*

Proventil® Inhaler *(Discontinued)* *see page 1042*

Proventil® Repetabs® [US] *see* albuterol *on page 25*

Proventil® Solution *(Discontinued)* *see page 1042*

Proventil® Tablet *(Discontinued)* *see page 1042*

Provera® [US/Can] *see* medroxyprogesterone acetate *on page 548*

Provigil® [US/Can] *see* modafinil *on page 587*

Proviodine [Can] *see* povidone-iodine *on page 718*

Provocholine® [US/Can] *see* methacholine *on page 561*

proxymetacaine *see* proparacaine *on page 738*

Prozac® [US/Can] *see* fluoxetine *on page 379*

Prozac® Weekly™ [US] *see* fluoxetine *on page 379*

PRP-D *see* *Haemophilus* B conjugate vaccine *on page 426*

Prudoxin™ [US] *see* doxepin *on page 292*

prymaccone *see* primaquine *on page 728*

23PS *see* pneumococcal polysaccharide vaccine (polyvalent) *on page 704*

PS-341 *see* bortezomib *on page 124*

pseudoephedrine (soo doe e FED rin)

Sound-Alike/Look-Alike Issues

Dimetapp® may be confused with Dermatop®, Dimetabs®, Dimetane®

Synonyms *d*-isoephedrine hydrochloride; pseudoephedrine hydrochloride; pseudoephedrine sulfate

U.S./Canadian Brand Names Balminil® Decongestant [Can]; Biofed [US-OTC]; Contac® Cold 12 Hour Relief Non Drowsy [Can]; Decofed® [US-OTC]; Dimetapp® 12-Hour Non-Drowsy Extentabs® [US-OTC]; Dimetapp® Decongestant [US-OTC]; Drixoral® ND [Can]; Eltor® [Can]; Genaphed® [US-OTC]; Kidkare Decongestant [US-OTC]; Kodet SE [US-OTC]; Oranyl [US-OTC]; PediaCare® Decongestant Infants [US-OTC]; PMS-Pseudoephedrine [Can]; Pseudofrin [Can]; Robidrine® [Can]; Silfedrine Children's [US-OTC]; Sudafed® 12 Hour [US-OTC]; Sudafed® 24 Hour [US-OTC]; Sudafed® Children's [US-OTC]; Sudafed® Decongestant [Can]; Sudafed® [US-OTC]; Sudodrin [US-OTC]; Triaminic® Allergy Congestion [US-OTC/Can]

Therapeutic Category Adrenergic Agonist Agent

Use Temporary symptomatic relief of nasal congestion due to common cold, upper respiratory allergies, and sinusitis; also promotes nasal or sinus drainage

Usual Dosage Oral:

Children:

<2 years: 4 mg/kg/day in divided doses every 6 hours

2-5 years: 15 mg every 6 hours; maximum: 60 mg/24 hours

6-12 years: 30 mg every 6 hours; maximum: 120 mg/24 hours

Adults: 30-60 mg every 4-6 hours, sustained release: 120 mg every 12 hours; maximum: 240 mg/24 hours

Dosage Forms

Gelcap (Dimetapp® Decongestant): 30 mg

Liquid, as hydrochloride:

Silfedrine Children's: 15 mg/5 mL (120 mL, 480 mL) [alcohol and sugar free; grape flavor]

Sudafed® Children's: 15 mg/5 mL (120 mL) [alcohol and sugar free; contains sodium benzoate; grape flavor]

Triaminic® Allergy Congestion: 15 mg/5 mL (120 mL) [contains benzoic acid]

Solution, oral drops, as hydrochloride:

Dimetapp® Decongestant Infant Drops: 7.5 mg/0.8 mL (15 mL) [alcohol free]

Kidkare Decongestant: 7.5 mg/0.8 mL (30 mL)

(Continued)

pseudoephedrine *(Continued)*

PediaCare® Decongestant: 7.5 mg/0.8 mL (15 mL) [contains benzoic acid, sodium benzoate; fruit flavor]

Syrup, as hydrochloride: 30 mg/5 mL (120 mL, 480 mL)

Biofed: 30 mg/5 mL (120 mL, 240 mL, 480 mL, 3840 mL) [alcohol free; contains sodium benzoate]

Decofed®: 30 mg/5 mL (120 mL, 480 mL) [raspberry flavor]

Tablet, as hydrochloride: 30 mg, 60 mg

Genaphed®, Kodet SE, Oranyl, Sudafed®, Sudodrin: 30 mg

Tablet, chewable, as hydrochloride:

Sudafed® Children's: 15 mg [sugar free; contains phenylalanine 0.78 mg (as aspartame)/tablet; orange flavor]

Triaminic® Allergy Congestion: 15 mg [contains phenylalanine 17.6 mg (as aspartame)/tablet, coconut oil]

Tablet, extended release, as hydrochloride:

Dimetapp® 12-Hour Non-Drowsy Extentabs®, Sudafed® 12 Hour: 120 mg

Sudafed® 24 Hour: 240 mg

pseudoephedrine, acetaminophen, and chlorpheniramine *see* acetaminophen, chlorpheniramine, and pseudoephedrine *on page 11*

pseudoephedrine, acetaminophen, and dextromethorphan *see* acetaminophen, dextromethorphan, and pseudoephedrine *on page 12*

pseudoephedrine and acetaminophen *see* acetaminophen and pseudoephedrine *on page 9*

pseudoephedrine and acrivastine *see* acrivastine and pseudoephedrine *on page 17*

pseudoephedrine and azatadine *see* azatadine and pseudoephedrine *on page 93*

pseudoephedrine and brompheniramine *see* brompheniramine and pseudoephedrine *on page 129*

pseudoephedrine and carbinoxamine *see* carbinoxamine and pseudoephedrine *on page 157*

pseudoephedrine and chlorpheniramine *see* chlorpheniramine and pseudoephedrine *on page 189*

pseudoephedrine and dexbrompheniramine *see* dexbrompheniramine and pseudoephedrine *on page 256*

pseudoephedrine and dextromethorphan

(soo doe e FED rin & deks troe meth OR fan)

Synonyms dextromethorphan and pseudoephedrine

U.S./Canadian Brand Names Balminil® DM D [Can]; Benylin® DM-D [Can]; Children's Sudafed® Cough & Cold [US-OTC]; Koffex DM-D [Can]; Novahistex® DM Decongestant [Can]; Novahistine® DM Decongestant [Can]; Pediacare® Decongestant Plus Cough [US-OTC]; Pediacare® Long Acting Cough Plus Cold [US-OTC]; Robitussin® Childrens Cough & Cold [Can]; Robitussin® Maximum Strength Cough & Cold [US-OTC]; Robitussin® Pediatric Cough & Cold [US-OTC]; Vicks® 44D Cough & Head Congestion [US-OTC]

Therapeutic Category Antitussive/Decongestant

Use Temporary symptomatic relief of nasal congestion due to common cold, upper respiratory allergies, and sinusitis; also promotes nasal or sinus drainage; symptomatic relief of coughs caused by minor viral upper respiratory tract infections or inhaled irritants; most effective for a chronic nonproductive cough

Usual Dosage Oral:

Children: Dose should be based on pseudoephedrine component

Adults: 5-10 mL every 6 hours

Dosage Forms

Liquid: Pseudoephedrine hydrochloride 15 mg and dextromethorphan hydrobromide 7.5 mg per 5 mL (120 mL)

Children's Sudafed® Cold & Cough: Pseudoephedrine hydrochloride 15 mg and dextromethorphan hydrobromide 5 mg per 5 mL (120 mL) [alcohol free, sugar free; contains sodium benzoate; cherry berry flavor]

Robitussin® Maximum Strength Cough & Cold: Pseudoephedrine hydrochloride 30 mg and dextromethorphan hydrobromide 15 mg per 5 mL (120 mL, 240 mL) [contains alcohol 1.4%]

Pediacare® Long Acting Cough Plus Cold: Pseudoephedrine hydrochloride 15 mg and dextromethorphan hydrobromide 7.5 mg per 5 mL (120 mL) [alcohol free; contains sodium benzoate; grape flavor]

Robitussin® Pediatric Cough & Cold: Pseudoephedrine hydrochloride 15 mg and dextromethorphan hydrobromide 7.5 mg per 5 mL (120 mL, 240 mL) [alcohol free; fruit punch flavor]

Vicks® 44D Cough & Head Congestion: Pseudoephedrine hydrochloride 20 mg and dextromethorphan hydrobromide 10 mg per 5 mL (120 mL, 240 mL) [contains alcohol 5%, sodium 31 mg/15 mL, and sodium benzoate; cherry flavor]

Liquid, oral drops: (Pediacare® Decongestant Plus Cough): Pseudoephedrine hydrochloride 7.5 mg and dextromethorphan hydrobromide 2.5 mg per 0.8 mL (15 mL) [alcohol free; contains sodium benzoate; cherry flavor]

Tablets, chewable (Pediacare® Long Acting Cough Plus Cold): Pseudoephedrine hydrochloride 7.5 mg and dextromethorphan hydrobromide 2.5 mg [contains phenylalanine 5.04 mg per tablet; grape flavor]

pseudoephedrine and diphenhydramine *see* diphenhydramine and pseudoephedrine *on page 279*

pseudoephedrine and fexofenadine *see* fexofenadine and pseudoephedrine *on page 366*

pseudoephedrine and guaifenesin *see* guaifenesin and pseudoephedrine *on page 419*

pseudoephedrine and hydrocodone *see* hydrocodone and pseudoephedrine *on page 446*

pseudoephedrine and ibuprofen

(soo doe e FED rin & eye byoo PROE fen)

Synonyms ibuprofen and pseudoephedrine

U.S./Canadian Brand Names Advil® Cold, Children's [US-OTC]; Advil® Cold & Sinus [US-OTC/Can]; Dristan® Sinus Tablet [US-OTC/Can]; Motrin® Cold and Sinus [US-OTC]; Motrin® Cold, Children's [US-OTC]; Sudafed® Sinus Advance [Can]

Therapeutic Category Decongestant/Analgesic

Use For temporary relief of cold, sinus and flu symptoms (including nasal congestion, headache, sore throat, minor body aches and pains, and fever)

Usual Dosage OTC labeling: Oral:

Children: Ibuprofen 100 mg and pseudoephedrine 15 mg per 5 mL: May repeat dose every 6 hours (maximum: 4 doses/24 hours); dose should be based on weight when possible. Contact healthcare provider if symptoms have not improved within 3 days (2 days if treating sore throat accompanied by fever).

2-5 years or 11 to <22 kg (24-47 pounds): 5 mL

6-11 years or 22-43 kg (48-95 pounds): 10 mL

Children ≥12 years and Adults: Ibuprofen 200 mg and pseudoephedrine 30 mg per dose: One dose every 4-6 hours as needed; may increase to 2 doses if necessary (maximum: 6 doses/24 hours). Contact healthcare provider if symptoms have not improved within 7 days when treating cold symptoms or within 3 days when treating fever.

(Continued)

pseudoephedrine and ibuprofen *(Continued)*

Dosage Forms

Caplet:

Advil® Cold and Sinus, Dristan® Sinus: Pseudoephedrine hydrochloride 30 mg and ibuprofen 200 mg [contains sodium benzoate]

Motrin® Cold and Sinus: Pseudoephedrine hydrochloride 30 mg and ibuprofen 200 mg

Capsule, liquid filled (Advil® Cold and Sinus Liqui-gel®): Pseudoephedrine hydrochloride 30 mg and ibuprofen 200 mg [solubilized ibuprofen as free and potassium salt; contains coconut oil]

Suspension:

Advil® Cold, Children's: Pseudoephedrine hydrochloride 15 mg and ibuprofen 100 mg per 5 mL (120 mL) [alcohol free; contains sodium benzoate; grape flavor]

Motrin® Cold, Children's: Pseudoephedrine hydrochloride 15 mg and ibuprofen 100 mg per 5 mL (120 mL) [contains sodium benzoate; berry, dye free berry, and grape flavors]

Tablet (Advil® Cold and Sinus): Pseudoephedrine hydrochloride 30 mg and ibuprofen 200 mg [contains sodium benzoate]

pseudoephedrine and loratadine *see* loratadine and pseudoephedrine *on page 530*

pseudoephedrine and triprolidine *see* triprolidine and pseudoephedrine *on page 889*

pseudoephedrine, carbinoxamine, and dextromethorphan *see* carbinoxamine, pseudoephedrine, and dextromethorphan *on page 159*

pseudoephedrine, chlorpheniramine, and acetaminophen *see* acetaminophen, chlorpheniramine, and pseudoephedrine *on page 11*

pseudoephedrine, chlorpheniramine, and codeine *see* chlorpheniramine, pseudoephedrine, and codeine *on page 193*

pseudoephedrine, dextromethorphan, and acetaminophen *see* acetaminophen, dextromethorphan, and pseudoephedrine *on page 12*

pseudoephedrine, dextromethorphan, and carbinoxamine *see* carbinoxamine, pseudoephedrine, and dextromethorphan *on page 159*

pseudoephedrine, dextromethorphan, and guaifenesin *see* guaifenesin, pseudoephedrine, and dextromethorphan *on page 422*

pseudoephedrine, guaifenesin, and codeine *see* guaifenesin, pseudoephedrine, and codeine *on page 422*

pseudoephedrine hydrochloride *see* pseudoephedrine *on page 745*

pseudoephedrine hydrochloride and cetirizine hydrochloride *see* cetirizine and pseudoephedrine *on page 178*

pseudoephedrine, hydrocodone, and guaifenesin *see* hydrocodone, pseudoephedrine, and guaifenesin *on page 447*

pseudoephedrine sulfate *see* pseudoephedrine *on page 745*

pseudoephedrine, triprolidine, and codeine pseudoephedrine, codeine, and triprolidine *see* triprolidine, pseudoephedrine, and codeine *on page 890*

Pseudoevent™ 400 [US] *see* guaifenesin and pseudoephedrine *on page 419*

Pseudofrin [Can] *see* pseudoephedrine *on page 745*

Pseudo-Gest Plus® Tablet *(Discontinued)* *see page 1042*

Pseudo GG TR [US] *see* guaifenesin and pseudoephedrine *on page 419*

pseudomonic acid A *see* mupirocin *on page 595*

Pseudovent™ [US] *see* guaifenesin and pseudoephedrine *on page 419*

Pseudovent™ DM [US] *see* guaifenesin, pseudoephedrine, and dextromethorphan *on page 422*

Pseudovent™-Ped [US] *see* guaifenesin and pseudoephedrine *on page 419*

P & S™ Liquid Phenol [Can] *see* phenol *on page 687*

Psorcon® [US/Can] *see* diflorasone *on page 269*

Psorcon® E™ [US] *see* diflorasone *on page 269*

Psoriatec™ [US] *see* anthralin *on page 60*

PsoriGel® [US-OTC] *see* coal tar *on page 219*

Psorion® Topical *(Discontinued)* *see page 1042*

psyllium (SIL i yum)

Sound-Alike/Look-Alike Issues

Fiberall® may be confused with Feverall®
Hydrocil® may be confused with Hydrocet®
Modane® may be confused with Matulane®, Moban®
Perdiem® may be confused with Pyridium®

Synonyms plantago seed; plantain seed; psyllium hydrophilic mucilloid

U.S./Canadian Brand Names Fiberall® [US]; Genfiber® [US-OTC]; Hydrocil® [US-OTC]; Konsyl-D® [US-OTC]; Konsyl® Easy Mix [US-OTC]; Konsyl® Orange [US-OTC]; Konsyl® [US-OTC]; Metamucil® [Can]; Metamucil® Smooth Texture [US-OTC]; Metamucil® [US-OTC]; Modane® Bulk [US-OTC]; Novo-Mucilax [Can]; Perdiem® Fiber Therapy [US-OTC]; Reguloid® [US-OTC]; Serutan® [US-OTC]

Therapeutic Category Laxative

Use Treatment of chronic atonic or spastic constipation and in constipation associated with rectal disorders; management of irritable bowel syndrome; labeled for OTC use as fiber supplement, treatment of constipation

Usual Dosage Oral (administer at least 2 hours before or after other drugs):

Children 6-11 years: Approximately ½ adult dosage

Children ≥12 years and Adults: Take 1 dose up to 3 times/day; all doses should be followed with 8 oz of water or liquid

- Capsule: 4 capsules/dose (range: 2-6); swallow capsules one at a time
- Powder: 1 rounded tablespoonful/dose (1 teaspoonful/dose for many sugar free or select concentrated products) mixed in 8 oz liquid
- Tablet: 1 tablet/dose
- Wafer: 2 wafers/dose

Dosage Forms

Capsule (Metamucil®): 0.52 g [provides 3 g dietary fiber per 6 capsules]

Granules:
- Perdiem® Fiber Therapy: 4 g/teaspoon (250 g)
- Serutan®: 2.5 g/teaspoon (510 g) [contains sodium benzoate]

Powder: 3.4 g/dose (unit-dose packets, 397 g)
- Fiberall®: 3.5 g/dose (454 g) [sugar free; contains phenylalanine; orange flavor]
- Genfiber®: 3.4 g/dose (397 g, 595 g) [regular and orange flavors]
- Hydrocil® Instant: 3.5 g/dose (300 g)
- Konsyl®: 6 g/dose (6 g unit-dose packets, 300 g, 450 g) [sodium and sugar free; regular and orange flavors]
- Konsyl-D®: 3.4 g/dose (6.5 g unit-dose packets, 325 g, 500 g) [contains dextrose]
- Konsyl® Easy Mix: 6 g/dose (6 g unit-dose packets, 250 g) [sodium and sugar free]
- Konsyl® Orange: 3.4 g/dose (12 g unit-dose packets, 425 g, 538 g) [contains sucrose]
- Metamucil®: 3.4 g/dose (390 g, 570 g, 870 g, 1254 g) [regular or orange flavor]
- Metamucil® Smooth Texture: 3.4 g/dose (unit-dose packets, 609 g, 912 g, 1368 g) [orange flavor]
- Metamucil® Smooth Texture: 3.4 g/dose (12 g unit-dose packets, 300 g, 450 g, 660 g, 699 g) [sugar free; contains phenylalanine 25 mg/teaspoon; regular or orange flavor]
- Modane® Bulk: 3.4 g/dose (390 g)
- Reguloid®: 3.4 g/dose (300 g, 390 g, 450 g, 570 g) [regular and orange flavor; also available sugar free]

Wafers (Metamucil®): 3.4 g/dose (24s) [apple crisp and cinnamon spice flavors]

psyllium hydrophilic mucilloid *see* psyllium *on previous page*

P.T.E.-4® [US] *see* trace metals *on page 874*

P.T.E.-5® [US] *see* trace metals *on page 874*

pteroylglutamic acid *see* folic acid *on page 385*

PTU *see* propylthiouracil *on page 743*

Pulmicort® [Can] *see* budesonide *on page 131*

Pulmicort Respules® [US] *see* budesonide *on page 131*

Pulmicort Turbuhaler® [US] *see* budesonide *on page 131*

Pulmophylline [Can] *see* theophylline *on page 854*

Pulmozyme® [US/Can] *see* dornase alfa *on page 289*

Puralube® Tears [US-OTC] *see* artificial tears *on page 78*

Purge® [US-OTC] *see* castor oil *on page 165*

purified chick embryo cell *see* rabies virus vaccine *on page 759*

Purinethol® [US/Can] *see* mercaptopurine *on page 555*

PVF® K [Can] *see* penicillin V potassium *on page 677*

P-V Tussin Tablet [US] *see* hydrocodone and pseudoephedrine *on page 446*

pyrantel pamoate (pi RAN tel PAM oh ate)

U.S./Canadian Brand Names Combantrin™ [Can]; Pin-X® [US-OTC]; Reese's® Pinworm Medicine [US-OTC]

Therapeutic Category Anthelmintic

Use Treatment of pinworms (*Enterobius vermicularis*) and roundworms (*Ascaris lumbricoides*)

Usual Dosage Children and Adults (purgation is not required prior to use): Oral: Roundworm, pinworm, or trichostrongyliasis: 11 mg/kg administered as a single dose; maximum dose: 1 g. (**Note:** For pinworm infection, dosage should be repeated in 2 weeks and all family members should be treated).

Dosage Forms

Suspension, oral as pamoate:
- Pin-X®: 144 mg/mL (30 mL, 60 mL) [contains sodium benzoate, caramel flavor]
- Reese's® Pinworm Medicine: 144 mg/mL (30 mL)

Tablet, as pamoate (Reese's® Pinworm Medicine): 180 mg

pyrazinamide (peer a ZIN a mide)

Synonyms pyrazinoic acid amide

U.S./Canadian Brand Names Tebrazid™ [Can]

Therapeutic Category Antitubercular Agent

Use Adjunctive treatment of tuberculosis in combination with other antituberculosis agents

Usual Dosage Oral (calculate dose on ideal body weight rather than total body weight): **Note:** A four-drug regimen (isoniazid, rifampin, pyrazinamide, and either streptomycin or ethambutol) is preferred for the initial, empiric treatment of TB. When the drug susceptibility results are available, the regimen should be altered as appropriate. For the treatment of latent TB infection (LTBI), combination pyrazinamide/rifampin therapy should not generally be offered (*MMWR* Aug 8, 2003).

Children and Adults:
- Daily therapy: 15-30 mg/kg/day (maximum: 2 g/day)
- Directly observed therapy (DOT):
  - Twice weekly: 50-70 mg/kg (maximum: 4 g)
  - Three times/week: 50-70 mg/kg (maximum: 3 g)

Dosage Forms Tablet: 500 mg

pyrazinamide, rifampin, and isoniazid *see* rifampin, isoniazid, and pyrazinamide *on page 776*

pyrazinoic acid amide *see* pyrazinamide *on previous page*

pyrethrins and piperonyl butoxide

(pye RE thrins & pi PER oh nil byo TOKS ide)

Synonyms piperonyl butoxide and pyrethrins

U.S./Canadian Brand Names A-200® Maximum Strength [US-OTC]; Pronto® Lice Control [Can]; Pronto® [US-OTC]; Pyrinyl Plus® [US-OTC]; Pyrinyl® [US-OTC]; R & C™ [Can]; R & C™ II [Can]; RID® Maximum Strength [US-OTC]; RID® Mousse [Can]; Tisit® Blue Gel [US-OTC]; Tisit® [US-OTC]

Therapeutic Category Scabicides/Pediculicides

Use Treatment of *Pediculus humanus* infestations (head lice, body lice, pubic lice and their eggs)

Usual Dosage Application of pyrethrins:

Topical products:

Apply enough solution to completely wet infested area, including hair
Allow to remain on area for 10 minutes
Wash and rinse with large amounts of warm water
Use fine-toothed comb to remove lice and eggs from hair
Shampoo hair to restore body and luster
Treatment may be repeated if necessary once in a 24-hour period
Repeat treatment in 7-10 days to kill newly hatched lice

Solution for furniture, bedding: Spray on entire area to be treated; allow to dry before use. Intended for use on items which cannot be laundered or dry cleaned. **Not for use on humans or animals.**

Dosage Forms

Foam, topical [mousse] (RID®): Pyrethrum extract 0.33% and piperonyl butoxide 4% (156 g)

Gel (Tisit® Blue Gel): Pyrethrum extract 0.33% and piperonyl butoxide 3% (30 g)

Liquid, topical (Tisit®): Pyrethrum extract 0.33% and piperonyl butoxide 2% (60 mL, 120 mL)

Shampoo: Pyrethrum extract 0.33% and piperonyl butoxide 4% (60 mL, 120 mL)

A-200® Maximum Strength: Pyrethrum extract 0.33% and piperonyl butoxide 4% (60 mL, 120 mL) [contains benzyl alcohol]

Pronto®: Pyrethrum extract 0.33% and piperonyl butoxide 4% (60 mL, 120 mL) [contains benzyl alcohol; supplied with comb; also available with creme rinse or in a kit containing shampoo, creme rinse, comb, gloves and furniture spray]

Pyrinyl Plus®: Pyrethrum extract 0.33% and piperonyl butoxide 4% (60 mL)

RID® Maximum Strength: Pyrethrum extract 0.33% and piperonyl butoxide 4% (60 mL, 120 mL, 240 mL) [also available in a kit containing shampoo, gel, and furniture spray]

Tisit®: Pyrethrum extract 0.33% and piperonyl butoxide 3% (60 mL, 120 mL) [also available in a kit containing shampoo, comb, and furniture spray]

Solution, spray [for furniture, garments, bedding; not for human or animal use] (Tisit®): Pyrethrum extract 0.4% and piperonyl butoxide 2% (150 mL)

2-pyridine aldoxime methochloride *see* pralidoxime *on page 719*

Pyridium® [US/Can] *see* phenazopyridine *on page 685*

Pyridium Plus® ***(Discontinued)*** *see page 1042*

pyridostigmine (peer id oh STIG meen)

Sound-Alike/Look-Alike Issues

pyridostigmine may be confused with physostigmine
Mestinon® may be confused with Metatensin®

Synonyms pyridostigmine bromide

U.S./Canadian Brand Names Mestinon® [US/Can]; Mestinon®-SR [Can]; Mestinon® Timespan® [US]

(Continued)

pyridostigmine *(Continued)*

Therapeutic Category Cholinergic Agent

Use Symptomatic treatment of myasthenia gravis; antidote for nondepolarizing neuromuscular blockers

Military use: Pretreatment for Soman nerve gas exposure

Usual Dosage

Myasthenia gravis:

Oral:

Children: 7 mg/kg/24 hours divided into 5-6 doses

Adults: Highly individualized dosing ranges: 60-1500 mg/day, usually 600 mg/day divided into 5-6 doses, spaced to provide maximum relief Sustained release formulation: Highly individualized dosing ranges: 180-540 mg once or twice daily (doses separated by at least 6 hours); **Note:** Most clinicians reserve sustained release dosage form for bedtime dose only.

I.M., slow I.V. push:

Children: 0.05-0.15 mg/kg/dose

Adults: To supplement oral dosage pre- and postoperatively during labor and postpartum, during myasthenic crisis, or when oral therapy is impractical: ~1/30th of oral dose; observe patient closely for cholinergic reactions **or** I.V. infusion: Initial: 2 mg/hour with gradual titration in increments of 0.5-1 mg/hour, up to a maximum rate of 4 mg/hour

Pretreatment for Soman nerve gas exposure (military use): Oral: Adults: 30 mg every 8 hours beginning several hours prior to exposure; discontinue at first sign of nerve agent exposure, then begin atropine and pralidoxime

Reversal of nondepolarizing muscle relaxants: **Note:** Atropine sulfate (0.6-1.2 mg) I.V. immediately prior to pyridostigmine to minimize side effects: I.V.:

Children: Dosing range: 0.1-0.25 mg/kg/dose*

Adults: 0.1-0.25 mg/kg/dose; 10-20 mg is usually sufficient*

*Full recovery usually occurs ≤15 minutes, but ≥30 minutes may be required

Dosage Forms

Injection, solution, as bromide (Mestinon®): 5 mg/mL (2 mL)

Syrup, as bromide (Mestinon®): 60 mg/5 mL (480 mL) [raspberry flavor; contains alcohol 5%, sodium benzoate]

Tablet, as bromide (Mestinon®): 60 mg

Tablet, sustained release, as bromide (Mestinon® Timespan®): 180 mg

pyridostigmine bromide *see* pyridostigmine *on previous page*

pyridoxine (peer i DOKS een)

Sound-Alike/Look-Alike Issues

pyridoxine may be confused with paroxetine, pralidoxime, Pyridium®

Synonyms pyridoxine hydrochloride; vitamin B_6

U.S./Canadian Brand Names Aminoxin® [US-OTC]

Therapeutic Category Vitamin, Water Soluble

Use Prevention and treatment of vitamin B_6 deficiency, pyridoxine-dependent seizures in infants; adjunct to treatment of acute toxicity from isoniazid, cycloserine, or hydralazine overdose

Usual Dosage

Recommended daily allowance (RDA):

Children:

1-3 years: 0.9 mg

4-6 years: 1.3 mg

7-10 years: 1.6 mg

Adults:

Male: 1.7-2.0 mg

Female: 1.4-1.6 mg

Pyridoxine-dependent Infants:
Oral: 2-100 mg/day
I.M., I.V., SubQ: 10-100 mg
Dietary deficiency: Oral:
Children: 5-25 mg/24 hours for 3 weeks, then 1.5-2.5 mg/day in multiple vitamin product
Adults: 10-20 mg/day for 3 weeks
Drug-induced neuritis (eg, isoniazid, hydralazine, penicillamine, cycloserine): Oral:
Children:
Treatment: 10-50 mg/24 hours
Prophylaxis: 1-2 mg/kg/24 hours
Adults:
Treatment: 100-200 mg/24 hours
Prophylaxis: 25-100 mg/24 hours
Treatment of seizures and/or coma from acute isoniazid toxicity, a dose of pyridoxine hydrochloride equal to the amount of INH ingested can be given I.M./I.V. in divided doses together with other anticonvulsants; if the amount INH ingested is not known, administer 5 g I.V. pyridoxine
Treatment of acute hydralazine toxicity, a pyridoxine dose of 25 mg/kg in divided doses I.M./I.V. has been used

Dosage Forms
Capsule, as hydrochloride: 250 mg
Injection, solution, as hydrochloride: 100 mg/mL (1 mL)
Tablet, as hydrochloride: 25 mg, 50 mg, 100 mg, 250 mg, 500 mg
Tablet, enteric coated, as hydrochloride (Aminoxin®): 20 mg

pyridoxine, folic acid, and cyanocobalamin *see* folic acid, cyanocobalamin, and pyridoxine *on page 386*

pyridoxine hydrochloride *see* pyridoxine *on previous page*

pyrimethamine (peer i METH a meen)

Sound-Alike/Look-Alike Issues
Daraprim® may be confused with Dantrium®, Daranide®

U.S./Canadian Brand Names Daraprim® [US/Can]

Therapeutic Category Folic Acid Antagonist (Antimalarial)

Use Prophylaxis of malaria due to susceptible strains of plasmodia; used in conjunction with quinine and sulfadiazine for the treatment of uncomplicated attacks of chloroquine-resistant *P. falciparum* malaria; used in conjunction with fast-acting schizonticide to initiate transmission control and suppression cure; synergistic combination with sulfonamide in treatment of toxoplasmosis

Usual Dosage
Malaria chemoprophylaxis (for areas where chloroquine-resistant *P. falciparum* exists):
Begin prophylaxis 2 weeks before entering endemic area:
Children: 0.5 mg/kg once weekly; not to exceed 25 mg/dose
or
Children:
<4 years: 6.25 mg once weekly
4-10 years: 12.5 mg once weekly
Children >10 years and Adults: 25 mg once weekly
Dosage should be continued for all age groups for at least 6-10 weeks after leaving endemic areas
Chloroquine-resistant *P. falciparum* malaria (when used in conjunction with quinine and sulfadiazine):
Children:
<10 kg: 6.25 mg/day once daily for 3 days
10-20 kg: 12.5 mg/day once daily for 3 days
20-40 kg: 25 mg/day once daily for 3 days
Adults: 25 mg twice daily for 3 days
(Continued)

pyrimethamine *(Continued)*

Toxoplasmosis:

Infants (congenital toxoplasmosis): Oral: 1 mg/kg once daily for 6 months with sulfadiazine then every other month with sulfa, alternating with spiramycin.

Children: Loading dose: 2 mg/kg/day divided into 2 equal daily doses for 1-3 days (maximum: 100 mg/day) followed by 1 mg/kg/day divided into 2 doses for 4 weeks; maximum: 25 mg/day

With sulfadiazine or trisulfapyrimidines: 2 mg/kg/day divided every 12 hours for 3 days, followed by 1 mg/kg/day once daily or divided twice daily for 4 weeks given with trisulfapyrimidines or sulfadiazine

Adults: 50-75 mg/day together with 1-4 g of a sulfonamide for 1-3 weeks depending on patient's tolerance and response, then reduce dose by 50% and continue for 4-5 weeks **or** 25-50 mg/day for 3-4 weeks

Prophylaxis for first episode of *Toxoplasma gondii*:

Children ≥1 month of age: 1 mg/kg/day once daily with dapsone, plus oral folinic acid 5 mg every 3 days

Adolescents and Adults: 50 mg once weekly with dapsone, plus oral folinic acid 25 mg once weekly

Prophylaxis to prevent recurrence of *Toxoplasma gondii:*

Children ≥1 month of age: 1 mg/kg/day once daily given with sulfadiazine or clindamycin, plus oral folinic acid 5 mg every 3 days

Adolescents and Adults: 25-50 mg once daily in combination with sulfadiazine or clindamycin, plus oral folinic acid 10-25 mg daily; atovaquone plus oral folinic acid has also been used in combination with pyrimethamine.

Dosage Forms Tablet: 25 mg

pyrimethamine and sulfadoxine *see* sulfadoxine and pyrimethamine *on page 831*

Pyrinyl Plus® [US-OTC] *see* pyrethrins and piperonyl butoxide *on page 751*

Pyrinyl® [US-OTC] *see* pyrethrins and piperonyl butoxide *on page 751*

pyrithione zinc (peer i THYE one zingk)

Sound-Alike/Look-Alike Issues

pyrithione may be confused with Pyridium®

U.S./Canadian Brand Names DHS™ Zinc [US-OTC]; Head & Shoulders® Classic Clean 2-In-1 [US-OTC]; Head & Shoulders® Classic Clean [US-OTC]; Head & Shoulders® Dry Scalp Care [US-OTC]; Head & Shoulders® Extra Fullness [US-OTC]; Head & Shoulders® Refresh [US-OTC]; Head & Shoulders® Smooth & Silky 2-In-1 [US-OTC]; Zincon® [US-OTC]; ZNP® Bar [US-OTC]

Therapeutic Category Antiseborrheic Agent, Topical

Use Relieves the itching, irritation and scalp flaking associated with dandruff and/or seborrheal dermatitis

Usual Dosage Adults: Products should be used at least twice weekly for best results, but may be used with each washing.

Bar: May be used on body and or scalp; wet area, massage in, and rinse.

Shampoo: Should be applied to wet hair and massaged into scalp; rinse. May be followed with conditioner

Dosage Forms

Bar, topical [soap] (ZNP® Bar): 2% (119 g)

Conditioner, topical (Head & Shoulders® Dry Scalp Care): 0.5% (405 mL)

Shampoo, topical:

DHS™ Zinc: 2% (240 mL, 360 mL)

Head & Shoulders® Classic Clean: 1% (405 mL, 762 mL)

Head & Shoulders® Classic Clean 2-In-1: 1% (204 mL, 405 mL)

Head & Shoulders® Dry Scalp Care: 1% (405 mL)

Head & Shoulders® Extra Fullness: 1% (405 mL)

Head & Shoulders® Refresh: 1% (405 mL, 762 mL)

Head & Shoulders® Smooth & Silky 2-In-1: 1% (405 mL)

Zincon®: 1% (120 mL, 240 mL)

Q-Tussin [US-OTC] *see* guaifenesin *on page 415*

quaternium-18 bentonite *see* bentoquatam *on page 106*

quazepam (KWAY ze pam)

Sound-Alike/Look-Alike Issues
quazepam may be confused with oxazepam

U.S./Canadian Brand Names Doral® [US/Can]

Therapeutic Category Benzodiazepine

Controlled Substance C-IV

Use Treatment of insomnia

Usual Dosage Adults: Oral: Initial: 15 mg at bedtime, in some patients the dose may be reduced to 7.5 mg after a few nights

Dosage Forms Tablet: 7.5 mg, 15 mg

Quelicin® [US/Can] *see* succinylcholine *on page 826*

Queltuss® *(Discontinued)* *see page 1042*

Questran® [US/Can] *see* cholestyramine resin *on page 196*

Questran® Light [US] *see* cholestyramine resin *on page 196*

Questran® Light Sugar Free [Can] *see* cholestyramine resin *on page 196*

Questran® Tablet *(Discontinued)* *see page 1042*

quetiapine (kwe TYE a peen)

Sound-Alike/Look-Alike Issues
Seroquel® may be confused with Serentil®, Serzone®, Sinequan®

Synonyms quetiapine fumarate

U.S./Canadian Brand Names Seroquel® [US/Can]

Therapeutic Category Antipsychotic Agent

Use Treatment of schizophrenia; treatment of acute manic episodes associated with bipolar disorder (as monotherapy or in combination with lithium or valproate)

Usual Dosage Oral: Adults:

Schizophrenia/psychoses: Initial: 25 mg twice daily; increase in increments of 25-50 mg 2-3 times/day on the second and third day, if tolerated, to a target dose of 300-400 mg in 2-3 divided doses by day 4. Make further adjustments as needed at intervals of at least 2 days in adjustments of 25-50 mg twice daily. Usual maintenance range: 300-800 mg/day

Mania: Initial: 50 mg twice daily on day 1, increase dose in increments of 100 mg/day to 200 mg twice daily on day 4; may increase to a target dose of 800 mg/day by day 6 at increments of ≤200 mg/day. Usual dosage range: 400-800 mg/day

Note: Dose reductions should be attempted periodically to establish lowest effective dose in patients with psychosis or to establish need to continue treating agitated symptoms in demented older adults. Patients being restarted after 1 week of no drug need to be titrated as above.

Dosage Forms Tablet, as fumarate: 25 mg, 100 mg, 200 mg, 300 mg [contains lactose]

quetiapine fumarate *see* quetiapine *on this page*

Quibron® [US] *see* theophylline and guaifenesin *on page 855*

Quibron®-T [US] *see* theophylline *on page 854*

Quibron®-T/SR [US/Can] *see* theophylline *on page 854*

Quiess® Injection *(Discontinued)* *see page 1042*

Quinaglute® Dura-Tabs® *(Discontinued)* *see page 1042*

quinagolide *(Discontinued)* *see page 1042*

Quinalan® *(Discontinued)* *see page 1042*

quinalbarbitone sodium *see* secobarbital *on page 797*

Quinamm® *(Discontinued)* *see page 1042*

quinapril (KWIN a pril)

Sound-Alike/Look-Alike Issues
Accupril® may be confused with Accolate®, Accutane®, Aciphex™, Monopril®

Synonyms quinapril hydrochloride

U.S./Canadian Brand Names Accupril® [US/Can]

Therapeutic Category Angiotensin-Converting Enzyme (ACE) Inhibitor

Use Management of hypertension; treatment of congestive heart failure

Usual Dosage Adults: Oral:
Hypertension: Initial: 10-20 mg once daily, adjust according to blood pressure response at peak and trough blood levels; initial dose may be reduced to 5 mg in patients receiving diuretic therapy if the diuretic is continued; usual dose range (JNC 7): 10-40 mg once daily
Congestive heart failure or post-MI: Initial: 5 mg once daily, titrated at weekly intervals to 20-40 mg daily in 2 divided doses

Dosage Forms Tablet, as hydrochloride: 5 mg, 10 mg, 20 mg, 40 mg

quinapril and hydrochlorothiazide
(KWIN a pril & hye droe klor oh THYE a zide)

Synonyms hydrochlorothiazide and quinapril

U.S./Canadian Brand Names Accuretic™ [US/Can]

Therapeutic Category Antihypertensive Agent, Combination

Use Treatment of hypertension (not for initial therapy)

Usual Dosage Oral:
Children: Safety and efficacy have not been established.
Adults: Initial:
Patients who have failed quinapril monotherapy:
Quinapril 10 mg/hydrochlorothiazide 12.5 mg **or**
Quinapril 20 mg/hydrochlorothiazide 12.5 mg once daily
Patients with adequate blood pressure control on hydrochlorothiazide 25 mg/day, but significant potassium loss:
Quinapril 10 mg/hydrochlorothiazide 12.5 mg **or**
Quinapril 20 mg/hydrochlorothiazide 12.5 mg once daily
Note: Clinical trials of quinapril/hydrochlorothiazide combinations used quinapril doses of 2.5-40 mg/day and hydrochlorothiazide doses of 6.25-25 mg/day.

Dosage Forms Tablet:
10/12.5: Quinapril hydrochloride 10 mg and hydrochlorothiazide 12.5 mg
20/12.5: Quinapril hydrochloride 20 mg and hydrochlorothiazide 12.5 mg
20/25: Quinapril hydrochloride 20 mg and hydrochlorothiazide 25 mg

quinapril hydrochloride *see* quinapril *on this page*

Quinate® [Can] *see* quinidine *on this page*

quinidine (KWIN i deen)

Sound-Alike/Look-Alike Issues
quinidine may be confused with clonidine, quinine, Quinora®

Synonyms quinidine gluconate; quinidine polygalacturonate; quinidine sulfate

U.S./Canadian Brand Names Apo-Quin-G® [Can]; Apo-Quinidine® [Can]; BioQuin® Durules™ [Can]; Novo-Quinidin [Can]; Quinate® [Can]

Therapeutic Category Antiarrhythmic Agent, Class I-A

Use Prophylaxis after cardioversion of atrial fibrillation and/or flutter to maintain normal sinus rhythm; prevent recurrence of paroxysmal supraventricular tachycardia, paroxysmal AV junctional rhythm, paroxysmal ventricular tachycardia, paroxysmal atrial fibrillation, and atrial or ventricular premature contractions; has activity against *Plasmodium falciparum* malaria

Usual Dosage **Dosage expressed in terms of the salt: 267 mg of quinidine gluconate = 200 mg of quinidine sulfate.**

Children: Test dose for idiosyncratic reaction (sulfate, oral or gluconate, I.M.): 2 mg/kg or 60 mg/m^2

Oral (quinidine sulfate): 15-60 mg/kg/day in 4-5 divided doses or 6 mg/kg every 4-6 hours; usual 30 mg/kg/day or 900 mg/m^2/day given in 5 daily doses

I.V. **not** recommended (quinidine gluconate): 2-10 mg/kg/dose given at a rate ≤10 mg/minute every 3-6 hours as needed

Adults: Test dose: Oral, I.M.: 200 mg administered several hours before full dosage (to determine possibility of idiosyncratic reaction)

Oral (for malaria):

Sulfate: 100-600 mg/dose every 4-6 hours; begin at 200 mg/dose and titrate to desired effect (maximum daily dose: 3-4 g)

Gluconate: 324-972 mg every 8-12 hours

I.M.: 400 mg/dose every 2-6 hours; initial dose: 600 mg (gluconate)

I.V.: 200-400 mg/dose diluted and given at a rate ≤10 mg/minute; may require as much as 500-750 mg

Dosage Forms [DSC] = Discontinued product

Injection, solution, as gluconate: 80 mg/mL (10 mL) [equivalent to quinidine base 50 mg]

Tablet, as sulfate: 200 mg, 300 mg

Tablet, extended release, as gluconate: 324 mg [equivalent to quinidine base 202 mg]

Quinaglute® Dura-Tabs: 324 mg [equivalent to quinidine base 202 mg] [DSC]

Tablet, extended release, as sulfate: 300 mg [equivalent to quinidine base 249 mg]

quinidine gluconate *see* quinidine *on previous page*

quinidine polygalacturonate *see* quinidine *on previous page*

quinidine sulfate *see* quinidine *on previous page*

quinine (KWYE nine)

Sound-Alike/Look-Alike Issues

quinine may be confused with quinidine

Synonyms quinine sulfate

U.S./Canadian Brand Names Quinine-Odan™ [Can]

Therapeutic Category Antimalarial Agent

Use In conjunction with other antimalarial agents, suppression or treatment of chloroquine-resistant *P. falciparum* malaria; treatment of *Babesia microti* infection in conjunction with clindamycin

Usual Dosage Oral:

Children:

Treatment of chloroquine-resistant malaria: 25-30 mg/kg/day in divided doses every 8 hours for 3-7 days with tetracycline (consider risk versus benefit in children <8 years of age)

Babesiosis: 25 mg/kg/day divided every 8 hours for 7 days

Adults:

Treatment of chloroquine-resistant malaria: 650 mg every 8 hours for 3-7 days with tetracycline

Suppression of malaria: 325 mg twice daily and continued for 6 weeks after exposure

Babesiosis: 650 mg every 6-8 hours for 7 days

Leg cramps: 200-300 mg at bedtime

Dosage Forms

Capsule, as sulfate: 200 mg, 325 mg

Tablet, as sulfate: 260 mg

Quinine-Odan™ [Can] *see* quinine *on this page*

quinine sulfate *see* quinine *on this page*

quinol *see* hydroquinone *on page 454*

Quinora® ***(Discontinued)*** *see page 1042*

Quintasa® [Can] *see* mesalamine *on page 556*

quinupristin and dalfopristin (kwi NYOO pris tin & dal FOE pris tin)

Synonyms pristinamycin; RP-59500

U.S./Canadian Brand Names Synercid® [US/Can]

Therapeutic Category Antibiotic, Streptogramin

Use Treatment of serious or life-threatening infections associated with vancomycin-resistant *Enterococcus faecium* bacteremia; treatment of complicated skin and skin structure infections caused by methcillin-susceptible *Staphylococcus aureus* or *Streptococcus pyogenes*

Has been studied in the treatment of a variety of infections caused by *Enterococcus faecium* (not *E. fecalis*) including vancomycin-resistant strains. May also be effective in the treatment of serious infections caused by *Staphylococcus* species including those resistant to methicillin.

Usual Dosage I.V.:

Children (limited information): Dosages similar to adult dosing have been used in the treatment of complicated skin/soft tissue infections and infections caused by vancomycin-resistant *Enterococcus faecium*

CNS shunt infection due to vancomycin-resistant *Enterococcus faecium*: 7.5 mg/kg/dose every 8 hours; concurrent intrathecal doses of 1-2 mg/day have been administered for up to 68 days

Adults:

Vancomycin-resistant *Enterococcus faecium:* 7.5 mg/kg every 8 hours

Complicated skin and skin structure infection: 7.5 mg/kg every 12 hours

Dosage Forms Injection, powder for reconstitution: 500 mg (dalfopristin 350 mg and quinupristin 150 mg)

Quiphile® ***(Discontinued)*** *see page 1042*

Quixin™ [US] *see* levofloxacin *on page 514*

QVAR® [US/Can] *see* beclomethasone *on page 102*

Q-vel® ***(Discontinued)*** *see page 1042*

R-3827 *see* abarelix *on page 2*

RabAvert® [US] *see* rabies virus vaccine *on next page*

rabeprazole (ra BE pray zole)

Sound-Alike/Look-Alike Issues

Aciphex® may be confused with Acephen®, Accupril®, Aricept®

Synonyms pariprazole

U.S./Canadian Brand Names Aciphex® [US/Can]; Pariet® [Can]

Therapeutic Category Gastric Acid Secretion Inhibitor

Use Short-term (4-8 weeks) treatment and maintenance of erosive or ulcerative gastroesophageal reflux disease (GERD); symptomatic GERD; short-term (up to 4 weeks) treatment of duodenal ulcers; long-term treatment of pathological hypersecretory conditions, including Zollinger-Ellison syndrome; *H. pylori* eradication (in combination with amoxicillin and clarithromycin)

Usual Dosage Oral: Adults >18 years and Elderly:

GERD: 20 mg once daily for 4-8 weeks; maintenance: 20 mg once daily

Duodenal ulcer: 20 mg/day before breakfast for 4 weeks

H. pylori eradication: 20 mg twice daily for 7 days; to be administered with amoxicillin 1000 mg and clarithromycin 500 mg, also given twice daily for 7 days.

Hypersecretory conditions: 60 mg once daily; dose may need to be adjusted as necessary. Doses as high as 100 mg once daily and 60 mg twice daily have been used.

Dosage Forms Tablet, delayed release, enteric coated: 20 mg

rabies immune globulin (human)

(RAY beez i MYUN GLOB yoo lin HYU man)

Synonyms RIG

U.S./Canadian Brand Names BayRab® [US/Can]; Imogam® Rabies Pasteurized [Can]; Imogam® [US]

Therapeutic Category Immune Globulin

Use Part of postexposure prophylaxis of persons with rabies exposure who lack a history of pre-exposure or postexposure prophylaxis with rabies vaccine or a recently documented neutralizing antibody response to previous rabies vaccination; although it is preferable to administer RIG with the first dose of vaccine, it can be given up to 8 days after vaccination

Usual Dosage Children and Adults: I.M.: 20 units/kg in a single dose (RIG should always be administered as part of rabies vaccine (HDCV)) regimen (as soon as possible after the first dose of vaccine, up to 8 days); infiltrate $^1/_2$ of the dose locally around the wound; administer the remainder I.M.

Note: Persons known to have an adequate titer or who have been completely immunized with rabies vaccine should not receive RIG, only booster doses of HDCV

Dosage Forms Injection, solution: 150 units/mL (2 mL, 10 mL)

rabies virus vaccine (RAY beez VYE rus vak SEEN)

Synonyms HDCV; human diploid cell cultures rabies vaccine; PCEC; purified chick embryo cell

U.S./Canadian Brand Names Imovax® Rabies [US/Can]; RabAvert® [US]

Therapeutic Category Vaccine, Inactivated Virus

Use Pre-exposure immunization: Vaccinate persons with greater than usual risk due to occupation or avocation including veterinarians, rangers, animal handlers, certain laboratory workers, and persons living in or visiting countries for longer than 1 month where rabies is a constant threat.

Postexposure prophylaxis: If a bite from a carrier animal is unprovoked, if it is not captured and rabies is present in that species and area, administer rabies immune globulin (RIG) and the vaccine as indicated

Usual Dosage

Pre-exposure prophylaxis: 1 mL I.M. on days 0, 7, and 21 to 28. **Note:** Prolonging the interval between doses does not interfere with immunity achieved after the concluding dose of the basic series.

Postexposure prophylaxis: All postexposure treatment should begin with immediate cleansing of the wound with soap and water

Persons not previously immunized as above: Rabies immune globulin 20 units/kg body weight, half infiltrated at bite site if possible, remainder I.M.; and 5 doses of rabies vaccine, 1 mL I.M., one each on days 0, 3, 7, 14, 28

Persons who have previously received postexposure prophylaxis with rabies vaccine, received a recommended I.M. pre-exposure series of rabies vaccine or have a previously documented rabies antibody titer considered adequate: 1 mL of either vaccine I.M. only on days 0 and 3; do not administer RIG

Booster (for occupational or other continuing risk): 1 mL I.M. every 2-5 years or based on antibody titers

Dosage Forms Injection, powder for reconstitution:

Imovax® Rabies: 2.5 int. units [HDCV; grown in human diploid cell culture; contains albumin <100 mg, neomycin <150 mcg]

RabAvert®: 2.5 int. units [PCEC; grown in chicken fibroblasts; contains amphotericin <2 ng, chlortetracycline <20 ng, and neomycin <1 mcg]

radiological/contrast media (ionic)

(ray deo LOG ik al/KON trast MEE dia eye ON ik)

Synonyms barium sulfate; diatrizoate meglumine; diatrizoate meglumine and diatrizoate sodium; diatrizoate meglumine and iodipamide meglumine; diatrizoate sodium; ethiodized oil; gadopentetate dimeglumine; iocetamic acid; iodamide meglumine; iodipamide

(Continued)

radiological/contrast media (ionic) *(Continued)*

meglumine; iopanoic acid; iothalamate meglumine and iothalamate sodium; iothalamate sodium; ipodate calcium; ipodate sodium; isosulfan blue; potassium perchlorate; propyliodone; tyropanoate sodium

U.S./Canadian Brand Names Anatrast® [US]; Angio Conray® [US]; Angiovist® [US]; Baricon® [US]; Barobag® [US]; Baro-CAT® [US]; Baroflave® [US]; Barosperse® [US]; Bar-Test® [US]; Cholebrine® [US]; Cholografin® Meglumine [US]; Conray® [US]; Cystografin® [US]; Dionosil Oily® [US]; Enecat® [US]; Entrobar® [US]; Epi-C® [US]; Ethiodol® [US]; Flo-Coat® [US]; Gastrografin® [US]; HD 85® [US]; HD 200 Plus® [US]; Hexabrix™ [US]; Hypaque-Cysto® [US]; Hypaque® Meglumine [US]; Hypaque® Sodium [US]; Liquid Barosperse® [US]; Liquipake® [US]; Lymphazurin® [US/Can]; Magnevist® [US/Can]; MD-Gastroview® [US]; Oragrafin® Calcium [US]; Oragrafin® Sodium [US]; Perchloracap® [US]; Prepcat® [US]; Reno-M-30® [US]; Reno-M-60® [US]; Reno-M-DIP® [US]; Renovue®-65 [US]; Renovue®-DIP [US]; Sinografin® [US]; Telepaque® [US]; Tomocat® [US]; Tonopaque® [US]; Urovist Cysto® [US]; Urovist® Meglumine [US]; Urovist® Sodium 300 [US]; Vascoray® [US]

Therapeutic Category Radiopaque Agents

Use Enhance visualization of structures during radiologic procedures

Dosage Forms [DSC] = Discontinued product

Oral cholecystographic agents:
- Iocetamic acid: Tablet (Cholebrine®): 750 mg
- Iopanoic acid: Tablet (Telepaque®): 500 mg
- Ipodate calcium: Granules for oral suspension (Oragrafin® Calcium): 3 g
- Ipodate sodium: Capsule (Bilivist®, Oragrafin® Sodium): 500 mg
- Tyropanoate sodium: Capsule (Bilopaque®): 750 mg [DSC]

GI contrast agents: **Barium sulfate**:
- Paste (Anatrast®): 100% (500 g)
- Powder:
  - Baroflave®: 100%
  - Baricon®, HD 200 Plus®: 98%
  - Barosperse®, Tonopaque®: 95%
- Suspension:
  - Baro-CAT®, Prepcat®: 1.5%
  - Enecat®, Tomocat®: 5%
  - Entrobar®: 50%
  - Liquid Barasperse®: 60%
  - HD 85®: 85%
  - Barobag®: 97%
  - Flo-Coat®, Liquipake®: 100%
  - Epi-C®: 150%
- Tablet (Bar-Test®): 650 mg

Parenteral agents: Injection:
- **Diatrizoate meglumine**:
  - Hypaque® Meglumine
  - Reno-M-DIP®
  - Urovist® Meglumine
  - Angiovist® 282
  - Hypaque® Meglumine
  - Reno-M-60®
- **Diatrizoate sodium**:
  - Hypaque® Sodium
  - Urovist® Sodium 300
- **Gadopentetate dimeglumine**: Magnevist®
- **Iodamide meglumine**:
  - Renovue®-DIP
  - Renovue®-65
- **Iodipamide meglumine**: Cholografin® meglumine

Iothalamate meglumine:
Conray® 30
Conray® 43
Conray®

Iothalamate sodium:
Angio Conray®
Conray® 325
Conray® 400

Diatrizoate meglumine and diatrizoate sodium:
Angiovist® 292
Angiovist® 370
Hypaque-76®
Hypaque-M®, 75%
Hypaque-M®, 90%
MD-60®
MD-76®
Renografin-60®
Renografin-76®
Renovist® II
Renovist®

Iothalamate meglumine and iothalamate sodium:
Vascoray®
Hexabrix™

Miscellaneous agents (**NOT** for intravascular use, for instillation into various cavities):

Diatrizoate meglumine: Urogenital solution, sterile:
Crystografin®
Crystografin® Dilute
Hypaque-Cysto®
Reno-M-30®
Urovist Cysto®

Diatrizoate meglumine and diatrizoate sodium: Solution, oral or rectal:
Gastrografin®
MD-Gastroview®

Diatrizoate sodium:
Solution, oral or rectal (Hypaque® sodium oral)
Solution, urogenital (Hypaque® sodium 20%)

Iothalamate meglumine: Solution, urogenital:
Cysto-Conray®
Cysto-Conray® II

Diatrizoate meglumine and iodipamide meglumine:
Injection, urogenital for intrauterine instillation (Sinografin®)
Ethiodized oil: Injection (Ethiodol®)
Propyliodone: Suspension (Dionosil Oily®)
Isosulfan blue: Injection (Lymphazurin® 1%)
Potassium perchlorate: Capsule (Perchloracap®): 200 mg

radiological/contrast media (nonionic)

(ray deo LOG ik al/KON trast MEE dia non eye ON ik)

Sound-Alike/Look-Alike Issues
Optiray® may be confused with Optivar™

Synonyms gadoteridol; iohexol; iopamidol; ioversol; metrizamide

U.S./Canadian Brand Names Isovue® [US]; Omnipaque® [US]; Optiray® [US]; ProHance® [US]

Therapeutic Category Radiopaque Agents

Use Enhance visualization of structures during radiologic procedures

(Continued)

radiological/contrast media (nonionic) *(Continued)*

Dosage Forms [DSC] = Discontinued product

Injection, solution:

Gadoteridol (ProHance®): 279.3 mg/mL (15 mL, 30 mL, 50 mL) [single use vial]; 279.3 mg/mL (20 mL) [prefilled syringe]

Iohexol (Omnipaque®): 140 mg/mL, 180 mg/mL, 210 mg/mL, 240 mg/mL, 300 mg/mL, 350 mg/mL

Iopamidol:

Isovue-128®

Isovue-200®

Isovue-300®

Isovue-370®

Isovue-M 200®

Isovue-M 300®

Ioversol:

Optiray® 160

Optiray® 240

Optiray® 320

Metrizamide: Amipaque® [DSC]

rAHF *see* antihemophilic factor (recombinant) *on page 63*

R-albuterol *see* levalbuterol *on page 510*

raloxifene (ral OX i feen)

Sound-Alike/Look-Alike Issues

Evista® may be confused with Avinza™

Synonyms keoxifene hydrochloride; raloxifene hydrochloride

U.S./Canadian Brand Names Evista® [US/Can]

Therapeutic Category Selective Estrogen Receptor Modulator (SERM)

Use Prevention and treatment of osteoporosis in postmenopausal women

Usual Dosage Adults: Female: Oral: 60 mg/day which may be administered any time of the day without regard to meals

Dosage Forms Tablet, as hydrochloride: 60 mg

raloxifene hydrochloride *see* raloxifene *on this page*

raltitrexed *(Canada only)* (ral ti TREX ed)

Synonyms ICI-D1694; NSC-639186; raltitrexed disodium; ZD1694

U.S./Canadian Brand Names Tomudex® [Can]

Therapeutic Category Antineoplastic Agent

Use Treatment of advanced colorectal neoplasms

Usual Dosage Refer to individual protocols.

I.V.: 3 mg/m^2 every 3 weeks

Dosage Forms Injection, powder for reconstitution, as disodium: 2 mg

raltitrexed disodium *see* raltitrexed *(Canada only)* *on this page*

ramipril (ra MI pril)

Sound-Alike/Look-Alike Issues

ramipril may be confused with enalapril, Monopril®

Altace® may be confused with alteplase, Amaryl®, Amerge®, Artane®

U.S./Canadian Brand Names Altace® [US/Can]

Therapeutic Category Angiotensin-Converting Enzyme (ACE) Inhibitor

Use Treatment of hypertension, alone or in combination with thiazide diuretics; treatment of congestive heart failure; treatment of left ventricular dysfunction after myocardial infarction; to reduce risk of heart attack, stroke, and death in patients at increased risk for these problems

Usual Dosage Adults: Oral:

Hypertension: 2.5-5 mg once daily, maximum: 20 mg/day

Reduction in risk of MI, stroke, and death from cardiovascular causes: Initial: 2.5 mg once daily for 1 week, then 5 mg once daily for the next 3 weeks, then increase as tolerated to 10 mg once daily (may be given as divided dose)

Heart failure postmyocardial infarction: Initial: 2.5 mg twice daily titrated upward, if possible, to 5 mg twice daily.

Note: The dose of any concomitant diuretic should be reduced. If the diuretic cannot be discontinued, initiate therapy with 1.25 mg. After the initial dose, the patient should be monitored carefully until blood pressure has stabilized.

Dosage Forms Capsule: 1.25 mg, 2.5 mg, 5 mg, 10 mg

Raniclor™ [US] *see* cefaclor *on page 165*

ranitidine hydrochloride (ra NI ti deen hye droe KLOR ide)

Sound-Alike/Look-Alike Issues

ranitidine may be confused with amantadine, rimantadine

Zantac® may be confused with Xanax®, Zarontin®, Zofran®, Zyrtec®

U.S./Canadian Brand Names Alti-Ranitidine [Can]; Apo-Ranitidine® [Can]; Gen-Ranitidine [Can]; Novo-Ranidine [Can]; Nu-Ranit [Can]; PMS-Ranitidine [Can]; Rhoxal-ranitidine [Can]; Zantac® [US/Can]; Zantac® 75 [US-OTC/Can]

Therapeutic Category Histamine H_2 Antagonist

Use

Zantac®: Short-term and maintenance therapy of duodenal ulcer, gastric ulcer, gastroesophageal reflux, active benign ulcer, erosive esophagitis, and pathological hypersecretory conditions; as part of a multidrug regimen for *H. pylori* eradication to reduce the risk of duodenal ulcer recurrence

Zantac® 75 [OTC]: Relief of heartburn, acid indigestion, and sour stomach

Usual Dosage

Children 1 month to 16 years:

Duodenal and gastric ulcer:

Oral: Treatment: 2-4 mg/kg/day divided twice daily; maximum treatment dose: 300 mg/day Maintenance: 2-4 mg/kg once daily; maximum maintenance dose: 150 mg/day

I.V.: 2-4 mg/kg/day divided every 6-8 hours; maximum: 150 mg/day

GERD and erosive esophagitis:

Oral: 5-10 mg/kg/day divided twice daily; maximum: GERD: 300 mg/day, erosive esophagitis: 600 mg/day

I.V.: 2-4 mg/kg/day divided every 6-8 hours; maximum: 150 mg/day **or as an alternative** Continuous infusion: Initial: 1 mg/kg/dose for one dose followed by infusion of 0.08-0.17 mg/kg/hour or 2-4 mg/kg/day

Children ≥12 years: Prevention of heartburn: Oral: Zantac® 75 [OTC]: 75 mg 30-60 minutes before eating food or drinking beverages which cause heartburn; maximum: 150 mg/24 hours; do not use for more than 14 days

Adults:

Duodenal ulcer: Oral: Treatment: 150 mg twice daily, or 300 mg once daily after the evening meal or at bedtime; maintenance: 150 mg once daily at bedtime

Helicobacter pylori eradication: 150 mg twice daily; requires combination therapy

Pathological hypersecretory conditions:

Oral: 150 mg twice daily; adjust dose or frequency as clinically indicated; doses of up to 6 g/day have been used

I.V.: Continuous infusion for Zollinger-Ellison: 1 mg/kg/hour; measure gastric acid output at 4 hours, if >10 mEq or if patient is symptomatic, increase dose in increments of 0.5 mg/kg/hour; doses of up to 2.5 mg/kg/hour have been used

Gastric ulcer, benign: Oral: 150 mg twice daily; maintenance: 150 mg once daily at bedtime

Erosive esophagitis: Oral: Treatment: 150 mg 4 times/day; maintenance: 150 mg twice daily

(Continued)

ranitidine hydrochloride *(Continued)*

Prevention of heartburn: Oral: Zantac® 75 [OTC]: 75 mg 30-60 minutes before eating food or drinking beverages which cause heartburn; maximum: 150 mg in 24 hours; do not use for more than 14 days

Patients not able to take oral medication:

I.M.: 50 mg every 6-8 hours

I.V.: Intermittent bolus or infusion: 50 mg every 6-8 hours

Continuous I.V. infusion: 6.25 mg/hour

Dosage Forms [DSC] = Discontinued product

Capsule, as hydrochloride: 150 mg, 300 mg

Granules, effervescent, as hydrochloride (Zantac® EFFERdose®): 150 mg (60s) [contains sodium 7.55 mEq/packet, phenylalanine 16.84 mg/packet, and sodium benzoate] [DSC]

Infusion, as hydrochloride [premixed in NaCl 0.45%; preservative free] (Zantac®): 50 mg (50 mL)

Injection, solution, as hydrochloride (Zantac®): 25 mg/mL (2 mL, 6 mL, 40 mL) [contains phenol 0.5% as preservative]

Syrup, as hydrochloride: 15 mg/mL (10 mL) [contains alcohol 7.5%; peppermint flavor]

Zantac®: 15 mg/mL (473 mL) [contains alcohol 7.5%; peppermint flavor]

Tablet, as hydrochloride: 75 mg [OTC], 150 mg, 300 mg

Zantac®: 150 mg, 300 mg

Zantac® 75: 75 mg

Tablet, effervescent, as hydrochloride (Zantac® EFFERdose®): 25 mg [contains sodium 1.33 mEq/tablet, phenylalanine 2.81 mg/tablet, and sodium benzoate]; 150 mg [contains sodium 7.96 mEq/tablet, phenylalanine 16.84 mg/tablet, and sodium benzoate]

Rapamune® [US/Can] *see* sirolimus *on page 807*

Raplon® *(Discontinued)* *see page 1042*

Raptiva™ [US] *see* efalizumab *on page 304*

rasburicase (ras BYOOR i kayse)

U.S./Canadian Brand Names Elitek™ [US]

Therapeutic Category Enzyme

Use Initial management of uric acid levels in pediatric patients with leukemia, lymphoma, and solid tumor malignancies receiving anticancer therapy expected to result in tumor lysis and elevation of plasma uric acid

Usual Dosage I.V.:

Children: Management of uric acid levels: 0.15 mg/kg or 0.2 mg/kg once daily for 5 days (manufacturer-recommended duration); begin chemotherapy 4-24 hours after the first dose

Limited data suggest that a single prechemotherapy dose (versus multiple-day administration) may be sufficiently efficacious. Monitoring electrolytes, hydration status, and uric acid concentrations are necessary to identify the need for additional doses. Other clinical manifestations of tumor lysis syndrome (eg, hyperphosphatemia, hypocalcemia, and hyperkalemia) may occur.

Adults and Elderly: Refer to pediatric dosing; insufficient data collected in adult/geriatric patients to determine response to treatment

Dosage Forms Injection, powder for reconstitution: 1.5 mg [packaged with three 1 mL ampules of diluent]

ratio-Acyclovir [Can] *see* acyclovir *on page 19*

ratio-AmoxiClav *see* amoxicillin and clavulanate potassium *on page 52*

ratio-Benzydamine [Can] *see* benzydamine *(Canada only) on page 112*

ratio-Brimonidine [Can] *see* brimonidine *on page 127*

ratio-Cefuroxime [Can] *see* cefuroxime *on page 173*

recombinant human platelet-derived growth factor B *see* becaplermin *on page 102*

recombinant interleukin-11 *see* oprelvekin *on page 647*

recombinant plasminogen activator *see* reteplase *on page 770*

Recombinate™ [US/Can] *see* antihemophilic factor (recombinant) *on page 63*

Recombivax HB® [US/Can] *see* hepatitis B vaccine *on page 433*

Rectacort® Suppository *(Discontinued)* *see page 1042*

Redisol® *(Discontinued)* *see page 1042*

Redutemp® [US-OTC] *see* acetaminophen *on page 5*

Redux® *(Discontinued)* *see page 1042*

Reese's® Pinworm Medicine [US-OTC] *see* pyrantel pamoate *on page 750*

ReFacto® [US/Can] *see* antihemophilic factor (recombinant) *on page 63*

Refenesen Plus [US-OTC] *see* guaifenesin and pseudoephedrine *on page 419*

Refludan® [US/Can] *see* lepirudin *on page 508*

Refresh® Liquigel [US-OTC] *see* carboxymethylcellulose *on page 161*

Refresh® Plus [US-OTC/Can] *see* carboxymethylcellulose *on page 161*

Refresh® Tears [US-OTC] *see* artificial tears *on page 78*

Refresh® [US-OTC] *see* artificial tears *on page 78*

Regitine® *(Discontinued)* *see page 1042*

Regitine® [Can] *see* phentolamine *on page 688*

Reglan® [US] *see* metoclopramide *on page 574*

Reglan® Syrup *(Discontinued)* *see page 1042*

Regonol® *(Discontinued)* *see page 1042*

Regranex® [US/Can] *see* becaplermin *on page 102*

Regulace® *(Discontinued)* *see page 1042*

Regular Iletin® II [US] *see* insulin preparations *on page 474*

Regular Iletin® I Insulin *(Discontinued)* *see page 1042*

regular, insulin *see* insulin preparations *on page 474*

Regulax SS® *(Discontinued)* *see page 1042*

Regulex® [Can] *see* docusate *on page 285*

Reguloid® [US-OTC] *see* psyllium *on page 749*

Regutol® *(Discontinued)* *see page 1042*

Rejuva-A® [Can] *see* tretinoin (topical) *on page 879*

Relacon-DM [US] *see* guaifenesin, pseudoephedrine, and dextromethorphan *on page 422*

Relafen® [US/Can] *see* nabumetone *on page 598*

Relefact® TRH *(Discontinued)* *see page 1042*

Relefact® TRH [Can] *see* protirelin *on page 744*

Relenza® [US/Can] *see* zanamivir *on page 937*

Relief® Ophthalmic Solution *(Discontinued)* *see page 1042*

Relief® [US-OTC] *see* phenylephrine *on page 689*

Relpax® [US] *see* eletriptan *on page 305*

Remeron® [US/Can] *see* mirtazapine *on page 584*

Remeron® SolTab® [US] *see* mirtazapine *on page 584*

Reme-T™ [US-OTC] *see* coal tar *on page 219*

Remicade® [US/Can] *see* infliximab *on page 472*

remifentanil (rem i FEN ta nil)

Sound-Alike/Look-Alike Issues
remifentanil may be confused with alfentanil

Synonyms GI87084B

U.S./Canadian Brand Names Ultiva™ [US/Can]

Therapeutic Category Analgesic, Narcotic

Use Analgesic for use during the induction and maintenance of general anesthesia; for continued analgesia into the immediate postoperative period; analgesic component of monitored anesthesia

Usual Dosage I.V. continuous infusion: Dose should be based on ideal body weight (IBW) in obese patients (>30% over IBW).

Children birth to 2 months: Maintenance of anesthesia with nitrous oxide (70%): 0.4 mcg/kg/minute (range: 0.4-1 mcg/kg/minute); supplemental bolus dose of 1 mcg/kg may be administered, smaller bolus dose may be required with potent inhalation agents, potent neuraxial anesthesia, significant comorbidities, significant fluid shifts, or without atropine pretreatment. Clearance in neonates is highly variable; dose should be carefully titrated.

Children 1-12 years: Maintenance of anesthesia with halothane, sevoflurane or isoflurane: 0.25 mcg/kg/minute (range 0.05-1.3 mcg/kg/minute); supplemental bolus dose of 1 mcg/kg may be administered every 2-5 minutes. Consider increasing concomitant anesthetics with infusion rate >1 mcg/kg/minute. Infusion rate can be titrated upward in increments up to 50% or titrated downward in decrements of 25% to 50%. May titrate every 2-5 minutes.

Adults:

Induction of anesthesia: 0.5-1 mcg/kg/minute; if endotracheal intubation is to occur in <8 minutes, an initial dose of 1 mcg/kg may be given over 30-60 seconds

Coronary bypass surgery: 1 mcg/kg/minute

Maintenance of anesthesia: **Note:** Supplemental bolus dose of 1 mcg/kg may be administered every 2-5 minutes. Consider increasing concomitant anesthetics with infusion rate >1 mcg/kg/minute. Infusion rate can be titrated upward in increments of 25% to 100% or downward in decrements of 25% to 50%. May titrate every 2-5 minutes.

With nitrous oxide (66%): 0.4 mcg/kg/minute (range: 0.1-2 mcg/kg/minute)

With isoflurane: 0.25 mcg/kg/minute (range: 0.05-2 mcg/kg/minute)

With propofol: 0.25 mcg/kg/minute (range: 0.05-2 mcg/kg/minute)

Coronary bypass surgery: 1 mcg/kg/minute (range: 0.125-4 mcg/kg/minute); supplemental dose: 0.5-1 mcg/kg

Continuation as an analgesic in immediate postoperative period: 0.1 mcg/kg/minute (range: 0.025-0.2 mcg/kg/minute). Infusion rate may be adjusted every 5 minutes in increments of 0.025 mcg/kg/minute. Bolus doses are not recommended. Infusion rates >0.2 mcg/kg/minute are associated with respiratory depression.

Coronary bypass surgery, continuation as an analgesic into the ICU: 1 mcg/kg/minute (range: 0.05-1 mcg/kg/minute)

Analgesic component of monitored anesthesia care: **Note:** Supplemental oxygen is recommended:

Single I.V. dose given 90 seconds prior to local anesthetic: Remifentanil alone: 1 mcg/kg over 30-60 seconds With midazolam: 0.5 mcg/kg over 30-60 seconds

Continuous infusion beginning 5 minutes prior to local anesthetic: Remifentanil alone: 0.1 mcg/kg minute With midazolam: 0.05 mcg/kg/minute

Continuous infusion given after local anesthetic: Remifentanil alone: 0.05 mcg/kg/minute (range: 0.025-0.2 mcg/kg/minute) With midazolam: 0.025 mcg/kg/minute (range: 0.025-0.2 mcg/kg/minute)

Note: Following local or anesthetic block, infusion rate should be decreased to 0.05 mcg/kg/minute; rate adjustments of 0.025 mcg/kg/minute may be done at 5-minute intervals

(Continued)

remifentanil *(Continued)*

Dosage Forms Injection, powder for reconstitution: 1 mg, 2 mg, 5 mg [contains glycine 15 mg]

Reminyl® [US/Can] *see* galantamine *on page 395*

Remodulin™ [US] *see* treprostinil *on page 878*

Renacidin® [US] *see* citric acid, magnesium carbonate, and glucono-delta-lactone *on page 206*

Renagel® [US/Can] *see* sevelamer *on page 802*

Renedil® [Can] *see* felodipine *on page 359*

Renese® [US] *see* polythiazide *on page 709*

Renografin-60® ***(Discontinued)*** *see page 1042*

Renografin-76® ***(Discontinued)*** *see page 1042*

Reno-M-30® [US] *see* radiological/contrast media (ionic) *on page 759*

Reno-M-60® [US] *see* radiological/contrast media (ionic) *on page 759*

Reno-M-DIP® [US] *see* radiological/contrast media (ionic) *on page 759*

Renoquid® ***(Discontinued)*** *see page 1042*

Renormax® ***(Discontinued)*** *see page 1042*

Renova® [US] *see* tretinoin (topical) *on page 879*

Renovist® ***(Discontinued)*** *see page 1042*

Renovist® II ***(Discontinued)*** *see page 1042*

Renovue®-65 [US] *see* radiological/contrast media (ionic) *on page 759*

Renovue®-DIP [US] *see* radiological/contrast media (ionic) *on page 759*

ReoPro® [US/Can] *see* abciximab *on page 3*

repaglinide (re PAG li nide)

Sound-Alike/Look-Alike Issues

Prandin® may be confused with Avandia®

U.S./Canadian Brand Names GlucoNorm® [Can]; Prandin® [US/Can]

Therapeutic Category Hypoglycemic Agent, Oral

Use Management of type 2 diabetes mellitus (noninsulin dependent, NIDDM); may be used in combination with metformin or thiazolidinediones

Usual Dosage Adults: Oral: Should be taken within 15 minutes of the meal, but time may vary from immediately preceding the meal to as long as 30 minutes before the meal

Initial: For patients not previously treated or whose Hb A_{1c} is <8%, the starting dose is 0.5 mg. For patients previously treated with blood glucose-lowering agents whose Hb A_{1c} is ≥8%, the initial dose is 1 or 2 mg before each meal.

Dose adjustment: Determine dosing adjustments by blood glucose response, usually fasting blood glucose. Double the preprandial dose up to 4 mg until satisfactory blood glucose response is achieved. At least 1 week should elapse to assess response after each dose adjustment.

Dose range: 0.5-4 mg taken with meals. Repaglinide may be dosed preprandial 2, 3 or 4 times/day in response to changes in the patient's meal pattern. Maximum recommended daily dose: 16 mg.

Patients receiving other oral hypoglycemic agents: When repaglinide is used to replace therapy with other oral hypoglycemic agents, it may be started the day after the final dose is given. Observe patients carefully for hypoglycemia because of potential overlapping of drug effects. When transferred from longer half-life sulfonylureas (eg, chlorpropamide), close monitoring may be indicated for up to ≥1 week.

Combination therapy: If repaglinide monotherapy does not result in adequate glycemic control, metformin or a thiazolidinedione may be added. Or, if metformin or thiazolidinedione therapy does not provide adequate control, repaglinide may be added. The starting dose and dose adjustments for combination therapy are the same as repaglinide monotherapy. Carefully adjust the dose of each drug to determine the minimal dose required to achieve the desired pharmacologic effect. Failure to do so could result in an increase in the incidence of hypoglycemic episodes. Use appropriate monitoring of FPG and Hb A_{1c} measurements to ensure that the patient is not subjected to excessive drug exposure or increased probability of secondary drug failure. If glucose is not achieved after a suitable trial of combination therapy, consider discontinuing these drugs and using insulin.

Dosage Forms Tablet: 0.5 mg, 1 mg, 2 mg

Repan® [US] *see* butalbital, acetaminophen, and caffeine *on page 138*

Reposans-10® Oral *(Discontinued)* *see page 1042*

Rep-Pred® *(Discontinued)* *see page 1042*

Repronex® [US/Can] *see* menotropins *on page 551*

ReQuip® [US/Can] *see* ropinirole *on page 784*

Resa® *(Discontinued)* *see page 1042*

Resaid® *(Discontinued)* *see page 1042*

Rescaps-D® S.R. Capsule *(Discontinued)* *see page 1042*

Rescon GG [US] *see* guaifenesin and phenylephrine *on page 418*

Rescon® Liquid *(Discontinued)* *see page 1042*

Rescriptor® [US/Can] *see* delavirdine *on page 248*

Rescula® [US] *see* unoprostone *on page 897*

Resectisol® [US] *see* mannitol *on page 542*

reserpine (re SER peen)

Sound-Alike/Look-Alike Issues

reserpine may be confused with Risperdal®, risperidone

Therapeutic Category Rauwolfia Alkaloid

Use Management of mild to moderate hypertension

Usual Dosage Note: When used for management of hypertension, full antihypertensive effects may take as long as 3 weeks.

Oral:

Children: Hypertension: 0.01-0.02 mg/kg/24 hours divided every 12 hours; maximum dose: 0.25 mg/day (not recommended in children)

Adults:

Hypertension: Initial: 0.5 mg/day for 1-2 weeks; usual dose range (JNC 7): 0.05-0.25 mg once daily; 0.1 mg every other day may be given to achieve 0.05 mg once daily

Dosage Forms Tablet: 0.1 mg, 0.25 mg

reserpine, hydralazine, and hydrochlorothiazide *see* hydralazine, hydrochlorothiazide, and reserpine *on page 441*

Respa-DM® [US] *see* guaifenesin and dextromethorphan *on page 416*

Respa-GF® *(Discontinued)* *see page 1042*

Respaire®-60 SR [US] *see* guaifenesin and pseudoephedrine *on page 419*

Respaire®-120 SR [US] *see* guaifenesin and pseudoephedrine *on page 419*

Respbid® *(Discontinued)* *see page 1042*

RespiGam® *(Discontinued)* *see page 1042*

respiratory syncytial virus immune globulin (intravenous)

(RES peer rah tor ee sin SISH al VYE rus i MYUN GLOB yoo lin in tra VEE nus)

Synonyms RSV-IGIV

Therapeutic Category Immune Globulin

(Continued)

respiratory syncytial virus immune globulin (intravenous) *(Continued)*

Use Orphan drug: Prevention of serious lower respiratory infection caused by respiratory syncytial virus (RSV) in children <24 months of age with bronchopulmonary dysplasia (BPD) or a history of premature birth (≤35 weeks gestation)

Usual Dosage I.V.: Children <24 months of age: Prevention of respiratory syncytial virus (RSV) infection: 750 mg/kg/month according to the following infusion schedule:

Initial infusion rate for the first 15 minutes: 1.5 mL/kg/hour; after 15 minutes increase to 3.6 mL/kg/hour (maximum infusion rate: 3.6 mL/kg/hour); rate should be decreased in patients at risk of renal dysfunction

Dosage Forms [DSC] = Discontinued product

Injection, solution [preservative free]: 50 mg/mL (50 mL) [contains sodium 1-1.5 mEq per 50 mL, sucrose 50 mg, human albumin 10 mg] [DSC]

Resporal® *(Discontinued)* *see page 1042*

Restall® *(Discontinued)* *see page 1042*

Restasis™ [US] *see* cyclosporine *on page 235*

Restoril® [US/Can] *see* temazepam *on page 843*

Retavase® [US/Can] *see* reteplase *on this page*

reteplase (RE ta plase)

Synonyms recombinant plasminogen activator; r-PA

U.S./Canadian Brand Names Retavase® [US/Can]

Therapeutic Category Fibrinolytic Agent

Use Management of acute myocardial infarction (AMI); improvement of ventricular function; reduction of the incidence of CHF and the reduction of mortality following AMI

Usual Dosage

Children: Not recommended

Adults: 10 units I.V. over 2 minutes, followed by a second dose 30 minutes later of 10 units I.V. over 2 minutes

Withhold second dose if serious bleeding or anaphylaxis occurs

Dosage Forms Injection, powder for reconstitution [preservative free]: 10.4 units [equivalent to reteplase 18.1 mg; packaged with sterile water for injection]

Retin-A® [US/Can] *see* tretinoin (topical) *on page 879*

Retin-A® Micro [US/Can] *see* tretinoin (topical) *on page 879*

retinoic acid *see* tretinoin (topical) *on page 879*

Retinova® [Can] *see* tretinoin (topical) *on page 879*

Retrovir® [US/Can] *see* zidovudine *on page 939*

Reversol® [US] *see* edrophonium *on page 303*

Revex® [US] *see* nalmefene *on page 601*

Rēv-Eyes™ [US] *see* dapiprazole *on page 244*

ReVia® [US/Can] *see* naltrexone *on page 603*

Revitalose C-1000® [Can] *see* ascorbic acid *on page 79*

Rexigen Forte® *(Discontinued)* *see page 1042*

Reyataz® [US] *see* atazanavir *on page 84*

Rezulin® *(Discontinued)* *see page 1042*

rFVIIa *see* factor VIIa (recombinant) *on page 354*

R-Gel® *(Discontinued)* *see page 1042*

R-Gen® *(Discontinued)* *see page 1042*

R-Gene® [US] *see* arginine *on page 76*

Rh_o(D) immune globulin (ar aych oh (dee) i MYUN GLOB yoo lin)

Synonyms RhIG; Rho(D) immune globulin (human); RhoIGIV; RhoIVIM

U.S./Canadian Brand Names BayRho-D® Full-Dose [US/Can]; BayRho-D® Mini-Dose [US]; MICRhoGAM® [US]; RhoGAM® [US]; Rhophylac® [US]; WinRho SDF® [US]

Therapeutic Category Immune Globulin

Use

Suppression of Rh isoimmunization: Use in the following situations when an Rh_o(D)-negative individual is exposed to Rh_o(D)-positive blood: During delivery of an Rh_o(D)-positive infant; abortion; amniocentesis; chorionic villus sampling; ruptured tubal pregnancy; abdominal trauma; transplacental hemorrhage. Used when the mother is Rh_o(D) negative, the father of the child is either Rh_o(D) positive or Rh_o(D) unknown, the baby is either either Rh_o(D) positive or Rh_o(D) unknown.

Transfusion: Suppression of Rh isoimmunization in Rh_o(D)-negative female children and female adults in their childbearing years transfused with Rh_o(D) antigen-positive RBCs or blood components containing Rh_o(D) antigen-positive RBCs

Treatment of idiopathic thrombocytopenic purpura (ITP): Used in the following nonsplenectomized Rh_o(D) positive individuals: Children with acute or chronic ITP, adults with chronic ITP, children and adults with ITP secondary to HIV infection

Usual Dosage

ITP: Children and Adults: WinRho SDF®: I.V.:

Initial: 50 mcg/kg as a single injection, or can be given as a divided dose on separate days. If hemoglobin is <10 g/dL: Dose should be reduced to 25-40 mcg/kg.

Subsequent dosing: 25-60 mcg/kg can be used if required to elevate platelet count

Maintenance dosing if patient **did respond** to initial dosing: 25-60 mcg/kg based on platelet and hemoglobin levels:

Maintenance dosing if patient **did not respond** to initial dosing:

- Hemoglobin 8-10 g/dL: Redose between 25-40 mcg/kg
- Hemoglobin >10 g/dL: Redose between 50-60 mcg/kg
- Hemoglobin <8 g/dL: Use with caution

(Continued)

Rh_0(D) immune globulin *(Continued)*

Rh_0(D) suppression: Adults: **Note:** One "full dose" (300 mcg) provides enough antibody to prevent Rh sensitization if the volume of RBC entering the circulation is ≤15 mL. When >15 mL is suspected, a fetal red cell count should be performed to determine the appropriate dose.

Pregnancy:

Antepartum prophylaxis: In general, dose is given at 28 weeks. If given early in pregnancy, administer every 12 weeks to ensure adequate levels of passively acquired anti-Rh BayRho-D® Full Dose, RhoGAM®: I.M.: 300 mcg Rhophylac®, WinRho SDF®: I.M., I.V.: 300 mcg

Postpartum prophylaxis: In general, dose is administered as soon as possible after delivery, preferably within 72 hours. Can be given up to 28 days following delivery BayRho-D® Full Dose, RhoGAM®: I.M.: 300 mcg Rhophylac®: I.M., I.V.: 300 mcg WinRho SDF®: I.M., I.V.: 120 mcg

Threatened abortion, any time during pregnancy (with continuation of pregnancy):

BayRho-D® Full Dose, RhoGAM®: I.M.: 300 mcg; administer as soon as possible

Rhophylac®, WinRho SDF®: I.M., I.V.: 300 mcg; administer as soon as possible

Abortion, miscarriage, termination of ectopic pregnancy:

BayRho-D®, RhoGAM®: I.M.: ≥13 weeks gestation: 300 mcg.

BayRho-D Mini Dose®, MICRhoGAM®: <13 weeks gestation: I.M.: 50 mcg

Rhophylac®: I.M., I.V.: 300 mcg

WinRho SDF®: I.M., I.V.: After 34 weeks gestation: 120 mcg; administer immediately or within 72 hours

Amniocentesis, chorionic villus sampling:

BayRho-D®, RhoGAM®: I.M.: At 15-18 weeks gestation or during the 3rd trimester: 300 mcg. If dose is given between 13-18 weeks, repeat at 26-28 weeks and within 72 hours of delivery.

Rhophylac®: I.M., I.V.: 300 mcg

WinRho SDF®: I.M., I.V.: Before 34 weeks gestation: 300 mcg; administer immediately, repeat dose every 12 weeks during pregnancy; After 34 weeks gestation: 120 mcg, administered immediately or within 72 hours

Abdominal trauma, manipulation:

BayRho-D®, RhoGAM®: I.M.: 2nd or 3rd trimester: 300 mcg. If dose is given between 13-18 weeks, repeat at 26-28 weeks and within 72 hours of delivery

WinRho SDF®: I.M./I.V.: After 34 weeks gestation: 120 mcg; administer immediately or within 72 hours

Transfusion:

Children and Adults: WinRho SDF®: Administer within 72 hours after exposure of incompatible blood transfusions or massive fetal hemorrhage.

I.V.: Calculate dose as follows; administer 600 mcg every 8 hours until the total dose is administered: Exposure to Rh_0(D) positive whole blood: 9 mcg/mL blood Exposure to Rh_0(D) positive red blood cells: 18 mcg/mL cells

I.M.: Calculate dose as follows; administer 1200 mcg every 12 hours until the total dose is administered: Exposure to Rh_0(D) positive whole blood: 12 mcg/mL blood Exposure to Rh_0(D) positive red blood cells: 24 mcg/mL cells

Adults:

BayRho-D®, RhoGAM®: I.M.: Multiply the volume of Rh positive whole blood administered by the hematocrit of the donor unit to equal the volume of RBCs transfused. The volume of RBCs is then divided by 15 mL, providing the number of 300 mcg doses (vials/syringes) to administer. If the dose calculated results in a fraction, round up to the next higher whole 300 mcg dose (vial/syringe).

Rhophylac®: I.M., I.V.: 20 mcg/2 mL transfused blood or 20 mcg/mL erythrocyte concentrate

Dosage Forms

Injection, solution [preservative free]:

BayRho-D® Full-Dose, RhoGAM®: 300 mcg [for I.M. use only]

BayRho-D® Mini-Dose, MICRhoGAM®: 50 mcg [for I.M. use only]

Rhophylac®: 300 mcg/2 mL (2 mL) [1500 int. units; for I.M. or I.V. use]

Injection, powder for reconstitution [preservative free] (WinRho SDF®): 120 mcg [600 int. units], 300 mcg [1500 int. units], 1000 mcg [5000 int. units] [for I.M. or I.V. use]

Rho(D) immune globulin (human) *see* Rh$_o$(D) immune globulin *on page 771*

Rhodis™ [Can] *see* ketoprofen *on page 495*

Rhodis-EC™ [Can] *see* ketoprofen *on page 495*

Rhodis SR™ [Can] *see* ketoprofen *on page 495*

RhoGAM® [US] *see* Rh$_o$(D) immune globulin *on page 771*

RhoIGIV *see* Rh$_o$(D) immune globulin *on page 771*

RhoIVIM *see* Rh$_o$(D) immune globulin *on page 771*

Rho®-Loperamine [Can] *see* loperamide *on page 528*

Rho®-Metformin [Can] *see* metformin *on page 560*

Rho®-Nitro [Can] *see* nitroglycerin *on page 623*

Rhophylac® [US] *see* Rh$_o$(D) immune globulin *on page 771*

Rho®-Sotalol [Can] *see* sotalol *on page 819*

Rhotral [Can] *see* acebutolol *on page 4*

Rhotrimine® [Can] *see* trimipramine *on page 888*

Rhovane® [Can] *see* zopiclone *(Canada only)* *on page 944*

Rhoxal-amiodarone [Can] *see* amiodarone *on page 47*

Rhoxal-atenolol [Can] *see* atenolol *on page 85*

Rhoxal-clozapine [Can] *see* clozapine *on page 219*

Rhoxal-cyclosporine [Can] *see* cyclosporine *on page 235*

Rhoxal-diltiazem CD [Can] *see* diltiazem *on page 273*

Rhoxal-diltiazem SR [Can] *see* diltiazem *on page 273*

Rhoxal-famotidine [Can] *see* famotidine *on page 356*

Rhoxal-fluoxetine [Can] *see* fluoxetine *on page 379*

Rhoxal-fluvoxamine [Can] *see* fluvoxamine *on page 385*

Rhoxal-metformin FC [Can] *see* metformin *on page 560*

Rhoxal-minocycline [Can] *see* minocycline *on page 583*

Rhoxal-nabumetone [Can] *see* nabumetone *on page 598*

Rhoxal-orphendrine [Can] *see* orphenadrine *on page 649*

Rhoxal-oxaprozin [Can] *see* oxaprozin *on page 652*

Rhoxal-ranitidine [Can] *see* ranitidine hydrochloride *on page 763*

Rhoxal-salbutamol [Can] *see* albuterol *on page 25*

Rhoxal-sertraline [Can] *see* sertraline *on page 801*

Rhoxal-ticlopidine [Can] *see* ticlopidine *on page 862*

Rhoxal-valproic [Can] *see* valproic acid and derivatives *on page 901*

rhPTH(1-34) *see* teriparatide *on page 847*

***r*HuEPO-α** *see* epoetin alfa *on page 314*

Rhulicaine® ***(Discontinued)*** *see page 1042*

Rhuli® Cream ***(Discontinued)*** *see page 1042*

rhuMAb-E25 *see* omalizumab *on page 643*

rhuMAb-VEGF *see* bevacizumab *on page 117*

Ribasphere™ [US] *see* ribavirin *on next page*

ribavirin (rye ba VYE rin)

Sound-Alike/Look-Alike Issues

ribavirin may be confused with riboflavin

Synonyms RTCA; tribavirin

U.S./Canadian Brand Names Copegus® [US]; Rebetol® [US]; Ribasphere™ [US]; Virazole® [US/Can]

Therapeutic Category Antiviral Agent

Use

Inhalation: Treatment of patients with respiratory syncytial virus (RSV) infections; specially indicated for treatment of severe lower respiratory tract RSV infections in patients with an underlying compromising condition (prematurity, bronchopulmonary dysplasia and other chronic lung conditions, congenital heart disease, immunodeficiency, immunosuppression), and recent transplant recipients

Oral capsule:

In combination with interferon alfa-2b (Intron® A) injection for the treatment of chronic hepatitis C in patients with compensated liver disease who have relapsed after alpha interferon therapy or were previously untreated with alpha interferons

In combination with peginterferon alfa-2b (PEG-Intron®) injection for the treatment of chronic hepatitis C in patients with compensated liver disease who were previously untreated with alpha interferons

Oral solution: In combination with interferon alfa 2b (Intron® A) injection for the treatment of chronic hepatitis C in patients ≥3 years of age with compensated liver disease who were previously untreated with alpha interferons or patients ≥18 years of age who have relapsed after alpha interferon therapy

Oral tablet: In combination with peginterferon alfa-2a (Pegasys®) injection for the treatment of chronic hepatitis C in patients with compensated liver disease who were previously untreated with alpha interferons

Usual Dosage

Aerosol inhalation: Infants and children: Use with Viratek® small particle aerosol generator (SPAG-2) at a concentration of 20 mg/mL (6 g reconstituted with 300 mL of sterile water without preservatives). Continuous aerosol administration: 12-18 hours/day for 3 days, up to 7 days in length

Oral capsule or solution: Children ≥3 years: Chronic hepatitis C (in combination with interferon alfa-2b):

Rebetol®: Oral: **Note:** Oral solution should be used in children 3-5 years of age, children ≤25 kg, or those unable to swallow capsules.

Capsule/solution: 15 mg/kg/day in 2 divided doses (morning and evening)

Capsule dosing recommendations: 25-36 kg: 400 mg/day (200 mg morning and evening). 37-49 kg: 600 mg/day (200 mg in the morning and two 200 mg capsules in the evening). 50-61 kg: 800 mg/day (two 200 mg capsules morning and evening). >61 kg: Refer to Adults dosing.

Note: Duration of therapy is 48 weeks in pediatric patients with genotype 1 and 24 weeks in patients with genotype 2,3. Discontinue treatment in any patient if HCV-RNA is not below the limit of detection of the assay after 24 weeks of therapy.

Note: Also refer to Interferon Alfa-2b/Ribavirin combination pack monograph.

Oral capsule:

Adults:

Chronic hepatitis C (in combination with interferon alfa-2b): ≤75 kg: 400 mg in the morning, then 600 mg in the evening. >75 kg: 600 mg in the morning, then 600 mg in the evening. **Note:** If HCV-RNA is undetectable at 24 weeks, duration of therapy is 48 weeks. In patients who relapse following interferon therapy, duration of dual therapy is 24 weeks. **Note:** Also refer to Interferon Alfa-2b/Ribavirin combination pack monograph.

Chronic hepatitis C (in combination with peginterferon alfa-2b): 400 mg twice daily; duration of therapy is 1 year; after 24 weeks of treatment, if serum HCV-RNA is not below the limit of detection of the assay, consider discontinuation.

Oral tablet: Adults:
Chronic hepatitis C, genotype 1,4 (in combination with peginterferon alfa-2a):
<75kg: 1000 mg/day in 2 divided doses for 48 weeks
≥75kg: 1200 mg/day in 2 divided doses for 48 weeks
Chronic hepatitis C, genotype 2,3 (in combination with peginterferon alfa-2a): 800 mg/day in 2 divided doses for 24 weeks
Note: Also refer to Peginterferon Alfa-2a monograph.

Dosage Forms
Capsule (Rebetol®, Ribasphere™): 200 mg
Powder for aerosol (Virazole®): 6 g
Solution, oral (Rebetol®): 40 mg/mL (100 mL) [contains sodium benzoate; bubblegum flavor]
Tablet (Copegus®): 200 mg

ribavirin and interferon alfa-2b combination pack *see* interferon alfa-2b and ribavirin combination pack *on page 477*

riboflavin (RYE boe flay vin)

Sound-Alike/Look-Alike Issues
riboflavin may be confused with ribavirin
Synonyms lactoflavin; vitamin B_2; vitamin G
Therapeutic Category Vitamin, Water Soluble
Use Prevention of riboflavin deficiency and treatment of ariboflavinosis
Usual Dosage Oral:
Riboflavin deficiency:
Children: 2.5-10 mg/day in divided doses
Adults: 5-30 mg/day in divided doses
Recommended daily allowance:
Children: 0.4-1.8 mg
Adults: 1.2-1.7 mg

Dosage Forms
Capsule: 100 mg
Tablet: 25 mg, 50 mg, 100 mg

RID® *(Discontinued)* *see page 1042*

Ridaura® [US/Can] *see* auranofin *on page 90*

RID® Maximum Strength [US-OTC] *see* pyrethrins and piperonyl butoxide *on page 751*

RID® Mousse [Can] *see* pyrethrins and piperonyl butoxide *on page 751*

Rid® Spray [US-OTC] *see* permethrin *on page 683*

rifabutin (rif a BYOO tin)

Sound-Alike/Look-Alike Issues
rifabutin may be confused with rifampin
Synonyms ansamycin
U.S./Canadian Brand Names Mycobutin® [US/Can]
Therapeutic Category Antibiotic, Miscellaneous
Use Prevention of disseminated *Mycobacterium avium* complex (MAC) in patients with advanced HIV infection
Usual Dosage Oral:
Children >1 year:
Prophylaxis: 5 mg/kg daily; higher dosages have been used in limited trials
Initial phase (2 weeks to 2 months): 10-20 mg/kg daily (maximum: 300 mg).
Second phase: 10-20 mg/kg daily (maximum: 300 mg) or twice weekly
Adults: Prophylaxis: 300 mg once daily (alone or in combination with azithromycin)
Dosage Forms Capsule: 150 mg

Rifadin® [US/Can] *see* rifampin *on this page*

Rifamate® [US/Can] *see* rifampin and isoniazid *on this page*

rifampicin *see* rifampin *on this page*

rifampin (RIF am pin)

Sound-Alike/Look-Alike Issues

rifampin may be confused with rifabutin, Rifamate®, rifapentine
Rifadin® may be confused with Ritalin®
Rimactane® may be confused with rimantadine

Synonyms rifampicin

U.S./Canadian Brand Names Rifadin® [US/Can]; Rimactane® [US]; Rofact™ [Can]

Therapeutic Category Antibiotic, Miscellaneous

Use Management of active tuberculosis in combination with other agents; eliminate meningococci from asymptomatic carriers

Usual Dosage Oral (I.V. infusion dose is the same as for the oral route):

Tuberculosis therapy: Note: A four-drug regimen (isoniazid, rifampin, pyrazinamide, and either streptomycin or ethambutol) is preferred for the initial, empiric treatment of TB. When the drug susceptibility results are available, the regimen should be altered as appropriate.

Infants and Children <12 years:

Daily therapy: 10-20 mg/kg/day usually as a single dose (maximum: 600 mg/day)

Directly observed therapy (DOT): Twice weekly: 10-20 mg/kg (maximum: 600 mg); 3 times/week: 10-20 mg/kg (maximum: 600 mg)

Adults:

Daily therapy: 10 mg/kg/day (maximum: 600 mg/day)

Directly observed therapy (DOT): Twice weekly: 10 mg/kg (maximum: 600 mg); 3 times/week: 10 mg/kg (maximum: 600 mg)

Latent tuberculosis infection (LTBI): As an alternative to isoniazid:

Children: 10-20 mg/kg/day (maximum: 600 mg/day)

Adults: 10 mg/kg/day (maximum: 600 mg/day) for 2 months. **Note:** Combination with pyrazinamide should not generally be offered (*MMWR*, Aug 8, 2003).

Meningococcal meningitis prophylaxis:

Infants <1 month: 10 mg/kg/day in divided doses every 12 hours for 2 days

Infants ≥1 month and Children: 20 mg/kg/day in divided doses every 12 hours for 2 days

Adults: 600 mg every 12 hours for 2 days

Dosage Forms

Capsule: 150 mg, 300 mg
Rifadin®: 150 mg, 300 mg
Rimactane®: 300 mg

Injection, powder for reconstitution (Rifadin®): 600 mg

rifampin and isoniazid (RIF am pin & eye soe NYE a zid)

Sound-Alike/Look-Alike Issues

Rifamate® may be confused with rifampin

Synonyms isoniazid and rifampin

U.S./Canadian Brand Names Rifamate® [US/Can]

Therapeutic Category Antibiotic, Miscellaneous

Use Management of active tuberculosis; see individual agents for additional information

Usual Dosage Oral: 2 capsules/day

Dosage Forms Capsule: Rifampin 300 mg and isoniazid 150 mg

rifampin, isoniazid, and pyrazinamide

(RIF am pin, eye soe NYE a zid, & peer a ZIN a mide)

Synonyms isoniazid, rifampin, and pyrazinamide; pyrazinamide, rifampin, and isoniazid

U.S./Canadian Brand Names Rifater® [US/Can]

Therapeutic Category Antibiotic, Miscellaneous

Use Management of active tuberculosis; see individual agents for additional information

Usual Dosage Adults: Oral: Patients weighing:

≤44 kg: 4 tablets

45-54 kg: 5 tablets

≥55 kg: 6 tablets

Doses should be administered in a single daily dose

Dosage Forms Tablet: Rifampin 120 mg, isoniazid 50 mg, and pyrazinamide 300 mg

rifapentine (RIF a pen teen)

Sound-Alike/Look-Alike Issues

rifapentine may be confused with rifampin

U.S./Canadian Brand Names Priftin® [US/Can]

Therapeutic Category Antitubercular Agent

Use Treatment of pulmonary tuberculosis; rifapentine must always be used in conjunction with at least one other antituberculosis drug to which the isolate is susceptible; it may also be necessary to add a third agent (either streptomycin or ethambutol) until susceptibility is known.

Usual Dosage

Children: No dosing information available

Adults: **Rifapentine should not be used alone**; initial phase should include a 3- to 4-drug regimen

Intensive phase (initial 2 months) of short-term therapy: 600 mg (four 150 mg tablets) given twice weekly (with an interval of not less than 72 hours between doses); following the intensive phase, treatment should continue with rifapentine 600 mg once weekly for 4 months in combination with INH or appropriate agent for susceptible organisms

Dosage Forms Tablet [film coated]: 150 mg

Rifater® [US/Can] *see* rifampin, isoniazid, and pyrazinamide *on previous page*

rifaximin (rif AX i min)

U.S./Canadian Brand Names Xifaxan™ [US]

Therapeutic Category Antibiotic, Miscellaneous

Use Treatment of travelers' diarrhea caused by noninvasive strains of *E. coli*

Usual Dosage Oral: Children ≥12 years and Adults: Travelers' diarrhea: 200 mg 3 times/day for 3 days

Dosage Forms Tablet: 200 mg

rIFN-A *see* interferon alfa-2a *on page 476*

rIFN beta-1a *see* interferon beta-1a *on page 479*

rIFN beta-1b *see* interferon beta-1b *on page 480*

RIG *see* rabies immune globulin (human) *on page 759*

rIL-11 *see* oprelvekin *on page 647*

Rilutek® [US/Can] *see* riluzole *on this page*

riluzole (RIL yoo zole)

Synonyms 2-amino-6-trifluoromethoxy-benzothiazole; RP-54274

U.S./Canadian Brand Names Rilutek® [US/Can]

Therapeutic Category Miscellaneous Product

Use **Orphan drug:** Treatment of amyotrophic lateral sclerosis (ALS); riluzole can extend survival or time to tracheostomy

Usual Dosage Adults: Oral: 50 mg every 12 hours; no increased benefit can be expected from higher daily doses, but adverse events are increased

Dosage adjustment in smoking: Cigarette smoking is known to induce CYP1A2; patients who smoke cigarettes would be expected to eliminate riluzole faster. There is

(Continued)

riluzole *(Continued)*

no information, however, on the effect of, or need for, dosage adjustment in these patients.

Dosage adjustment in special populations: Females and Japanese patients may possess a lower metabolic capacity to eliminate riluzole compared with male and Caucasian subjects, respectively

Dosage Forms Tablet: 50 mg

Rimactane® [US] *see* rifampin *on page 776*

rimantadine (ri MAN ta deen)

Sound-Alike/Look-Alike Issues

rimantadine may be confused with amantadine, ranitidine, Rimactane®

Flumadine® may be confused with fludarabine, flunisolide, flutamide

Synonyms rimantadine hydrochloride

U.S./Canadian Brand Names Flumadine® [US/Can]

Therapeutic Category Antiviral Agent

Use Prophylaxis (adults and children >1 year of age) and treatment (adults) of influenza A viral infection

Usual Dosage Oral:

Prophylaxis:

Children <10 years: 5 mg/kg once daily; maximum: 150 mg

Children >10 years and Adults: 100 mg twice daily; decrease to 100 mg/day in elderly or in patients with severe hepatic or renal impairment (Cl_{cr} ≤10 mL/minute)

Treatment: Adults: 100 mg twice daily; decrease to 100 mg/day in elderly or in patients with severe hepatic or renal impairment (Cl_{cr} ≤10 mL/minute)

Dosage Forms

Syrup, as hydrochloride: 50 mg/5 mL (240 mL) [raspberry flavor]

Tablet, as hydrochloride: 100 mg

rimantadine hydrochloride *see* rimantadine *on this page*

rimexolone (ri MEKS oh lone)

Sound-Alike/Look-Alike Issues

Vexol® may be confused with VoSol®

U.S./Canadian Brand Names Vexol® [US/Can]

Therapeutic Category Adrenal Corticosteroid

Use Treatment of inflammation after ocular surgery and the treatment of anterior uveitis

Usual Dosage Adults: Ophthalmic: Instill 1 drop in conjunctival sac 2-4 times/day up to every 4 hours; may use every 1-2 hours during first 1-2 days

Dosage Forms Suspension, ophthalmic: 1% (5 mL, 10 mL) [contains benzalkonium chloride]

Rimso®-50 [US/Can] *see* dimethyl sulfoxide *on page 275*

Riobin® ***(Discontinued)*** *see page 1042*

Riopan® ***(Discontinued)*** *see page 1042*

Riopan® Plus ***(Discontinued)*** *see page 1042*

Riopan® Plus Double Strength ***(Discontinued)*** *see page 1042*

risedronate (ris ED roe nate)

Synonyms risedronate sodium

U.S./Canadian Brand Names Actonel® [US/Can]

Therapeutic Category Bisphosphonate Derivative

Use Paget disease of the bone; treatment and prevention of glucocorticoid-induced osteoporosis; treatment and prevention of osteoporosis in postmenopausal women

Usual Dosage Risedronate should be taken at least 30 minutes before the first food or drink of the day other than water. Oral:

Adults (patients should receive supplemental calcium and vitamin D if dietary intake is inadequate):

Paget disease of bone: 30 mg once daily for 2 months

Retreatment may be considered (following post-treatment observation of at least 2 months) if relapse occurs, or if treatment fails to normalize serum alkaline phosphatase. For retreatment, the dose and duration of therapy are the same as for initial treatment. No data are available on more than one course of retreatment.

Osteoporosis (postmenopausal) prevention and treatment: 5 mg once daily; efficacy for use longer than 1 year has not been established; **alternatively,** a dose of 35 mg once weekly has been demonstrated to be effective

Osteoporosis (glucocorticoid-induced) prevention and treatment: 5 mg once daily

Dosage Forms Tablet, as sodium: 5 mg, 30 mg, 35 mg

risedronate sodium *see* risedronate *on previous page*

Risperdal® [US/Can] *see* risperidone *on this page*

Risperdal Consta™ [US] *see* risperidone *on this page*

Risperdal M-Tab™ *see* risperidone *on this page*

risperidone (ris PER i done)

Sound-Alike/Look-Alike Issues

risperidone may be confused with buspirone, reserpine, Risperdal®

Risperdal® may be confused with lisinopril, reserpine, risperidone

Synonyms Risperdal M-Tab™

U.S./Canadian Brand Names Risperdal® [US/Can]; Risperdal Consta™ [US]

Therapeutic Category Antipsychotic Agent, Benzisoxazole

Use Treatment of schizophrenia; treatment of acute mania or mixed episodes associated with bipolar I disorder (as monotherapy or in combination with lithium or valproate)

Usual Dosage

Oral:

Adults:

Schizophrenia: Recommended starting dose: 0.5-1 mg twice daily; slowly increase to the optimum range of 3-6 mg/day; may be given as a single daily dose once maintenance dose is achieved; daily dosages >10 mg does not appear to confer any additional benefit, and the incidence of extrapyramidal symptoms is higher than with lower doses

Bipolar mania: Recommended starting dose: 2-3 mg once daily; if needed, adjust dose by 1 mg/day in intervals ≥24 hours; dosing range: 1-6 mg/day

Elderly: A starting dose of 0.25-1 mg in 1-2 divided doses, and titration should progress slowly. Additional monitoring of renal function and orthostatic blood pressure may be warranted. If once-a-day dosing in the elderly or debilitated patient is considered, a twice daily regimen should be used to titrate to the target dose, and this dose should be maintained for 2-3 days prior to attempts to switch to a once-daily regimen.

I.M.: Adults: Schizophrenia (Risperdal® Consta™): 25 mg every 2 weeks; some patients may benefit from larger doses; maximum dose not to exceed 50 mg every 2 weeks. Dosage adjustments should not be made more frequently than every 4 weeks.

Note: Oral risperidone (or other antipsychotic) should be administered with the initial injection of Risperdal® Consta™ and continued for 3 weeks (then discontinued) to maintain adequate therapeutic plasma concentrations prior to main release phase of risperidone from injection site.

Dosage Forms

Injection, microspheres for reconstitution, extended release (Risperdal® Consta™): 25 mg, 37.5 mg, 50 mg [supplied in a dose-pack containing vial with active ingredient in microsphere formulation, prefilled syringe with diluent, needle-free vial access device, and safety needle]

Solution, oral: 1 mg/mL (30 mL) [contains benzoic acid]

Tablet: 0.25 mg, 0.5 mg, 1 mg, 2 mg, 3 mg, 4 mg

(Continued)

risperidone *(Continued)*

Tablet, orally disintegrating (Risperdal® M-Tabs™): 0.5 mg [contains phenylalanine 0.14 mg]; 1 mg [contains phenylalanine 0.28 mg]; 2 mg [contains phenylalanine 0.56 mg]

Ritalin® [US/Can] *see* methylphenidate *on page 571*

Ritalin® LA [US] *see* methylphenidate *on page 571*

Ritalin-SR® [US/Can] *see* methylphenidate *on page 571*

ritonavir (rye TON a veer)

Sound-Alike/Look-Alike Issues

ritonavir may be confused with Retrovir®

Norvir® may be confused with Norvasc®

U.S./Canadian Brand Names Norvir® SEC [Can]; Norvir® [US/Can]

Therapeutic Category Antiviral Agent

Use Treatment of HIV infection; should always be used as part of a multidrug regimen (at least three antiretroviral agents)

Usual Dosage Oral:

Children ≥2 years: 250 mg/m^2 twice daily; titrate dose upward to 400 mg/m^2 twice daily (maximum: 600 mg twice daily)

Adults: 600 mg twice daily; dose escalation tends to avoid nausea that many patients experience upon initiation of full dosing. Escalate the dose as follows: 300 mg twice daily for 1 day, 400 mg twice daily for 2 days, 500 mg twice daily for 1 day, then 600 mg twice daily. Ritonavir may be better tolerated when used in combination with other antiretrovirals by initiating the drug alone and subsequently adding the second agent within 2 weeks.

Note: Dosage adjustments for ritonavir when administered in combination therapy:

Amprenavir: Adjustments necessary for each agent: Amprenavir 1200 mg with ritonavir 200 mg once daily **or** Amprenavir 600 mg with ritonavir 100 mg twice daily

Amprenavir plus efavirenz (3-drug regimen): Amprenavir 1200 mg twice daily plus ritonavir 200 mg twice daily plus efavirenz at standard dose

Indinavir: Adjustments necessary for both agents: Indinavir 800 mg twice daily plus ritonavir 100-200 mg twice daily **or** Indinavir 400 mg twice daily plus ritonavir 400 mg twice daily

Nelfinavir or saquinavir: Ritonavir 400 mg twice daily

Rifabutin: Decrease rifabutin dose to 150 mg every other day

Dosage Forms

Capsule: 100 mg [contains ethanol and polyoxyl 35 castor oil]

Solution: 80 mg/mL (240 mL) [contains ethanol and polyoxyl 35 castor oil]

ritonavir and lopinavir *see* lopinavir and ritonavir *on page 529*

Rituxan® [US/Can] *see* rituximab *on this page*

rituximab (ri TUK si mab)

Synonyms anti-CD20 monoclonal antibody; C2B8; C2B8 monoclonal antibody; IDEC-C2B8; pan-B antibody

U.S./Canadian Brand Names Rituxan® [US/Can]

Therapeutic Category Antineoplastic Agent

Use Treatment of relapsed or refractory CD20 positive, B-cell non-Hodgkin lymphoma

Usual Dosage Refer to individual protocols. Adults: I.V. infusion:

Manufacturer's labeling: 375 mg/m^2 once weekly for 4-8 weeks

or

100 mg/m^2 I.V. day 1, then 375 mg/m^2 3 times/week for 11 doses has also been reported (cycles may be repeated in patients with refractory or relapsed disease)

Retreatment following disease progression: 375 mg/m^2 once weekly for 4 doses

Combination therapy with ibritumomab: 250 mg/m^2 I.V. day 1; repeat in 7-9 days with ibritumomab (also see Ibritumomab monograph)

Rituximab dose in combination with ibritumomab:

Step 1: 250 mg/m^2 at an initial rate of 50 mg/hour. If hypersensitivity or infusion-related events do not occur, increase infusion in increments of 50 mg/hour every 30 minutes, to a maximum of 400 mg/hour. Infusions should be temporarily slowed or interrupted if hypersensitivity or infusion related events occur. The infusion may be resumed at 1/2 the previous rate upon improvement of symptoms.

Step 2: 250 mg/m^2 at an initial rate of 100 mg/hour (50 mg/hour if infusion-related events occurred with the first infusion). If hypersensitivity or infusion-related events do not occur, increase infusion in increments of 100 mg/hour every 30 minutes, to a maximum of 400 mg/hour, as tolerated.

Dosage Forms Injection, solution [preservative free]: 10 mg/mL (10 mL, 50 mL)

Riva-Cloxacillin [Can] *see* cloxacillin *on page 218*

Riva-Diclofenac [Can] *see* diclofenac *on page 266*

Riva-Diclofenac-K [Can] *see* diclofenac *on page 266*

Riva-Famotidine [Can] *see* famotidine *on page 356*

Riva-Loperamine [Can] *see* loperamide *on page 528*

Riva-Lorazepam [Can] *see* lorazepam *on page 530*

Riva-Naproxen [Can] *see* naproxen *on page 605*

Rivanase AQ [Can] *see* beclomethasone *on page 102*

Riva-Norfloxacin [Can] *see* norfloxacin *on page 628*

Riva-Simvastatin [Can] *see* simvastatin *on page 805*

Rivasol [Can] *see* zinc sulfate *on page 941*

rivastigmine (ri va STIG meen)

Synonyms ENA 713; SDZ ENA 713

U.S./Canadian Brand Names Exelon® [US/Can]

Therapeutic Category Acetylcholinesterase Inhibitor; Cholinergic Agent

Use Mild to moderate dementia from Alzheimer's disease

Usual Dosage Adults: Mild to moderate Alzheimer's dementia: Oral: Initial: 1.5 mg twice daily to start; if dose is tolerated for at least 2 weeks then it may be increased to 3 mg twice daily; increases to 4.5 mg twice daily and 6 mg twice daily should only be attempted after at least 2 weeks at the previous dose; maximum dose: 6 mg twice daily. If adverse events such as nausea, vomiting, abdominal pain, or loss of appetite occur, the patient should be instructed to discontinue treatment for several doses then restart at the same or next lower dosage level; antiemetics have been used to control GI symptoms. If treatment is interrupted for longer than several days, restart the treatment at the lowest dose and titrate as previously described.

Dosage Forms

Capsule, as tartrate: 1.5 mg, 3 mg, 4.5 mg, 6 mg

Solution, oral, as tartrate: 2 mg/mL (120 mL) [contains sodium benzoate]

Riva-Zide [Can] *see* hydrochlorothiazide and triamterene *on page 443*

Rivotril® [Can] *see* clonazepam *on page 215*

rizatriptan (rye za TRIP tan)

Synonyms MK462

U.S./Canadian Brand Names Maxalt® [US/Can]; Maxalt-MLT® [US]; Maxalt RPD™ [Can]

Therapeutic Category Antimigraine Agent; Serotonin Agonist

Use Acute treatment of migraine with or without aura

Usual Dosage Note: In patients with risk factors for coronary artery disease, following adequate evaluation to establish the absence of coronary artery disease, the initial dose should be administered in a setting where response may be evaluated (physician's office or similarly staffed setting). ECG monitoring may be considered.

(Continued)

rizatriptan *(Continued)*

Oral: 5-10 mg, repeat after 2 hours if significant relief is not attained; maximum: 30 mg in a 24-hour period (use 5 mg dose in patients receiving propranolol with a maximum of 15 mg in 24 hours)

Note: For orally-disintegrating tablets (Maxalt-MLT™): Patient should be instructed to place tablet on tongue and allow to dissolve. Dissolved tablet will be swallowed with saliva.

Dosage Forms

Tablet, as benzoate (Maxalt®): 5 mg, 10 mg

Tablet, orally-disintegrating, as benzoate (Maxalt-MLT®): 5 mg [contains phenylalanine 1.05 mg/tablet; peppermint flavor]; 10 mg [contains phenylalanine 2.1 mg/tablet; peppermint flavor]

rLFN-α2 *see* interferon alfa-2b *on page 477*

RMS® [US] *see* morphine sulfate *on page 591*

Ro 11-1163 *see* moclobemide *(Canada only) on page 587*

Robafen® AC [US] *see* guaifenesin and codeine *on page 416*

Robafen® CF *(Discontinued)* *see page 1042*

Robaxin® [US/Can] *see* methocarbamol *on page 564*

Robaxisal® *(Discontinued)* *see page 1042*

Robicillin® Tablet *(Discontinued)* *see page 1042*

Robidrine® [Can] *see* pseudoephedrine *on page 745*

Robinul® [US] *see* glycopyrrolate *on page 411*

Robinul® Forte [US] *see* glycopyrrolate *on page 411*

Robitet® *(Discontinued)* *see page 1042*

Robitussin® A-C *(Discontinued)* *see page 1042*

Robitussin® CF [US-OTC] *see* guaifenesin, pseudoephedrine, and dextromethorphan *on page 422*

Robitussin® Childrens Cough & Cold [Can] *see* pseudoephedrine and dextromethorphan *on page 746*

Robitussin® Cold and Congestion [US-OTC] *see* guaifenesin, pseudoephedrine, and dextromethorphan *on page 422*

Robitussin® Cough and Cold Infant [US-OTC] *see* guaifenesin, pseudoephedrine, and dextromethorphan *on page 422*

Robitussin® Cough & Cold® [Can] *see* guaifenesin, pseudoephedrine, and dextromethorphan *on page 422*

Robitussin® CoughGels™ [US-OTC] *see* dextromethorphan *on page 261*

Robitussin®-DAC *(Discontinued)* *see page 1042*

Robitussin® DM [US-OTC/Can] *see* guaifenesin and dextromethorphan *on page 416*

Robitussin® Honey Cough [US-OTC] *see* dextromethorphan *on page 261*

Robitussin® Maximum Strength Cough & Cold [US-OTC] *see* pseudoephedrine and dextromethorphan *on page 746*

Robitussin® Maximum Strength Cough [US-OTC] *see* dextromethorphan *on page 261*

Robitussin® Pediatric Cough & Cold [US-OTC] *see* pseudoephedrine and dextromethorphan *on page 746*

Robitussin® Pediatric Cough [US-OTC] *see* dextromethorphan *on page 261*

Robitussin® Pediatric [US-OTC] *see* dextromethorphan *on page 261*

Robitussin-PE® [US-OTC] *see* guaifenesin and pseudoephedrine *on page 419*

Robitussin® Severe Congestion [US-OTC] *see* guaifenesin and pseudoephedrine *on page 419*

Robitussin® Sugar Free Cough [US-OTC] *see* guaifenesin and dextromethorphan *on page 416*

Robitussin® [US-OTC/Can] *see* guaifenesin *on page 415*

Rocaltrol® [US/Can] *see* calcitriol *on page 143*

Rocephin® [US/Can] *see* ceftriaxone *on page 172*

rocuronium (roe kyoor OH nee um)

Sound-Alike/Look-Alike Issues
Zemuron® may be confused with Remeron®

Synonyms ORG 946; rocuronium bromide

U.S./Canadian Brand Names Zemuron® [US/Can]

Therapeutic Category Skeletal Muscle Relaxant

Use Adjunct to general anesthesia to facilitate both rapid sequence and routine endotracheal intubation and to relax skeletal muscles during surgery; to facilitate mechanical ventilation in ICU patients; does not relieve pain or produce sedation

Usual Dosage Administer I.V.; dose to effect; doses will vary due to interpatient variability; use ideal body weight for obese patients

Children:

Initial: 0.6 mg/kg under halothane anesthesia produce excellent to good intubating conditions within 1 minute and will provide a median time of 41 minutes of clinical relaxation in children 3 months to 1 year of age, and 27 minutes in children 1-12 years

Maintenance: 0.075-0.125 mg/kg administered upon return of T_1 to 25% of control provides clinical relaxation for 7-10 minutes

Adults:

Tracheal intubation: I.V.:

Initial: 0.6 mg/kg is expected to provide approximately 31 minutes of clinical relaxation under opioid/nitrous oxide/oxygen anesthesia with neuromuscular block sufficient for intubation attained in 1-2 minutes; lower doses (0.45 mg/kg) may be used to provide 22 minutes of clinical relaxation with median time to neuromuscular block of 1-3 minutes; maximum blockade is achieved in <4 minutes

Maximum: 0.9-1.2 mg/kg may be given during surgery under opioid/nitrous oxide/oxygen anesthesia without adverse cardiovascular effects and is expected to provide 58-67 minutes of clinical relaxation; neuromuscular blockade sufficient for intubation is achieved in <2 minutes with maximum blockade in <3 minutes

Maintenance: 0.1, 0.15, and 0.2 mg/kg administered at 25% recovery of control T_1 (defined as 3 twitches of train-of-four) provides a median of 12, 17, and 24 minutes of clinical duration under anesthesia

Rapid sequence intubation: 0.6-1.2 mg/kg in appropriately premedicated and anesthetized patients with excellent or good intubating conditions within 2 minutes

Continuous infusion: Initial: 0.01-0.012 mg/kg/minute only after early evidence of spontaneous recovery of neuromuscular function is evident; infusion rates have ranged from 4-16 mcg/kg/minute

ICU: 10 mcg/kg/minute; adjust dose to maintain appropriate degree of neuromuscular blockade (eg, 1 or 2 twitches on train-of-four)

Dosage Forms Injection, solution, as bromide: 10 mg/mL (5 mL, 10 mL)

rocuronium bromide *see* rocuronium *on this page*

Rofact™ [Can] *see* rifampin *on page 776*

rofecoxib (roe fe COX ib)

Sound-Alike/Look-Alike Issues
Vioxx® may be confused with Zyvox™

Therapeutic Category Nonsteroidal Antiinflammatory Drug (NSAID), COX-2 Selective

(Continued)

rofecoxib *(Continued)*

Use

Rofecoxib Withdrawal Announced - September 30, 2004

Merck & Co has announced that rofecoxib (Vioxx®) has been withdrawn from the market. The withdrawal is voluntary and is based on results from a recent clinical trial designed to evaluate rofecoxib's effectiveness in preventing the recurrence of colorectal polyps. The study noted an increased relative risk for cardiovascular events and was stopped early for safety reasons. Patients taking rofecoxib chronically were noted to have twice the risk of heart attack when compared to patients taking placebo. The Food and Drug Administration (FDA) has acknowledged the withdrawal and is working with Merck to safely remove this product from the market. Patients should contact their healthcare providers for alternative therapies as Merck will no longer be providing this medication to pharmacies worldwide.

A complete copy of the press announcement can be found at: http://www.vioxx.com/

Additional information can also be found on the following websites:
http://www.fda.gov/bbs/topics/news/2004/NEW01122.html
http://www.hc-sc.gc.ca/english/protection/warnings/2004/2004_50.htm

Roferon-A® [US/Can] *see* interferon alfa-2a *on page 476*

Rogaine® [Can] *see* minoxidil *on page 584*

Rogaine® Extra Strength for Men [US-OTC] *see* minoxidil *on page 584*

Rogaine® for Men [US-OTC] *see* minoxidil *on page 584*

Rogaine® for Women [US-OTC] *see* minoxidil *on page 584*

Rogitine® [Can] *see* phentolamine *on page 688*

Rolaids®, Extra Strength [US-OTC] *see* calcium carbonate and magnesium hydroxide *on page 146*

Rolaids® [US-OTC] *see* calcium carbonate and magnesium hydroxide *on page 146*

Rolatuss® Plain Liquid *(Discontinued)* *see page 1042*

Romazicon® [US/Can] *see* flumazenil *on page 373*

Romilar® AC [US] *see* guaifenesin and codeine *on page 416*

Romycin® [US] *see* erythromycin *on page 320*

Rondec®-DM Drops [US] *see* carbinoxamine, pseudoephedrine, and dextromethorphan *on page 159*

Rondec® Drops [US] *see* carbinoxamine and pseudoephedrine *on page 157*

Rondec® Syrup [US] *see* brompheniramine and pseudoephedrine *on page 129*

Rondec® Tablets [US] *see* carbinoxamine and pseudoephedrine *on page 157*

Rondec-TR® [US] *see* carbinoxamine and pseudoephedrine *on page 157*

Rondomycin® Capsule *(Discontinued)* *see page 1042*

ropinirole (roe PIN i role)

Synonyms ropinirole hydrochloride

U.S./Canadian Brand Names ReQuip® [US/Can]

Therapeutic Category Anti-Parkinson Agent

Use Treatment of idiopathic Parkinson disease; in patients with early Parkinson's disease who were not receiving concomitant levodopa therapy as well as in patients with advanced disease on concomitant levodopa

Usual Dosage Adults: Oral: The dosage should be increased to achieve a maximum therapeutic effect, balanced against the principal side effects of nausea, dizziness, somnolence and dyskinesia

Recommended starting dose is 0.25 mg 3 times/day; based on individual patient response, the dosage should be titrated with weekly increments as described below:
- Week 1: 0.25 mg 3 times/day; total daily dose: 0.75 mg
- Week 2: 0.5 mg 3 times/day; total daily dose: 1.5 mg
- Week 3: 0.75 mg 3 times/day; total daily dose: 2.25 mg
- Week 4: 1 mg 3 times/day; total daily dose: 3 mg

After week 4, if necessary, daily dosage may be increased by 1.5 mg per day on a weekly basis up to a dose of 9 mg/day, and then by up to 3 mg/day weekly to a total of 24 mg/day

Removal by hemodialysis is unlikely.

Dosage Forms Tablet, as hydrochloride: 0.25 mg, 0.5 mg, 1 mg, 2 mg, 3 mg, 4 mg, 5 mg

ropinirole hydrochloride *see* ropinirole *on previous page*

ropivacaine (roe PIV a kane)

Sound-Alike/Look-Alike Issues

ropivacaine may be confused with bupivacaine

Synonyms ropivacaine hydrochloride

U.S./Canadian Brand Names Naropin® [US/Can]

Therapeutic Category Local Anesthetic

Use Local anesthetic for use in surgery, postoperative pain management, and obstetrical procedures when local or regional anesthesia is needed

Usual Dosage Dose varies with procedure, onset and depth of anesthesia desired, vascularity of tissues, duration of anesthesia, and condition of patient: Adults:

Surgical anesthesia:
- Lumbar epidural: 15-30 mL of 0.5% to 1% solution
- Lumbar epidural block for cesarean section:
  - 20-30 mL dose of 0.5% solution
  - 15-20 mL dose of 0.75% solution
- Thoracic epidural block: 5-15 mL dose of 0.5% to 0.75% solution
- Major nerve block:
  - 35-50 mL dose of 0.5% solution (175-250 mg)
  - 10-40 mL dose of 0.75% solution (75-300 mg)
- Field block: 1-40 mL dose of 0.5% solution (5-200 mg)

Labor pain management: Lumbar epidural: Initial: 10-20 mL 0.2% solution; continuous infusion dose: 6-14 mL/hour of 0.2% solution with incremental injections of 10-15 mL/hour of 0.2% solution

Postoperative pain management:
- Lumbar or thoracic epidural: Continuous infusion dose: 6-14 mL/hour of 0.2% solution
- Infiltration/minor nerve block:
  - 1-100 mL dose of 0.2% solution
  - 1-40 mL dose of 0.5% solution

Dosage Forms

Infusion, as hydrochloride: 2 mg/mL (100 mL, 200 mL)

Injection, solution, as hydrochloride [single dose]: 2 mg/mL (10 mL, 20 mL); 5 mg/mL (10 mL, 20 mL, 30 mL); 7.5 mg/mL (10 mL, 20 mL); 10 mg/mL (10 mL, 20 mL)

ropivacaine hydrochloride *see* ropivacaine *on this page*

Rosanil™ [US] *see* sulfur and sulfacetamide *on page 834*

rosiglitazone (roe si GLI ta zone)

Sound-Alike/Look-Alike Issues

Avandia® may be confused with Avalide®, Coumadin®, Prandin™

U.S./Canadian Brand Names Avandia® [US/Can]

Therapeutic Category Hypoglycemic Agent, Oral; Thiazolidinedione Derivative

Use Type 2 diabetes mellitus (noninsulin dependent, NIDDM):

Monotherapy: Improve glycemic control as an adjunct to diet and exercise

(Continued)

rosiglitazone *(Continued)*

Combination therapy: In combination with a sulfonylurea, metformin, or insulin when diet, exercise, and a single agent do not result in adequate glycemic control

Usual Dosage Oral: Adults:

Monotherapy: Initial: 4 mg daily as a single daily dose or in divided doses twice daily. If response is inadequate after 12 weeks of treatment, the dosage may be increased to 8 mg daily as a single daily dose or in divided doses twice daily. In clinical trials, the 4 mg twice-daily regimen resulted in the greatest reduction in fasting plasma glucose and Hb A_{1c}.

Combination therapy:

With sulfonylureas: Initial: 4 mg daily as a single daily dose or in divided doses twice daily; dose of sulfonylurea should be reduced if the patient reports hypoglycemia. Doses of rosiglitazone >4 mg/day are not indicated in combination with sulfonylureas.

With metformin: Initial: 4 mg daily as a single daily dose or in divided doses twice daily. If response is inadequate after 12 weeks of treatment, the dosage may be increased to 8 mg daily as a single daily dose or in divided doses twice daily. It is unlikely that the dose of metformin will need to be reduced due to hypoglycemia

With insulin: Initial: 4 mg daily as a single daily dose or in divided doses twice daily. Dose of insulin should be reduced by 10% to 25% if the patient reports hypoglycemia or if the plasma glucose falls to <100 mg/dL. Doses of rosiglitazone >4 mg/day are not indicated in combination with insulin.

Dosage Forms Tablet: 2 mg, 4 mg, 8 mg

rosiglitazone and metformin (roh si GLI ta zone & met FOR min)

Synonyms metformin and rosiglitazone; metformin hydrochloride and rosiglitazone maleate; rosiglitazone maleate and metformin hydrochloride

U.S./Canadian Brand Names Avandamet™ [US/Can]

Therapeutic Category Antidiabetic Agent (Biguanide); Antidiabetic Agent (Thiazolidinedione)

Use Management of type 2 diabetes mellitus (noninsulin dependent, NIDDM) in patients who are already treated with the combination of rosiglitazone and metformin, or who are not adequately controlled on metformin alone. Used as an adjunct to diet and exercise to lower the blood glucose when hyperglycemia cannot be controlled satisfactorily by diet and exercise alone

Usual Dosage Oral: Adults: Type 2 diabetes mellitus: Initial dose should be based on current dose of rosiglitazone and/or metformin; daily dose should be divided and given with meals

Patients inadequately controlled on **metformin alone**: Initial dose: Rosiglitazone 4 mg/day plus current dose of metformin

Patients inadequately controlled on **rosiglitazone alone**: Initial dose: Metformin 1000 mg/day plus current dose of rosiglitazone

Note: When switching from combination rosiglitazone and metformin as separate tablets: Use current dose

Dose adjustment: Doses may be increased as increments of rosiglitazone 4 mg and/or metformin 500 mg, up to the maximum dose; doses should be titrated gradually.
After a change in the metformin dosage, titration can be done after 1-2 weeks
After a change in the rosiglitazone dosage, titration can be done after 8-12 weeks
Maximum dose: Rosiglitazone 8 mg/metformin 2000 mg daily

Dosage Forms Tablet [film coated]:

1/500: Rosiglitazone 1 mg and metformin 500 mg
2/500: Rosiglitazone 2 mg and metformin 500 mg
4/500: Rosiglitazone 4 mg and metformin 500 mg
2/1000: Rosiglitazone 2 mg and metformin 1000 mg
4/1000: Rosiglitazone 4 mg and metformin 1000 mg

rosiglitazone maleate and metformin hydrochloride *see* rosiglitazone and metformin *on this page*

Rosula® [US] *see* sulfur and sulfacetamide *on page 834*

rosuvastatin (roe SOO va sta tin)

Synonyms rosuvastatin calcium

U.S./Canadian Brand Names Crestor® [US/Can]

Therapeutic Category Antilipemic Agent, HMG-CoA Reductase Inhibitor

Use Used with dietary therapy for hyperlipidemias to reduce elevations in total cholesterol (TC), LDL-C, apolipoprotein B, and triglycerides (TG) in patients with primary hypercholesterolemia (elevations of 1 or more components are present in Fredrickson type IIa, IIb, and IV hyperlipidemias); treatment of homozygous familial hypercholesterolemia (FH)

Usual Dosage Adults: Oral:

Heterozygous familial and nonfamilial hypercholesterolemia; mixed dyslipidemia: Initial: 10 mg once daily (20 mg in patients with severe hypercholesterolemia); after 2 weeks, may be increased to 20 mg once daily; dosing range: 5-40 mg/day (maximum dose: 40 mg once daily)

Homozygous FH: Initial: 20 mg once daily (maximum dose: 40 mg/day)

Dosage adjustment with concomitant medications:

Cyclosporine: Rosuvastatin dose should not exceed 5 mg/day

Gemfibrozil: Rosuvastatin dose should not exceed 10 mg/day

Dosage Forms Tablet, as calcium: 5 mg, 10 mg, 20 mg, 40 mg

rosuvastatin calcium *see* rosuvastatin *on this page*

RotaShield® ***(Discontinued)*** *see page 1042*

Rovamycine® [Can] *see* spiramycin *(Canada only) on page 821*

Rowasa® [US/Can] *see* mesalamine *on page 556*

Roxanol® [US] *see* morphine sulfate *on page 591*

Roxanol 100® [US] *see* morphine sulfate *on page 591*

Roxanol SR™ Oral ***(Discontinued)*** *see page 1042*

Roxanol®-T [US] *see* morphine sulfate *on page 591*

Roxicet™ [US] *see* oxycodone and acetaminophen *on page 656*

Roxicet® 5/500 [US] *see* oxycodone and acetaminophen *on page 656*

Roxicodone™ [US] *see* oxycodone *on page 656*

Roxicodone™ Intensol™ [US] *see* oxycodone *on page 656*

Roxiprin® ***(Discontinued)*** *see page 1042*

Roychlor® [Can] *see* potassium chloride *on page 713*

Rozex™ [US] *see* metronidazole *on page 576*

RP-6976 *see* docetaxel *on page 284*

RP-54274 *see* riluzole *on page 777*

RP-59500 *see* quinupristin and dalfopristin *on page 758*

r-PA *see* reteplase *on page 770*

rPDGF-BB *see* becaplermin *on page 102*

RS-25259 *see* palonosetron *on page 661*

RS-25259-197 *see* palonosetron *on page 661*

RSV-IGIV *see* respiratory syncytial virus immune globulin (intravenous) *on page 769*

RTCA *see* ribavirin *on page 774*

RU-486 *see* mifepristone *on page 581*

RU-23908 *see* nilutamide *on page 620*

RU-38486 *see* mifepristone *on page 581*

rubella, measles and mumps vaccines, combined *see* measles, mumps, and rubella vaccines, combined *on page 544*

rubella virus vaccine (live) (rue BEL a VYE rus vak SEEN live)

Sound-Alike/Look-Alike Issues

Meruvax® II may be confused with Attenuvax®

Synonyms german measles vaccine

U.S./Canadian Brand Names Meruvax® II [US]

Therapeutic Category Vaccine, Live Virus

Use Selective active immunization against rubella; vaccination is routinely recommended for persons from 12 months of age to puberty. All adults, both male and female, lacking documentation of live vaccine on or after first birthday, or laboratory evidence of immunity (particularly women of childbearing age and young adults who work in or congregate in hospitals, colleges, and on military bases) should be vaccinated. Susceptible travelers should be vaccinated.

Note: Trivalent measles - mumps - rubella (MMR) vaccine is the preferred immunizing agent for most children and many adults.

Usual Dosage Children ≥12 months and Adults: SubQ: 0.5 mL in outer aspect of upper arm; children vaccinated before 12 months of age should be revaccinated. Recommended age for primary immunization is 12-15 months; revaccination with MMR-II is recommended prior to elementary school.

Dosage Forms Injection, powder for reconstitution [single dose]: 1000 $TCID_{50}$ (Wistar RA 27/3 Strain) [contains gelatin, human albumin, and neomycin]

rubeola vaccine *see* measles virus vaccine (live) *on page 545*

Rubex® [US] *see* doxorubicin *on page 293*

rubidomycin hydrochloride *see* daunorubicin hydrochloride *on page 246*

Rubramin-PC® *(Discontinued)* *see page 1042*

Rufen® *(Discontinued)* *see page 1042*

Rulox [US] *see* aluminum hydroxide and magnesium hydroxide *on page 40*

Rulox No. 1 [US] *see* aluminum hydroxide and magnesium hydroxide *on page 40*

Rum-K® [US] *see* potassium chloride *on page 713*

Ru-Tuss® Liquid *(Discontinued)* *see page 1042*

Ru-Tuss® Tablet *(Discontinued)* *see page 1042*

Ru-Vert-M® *(Discontinued)* *see page 1042*

Rymed® *(Discontinued)* *see page 1042*

Rymed-TR® *(Discontinued)* *see page 1042*

Ryna® *(Discontinued)* *see page 1042*

Ryna-C® *(Discontinued)* *see page 1042*

Rynatan® [US] *see* chlorpheniramine and phenylephrine *on page 188*

Rynatan® Pediatric Suspension [US] *see* chlorpheniramine and phenylephrine *on page 188*

Rynatuss® [US] *see* chlorpheniramine, ephedrine, phenylephrine, and carbetapentane *on page 190*

Rynatuss® Pediatric [US] *see* chlorpheniramine, ephedrine, phenylephrine, and carbetapentane *on page 190*

Rythmodan® [Can] *see* disopyramide *on page 283*

Rythmodan®-LA [Can] *see* disopyramide *on page 283*

Rythmol® [US/Can] *see* propafenone *on page 737*

Rythmol® SR [US] *see* propafenone *on page 737*

SAB-Gentamicin [Can] *see* gentamicin *on page 403*

Sab-Prenase® [Can] *see* prednisolone (ophthalmic) *on page 723*

Sabril® [Can] *see* vigabatrin *(Canada only)* *on page 911*

sacrosidase (sak RO se dase)

U.S./Canadian Brand Names Sucraid™ [US/Can]

Therapeutic Category Enzyme

Use **Orphan drug:** Oral replacement therapy in sucrase deficiency, as seen in congenital sucrase-isomaltase deficiency (CSID)

Usual Dosage Oral:

Infants ≥5 months and Children <15 kg: 8500 int. units (1 mL) per meal or snack

Children >15 kg and Adults: 17,000 int. units (2 mL) per meal or snack

Doses should be diluted with 2-4 oz of water, milk, or formula with each meal or snack. Approximately one-half of the dose may be taken before, and the remainder of a dose taken at the completion of each meal or snack.

Dosage Forms Solution, oral: 8500 int. units per mL (118 mL)

Safe Tussin® 30 [US-OTC] *see* guaifenesin and dextromethorphan *on page 416*

Saizen® [US/Can] *see* human growth hormone *on page 437*

Salacid® Ointment *(Discontinued)* *see* *page 1042*

Sal-Acid® [US-OTC] *see* salicylic acid *on this page*

Salactic® [US-OTC] *see* salicylic acid *on this page*

SalAc® [US-OTC] *see* salicylic acid *on this page*

Salagen® [US/Can] *see* pilocarpine *on page 694*

Salazopyrin® [Can] *see* sulfasalazine *on page 833*

Salazopyrin En-Tabs® [Can] *see* sulfasalazine *on page 833*

Salbu-2 [Can] *see* albuterol *on page 25*

Salbu-4 [Can] *see* albuterol *on page 25*

salbutamol *see* albuterol *on page 25*

Saleto-200® *(Discontinued)* *see* *page 1042*

Saleto-400® *(Discontinued)* *see* *page 1042*

Salflex® [US/Can] *see* salsalate *on page 793*

Salgesic® *(Discontinued)* *see* *page 1042*

salicylazosulfapyridine *see* sulfasalazine *on page 833*

salicylic acid (sal i SIL ik AS id)

U.S./Canadian Brand Names Compound W® One Step Wart Remover [US-OTC]; Compound W® [US-OTC]; DHS™ Sal [US-OTC]; Dr. Scholl's® Callus Remover [US-OTC]; Dr. Scholl's® Clear Away [US-OTC]; DuoFilm® [US-OTC/Can]; Duoforte® 27 [Can]; Freezone® [US-OTC]; Fung-O® [US-OTC]; Gordofilm® [US-OTC]; Hydrisalic™ [US-OTC]; Ionil® Plus [US-OTC]; Ionil® [US-OTC]; Keralyt® [US-OTC]; LupiCare™ Dandruff [US-OTC]; LupiCare™ II Psoriasis [US-OTC]; LupiCare™ Psoriasis [US-OTC]; Mediplast® [US-OTC]; MG217 Sal-Acid® [US-OTC]; Mosco® Corn and Callus Remover [US-OTC]; NeoCeuticals™ Acne Spot Treatment [US-OTC]; Neutrogena® Acne Wash [US-OTC]; Neutrogena® Body Clear™ [US-OTC]; Neutrogena® Clear Pore Shine Control [US-OTC]; Neutrogena® Clear Pore [US-OTC]; Neutrogena® Healthy Scalp [US-OTC]; Neutrogena® Maximum Strength T/Sal® [US-OTC]; Neutrogena® On The Spot® Acne Patch [US-OTC]; Occlusal™ [Can]; Occlusal®-HP [US/Can]; Oxy® Balance Deep Pore [US-OTC]; Oxy® Balance [US-OTC]; Palmer's® Skin Success Acne Cleanser [US-OTC]; Pedisilk® [US-OTC]; Propa pH [US-OTC]; Sal-Acid® [US-OTC]; Salactic® [US-OTC]; SalAc® [US-OTC]; Sal-Plant® [US-OTC]; Sebcur® [Can]; Soluver® [Can]; Soluver® Plus [Can]; Stri-dex® Body Focus [US-OTC]; Stri-dex® Facewipes To Go™ [US-OTC]; Stri-dex® Maximum Strength [US-OTC]; Stri-dex® [US-OTC]; Tinamed® [US-OTC]; Tiseb® [US-OTC]; Trans-Plantar® [Can]; Trans-Ver-Sal® [US-OTC/Can]; (Continued)

salicylic acid *(Continued)*

Wart-Off® Maximum Strength [US-OTC]; Zapzyt® Acne Wash [US-OTC]; Zapzyt® Pore Treatment [US-OTC]

Therapeutic Category Keratolytic Agent

Use Topically for its keratolytic effect in controlling seborrheic dermatitis or psoriasis of body and scalp, dandruff, and other scaling dermatoses; also used to remove warts, corns, and calluses; acne

Usual Dosage Children and Adults (consult specific product labeling for use in children <12 years):

Acne:

Cream, cloth, foam, or liquid cleansers (2%): Use to cleanse skin once or twice daily. Massage gently into skin, work into lather and rinse thoroughly. Cloths should be wet with water prior to using and disposed of (not flushed) after use.

Gel (0.5% or 2%): Apply small amount to face in the morning or evening; if peeling occurs, may be used every other day. Some products may be labeled for OTC use up to 3 or 4 times per day. Apply to clean, dry skin

Pads (0.5% or 2%): Use pad to cover affected area with thin layer of salicylic acid one to three times a day. Apply to clean, dry skin. Do not leave pad on skin.

Patch (2%): At bedtime, after washing face, allow skin to dry at least 5 minutes. Apply patch directly over pimple being treated. Remove in the morning.

Shower/bath gels or soap (2%): Use once daily in shower or bath to massage over skin prone to acne. Rinse well.

Callus, corns, or warts:

Gel or liquid (17%): Apply to each wart and allow to dry. May repeat once or twice daily, up to 12 weeks. Apply to clean dry area.

Gel (6%): Apply to affected area once daily, generally used at night and rinsed off in the morning.

Plaster or transdermal patch (40%): Apply directly over affected area, leave in place for 48 hours. Some products may be cut to fit area or secured with adhesive strips. May repeat procedure for up to 12 weeks. Apply to clean, dry skin

Transdermal patch (15%): Apply directly over affected area at bedtime, leave in place overnight and remove in the morning. Patch should be trimmed to cover affected area. May repeat daily for up to 12 weeks.

Dandruff, psoriasis, or seborrheic dermatitis:

Cream (2.5%): Apply to affected area 3-4 times daily. Apply to clean, dry skin. Some products may be left in place overnight.

Ointment (3%): Apply to scales or plaques on skin up to 4 times per day (not for scalp or face)

Shampoo (1.8% to 3%): Massage into wet hair or affected area; leave in place for several minutes; rinse thoroughly. Labeled for OTC use 2-3 times a week, or as directed by healthcare provider. Some products may be left in place overnight.

Dosage Forms [DSC] = Discontinued product

Cream:

LupiCare® Dandruff, LupiCare® Psoriasis: 2.5% (120 g, 240 g) [contains alcohol]

LupiCare® II Psoriasis: 2.5% (60 g, 240 g) [contains alcohol]

Neutrogena® Acne Wash: 2% (200 mL) [contains alcohol]

Cloths: Neutrogena® Acne Wash: 2% (30s) [disposable cloths]

Foam:

Neutrogena® Acne Wash: 2% (150 mL) [foaming cleanser]

SalAc®: 2% (100 g)

Gel: 17% (15 g)

Compound W®: 17% (7 g) [contains alcohol]

DuoPlant® [DSC]: 17% (15 g)

Hydrisalic™: 6% (28 g) [contains alcohol and propylene glycol]

Keralyt®: 6% (30 g) [contains alcohol and propylene glycol]

NeoCeuticals™ Acne Spot Treatment: 2% (15 g) [contains alcohol]

Neutrogena® Clear Pore: 2% (60 g) [contains alcohol]

Neutrogena® Clear Pore Shine Control: 0.5% (10 g)

Oxy® Balance: 2% (240 mL) [shower gel]
Sal-Plant®: 17% (14 g) [contains alcohol]
Stri-dex® Body Focus™: 2% (300 mL)
Zapzyt® Acne Wash: 2% (190 g) [alcohol free]
Zapzyt® Pore Treatment: 2% (23 g) [alcohol free]

Liquid, topical:
Compound W®: 17% (9 mL) [contains alcohol]
DuoFilm®: 17% (15 mL) [contains alcohol]
Freezone®: 17.6% (9.3 mL) [contains alcohol]
Fung-O®: 17% (15 mL)
Gordofilm®: 16.7% (15 mL)
Mosco® Corn and Callus Remover: 17.6% (10 mL)
NeoCeuticals™ Acne Spot Treatment: 2% (60 mL) [contains alcohol]
Neutrogena® Acne Wash: 2% (180 mL) [contains tartrazine]
Neutrogena® Body Clear™ [body scrub with microbeads]: 2% (250 mL) [contains tartrazine]
Neutrogena® Body Clear™ [body wash]: 2% (250 mL) [contains tartrazine]
Occlusal®-HP: 17% (10 mL)
Palmer's® Skin Success Acne Cleanser: 0.5% (240 mL)
Pedisilk®: 17% (15 mL)
Propa pH: 2% (80 mL) [alcohol free; contains aloe vera]
SalAc®: 2% (180 mL)
Salactic®: 17% (15 mL) [contains alcohol]
Tinamed®: 17% (15 mL)
Wart-Off®: 17% (13 mL) [contains alcohol]

Ointment (MG217 Sal-Acid®): 3% (56 g) [contains vitamin E]

Pads:
Oxy® Balance, Oxy® Balance Deep Pore: 0.5% (55s, 90s) [contains alcohol]
Stri-dex®: 0.5% (55s)
Stri-dex® Facewipes To Go™ : 0.5% (32s) [contains alcohol]
Stri-dex® Maximum Strength: 2% (32s, 55s, 90s)

Patch, transdermal:
Compound W® One Step Wart Remover: 40% (12s, 14s)
Dr. Scholl's® Callus Remover: 40% (4s)
Dr. Scholl's® Clear Away: 40% (14s, 16s, 18s, 24s)
DuoFilm®: 40% (18s)
Neutrogena® On The Spot® Acne Patch: 2% (27s)
Trans-Ver-Sal®: 15% [6 mm PediaPatch, 12 mm AdultPatch, 20 mm PlantarPatch] (10s, 12s, 15s, 25s, 40s)

Plaster:
Mediplast®: 40% (25s)
Sal-Acid®: 40% (14s)
Tinamed®: 40% (24s)

Shampoo:
DHS™ Sal: 3% (120 mL)
Ionil®: 2% (240 mL, 480 mL, 960 mL)
Ionil® Plus: 2% (240 mL) [conditioning shampoo]
LupiCare® Dandruff, LupiCare® Psoriasis: 2% (120 mL, 240 mL)
Neutrogena® Healthy Scalp: 1.8% (90 mL, 180 mL)
Neutrogena® Maximum Strength T/Sal®: 3% (135 mL)
Tiseb®: 2% (240 mL)

Soap: 2% (114 g)

salicylic acid and coal tar *see* coal tar and salicylic acid *on page 220*

salicylic acid and lactic acid (sal i SIL ik AS id & LAK tik AS id)

Synonyms lactic acid and salicylic acid
Therapeutic Category Keratolytic Agent
Use Treatment of benign epithelial tumors such as warts
(Continued)

salicylic acid and lactic acid *(Continued)*

Usual Dosage Topical: Apply a thin layer directly to wart once daily (may be useful to apply at bedtime and wash off in morning)

Dosage Forms Solution, topical: Salicylic acid 16.7% and lactic acid 16.7% in flexible collodion (15 mL)

salicylic acid and propylene glycol

(sal i SIL ik AS id & PROE pi leen GLYE cole)

Synonyms propylene glycol and salicylic acid

Therapeutic Category Keratolytic Agent

Use Removal of excessive keratin in hyperkeratotic skin disorders, including various ichthyosis, keratosis palmaris and plantaris and psoriasis; may be used to remove excessive keratin in dorsal and plantar hyperkeratotic lesions

Usual Dosage Topical: Apply to area at night after soaking region for at least 5 minutes to hydrate area, and place under occlusion; medication is washed off in morning

Dosage Forms Gel, topical: Salicylic acid 6% and propylene glycol 60% in ethyl alcohol 19.4% with hydroxypropyl methylcellulose and water (30 g)

salicylic acid and sulfur *see* sulfur and salicylic acid *on page 834*

salicylsalicylic acid *see* salsalate *on next page*

SalineX® [US-OTC] *see* sodium chloride *on page 810*

Salivart® [US-OTC] *see* saliva substitute *on this page*

saliva substitute (sa LYE va SUB stee tute)

U.S./Canadian Brand Names Entertainer's Secret® [US-OTC]; Moi-Stir® [US-OTC]; MouthKote® [US-OTC]; Salivart® [US-OTC]; Saliva Substitute™ [US-OTC]; Salix® [US-OTC]

Therapeutic Category Gastrointestinal Agent, Miscellaneous

Use Relief of dry mouth and throat in xerostomia

Usual Dosage Use as needed

Dosage Forms

Lozenge (Salix®): Sorbitol, malic acid, sodium citrate, citric acid, dibasic calcium phosphate, sodium carboxymethylcellulose, propylene glycol, hydrogenated cottonseed oil, silicon dioxide, magnesium stearate [fruit flavor]

Solution, oral:

Entertainer's Secret®: Sodium carboxymethylcellulose, aloe vera gel, glycerin (60 mL) [honey-apple flavor]

Saliva Substitute®: Sorbitol, sodium carboxymethylcellulose, methylparaben (5 mL, 120 mL)

Spray, oral:

Moi-Stir®: Water, sorbitol, sodium carboxymethylcellulose, methylparaben, propylparaben, potassium chloride, dibasic sodium phosphate, calcium chloride, magnesium chloride, sodium chloride (120 mL)

Mouthkote®: Water, xylitol, sorbitol, yerba santa, citric acid, ascorbic acid, sodium saccharin, sodium benzoate (60 mL, 240 mL) [lemon-lime flavor]

Salivart™: Water, sodium carboxymethylcellulose, sorbitol, sodium chloride, potassium chloride, calcium chloride, magnesium chloride, potassium phosphate (70 mL)

Swabsticks, oral (Moi-Stir®): Water, sorbitol, sodium carboxymethylcellulose, methylparaben, propylparaben, potassium chloride, dibasic sodium phosphate, calcium chloride, magnesium chloride, sodium chloride (300s)

Saliva Substitute™ [US-OTC] *see* saliva substitute *on this page*

Salix® [US-OTC] *see* saliva substitute *on this page*

salk vaccine *see* poliovirus vaccine (inactivated) *on page 705*

salmeterol (sal ME te role)

Sound-Alike/Look-Alike Issues

salmeterol may be confused with salbutamol

Serevent® may be confused with Serentil®

Synonyms salmeterol xinafoate

U.S./Canadian Brand Names Serevent® [Can]; Serevent® Diskus® [US]

Therapeutic Category Adrenergic Agonist Agent

Use Maintenance treatment of asthma and in prevention of bronchospasm with reversible obstructive airway disease, including patients with symptoms of nocturnal asthma, who require regular treatment with inhaled, short-acting $beta_2$ agonists; prevention of exercise-induced bronchospasm; maintenance treatment of bronchospasm associated with COPD

Usual Dosage Inhalation, powder (Serevent® Diskus®):

Asthma, maintenance and prevention: Children ≥4 years and Adults: One inhalation (50 mcg) twice daily (~12 hours apart)

Exercise-induced asthma, prevention: Children ≥4 years and Adults: One inhalation (50 mcg) at least 30 minutes prior to exercise; additional doses should not be used for 12 hours; should not be used in individuals already receiving salmeterol twice daily

COPD (maintenance treatment of associated bronchospasm): Adults: One inhalation (50 mcg) twice daily (~12 hours apart)

Dosage Forms Powder for oral inhalation (Serevent® Diskus®): 50 mcg (28s, 60s) [delivers 46 mcg/inhalation; contains lactose]

salmeterol and fluticasone *see* fluticasone and salmeterol *on page 382*

salmeterol xinafoate *see* salmeterol *on this page*

Salmonella typhi Vi capsular polysaccharide vaccine *(Canada only)* (sal mo NEL la TI fi vi CAP su lar po le SAK ar ide VAK seen)

Therapeutic Category Vaccine

Use For active immunization against typhoid fever in persons 2 years of age and older.

Usual Dosage One dose administered I.M. ensures protection for at least 3 years. The vaccine must be given at least 2 weeks prior to travel to endemic areas.

Dosage Forms Injection: Vi polysaccharide vaccine of *S. typhi* 25 mcg (0.5 mL)

Salmonine® ***(Discontinued)*** *see page 1042*

Salofalk® [Can] *see* mesalamine *on page 556*

Sal-Plant® [US-OTC] *see* salicylic acid *on page 789*

salsalate (SAL sa late)

Sound-Alike/Look-Alike Issues

salsalate may be confused with sucralfate, sulfasalazine

Synonyms disalicylic acid; salicylsalicylic acid

U.S./Canadian Brand Names Amigesic® [US/Can]; Mono-Gesic® [US]; Salflex® [US/Can]

Therapeutic Category Analgesic, Nonnarcotic; Antipyretic; Nonsteroidal Antiinflammatory Drug (NSAID)

Use Treatment of minor pain or fever; arthritis

Usual Dosage Adults: Oral: 3 g/day in 2-3 divided doses

Dosage Forms [DSC] = Discontinued product

Tablet: 500 mg, 750 mg

Amigesic®, Disalcid® [DSC]: 500 mg, 750 mg

Mono-Gesic®, Salflex®: 750 mg

Salsitab® ***(Discontinued)*** *see page 1042*

salt *see* sodium chloride *on page 810*

salt poor albumin *see* albumin *on page 25*

Sal-Tropine™ [US] *see* atropine *on page 88*

Saluron® *(Discontinued)* *see page 1042*

Salutensin® *(Discontinued)* *see page 1042*

Salutensin-Demi® *(Discontinued)* *see page 1042*

Sanctura™ [US] *see* trospium *on page 892*

Sandimmune® [US] *see* cyclosporine *on page 235*

Sandimmune® I.V. [Can] *see* cyclosporine *on page 235*

Sandomigran® [Can] *see* pizotifen *(Canada only) on page 699*

Sandomigran DS® [Can] *see* pizotifen *(Canada only) on page 699*

Sandostatin® [US/Can] *see* octreotide *on page 639*

Sandostatin LAR® [US/Can] *see* octreotide *on page 639*

SangCya™ *(Discontinued)* *see page 1042*

Sani-Supp® [US-OTC] *see* glycerin *on page 410*

Sanorex® *(Discontinued)* *see page 1042*

Sans Acne® [Can] *see* erythromycin *on page 320*

Sansert® *(Discontinued)* *see page 1042*

Santyl® [US/Can] *see* collagenase *on page 225*

saquinavir (sa KWIN a veer)

Sound-Alike/Look-Alike Issues

saquinavir may be confused with Sinequan®
Fortovase® may be confused with Invirase®
Invirase® may be confused with Fortovase®

Synonyms saquinavir mesylate

U.S./Canadian Brand Names Fortovase® [US/Can]; Invirase® [US/Can]

Therapeutic Category Antiviral Agent

Use Treatment of HIV infection; used in combination with at least two other antiretroviral agents

Usual Dosage Oral:

Children and Adolescents <16 years: Safety and efficacy have not been established; dosages of 50 mg/kg/dose 3 times/day are under study

Children ≥16 years and Adults: **Note:** Fortovase® and Invirase® are not bioequivalent and should not be used interchangeably; only Fortovase® should be used to initiate therapy:

Fortovase®: 1200 mg (six 200 mg capsules) 3 times/day within 2 hours after a meal in combination with a nucleoside analog or 1000 mg (five 200 mg capsules) twice daily in combination with ritonavir 100 mg twice daily

Invirase®: 1000 mg (five 200 mg capsules) twice daily given in combination with ritonavir 100 mg twice daily; this combination should be given together and within 2 hours after a full meal in combination with a nucleoside analog

Note: Dosage adjustments of Fortovase® when administered in combination therapy:

Delavirdine: Fortovase® 800 mg 3 times/day
Lopinavir and ritonavir (Kaletra™): Fortovase® 800 mg twice daily
Nelfinavir: Fortovase® 1200 mg twice daily

Dosage Forms

Capsule, as mesylate (Invirase®): 200 mg [contains lactose 63.3 mg/capsule]
Capsule, soft gelatin, as base (Fortovase®): 200 mg

saquinavir mesylate *see* saquinavir *on this page*

Sarafem™ [US] *see* fluoxetine *on page 379*

sargramostim (sar GRAM oh stim)

Sound-Alike/Look-Alike Issues

Leukine™ may be confused with Leukeran®

Synonyms GM-CSF; granulocyte-macrophage colony stimulating factor; rGM-CSF

U.S./Canadian Brand Names Leukine™ [US/Can]

Therapeutic Category Colony-Stimulating Factor

Use

Myeloid reconstitution after autologous bone marrow transplantation: Non-Hodgkin lymphoma (NHL), acute lymphoblastic leukemia (ALL), Hodgkin lymphoma, metastatic breast cancer

Myeloid reconstitution after allogeneic bone marrow transplantation

Peripheral stem cell transplantation: Metastatic breast cancer, non-Hodgkin lymphoma, Hodgkin lymphoma, multiple myeloma

Orphan drug:

Acute myelogenous leukemia (AML) following induction chemotherapy in older adults to shorten time to neutrophil recovery and to reduce the incidence of severe and life-threatening infections and infections resulting in death

Bone marrow transplant (allogeneic or autologous) failure or engraftment delay

Safety and efficacy of GM-CSF given simultaneously with cytotoxic chemotherapy have not been established. Concurrent treatment may increase myelosuppression.

Usual Dosage

Children and Adults: I.V. infusion over ≥2 hours or SubQ

Existing clinical data suggest that starting GM-CSF between 24 and 72 hours subsequent to chemotherapy may provide optimal neutrophil recover; continue therapy until the occurrence of an absolute neutrophil count of 10,000/µL after the neutrophil nadir

The available data suggest that rounding the dose to the nearest vial size may enhance patient convenience and reduce costs without clinical detriment

Myeloid reconstitution after peripheral stem cell, allogeneic or autologous bone marrow transplant: I.V.: 250 mcg/m^2/day for 21 days to begin 2-4 hours after the marrow infusion on day 0 of autologous bone marrow transplant or ≥24 hours after chemotherapy or 12 hours after last dose of radiotherapy

If a severe adverse reaction occurs, reduce or temporarily discontinue the dose until the reaction abates

If blast cells appear or progression of the underlying disease occurs, disrupt treatment

Interrupt or reduce the dose by half if ANC is >20,000 cells/mm^3

Patients should not receive sargramostim until the postmarrow infusion ANC is <500 cells/mm^3

Neutrophil recovery following chemotherapy in AML: I.V.: 250 mcg/m^2/day over a 4-hour period starting approximately day 11 or 4 days following the completion of induction chemotherapy, if day 10 bone marrow is hypoblastic with <5% blasts

If a second cycle of chemotherapy is necessary, administer ~4 days after the completion of chemotherapy if the bone marrow is hypoblastic with <5% blasts

Continue sargramostim until ANC is >1500 cells/mm^3 for consecutive days or a maximum of 42 days

Discontinue sargramostim immediately if leukemic regrowth occurs

If a severe adverse reaction occurs, reduce the dose by 50% or temporarily discontinue the dose until the reaction abates

Mobilization of peripheral blood progenitor cells: I.V.: 250 mcg/m^2/day over 24 hours or SubQ once daily

Continue the same dose through the period of PBPC collection

The optimal schedule for PBPC collection has not been established (usually begun by day 5 and performed daily until protocol specified targets are achieved)

If WBC >50,000 cells/mm^3, reduce the dose by 50%

If adequate numbers of progenitor cells are not collected, consider other mobilization therapy

(Continued)

sargramostim *(Continued)*

Postperipheral blood progenitor cell transplantation: I.V.: 250 mcg/m^2/day over 24 hours or SubQ once daily beginning immediately following infusion of progenitor cells and continuing until ANC is >1500 for 3 consecutive days is attained

BMT failure or engraftment delay: I.V.: 250 mcg/m^2/day for 14 days as a 2-hour infusion

The dose can be repeated after 7 days off therapy if engraftment has not occurred

If engraftment still has not occurred, a third course of 500 mcg/m^2/day for 14 days may be tried after another 7 days off therapy; if there is still no improvement, it is unlikely that further dose escalation will be beneficial

If a severe adverse reaction occurs, reduce or temporarily discontinue the dose until the reaction abates

If blast cells appear or disease progression occurs, discontinue treatment

Dosage Forms

Injection, powder for reconstitution: 250 mcg

Injection, solution: 500 mcg/mL (1 mL) [contains benzyl alcohol]

Sarnol®-HC [US] *see* hydrocortisone (topical) *on page 451*

SB-265805 *see* gemifloxacin *on page 400*

SC 33428 *see* idarubicin *on page 464*

Scabene® ***(Discontinued)*** *see page 1042*

SCH 13521 *see* flutamide *on page 382*

Scheinpharm B12 [Can] *see* cyanocobalamin *on page 232*

S-citalopram *see* escitalopram *on page 322*

Sclavo Test - PPD® ***(Discontinued)*** *see page 1042*

Scleromate™ [US] *see* morrhuate sodium *on page 593*

Scopace™ [US] *see* scopolamine *on this page*

scopolamine (skoe POL a meen)

Synonyms hyoscine; scopolamine hydrobromide

U.S./Canadian Brand Names Buscopan® [Can]; Isopto® Hyoscine [US]; Scopace™ [US]; Transderm Scōp® [US]; Transderm-V® [Can]

Therapeutic Category Anticholinergic Agent

Use Preoperative medication to produce amnesia and decrease salivary and respiratory secretions; to produce cycloplegia and mydriasis; treatment of iridocyclitis; prevention of motion sickness; prevention of nausea/vomiting associated with anesthesia or opiate analgesia (patch); symptomatic treatment of postencephalitic parkinsonism and paralysis agitans (oral); inhibits excessive motility and hypertonus of the genitourinary or gastrointestinal tract in such conditions as the irritable colon syndrome, mild dysentery, diverticulitis, pylorospasm, and cardiospasm

Usual Dosage

Preoperatively:

Children: I.M., SubQ: 6 mcg/kg/dose (maximum: 0.3 mg/dose) or 0.2 mg/m^2 may be repeated every 6-8 hours **or** alternatively:

4-7 months: 0.1 mg

7 months to 3 years: 0.15 mg

3-8 years: 0.2 mg

8-12 years: 0.3 mg

Adults:

I.M., I.V., SubQ: 0.3-0.65 mg; may be repeated every 4-6 hours

Transdermal patch: Apply 2.5 cm^2 patch to hairless area behind ear the night before surgery or 1 hour prior to cesarean section (the patch should be applied no sooner than 1 hour before surgery for best results and removed 24 hours after surgery)

Motion sickness: Transdermal: Children >12 years and Adults: Apply 1 disc behind the ear at least 4 hours prior to exposure and every 3 days as needed; effective if applied as soon as 2-3 hours before anticipated need, best if 12 hours before

Ophthalmic:

Refraction:

Children: Instill 1 drop of 0.25% to eye(s) twice daily for 2 days before procedure

Adults: Instill 1-2 drops of 0.25% to eye(s) 1 hour before procedure

Iridocyclitis:

Children: Instill 1 drop of 0.25% to eye(s) up to 3 times/day

Adults: Instill 1-2 drops of 0.25% to eye(s) up to 4 times/day

Parkinsonism, spasticity, motion sickness: Oral: 0.4-0.8 mg as a range; the dosage may be cautiously increased in parkinsonism and spastic states.

Gastrointestinal/genitourinary spasm (Buscopan® [available in Canada; not available in the U.S.]): Adults:

Oral: 10-20 mg daily (1-2 tablets); maximum: 6 tablets/day

I.M., I.V., SubQ: 10-20 mg; maximum: 100 mg/day

Dosage Forms

Injection, solution, as hydrobromide: 0.4 mg/mL (1 mL)

Injection, solution, as hyoscine-N-butylbromide (Buscopan® [available in Canada; not available in U.S.]): 20 mg/mL

Solution, ophthalmic, as hydrobromide (Isopto® Hyoscine): 0.25% (5 mL, 15 mL) [contains benzalkonium chloride]

Tablet, as hyoscine-N-butylbromide (Buscopan® [available in Canada; not available in U.S.]): 10 mg

Tablet, soluble, as hydrobromide (Scopace™): 0.4 mg

Transdermal system (Transderm Scōp®): 1.5 mg (4s) [releases ~1 mg over 72 hours]

scopolamine and phenylephrine *see* phenylephrine and scopolamine *on page 690*

scopolamine hydrobromide *see* scopolamine *on previous page*

scopolamine, hyoscyamine, atropine, and phenobarbital *see* hyoscyamine, atropine, scopolamine, and phenobarbital *on page 460*

Scot-Tussin DM® Cough Chasers [US-OTC] *see* dextromethorphan *on page 261*

Scot-Tussin® Expectorant [US-OTC] *see* guaifenesin *on page 415*

SDZ ENA 713 *see* rivastigmine *on page 781*

SeaMist® [US-OTC] *see* sodium chloride *on page 810*

Seasonale® [US] *see* ethinyl estradiol and levonorgestrel *on page 339*

Seba-Gel™ [US] *see* benzoyl peroxide *on page 109*

Sebcur® [Can] *see* salicylic acid *on page 789*

Sebcur/T® [Can] *see* coal tar and salicylic acid *on page 220*

Sebizon® *(Discontinued)* *see page 1042*

secobarbital (see koe BAR bi tal)

Sound-Alike/Look-Alike Issues

Seconal® may be confused with Sectral®

Synonyms quinalbarbitone sodium; secobarbital sodium

U.S./Canadian Brand Names Seconal® [US]

Therapeutic Category Barbiturate

Controlled Substance C-II

Use Preanesthetic agent; short-term treatment of insomnia

Usual Dosage Oral:

Children:

Preoperative sedation: 2-6 mg/kg (maximum dose: 100 mg/dose) 1-2 hours before procedure

(Continued)

secobarbital *(Continued)*

Sedation: 6 mg/kg/day divided every 8 hours

Adults:

Hypnotic: Usual: 100 mg/dose at bedtime; range 100-200 mg/dose

Preoperative sedation: 100-300 mg 1-2 hours before procedure

Dosage Forms Capsule, as sodium: 100 mg

secobarbital and amobarbital *see* amobarbital and secobarbital *on page 51*

secobarbital sodium *see* secobarbital *on previous page*

Seconal® [US] *see* secobarbital *on previous page*

Secran® ***(Discontinued)*** *see page 1042*

SecreFlo™ [US] *see* secretin *on this page*

secretin (SEE kre tin)

Synonyms secretin, human; secretin, porcine

U.S./Canadian Brand Names SecreFlo™ [US]

Therapeutic Category Diagnostic Agent

Use Secretin-stimulation testing to aid in diagnosis of pancreatic exocrine dysfunction; diagnosis of gastrinoma (Zollinger-Ellison syndrome); facilitation of ERCP visualization

Usual Dosage I.V.: Adults: **Note:** A test dose of 0.2 mcg (0.1 mL) is injected to test for possible allergy. Dosing may be completed if no reaction occurs after 1 minute.

Diagnosis of pancreatic dysfunction, facilitation of ERCP: 0.2 mcg/kg over 1 minute

Diagnosis of gastrinoma: 0.4 mcg/kg over 1 minute

Dosage Forms

Injection, powder for reconstitution [human]: 16 mcg

Injection, powder for reconstitution [porcine] (SecreFlo™): 16 mcg

secretin, human *see* secretin *on this page*

secretin, porcine *see* secretin *on this page*

Sectral® [US/Can] *see* acebutolol *on page 4*

Selax® [Can] *see* docusate *on page 285*

Seldane® ***(Discontinued)*** *see page 1042*

Seldane-D® ***(Discontinued)*** *see page 1042*

Selecor® ***(Discontinued)*** *see page 1042*

Select™ 1/35 [Can] *see* ethinyl estradiol and norethindrone *on page 342*

Selectol® ***(Discontinued)*** *see page 1042*

selegiline (seh LEDGE ah leen)

Sound-Alike/Look-Alike Issues

selegiline may be confused with Serentil®, sertraline, Serzone®, Stelazine®

Eldepryl® may be confused with Elavil®, enalapril

Synonyms deprenyl; L-deprenyl; selegiline hydrochloride

U.S./Canadian Brand Names Apo-Selegiline® [Can]; Eldepryl® [US/Can]; Gen-Selegiline [Can]; Novo-Selegiline [Can]; Nu-Selegiline [Can]

Therapeutic Category Anti-Parkinson Agent; Dopaminergic Agent (Anti-Parkinson)

Use Adjunct in the management of parkinsonian patients in which levodopa/carbidopa therapy is deteriorating

Usual Dosage Oral: Adults: Parkinson disease: 5 mg twice daily with breakfast and lunch or 10 mg in the morning

Dosage Forms

Capsule, as hydrochloride (Eldepryl®): 5 mg

Tablet, as hydrochloride: 5 mg

selegiline hydrochloride *see* selegiline *on this page*

selenium *see* trace metals *on page 874*

selenium sulfide (se LEE nee um SUL fide)

U.S./Canadian Brand Names Head & Shoulders® Intensive Treatment [US-OTC]; Selsun® [US]; Selsun Blue® 2-in-1 Treatment [US-OTC]; Selsun Blue® Balanced Treatment [US-OTC]; Selsun Blue® Medicated Treatment [US-OTC]; Selsun Blue® Moisturizing Treatment [US-OTC]; Versel® [Can]

Therapeutic Category Antiseborrheic Agent, Topical

Use Treatment of itching and flaking of the scalp associated with dandruff, to control scalp seborrheic dermatitis; treatment of tinea versicolor

Usual Dosage Topical:

Dandruff, seborrhea: Massage 5-10 mL into wet scalp, leave on scalp 2-3 minutes, rinse thoroughly

Tinea versicolor: Apply the 2.5% lotion to affected area and lather with small amounts of water; leave on skin for 10 minutes, then rinse thoroughly; apply every day for 7 days

Dosage Forms [DSC] = Discontinued product

Lotion, topical: 2.5% (120 mL)

Shampoo, topical: 1% (210 mL)

Exsel® [DSC], Selsun®: 2.5% (120 mL)

Head & Shoulders® Intensive Treatment: 1% (400 mL)

Selsun Blue® Balanced Treatment, Selsun Blue® Medicated Treatment, Selsun Blue® Moisturizing Treatment, Selsun Blue® 2-in-1 Treatment: 1% (120 mL, 210 mL, 330 mL)

Selepen® [US] *see* trace metals *on page 874*

Selestoject® ***(Discontinued)*** *see page 1042*

Selpak® ***(Discontinued)*** *see page 1042*

Selsun® [US] *see* selenium sulfide *on this page*

Selsun Blue® 2-in-1 Treatment [US-OTC] *see* selenium sulfide *on this page*

Selsun Blue® Balanced Treatment [US-OTC] *see* selenium sulfide *on this page*

Selsun Blue® Medicated Treatment [US-OTC] *see* selenium sulfide *on this page*

Selsun Blue® Moisturizing Treatment [US-OTC] *see* selenium sulfide *on this page*

Selsun Gold® for Women ***(Discontinued)*** *see page 1042*

Semicid® [US-OTC] *see* nonoxynol 9 *on page 626*

Semprex®-D [US] *see* acrivastine and pseudoephedrine *on page 17*

Senexon® [US-OTC] *see* senna *on this page*

senna (SEN na)

Sound-Alike/Look-Alike Issues

Senexon® may be confused with Cenestin®

Senokot® may be confused with Depakote®

U.S./Canadian Brand Names Agoral® Maximum Strength Laxative [US-OTC]; Evac-U-Gen [US-OTC]; ex-lax® Maximum Strength [US-OTC]; ex-lax® [US-OTC]; Fletcher's® Castoria® [US-OTC]; Senexon® [US-OTC]; Senna-Gen® [US-OTC]; Sennatural™ [US-OTC]; Senokot® Children's [US-OTC]; Senokot® [US-OTC]; SenokotXTRA® [US-OTC]; X-Prep® [US-OTC]

Therapeutic Category Laxative

Use Short-term treatment of constipation; evacuate the colon for bowel or rectal examinations

(Continued)

senna *(Continued)*

Usual Dosage Oral:

Bowel evacuation: OTC labeling: Children ≥12 years and Adults: Usual dose: Sennosides 130 mg (X-Prep® 75 mL) between 2-4 PM the afternoon of the day prior to procedure

Constipation: OTC ranges:

Children :

2-6 years: Sennosides: Initial: 3.75 mg once daily (maximum: 15 mg/day, divided twice daily) Senna concentrate: 33.3 mg/mL: 5-10 mL up to twice daily

6-12 years: Sennosides: Initial: 8.6 mg once daily (maximum: 50 mg/day, divided twice daily) Senna concentrate: 33.3 mg/mL: 10-30 mL up to twice daily

Children ≥12 years and Adults: Sennosides 15 mg once daily (maximum: 70-100 mg/day, divided twice daily)

Dosage Forms

Granules (Senokot®): Sennosides 15 mg/teaspoon (60 g, 180 g, 360 g) [cocoa flavor]

Liquid:

Agoral® Maximum Strength Laxative: Sennosides 25 mg/15 mL (480 mL) [contains sodium 19.6 mg/15 mL; marshmallow and raspberry flavors]

X-Prep®: Sennosides 8.8 mg/5 mL (75 mL) [alcohol free; contains sugar 50 g/75 mL; available individually or in a kit]

Liquid concentrate:

Fletcher's® Castoria®: Senna concentrate 33.3 mg/mL (75 mL) [alcohol free; contains sodium benzoate; root beer flavor]

Syrup:

Senokot®: Sennosides 8.8 mg/5 mL (240 mL) [alcohol free; cocoa flavor]

Senokot® Children's: Sennosides 8.8 mg/5 mL (74 mL) [alcohol free; chocolate flavor]

Tablet: Sennosides 8.6 mg

ex-lax®: Sennosides USP 15 mg [contains sodium benzoate]

ex-lax® Maximum Strength: Sennosides USP 25 mg [contains sodium benzoate]

Sennatural™, Senokot®, Senexon®, Senna-Gen®: Sennosides 8.6 mg

SenokotXTRA®: Sennosides 17 mg

Tablet, chewable:

ex-lax®: Sennosides USP 15 mg [chocolate flavor]

Evac-U-Gen: Sennosides 10 mg

senna and docusate *see* docusate and senna *on page 286*

Senna-Gen® [US-OTC] *see* senna *on previous page*

senna-S *see* docusate and senna *on page 286*

Sennatural™ [US-OTC] *see* senna *on previous page*

Senokot® Children's [US-OTC] *see* senna *on previous page*

Senokot-S® [US-OTC] *see* docusate and senna *on page 286*

Senokot® [US-OTC] *see* senna *on previous page*

SenokotXTRA® [US-OTC] *see* senna *on previous page*

Senolax® *(Discontinued)* *see page 1042*

Sensipar™ [US] *see* cinacalcet *on page 200*

Sensorcaine® [US/Can] *see* bupivacaine *on page 133*

Sensorcaine®-MPF [US] *see* bupivacaine *on page 133*

Septa® Topical Ointment *(Discontinued)* *see page 1042*

Septisol® *(Discontinued)* *see page 1042*

Septra® [US/Can] *see* sulfamethoxazole and trimethoprim *on page 831*

Septra® DS [US/Can] *see* sulfamethoxazole and trimethoprim *on page 831*

Septra® Injection [Can] *see* sulfamethoxazole and trimethoprim *on page 831*

Ser-A-Gen® *(Discontinued)* *see page 1042*

Ser-Ap-Es® *(Discontinued)* *see page 1042*

Serax® [US] *see* oxazepam *on page 653*

Serc® [Can] *see* betahistine *(Canada only)* *on page 114*

Serentil® *(Discontinued)* *see page 1042*

Serentil® [Can] *see* mesoridazine *on page 557*

Serevent® *(Discontinued)* *see page 1042*

Serevent® [Can] *see* salmeterol *on page 793*

Serevent® Diskus® [US] *see* salmeterol *on page 793*

sermorelin acetate (ser moe REL in AS e tate)

U.S./Canadian Brand Names Geref® Diagnostic [US]

Therapeutic Category Diagnostic Agent

Use

Geref® Diagnostic: For evaluation of the ability of the pituitary gland to secrete growth hormone (GH)

Geref® injection: Treatment of idiopathic growth hormone deficiency in children

Orphan drug: Sermorelin has been designated an orphan product for AIDS-associated catabolism or weight loss, and as an adjunct to gonadotropin on ovulation induction.

Usual Dosage

Children: Treatment of idiopathic growth hormone deficiency: SubQ: 30 mcg/kg at bedtime; discontinue when epiphyses are fused

Children and Adults: Diagnostic: I.V.: 1 mcg/kg as a single dose in the morning following an overnight fast

Note: Response to diagnostic test may be decreased in patients >40 years

Dosage Forms [DSC] = Discontinued product

Injection, powder for reconstitution:

Geref® [DSC]: 0.5 mg, 1 mg

Geref® Diagnostic: 50 mcg

Seromycin® [US] *see* cycloserine *on page 235*

Serophene® [US/Can] *see* clomiphene *on page 214*

Seroquel® [US/Can] *see* quetiapine *on page 755*

Serostim® [US/Can] *see* human growth hormone *on page 437*

Serpalan® *(Discontinued)* *see page 1042*

Serpasil® *(Discontinued)* *see page 1042*

Serpatabs® *(Discontinued)* *see page 1042*

sertaconazole (ser ta KOE na zole)

Synonyms sertaconazole nitrate

U.S./Canadian Brand Names Ertaczo™ [US]

Therapeutic Category Antifungal Agent, Topical

Use Topical treatment of tinea pedis (athlete's foot)

Usual Dosage Topical: Children ≥12 years and Adults: Apply between toes and to surrounding healthy skin twice daily for 4 weeks

Dosage Forms Cream, topical, as nitrate: 2% (15 g, 30 g)

sertaconazole nitrate *see* sertaconazole *on this page*

sertraline (SER tra leen)

Sound-Alike/Look-Alike Issues

sertraline may be confused with Serentil®

Zoloft® may be confused with Zocor®

Synonyms sertraline hydrochloride

(Continued)

sertraline *(Continued)*

U.S./Canadian Brand Names Apo-Sertraline® [Can]; Gen-Sertraline [Can]; Novo-Sertraline [Can]; Nu-Sertraline [Can]; PMS-Sertraline [Can]; ratio-Sertraline [Can]; Rhoxal-sertraline [Can]; Zoloft® [US/Can]

Therapeutic Category Antidepressant, Selective Serotonin Reuptake Inhibitor

Use Treatment of major depression; obsessive-compulsive disorder (OCD); panic disorder; post-traumatic stress disorder (PTSD); premenstrual dysphoric disorder (PMDD); social anxiety disorder

Usual Dosage Oral:

Children and Adolescents: OCD:

6-12 years: Initial: 25 mg once daily

13-17 years: Initial: 50 mg once daily

Note: May increase daily dose, at intervals of not less than 1 week, to a maximum of 200 mg/day. If somnolence is noted, give at bedtime.

Adults:

Depression/OCD: Oral: Initial: 50 mg/day (see "Note" above)

Panic disorder, PTSD, social anxiety disorder: Initial: 25 mg once daily; increase to 50 mg once daily after 1 week (see "Note" above)

PMDD: 50 mg/day either daily throughout menstrual cycle **or** limited to the luteal phase of menstrual cycle, depending on physician assessment. Patients not responding to 50 mg/day may benefit from dose increases (50 mg increments per menstrual cycle) up to 150 mg/day when dosing throughout menstrual cycle **or** up to 100 mg day when dosing during luteal phase only. If a 100 mg/day dose has been established with luteal phase dosing, a 50 mg/day titration step for 3 days should be utilized at the beginning of each luteal phase dosing period.

Dosage Forms Note: Available as sertraline hydrochloride; mg strength refers to sertraline

Solution, oral concentrate: 20 mg/mL (60 mL) [contains alcohol 12%]

Tablet: 25 mg, 50 mg, 100 mg

sertraline hydrochloride *see* sertraline *on previous page*

Serutan® [US-OTC] *see* psyllium *on page 749*

Serzone® ***(Discontinued)*** *see page 1042*

sevelamer (se VEL a mer)

Sound-Alike/Look-Alike Issues

Renagel® may be confused with Reglan®, Regonol®

Synonyms sevelamer hydrochloride

U.S./Canadian Brand Names Renagel® [US/Can]

Therapeutic Category Phosphate Binder

Use Reduction of serum phosphorous in patients with end-stage renal disease

Usual Dosage Adults: Oral: Patients not taking a phosphate binder: 800-1600 mg 3 times/day with meals; the initial dose may be based on serum phosphorous:

(Phosphorous: Initial Dose:)

>6 mg/dL and <7.5 mg/dL: 800 mg 3 times/day

≥7.5 mg/dL and <9 mg/dL: 1200-1600 mg 3 times/day

≥9.0 mg/dL: 1600 mg 3 times/day

Dosage should be adjusted based on serum phosphorous concentration, with a goal of lowering to <6 mg/dL; maximum daily dose studied was equivalent to 30 capsules/day

Dosage Forms

Capsule, as hydrochloride: 403 mg

Tablet, as hydrochloride: 400 mg, 800 mg

sevelamer hydrochloride *see* sevelamer *on this page*

sevoflurane (see voe FLOO rane)

Sound-Alike/Look-Alike Issues

Ultane® may be confused with Ultram®

U.S./Canadian Brand Names Sevorane AF™ [Can]; Ultane® [US]

Therapeutic Category General Anesthetic

Use Induction and maintenance of general anesthesia in pediatric and adult patients (inhalation); sevoflurane is less irritating to the airway and therefore is useful to induce general anesthesia

Usual Dosage Minimum alveolar concentration (MAC), the concentration at which 50% of patients do not respond to surgical incision, is 2.6% (25 years of age) for sevoflurane. The concentration at which amnesia and loss of awareness occur (MAC - awake) is 0.6%. MAC is reduced in the elderly (50% reduction by age 80).

Dosage Forms Liquid for inhalation: 250 mL

Sevorane AF™ [Can] *see* sevoflurane *on this page*

Shur-Seal® [US-OTC] *see* nonoxynol 9 *on page 626*

Siblin® *(Discontinued)* *see page 1042*

sibutramine (si BYOO tra meen)

Synonyms sibutramine hydrochloride monohydrate

U.S./Canadian Brand Names Meridia® [US/Can]

Therapeutic Category Anorexiant

Use Management of obesity, including weight loss and maintenance of weight loss, and should be used in conjunction with a reduced calorie diet

Usual Dosage Adults ≥16 years: Initial: 10 mg once daily; after 4 weeks may titrate up to 15 mg once daily as needed and tolerated (may be used for up to 2 years, per manufacturer labeling)

Dosage Forms Capsule, as hydrochloride: 5 mg, 10 mg, 15 mg

sibutramine hydrochloride monohydrate *see* sibutramine *on this page*

Silace [US-OTC] *see* docusate *on page 285*

Siladryl® Allergy [US-OTC] *see* diphenhydramine *on page 277*

Silafed® [US-OTC] *see* triprolidine and pseudoephedrine *on page 889*

Silain® *(Discontinued)* *see page 1042*

Silaminic® Cold Syrup *(Discontinued)* *see page 1042*

Silaminic® Expectorant *(Discontinued)* *see page 1042*

Silapap® Children's [US-OTC] *see* acetaminophen *on page 5*

Silapap® Infants [US-OTC] *see* acetaminophen *on page 5*

Sildec [US] *see* carbinoxamine and pseudoephedrine *on page 157*

sildenafil (sil DEN a fil)

Sound-Alike/Look-Alike Issues

Viagra® may be confused with Allegra®, Vaniqa™

Synonyms UK92480

U.S./Canadian Brand Names Viagra® [US/Can]

Therapeutic Category Phosphodiesterase (Type 5) Enzyme Inhibitor

Use Treatment of erectile dysfunction

Usual Dosage Adults: Oral: Erectile dysfunction: For most patients, the recommended dose is 50 mg taken as needed, approximately 1 hour before sexual activity. However, sildenafil may be taken anywhere from 30 minutes to 4 hours before sexual activity. Based on effectiveness and tolerance, the dose may be increased to a maximum recommended dose of 100 mg or decreased to 25 mg. The maximum recommended dosing frequency is once daily.

Dosage Forms Tablet, as citrate: 25 mg, 50 mg, 100 mg

Sildicon-E® *(Discontinued)* *see page 1042*

Silexin® [US-OTC] *see* guaifenesin and dextromethorphan *on page 416*

Silfedrine Children's [US-OTC] *see* pseudoephedrine *on page 745*

Silphen DM® [US-OTC] *see* dextromethorphan *on page 261*

Silphen® [US-OTC] *see* diphenhydramine *on page 277*

Sil-Tex [US] *see* guaifenesin and phenylephrine *on page 418*

Siltussin-CF® *(Discontinued)* *see page 1042*

Siltussin DAS [US-OTC] *see* guaifenesin *on page 415*

Siltussin SA [US-OTC] *see* guaifenesin *on page 415*

Silvadene® [US] *see* silver sulfadiazine *on this page*

silver nitrate (SIL ver NYE trate)

Synonyms $AgNO_3$

Therapeutic Category Topical Skin Product

Use Cauterization of wounds and sluggish ulcers, removal of granulation tissue and warts; aseptic prophylaxis of burns

Usual Dosage Children and Adults:

Sticks: Apply to mucous membranes and other moist skin surfaces only on area to be treated 2-3 times/week for 2-3 weeks

Topical solution: Apply a cotton applicator dipped in solution on the affected area 2-3 times/week for 2-3 weeks

Dosage Forms

Applicator sticks, topical: Silver nitrate 75% and potassium nitrate 25% (6", 12", 18")

Solution, topical: 10% (30 mL); 25% (30 mL); 50% (30 mL)

silver sulfadiazine (SIL ver sul fa DYE a zeen)

U.S./Canadian Brand Names Dermazin™ [Can]; Flamazine® [Can]; Silvadene® [US]; SSD® [US/Can]; SSD® AF [US]; Thermazene® [US]

Therapeutic Category Antibacterial, Topical

Use Prevention and treatment of infection in second- and third-degree burns

Usual Dosage Children and Adults: Topical: Apply once or twice daily with a sterile-gloved hand; apply to a thickness of $^1/_{16}$"; burned area should be covered with cream at all times

Dosage Forms

Cream, topical: 1% [10 mg/g] (25 g, 85 g, 400 g)

Silvadene®, Thermazene®: 1% (20 g, 50 g, 85 g, 400 g, 1000 g)

SSD®: 1% (25 g, 50 g, 85 g, 400 g)

SSD AF®: 1% (50 g, 400 g)

simethicone (sye METH i kone)

Sound-Alike/Look-Alike Issues

simethicone may be confused with cimetidine

Mylicon® may be confused with Modicon®, Myleran®

Phazyme® may be confused with Pherazine®

Synonyms activated dimethicone; activated methylpolysiloxane

U.S./Canadian Brand Names Alka-Seltzer® Gas Relief [US-OTC]; Baby Gasz [US-OTC]; Flatulex® [US-OTC]; Gas-X® Extra Strength [US-OTC]; Gas-X® [US-OTC]; Genasyme® [US-OTC]; Mylanta® Gas Maximum Strength [US-OTC]; Mylanta® Gas [US-OTC]; Mylicon® Infants [US-OTC]; Ovol® [Can]; Phazyme™ [Can]; Phazyme® Quick Dissolve [US-OTC]; Phazyme® Ultra Strength [US-OTC]

Therapeutic Category Antiflatulent

Use Relieves flatulence and functional gastric bloating, and postoperative gas pains

Usual Dosage Oral:

Infants: 20 mg 4 times/day

Children <12 years: 40 mg 4 times/day

Children >12 years and Adults: 40-120 mg after meals and at bedtime as needed, not to exceed 500 mg/day

Dosage Forms

Softgels:

Alka-Seltzer® Gas Relief, Gas-X® Extra Strength, Mylanta® Gas Maximum Strength: 125 mg

Phazyme® Ultra Strength: 180 mg

Suspension, oral drops: 40 mg/0.6 mL (30 mL)

Baby Gasz, Genasym®: 40 mg/0.6 mL (30 mL)

Flatulex®: 40 mg/0.6 mL (30 mL) [fruit flavor]

Mylicon® Infants: 40 mg/0.6 mL (30 mL) [alcohol free; contains sodium benzoate; available in a non-staining formula]

Tablet, chewable: 80 mg, 125 mg

Gas-X®: 80 mg [peppermint crème or sodium free cherry crème flavor]

Gas-X® Extra Strength: 125 mg [peppermint crème or cherry crème flavor]

Genasyme®: 80 mg

Mylanta® Gas: 80 mg [mint flavor]

Mylanta® Gas Extra Strength: 125 mg [cherry and mint flavors]

Phazyme® Quick Dissolve: 125 mg [contains 0.4 mg phenylalanine (as aspartame)/tablet; mint flavor]

simethicone, aluminum hydroxide, and magnesium hydroxide *see* aluminum hydroxide, magnesium hydroxide, and simethicone *on page 40*

simethicone and calcium carbonate *see* calcium carbonate and simethicone *on page 146*

simethicone and magaldrate *see* magaldrate and simethicone *on page 536*

Simply Cough® [US-OTC] *see* dextromethorphan *on page 261*

Simply Saline™ [US-OTC] *see* sodium chloride *on page 810*

Simply Sleep® [Can] *see* diphenhydramine *on page 277*

Simulect® [US/Can] *see* basiliximab *on page 100*

simvastatin (SIM va stat in)

Sound-Alike/Look-Alike Issues

Zocor® may be confused with Cozaar®, Yocon®, Zoloft®

U.S./Canadian Brand Names Apo-Simvastatin® [Can]; Gen-Simvastatin [Can]; ratio-Simvastatin [Can]; Riva-Simvastatin [Can]; Zocor® [US/Can]

Therapeutic Category HMG-CoA Reductase Inhibitor

Use Used with dietary therapy for the following:

Secondary prevention of cardiovascular events in hypercholesterolemic patients with established coronary heart disease (CHD) or at high risk for CHD: To reduce cardiovascular morbidity (myocardial infarction, coronary revascularization procedures) and mortality; to reduce the risk of stroke and transient ischemic attacks

Hyperlipidemias: To reduce elevations in total cholesterol, LDL-C, apolipoprotein B, and triglycerides in patients with primary hypercholesterolemia (elevations of 1 or more components are present in Fredrickson type IIa, IIb, III, and IV hyperlipidemias); treatment of homozygous familial hypercholesterolemia

Heterozygous familial hypercholesterolemia (HeFH): In adolescent patients (10-17 years of age, females >1 year postmenarche) with HeFH having LDL-C ≥190 mg/dL **or** LDL ≥160 mg/dL with positive family history of premature cardiovascular disease (CVD), or 2 or more CVD risk factors in the adolescent patient

Usual Dosage Oral: **Note:** Doses should be individualized according to the baseline LDL-cholesterol levels, the recommended goal of therapy, and the patient's response; adjustments should be made at intervals of 4 weeks or more; doses may need adjusted based on concomitant medications

Children 10-17 years (females >1 year postmenarche): HeFH: 10 mg once daily in the evening; range: 10-40 mg/day (maximum: 40 mg/day)

(Continued)

simvastatin *(Continued)*

Dosage adjustment for simvastatin with concomitant cyclosporine, fibrates, niacin, amiodarone, or verapamil: Refer to drug-specific dosing in Adults dosing section

Adults:

Homozygous familial hypercholesterolemia: 40 mg once daily in the evening **or** 80 mg/day (given as 20 mg, 20 mg, and 40 mg evening dose)

Prevention of cardiovascular events, hyperlipidemias: 20-40 mg once daily in the evening; range: 5-80 mg/day

Patients requiring only moderate reduction of LDL-cholesterol may be started at 10 mg once daily

Patients requiring reduction of >45% in low-density lipoprotein (LDL) cholesterol may be started at 40 mg once daily in the evening

Patients with CHD or at high risk for CHD: Dosing should be started at 40 mg once daily in the evening; simvastatin may be started simultaneously with diet

Dosage adjustment with concomitant medications:

Cyclosporine: Initial: 5 mg simvastatin, should **not** exceed 10 mg/day

Fibrates or niacin: Simvastatin dose should **not** exceed 10 mg/day

Amiodarone or verapamil: Simvastatin dose should **not** exceed 20 mg/day

Dosage Forms Tablet: 5 mg, 10 mg, 20 mg, 40 mg, 80 mg

Sina-12X [US] *see* guaifenesin and phenylephrine *on page 418*

sincalide (SIN ka lide)

Synonyms C8-CCK; OP-CCK

U.S./Canadian Brand Names Kinevac® [US]

Therapeutic Category Diagnostic Agent

Use Postevacuation cholecystography; gallbladder bile sampling; stimulate pancreatic secretion for analysis

Usual Dosage Adults: I.V.:

Contraction of gallbladder: 0.02 mcg/kg over 30 seconds to 1 minute, may repeat in 15 minutes a 0.04 mcg/kg dose

Pancreatic function: 0.02 mcg/kg over 30 minutes administered after secretin

Dosage Forms Injection, powder for reconstitution: 5 mcg

Sine-Aid® IB *(Discontinued)* *see page 1042*

Sinemet® [US/Can] *see* levodopa and carbidopa *on page 513*

Sinemet® CR [US/Can] *see* levodopa and carbidopa *on page 513*

Sinequan® [US/Can] *see* doxepin *on page 292*

Singulair® [US/Can] *see* montelukast *on page 590*

Sinografin® [US] *see* radiological/contrast media (ionic) *on page 759*

Sinubid® *(Discontinued)* *see page 1042*

Sinufed® Timecelles® *(Discontinued)* *see page 1042*

Sinumed® *(Discontinued)* *see page 1042*

Sinumist®-SR Capsulets® *(Discontinued)* *see page 1042*

Sinus-Relief® [US-OTC] *see* acetaminophen and pseudoephedrine *on page 9*

Sinutab® Non Drowsy [Can] *see* acetaminophen and pseudoephedrine *on page 9*

Sinutab® Sinus & Allergy [Can] *see* acetaminophen, chlorpheniramine, and pseudoephedrine *on page 11*

Sinutab® Sinus Allergy Maximum Strength [US-OTC] *see* acetaminophen, chlorpheniramine, and pseudoephedrine *on page 11*

Sinutab® Sinus [US-OTC] *see* acetaminophen and pseudoephedrine *on page 9*

SINUvent® PE [US] *see* guaifenesin and phenylephrine *on page 418*

Sirdalud® *see* tizanidine *on page 866*

sirolimus (sir OH li mus)

U.S./Canadian Brand Names Rapamune® [US/Can]

Therapeutic Category Immunosuppressant Agent

Use Prophylaxis of organ rejection in patients receiving renal transplants, in combination with corticosteroids and cyclosporine (cyclosporine may be withdrawn in low-to-moderate immunological risk patients after 2-4 months, in conjunction with an increase in sirolimus dosage)

Usual Dosage Oral:

Children ≥13 years or Adults <40 kg: Loading dose: 3 mg/m^2 (day 1); followed by a maintenance of 1 mg/m^2/day.

Adults ≥40 kg: Loading dose: For *de novo* transplant recipients, a loading dose of 3 times the daily maintenance dose should be administered on day 1 of dosing. Maintenance dose: 2 mg/day. Doses should be taken 4 hours after cyclosporine, and should be taken consistently either with or without food.

Withdrawal of cyclosporine:

Following 2-4 months of combined therapy, withdrawal of cyclosporine may be considered in low-to-moderate risk patients. Cyclosporine withdrawal in not recommended in high immunological risk patients. Cyclosporine should be discontinued over 4-8 weeks, and a necessary increase in the dosage of sirolimus (up to fourfold) should be anticipated due to removal of metabolic inhibition by cyclosporine and to maintain adequate immunosuppressive effects.

Sirolimus dosages should be adjusted to maintain trough concentrations of 12-24 ng/mL. Dosage should be adjusted at intervals of 7-14 days to account for the long half-life of sirolimus. Considerable increases in dosage may require an additional loading dose, calculated as the difference between the target concentration and the current concentration, multiplied by a factor of 3. Loading doses >40 mg may be administered over two days. Serum concentrations should not be used as the sole basis for dosage adjustment (monitor clinical signs/symptoms, tissue biopsy, and laboratory parameters).

Dosage Forms

Solution, oral [bottle]: 1 mg/mL (60 mL, 150 mL) [contains ethanol 1.5% to 2.5%; packaged with 1 mL, 2 mL, or 5 mL oral syringes]

Solution, oral [unit-dose pouch]: 1 mg/mL (1 mL, 2 mL, 5 mL) [contains ethanol 1.5% to 2.5%; packaged in cartons of 30]

Tablet: 1 mg, 2 mg, 5 mg

SK *see* streptokinase *on page 823*

SK and F 104864 *see* topotecan *on page 872*

Skelaxin® [US/Can] *see* metaxalone *on page 560*

Skelex® ***(Discontinued)*** *see page 1042*

Skelid® [US] *see* tiludronate *on page 863*

SKF 104864 *see* topotecan *on page 872*

SKF 104864-A *see* topotecan *on page 872*

Sleep-eze 3® Oral ***(Discontinued)*** *see page 1042*

Sleepinal® [US-OTC] *see* diphenhydramine *on page 277*

Sleepwell 2-nite® ***(Discontinued)*** *see page 1042*

Slidec-DM [US] *see* carbinoxamine, pseudoephedrine, and dextromethorphan *on page 159*

Slim-Mint® ***(Discontinued)*** *see page 1042*

Slo-bid™ ***(Discontinued)*** *see page 1042*

Slo-Niacin® [US-OTC] *see* niacin *on page 616*

Slo-Phyllin® (all products) ***(Discontinued)*** *see page 1042*

Slo-Phyllin® GG ***(Discontinued)*** *see page 1042*

Slo-Salt® ***(Discontinued)*** *see page 1042*

Slow FE® [US-OTC] *see* ferrous sulfate *on page 364*

Slow-K® ***(Discontinued)*** *see page 1042*

Slow-K® [Can] *see* potassium chloride *on page 713*

Slow-Mag® [US-OTC] *see* magnesium chloride *on page 536*

Slow-Trasicor® [Can] *see* oxprenolol *(Canada only) on page 654*

smallpox vaccine (SMAL poks vak SEEN)

Synonyms dried smallpox vaccine; vaccinia vaccine

U.S./Canadian Brand Names Dryvax® [US]

Therapeutic Category Vaccine

Use Active immunization against vaccinia virus, the causative agent of smallpox. The ACIP recommends vaccination of laboratory workers at risk of exposure from cultures or contaminated animals which may be a source of vaccinia or related Orthopoxviruses capable of causing infections in humans (monkeypox, cowpox, or variola). Revaccination is recommended every 10 years. The Armed Forces recommend vaccination of certain personnel categories. Recommendations for use in response to bioterrorism are regularly updated by the CDC, and may be found at www.cdc.gov.

Usual Dosage Not for I.M., I.V., or SubQ injection: Vaccination by scarification (multiple-puncture technique) only: **Note:** A trace of blood should appear at vaccination site after 15-20 seconds; if no trace of blood is visible, an additional 3 insertions should be made using the same needle, without reinserting the needle into the vaccine bottle.

Adults (children ≥12 months in emergency conditions only):

Primary vaccination: Use a single drop of vaccine suspension and 2 or 3 needle punctures (using the same needle) into the superficial skin

Revaccination: Use a single drop of vaccine suspension and 15 needle punctures (using the same needle) into the superficial skin

Dosage Forms Injection, powder for reconstitution [calf liver source]: ~100 million vaccinia virions per mL following reconstitution [contains polymyxin B, neomycin, dihydrostreptomycin sulfate, and chlortetracycline (trace amounts); packed with diluent, venting needle, and 100 bifurcated needles]

smelling salts *see* ammonia spirit (aromatic) *on page 50*

SMZ-TMP *see* sulfamethoxazole and trimethoprim *on page 831*

snake (pit viper) antivenin *see* antivenin *(Crotalidae)* polyvalent *on page 67*

Snaplets-EX® ***(Discontinued)*** *see page 1042*

sodium 2-mercaptoethane sulfonate *see* mesna *on page 557*

sodium 4-hydroxybutyrate *see* sodium oxybate *on page 813*

sodium acetate (SOW dee um AS e tate)

Therapeutic Category Alkalinizing Agent; Electrolyte Supplement, Oral

Use Sodium source in large volume I.V. fluids to prevent or correct hyponatremia in patients with restricted intake; used to counter acidosis through conversion to bicarbonate

Usual Dosage Sodium acetate is metabolized to bicarbonate on an equimolar basis outside the liver; administer in large volume I.V. fluids as a sodium source. Refer to Sodium Bicarbonate monograph.

Maintenance electrolyte requirements of sodium in parenteral nutrition solutions:

Daily requirements: 3-4 mEq/kg/24 hours or 25-40 mEq/1000 kcal/24 hours

Maximum: 100-150 mEq/24 hours

Dosage Forms Injection, solution: 2 mEq/mL (20 mL, 50 mL, 100 mL, 250 mL); 4 mEq/mL (50 mL, 100 mL)

sodium acid carbonate *see* sodium bicarbonate *on this page*

sodium ascorbate (SOW dee um a SKOR bate)

Therapeutic Category Vitamin, Water Soluble

Use Prevention and treatment of scurvy and to acidify the urine; large doses may decrease the severity of "colds"

Usual Dosage Oral, I.V.:

Children:

Scurvy: 100-300 mg/day in divided doses for at least 2 weeks

Urinary acidification: 500 mg every 6-8 hours

Dietary supplement: 35-45 mg/day

Adults:

Scurvy: 100-250 mg 1-2 times/day for at least 2 weeks

Urinary acidification: 4-12 g/day in divided doses

Dietary supplement: 50-60 mg/day

Prevention and treatment of cold: 1-3 g/day

Dosage Forms Injection: 562.5 mg/mL [ascorbic acid 500 mg/mL] (1 mL, 2 mL)

sodium benzoate and caffeine *see* caffeine and sodium benzoate *on page 141*

sodium benzoate and sodium phenylacetate *see* sodium phenylacetate and sodium benzoate *on page 814*

sodium bicarbonate (SOW dee um bye KAR bun ate)

Synonyms baking soda; $NaHCO_3$; sodium acid carbonate; sodium hydrogen carbonate

U.S./Canadian Brand Names Brioschi® [US-OTC]; Neut® [US]

Therapeutic Category Alkalinizing Agent; Antacid; Electrolyte Supplement, Oral

Use Management of metabolic acidosis; gastric hyperacidity; as an alkalinization agent for the urine; treatment of hyperkalemia; management of overdose of certain drugs, including tricyclic antidepressants and aspirin

Usual Dosage

Cardiac arrest: **Routine use of $NaHCO_3$ is not recommended and should be given only after adequate alveolar ventilation has been established and effective cardiac compressions are provided**

Infants and Children: I.V.: 0.5-1 mEq/kg/dose repeated every 10 minutes or as indicated by arterial blood gases; rate of infusion should not exceed 10 mEq/minute; neonates and children <2 years of age should receive 4.2% (0.5 mEq/mL) solution

Adults: I.V.: Initial: 1 mEq/kg/dose one time; maintenance: 0.5 mEq/kg/dose every 10 minutes or as indicated by arterial blood gases

Metabolic acidosis: Infants, Children, and Adults: Dosage should be based on the following formula if blood gases and pH measurements are available:

HCO_3^-(mEq) = 0.3 x weight (kg) x base deficit (mEq/L)

Administer ½ dose initially, then remaining ½ dose over the next 24 hours; monitor pH, serum HCO_3^-, and clinical status

Note: If acid-base status is not available: Dose for older Children and Adults: 2-5 mEq/kg I.V. infusion over 4-8 hours; subsequent doses should be based on patient's acid-base status

Chronic renal failure: Oral: Initiate when plasma HCO_3^- <15 mEq/L

Children: 1-3 mEq/kg/day

Adults: Start with 20-36 mEq/day in divided doses, titrate to bicarbonate level of 18-20 mEq/L

Hyperkalemia: Adults: I.V.: 1 mEq/kg over 5 minutes

Renal tubular acidosis: Oral:

Distal:

Children: 2-3 mEq/kg/day

Adults: 0.5-2 mEq/kg/day in 4-5 divided doses

Proximal: Children and Adults: Initial: 5-10 mEq/kg/day; maintenance: Increase as required to maintain serum bicarbonate in the normal range

(Continued)

sodium bicarbonate *(Continued)*

Urine alkalinization: Oral:

Children: 1-10 mEq (84-840 mg)/kg/day in divided doses every 4-6 hours; dose should be titrated to desired urinary pH

Adults: Initial: 48 mEq (4 g), then 12-24 mEq (1-2 g) every 4 hours; dose should be titrated to desired urinary pH; doses up to 16 g/day (200 mEq) in patients <60 years and 8 g (100 mEq) in patients >60 years

Antacid: Adults: Oral: 325 mg to 2 g 1-4 times/day

Dosage Forms

Granules, effervescent (Brioschi®): 6 g, 120 g, 240 g [lemon flavor]

Infusion [premixed in sterile water]: 5% (500 mL)

Injection, solution:

4.2% [42 mg/mL = 5 mEq/10 mL] (10 mL)

5% [50 mg/mL = 5.95 mEq/10 mL] (500 mL)

7.5% [75 mg/mL = 8.92 mEq/10 mL] (50 mL)

8.4% [84 mg/mL = 10 mEq/10 mL] (10 mL, 50 mL)

Neut®: 4% [40 mg/mL = 2.4 mEq/5 mL] (5 mL)

Powder: 120 g, 480 g

Tablet: 325 mg [3.8 mEq]; 650 mg [7.6 mEq]

sodium cellulose phosphate *see* cellulose sodium phosphate *on page 175*

sodium chloride (SOW dee um KLOR ide)

Synonyms NaCl; normal saline; salt

U.S./Canadian Brand Names Altamist [US-OTC]; Ayr® Baby Saline [US-OTC]; Ayr® Saline Mist [US-OTC]; Ayr® Saline [US-OTC]; Breathe Right® Saline [US-OTC]; Broncho Saline® [US-OTC]; Entsol® [US-OTC]; Muro 128® [US-OTC]; Nasal Moist® [US-OTC]; NaSal™ [US-OTC]; Na-Zone® [US-OTC]; Ocean® [US-OTC]; Pediamist® [US-OTC]; Pretz® Irrigation [US-OTC]; SalineX® [US-OTC]; SeaMist® [US-OTC]; Simply Saline™ [US-OTC]; Wound Wash Saline™ [US-OTC]

Therapeutic Category Electrolyte Supplement, Oral; Lubricant, Ocular

Use

Parenteral: Restores sodium ion in patients with restricted oral intake (especially hyponatremia states or low salt syndrome). In general, parenteral saline uses:

Bacteriostatic sodium chloride: Dilution or dissolving drugs for I.M., I.V., or SubQ injections

Concentrated sodium chloride: Additive for parenteral fluid therapy

Hypertonic sodium chloride: For severe hyponatremia and hypochloremia

Hypotonic sodium chloride: Hydrating solution

Normal saline: Restores water/sodium losses

Pharmaceutical aid/diluent for infusion of compatible drug additives

Ophthalmic: Reduces corneal edema

Oral: Restores sodium losses

Inhalation: Restores moisture to pulmonary system; loosens and thins congestion caused by colds or allergies; diluent for bronchodilator solutions that require dilution before inhalation

Intranasal: Restores moisture to nasal membranes

Irrigation: Wound cleansing, irrigation, and flushing

Usual Dosage

Newborn electrolyte requirement:

Premature: 2-8 mEq/kg/24 hours

Term:

0-48 hours: 0-2 mEq/kg/24 hours

>48 hours: 1-4 mEq/kg/24 hours

Children: I.V.: Hypertonic solutions (>0.9%) should only be used for the initial treatment of acute serious symptomatic hyponatremia; maintenance: 3-4 mEq/kg/day; maximum: 100-150 mEq/day; dosage varies widely depending on clinical condition

Replacement: Determined by laboratory determinations mEq

Sodium deficiency (mEq/kg) = [% dehydration (L/kg)/100 x 70 (mEq/L) = [0.6 (L/kg) x (140 - serum sodium) (mEq/L)]

Nasal: Use as often as needed

Adults:

GI irrigant: 1-3 L/day by intermittent irrigation

Heat cramps: Oral: 0.5-1 g with full glass of water, up to 4.8 g/day

Replacement I.V.: Determined by laboratory determinations mEq

Sodium deficiency (mEq/kg) = [% dehydration (L/kg)/100 x 70 (mEq/L)] + [0.6 (L/kg) x (140 - serum sodium) (mEq/L)]

To correct acute, serious hyponatremia: mEq sodium = (desired sodium (mEq/L) - actual sodium (mEq/L) x 0.6 x wt (kg)); for acute correction use 125 mEq/L as the desired serum sodium; acutely correct serum sodium in 5 mEq/L/dose increments; more gradual correction in increments of 10 mEq/L/day is indicated in the asymptomatic patient

Chloride maintenance electrolyte requirement in parenteral nutrition: 2-4 mEq/kg/24 hours or 25-40 mEq/1000 kcals/24 hours; maximum: 100-150 mEq/24 hours

Sodium maintenance electrolyte requirement in parenteral nutrition: 3-4 mEq/kg/24 hours or 25-40 mEq/1000 kcals/24 hours; maximum: 100-150 mEq/24 hours.

Nasal: Use as often as needed

Ophthalmic:

Ointment: Apply once daily or more often

Solution: Instill 1-2 drops into affected eye(s) every 3-4 hours

Abortifacient: 20% (250 mL) administered by transabdominal intra-amniotic instillation

Dosage Forms

Gel, intranasal (Nasal Moist®): 0.65% (30 g)

Injection, solution: 0.45% (25 mL, 50 mL, 100 mL, 250 mL, 500 mL, 1000 mL, 1500 mL, 2000 mL); 0.9% (1 mL, 2 mL, 3 mL, 5 mL, 10 mL, 20 mL, 25 mL, 30 mL, 50 mL, 100 mL, 150 mL, 250 mL, 500 mL, 1000 mL); 2.5 % (250 mL); 3% (500 mL); 5% (500 mL)

Injection, solution [preservative free]: 0.9% (2 mL, 3 mL, 5 mL, 10 mL, 20 mL, 50 mL, 100 mL)

Injection, solution, bacteriostatic: 0.9% (10 mL, 20 mL, 30 mL)

Injection, solution, concentrate: 14.6% [2.5 mEq/mL] (20 mL, 40 mL, 250 mL); 23.4% [4 mEq/mL] (30 mL, 50 mL, 100 mL, 200 mL, 250 mL)

Ointment, ophthalmic (Muro-128®): 5% (3.5 g)

Powder, for nasal solution:

Broncho Saline®: 0.9% (90 mL, 240 mL)

Entsol®: 3% (10.5 g)

Solution, for inhalation: 0.45% (3 mL, 5 mL); 0.9% (3 mL, 5 mL, 15 mL); 3% (15 mL); 10% (15 mL)

Solution, intranasal: 0.65% (45 mL)

Altamist: 0.65% (60 mL) [spray]

Ayr® Baby Saline: 0.65% (30 mL) [spray/drops]

Ayr® Saline: 0.65% (50 mL) [drops]

Ayr® Saline Mist: 0.65% (50 mL) [spray]

Breathe Right® Saline: 0.65% (44 mL) [spray]

Entsol® [preservative free]: 3% (100 mL) [spray]

Entsol® Mist: 3% (30 mL) [spray]

Enstol® Single Use [preservative free]: 3% (240 mL) [nasal wash]

Na-Zone®: 0.75% (60 mL) [spray]

NāSal™: 0.65% (15 mL) [drops]; (30 mL) [spray]

Nasal Moist®: 0.65% (15 mL, 45 mL) [spray]

Ocean®: 0.65% (45 mL) [spray/drops]

Pediamist®: 0.5% (15 mL) [spray]

Pretz® Irrigation: 0.75% (240 mL)

SalineX®: 0.4% (15 mL) [drops]; (50 mL) [spray]

SeaMist®: 0.65% (15 mL) [spray]

Simply Saline™: 0.9% (44 mL) [mist]

Solution for irrigation: 0.45% (2000 mL); 0.9% (250 mL, 500 mL, 1000 mL, 1500 mL, 2000 mL, 3000 mL, 4000 mL, 5000 mL)

(Continued)

sodium chloride *(Continued)*

Wound Wash Saline™: 0.9% (90 mL, 210 mL)
Solution, ophthalmic: 5% (15 mL)
Muro-128®: 2% (15 mL), 5% (15 mL, 30 mL)
Tablet: 1 g

sodium citrate, citric acid, and potassium citrate *see* citric acid, sodium citrate, and potassium citrate *on page 206*

sodium edetate *see* edetate disodium *on page 303*

sodium etidronate *see* etidronate disodium *on page 350*

sodium ferric gluconate *see* ferric gluconate *on page 363*

sodium fluoride *see* fluoride *on page 376*

sodium fusidate *see* fusidic acid *(Canada only) on page 394*

sodium hyaluronate (SOW dee um hye al yoor ON nate)

Synonyms hyaluronic acid

Therapeutic Category Ophthalmic Agent, Viscoelastic

Use Surgical aid in cataract extraction, intraocular implantation, corneal transplant, glaucoma filtration, and retinal attachment surgery

Intraarticular injection (Hyalgan®, Suppartz™): Treatment of pain in osteoarthritis in knee in patients who have failed nonpharmacologic treatment and simple analgesics

Usual Dosage Depends upon procedure

Dosage Forms

Gel, topical (IPM Wound Gel™): 2.5% (10 g)
Injection, solution, intraarticular:
Hyalgan®: 10 mg/mL (2 mL)
Supartz™: 10 mg/mL (2.5 mL)
Injection, solution, intraocular:
Biolon™: 10 mg/mL (0.5 mL, 1 mL)
Healon GV®: 14 mg/mL (0.55 mL, 0.85 mL)
Provisc®: 10 mg/mL (0.4 mL, 0.55 mL, 0.8 mL) [prefilled syringe]
Vitrax®: 30 mg/mL (0.65 mL)

sodium hyaluronate-chrondroitin sulfate *see* chondroitin sulfate and sodium hyaluronate *on page 197*

sodium hyaluronate/hylan G-F 20

(SOW dee um hye al yoor ON ate/HYE lan gee-eff TWEN tee)

U.S./Canadian Brand Names Synvisc® [US/Can]

Therapeutic Category Miscellaneous Product

Use Treatment of pain in osteoarthritis of the knee in patients who have failed to respond adequately to conservative nonpharmacologic therapy and simple analgesics

Usual Dosage The recommended treatment regimen is 3 injections in the knee, 1 week apart. To achieve maximum effect, it is essential to administer all 3 injections. The maximum recommended dosage is 6 injections within 6 months, with a minimum of 4 weeks between treatment regimens. The duration of effect for those patients who respond to treatment is generally 12 to 26 weeks, although shorter and longer periods have also been observed. Synvisc® does not produce a general systemic effect.

Dosage Forms Injection: Hylan polymers 16 mg/2 mL; Each mL contains: hylan 8 mg, sodium chloride 8.5 mg, disodium hydrogen phosphate 0.16 mg, sodium dihydrogen phosphate hydrate 0.04 mg, sterile water for injection USP q.s.

sodium hydrogen carbonate *see* sodium bicarbonate *on page 809*

sodium hypochlorite solution

(SOW dee um hye poe KLOR ite soe LOO shun)

Synonyms modified Dakin's solution

U.S./Canadian Brand Names Dakin's Solution [US]

Therapeutic Category Disinfectant

Use Treatment of athlete's foot (0.5%); wound irrigation (0.5%); disinfection of utensils and equipment (5%)

Usual Dosage Topical irrigation

Dosage Forms Solution, topical (Dakin's): 0.25% (480 mL); 0.5% (480 mL, 3840 mL)

sodium hyposulfate *see* sodium thiosulfate *on page 817*

sodium lactate (SOW dee um LAK tate)

Therapeutic Category Alkalinizing Agent

Use Source of bicarbonate for prevention and treatment of mild to moderate metabolic acidosis

Usual Dosage Dosage depends on degree of acidosis

Dosage Forms Injection, solution:

560 mg/mL [sodium 5 mEq and lactate 5 mEq per mL] (10 mL)

1.87 g/100 mL [sodium 16.7 mEq and lactate 16.7 mEq per 100 mL] (500 mL, 1000 mL)

sodium *L*-triiodothyronine *see* liothyronine *on page 523*

sodium nafcillin *see* nafcillin *on page 600*

sodium nitrite, sodium thiosulfate, and amyl nitrite

(SOE dee um NYE trite, SOE dee um thy oh SUL fate, & A mil NYE trite)

Synonyms amyl nitrite, sodium thiosulfate, and sodium nitrite; sodium thiosulfate, sodium nitrite, and amyl nitrite

U.S./Canadian Brand Names Cyanide Antidote Package

Therapeutic Category Antidote

Use Treatment of cyanide poisoning

Usual Dosage Cyanide poisoning:

Children: 0.3 mL ampul of amyl nitrite is crushed every minute and vapor is inhaled for 15-30 seconds until an I.V. sodium nitrite infusion is available. Following administration of sodium nitrite I.V. 6-8 mL/m^2 (~0.2 mL/kg, maximum: 10 mL), inject sodium thiosulfate I.V. 7 g/m^2 (maximum 12.5 g) over ~10 minutes, if needed; injection of both may be repeated at ½ the original dose.

Adults: 0.3 mL ampul of amyl nitrite is crushed every minute and vapor is inhaled for 15-30 seconds until an I.V. sodium nitrite infusion is available. Following administration of 300 mg I.V. sodium nitrite, inject 12.5 g sodium thiosulfate I.V. (over ~10 minutes), if needed; injection of both may be repeated at ½ the original dose.

Dosage Forms

Kit [each kit contains] (Cyanide Antidote Package):

Injection, solution:

Sodium nitrite 300 mg/10 mL (2)

Sodium thiosulfate 12.5 g/50 mL (2)

Inhalant: Amyl nitrite 0.3 mL (12)

[kit also includes disposable syringes, stomach tube, tourniquet, and instructions]

sodium nitroferricyanide *see* nitroprusside *on page 624*

sodium nitroprusside *see* nitroprusside *on page 624*

sodium oxybate (SOW dee um ox i BATE)

Synonyms gamma hydroxybutyric acid; GHB; 4-hydroxybutyrate; sodium 4-hydroxybutyrate

U.S./Canadian Brand Names Xyrem® [US]

Therapeutic Category Central Nervous System Depressant

(Continued)

sodium oxybate *(Continued)*

Controlled Substance C-I (illicit use); C-III (medical use)

Sodium oxybate oral solution will be available only to prescribers enrolled in the Xyrem® Success Program℠ and dispensed to the patient through the designated centralized pharmacy. Prior to dispensing the first prescription, prescribers will be sent educational materials to be reviewed with the patient and enrollment forms for the postmarketing surveillance program. Patients must be seen at least every 3 months; prescriptions can be written for a maximum of 3 months (the first prescription may only be written for a 1-month supply).

Use **Orphan drug:** Treatment of cataplexy in patients with narcolepsy

Usual Dosage Oral: Children ≥16 years and Adults: Treatment of cataplexy in patients with narcolepsy: Initial: 4.5 g/day, in 2 equal doses; first dose to be given at bedtime after the patient is in bed, and second dose to be given 2.5-4 hours later. Dose may be increased or adjusted in 2-week intervals; average dose: 6-9 g/day (maximum: 9 g/day)

Dosage Forms Solution, oral: 500 mg/mL (180 mL) [supplied in a kit containing two dosing cups and measuring device]

Sodium P.A.S.® *(Discontinued)* *see page 1042*

sodium-PCA and lactic acid *see* lactic acid *on page 500*

sodium phenylacetate and sodium benzoate

(SOW dee um fen il AS e tate & SOW dee um BENZ oh ate)

Synonyms sodium benzoate and sodium phenylacetate

U.S./Canadian Brand Names Ucephan® [US]

Therapeutic Category Ammonium Detoxicant

Use **Orphan drug:** Adjunctive therapy to prevention/treatment of hyperammonemia in patients with urea cycle enzymopathy involving partial or complete deficiencies of carbamoyl-phosphate synthetase, ornithine transcarbamoylase, or argininosuccinate synthetase

Usual Dosage Infants and Children: Oral: 2.5 mL (250 mg sodium benzoate and 250 mg sodium phenylacetate)/kg/day divided 3-6 times/day; total daily dose should not exceed 100 mL

Dosage Forms Solution, oral: Sodium phenylacetate 100 mg and sodium benzoate 100 mg per mL (100 mL)

sodium phenylbutyrate (SOW dee um fen il BYOO ti rate)

Synonyms ammonapse

U.S./Canadian Brand Names Buphenyl® [US]

Therapeutic Category Miscellaneous Product

Use **Orphan drug:** Adjunctive therapy in the chronic management of patients with urea cycle disorder involving deficiencies of carbamoylphosphate synthetase, ornithine transcarbamylase, or argininosuccinic acid synthetase

Usual Dosage Oral:

Powder: Patients weighing <20 kg: 450-600 mg/kg/day or 9.9-13 g/m^2/day, administered in equally divided amounts with each meal or feeding, four to six times daily; safety and efficacy of doses >20 g/day has not been established

Tablet: Children >20 kg and Adults: 450-600 mg/kg/day or 9.9-13 g/m^2/day, administered in equally divided amounts with each meal; safety and efficacy of doses >20 g/day have not been established

Dosage Forms

Powder, for oral solution: 250 mg

Tablet: 500 mg

sodium phosphate and potassium phosphate *see* potassium phosphate and sodium phosphate *on page 717*

sodium phosphates (SOW dee um FOS fates)

U.S./Canadian Brand Names Fleet® Enema [US-OTC/Can]; Fleet® Phospho®-Soda Accu-Prep™ [US-OTC]; Fleet® Phospho®-Soda Oral Laxative [Can]; Fleet® Phospho®-Soda [US-OTC]; Visicol™ [US]

Therapeutic Category Electrolyte Supplement, Oral; Laxative

Use

Oral, rectal: Short-term treatment of constipation and to evacuate the colon for rectal and bowel exams

I.V.: Source of phosphate in large volume I.V. fluids and parenteral nutrition; treatment and prevention of hypophosphatemia

Usual Dosage

Normal requirements elemental phosphorus: Oral:

0-6 months: Adequate intake: 100 mg/day
6-12 months: Adequate intake: 275 mg/day
1-3 years: RDA: 460 mg
4-8 years: RDA: 500 mg
9-18 years: RDA: 1250 mg
≥19 years: RDA: 700 mg

Hypophosphatemia: It is difficult to provide concrete guidelines for the treatment of severe hypophosphatemia because the extent of total body deficits and response to therapy are difficult to predict. Aggressive doses of phosphate may result in a transient serum elevation followed by redistribution into intracellular compartments or bone tissue. Intermittent I.V. infusion should be reserved for severe depletion situations (<1 mg/dL in adults); large doses of oral phosphate may cause diarrhea and intestinal absorption may be unreliable. I.V. solutions should be infused slowly. Use caution when mixing with calcium and magnesium, precipitate may form. The following dosages are empiric guidelines. **Note:** 1 mmol phosphate = 31 mg phosphorus; 1 mg phosphorus = 0.032 mmol phosphate

Hypophosphatemia treatment: Doses listed as mmol of phosphate:

Intermittent I.V. infusion: Acute repletion or replacement:

Children: Low dose: 0.08 mmol/kg over 6 hours; use if losses are recent and uncomplicated Intermediate dose: 0.16-0.24 mmol/kg over 4-6 hours; use if serum phosphorus level 0.5-1 mg/dL High dose: 0.36 mmol/kg over 6 hours; use if serum phosphorus <0.5 mg/dL

Adults: Varying dosages: 0.15-0.3 mmol/kg/dose over 12 hours; may repeat as needed to achieve desired serum level **or** 15 mmol/dose over 2 hours; use if serum phosphorus <2 mg/dL **or** Low dose: 0.16 mmol/kg over 4-6 hours; use if serum phosphorus level 2.3-3 mg/dL Intermediate dose: 0.32 mmol/kg over 4-6 hours; use if serum phosphorus level 1.6-2.2 mg/dL High dose: 0.64 mmol/kg over 8-12 hours; use if serum phosphorus <1.5 mg/dL

Oral: Adults: 0.5-1 g elemental phosphorus 2-3 times/day may be used when serum phosphorus level is 1-2.5 mg/dL

Maintenance: Doses listed as mmol of phosphate:

Children:

Oral: 2-3 mmol/kg/day in divided doses
I.V.: 0.5-1.5 mmol/kg/day

Adults:

Oral: 50-150 mmol/day in divided doses
I.V.: 50-70 mmol/day

Laxative (Fleet®): Rectal:

Children 2-<5 years: One-half contents of one 2.25 oz pediatric enema
Children 5-12 years: Contents of one 2.25 oz pediatric enema, may repeat
Children ≥12 years and Adults: Contents of one 4.5 oz enema as a single dose, may repeat

Laxative (Fleet® Phospho®-Soda): Oral: Take on an empty stomach; dilute dose with 4 ounces cool water, then follow dose with 8 ounces water; **do not repeat dose within 24 hours**

(Continued)

sodium phosphates *(Continued)*

Children 5-9 years: 5-10 mL as a single dose
Children 10-12 years: 10-20 mL as a single dose
Children ≥12 years and Adults: 20-45 mL as a single dose

Bowel cleansing prior to colonoscopy: Adults:

Fleet® Phospho-Soda® Accu-Prep™: Oral: Prior to procedure (timing of doses determined by prescriber): One dose is equal to 45 mL (2 doses are recommended): Each dose is diluted as follows:

Mix 45 mL with 120 mL clear liquid; drink, then follow with at least 240 mL of clear liquid; **or**

Mix 15 mL with 240 mL clear liquid; drink, then follow with 240 mL clear liquid; repeat every 10 minutes for a total of 45 mL

Visicol™: Oral: Adults: A total of 40 tablets divided as follows:

Evening before colonoscopy: 3 tablets every 15 minutes for 6 doses, then 2 additional tablets in 15 minutes (total of 20 tablets)

3-5 hours prior to colonoscopy: 3 tablets every 15 minutes for 6 doses, then 2 additional tablets in 15 minutes (total of 20 tablets)

Note: Each dose should be taken with a minimum of 8 ounces of clear liquids. Do not repeat treatment within 7 days. Do not use additional agents, especially sodium phosphate products.

Dosage Forms

Enema: Monobasic sodium phosphate 19 g and dibasic sodium phosphate 7 g per 118 mL delivered dose (135 mL)

Fleet® Enema: Monobasic sodium phosphate 19 g and dibasic sodium phosphate 7 g per 118 mL delivered dose (135 mL)

Fleet® Enema for Children: Monobasic sodium phosphate 9.5 g and dibasic sodium phosphate 3.5 g per 59 mL delivered dose (68 mL)

Injection, solution [preservative free]: Phosphate 3 mmol and sodium 4 mEq per mL (5 mL, 15 mL, 50 mL)

Solution, oral:

Fleet® Phospho®-Soda: Monobasic sodium phosphate monohydrate 2.4 g and dibasic sodium phosphate heptahydrate 0.9 g per 5 mL (45 mL, 90 mL) [contains sodium benzoate; unflavored or ginger-lemon flavor]

Fleet® Phospho-Soda® Accu-Prep™ [kit]: Monobasic sodium phosphate monohydrate 2.4 g and dibasic sodium phosphate heptahydrate 0.9 g per 5 mL (15 mL) [solution contains sodium benzoate; kit contains solution in six 15 mL unit-dose containers (equal to two 45 mL doses) plus 4 anorectal pads containing pramoxine hydrochloride 1% and glycerin 12%]

Tablet, oral (Visicol™): Sodium phosphate monobasic monohydrate 1.102 g and sodium phosphate dibasic anhydrous 0.398 g [1.5 g total sodium phosphate per tablet]

sodium polystyrene sulfonate

(SOW dee um pol ee STYE reen SUL fon ate)

Sound-Alike/Look-Alike Issues

Kayexalate® may be confused with Kaopectate®

U.S./Canadian Brand Names Kayexalate® [US/Can]; Kionex™ [US]; PMS-Sodium Polystyrene Sulfonate [Can]; SPS® [US]

Therapeutic Category Antidote

Use Treatment of hyperkalemia

Usual Dosage

Children:

Oral: 1 g/kg/dose every 6 hours

Rectal: 1 g/kg/dose every 2-6 hours (In small children and infants, employ lower doses by using the practical exchange ratio of 1 mEq K^+/g of resin as the basis for calculation)

Adults: Hyperkalemia:

Oral: 15 g (60 mL) 1-4 times/day

Rectal: 30-50 g every 6 hours

Dosage Forms

Powder for suspension, oral/rectal:

Kayexalate®: 480 g

Kionex™: 454 g

Suspension, oral/rectal: 15 g/60 mL (60 mL, 120 mL, 200 mL, 500 mL) [with sorbitol and alcohol]

SPS®: 15 g/60 mL (60 mL, 120 mL, 480 mL) [contains alcohol 0.3% and sorbitol; cherry flavor]

sodium salicylate (SOW dee um sa LIS i late)

Therapeutic Category Analgesic, Nonnarcotic; Antipyretic

Use Treatment of minor pain or fever; arthritis

Usual Dosage Adults: Oral: 325-650 mg every 4 hours

Dosage Forms Tablet, enteric coated: 325 mg, 650 mg

Sodium Sulamyd® [US/Can] *see* sulfacetamide *on page 829*

sodium sulfacetamide *see* sulfacetamide *on page 829*

sodium sulfacetamide and sulfur *see* sulfur and sulfacetamide *on page 834*

sodium tetradecyl *(Discontinued)* *see page 1042*

sodium thiosulfate (SOW dee um thye oh SUL fate)

Synonyms disodium thiosulfate pentahydrate; pentahydrate; sodium hyposulfate; sodium thiosulphate; thiosulfuric acid disodium salt

U.S./Canadian Brand Names Versiclear™ [US]

Therapeutic Category Antidote; Antifungal Agent

Use

Parenteral: Used alone or with sodium nitrite or amyl nitrite in cyanide poisoning or arsenic poisoning; reduce the risk of nephrotoxicity associated with cisplatin therapy

Topical: Treatment of tinea versicolor

Usual Dosage I.V.:

Cyanide and nitroprusside antidote:

Children <25 kg: 50 mg/kg after receiving 4.5-10 mg/kg sodium nitrite; a half dose of each may be repeated if necessary

Children >25 kg and Adults: 12.5 g after 300 mg of sodium nitrite; a half dose of each may be repeated if necessary

Cyanide poisoning: Dose should be based on determination as with nitrite, at rate of 2.5-5 mL/minute to maximum of 50 mL

Dosage Forms

Injection, solution [preservative free]: 100 mg/mL (10 mL); 250 mg/mL (50 mL)

Lotion (Versiclear™): Sodium thiosulfate 25% and salicylic acid 1% (120 mL) [contains isopropyl alcohol 10%]

sodium thiosulfate, sodium nitrite, and amyl nitrite *see* sodium nitrite, sodium thiosulfate, and amyl nitrite *on page 813*

sodium thiosulphate *see* sodium thiosulfate *on this page*

Sofarin® *(Discontinued)* *see page 1042*

Soflax™ [Can] *see* docusate *on page 285*

Soft Plug® [US] *see* collagen implants *on page 225*

Solagé™ [US/Can] *see* mequinol and tretinoin *on page 555*

Solaquin Forte® [US/Can] *see* hydroquinone *on page 454*

Solaquin® [US-OTC/Can] *see* hydroquinone *on page 454*

Solaraze™ [US] *see* diclofenac *on page 266*

Solarcaine® Aloe Extra Burn Relief [US-OTC] *see* lidocaine *on page 518*

Solarcaine® [US-OTC] *see* benzocaine *on page 107*

Solatene® *(Discontinued)* *see page 1042*

Solfoton® *(Discontinued)* *see page 1042*

Solganal® *(Discontinued)* *see page 1042*

Solia™ [US] *see* ethinyl estradiol and desogestrel *on page 335*

soluble fluorescein *see* fluorescein sodium *on page 375*

Solu-Cortef® [US/Can] *see* hydrocortisone (systemic) *on page 449*

Solugel® [Can] *see* benzoyl peroxide *on page 109*

Solu-Medrol® [US/Can] *see* methylprednisolone *on page 572*

Soluver® [Can] *see* salicylic acid *on page 789*

Soluver® Plus [Can] *see* salicylic acid *on page 789*

Soluvite-F [US] *see* vitamins (multiple/pediatric) *on page 927*

Soma® [US/Can] *see* carisoprodol *on page 162*

Soma® Compound [US] *see* carisoprodol and aspirin *on page 162*

Soma® Compound w/Codeine [US] *see* carisoprodol, aspirin, and codeine *on page 162*

somatostatin *(Canada only)* (soe mat oh STA tin)

U.S./Canadian Brand Names Stilamin® [Can]

Therapeutic Category Variceal Bleeding (Acute) Agent

Use For the symptomatic treatment of acute bleeding from esophageal varices. Other treatment options for long-term management of the condition may be considered if necessary, once initial control has been established.

Usual Dosage Slow 250 mcg I.V. bolus injection over 3 to 5 minutes, followed by a continuous infusion at a rate of 250 mcg/hour until bleeding from the varices has stopped (usually within 12 to 24 hours). Once bleeding has been controlled, it is recommended that the infusion be continued for at least another 48 to 72 hours, or out to a maximum of 120 hours to prevent recurrent bleeding.

Dosage Forms Injection: 250 mcg, 3 mg

somatrem *see* human growth hormone *on page 437*

somatropin *see* human growth hormone *on page 437*

Somavert® [US] *see* pegvisomant *on page 672*

Sominex® Maximum Strength [US-OTC] *see* diphenhydramine *on page 277*

Sominex® [US-OTC] *see* diphenhydramine *on page 277*

Somnote™ [US] *see* chloral hydrate *on page 181*

Sonata® [US/Can] *see* zaleplon *on page 937*

sorbitol (SOR bi tole)

Therapeutic Category Genitourinary Irrigant; Laxative

Use Genitourinary irrigant in transurethral prostatic resection or other transurethral resection or other transurethral surgical procedures; diuretic; humectant; sweetening agent; hyperosmotic laxative; facilitate the passage of sodium polystyrene sulfonate through the intestinal tract

Usual Dosage Hyperosmotic laxative (as single dose, at infrequent intervals):

Children 2-11 years:

- Oral: 2 mL/kg (as 70% solution)
- Rectal enema: 30-60 mL as 25% to 30% solution

Children >12 years and Adults:

- Oral: 30-150 mL (as 70% solution)
- Rectal enema: 120 mL as 25% to 30% solution

Adjunct to sodium polystyrene sulfonate: 15 mL as 70% solution orally until diarrhea occurs (10-20 mL/2 hours) or 20-100 mL as an oral vehicle for the sodium polystyrene sulfonate resin

When administered with charcoal:

Oral:

Children: 4.3 mL/kg of 35% sorbitol with 1 g/kg of activated charcoal

Adults: 4.3 mL/kg of 70% sorbitol with 1 g/kg of activated charcoal every 4 hours until first stool containing charcoal is passed

Topical: 3% to 3.3% as transurethral surgical procedure irrigation

Dosage Forms

Solution, genitourinary irrigation: 3% (1500 mL, 3000 mL); 3.3% (2000 mL, 4000 mL)

Solution, oral: 70% (480 mL, 3840 mL)

Sorbitrate® *(Discontinued)* *see page 1042*

Soriatane® [US/Can] *see* acitretin *on page 17*

Sorine® [US] *see* sotalol *on this page*

Sotacor® [Can] *see* sotalol *on this page*

sotalol (SOE ta lole)

Sound-Alike/Look-Alike Issues

sotalol may be confused with Stadol®

Betapace® may be confused with Betapace AF®

Betapace AF® may be confused with Betapace®

Synonyms sotalol hydrochloride

U.S./Canadian Brand Names Alti-Sotalol [Can]; Apo-Sotalol® [Can]; Betapace® [US]; Betapace AF® [US/Can]; Gen-Sotalol [Can]; Lin-Sotalol [Can]; Novo-Sotalol [Can]; Nu-Sotalol [Can]; PMS-Sotalol [Can]; Rho®-Sotalol [Can]; Sorine® [US]; Sotacor® [Can]

Therapeutic Category Antiarrhythmic Agent, Class II; Antiarrhythmic Agent, Class III; Beta-Adrenergic Blocker, Nonselective

Use Treatment of documented ventricular arrhythmias (ie, sustained ventricular tachycardia), that in the judgment of the physician are life-threatening; maintenance of normal sinus rhythm in patients with symptomatic atrial fibrillation and atrial flutter who are currently in sinus rhythm. Manufacturer states substitutions should not be made for Betapace AF® since Betapace AF® is distributed with a patient package insert specific for atrial fibrillation/flutter.

Usual Dosage Sotalol should be initiated and doses increased in a hospital with facilities for cardiac rhythm monitoring and assessment. Proarrhythmic events can occur after initiation of therapy and with each upward dosage adjustment.

Children: Oral: The safety and efficacy of sotalol in children have not been established

Note: Dosing per manufacturer, based on pediatric pharmacokinetic data; wait at least 36 hours between dosage adjustments to allow monitoring of QT intervals

≤2 years: Dosage should be adjusted (decreased) by plotting of the child's age on a logarithmic scale; refer to manufacturer's package labeling.

>2 years: Initial: 90 mg/m^2/day in 3 divided doses; may be incrementally increased to a maximum of 180 mg/m^2/day

Adults: Oral:

Ventricular arrhythmias (Betapace®, Sorine®):

Initial: 80 mg twice daily

Dose may be increased gradually to 240-320 mg/day; allow 3 days between dosing increments in order to attain steady-state plasma concentrations and to allow monitoring of QT intervals

Most patients respond to a total daily dose of 160-320 mg/day in 2-3 divided doses.

Some patients, with life-threatening refractory ventricular arrhythmias, may require doses as high as 480-640 mg/day; however, these doses should only be prescribed when the potential benefit outweighs the increased of adverse events.

Atrial fibrillation or atrial flutter (Betapace AF®): Initial: 80 mg twice daily

(Continued)

sotalol *(Continued)*

If the initial dose does not reduce the frequency of relapses of atrial fibrillation/flutter and is tolerated without excessive QT prolongation (not >520 msec) after 3 days, the dose may be increased to 120 mg twice daily. This may be further increased to 160 mg twice daily if response is inadequate and QT prolongation is not excessive.

Dosage Forms Tablet, as hydrochloride: 80 mg, 80 mg [AF], 120 mg, 120 mg [AF], 160 mg, 160 mg [AF], 240 mg

Betapace® [light blue]: 80 mg, 120 mg, 160 mg, 240 mg

Betapace AF® [white]: 80 mg, 120 mg, 160 mg

Sorine® [white]: 80 mg, 120 mg, 160 mg, 240 mg

sotalol hydrochloride *see* sotalol *on previous page*

Sotradecol® ***(Discontinued)*** *see page 1042*

Sotret® [US] *see* isotretinoin *on page 489*

Soyacal® ***(Discontinued)*** *see page 1042*

SPA *see* albumin *on page 25*

Spacol [US] *see* hyoscyamine *on page 459*

Spacol T/S [US] *see* hyoscyamine *on page 459*

Span-FF® ***(Discontinued)*** *see page 1042*

sparfloxacin (spar FLOKS a sin)

Sound-Alike/Look-Alike Issues

Zagam® may be confused with Zyban™

U.S./Canadian Brand Names Zagam® [US]

Therapeutic Category Quinolone

Use Treatment of adults with community-acquired pneumonia caused by *C. pneumoniae, H. influenzae, H. parainfluenzae, M. catarrhalis, M. pneumoniae* or *S. pneumoniae*; treatment of acute bacterial exacerbations of chronic bronchitis caused by *C. pneumoniae, E. cloacae, H. influenzae, H. parainfluenzae, K. pneumoniae, M. catarrhalis, S. aureus* or *S. pneumoniae*

Usual Dosage Adults: Oral:

Loading dose: 400 mg on day 1

Maintenance: 200 mg/day for 10 days total therapy

Dosage Forms Tablet [film coated]: 200 mg

Sparine® ***(Discontinued)*** *see page 1042*

Spasmoject® ***(Discontinued)*** *see page 1042*

Spasmolin® ***(Discontinued)*** *see page 1042*

Spec-T® ***(Discontinued)*** *see page 1042*

Spectazole® [US/Can] *see* econazole *on page 301*

spectinomycin (spek ti noe MYE sin)

Sound-Alike/Look-Alike Issues

Trobicin® may be confused with tobramycin

Synonyms spectinomycin hydrochloride

U.S./Canadian Brand Names Trobicin® [US]

Therapeutic Category Antibiotic, Miscellaneous

Use Treatment of uncomplicated gonorrhea

Usual Dosage I.M.:

Children:

<45 kg: 40 mg/kg/dose 1 time (ceftriaxone preferred)

≥45 kg: Refer to adult dosing.

Children >8 years who are allergic to PCNS/cephalosporins may be treated with oral tetracycline

Adults:

Uncomplicated urethral, cervical, pharyngeal, or rectal gonorrhea: 2 g deep I.M. or 4 g where antibiotic resistance is prevalent 1 time; 4 g (10 mL) dose should be given as two 5 mL injections, followed by adequate chlamydial treatment (doxycycline 100 mg twice daily for 7 days)

Disseminated gonococcal infection: 2 g every 12 hours

Dosage Forms Injection, powder for reconstitution, as hydrochloride: 2 g [diluent contains benzyl alcohol]

spectinomycin hydrochloride *see* spectinomycin *on previous page*

Spectracef™ [US] *see* cefditoren *on page 167*

Spectrobid® Tablet *(Discontinued)* *see page 1042*

SpectroGram 2™ [Can] *see* chlorhexidine gluconate *on page 183*

SpectroTar Skin Wash™ [Can] *see* coal tar *on page 219*

Spherulin® *(Discontinued)* *see page 1042*

spiramycin *(Canada only)* (speer a MYE sin)

U.S./Canadian Brand Names Rovamycine® [Can]

Therapeutic Category Antibiotic, Macrolide

Use Treatment of infections of the respiratory tract, buccal cavity, skin and soft tissues due to susceptible organisms. *N. gonorrhoeae*: as an alternate choice of treatment for gonorrhea in patients allergic to the penicillins. Before treatment of gonorrhea, the possibility of concomitant infection due to *T. pallidum* should be excluded.

Usual Dosage Oral:

Children: Dosage by body weight; usual dosage 150,000 int. units/kg; expressed as the number of 750,000 int. unit (Rovamycine® "250") capsules per day. Daily dose should be administered in 2-3 divided doses.

15 kg = 3 capsules per day

20 kg = 4 capsules per day

30 kg = 6 capsules per day

Note: In severe infections, dosage may be increased by 50%.

Adults:

Mild to moderate infections: 6,000,000 to 9,000,000 int. units (4-6 capsules of Rovamycine® "500" per day) in 2 divided doses

Severe infections: 12,000,000 to 15,000,000 int. units (8-10 capsules of Rovamycine® "500" per day) in 2 divided doses

Gonorrhea: 12,000,000 to 13,500,000 int. units (8-9 capsules of Rovamycine® "500") as a single dose

Dosage Forms Capsule:

Rovamycine® "250": 750,000 int. units

Rovamycine® "500": 1,500,000 int. units

spirapril (SPYE ra pril)

Therapeutic Category Angiotensin-Converting Enzyme (ACE) Inhibitor

Use Management of mild to severe hypertension; treatment of left ventricular dysfunction after myocardial infarction

Usual Dosage Adults: Oral: 12-48 mg once daily

Dosage Forms Tablet: 3 mg, 6 mg, 12 mg, 24 mg

Spiriva® [US/Can] *see* tiotropium *on page 865*

Spironazide® *(Discontinued)* *see page 1042*

spironolactone (speer on oh LAK tone)

Sound-Alike/Look-Alike Issues

Aldactone® may be confused with Aldactazide®

U.S./Canadian Brand Names Aldactone® [US/Can]; Novo-Spiroton [Can]

(Continued)

spironolactone *(Continued)*

Therapeutic Category Diuretic, Potassium Sparing

Use Management of edema associated with excessive aldosterone excretion; hypertension; primary hyperaldosteronism; hypokalemia; treatment of hirsutism; cirrhosis of liver accompanied by edema or ascites

Usual Dosage To reduce delay in onset of effect, a loading dose of 2 or 3 times the daily dose may be administered on the first day of therapy. Oral:

Adults:

Edema, hypokalemia: 25-200 mg/day in 1-2 divided doses

Hypertension (JNC 7): 25-50 mg/day in 1-2 divided doses

Diagnosis of primary aldosteronism: 100-400 mg/day in 1-2 divided doses

CHF, severe (with ACE inhibitor and a loop diuretic ± digoxin): 25 mg/day, increased or reduced depending on individual response and evidence of hyperkalemia

Dosage Forms Tablet: 25 mg, 50 mg, 100 mg

spironolactone and hydrochlorothiazide *see* hydrochlorothiazide and spironolactone *on page 443*

Spirozide® *(Discontinued)* *see page 1042*

Sporanox® [US/Can] *see* itraconazole *on page 490*

Sportscreme® [US-OTC] *see* triethanolamine salicylate *on page 884*

Sprintec™ [US] *see* ethinyl estradiol and norgestimate *on page 346*

SPS® [US] *see* sodium polystyrene sulfonate *on page 816*

SRC® Expectorant *(Discontinued)* *see page 1042*

SSD® [US/Can] *see* silver sulfadiazine *on page 804*

SSD® AF [US] *see* silver sulfadiazine *on page 804*

SSKI® [US] *see* potassium iodide *on page 715*

Stadol® [US] *see* butorphanol *on page 140*

Stadol NS™ [Can] *see* butorphanol *on page 140*

Stadol® NS *(Discontinued)* *see page 1042*

Stagesic® [US] *see* hydrocodone and acetaminophen *on page 443*

Stahist® *(Discontinued)* *see page 1042*

Stalevo™ [US] *see* levodopa, carbidopa, and entacapone *on page 513*

Stan-Gard® [US] *see* fluoride *on page 376*

stannous fluoride *see* fluoride *on page 376*

stanozolol (stan OH zoe lole)

U.S./Canadian Brand Names Winstrol® [US]

Therapeutic Category Anabolic Steroid

Controlled Substance C-III

Use Prophylactic use against hereditary angioedema

Usual Dosage

Children: Acute attacks:

<6 years: 1 mg/day

6-12 years: 2 mg/day

Adults: Oral: Initial: 2 mg 3 times/day, may then reduce to a maintenance dose of 2 mg/day or 2 mg every other day after 1-3 months

Dosage Forms Tablet: 2 mg

Staphcillin® *(Discontinued)* *see page 1042*

Starlix® [US/Can] *see* nateglinide *on page 607*

Starnoc® [Can] *see* zaleplon *on page 937*

Statex® [Can] *see* morphine sulfate *on page 591*

Staticin® ***(Discontinued)*** *see page 1042*

Statobex® ***(Discontinued)*** *see page 1042*

Statobex® [Can] *see* phendimetrazine *on page 685*

stavudine (STAV yoo deen)

Sound-Alike/Look-Alike Issues

Zerit® may be confused with Ziac®

Synonyms d4T

U.S./Canadian Brand Names Zerit® [US/Can]

Therapeutic Category Antiviral Agent

Use Treatment of HIV infection in combination with other antiretroviral agents

Usual Dosage Oral:

Newborns (Birth to 13 days): 0.5 mg/kg every 12 hours

Children:

>14 days and <30 kg: 1 mg/kg every 12 hours

≥30 kg: Refer to Adults dosing

Adults:

≥60 kg: 40 mg every 12 hours

<60 kg: 30 mg every 12 hours

Dosage Forms

Capsule: 15 mg, 20 mg, 30 mg, 40 mg

Powder, for oral solution: 1 mg/mL (200 mL) [dye-free; fruit flavor]

Stelazine® ***(Discontinued)*** *see page 1042*

Stemetil® [Can] *see* prochlorperazine *on page 731*

Stemex® ***(Discontinued)*** *see page 1042*

Sterapred® [US] *see* prednisone *on page 725*

Sterapred® DS [US] *see* prednisone *on page 725*

STI571 *see* imatinib *on page 465*

Stilamin® [Can] *see* somatostatin *(Canada only) on page 818*

Stilphostrol® ***(Discontinued)*** *see page 1042*

Stimate™ [US] *see* desmopressin acetate *on page 252*

St Joseph® Adult Aspirin [US-OTC] *see* aspirin *on page 80*

St. Joseph® Cough Suppressant ***(Discontinued)*** *see page 1042*

St. Joseph® Measured Dose Nasal Solution ***(Discontinued)*** *see page 1042*

Stop® [US] *see* fluoride *on page 376*

Strattera™ [US] *see* atomoxetine *on page 86*

Streptase® [US/Can] *see* streptokinase *on this page*

streptokinase (strep toe KYE nase)

Synonyms SK

U.S./Canadian Brand Names Streptase® [US/Can]

Therapeutic Category Fibrinolytic Agent

Use Thrombolytic agent used in treatment of recent severe or massive deep vein thrombosis, pulmonary emboli, myocardial infarction, and occluded arteriovenous cannulas

Usual Dosage I.V.:

Children: Safety and efficacy have not been not established. Limited studies have used 3500-4000 units/kg over 30 minutes followed by 1000-1500 units/kg/hour.

Clotted catheter: I.V.: **Note:** Not recommended due to possibility of allergic reactions with repeated doses: 10,000-25,000 units diluted in NS to a final volume equivalent to catheter volume; instill into catheter and leave in place for 1 hour, then aspirate contents out of catheter and flush catheter with normal saline.

(Continued)

streptokinase *(Continued)*

Adults: Antibodies to streptokinase remain for at least 3-6 months after initial dose: Administration requires the use of an infusion pump.

An intradermal skin test of 100 units has been suggested to predict allergic response to streptokinase. If a positive reaction is not seen after 15-20 minutes, a therapeutic dose may be administered.

Guidelines for acute myocardial infarction (AMI): 1.5 million units over 60 minutes

Administration:

Dilute two 750,000 unit vials of streptokinase with 5 mL dextrose 5% in water (D_5W) each, gently swirl to dissolve.

Add this dose of the 1.5 million units to 150 mL D_5W.

This should be infused over 60 minutes; an in-line filter ≥0.45 micron should be used.

Monitor for the first few hours for signs of anaphylaxis or allergic reaction. **Infusion should be slowed if blood pressure falls by 25 mm Hg or terminated if asthmatic symptoms appear.**

Following completion of streptokinase, initiate heparin, if directed, when aPTT returns to less than 2 times the upper limit of control; do not use a bolus, but initiate infusion adjusted to a target aPTT of 1.5-2 times the upper limit of control. If prolonged (>48 hours) heparin is required, infusion may be switched to subcutaneous therapy.

Guidelines for acute pulmonary embolism (APE): 3 million unit dose over 24 hours

Administration:

Dilute four 750,000 unit vials of streptokinase with 5 mL dextrose 5% in water (D_5W) each, gently swirl to dissolve.

Add this dose of 3 million units to 250 mL D_5W, an in-line filter ≥0.45 micron should be used.

Administer 250,000 units (23 mL) over 30 minutes followed by 100,000 units/hour (9 mL/hour) for 24 hours.

Monitor for the first few hours for signs of anaphylaxis or allergic reaction. **Infusion should be slowed if blood pressure is lowered by 25 mm Hg or if asthmatic symptoms appear.**

Begin heparin 1000 units/hour about 3-4 hours after completion of streptokinase infusion or when PTT is <100 seconds.

Monitor PT, PTT, and fibrinogen levels during therapy.

Thromboses: 250,000 units to start, then 100,000 units/hour for 24-72 hours depending on location.

Cannula occlusion: 250,000 units into cannula, clamp for 2 hours, then aspirate contents and flush with normal saline; **Not recommended**

Dosage Forms Injection, powder for reconstitution: 250,000 units, 750,000 units, 1,500,000 units

streptomycin (strep toe MYE sin)

Sound-Alike/Look-Alike Issues

streptomycin may be confused with streptozocin

Synonyms streptomycin sulfate

Therapeutic Category Antibiotic, Aminoglycoside; Antitubercular Agent

Use Part of combination therapy of active tuberculosis; used in combination with other agents for treatment of streptococcal or enterococcal endocarditis, mycobacterial infections, plague, tularemia, and brucellosis

Usual Dosage

Children: Tuberculosis:

Daily therapy: 20-40 mg/kg/day (maximum: 1 g/day)

Directly observed therapy (DOT): Twice weekly: 20-40 mg/kg (maximum: 1 g)

DOT: 3 times/week: 25-30 mg/kg (maximum: 1 g)

Adults:

Tuberculosis:

Daily therapy: 15 mg/kg/day (maximum: 1 g)

Directly observed therapy (DOT): Twice weekly: 25-30 mg/kg (maximum: 1.5 g)

DOT: 3 times/week: 25-30 mg/kg (maximum: 1 g)

Enterococcal endocarditis: 1 g every 12 hours for 2 weeks, 500 mg every 12 hours for 4 weeks in combination with penicillin

Streptococcal endocarditis: 1 g every 12 hours for 1 week, 500 mg every 12 hours for 1 week

Tularemia: 1-2 g/day in divided doses for 7-10 days or until patient is afebrile for 5-7 days

Plague: 2-4 g/day in divided doses until the patient is afebrile for at least 3 days

Dosage Forms Injection, powder for reconstitution, as sulfate: 1 g

streptomycin sulfate *see* streptomycin *on previous page*

streptozocin (strep toe ZOE sin)

Sound-Alike/Look-Alike Issues

streptozocin may be confused with streptomycin

Synonyms NSC-85998

U.S./Canadian Brand Names Zanosar® [US/Can]

Therapeutic Category Antineoplastic Agent

Use Treatment of metastatic islet cell carcinoma of the pancreas, carcinoid tumor and syndrome, Hodgkin disease, palliative treatment of colorectal cancer

Usual Dosage Refer to individual protocols. I.V.: Children and Adults:

Single agent therapy: 1-1.5 g/m^2 weekly for 6 weeks followed by a 4-week rest period

Combination therapy: 0.5-1 g/m^2 for 5 consecutive days followed by a 4- to 6-week rest period

Dosage Forms Injection, powder for reconstitution: 1 g

Stresstabs® B-Complex + Iron [US-OTC] *see* vitamin B complex combinations *on page 915*

Stresstabs® B-Complex [US-OTC] *see* vitamin B complex combinations *on page 915*

Stresstabs® B-Complex + Zinc [US-OTC] *see* vitamin B complex combinations *on page 915*

Striant™ [US] *see* testosterone *on page 848*

Stri-dex® Body Focus [US-OTC] *see* salicylic acid *on page 789*

Stri-dex® Facewipes To Go™ [US-OTC] *see* salicylic acid *on page 789*

Stri-dex® Maximum Strength [US-OTC] *see* salicylic acid *on page 789*

Stri-dex® [US-OTC] *see* salicylic acid *on page 789*

Strifon Forte® [Can] *see* chlorzoxazone *on page 196*

Stromectol® [US] *see* ivermectin *on page 491*

strong iodine solution *see* potassium iodide *on page 715*

StrongStart™ [US] *see* vitamins (multiple/prenatal) *on page 927*

strontium-89 (STRON shee um-atey nine)

Synonyms strontium-89 chloride

U.S./Canadian Brand Names Metastron® [US/Can]

Therapeutic Category Radiopharmaceutical

Use Relief of bone pain in patients with skeletal metastases

Usual Dosage Adults: I.V.: 148 megabecquerel (4 millicurie) administered by slow I.V. injection over 1-2 minutes or 1.5-2.2 megabecquerel (40-60 microcurie)/kg; repeated doses are generally not recommended at intervals <90 days; measure the patient dose by a suitable radioactivity calibration system immediately prior to administration

Dosage Forms Injection, solution, as chloride [preservative free]: 10.9-22.6 mg/mL [148 megabecquerel, 4 millicurie] (10 mL)

strontium-89 chloride *see* strontium-89 *on this page*

Stuartnatal® Plus 3™ [US-OTC] *see* vitamins (multiple/prenatal) *on page 927*

Stuart Prenatal® [US-OTC] *see* vitamins (multiple/prenatal) *on page 927*

Sublimaze® [US] *see* fentanyl *on page 361*

Suboxone® [US] *see* buprenorphine and naloxone *on page 135*

Subutex® [US] *see* buprenorphine *on page 134*

succimer (SUKS i mer)

Synonyms DMSA

U.S./Canadian Brand Names Chemet® [US/Can]

Therapeutic Category Chelating Agent

Use **Orphan drug:** Treatment of lead poisoning in children with blood levels >45 mcg/dL. It is not indicated for prophylaxis of lead poisoning in a lead-containing environment. Following oral administration, succimer is generally well tolerated and produces a linear dose-dependent reduction in serum lead concentrations. This agent appears to offer advantages over existing lead chelating agents.

Usual Dosage Children and Adults: Oral: 10 mg/kg/dose every 8 hours for 5 days followed by 10 mg/kg/dose every 12 hours for 14 days

Concomitant iron therapy has been reported in a small number of children without the formation of a toxic complex with iron (as seen with dimercaprol); courses of therapy may be repeated if indicated by weekly monitoring of blood lead levels; lead levels should be stabilized <15 mcg/dL; 2 weeks between courses is recommended unless more timely treatment is indicated by lead levels

Dosage Forms Capsule: 100 mg

succinate *see* hydrocortisone (topical) *on page 451*

succinylcholine (suks in il KOE leen)

Synonyms succinylcholine chloride; suxamethonium chloride

U.S./Canadian Brand Names Quelicin® [US/Can]

Therapeutic Category Skeletal Muscle Relaxant

Use Adjunct to general anesthesia to facilitate both rapid sequence and routine endotracheal intubation and to relax skeletal muscles during surgery; to reduce the intensity of muscle contractions of pharmacologically- or electrically-induced convulsions; does not relieve pain or produce sedation

Usual Dosage I.M., I.V.: Dose to effect; doses will vary due to interpatient variability; use ideal body weight for obese patients

I.M.: 2.5-4 mg/kg, total dose should not exceed 150 mg

I.V.:

Children: Initial: 1-2 mg/kg; maintenance: 0.3-0.6 mg/kg every 5-10 minutes as needed; because of the risk of malignant hyperthermia, use of continuous infusions is not recommended in infants and children

Adults: 1-1.5 mg/kg, up to 150 mg total dose

Maintenance: 0.04-0.07 mg/kg every 5-10 minutes as needed

Continuous infusion: 10-100 mcg/kg/minute (or 0.5-10 mg/minute); dilute to concentration of 1-2 mg/mL in D_5W or NS

Note: Initial dose of succinylcholine must be increased when nondepolarizing agent pretreatment used because of the antagonism between succinylcholine and nondepolarizing neuromuscular blocking agents

Dosage Forms [DSC] = Discontinued product

Injection, solution, as chloride: 20 mg/mL (10 mL) [may contain benzyl alcohol]

Anectine® [DSC]: 20 mg/mL (10 mL)

Quelicin®: 20 mg/mL (5 mL, 10 mL); 50 mg/mL (10 mL); 100 mg/mL (10 mL)

succinylcholine chloride *see* succinylcholine *on this page*

Sucostrin® ***(Discontinued)*** *see page 1042*

Sucraid™ [US/Can] *see* sacrosidase *on page 789*

sucralfate (soo KRAL fate)

Sound-Alike/Look-Alike Issues

sucralfate may be confused with salsalate

Carafate® may be confused with Cafergot®

Synonyms aluminum sucrose sulfate, basic

U.S./Canadian Brand Names Apo-Sucralate® [Can]; Carafate® [US]; Novo-Sucralate [Can]; Nu-Sucralate [Can]; PMS-Sucralate [Can]; Sulcrate® [Can]; Sulcrate® Suspension Plus [Can]

Therapeutic Category Gastrointestinal Agent, Gastric or Duodenal Ulcer Treatment

Use Short-term management of duodenal ulcers; maintenance of duodenal ulcers

Usual Dosage Oral:

Children: Dose not established, doses of 40-80 mg/kg/day divided every 6 hours have been used

Adults:

Stress ulcer prophylaxis: 1 g 4 times/day

Stress ulcer treatment: 1 g every 4 hours

Duodenal ulcer:

Treatment: 1 g 4 times/day on an empty stomach and at bedtime for 4-8 weeks, or alternatively 2 g twice daily; treatment is recommended for 4-8 weeks in adults, the elderly may require 12 weeks

Maintenance: Prophylaxis: 1 g twice daily

Dosage Forms

Suspension, oral: 1 g/10 mL (10 mL)

Carafate®: 1 g/10 mL (420 mL)

Tablet (Carafate®): 1 g

Sucrets® Cough Calmers *(Discontinued)* *see page 1042*

Sucrets® Original [US-OTC] *see* hexylresorcinol *on page 435*

Sucrets® [US-OTC] *see* dyclonine *on page 300*

Sudafed® 12 Hour [US-OTC] *see* pseudoephedrine *on page 745*

Sudafed® 24 Hour [US-OTC] *see* pseudoephedrine *on page 745*

Sudafed® Children's [US-OTC] *see* pseudoephedrine *on page 745*

Sudafed® Cold & Cough Extra Strength [Can] *see* acetaminophen, dextromethorphan, and pseudoephedrine *on page 12*

Sudafed® Cough *(Discontinued)* *see page 1042*

Sudafed® Decongestant [Can] *see* pseudoephedrine *on page 745*

Sudafed® Head Cold and Sinus Extra Strength [Can] *see* acetaminophen and pseudoephedrine *on page 9*

Sudafed® Non-Drying Sinus [US-OTC] *see* guaifenesin and pseudoephedrine *on page 419*

Sudafed® Plus Liquid *(Discontinued)* *see page 1042*

Sudafed® Severe Cold [US-OTC] *see* acetaminophen, dextromethorphan, and pseudoephedrine *on page 12*

Sudafed® Sinus Advance [Can] *see* pseudoephedrine and ibuprofen *on page 747*

Sudafed® Sinus & Allergy [US-OTC] *see* chlorpheniramine and pseudoephedrine *on page 189*

Sudafed® Sinus and Cold [US-OTC] *see* acetaminophen and pseudoephedrine *on page 9*

Sudafed® Sinus Headache [US-OTC] *see* acetaminophen and pseudoephedrine *on page 9*

Sudafed® [US-OTC] *see* pseudoephedrine *on page 745*

Sudex® *(Discontinued)* *see page 1042*

Sudodrin [US-OTC] *see* pseudoephedrine *on page 745*

SudoGest Sinus [US-OTC] *see* acetaminophen and pseudoephedrine *on page 9*

Sufedrin® *(Discontinued)* *see* *page 1042*

Sufenta® [US/Can] *see* sufentanil *on this page*

sufentanil (soo FEN ta nil)

Sound-Alike/Look-Alike Issues

sufentanil may be confused with alfentanil, fentanyl

Sufenta® may be confused with Alfenta®, Sublimaze®, Sudafed®, Survanta®

Synonyms sufentanil citrate

U.S./Canadian Brand Names Sufenta® [US/Can]

Therapeutic Category Analgesic, Narcotic; General Anesthetic

Controlled Substance C-II

Use Analgesic supplement in maintenance of balanced general anesthesia

Usual Dosage

Children 2-12 years: 10-25 mcg/kg (10-15 mcg/kg most common dose) with 100% O_2, maintenance: up to 1-2 mcg/kg total dose

Adults: Dose should be based on body weight. **Note:** In obese patients (ie, >20% above ideal body weight), use lean body weight to determine dosage.

1-2 mcg/kg with N_2O/O_2 for endotracheal intubation; maintenance: 10-25 mcg as needed

2-8 mcg/kg with N_2O/O_2 more complicated major surgical procedures; maintenance: 10-50 mcg as needed

8-30 mcg/kg with 100% O_2 and muscle relaxant produces sleep; at doses ≥8 mcg/kg maintains a deep level of anesthesia; maintenance: 10-50 mcg as needed

Dosage Forms Injection, solution, as citrate [preservative free]: 50 mcg/mL (1 mL, 2 mL, 5 mL)

sufentanil citrate *see* sufentanil *on this page*

Sular® [US] *see* nisoldipine *on page 621*

sulbactam and ampicillin *see* ampicillin and sulbactam *on page 57*

sulconazole (sul KON a zole)

Synonyms sulconazole nitrate

U.S./Canadian Brand Names Exelderm® [US/Can]

Therapeutic Category Antifungal Agent

Use Treatment of superficial fungal infections of the skin, including tinea cruris (jock itch), tinea corporis (ringworm), tinea versicolor, and possibly tinea pedis (athlete's foot, cream only)

Usual Dosage Adults: Topical: Apply a small amount to the affected area and gently massage once or twice daily for 3 weeks (tinea cruris, tinea corporis, tinea versicolor) to 4 weeks (tinea pedis).

Dosage Forms

Cream, as nitrate: 1% (15 g, 30 g, 60 g)

Solution, topical, as nitrate: 1% (30 mL)

sulconazole nitrate *see* sulconazole *on this page*

Sulcrate® [Can] *see* sucralfate *on previous page*

Sulcrate® Suspension Plus [Can] *see* sucralfate *on previous page*

Sulf-10® [US] *see* sulfacetamide *on next page*

sulfabenzamide, sulfacetamide, and sulfathiazole

(sul fa BENZ a mide, sul fa SEE ta mide, & sul fa THYE a zole)

Synonyms triple sulfa

U.S./Canadian Brand Names V.V.S.® [US]

Therapeutic Category Antibiotic, Vaginal

Use Treatment of *Haemophilus vaginalis* vaginitis

Usual Dosage Intravaginal: Adults: Female: Insert one applicatorful into vagina twice daily for 4-6 days; dosage may then be decreased to 1/2 to 1/4 of an applicatorful twice daily

Dosage Forms Cream, vaginal: Sulfabenzamide 3.7%, sulfacetamide 2.86%, and sulfathiazole 3.42% (78 g with applicator)

sulfacetamide (sul fa SEE ta mide)

Sound-Alike/Look-Alike Issues

Bleph®-10 may be confused with Blephamide®
Klaron® may be confused with Klor-Con®

Synonyms sodium sulfacetamide; sulfacetamide sodium

U.S./Canadian Brand Names AK-Sulf® [US]; Bleph®-10 [US]; Carmol® Scalp [US]; Cetamide™ [Can]; Diosulf™ [Can]; Klaron® [US]; Ocusulf-10 [US]; Ovace™ [US]; Sodium Sulamyd® [US/Can]; Sulf-10® [US]

Therapeutic Category Antibiotic, Ophthalmic

Use

Ophthalmic: Treatment and prophylaxis of conjunctivitis due to susceptible organisms; corneal ulcers; adjunctive treatment with systemic sulfonamides for therapy of trachoma

Dermatologic: Scaling dermatosis (seborrheic); bacterial infections of the skin; acne vulgaris

Usual Dosage

Children >2 months and Adults: Ophthalmic:

Ointment: Apply to lower conjunctival sac 1-4 times/day and at bedtime

Solution: Instill 1-2 drops several times daily up to every 2-3 hours in lower conjunctival sac during waking hours and less frequently at night; increase dosing interval as condition responds. Usual duration of treatment: 7-10 days

Trachoma: Instill 2 drops into the conjunctival sac every 2 hours; must be used in conjunction with systemic therapy

Children >12 years and Adults: Topical:

Acne: Apply thin film to affected area twice daily

Seborrheic dermatitis: Apply at bedtime and allow to remain overnight; in severe cases, may apply twice daily. Duration of therapy is usually 8-10 applications; dosing interval may be increased as eruption subsides. Applications once or twice weekly, or every other week may be used to prevent eruptions.

Secondary cutaneous bacterial infections: Apply 2-4 times/day until infection clears

Dosage Forms

Lotion, as sodium:

Carmol® Scalp: 10% (85 g) [contains urea 10%]
Klaron®: 10% (120 mL) [contains sodium metabisulfite]
Ovace™: 10% (180 mL, 360 mL)

Ointment, ophthalmic, as sodium (AK-Sulf®): 10% (3.5 g)

Solution, ophthalmic, as sodium: 10% (15 mL)

Bleph®-10: 10% (5 mL, 15 mL) [contains benzalkonium chloride]
Ocusulf-10: 10% (15 mL)
Sulf-10®: 10% (1 mL)

sulfacetamide and prednisolone (sul fa SEE ta mide & pred NIS oh lone)

Sound-Alike/Look-Alike Issues

Blephamide® may be confused with Bleph®-10
Vasocidin® may be confused with Vasodilan®

Synonyms prednisolone and sulfacetamide

(Continued)

sulfacetamide and prednisolone *(Continued)*

U.S./Canadian Brand Names Blephamide® [US/Can]; Dioptimyd® [Can]; Vasocidin® [US/Can]

Therapeutic Category Antibiotic/Corticosteroid, Ophthalmic

Use Steroid-responsive inflammatory ocular conditions where infection is present or there is a risk of infection; ophthalmic suspension may be used as an otic preparation

Usual Dosage Children >2 months and Adults: Ophthalmic:

Ointment: Apply to lower conjunctival sac 1-4 times/day

Solution: Instill 1-3 drops every 2-3 hours while awake

Dosage Forms

Ointment, ophthalmic:

Blephamide®: Sulfacetamide sodium 10% and prednisolone acetate 0.2% (3.5 g)

Vasocidin®: Sulfacetamide sodium 10% and prednisolone acetate 0.5% (3.5 g)

Suspension, ophthalmic: Sulfacetamide sodium 10% and prednisolone sodium phosphate 0.25% (5 mL, 10 mL)

Blephamide®: Sulfacetamide sodium 10% and prednisolone acetate 0.2% (5 mL, 10 mL) [contains benzalkonium chloride]

Vasocidin®: Sulfacetamide sodium 10% and prednisolone sodium phosphate: 0.25% (5 mL, 10 mL)

sulfacetamide and sulfur *see* sulfur and sulfacetamide *on page 834*

sulfacetamide sodium *see* sulfacetamide *on previous page*

sulfacetamide sodium and fluorometholone

(sul fa SEE ta mide SOW dee um & flure oh METH oh lone)

Synonyms fluorometholone and sulfacetamide

U.S./Canadian Brand Names FML-S® [US]

Therapeutic Category Antibiotic/Corticosteroid, Ophthalmic

Use Steroid-responsive inflammatory ocular conditions where infection is present or there is a risk of infection

Usual Dosage Children >2 months and Adults: Ophthalmic: Instill 1-3 drops every 2-3 hours while awake

Dosage Forms Suspension, ophthalmic: Sulfacetamide sodium 10% and fluorometholone 0.1% (5 mL, 10 mL) [contains benzalkonium chloride]

Sulfacet-R® [US/Can] *see* sulfur and sulfacetamide *on page 834*

sulfadiazine (sul fa DYE a zeen)

Sound-Alike/Look-Alike Issues

sulfadiazine may be confused with sulfasalazine, sulfisoxazole

Tall-Man sulfa**DIAZINE**

Therapeutic Category Sulfonamide

Use Treatment of urinary tract infections and nocardiosis; adjunctive treatment in toxoplasmosis; uncomplicated attack of malaria

Usual Dosage Oral:

Asymptomatic meningococcal carriers:

Infants 1-12 months: 500 mg once daily for 2 days

Children 1-12 years: 500 mg twice daily for 2 days

Adults: 1 g twice daily for 2 days

Congenital toxoplasmosis:

Newborns and Children <2 months: 100 mg/kg/day divided every 6 hours in conjunction with pyrimethamine 1 mg/kg/day once daily and supplemental folinic acid 5 mg every 3 days for 6 months

Children >2 months: 25-50 mg/kg/dose 4 times/day

Nocardiosis: 4-8 g/day for a minimum of 6 weeks

Toxoplasmosis:

Children >2 months: Loading dose: 75 mg/kg; maintenance dose: 120-150 mg/kg/day, maximum dose: 6 g/day; divided every 4-6 hours in conjunction with pyrimethamine 2 mg/kg/day divided every 12 hours for 3 days followed by 1 mg/kg/day once daily with supplemental folinic acid

Adults: 2-6 g/day in divided doses every 6 hours in conjunction with pyrimethamine 50-75 mg/day and with supplemental folinic acid

Dosage Forms Tablet: 500 mg

sulfadoxine and pyrimethamine (sul fa DOKS een & peer i METH a meen)

Synonyms pyrimethamine and sulfadoxine

U.S./Canadian Brand Names Fansidar® [US]

Therapeutic Category Antimalarial Agent

Use Treatment of *Plasmodium falciparum* malaria in patients in whom chloroquine resistance is suspected; malaria prophylaxis for travelers to areas where chloroquine-resistant malaria is endemic

Usual Dosage Children and Adults: Oral:

Treatment of acute attack of malaria: A single dose of the following number of Fansidar® tablets is used in sequence with quinine or alone:

2-11 months: 1/4 tablet

1-3 years: 1/2 tablet

4-8 years: 1 tablet

9-14 years: 2 tablets

>14 years: 3 tablets

Malaria prophylaxis: A single dose should be carried for self-treatment in the event of febrile illness when medical attention is not immediately available:

2-11 months: 1/4 tablet

1-3 years: 1/2 tablet

4-8 years: 1 tablet

9-14 years: 2 tablets

>14 years and Adults: 3 tablets

Dosage Forms Tablet: Sulfadoxine 500 mg and pyrimethamine 25 mg

Sulfa-Gyn® ***(Discontinued)*** *see page 1042*

Sulfamethoprim® ***(Discontinued)*** *see page 1042*

sulfamethoxazole and trimethoprim

(sul fa meth OKS a zole & trye METH oh prim)

Sound-Alike/Look-Alike Issues

Bactrim™ may be confused with bacitracin, Bactine®

co-trimoxazole may be confused with clotrimazole

Septra® may be confused with Ceptaz®, Sectral®, Septa®

Synonyms co-trimoxazole; SMZ-TMP; sulfatrim; TMP-SMZ; trimethoprim and sulfamethoxazole

U.S./Canadian Brand Names Apo-Sulfatrim® [Can]; Bactrim™ [US]; Bactrim™ DS [US]; Novo-Trimel [Can]; Novo-Trimel D.S. [Can]; Nu-Cotrimox® [Can]; Septra® [US/Can]; Septra® DS [US/Can]; Septra® Injection [Can]

Therapeutic Category Sulfonamide

Use

Oral treatment of urinary tract infections due to *E. coli*, *Klebsiella* and *Enterobacter* sp, *M. morganii*, *P. mirabilis* and *P. vulgaris*; acute otitis media in children and acute exacerbations of chronic bronchitis in adults due to susceptible strains of *H. influenzae* or *S. pneumoniae*; treatment and prophylaxis of *Pneumocystis carinii* pneumonitis (PCP), traveler's diarrhea due to enterotoxigenic *E. coli*; treatment of enteritis caused by *Shigella flexneri* or *Shigella sonnei*

(Continued)

sulfamethoxazole and trimethoprim *(Continued)*

I.V. treatment or severe or complicated infections when oral therapy is not feasible, for documented PCP, empiric treatment of PCP in immune compromised patients; treatment of documented or suspected shigellosis, typhoid fever, *Nocardia asteroides* infection, or other infections caused by susceptible bacteria

Usual Dosage Dosage recommendations are based on the trimethoprim component. Double-strength tablets are equivalent to sulfamethoxazole 800 mg and trimethoprim 160 mg.

Children >2 months:

General dosing guidelines:

Mild-to-moderate infections: Oral: 8-12 mg TMP/kg/day in divided doses every 12 hours

Serious infection:

Oral: 20 mg TMP/kg/day in divided doses every 6 hours

I.V.: 8-12 mg TMP/kg/day in divided doses every 6 hours

Acute otitis media: Oral: 8 mg TMP/kg/day in divided doses every 12 hours for 10 days

Urinary tract infection:

Treatment: Oral: 6-12 mg TMP/kg/day in divided doses every 12 hours I.V.: 8-10 mg TMP/kg/day in divided doses every 6, 8, or 12 hours for up to 4 days with serious infections

Prophylaxis: Oral: 2 mg TMP/kg/dose daily or 5 mg TMP/kg/dose twice weekly

Pneumocystis:

Treatment: Oral, I.V.: 15-20 mg TMP/kg/day in divided doses every 6-8 hours

Prophylaxis: Oral, 150 mg TMP/m^2/day in divided doses every 12 hours for 3 days/week; dose should not exceed trimethoprim 320 mg and sulfamethoxazole 1600 mg daily

Alternative prophylaxis dosing schedules include: 150 mg TMP/m$_2$/day as a single daily dose 3 times/week on consecutive days **or** 150 mg TMP/m$_2$/day in divided doses every 12 hours administered 7 days/week **or** 150 mg TMP/m$_2$/day in divided doses every 12 hours administered 3 times/week on alternate days

Shigellosis:

Oral: 8 mg TMP/kg/day in divided doses every 12 hours for 5 days

I.V.: 8-10 mg TMP/kg/day in divided doses every 6, 8, or 12 hours for up to 5 days

Adults:

Urinary tract infection:

Oral: One double-strength tablet every 12 hours for 10-14 days

I.V.: 8-10 mg TMP/kg/day in divided doses every 6, 8, or 12 hours for up to 14 days with severe infections

Chronic bronchitis: Oral: One double-strength tablet every 12 hours for 10-14 days

Shigellosis:

Oral: One double strength tablet every 12 hours for 5 days

I.V.: 8-10 mg TMP/kg/day in divided doses every 6, 8, or 12 hours for up to 5 days

Travelers' diarrhea: Oral: One double strength tablet every 12 hours for 5 days

Sepsis: I.V.: 20 TMP/kg/day divided every 6 hours

Pneumocystis carinii:

Prophylaxis: Oral: 1 double strength tablet daily or 3 times/week

Treatment: Oral, I.V.: 15-20 mg TMP/kg/day in 3-4 divided doses

Dosage Forms Note: The 5:1 ratio (SMX:TMP) remains constant in all dosage forms.

Injection, solution: Sulfamethoxazole 80 mg and trimethoprim 16 mg per mL (5 mL, 10 mL, 30 mL, 50 mL) [contains propylene glycol ~400 mg/mL, alcohol, benzyl alcohol, and sodium metabisulfite]

Suspension, oral: Sulfamethoxazole 200 mg and trimethoprim 40 mg per 5 mL (20 mL, 480 mL) [contains alcohol]

Septra®: Sulfamethoxazole 200 mg and trimethoprim 40 mg per 5 mL (100 mL, 480 mL) [contains alcohol 0.26% and sodium benzoate; cherry and grape flavors]

Tablet: Sulfamethoxazole 400 mg and trimethoprim 80 mg

Bactrim™: Sulfamethoxazole 400 mg and trimethoprim 80 mg [contains sodium benzoate]

Septra®: Sulfamethoxazole 400 mg and trimethoprim 80 mg
Tablet, double strength: Sulfamethoxazole 800 mg and trimethoprim 160 mg
Bactrim™ DS: Sulfamethoxazole 800 mg and trimethoprim 160 mg [contains sodium benzoate]
Septra® DS: Sulfamethoxazole 800 mg and trimethoprim 160 mg

Sulfamylon® [US] *see* mafenide *on page 536*

sulfasalazine (sul fa SAL a zeen)

Sound-Alike/Look-Alike Issues
sulfasalazine may be confused with salsalate, sulfadiazine, sulfisoxazole
Azulfidine® may be confused with Augmentin®, azathioprine

Synonyms salicylazosulfapyridine

U.S./Canadian Brand Names Alti-Sulfasalazine [Can]; Azulfidine® [US]; Azulfidine® EN-tabs® [US]; Salazopyrin® [Can]; Salazopyrin En-Tabs® [Can]

Therapeutic Category 5-Aminosalicylic Acid Derivative

Use Management of ulcerative colitis; enteric coated tablets are also used for rheumatoid arthritis (including juvenile rheumatoid arthritis) in patients who inadequately respond to analgesics and NSAIDs

Usual Dosage Oral:
Children ≥2 years: Ulcerative colitis: Initial: 40-60 mg/kg/day in 3-6 divided doses; maintenance dose: 20-30 mg/kg/day in 4 divided doses
Children ≥6 years: Juvenile rheumatoid arthritis: Enteric coated tablet: 30-50 mg/kg/day in 2 divided doses; Initial: Begin with $1/4$ to $1/3$ of expected maintenance dose; increase weekly; maximum: 2 g/day typically
Adults:
Ulcerative colitis: Initial: 1 g 3-4 times/day, 2 g/day maintenance in divided doses; may initiate therapy with 0.5-1 g/day
Rheumatoid arthritis: Enteric coated tablet: Initial: 0.5-1 g/day; increase weekly to maintenance dose of 2 g/day in 2 divided doses; maximum: 3 g/day (if response to 2 g/day is inadequate after 12 weeks of treatment)

Dosage Forms
Tablet (Azulfidine®): 500 mg
Tablet, delayed release, enteric coated (Azulfidine® EN-tabs®): 500 mg

sulfatrim *see* sulfamethoxazole and trimethoprim *on page 831*

Sulfa-Trip® ***(Discontinued)*** *see page 1042*

sulfinpyrazone (sul fin PEER a zone)

U.S./Canadian Brand Names Apo-Sulfinpyrazone® [Can]; Nu-Sulfinpyrazone [Can]

Therapeutic Category Uricosuric Agent

Use Treatment of chronic gouty arthritis and intermittent gouty arthritis

Usual Dosage Adults: Oral: 100-200 mg twice daily; maximum daily dose: 800 mg

Dosage Forms Tablet: 100 mg

sulfisoxazole (sul fi SOKS a zole)

Sound-Alike/Look-Alike Issues
sulfisoxazole may be confused with sulfadiazine, sulfamethoxazole, sulfasalazine
Gantrisin® may be confused with Gastrosed™

Synonyms sulfisoxazole acetyl; sulphafurazole

Tall-Man sulfi**SOXAZOLE**

U.S./Canadian Brand Names Gantrisin® [US]; Novo-Soxazole® [Can]; Sulfizole® [Can]

Therapeutic Category Sulfonamide

Use Treatment of urinary tract infections, otitis media, *Chlamydia*; nocardiosis

Usual Dosage Oral: Not for use in patients <2 months of age:
Children >2 months: Initial: 75 mg/kg, followed by 120-150 mg/kg/day in divided doses every 4-6 hours; not to exceed 6 g/day
Adults: Initial: 2-4 g, then 4-8 g/day in divided doses every 4-6 hours
(Continued)

sulfisoxazole *(Continued)*

Dosage Forms

Suspension, oral, pediatric, as acetyl (Gantrisin®): 500 mg/5 mL (480 mL) [contains alcohol 0.3%; raspberry flavor]

Tablet: 500 mg

sulfisoxazole acetyl *see* sulfisoxazole *on previous page*

sulfisoxazole and erythromycin *see* erythromycin and sulfisoxazole *on page 321*

Sulfizole® [Can] *see* sulfisoxazole *on previous page*

sulfur and salicylic acid (SUL fur & sal i SIL ik AS id)

Synonyms salicylic acid and sulfur

Therapeutic Category Antiseborrheic Agent, Topical

Use Therapeutic shampoo for dandruff and seborrheal dermatitis; acne skin cleanser

Usual Dosage Children and Adults: Topical:

Shampoo: Initial: Use daily or every other day; 1-2 treatments/week will usually maintain control

Soap: Use daily or every other day

Dosage Forms

Cake: Sulfur 2% and salicylic acid 2% (123 g)

Cleanser: Sulfur 2% and salicylic acid 1.5% (60 mL, 120 mL)

Shampoo: Micropulverized sulfur 2% and salicylic acid 2% (120 mL, 240 mL)

Soap: Micropulverized sulfur 2% and salicylic acid 2% (113 g)

Wash: Sulfur 1.6% and salicylic acid 1.6% (75 mL)

sulfur and sulfacetamide (SUL fur & sul fa SEE ta mide)

Synonyms sodium sulfacetamide and sulfur; sulfacetamide and sulfur; sulfur and sulfacetamide sodium

U.S./Canadian Brand Names AVAR™ [US]; AVAR™ Cleanser [US]; AVAR™ Green [US]; Clenia™ [US]; Nocosyn™ [US]; Plexion® [US]; Plexion SCT™ [US]; Plexion TS™ [US]; Rosanil™ [US]; Rosula® [US]; Sulfacet-R® [US/Can]; Zetacet® [US]

Therapeutic Category Antiseborrheic Agent, Topical

Use Aid in the treatment of acne vulgaris, acne rosacea, and seborrheic dermatitis

Usual Dosage Topical: Children ≥12 years and Adults: Apply in a thin film 1-3 times/day. Cleansing products should be used 1-2 times/day.

Dosage Forms

Cream, topical:

Clenia™: Sulfur 5% and sulfacetamide sodium 10% (28 g)

Plexion SCT™: Sulfur 5% and sulfacetamide sodium 10% (120 g) [contains benzyl alcohol]

Rosanil™: Sulfur 5% and sulfacetamide sodium 10% (170 g) [cleanser]

Gel, topical:

AVAR™: Sulfur 5% and sulfacetamide sodium 10% (45 g) [contains benzyl alcohol]

AVAR™ Green: Sulfur 5% and sulfacetamide sodium 10% (45 g) [contains benzyl alcohol; color corrective gel]

Rosula®: Sulfur 5% and sulfacetamide sodium 10% (45 g) [contains urea 10% and benzyl alcohol]

Liquid soap (Clenia™): Sulfur 5% and sulfacetamide sodium 10% (170 g, 340 g)

Lotion, topical: Sulfur 5% and sulfacetamide sodium 10% (25 g)

AVAR™ Cleanser: Sulfur 5% and sulfacetamide sodium 10% (228 g)

Nicosyn™: Sulfur 5% and sulfacetamide sodium 10% (45 g) [contains benzyl alcohol]

Plexion™: Sulfur 5% and sulfacetamide sodium 10% (170 g, 340 g) [cleanser]

Rosula®: Sulfur 5% and sulfacetamide sodium 10% (45 g) [contains urea 10% and benzyl alcohol]

Sulfacet-R®: Sulfur 5% and sulfacetamide sodium 10% (25 g) [contains sodium metabisulfate; available with tint or tint-free formulations]

Suspension, topical (Plexion TS™, Zetacet®): Sulfur 5% and sulfacetamide sodium 10% (30 g) [contains benzyl alcohol]

sulfur and sulfacetamide sodium *see* sulfur and sulfacetamide *on previous page*

sulindac (sul IN dak)

Sound-Alike/Look-Alike Issues

Clinoril® may be confused with Cleocin®, Clozaril®, Oruvail®

U.S./Canadian Brand Names Apo-Sulin® [Can]; Clinoril® [US]; Novo-Sundac [Can]; Nu-Sundac [Can]

Therapeutic Category Analgesic, Nonnarcotic; Nonsteroidal Antiinflammatory Drug (NSAID)

Use Management of inflammatory disease, rheumatoid disorders, acute gouty arthritis, ankylosing spondylitis, bursitis, tendonitis

Usual Dosage Maximum therapeutic response may not be realized for up to 3 weeks

Oral:

Children: Dose not established

Adults: 150-200 mg twice daily or 300-400 mg once daily; not to exceed 400 mg/day

Dosage Forms Tablet: 150 mg, 200 mg

sulphafurazole *see* sulfisoxazole *on page 833*

Sultrin™ *(Discontinued)* *see page 1042*

sumatriptan succinate (SOO ma trip tan SUKS i nate)

Sound-Alike/Look-Alike Issues

sumatriptan may be confused with somatropin, zolmitriptan

U.S./Canadian Brand Names Imitrex® [US/Can]

Therapeutic Category Antimigraine Agent

Use

Oral, SubQ: Acute treatment of migraine with or without aura

SubQ: Acute treatment of cluster headache episodes

Usual Dosage Adults:

Oral: A single dose of 25 mg, 50 mg, or 100 mg (taken with fluids). If a satisfactory response has not been obtained at 2 hours, a second dose may be administered. Results from clinical trials show that initial doses of 50 mg and 100 mg are more effective than doses of 25 mg, and that 100 mg doses do not provide a greater effect than 50 mg and may have increased incidence of side effects. Although doses of up to 300 mg/day have been studied, the total daily dose should not exceed 200 mg. The safety of treating an average of >4 headaches in a 30-day period have not been established.

Intranasal: A single dose of 5 mg, 10 mg, or 20 mg administered in one nostril. A 10 mg dose may be achieved by administering a single 5 mg dose in each nostril. If headache returns, the dose may be repeated once after 2 hours, not to exceed a total daily dose of 40 mg. The safety of treating an average of >4 headaches in a 30-day period has not been established.

SubQ: 6 mg; a second injection may be administered at least 1 hour after the initial dose, but not more than 2 injections in a 24-hour period. If side effects are dose-limiting, lower doses may be used.

Dosage Forms Note: Expressed as sumatriptan base

Injection, solution, as succinate: 12 mg/mL (0.5 mL)

Solution, intranasal spray: 5 mg (100 μL unit dose spray device); 20 mg (100 μL unit dose spray device)

Tablet, as succinate: 25 mg, 50 mg, 100 mg

Summer's Eve® Medicated Douche [US-OTC] *see* povidone-iodine *on page 718*

Summer's Eve® SpecialCare™ Medicated Anti-Itch Cream [US] *see* hydrocortisone (topical) *on page 451*

Sumycin® [US] *see* tetracycline *on page 851*
Sun-Benz® [Can] *see* benzydamine *(Canada only) on page 112*
sunscreen (paba-free) *see* methoxycinnamate and oxybenzone *on page 567*
Superchar® ***(Discontinued)*** *see page 1042*
Superchar® With Sorbitol ***(Discontinued)*** *see page 1042*
Superdophilus® [US-OTC] *see* Lactobacillus *on page 501*
Supeudol® [Can] *see* oxycodone *on page 656*
Supprelin® ***(Discontinued)*** *see page 1042*
Suppress® ***(Discontinued)*** *see page 1042*
Suprane® [US/Can] *see* desflurane *on page 250*
Suprax® [US/Can] *see* cefixime *on page 168*
Surbex-T® [US-OTC] *see* vitamin B complex combinations *on page 915*
Sureprin 81™ [US-OTC] *see* aspirin *on page 80*
Surfak® [US-OTC] *see* docusate *on page 285*
Surgam® [Can] *see* tiaprofenic acid *(Canada only) on page 861*
Surgam® SR [Can] *see* tiaprofenic acid *(Canada only) on page 861*
Surgical® Fibrillar [US] *see* cellulose, oxidized regenerated *on page 174*
Surgicel® [US] *see* cellulose, oxidized regenerated *on page 174*
Surgicel® NuKnit [US] *see* cellulose, oxidized regenerated *on page 174*
Surital® ***(Discontinued)*** *see page 1042*
Surmontil® [US/Can] *see* trimipramine *on page 888*
Survanta® [US/Can] *see* beractant *on page 113*
Sus-Phrine® ***(Discontinued)*** *see page 1042*
Sustaire® ***(Discontinued)*** *see page 1042*
Sustiva® [US/Can] *see* efavirenz *on page 304*
Su-Tuss®-HD [US] *see* hydrocodone, pseudoephedrine, and guaifenesin *on page 447*
suxamethonium chloride *see* succinylcholine *on page 826*
Sween Cream® [US-OTC] *see* vitamin A and vitamin D *on page 915*
Symadine® ***(Discontinued)*** *see page 1042*
Symax SL [US] *see* hyoscyamine *on page 459*
Symax SR [US] *see* hyoscyamine *on page 459*
Symbicort® [Can] *see* budesonide and formoterol *(Canada only) on page 132*
Symbyax™ [US] *see* olanzapine and fluoxetine *on page 642*
Symmetrel® [US/Can] *see* amantadine *on page 41*
Symmetrel® Capsule ***(Discontinued)*** *see page 1042*
synacthen *see* cosyntropin *on page 229*
Synagis® [US/Can] *see* palivizumab *on page 661*
Synalar® [US/Can] *see* fluocinolone *on page 374*
Synalar-HP® Topical ***(Discontinued)*** *see page 1042*
Synalgos®-DC [US] *see* dihydrocodeine, aspirin, and caffeine *on page 271*
Synarel® [US/Can] *see* nafarelin *on page 599*
Syn-Diltiazem® [Can] *see* diltiazem *on page 273*
Synemol® Topical ***(Discontinued)*** *see page 1042*
Synercid® [US/Can] *see* quinupristin and dalfopristin *on page 758*

Synkayvite® ***(Discontinued)*** *see page 1042*

Synphasic® [Can] *see* ethinyl estradiol and norethindrone *on page 342*

Synthroid® [US/Can] *see* levothyroxine *on page 516*

Syntocinon® [Can] *see* oxytocin *on page 660*

Syntocinon® Nasal ***(Discontinued)*** *see page 1042*

Synvisc® [US/Can] *see* sodium hyaluronate/hylan G-F 20 *on page 812*

Syprine® [US/Can] *see* trientine *on page 884*

SyringeAvitene™ [US] *see* collagen hemostat *on page 225*

syrup of ipecac *see* ipecac syrup *on page 482*

Sytobex® ***(Discontinued)*** *see page 1042*

T_3 sodium *see* liothyronine *on page 523*

T_3/T_4 liotrix *see* liotrix *on page 523*

T_4 *see* levothyroxine *on page 516*

T-20 *see* enfuvirtide *on page 309*

642® Tablet [Can] *see* propoxyphene *on page 739*

Tabron® ***(Discontinued)*** *see page 1042*

Tac™-40 Injection ***(Discontinued)*** *see page 1042*

Tacaryl® ***(Discontinued)*** *see page 1042*

TACE® ***(Discontinued)*** *see page 1042*

tacrine (TAK reen)

Sound-Alike/Look-Alike Issues

Cognex® may be confused with Corgard®

Synonyms tacrine hydrochloride; tetrahydroaminoacrine; THA

U.S./Canadian Brand Names Cognex® [US]

Therapeutic Category Acetylcholinesterase Inhibitor; Cholinergic Agent

Use Treatment of mild to moderate dementia of the Alzheimer's type

Usual Dosage Adults: Initial: 10 mg 4 times/day; may increase by 40 mg/day adjusted every 6 weeks; maximum: 160 mg/day; best administered separate from meal times.

Dose adjustment based upon transaminase elevations:

ALT ≤3 times ULN*: Continue titration

ALT >3 to ≤5 times ULN*: Decrease dose by 40 mg/day, resume when ALT returns to normal

ALT >5 times ULN*: Stop treatment, may rechallenge upon return of ALT to normal

*ULN = upper limit of normal

Patients with clinical jaundice confirmed by elevated total bilirubin (>3 mg/dL) should not be rechallenged with tacrine

Dosage Forms Capsule, as hydrochloride: 10 mg, 20 mg, 30 mg, 40 mg

tacrine hydrochloride *see* tacrine *on this page*

tacrolimus (ta KROE li mus)

Sound-Alike/Look-Alike Issues

Prograf® may be confused with Gengraf®

Synonyms FK506

U.S./Canadian Brand Names Prograf® [US/Can]; Protopic® [US/Can]

Therapeutic Category Immunosuppressant Agent

Use

Oral/injection: Potent immunosuppressive drug used in liver or kidney transplant recipients

Topical: Moderate to severe atopic dermatitis in patients not responsive to conventional therapy or when conventional therapy is not appropriate

(Continued)

tacrolimus *(Continued)*

Usual Dosage

Children:

Liver transplant: Patients without pre-existing renal or hepatic dysfunction have required and tolerated higher doses than adults to achieve similar blood concentrations. It is recommended that therapy be initiated at high end of the recommended adult I.V. and oral dosing ranges; dosage adjustments may be required.

Oral: Initial dose: 0.15-0.20 mg/kg/day in 2 divided doses, given every 12 hours; begin oral dose no sooner than 6 hours post-transplant; adjunctive therapy with corticosteroids is recommended; if switching from I.V. to oral, the oral dose should be started 8-12 hours after stopping the infusion Typical whole blood trough concentrations: Months 1-12: 5-20 ng/mL

I.V.: **Note:** I.V. route should only be used in patients not able to take oral medications, anaphylaxis has been reported. Initial dose: 0.03-0.05 mg/kg/day as a continuous infusion; begin no sooner than 6 hours post-transplant; adjunctive therapy with corticosteroids is recommended; continue only until oral medication can be tolerated

Children ≥2 years: Moderate to severe atopic dermatitis: Topical: Apply 0.03% ointment to affected area twice daily; rub in gently and completely; continue applications for 1 week after symptoms have cleared

Adults:

Kidney transplant:

Oral: Initial dose: 0.2 mg/kg/day in 2 divided doses, given every 12 hours; initial dose may be given within 24 hours of transplant, but should be delayed until renal function has recovered; African-American patients may require larger doses to maintain trough concentration Typical whole blood trough concentrations: Months 1-3: 7- 20 ng/mL; months 4-12: 5-15 ng/mL

I.V.: **Note:** I.V. route should only be used in patients not able to take oral medications, anaphylaxis has been reported. Initial dose: 0.03-0.05 mg/kg/day as a continuous infusion; begin no sooner than 6 hours post-transplant, starting at lower end of the dosage range; adjunctive therapy with corticosteroids is recommended; continue only until oral medication can be tolerated

Liver transplant:

Oral: Initial dose: 0.1-0.15 mg/kg/day in 2 divided doses, given every 12 hours; begin oral dose no sooner than 6 hours post-transplant; adjunctive therapy with corticosteroids is recommended; if switching from I.V. to oral, the oral dose should be started 8-12 hours after stopping the infusion Typical whole blood trough concentrations: Months 1-12: 5-20 ng/mL

I.V.: **Note:** I.V. route should only be used in patients not able to take oral medications, anaphylaxis has been reported. Initial dose: 0.03-0.05 mg/kg/day as a continuous infusion; begin no sooner than 6 hours post-transplant starting at lower end of the dosage range; adjunctive therapy with corticosteroids is recommended; continue only until oral medication can be tolerated

Prevention of graft-vs-host disease: I.V.: 0.03 mg/kg/day as continuous infusion

Moderate to severe atopic dermatitis: Topical: Apply 0.03% or 0.1% ointment to affected area twice daily; rub in gently and completely; continue applications for 1 week after symptoms have cleared

Dosage Forms

Capsule (Prograf®): 0.5 mg, 1 mg, 5 mg

Injection, solution (Prograf®): 5 mg/mL (1 mL) [contains dehydrated alcohol 80% and polyoxyl 60 hydrogenated castor oil]

Ointment, topical (Protopic®): 0.03% (30 g, 60 g, 100 g); 0.1% (30 g, 60 g, 100 g)

tadalafil (tah DA la fil)

Synonyms GF196960

U.S./Canadian Brand Names Cialis® [US]

Therapeutic Category Phosphodiesterase-5 Enzyme Inhibitor

Use Treatment of erectile dysfunction

Usual Dosage Oral: Adults: Erectile dysfunction: 10 mg prior to anticipated sexual activity (dosing range: 5-20 mg); to be given as one single dose and not given more than once daily. **Note:** Erectile function may be improved for up to 36 hours following a single dose; adjust dose.

Dosage Forms Tablet: 5 mg, 10 mg, 20 mg

Tagamet® [US] *see* cimetidine *on page 199*

Tagamet® 800 mg *(Discontinued)* *see page 1042*

Tagamet® HB 200 [US-OTC/Can] *see* cimetidine *on page 199*

Talwin® [US/Can] *see* pentazocine *on page 678*

Talwin® Compound *(Discontinued)* *see page 1042*

Talwin® NX [US] *see* pentazocine *on page 678*

TAM *see* tamoxifen *on this page*

Tambocor™ [US/Can] *see* flecainide *on page 369*

Tamiflu™ [US/Can] *see* oseltamivir *on page 650*

Tamine® *(Discontinued)* *see page 1042*

Tamofen® [Can] *see* tamoxifen *on this page*

tamoxifen (ta MOKS i fen)

Sound-Alike/Look-Alike Issues

tamoxifen may be confused with pentoxifylline, Tambocor™

Synonyms ICI-46474; NSC-180973; TAM; tamoxifen citrate

U.S./Canadian Brand Names Apo-Tamox® [Can]; Gen-Tamoxifen [Can]; Nolvadex® [US/Can]; Nolvadex®-D [Can]; Novo-Tamoxifen [Can]; PMS-Tamoxifen [Can]; Tamofen® [Can]

Therapeutic Category Antineoplastic Agent

Use Palliative or adjunctive treatment of advanced breast cancer; reduce the incidence of breast cancer in women at high risk; reduce risk of invasive breast cancer in women with ductal carcinoma *in situ* (DCIS); metastatic male breast cancer; treatment of melanoma, desmoid tumors

Usual Dosage Refer to individual protocols. Oral: Adults: Breast cancer:

Metastatic (males and females) or adjuvant therapy (females): 20-40 mg/day

Prevention (high-risk females): 20 mg/day for 5 years

DCIS (females): 20 mg once daily for 5 years

Note: Higher dosages (up to 700 mg/day) have been investigated for use in modulation of multidrug resistance (MDR), but are not routinely used in clinical practice

Dosage Forms Tablet, as citrate: 10 mg, 20 mg

tamoxifen citrate *see* tamoxifen *on this page*

tamsulosin (tam SOO loe sin)

Sound-Alike/Look-Alike Issues

Flomax® may be confused with Fosamax®, Volmax®

Synonyms tamsulosin hydrochloride

U.S./Canadian Brand Names Flomax® [US/Can]

Therapeutic Category Alpha-Adrenergic Blocking Agent

Use Treatment of signs and symptoms of benign prostatic hyperplasia (BPH)

Usual Dosage Oral: Adults: 0.4 mg once daily, ~30 minutes after the same meal each day; dose may be increased after 2-4 weeks to 0.8 mg once daily in patients who fail to respond. If therapy is interrupted for several days, restart with 0.4 mg once daily.

Dosage Forms Capsule, as hydrochloride: 0.4 mg

tamsulosin hydrochloride *see* tamsulosin *on this page*

Tanac® *(Discontinued)* *see page 1042*

Tanafed® [US] *see* chlorpheniramine and pseudoephedrine *on page 189*

Tanafed DP™ [US] *see* chlorpheniramine and pseudoephedrine *on page 189*

Tannic-12 [US] *see* carbetapentane and chlorpheniramine *on page 156*

Tannic-12 S [US] *see* carbetapentane and chlorpheniramine *on page 156*

Tannihist-12 RF [US] *see* carbetapentane and chlorpheniramine *on page 156*

Tanoral® Tablet *(Discontinued)* *see page 1042*

Tantum® [Can] *see* benzydamine *(Canada only) on page 112*

Tao® [US] *see* troleandomycin *on page 891*

TAP-144 *see* leuprolide acetate *on page 509*

Tapazole® [US/Can] *see* methimazole *on page 564*

Tarabine® PFS *(Discontinued)* *see page 1042*

Taractan® *(Discontinued)* *see page 1042*

Targel® [Can] *see* coal tar *on page 219*

Targretin® [US/Can] *see* bexarotene *on page 118*

Tarka® [US/Can] *see* trandolapril and verapamil *on page 876*

Taro-Carbamzepine Chewable [Can] *see* carbamazepine *on page 155*

Taro-Desoximetasone [Can] *see* desoximetasone *on page 253*

Taro-Sone® [Can] *see* betamethasone (topical) *on page 116*

Taro-Warfarin [Can] *see* warfarin *on page 933*

Tarsum® [US-OTC] *see* coal tar and salicylic acid *on page 220*

Tasmar® [US] *see* tolcapone *on page 869*

TAT *see* tetanus antitoxin *on page 849*

Tavist® Allergy [US-OTC] *see* clemastine *on page 209*

Tavist-D® *(Discontinued)* *see page 1042*

Tavist® ND [US-OTC] *see* loratadine *on page 530*

Taxol® [US/Can] *see* paclitaxel *on page 660*

Taxotere® [US/Can] *see* docetaxel *on page 284*

tazarotene (taz AR oh teen)

U.S./Canadian Brand Names Avage™ [US]; Tazorac® [US/Can]

Therapeutic Category Keratolytic Agent

Use Topical treatment of facial acne vulgaris; topical treatment of stable plaque psoriasis of up to 20% body surface area involvement; mitigation (palliation) of facial skin wrinkling, facial mottled hyper/hypopigmentation, and benign facial lentigines

Usual Dosage Topical: **Note:** In patients experiencing excessive pruritus, burning, skin redness, or peeling, discontinue until integrity of the skin is restored, or reduce dosing to an interval the patient is able to tolerate.

Children ≥12 years and Adults:

Acne: Tazorac® cream/gel 0.1%: Cleanse the face gently. After the skin is dry, apply a thin film of tazarotene (2 mg/cm^2) once daily, in the evening, to the skin where the acne lesions appear; use enough to cover the entire affected area

Psoriasis: Tazorac® gel 0.05% or 0.1%: Apply once daily, in the evening, to psoriatic lesions using enough (2 mg/cm^2) to cover only the lesion with a thin film to no more than 20% of body surface area. If a bath or shower is taken prior to application, dry the skin before applying. Unaffected skin may be more susceptible to irritation, avoid application to these areas.

Children ≥17 years and Adults: Palliation of fine facial wrinkles, facial mottled hyper/hypopigmentation, benign facial lentigines: Avage™: Apply a pea-sized amount once daily to clean dry face at bedtime; lightly cover entire face including eyelids if desired. Emollients or moisturizers may be applied before or after; if applied before tazarotene, ensure cream or lotion has absorbed into the skin and has dried completely.

Adults: Psoriasis: Tazorac® cream 0.05% or 0.1%: Apply once daily, in the evening, to psoriatic lesions using enough (2 mg/cm²) to cover only the lesion with a thin film to no more than 20% of body surface area. If a bath or shower is taken prior to application, dry the skin before applying. Unaffected skin may be more susceptible to irritation, avoid application to these areas.

Dosage Forms

Cream:

Avage™: 0.1% (15 g, 30 g) [contains benzyl alcohol]

Tazorac®: 0.05% (15 g, 30 g, 60 g); 0.1% (15 g, 30 g, 60 g) [contains benzyl alcohol]

Gel (Tazorac®): 0.05% (30 g, 100 g); 0.1% (30 g, 100 g) [contains benzyl alcohol]

Tazicef® [US] *see* ceftazidime *on page 171*

Tazocin® [Can] *see* piperacillin and tazobactam sodium *on page 697*

Tazorac® [US/Can] *see* tazarotene *on previous page*

Taztia XT™ [US] *see* diltiazem *on page 273*

3TC *see* lamivudine *on page 502*

3TC® [Can] *see* lamivudine *on page 502*

3TC, abacavir, and zidovudine *see* abacavir, lamivudine, and zidovudine *on page 2*

T-Caine® Lozenge *(Discontinued)* *see page 1042*

T-cell growth factor *see* aldesleukin *on page 28*

TCGF *see* aldesleukin *on page 28*

TCN *see* tetracycline *on page 851*

Td *see* diphtheria and tetanus toxoid *on page 280*

TDF *see* tenofovir *on page 845*

Teardrops® [Can] *see* artificial tears *on page 78*

Tear Drop® Solution *(Discontinued)* *see page 1042*

TearGard® Ophthalmic Solution *(Discontinued)* *see page 1042*

Teargen® II [US-OTC] *see* artificial tears *on page 78*

Teargen® [US-OTC] *see* artificial tears *on page 78*

Tearisol® [US-OTC] *see* artificial tears *on page 78*

Tears Again® Gel Drops™ [US-OTC] *see* carboxymethylcellulose *on page 161*

Tears Again® MC [US-OTC] *see* hydroxypropyl methylcellulose *on page 457*

Tears Again® Night and Day™ [US-OTC] *see* carboxymethylcellulose *on page 161*

Tears Again® [US-OTC] *see* artificial tears *on page 78*

Tears Naturale® Free [US-OTC] *see* artificial tears *on page 78*

Tears Naturale® II [US-OTC] *see* artificial tears *on page 78*

Tears Naturale® [US-OTC] *see* artificial tears *on page 78*

Tears Plus® [US-OTC] *see* artificial tears *on page 78*

Tears Renewed® [US-OTC] *see* artificial tears *on page 78*

Tebamide® *(Discontinued)* *see page 1042*

Tebrazid™ [Can] *see* pyrazinamide *on page 750*

Tecnal C 1/2 [Can] *see* butalbital, aspirin, caffeine, and codeine *on page 139*

Tecnal C 1/4 [Can] *see* butalbital, aspirin, caffeine, and codeine *on page 139*

Teczem® *(Discontinued)* *see page 1042*

Tedral® *(Discontinued)* *see page 1042*

tegaserod (teg a SER od)

Synonyms HTF919; tegaserod maleate

U.S./Canadian Brand Names Zelnorm® [US/Can]

Therapeutic Category Serotonin 5-HT_4 Receptor Agonist

Use Short-term treatment of constipation-predominate irritable bowel syndrome (IBS) in women; treatment of chronic idiopathic constipation

Usual Dosage Oral: Adults:

IBS with constipation (females): 6 mg twice daily, before meals, for 4-6 weeks; may consider continuing treatment for an additional 4-6 weeks in patients who respond initially

Chronic idiopathic constipation: 6 mg twice daily, before meals; the need for continued therapy should be reassessed periodically

Dosage Forms Tablet: 2 mg, 6 mg

tegaserod maleate *see* tegaserod *on this page*

Tega-Vert® Oral *(Discontinued)* *see page 1042*

Tegison® *(Discontinued)* *see page 1042*

Tegopen® *(Discontinued)* *see page 1042*

Tegretol® [US/Can] *see* carbamazepine *on page 155*

Tegretol®-XR [US] *see* carbamazepine *on page 155*

Tegrin® [US-OTC] *see* coal tar *on page 219*

Telachlor® Oral *(Discontinued)* *see page 1042*

Teladar® Topical *(Discontinued)* *see page 1042*

Teldrin® Oral *(Discontinued)* *see page 1042*

Telepaque® [US] *see* radiological/contrast media (ionic) *on page 759*

Teline® *(Discontinued)* *see page 1042*

telithromycin (tel ith roe MYE sin)

Synonyms HMR 3647

U.S./Canadian Brand Names Ketek™ [US/Can]

Therapeutic Category Antibiotic, Ketolide

Use Treatment of community-acquired pneumonia (mild to moderate) caused by susceptible strains of *Streptococcus pneumoniae* (including multidrug-resistant isolates), *Haemophilus influenzae, Chlamydia pneumoniae, Moraxella catarrhalis,* and *Mycoplasma pneumoniae*; treatment of bacterial exacerbation of chronic bronchitis caused by susceptible strains of *S. pneumoniae, H. influenzae,* and *Moraxella catarrhalis*; treatment of acute bacterial sinusitis caused by *Streptococcus pneumoniae, Haemophilus influenza,* and *Moraxella catarrhalis*

Usual Dosage Oral: Adults:

Acute exacerbation of chronic bronchitis, acute bacterial sinusitis: 800 mg once daily for 5 days

Community-acquired pneumonia: 800 mg once daily for 7-10 days

Dosage Forms Tablet [film coated]: 400 mg

Ketek Pak™ [blister pack]: 400 mg (10s) [packaged as 10 tablets/card; 2 tablets/blister]

telmisartan (tel mi SAR tan)

U.S./Canadian Brand Names Micardis® [US/Can]

Therapeutic Category Angiotensin II Receptor Antagonist

Use Treatment of hypertension; may be used alone or in combination with other antihypertensive agents

Usual Dosage Adults: Oral: Initial: 40 mg once daily; usual maintenance dose range: 20-80 mg/day. Patients with volume depletion should be initiated on the lower dosage with close supervision.

Dosage Forms Tablet: 20 mg, 40 mg, 80 mg

telmisartan and HCTZ *see* telmisartan and hydrochlorothiazide *on this page*

telmisartan and hydrochlorothiazide

(tel mi SAR tan & hye droe klor oh THYE a zide)

Synonyms HCTZ and telmisartan; hydrochlorothiazide and telmisartan; telmisartan and HCTZ

U.S./Canadian Brand Names Micardis® HCT [US]; Micardis® Plus [Can]

Therapeutic Category Antihypertensive Agent, Combination

Use Treatment of hypertension; combination product should not be used for initial therapy

Usual Dosage Adults: Oral: Replacement therapy: Combination product can be substituted for individual titrated agents. Initiation of combination therapy when monotherapy has failed to achieve desired effects:

Patients currently on telmisartan: Initial dose if blood pressure is not currently controlled on monotherapy of 80 mg telmisartan: Telmisartan 80 mg/hydrochlorothiazide 12.5 mg once daily; may titrate up to telmisartan 160 mg/hydrochlorothiazide 25 mg if needed

Patients currently on HCTZ: Initial dose if blood pressure is not currently controlled on monotherapy of 25 mg once daily: Telmisartan 80 mg/hydrochlorothiazide 12.5 mg once daily or telmisartan 80 mg/hydrochlorothiazide 25 mg once daily; may titrate up to telmisartan 160 mg/hydrochlorothiazide 25 mg if blood pressure remains uncontrolled after 2-4 weeks of therapy. Patients who develop hypokalemia may be switched to telmisartan 80 mg/hydrochlorothiazide 12.5 mg.

Dosage Forms Tablet:

40/12.5: Telmisartan 40 mg and hydrochlorothiazide 12.5 mg
80/12.5: Telmisartan 80 mg and hydrochlorothiazide 12.5 mg
80/25: Telmisartan 80 mg and hydrochlorothiazide 25 mg

Temaril® *(Discontinued)* *see page 1042*

temazepam (te MAZ e pam)

Sound-Alike/Look-Alike Issues

temazepam may be confused with flurazepam, lorazepam
Restoril® may be confused with Vistaril®, Zestril®

U.S./Canadian Brand Names Apo-Temazepam® [Can]; CO Temazepam [Can]; Gen-Temazepam [Can]; Novo-Temazepam [Can]; Nu-Temazepam [Can]; PMS-Temazepam [Can]; ratio-Temazepam [Can]; Restoril® [US/Can]

Therapeutic Category Benzodiazepine

Controlled Substance C-IV

Use Short-term treatment of insomnia

Usual Dosage Oral:

Adults: 15-30 mg at bedtime
Elderly or debilitated patients: 15 mg

Dosage Forms Capsule: 15 mg, 30 mg

Restoril®: 7.5 mg, 15 mg, 30 mg

Temazin® Cold Syrup *(Discontinued)* *see page 1042*

Temodal™ [Can] *see* temozolomide *on this page*

Temodar® [US/Can] *see* temozolomide *on this page*

Temovate® [US] *see* clobetasol *on page 212*

Temovate E® [US] *see* clobetasol *on page 212*

temozolomide (te mo ZOLE oh mide)

Synonyms NSC-362856; TMZ

U.S./Canadian Brand Names Temodal™ [Can]; Temodar® [US/Can]

Therapeutic Category Antineoplastic Agent, Alkylating Agent

(Continued)

temozolomide *(Continued)*

Use Treatment of adult patients with refractory (first relapse) anaplastic astrocytoma who have experienced disease progression on nitrosourea and procarbazine

Usual Dosage Refer to individual protocols. Oral:

Adults: Initial dose: 150 mg/m²/day for 5 days; repeat every 28 days. Subsequent doses of 100-200 mg/m²/day; based upon hematologic tolerance. This monthly-cycle regimen may be preceded by a 6- to 7-week regimen of 75 mg/m²/day.

ANC <1000/mm³ or platelets <50,000/mm³ (day 22 or 29): Postpone therapy until ANC >1500/mm³ and platelets >100,000/mm³; reduce dose by 50 mg/m²/day for subsequent cycle

ANC 1000-1500/mm³ or platelets 50,000-100,000/mm³ (day 22 and 29): Postpone therapy until ANC >1500/mm³ and platelets >100,000/mm³; maintain initial dose

ANC >1500/mm³ and platelets >100,000/mm³ (day 22 and 29): Increase dose to or maintain dose at 200 mg/m²/day for 5 days for subsequent cycle

Dosage Forms Capsule: 5 mg, 20 mg, 100 mg, 250 mg

Tempra® [Can] *see* acetaminophen *on page 5*

Tempra® *(Discontinued)* *see page 1042*

tenecteplase (ten EK te plase)

Sound-Alike/Look-Alike Issues

TNKase™ may be confused with t-PA

U.S./Canadian Brand Names TNKase™ [US/Can]

Therapeutic Category Thrombolytic Agent

Use Thrombolytic agent used in the management of acute myocardial infarction for the lysis of thrombi in the coronary vasculature to restore perfusion and reduce mortality.

Usual Dosage I.V.:

Adult: Recommended total dose should not exceed 50 mg and is based on patient's weight; administer as a bolus over 5 seconds

If patient's weight:

<60 kg, dose: 30 mg

≥60 to <70 kg, dose: 35 mg

≥70 to <80 kg, dose: 40 mg

≥80 to <90 kg, dose: 45 mg

≥90 kg, dose: 50 mg

All patients received 150-325 mg of aspirin as soon as possible and then daily. Intravenous heparin was initiated as soon as possible and aPTT was maintained between 50-70 seconds.

Dosage Forms Injection, powder for reconstitution, recombinant: 50 mg [packaged with diluent and syringe]

Tenex® [US/Can] *see* guanfacine *on page 425*

teniposide (ten i POE side)

Synonyms EPT; VM-26

U.S./Canadian Brand Names Vumon® [US/Can]

Therapeutic Category Antineoplastic Agent

Use Treatment of acute lymphocytic leukemia, small cell lung cancer

Usual Dosage I.V.:

Children: 130 mg/m²/week, increasing to 150 mg/m² after 3 weeks and up to 180 mg/m² after 6 weeks

Acute lymphoblastic leukemia (ALL): 165 mg/m² twice weekly for 8-9 doses **or** 250 mg/m² weekly for 4-8 weeks

Adults: 50-180 mg/m² once or twice weekly for 4-6 weeks or 20-60 mg/m²/day for 5 days

Small cell lung cancer: 80-90 mg/m²/day for 5 days every 4-6 weeks

Dosage Forms Injection, solution: 10 mg/mL (5 mL) [contains benzyl alcohol, dehydrated alcohol, and polyoxyethylated castor oil]

Ten-K® *(Discontinued)* *see page 1042*

tenofovir (te NOE fo veer)

Synonyms PMPA; TDF; tenofovir disoproxil fumarate

U.S./Canadian Brand Names Viread™ [US]

Therapeutic Category Antiretroviral Agent, Reverse Transcriptase Inhibitor (Nucleotide)

Use Management of HIV infections in combination with at least two other antiretroviral agents

Usual Dosage Oral: Adults: HIV infection: 300 mg once daily

Dosage Forms Tablet, as disoproxil fumarate: 300 mg [equivalent to 245 mg tenofovir disoproxil]

tenofovir and emtricitabine *see* emtricitabine and tenofovir *on page 307*

tenofovir disoproxil fumarate *see* tenofovir *on this page*

Tenolin [Can] *see* atenolol *on page 85*

Tenoretic® [US/Can] *see* atenolol and chlorthalidone *on page 85*

Tenormin® [US/Can] *see* atenolol *on page 85*

Tenuate® [US/Can] *see* diethylpropion *on page 269*

Tenuate® Dospan® [US/Can] *see* diethylpropion *on page 269*

Tepanil® *(Discontinued)* *see page 1042*

Tepanil® TenTabs® *(Discontinued)* *see page 1042*

Tequin® [US/Can] *see* gatifloxacin *on page 397*

Terazol® [Can] *see* terconazole *on next page*

Terazol® 3 [US] *see* terconazole *on next page*

Terazol® 7 [US] *see* terconazole *on next page*

terazosin (ter AY zoe sin)

U.S./Canadian Brand Names Alti-Terazosin [Can]; Apo-Terazosin® [Can]; Hytrin® [US/Can]; Novo-Terazosin [Can]; Nu-Terazosin [Can]; PMS-Terazosin [Can]

Therapeutic Category Alpha-Adrenergic Blocking Agent

Use Management of mild to moderate hypertension; alone or in combination with other agents such as diuretics or beta-blockers; benign prostate hyperplasia (BPH)

Usual Dosage Oral: Adults:

Hypertension: Initial: 1 mg at bedtime; slowly increase dose to achieve desired blood pressure, up to 20 mg/day; usual dose range (JNC 7): 1-20 mg once daily

Dosage reduction may be needed when adding a diuretic or other antihypertensive agent; if drug is discontinued for greater than several days, consider beginning with initial dose and retitrate as needed; dosage may be given on a twice daily regimen if response is diminished at 24 hours and hypotensive is observed at 2-4 hours following a dose

Benign prostatic hyperplasia: Initial: 1 mg at bedtime, increasing as needed; most patients require 10 mg day; if no response after 4-6 weeks of 10 mg/day, may increase to 20 mg/day

Dosage Forms

Capsule (Hytrin®): 1 mg, 2 mg, 5 mg, 10 mg

Tablet: 1 mg, 2 mg, 5 mg, 10 mg

terbinafine (oral) (TER bin a feen OR al)

U.S./Canadian Brand Names Lamisil® Oral

Therapeutic Category Antifungal Agent

(Continued)

terbinafine (oral) *(Continued)*

Use Treatment of onychomycosis infections of the toenail or fingernail

Usual Dosage Adults: Oral:

Fingernail onychomycosis: 250 mg once daily for 6 weeks

Toenail onychomycosis: 250 mg once daily for 12 weeks

Dosage Forms Tablet: 250 mg

terbinafine (topical) (TER bin a feen TOP i kal)

Sound-Alike/Look-Alike Issues

Lamisil® may be confused with Lamictal®

U.S./Canadian Brand Names Lamisil® Topical

Therapeutic Category Antifungal Agent

Use Topical antifungal for the treatment of tinea pedis (athlete's foot), tinea cruris (jock itch), and tinea corporis (ring worm); tinea versicolor (lotion)

Usual Dosage Adults: Topical:

Athlete's foot: Apply to affected area twice daily for at least 1 week, not to exceed 4 weeks

Ringworm and jock itch: Apply to affected area once or twice daily for at least 1 week, not to exceed 4 weeks

Dosage Forms

Cream: 1% (15 g, 30 g)

Lotion: 1%

terbutaline (ter BYOO ta leen)

Sound-Alike/Look-Alike Issues

terbutaline may be confused with terbinafine, tolbutamide

U.S./Canadian Brand Names Brethine® [US]

Therapeutic Category Adrenergic Agonist Agent

Use Bronchodilator in reversible airway obstruction and bronchial asthma; tocolytic agent

Usual Dosage

Children <12 years: Bronchoconstriction:

Oral: Initial: 0.05 mg/kg/dose 3 times/day, increased gradually as required; maximum: 0.15 mg/kg/dose 3-4 times/day or a total of 5 mg/24 hours

SubQ: 0.005-0.01 mg/kg/dose to a maximum of 0.3 mg/dose every 15-20 minutes for 3 doses

Children >12 years and Adults: Bronchoconstriction:

Oral:

12-15 years: 2.5 mg every 6 hours 3 times/day; not to exceed 7.5 mg in 24 hours

>15 years: 5 mg/dose every 6 hours 3 times/day; if side effects occur, reduce dose to 2.5 mg every 6 hours; not to exceed 15 mg in 24 hours

SubQ: 0.25 mg/dose repeated in 15-30 minutes for one time only; a total dose of 0.5 mg should not be exceeded within a 4-hour period inhalations

Dosage Forms

Injection, solution, as sulfate: 1 mg/mL (1 mL)

Tablet, as sulfate: 2.5 mg, 5 mg

terconazole (ter KONE a zole)

Sound-Alike/Look-Alike Issues

terconazole may be confused with tioconazole

Synonyms triaconazole

U.S./Canadian Brand Names Terazol® [Can]; Terazol® 3 [US]; Terazol® 7 [US]

Therapeutic Category Antifungal Agent

Use Local treatment of vulvovaginal candidiasis

Usual Dosage Adults: Female:

Terazol® 3 vaginal cream: Insert 1 applicatorful intravaginally at bedtime for 3 consecutive days

Terazol® 7 vaginal cream: Insert 1 applicatorful intravaginally at bedtime for 7 consecutive days

Terazol® 3 vaginal suppository: Insert 1 suppository intravaginally at bedtime for 3 consecutive days

Dosage Forms

Cream, vaginal:

Terazol® 7: 0.4% (45 g) [packaged with measured-dose applicator]

Terazol® 3: 0.8% (20 g) [packaged with measured-dose applicator]

Suppository, vaginal (Terazol® 3): 80 mg (3s) [may contain coconut and/or palm kernel oil]

Terfluzine [Can] *see* trifluoperazine *on page 885*

teriparatide (ter i PAR a tide)

Synonyms parathyroid hormone (1-34); recombinant human parathyroid hormone (1-34); rhPTH(1-34)

U.S./Canadian Brand Names Forteo™ [US]

Therapeutic Category Diagnostic Agent

Use Treatment of osteoporosis in postmenopausal women at high risk of fracture; treatment of primary or hypogonadal osteoporosis in men at high risk of fracture

Usual Dosage SubQ: Adults: 20 mcg once daily; **Note:** Initial administration should occur under circumstances in which the patient may sit or lie down, in the event of orthostasis.

Dosage Forms Injection, solution: 250 mcg/mL (3 mL) [prefilled syringe, delivers teriparatide 20 mcg/dose]

terpin hydrate *(Discontinued)* *see page 1042*

terpin hydrate and codeine *(Discontinued)* *see page 1042*

Terra-Cortril® Ophthalmic Suspension *(Discontinued)* *see page 1042*

Terramycin® [Can] *see* oxytetracycline *on page 659*

Terramycin® I.M. [US] *see* oxytetracycline *on page 659*

Terramycin® Oral *(Discontinued)* *see page 1042*

Terramycin® w/Polymyxin B Ophthalmic [US] *see* oxytetracycline and polymyxin B *on page 659*

Tesamone® Injection *(Discontinued)* *see page 1042*

Teslac® [US/Can] *see* testolactone *on this page*

TESPA *see* thiotepa *on page 858*

Tessalon® [US/Can] *see* benzonatate *on page 109*

Tes-Tape® *(Discontinued)* *see page 1042*

Testim™ [US] *see* testosterone *on next page*

Testoderm® *(Discontinued)* *see page 1042*

Testoderm® [Can] *see* testosterone *on next page*

Testoderm® TTS *(Discontinued)* *see page 1042*

Testoderm® with Adhesive *(Discontinued)* *see page 1042*

testolactone (tes toe LAK tone)

Sound-Alike/Look-Alike Issues

testolactone may be confused with testosterone

U.S./Canadian Brand Names Teslac® [US/Can]

Therapeutic Category Androgen

Use Palliative treatment of advanced or disseminated breast carcinoma

Usual Dosage Adults: Female: Oral: 250 mg 4 times/day for at least 3 months; desired response may take as long as 3 months

Dosage Forms Tablet: 50 mg

Testomar® *(Discontinued)* *see page 1042*

Testopel® [US] *see* testosterone *on this page*

Testopel® Pellet *(Discontinued)* *see page 1042*

testosterone (tes TOS ter one)

Sound-Alike/Look-Alike Issues

testosterone may be confused with testolactone
Testoderm® may be confused with Estraderm®

Synonyms testosterone cypionate; testosterone enanthate

U.S./Canadian Brand Names Andriol® [Can]; Androderm® [US/Can]; AndroGel® [US/Can]; Andropository [Can]; Delatestryl® [US/Can]; Depotest® 100 [Can]; Depo®-Testosterone [US]; Everone® 200 [Can]; Striant™ [US]; Testim™ [US]; Testoderm® [Can]; Testopel® [US]

Therapeutic Category Androgen

Controlled Substance C-III

Use

Injection: Androgen replacement therapy in the treatment of delayed male puberty; male hypogonadism (primary or hypogonadotropic); inoperable female breast cancer (enanthate only)

Pellet: Androgen replacement therapy in the treatment of delayed male puberty; male hypogonadism (primary or hypogonadotropic)

Buccal, topical: Male hypogonadism (primary or hypogonadotropic)

Usual Dosage

Adolescents: I.M.:

Male hypogonadism:

Initiation of pubertal growth: 40-50 mg/m^2/dose (cypionate or enanthate ester) monthly until the growth rate falls to prepubertal levels

Terminal growth phase: 100 mg/m^2/dose (cypionate or enanthate ester) monthly until growth ceases

Maintenance virilizing dose: 100 mg/m^2/dose (cypionate or enanthate ester) twice monthly

Delayed male puberty: 40-50 mg/m^2/dose monthly (cypionate or enanthate ester) for 6 months

Adolescents and Adults: Pellet (for subcutaneous implantation): Delayed male puberty, male hypogonadism: 150-450 mg every 3-6 months

Adults:

I.M.:

Female: Inoperable breast cancer: Testosterone enanthate: 200-400 mg every 2-4 weeks

Male: Long-acting formulations: Testosterone enanthate (in oil)/testosterone cypionate (in oil): Hypogonadism: 50-400 mg every 2-4 weeks Delayed puberty: 50-200 mg every 2-4 weeks for a limited duration

Transdermal: Primary male hypogonadism **or** hypogonadotropic hypogonadism:

Testoderm®: Apply 6 mg patch daily to scrotum (if scrotum is inadequate, use a 4 mg daily system)

Androderm®: Initial: Apply 5 mg/day once nightly to clean, dry area on the back, abdomen, upper arms, or thighs; dosing range: 2.5-7.5 mg/day; in nonvirilized patients, dose may be initiated at 2.5 mg/day

AndroGel®, Testim™: 5 g (to deliver 50 mg of testosterone with 5 mg systemically absorbed) applied once daily (preferably in the morning) to clean, dry, intact skin of the shoulder and upper arms. AndroGel® may also be applied to the abdomen. Dosage may be increased to a maximum of 10 g (100 mg). **Do not apply testosterone gel to the genitals.**

Oral (buccal): Hypogonadism or hypogonadotropic hypogonadism: 30 mg twice daily (every 12 hours) applied to the gum region above the incisor tooth

Dosage Forms [DSC] = Discontinued product

Gel, topical:

AndroGel®: 25 mg/2.5 g (30s); 50 mg/5 g (30s) [1% unit-dose packet]

Testim™: 50 mg/5 g (30s) [1% unit-dose tube]

Injection, in oil, as cypionate (Depo® Testosterone): 100 mg/mL (10 mL); 200 mg/mL (1 mL, 10 mL) [contains benzyl alcohol, benzyl benzoate, and cottonseed oil]

Injection, in oil, as enanthate (Delatestryl®): 200 mg/mL (1 mL [prefilled syringe; contains sesame oil]; 5 mL [multidose vial; contains sesame oil])

Mucoadhesive, for buccal application [buccal system] (Striant™): 30 mg

Pellet, for subcutaneous implantation (Testopel®): 75 mg (1 pellet/vial)

Transdermal system:

Androderm®: 2.5 mg/day (60s); 5 mg/day (30s)

Testoderm®: 4 mg/day (30s); 6 mg/day (30s) [DSC]

Testoderm® with Adhesive: 6 mg/day (30s) [DSC]

testosterone cypionate *see* testosterone *on previous page*

testosterone enanthate *see* testosterone *on previous page*

Testred® [US] *see* methyltestosterone *on page 573*

tetanus and diphtheria toxoid *see* diphtheria and tetanus toxoid *on page 280*

tetanus antitoxin (TET a nus an tee TOKS in)

Synonyms TAT

Therapeutic Category Antitoxin

Use Tetanus prophylaxis or treatment of active tetanus only when tetanus immune globulin (TIG) is not available; tetanus immune globulin (Hyper-Tet®) is the preferred tetanus immunoglobulin for the treatment of active tetanus; may be given concomitantly with tetanus toxoid adsorbed when immediate treatment is required, but active immunization is desirable

Usual Dosage

Prophylaxis: I.M., SubQ:

Children <30 kg: 1500 units

Children and Adults ≥30 kg: 3000-5000 units

Treatment: Children and Adults: Inject 10,000-40,000 units into wound; administer 40,000-100,000 units

Dosage Forms Injection, equine: Not less than 400 units/mL (12.5 mL, 50 mL)

tetanus immune globulin (human)

(TET a nus i MYUN GLOB yoo lin HYU man)

Synonyms TIG

U.S./Canadian Brand Names BayTet™ [US/Can]

Therapeutic Category Immune Globulin

Use Passive immunization against tetanus; tetanus immune globulin is preferred over tetanus antitoxin for treatment of active tetanus; part of the management of an unclean, wound in a person whose history of previous receipt of tetanus toxoid is unknown or who has received less than three doses of tetanus toxoid; elderly may require TIG more often than younger patients with tetanus infection due to declining antibody titers with age

Usual Dosage I.M.:

Prophylaxis of tetanus:

Children: 4 units/kg; some recommend administering 250 units to small children

Adults: 250 units

Treatment of tetanus:

Children: 500-3000 units; some should infiltrate locally around the wound

Adults: 3000-6000 units

(Continued)

tetanus immune globulin (human) *(Continued)*

Dosage Forms Injection, solution [preservative free]: 250 units/mL (1 mL) [prefilled syringe]

tetanus toxoid (adsorbed) (TET a nus TOKS oyd ad SORBED)

Therapeutic Category Toxoid

Use Selective induction of active immunity against tetanus in selected patients. **Note:** Tetanus and diphtheria toxoids for adult use (Td) is the preferred immunizing agent for most adults and for children after their seventh birthday. Young children should receive trivalent DTwP or DTaP (diphtheria/tetanus/pertussis - whole cell or acellular), as part of their childhood immunization program, unless pertussis is contraindicated, then TD is warranted.

Usual Dosage Adults: I.M.:

Primary immunization: 0.5 mL; repeat 0.5 mL at 4-8 weeks after first dose and at 6-12 months after second dose

Routine booster doses are recommended only every 5-10 years

Dosage Forms Injection, suspension: Tetanus 5 Lf units per 0.5 mL (5 mL) [contains thimerosal]

tetanus toxoid (fluid) (TET a nus TOKS oyd FLOO id)

Synonyms tetanus toxoid plain

Therapeutic Category Toxoid

Use Indicated as booster dose in the active immunization against tetanus in the rare adult or child who is allergic to the aluminum adjuvant (a product containing adsorbed tetanus toxoid is preferred); not indicated for primary immunization

Usual Dosage

Primary immunization: Not indicated for this use.

Booster doses: I.M., SubQ: 0.5 mL every 10 years

Dosage Forms Injection, solution: Tetanus 4 Lf units per 0.5 mL (7.5 mL) [contains thimerosal; vial stopper contains dry natural latex rubber]

tetanus toxoid plain *see* tetanus toxoid (fluid) *on this page*

tetrabenazine *(Canada only)* (tet ra BENZ a zeen)

Therapeutic Category Monoamine Depleting Agent

Use Treatment of hyperkinetic movement disorders such as Huntington chorea, hemiballismus, senile chorea, tic and Gilles de la Tourette syndrome and tardive dyskinesia; not indicated for the treatment of levodopa-induced dyskinetic/choreiform movements; should only be used by (or in consultation with) physicians who are experienced in the treatment of hyperkinetic movement disorders.

Usual Dosage Oral:

Children: No adequately controlled clinical studies have been performed in children. Limited clinical experience suggests that treatment should be started at approximately half the adult dose, and titrated slowly and carefully according to tolerance and individual response.

Adults: Initial starting dose: 12.5 mg 2-3 times/day is recommended. This can be increased by 12.5 mg/day every 3-5 days until the maximal tolerated and effective dose is reached for the individual, and may have to be up/down titrated depending on individual tolerance. In most cases the maximal tolerated dose will be 25 mg 3 times/day. In very rare cases, a 200 mg dose has been reached (the maximum recommended dose in some publications). If there is no improvement at the maximal tolerated dose in 7 days, it is unlikely that Nitoman® will be of benefit to the patient, either by increasing the dose or by extending the duration of treatment.

Dosage Forms Tablet: 25 mg

tetracaine (TET ra kane)

Synonyms amethocaine hydrochloride; tetracaine hydrochloride

U.S./Canadian Brand Names AK-T-Caine™ [US]; Ametop™ [Can]; Cēpacol Viractin® [US-OTC]; Opticaine® [US]; Pontocaine® [US/Can]

Therapeutic Category Local Anesthetic

Use Spinal anesthesia; local anesthesia in the eye for various diagnostic and examination purposes; topically applied to nose and throat for various diagnostic procedures; topical gel [OTC] for treatment of pain associated with cold sores and fever blisters

Usual Dosage

Children ≥2 years and Adults: Topical gel [OTC]: Cold sores and fever blisters: Apply to affected area up to 3-4 times/day for up to 7 days

Adults:

Ophthalmic solution (not for prolonged use): Instill 1-2 drops

Spinal anesthesia:

High, medium, low, and saddle blocks: 0.2% to 0.3% solution

Prolonged (2-3 hours): 1% solution

Subarachnoid injection: 5-20 mg

Saddle block: 2-5 mg; a 1% solution should be diluted with equal volume of CSF before administration

Topical mucous membranes (2% solution): Apply as needed; dose should not exceed 20 mg

Dosage Forms

Gel, as hydrochloride (Cēpacol Viractin®): 2% (7.1 g)

Injection, solution, as hydrochloride (Pontocaine®): 1% [10 mg/mL] (2 mL) [contains sodium bisulfite]

Injection, solution, as hydrochloride [premixed in dextrose 6%] (Pontocaine®): 0.3% [3 mg/mL] (5 mL)

Injection, powder for reconstitution, as hydrochloride (Pontocaine®): 20 mg

Solution, ophthalmic, as hydrochloride: 0.5% [5 mg/mL] (15 mL)

AK-T-Caine™, Opticaine®: 0.5% (15 mL)

Pontocaine®: 0.5% (15 mL, 59 mL)

Solution, topical, as hydrochloride (Pontocaine®): 2% [20 mg/mL] (30 mL, 118 mL)

tetracaine and dextrose (TET ra kane & DEKS trose)

Synonyms dextrose and tetracaine

U.S./Canadian Brand Names Pontocaine® With Dextrose [US]

Therapeutic Category Local Anesthetic

Use Spinal anesthesia (saddle block)

Usual Dosage Dose varies with procedure, depth of anesthesia, duration desired and physical condition of patient

Dosage Forms Injection, as hydrochloride [premixed in dextrose 6%] (Pontocaine®): Tetracaine hydrochloride 0.3% and dextrose 6% (5 mL)

tetracaine hydrochloride *see* tetracaine *on this page*

tetracaine hydrochloride, benzocaine butyl aminobenzoate, and benzalkonium chloride *see* benzocaine, butyl aminobenzoate, tetracaine, and benzalkonium chloride *on page 109*

Tetracap® ***(Discontinued)*** *see page 1042*

tetracosactide *see* cosyntropin *on page 229*

tetracycline (tet ra SYE kleen)

Sound-Alike/Look-Alike Issues

tetracycline may be confused with tetradecyl sulfate

Synonyms achromycin; TCN; tetracycline hydrochloride

U.S./Canadian Brand Names Apo-Tetra® [Can]; Novo-Tetra [Can]; Nu-Tetra [Can]; Sumycin® [US]; Wesmycin® [US]

(Continued)

tetracycline *(Continued)*

Therapeutic Category Antibiotic, Ophthalmic; Antibiotic, Topical; Tetracycline Derivative

Use Treatment of susceptible bacterial infections of both gram-positive and gram-negative organisms; also infections due to *Mycoplasma*, *Chlamydia*, and *Rickettsia*; indicated for acne, exacerbations of chronic bronchitis, and treatment of gonorrhea and syphilis in patients that are allergic to penicillin; as part of a multidrug regimen for *H. pylori* eradication to reduce the risk of duodenal ulcer recurrence

Usual Dosage Oral:

Children >8 years: 25-50 mg/kg/day in divided doses every 6 hours

Adults: 250-500 mg/dose every 6 hours

Helicobacter pylori eradication: 500 mg 2-4 times/day depending on regimen; requires combination therapy with at least one other antibiotic and an acid-suppressing agent (proton pump inhibitor or H_2 blocker)

Dosage Forms

Capsule, as hydrochloride: 250 mg, 500 mg

Wesmycin®: 250 mg

Suspension, oral, as hydrochloride (Sumycin®): 125 mg/5 mL (480 mL) [contains sodium benzoate and sodium metabisulfite; fruit flavor]

Tablet, as hydrochloride (Sumycin®): 250 mg, 500 mg

tetracycline, bismuth subsalicylate, and metronidazole *see* bismuth subsalicylate, metronidazole, and tetracycline *on page 121*

tetracycline hydrochloride *see* tetracycline *on previous page*

tetracycline, metronidazole, and bismuth subsalicylate *see* bismuth subsalicylate, metronidazole, and tetracycline *on page 121*

tetrahydroaminoacrine *see* tacrine *on page 837*

tetrahydrocannabinol *see* dronabinol *on page 297*

tetrahydrozoline (tet ra hye DROZ a leen)

Sound-Alike/Look-Alike Issues

Visine® may be confused with Visken®

Synonyms tetrahydrozoline hydrochloride; tetryzoline

U.S./Canadian Brand Names Eye-Sine™ [US-OTC]; Geneye® [US-OTC]; Murine® Tears Plus [US-OTC]; Optigene® 3 [US-OTC]; Tyzine® [US]; Tyzine® Pediatric [US]; Visine® Advanced Relief [US-OTC]; Visine® Original [US-OTC]

Therapeutic Category Adrenergic Agonist Agent

Use Symptomatic relief of nasal congestion and conjunctival congestion

Usual Dosage

Nasal congestion: Intranasal:

Children 2-6 years: Instill 2-3 drops of 0.05% solution every 4-6 hours as needed, no more frequent than every 3 hours

Children >6 years and Adults: Instill 2-4 drops or 3-4 sprays of 0.1% solution every 3-4 hours as needed, no more frequent than every 3 hours

Conjunctival congestion: Ophthalmic: Adults: Instill 1-2 drops in each eye 2-4 times/day

Dosage Forms

Solution, intranasal, as hydrochloride:

Tyzine®: 0.1% (15 mL) [spray bottle; contains benzalkonium chloride]; (30 mL) [dropper bottle; contains benzalkonium chloride]

Tyzine® Pediatric: 0.05% (15 mL) [spray bottle; contains benzalkonium chloride]

Solution, ophthalmic, as hydrochloride: 0.05% (15 mL)

Eye-Sine™, Geneye®, Optigene® 3: 0.05% (15 mL) [may contain benzalkonium chloride]

Murine® Tears Plus: 0.05% (15 mL, 30 mL) [contains benzalkonium chloride]

Visine® Advanced Relief: 0.05% (30 mL) [contains benzalkonium chloride and polyethylene glycol]

Visine® Original: 0.05% (15 mL, 30 mL) [contains benzalkonium chloride; 15 mL size also available with dropper]

tetrahydrozoline hydrochloride *see* tetrahydrozoline *on previous page*

Tetralan® *(Discontinued)* *see page 1042*

Tetram® *(Discontinued)* *see page 1042*

Tetramune® *(Discontinued)* *see page 1042*

Tetrasine® Extra Ophthalmic *(Discontinued)* *see page 1042*

Tetrasine® Ophthalmic *(Discontinued)* *see page 1042*

Tetra Tannate Pediatric [US] *see* chlorpheniramine, ephedrine, phenylephrine, and carbetapentane *on page 190*

tetryzoline *see* tetrahydrozoline *on previous page*

Tevetan® HCT [US/Can] *see* eprosartan and hydrochlorothiazide *on page 316*

Teveten® [US/Can] *see* eprosartan *on page 316*

Texacort® [US] *see* hydrocortisone (topical) *on page 451*

TG *see* thioguanine *on page 857*

6-TG *see* thioguanine *on page 857*

T-Gen® *(Discontinued)* *see page 1042*

THA *see* tacrine *on page 837*

thalidomide (tha LI doe mide)

U.S./Canadian Brand Names Thalomid® [US/Can]

Therapeutic Category Immunosuppressant Agent

Use Treatment and maintenance of cutaneous manifestations of erythema nodosum leprosum

Usual Dosage Oral:

Cutaneous ENL:

Initiate dosing at 100-300 mg/day taken once daily at bedtime with water (at least 1 hour after evening meal)

Patients weighing <50 kg: Initiate at lower end of the dosing range

Severe cutaneous reaction or previously requiring high dose may be initiated at 400 mg/day; doses may be divided, but taken 1 hour after meals

Dosing should continue until active reaction subsides (usually at least 2 weeks), then tapered in 50 mg decrements every 2-4 weeks

Patients who flare during tapering or with a history or requiring prolonged maintenance should be maintained on the minimum dosage necessary to control the reaction. Efforts to taper should be repeated every 3-6 months, in increments of 50 mg every 2-4 weeks.

Dosage Forms Capsule: 50 mg

Thalitone® [US] *see* chlorthalidone *on page 195*

Thalomid® [US/Can] *see* thalidomide *on this page*

THAM® [US] *see* tromethamine *on page 891*

THC *see* dronabinol *on page 297*

Theelin® Aqueous Injection *(Discontinued)* *see page 1042*

Theobid® *(Discontinued)* *see page 1042*

Theobid® Jr Duracaps® *(Discontinued)* *see page 1042*

Theochron® [US] *see* theophylline *on next page*

Theochron® SR [Can] *see* theophylline *on next page*

Theoclear-80® *(Discontinued)* *see page 1042*

Theoclear®-L.A. *(Discontinued)* *see page 1042*

Theo-Dur® [Can] *see* theophylline *on this page*

Theo-Dur® (all products) *(Discontinued)* *see page 1042*

Theo-Dur® Sprinkle® *(Discontinued)* *see page 1042*

Theolair™ [US/Can] *see* theophylline *on this page*

Theolair-SR® *(Discontinued)* *see page 1042*

Theolate® [US] *see* theophylline and guaifenesin *on next page*

Theo-Organidin® *(Discontinued)* *see page 1042*

theophylline (thee OF i lin)

Sound-Alike/Look-Alike Issues

Theolair™ may be confused with Thiola™, Thyrolar®

Synonyms theophylline anhydrous

U.S./Canadian Brand Names Apo-Theo LA® [Can]; Elixophyllin® [US]; Novo-Theophyl SR [Can]; PMS-Theophylline [Can]; Pulmophylline [Can]; Quibron®-T [US]; Quibron®-T/SR [US/Can]; ratio-Theo-Bronc [Can]; Theochron® [US]; Theochron® SR [Can]; Theo-Dur® [Can]; Theolair™ [US/Can]; T-Phyl® [US]; Uniphyl® [US]; Uniphyl® SRT [Can]

Therapeutic Category Theophylline Derivative

Use Treatment of symptoms and reversible airway obstruction due to chronic asthma, chronic bronchitis, or COPD

Usual Dosage

Apnea: Dosage should be determined by plasma level monitoring; each 0.5 mg/kg of theophylline administered as a loading dose will result in a 1 mcg/mL increase in serum theophylline concentration

Loading dose: 5 mg/kg; dilute dose in 1-hour I.V. fluid via syringe pump over 1 hour

Maintenance: 2 mg/kg every 8-12 hours or 1-3 mg/kg/dose every 8-12 hours; administer I.V. push 1 mL/minute (2 mg/minute)

Treatment of acute bronchospasm in older patients: (>6 months of age): Loading dose (in patients not currently receiving theophylline): 6 mg/kg (based on aminophylline) administered I.V. over 20-30 minutes; 4.7 mg/kg (based on theophylline) administered I.V. over 20-30 minutes; administration rate should not exceed 20 mg (1 mL)/minute (theophylline) or 25 mg (1 mL)/minute (aminophylline)

Approximate maintenance dosage for treatment of acute bronchospasm:

Children:

6 months to 9 years: 1.2 mg/kg/hour (aminophylline); 0.95 mg/kg/hour (theophylline)

9-16 years and young adult smokers: 1 mg/kg/hour (aminophylline); 0.79 mg/kg/hour (theophylline)

Adults (healthy, nonsmoking): 0.7 mg/kg/hour (aminophylline); 0.55 mg/kg/hour (theophylline)

Older patients and patients with cor pulmonale: 0.6 mg/kg/hour (aminophylline); 0.47 mg/kg/hour (theophylline)

Patients with CHF or liver failure: 0.5 mg/kg/hour (aminophylline); 0.39 mg/kg/hour (theophylline)

Chronic therapy: Slow clinical titration is generally preferred

Initial dose: 16 mg/kg/24 hours or 400 mg/24 hours, whichever is less

Increasing dose: The above dosage may be increased in ~25% increments at 2- to 3-day intervals so long as the drug is tolerated or until the maximum dose is reached; monitor serum levels

Exercise caution in younger children who cannot complain of minor side effects, older adults, and those with cor pulmonale; CHF or liver disease may have unusually low dosage requirements

Dosage Forms [DSC] = Discontinued product

Capsule, extended release (Theo-24®): 100 mg, 200 mg, 300 mg, 400 mg [24 hours]

Elixir (Elixophyllin®): 80 mg/15 mL (480 mL) [contains alcohol 20%; fruit flavor]

Infusion [premixed in D_5W]: 0.8 mg/mL (500 mL, 1000 mL); 1.6 mg/mL (250 mL, 500 mL); 2 mg/mL (100 mL); 3.2 mg/mL (250 mL); 4 mg/mL (50 mL, 100 mL)

Solution, oral: 80 mg/15 mL (15 mL, 18.75 mL, 500 mL) [dye free, sugar free; contains alcohol 0.4% and benzoic acid; orange flavor]
Tablet, controlled release:
T-Phyl®: 200 mg [12 hours; contains cetostearyl alcohol]
Uniphyl®: 400 mg, 600 mg [24 hours; contains cetostearyl alcohol]
Tablet, extended release: 100 mg, 200 mg, 300 mg, 450 mg
Theochron®: 100 mg, 200 mg, 300 mg [12-24 hours]
Tablet, immediate release:
Quibron®-T: 300 mg
Theolair™: 125 mg, 250 mg
Tablet, sustained release (Quibron®-T/SR): 300 mg [8-12 hours]
Tablet, timed release (Theolair™-SR [DSC]): 300 mg, 500 mg

theophylline and guaifenesin (thee OF i lin & gwye FEN e sin)

Synonyms guaifenesin and theophylline

U.S./Canadian Brand Names Elixophyllin-GG® [US]; Quibron® [US]; Theolate® [US]

Therapeutic Category Theophylline Derivative

Use Symptomatic treatment of bronchospasm associated with bronchial asthma, chronic bronchitis, and pulmonary emphysema

Usual Dosage Adults: Oral: 16 mg/kg/day or 400 mg theophylline/day, in divided doses, every 6-8 hours

Dosage Forms
Capsule (Quibron®): Theophylline 150 mg and guaifenesin 90 mg
Liquid:
Elixophyllin-GG®: Theophylline 100 mg and guaifenesin 100 mg per 15 mL (240 mL, 480 mL) [alcohol free, dye free, sugar free; cherry-berry flavor]
Theolate: Theophylline 150 mg and guaifenesin 90 mg per 15 mL (480 mL) [alcohol free, dye free]

theophylline anhydrous *see* theophylline *on previous page*

theophylline ethylenediamine *see* aminophylline *on page 46*

Theo-Sav® *(Discontinued)* *see page 1042*

Theospan®-SR *(Discontinued)* *see page 1042*

Theostat-80® *(Discontinued)* *see page 1042*

Theovent® *(Discontinued)* *see page 1042*

Theo-X® *(Discontinued)* *see page 1042*

Therabid® *(Discontinued)* *see page 1042*

Theracort® [US] *see* hydrocortisone (topical) *on page 451*

TheraCys® [US] *see* BCG vaccine *on page 101*

Thera-Flu® Cold and Sore Throat Night Time [US-OTC] *see* acetaminophen, chlorpheniramine, and pseudoephedrine *on page 11*

Thera-Flur® *(Discontinued)* *see page 1042*

Thera-Flur-N® [US] *see* fluoride *on page 376*

Thera-Flu® Severe Cold Non-Drowsy *(Discontinued)* *see page 1042*

Theragran® Heart Right™ [US-OTC] *see* vitamins (multiple/oral) *on page 927*

Theragran-M® Advanced Formula [US-OTC] *see* vitamins (multiple/oral) *on page 927*

Thera-Hist® Syrup *(Discontinued)* *see page 1042*

Theramine® Expectorant *(Discontinued)* *see page 1042*

Theramycin Z® [US] *see* erythromycin *on page 320*

TheraPatch® Warm *(Discontinued)* *see page 1042*

therapeutic multivitamins *see* vitamins (multiple/oral) *on page 927*

Theratears® [US] *see* carboxymethylcellulose *on page 161*

Thermazene® [US] *see* silver sulfadiazine *on page 804*

thiabendazole (thye a BEN da zole)

Synonyms tiabendazole

U.S./Canadian Brand Names Mintezol® [US]

Therapeutic Category Anthelmintic

Use Treatment of strongyloidiasis, cutaneous larva migrans, visceral larva migrans, dracunculiasis, trichinosis, and mixed helminthic infections

Usual Dosage Purgation is not required prior to use; drinking of fruit juice aids in expulsion of worms by removing the mucous to which the intestinal tapeworms attach themselves.

Children and Adults:

Oral: 50 mg/kg/day divided every 12 hours (if >68 kg: 1.5 g/dose); maximum dose: 3 g/day

Treatment duration: Strongyloidiasis, ascariasis, uncinariasis: For 2 consecutive days Cutaneous larva migrans: For 2 consecutive days; if active lesions are still present 2 days after completion, a second course of treatment is recommended. Visceral larva migrans: For 7 consecutive days Trichinosis: For 2-4 consecutive days; optimal dosage not established Dracunculosis: 50-75 mg/kg/day divided every 12 hours for 3 days

Dosage Forms

Suspension, oral: 500 mg/5 mL (120 mL)

Tablet, chewable: 500 mg [orange flavor]

Thiacide® *(Discontinued)* *see page 1042*

thiamazole *see* methimazole *on page 564*

Thiamilate® [US-OTC] *see* thiamine *on this page*

thiamine (THYE a min)

Sound-Alike/Look-Alike Issues

thiamine may be confused with Tenormin®, Thorazine®

Synonyms aneurine hydrochloride; thiamine hydrochloride; thiaminium chloride hydrochloride; vitamin B_1

U.S./Canadian Brand Names Betaxin® [Can]; Thiamilate® [US-OTC]

Therapeutic Category Vitamin, Water Soluble

Use Treatment of thiamine deficiency including beriberi, Wernicke encephalopathy syndrome, and peripheral neuritis associated with pellagra, alcoholic patients with altered sensorium; various genetic metabolic disorders

Usual Dosage

Recommended daily allowance:

<6 months: 0.3 mg
6 months to 1 year: 0.4 mg
1-3 years: 0.7 mg
4-6 years: 0.9 mg
7-10 years: 1 mg
11-14 years: 1.1-1.3 mg
>14 years: 1-1.5 mg

Thiamine deficiency (beriberi):

Children: 10-25 mg/dose I.M. or I.V. daily (if critically ill), or 10-50 mg/dose orally every day for 2 weeks, then 5-10 mg/dose orally daily for 1 month

Adults: 5-30 mg/dose I.M. or I.V. 3 times/day (if critically ill); then orally 5-30 mg/day in single or divided doses 3 times/day for 1 month

Wernicke's encephalopathy: Adults: Initial: 100 mg I.V., then 50-100 mg/day I.M. or I.V. until consuming a regular, balanced diet

Dietary supplement (depends on caloric or carbohydrate content of the diet):

Infants: 0.3-0.5 mg/day

Children: 0.5-1 mg/day
Adults: 1-2 mg/day
Note: The above doses can be found in multivitamin preparations
Metabolic disorders: Oral: Adults: 10-20 mg/day (dosages up to 4 g/day in divided doses have been used)

Dosage Forms
Injection, solution, as hydrochloride: 100 mg/mL (2 mL)
Tablet, as hydrochloride: 50 mg, 100 mg, 250 mg, 500 mg
Tablet, enteric coated, as hydrochloride (Thiamilate®): 20 mg

thiamine hydrochloride *see* thiamine *on previous page*

thiaminium chloride hydrochloride *see* thiamine *on previous page*

thimerosal (thye MER oh sal)

U.S./Canadian Brand Names Mersol® [US-OTC]; Merthiolate® [US-OTC]
Therapeutic Category Antibacterial, Topical
Use Organomercurial antiseptic with sustained bacteriostatic and fungistatic activity
Usual Dosage Apply 1-3 times/day
Dosage Forms
Solution, topical (Merthiolate®): 0.1% [1 mg/mL = 1:1000] (30 mL)
Solution, topical spray (Merthiolate®): 0.1% [1 mg/mL = 1:1000] (60 g)
Tincture, topical (Mersol®): 0.1% [1 mg/mL = 1:1000] (120 mL, 480 mL, 4000 mL)

thioguanine (thye oh GWAH neen)

Synonyms 2-amino-6-mercaptopurine; NSC-752; TG; 6-TG; 6-thioguanine; tioguanine
U.S./Canadian Brand Names Lanvis® [Can]
Therapeutic Category Antineoplastic Agent
Use Treatment of acute myelogenous (nonlymphocytic) leukemia; treatment of chronic myelogenous leukemia and granulocytic leukemia
Usual Dosage Total daily dose can be given at one time; is sometimes ordered as 6-thioguanine, with 6 being part of the drug name and not a unit or strength

Oral (refer to individual protocols):
Infants and Children <3 years: Combination drug therapy for acute nonlymphocytic leukemia: 3.3 mg/kg/day in divided doses twice daily for 4 days
Children and Adults: 2-3 mg/kg/day calculated to nearest 20 mg or 75-200 mg/m^2/day in 1-2 divided doses for 5-7 days or until remission is attained

Dosage Forms
Injection, powder for reconstitution: 75 mg [investigational in U.S.]
Tablet [scored]: 40 mg

6-thioguanine *see* thioguanine *on this page*

Thiola® [US/Can] *see* tiopronin *on page 865*

thiopental (thye oh PEN tal)

Synonyms thiopental sodium
U.S./Canadian Brand Names Pentothal® [US/Can]
Therapeutic Category Barbiturate
Controlled Substance C-III
Use Induction of anesthesia; adjunct for intubation in head injury patients; control of convulsive states; treatment of elevated intracranial pressure
Usual Dosage I.V.:
Induction anesthesia:
Infants: 5-8 mg/kg
Children 1-12 years: 5-6 mg/kg
Adults: 3-5 mg/kg
Maintenance anesthesia:
Children: 1 mg/kg as needed
(Continued)

thiopental *(Continued)*

Adults: 25-100 mg as needed

Increased intracranial pressure: Children and Adults: 1.5-5 mg/kg/dose; repeat as needed to control intracranial pressure

Seizures:

Children: 2-3 mg/kg/dose; repeat as needed

Adults: 75-250 mg/dose; repeat as needed

Note: Accumulation may occur with chronic dosing due to lipid solubility; prolonged recovery may result from redistribution of thiopental from fat stores

Dosage Forms Injection, powder for reconstitution, as sodium: 500 mg, 2.5 g, 5 g

Pentothal®: 250 mg, 400 mg, 500 mg, 1 g, 2.5 g, 5 g

thiopental sodium *see* thiopental *on previous page*

thiophosphoramide *see* thiotepa *on this page*

Thioplex® ***(Discontinued)*** *see page 1042*

thioproperazine *(Canada only)* (thye oh pro PER a zeen)

Therapeutic Category Neuroleptic Agent

Use All types of acute and chronic schizophrenia, including those which did not respond to the usual neuroleptics; manic syndromes.

Usual Dosage Initial treatment: Adults: It is recommended to start treatment at a low dosage of about 5 mg/day in a single dose or in divided doses. This initial dosage is gradually increased by the same amount every 2-3 days until the usual effective dosage of 30-40 mg/day is reached. In some cases, higher dosages of 90 mg or more per day, are necessary to control the psychotic manifestations.

Children >10 years of age: Start treatment with a daily dosage of 1-3 mg following the method of treatment described for adults

Maintenance therapy: Adults and Children: Dosage should be reduced gradually to the lowest effective level, which may be as low as a few mg per day and maintained as long as necessary

Dosage Forms Tablet, as mesylate: 10 mg

thiosulfuric acid disodium salt *see* sodium thiosulfate *on page 817*

thiotepa (thye oh TEP a)

Synonyms TESPA; thiophosphoramide; triethylenethiophosphoramide; TSPA

Therapeutic Category Antineoplastic Agent

Use Treatment of superficial tumors of the bladder; palliative treatment of adenocarcinoma of breast or ovary; lymphomas and sarcomas; controlling intracavitary effusions caused by metastatic tumors; I.T. use: CNS leukemia/lymphoma, CNS metastases

Usual Dosage Refer to individual protocols; dosing must be based on the clinical and hematologic response of the patient

Children: Sarcomas: I.V.: 25-65 mg/m^2 as a single dose every 21 days

Adults:

I.M., I.V., SubQ: 30-60 mg/m^2 once weekly

I.V.: 0.3-0.4 mg/kg by rapid I.V. administration every 1-4 weeks, **or** 0.2 mg/kg or 6-8 mg/m^2/day for 4-5 days every 2-4 weeks

High-dose therapy for bone marrow transplant: I.V.: 500 mg/m^2, up to 900 mg/m^2

I.M.: 15-30 mg in various schedules have been given

Intracavitary: 0.6-0.8 mg/kg or 30-60 mg weekly

Intrapericardial: 15-30 mg

Intrathecal: 10-15 mg or 5-11.5 mg/m^2

Dosage Forms Injection, powder for reconstitution: 15 mg

thiothixene (thye oh THIKS een)

Sound-Alike/Look-Alike Issues
thiothixene may be confused with thioridazine
Navane® may be confused with Norvasc®, Nubain®

Synonyms tiotixene

U.S./Canadian Brand Names Navane® [US/Can]

Therapeutic Category Thioxanthene Derivative

Use Management of schizophrenia

Usual Dosage Oral: Children >12 years and Adults:
Mild to moderate psychosis: 2 mg 3 times/day, up to 20-30 mg/day; more severe psychosis: Initial: 5 mg 2 times/day, may increase gradually, if necessary; maximum: 60 mg/day
Rapid tranquilization of the agitated patient (administered every 30-60 minutes): 5-10 mg; average total dose for tranquilization: 15-30 mg

Dosage Forms [DSC] = Discontinued product
Capsule: 1 mg, 2 mg, 5 mg, 10 mg
Navane®: 1 mg, 2 mg, 5 mg, 10 mg, 20 mg
Solution, oral concentrate, as hydrochloride [DSC]: 5 mg/mL (120 mL) [fruit flavor]

thonzonium, neomycin, colistin, and hydrocortisone *see* neomycin, colistin, hydrocortisone, and thonzonium *on page 610*

Thorazine® ***(Discontinued)*** *see page 1042*

Thrombate III® [US/Can] *see* antithrombin III *on page 65*

Thrombinar® ***(Discontinued)*** *see page 1042*

Thrombin-JMI® [US] *see* thrombin (topical) *on this page*

thrombin (topical) (THROM bin TOP i kal)

U.S./Canadian Brand Names Thrombin-JMI® [US]; Thrombogen® [US]; Thrombostat™ [Can]

Therapeutic Category Hemostatic Agent

Use Hemostasis whenever minor bleeding from capillaries and small venules is accessible

Usual Dosage Use 1000-2000 units/mL of solution where bleeding is profuse; apply powder directly to the site of bleeding or on oozing surfaces; use 100 units/mL for bleeding from skin or mucosal surfaces

Dosage Forms Powder for reconstitution, topical:
Thrombin-JMI®: 1000 units, 5000 units, 10,000 units, 20,000 units, 50,000 units
Thrombin-JMI® Spray Kit: 5000 unit, 10,000 units, 20,000 units
Thrombin-JMI® Syringe Spray Kit: 10,000 units, 20,000 units
Thrombogen®: 5000 units, 20,000 units
Thrombogen® Spray Kit: 10,000 units, 20,000 units

Thrombogen® [US] *see* thrombin (topical) *on this page*

Thrombostat® ***(Discontinued)*** *see page 1042*

Thrombostat™ [Can] *see* thrombin (topical) *on this page*

thymocyte stimulating factor *see* aldesleukin *on page 28*

Thymoglobulin® [US] *see* antithymocyte globulin (rabbit) *on page 66*

Thypinone® ***(Discontinued)*** *see page 1042*

Thyrar® ***(Discontinued)*** *see page 1042*

Thyrel® TRH ***(Discontinued)*** *see page 1042*

Thyro-Block® ***(Discontinued)*** *see page 1042*

Thyrogen® [US/Can] *see* thyrotropin alpha *on next page*

thyroid (THYE royd)

Synonyms desiccated thyroid; thyroid extract; thyroid USP

U.S./Canadian Brand Names Armour® Thyroid [US]; Nature-Throid® NT [US]; Westhroid® [US]

Therapeutic Category Thyroid Product

Use Replacement or supplemental therapy in hypothyroidism; pituitary TSH suppressants (thyroid nodules, thyroiditis, multinodular goiter, thyroid cancer), thyrotoxicosis, diagnostic suppression tests

Usual Dosage Adults: Oral: Start at 30 mg/day and titrate by 30 mg/day in increments of 2- to 3-week intervals; usual maintenance dose: 60-120 mg/day

Dosage Forms

Capsule: 15 mg, 30 mg, 60 mg, 90 mg, 120 mg, 180 mg, 240 mg

Tablet: 30 mg, 32.5 mg, 60 mg, 65 mg, 120 mg, 130 mg, 180 mg

Armour® Thyroid: 15 mg, 30 mg, 60 mg, 90 mg, 120 mg, 180 mg, 240 mg, 300 mg

Nature-Throid® NT, Westhroid®: 32.4 mg, 64.8 mg, 129.6 mg, 194.4 mg

thyroid extract *see* thyroid *on this page*

Thyroid Strong® ***(Discontinued)*** *see page 1042*

thyroid USP *see* thyroid *on this page*

Thyrolar® [US/Can] *see* liotrix *on page 523*

thyrotropin alpha (thye roe TROE pin AL fa)

Sound-Alike/Look-Alike Issues

Thyrogen® may be confused with Thyrolar®

Synonyms human thyroid stimulating hormone; TSH

U.S./Canadian Brand Names Thyrogen® [US/Can]

Therapeutic Category Diagnostic Agent

Use As an adjunctive diagnostic tool for serum thyroglobulin (Tg) testing with or without radioiodine imaging in the follow-up of patients with well-differentiated thyroid cancer

Potential clinical use:

1. Patients with an undetectable Tg on thyroid hormone suppressive therapy to exclude the diagnosis of residual or recurrent thyroid cancer
2. Patients requiring serum Tg testing and radioiodine imaging who are unwilling to undergo thyroid hormone withdrawal testing and whose treating physician believes that use of a less sensitive test is justified
3. Patients who are either unable to mount an adequate endogenous TSH response to thyroid hormone withdrawal or in whom withdrawal is medically contraindicated

Usual Dosage Children >16 years and Adults: I.M.: 0.9 mg every 24 hours for 2 doses or every 72 hours for 3 doses

For radioiodine imaging, radioiodine administration should be given 24 hours following the final Thyrogen® injection. Scanning should be performed 48 hours after radioiodine administration (72 hours after the final injection of Thyrogen®).

For serum testing, serum Tg should be obtained 72 hours after final injection.

Dosage Forms Injection, powder for reconstitution:

Two-vial kit: 1.1 mg [supplied as two vials of Thyrogen® and two 10 mL vials of SWFI]

Four-vial kit: 1.1 mg [supplied as four vials of Thyrogen® and two 10 mL vials of SWFI]

thyrotropin releasing hormone *see* protirelin *on page 744*

Thytropar® ***(Discontinued)*** *see page 1042*

tiabendazole *see* thiabendazole *on page 856*

tiagabine (tye AG a bene)

Sound-Alike/Look-Alike Issues

tiagabine may be confused with tizanidine

Synonyms tiagabine hydrochloride

U.S./Canadian Brand Names Gabitril® [US/Can]

Therapeutic Category Anticonvulsant

Use Adjunctive therapy in adults and children ≥12 years of age in the treatment of partial seizures

Usual Dosage Oral (administer with food):

Children 12-18 years: 4 mg once daily for 1 week; may increase to 8 mg daily in 2 divided doses for 1 week; then may increase by 4-8 mg weekly to response or up to 32 mg daily in 2-4 divided doses

Adults: 4 mg once daily for 1 week; may increase by 4-8 mg weekly to response or up to 56 mg daily in 2-4 divided doses

Dosage Forms Tablet, as hydrochloride: 2 mg, 4 mg, 12 mg, 16 mg

tiagabine hydrochloride *see* tiagabine *on previous page*

Tiamate® *(Discontinued)* *see page 1042*

Tiamol® [Can] *see* fluocinonide *on page 375*

Tiaprofenic-200 [Can] *see* tiaprofenic acid *(Canada only)* *on this page*

Tiaprofenic-300 [Can] *see* tiaprofenic acid *(Canada only)* *on this page*

tiaprofenic acid *(Canada only)* (tye ah PRO fen ik AS id)

U.S./Canadian Brand Names Albert® Tiafen [Can]; Apo-Tiaprofenic® [Can]; Dom-Tiaprofenic® [Can]; Novo-Tiaprofenic [Can]; Nu-Tiaprofenic [Can]; PMS-Tiaprofenic [Can]; Surgam® [Can]; Surgam® SR [Can]; Tiaprofenic-200 [Can]; Tiaprofenic-300 [Can]

Therapeutic Category Nonsteroidal Antiinflammatory Drug (NSAID)

Use Relief of signs and symptoms of rheumatoid arthritis and osteoarthritis (degenerative joint disease)

Usual Dosage Oral: Adults:

Rheumatoid arthritis:

Tablet: Usual initial and maintenance dose: 600 mg/day in 3 divided doses; some patients may do well on 300 mg twice daily; maximum daily dose: 600 mg

Sustained release capsule: Initial and maintenance dose: 2 sustained release capsules of 300 mg once daily; Surgam® SR capsules should be swallowed whole

Osteoarthritis:

Tablet: Usual initial and maintenance dose: 600 mg/day in 2 or 3 divided doses; in rare instances patients may be maintained on 300 mg/day in divided doses; maximum daily dose: 600 mg

Sustained release capsule: Initial and maintenance dose: 2 sustained release capsules of 300 mg once daily; Surgam® SR capsules should be swallowed whole

Dosage Forms

Capsule, sustained release: 300 mg

Tablet: 200 mg, 300 mg

Tiazac® [US/Can] *see* diltiazem *on page 273*

Ticar® [US] *see* ticarcillin *on this page*

ticarcillin (tye kar SIL in)

Sound-Alike/Look-Alike Issues

Ticar® may be confused with Tigan®

Synonyms ticarcillin disodium

U.S./Canadian Brand Names Ticar® [US]

Therapeutic Category Penicillin

Use Treatment of susceptible infections such as septicemia, acute and chronic respiratory tract infections, skin and soft tissue infections, and urinary tract infections due to susceptible strains of *Pseudomonas*, and other gram-negative bacteria

Usual Dosage Ticarcillin is generally given I.V., I.M. injection is only for the treatment of uncomplicated urinary tract infections and dose should not exceed 2 g/injection when administered I.M.

(Continued)

ticarcillin *(Continued)*

Neonates: I.M., I.V.:
Postnatal age <7 days:
<2000 g: 75 mg/kg/dose every 12 hours
>2000 g: 75 mg/kg/dose every 8 hours
Postnatal age >7 days:
<1200 g: 75 mg/kg/dose every 12 hours
1200-2000 g: 75 mg/kg/dose every 8 hours
>2000 g: 75 mg/kg/dose every 6 hours
Infants and Children:
Systemic infections: I.V.: 200-300 mg/kg/day in divided doses every 4-6 hours
Urinary tract infections: I.M., I.V.: 50-100 mg/kg/day in divided doses every 6-8 hours
Maximum dose: 24 g/day
Adults: I.M., I.V.: 1-4 g every 4-6 hours, usual dose: 3 g I.V. every 4-6 hours

Dosage Forms Injection, powder for reconstitution, as disodium: 3 g, 20 g

ticarcillin and clavulanate potassium

(tye kar SIL in & klav yoo LAN ate poe TASS ee um)

Synonyms ticarcillin and clavulanic acid

U.S./Canadian Brand Names Timentin® [US/Can]

Therapeutic Category Penicillin

Use Treatment of infections of lower respiratory tract, urinary tract, skin and skin structures, bone and joint, and septicemia caused by susceptible organisms. Clavulanate expands activity of ticarcillin to include beta-lactamase producing strains of *S. aureus*, *H. influenzae*, *Bacteroides* species, and some other gram-negative bacilli

Usual Dosage I.V.:
Children and Adults <60 kg: 200-300 mg of ticarcillin component/kg/day in divided doses every 4-6 hours
Children >60 kg and Adults: 3.1 g (ticarcillin 3 g plus clavulanic acid 0.1 g) every 4-6 hours; maximum: 24 g/day
Urinary tract infections: 3.1 g every 6-8 hours

Dosage Forms
Infusion [premixed, frozen]: Ticarcillin disodium 3 g and clavulanate potassium 0.1 g (100 mL)
Injection, powder for reconstitution: Ticarcillin disodium 3 g and clavulanate potassium 0.1 g (3.1 g, 31 g)

ticarcillin and clavulanic acid *see* ticarcillin and clavulanate potassium *on this page*

ticarcillin disodium *see* ticarcillin *on previous page*

TICE® BCG [US] *see* BCG vaccine *on page 101*

Ticlid® [US/Can] *see* ticlopidine *on this page*

ticlopidine (tye KLOE pi deen)

Synonyms ticlopidine hydrochloride

U.S./Canadian Brand Names Alti-Ticlopidine [Can]; Apo-Ticlopidine® [Can]; Gen-Ticlopidine [Can]; Novo-Ticlopidine [Can]; Nu-Ticlopidine [Can]; PMS-Ticlopidine [Can]; Rhoxal-ticlopidine [Can]; Ticlid® [US/Can]

Therapeutic Category Antiplatelet Agent

Use Platelet aggregation inhibitor that reduces the risk of thrombotic stroke in patients who have had a stroke or stroke precursors. **Note:** Due to its association with life-threatening hematologic disorders, ticlopidine should be reserved for patients who are intolerant to aspirin, or who have failed aspirin therapy. Adjunctive therapy (with aspirin) following successful coronary stent implantation to reduce the incidence of subacute stent thrombosis.

Usual Dosage Oral: Adults:
Stroke prevention: 250 mg twice daily with food

Coronary artery stenting (initiate after successful implantation): 250 mg twice daily with food (in combination with antiplatelet doses of aspirin) for up to 30 days

Dosage Forms Tablet, as hydrochloride: 250 mg

ticlopidine hydrochloride *see* ticlopidine *on previous page*

Ticon® *(Discontinued)* *see page 1042*

TIG *see* tetanus immune globulin (human) *on page 849*

Tigan® [US/Can] *see* trimethobenzamide *on page 887*

Tiject-20® *(Discontinued)* *see page 1042*

Tikosyn™ [US/Can] *see* dofetilide *on page 286*

Tilade® [US/Can] *see* nedocromil (inhalation) *on page 608*

tiludronate (tye LOO droe nate)

Synonyms tiludronate disodium

U.S./Canadian Brand Names Skelid® [US]

Therapeutic Category Bisphosphonate Derivative

Use Treatment of Paget disease of the bone in patients who have a level of serum alkaline phosphatase (SAP) at least twice the upper limit of normal, or who are symptomatic, or who are at risk for future complications of their disease

Usual Dosage Tiludronate should be taken with 6-8 oz of plain water and not taken within 2 hours of food

Adults: Oral: 400 mg (2 tablets of tiludronic acid) daily for a period of 3 months; allow an interval of 3 months to assess response

Dosage Forms Tablet, tiludronic acid: 200 mg [equivalent to 240 mg tiludronate disodium]

tiludronate disodium *see* tiludronate *on this page*

Tim-AK [Can] *see* timolol *on this page*

Timecelles® *(Discontinued)* *see page 1042*

Timentin® [US/Can] *see* ticarcillin and clavulanate potassium *on previous page*

timolol (TYE moe lole)

Sound-Alike/Look-Alike Issues

timolol may be confused with atenolol, Tylenol®

Timoptic® may be confused with Talacen®, Viroptic®

Synonyms timolol hemihydrate; timolol maleate

U.S./Canadian Brand Names Alti-Timolol [Can]; Apo-Timol® [Can]; Apo-Timop® [Can]; Betimol® [US]; Blocadren® [US]; Gen-Timolol [Can]; Istalol™ [US]; Nu-Timolol [Can]; Phoxal-timolol [Can]; PMS-Timolol [Can]; Tim-AK [Can]; Timoptic® [US/Can]; Timoptic® OcuDose® [US]; Timoptic-XE® [US/Can]

Therapeutic Category Beta-Adrenergic Blocker

Use Ophthalmic dosage form used in treatment of elevated intraocular pressure such as glaucoma or ocular hypertension; oral dosage form used for treatment of hypertension and angina, to reduce mortality following myocardial infarction, and for prophylaxis of migraine

Usual Dosage

Ophthalmic:

Children and Adults:

Solution: Initial: Instill 1 drop (0.25% solution) twice daily; increase to 0.5% solution if response not adequate; decrease to 1 drop/day if controlled; do not exceed 1 drop twice daily of 0.5% solution

Gel-forming solution (Timoptic-XE®): Instill 1 drop (either 0.25% or 0.5% solution) once daily

Adults: Solution (Istalol®): Instill 1 drop (0.5% solution) once daily in the morning

(Continued)

timolol *(Continued)*

Oral: Adults:

Hypertension: Initial: 10 mg twice daily, increase gradually every 7 days, usual dosage: 20-40 mg/day in 2 divided doses; maximum: 60 mg/day

Prevention of myocardial infarction: 10 mg twice daily initiated within 1-4 weeks after infarction

Migraine headache: Initial: 10 mg twice daily, increase to maximum of 30 mg/day

Dosage Forms Note: Strength expressed as base.

Gel-forming solution, ophthalmic, as maleate: 0.25% (5 mL); 0.5% (2.5 mL, 5 mL)

Timoptic-XE®: 0.25% (2.5 mL, 5 mL); 0.5% (2.5 mL, 5 mL)

Solution, ophthalmic, as hemihydrate (Betimol®): 0.25% (5 mL, 10 mL, 15 mL); 0.5% (5 mL, 10 mL, 15 mL) [contains benzalkonium chloride]

Solution, ophthalmic, as maleate: 0.25% (5 mL, 10 mL, 15 mL); 0.5% (5 mL, 10 mL, 15 mL) [contains benzalkonium chloride]

Istalol™: 0.5% (10 mL) [contains benzalkonium chloride and potassium sorbate]

Timoptic®: 0.25% (5 mL, 10 mL); 0.5% (5 mL, 10 mL) [contains benzalkonium chloride]

Solution, ophthalmic, as maleate [preservative free] (Timoptic® OcuDose®): 0.25% (0.2 mL); 0.5% (0.2 mL) [single use]

Tablet, as maleate (Blocadren®): 5 mg, 10 mg, 20 mg

timolol and dorzolamide *see* dorzolamide and timolol *on page 290*

timolol hemihydrate *see* timolol *on previous page*

timolol maleate *see* timolol *on previous page*

Timoptic® [US/Can] *see* timolol *on previous page*

Timoptic® OcuDose® [US] *see* timolol *on previous page*

Timoptic-XE® [US/Can] *see* timolol *on previous page*

Tinactin® Antifungal Jock Itch [US-OTC] *see* tolnaftate *on page 870*

Tinactin® Antifungal [US-OTC] *see* tolnaftate *on page 870*

Tinaderm [US-OTC] *see* tolnaftate *on page 870*

Tinamed® [US-OTC] *see* salicylic acid *on page 789*

TinBen® *(Discontinued)* *see page 1042*

Tindal® *(Discontinued)* *see page 1042*

Tindamax™ [US] *see* tinidazole *on this page*

tine test *see* tuberculin tests *on page 893*

Ting® [US-OTC] *see* tolnaftate *on page 870*

tinidazole (tye NI da zole)

U.S./Canadian Brand Names Tindamax™ [US]

Therapeutic Category Amebicide; Antibiotic, Miscellaneous; Antiprotozoal, Nitroimidazole

Use Treatment of trichomoniasis caused by *T. vaginalis*; treatment of giardiasis caused by *G. duodenalis (G. lamblia)*; treatment of intestinal amebiasis and amebic liver abscess caused by *E. histolytica*

Usual Dosage Oral:

Children >3 years:

Amebiasis, intestinal: 50 mg/kg/day for 3 days (maximum dose: 2 g/day)

Amebiasis, liver abscess: 50 mg/kg/day for 3-5 days (maximum dose: 2 g/day)

Giardiasis: 50 mg/kg as a single dose (maximum dose: 2 g)

Adults:

Amebiasis, intestinal: 2 g/day for 3 days

Amebiasis, liver abscess: 2 g/day for 3-5 days

Giardiasis: 2 g as a single dose

Trichomoniasis: Oral: 2 g as a single dose; sexual partners should be treated at the same time

Dosage Forms Tablet, scored: 250 mg, 500 mg

Tinver® ***(Discontinued)*** *see page 1042*

tinzaparin (tin ZA pa rin)

Synonyms tinzaparin sodium

U.S./Canadian Brand Names Innohep® [US/Can]

Therapeutic Category Anticoagulant (Other)

Use Treatment of acute symptomatic deep vein thrombosis, with or without pulmonary embolism, in conjunction with warfarin sodium

Usual Dosage SubQ:

Adults: 175 anti-Xa int. units/kg of body weight once daily. Warfarin sodium should be started when appropriate. Administer tinzaparin for at least 6 days and until patient is adequately anticoagulated with warfarin.

Note: To calculate the volume of solution to administer per dose: Volume to be administered (mL) = patient weight (kg) x 0.00875 mL/kg (may be rounded off to the nearest 0.05 mL)

Dosage Forms Injection, solution: 20,000 anti-Xa int. units/mL (2 mL) [contains benzyl alcohol and sodium metabisulfite]

tinzaparin sodium *see* tinzaparin *on this page*

tioconazole (tye oh KONE a zole)

Sound-Alike/Look-Alike Issues

tioconazole may be confused with terconazole

U.S./Canadian Brand Names 1-Day™ [US-OTC]; Vagistat®-1 [US-OTC]

Therapeutic Category Antifungal Agent

Use Local treatment of vulvovaginal candidiasis

Usual Dosage Adults: Vaginal: Insert 1 applicatorful in vagina, just prior to bedtime, as a single dose

Dosage Forms Ointment, vaginal: 6.5% (4.6 g) [with applicator]

tioguanine *see* thioguanine *on page 857*

tiopronin (tye oh PROE nin)

Sound-Alike/Look-Alike Issues

Thiola® may be confused with Theolair™

U.S./Canadian Brand Names Thiola® [US/Can]

Therapeutic Category Urinary Tract Product

Use Prevention of kidney stone (cystine) formation in patients with severe homozygous cystinuric who have urinary cystine >500 mg/day who are resistant to treatment with high fluid intake, alkali, and diet modification, or who have had adverse reactions to penicillamine

Usual Dosage Adults: Initial dose is 800 mg/day, average dose is 1000 mg/day

Dosage Forms Tablet: 100 mg

tiotixene *see* thiothixene *on page 859*

tiotropium (ty oh TRO pee um)

Synonyms tiotropium bromide monohydrate

U.S./Canadian Brand Names Spiriva® [US/Can]

Therapeutic Category Anticholinergic Agent

Use Maintenance treatment of bronchospasm associated with COPD (bronchitis and emphysema)

Usual Dosage Oral inhalation: Adults: Contents of 1 capsule (18 mcg) inhaled once daily using HandiHaler® device

Dosage Forms Powder for oral inhalation [capsule]: 18 mcg/capsule [contains lactose; packaged in 6s or 30s with HandiHaler® device

tiotropium bromide monohydrate *see* tiotropium *on previous page*

Tip Tap Toe [US-OTC] *see* tolnaftate *on page 870*

tirofiban (tye roe FYE ban)

Sound-Alike/Look-Alike Issues

Aggrastat® may be confused with Aggrenox™

Synonyms MK383; tirofiban hydrochloride

U.S./Canadian Brand Names Aggrastat® [US/Can]

Therapeutic Category Antiplatelet Agent

Use In combination with heparin, is indicated for the treatment of acute coronary syndrome, including patients who are to be managed medically and those undergoing PTCA or atherectomy. In this setting, it has been shown to decrease the rate of a combined endpoint of death, new myocardial infarction or refractory ischemia/repeat cardiac procedure.

Usual Dosage Adults: I.V.: Initial rate of 0.4 mcg/kg/minute for 30 minutes and then continued at 0.1 mcg/kg/minute

Dosage Forms

Infusion, as hydrochloride [premixed in sodium chloride]: 50 mcg/mL (100 mL, 250 mL)

Injection, solution, as hydrochloride: 250 mcg/mL (25 mL, 50 mL)

tirofiban hydrochloride *see* tirofiban *on this page*

Tiseb® [US-OTC] *see* salicylic acid *on page 789*

Tisit® Blue Gel [US-OTC] *see* pyrethrins and piperonyl butoxide *on page 751*

Tisit® [US-OTC] *see* pyrethrins and piperonyl butoxide *on page 751*

Tisseel® VH [US/Can] *see* fibrin sealant kit *on page 367*

Titralac™ Extra Strength [US-OTC] *see* calcium carbonate *on page 144*

Titralac™ Plus [US-OTC] *see* calcium carbonate and simethicone *on page 146*

Titralac™ [US-OTC] *see* calcium carbonate *on page 144*

Ti-U-Lac® H [Can] *see* urea and hydrocortisone *on page 898*

tizanidine (tye ZAN i deen)

Sound-Alike/Look-Alike Issues

tizanidine may be confused with tiagabine

Synonyms Sirdalud®

U.S./Canadian Brand Names Zanaflex® [US/Can]

Therapeutic Category Alpha$_2$-Adrenergic Agonist Agent

Use Skeletal muscle relaxant used for treatment of muscle spasticity

Usual Dosage Adults: 2-4 mg 3 times/day

Usual initial dose: 4 mg, may increase by 2-4 mg as needed for satisfactory reduction of muscle tone every 6-8 hours to a maximum of three doses in any 24 hour period

Maximum dose: 36 mg/day

Dosage Forms Tablet: 2 mg, 4 mg

TMP *see* trimethoprim *on page 887*

TMP-SMZ *see* sulfamethoxazole and trimethoprim *on page 831*

TMZ *see* temozolomide *on page 843*

TNKase™ [US/Can] *see* tenecteplase *on page 844*

TOBI® [US/Can] *see* tobramycin *on this page*

TobraDex® [US/Can] *see* tobramycin and dexamethasone *on page 868*

tobramycin (toe bra MYE sin)

Sound-Alike/Look-Alike Issues

tobramycin may be confused with Trobicin®

AKTob® may be confused with AK-Trol®
Nebcin® may be confused with Inapsine®, Naprosyn®, Nubain®
Tobrex® may be confused with TobraDex®

Synonyms tobramycin sulfate

U.S./Canadian Brand Names AKTob® [US]; Apo-Tobramycin® [Can]; Nebcin® [Can]; PMS-Tobramycin [Can]; TOBI® [US/Can]; Tobrex® [US/Can]; Tomycine™ [Can]

Therapeutic Category Aminoglycoside (Antibiotic); Antibiotic, Ophthalmic

Use Treatment of documented or suspected infections caused by susceptible gram-negative bacilli including *Pseudomonas aeruginosa*; topically used to treat superficial ophthalmic infections caused by susceptible bacteria. Tobramycin solution for inhalation is indicated for the management of cystic fibrosis patients (>6 years of age) with *Pseudomonas aeruginosa*.

Usual Dosage Individualization is critical because of the low therapeutic index

Use of ideal body weight (IBW) for determining the mg/kg/dose appears to be more accurate than dosing on the basis of total body weight (TBW)

In morbid obesity, dosage requirement may best be estimated using a dosing weight of IBW + 0.4 (TBW - IBW)

Initial and periodic peak and trough plasma drug levels should be determined, particularly in critically-ill patients with serious infections or in disease states known to significantly alter aminoglycoside pharmacokinetics (eg, cystic fibrosis, burns, or major surgery). Two to three serum level measurements should be obtained after the initial dose to measure the half-life in order to determine the frequency of subsequent doses.

Once daily dosing: Higher peak serum drug concentration to MIC ratios, demonstrated aminoglycoside postantibiotic effect, decreased renal cortex drug uptake, and improved cost-time efficiency are supportive reasons for the use of once daily dosing regimens for aminoglycosides. Current research indicates these regimens to be as effective for nonlife-threatening infections, with no higher incidence of nephrotoxicity, than those requiring multiple daily doses. Doses are determined by calculating the entire day's dose via usual multiple dose calculation techniques and administering this quantity as a single dose. Doses are then adjusted to maintain mean serum concentrations above the MIC(s) of the causative organism(s). (Example: 2.5-5 mg/kg as a single dose; expected Cp_{max}: 10-20 mcg/mL and Cp_{min}: <1 mcg/mL). Further research is needed for universal recommendation in all patient populations and gram-negative disease; exceptions may include those with known high clearance (eg, children, patients with cystic fibrosis, or burns who may require shorter dosage intervals) and patients with renal function impairment for whom longer than conventional dosage intervals are usually required.

Some clinicians suggest a daily dose of 4-7 mg/kg for all patients with normal renal function. This dose is at least as efficacious with similar, if not less, toxicity than conventional dosing.

I.M., I.V.:
Infants and Children <5 years: 2.5 mg/kg/dose every 8 hours
Children >5 years: 1.5-2.5 mg/kg/dose every 8 hours
Note: Some patients may require larger or more frequent doses if serum levels document the need (ie, cystic fibrosis or febrile granulocytopenic patients).
Adults:
Severe life-threatening infections: 2-2.5 mg/kg/dose
Urinary tract infection: 1.5 mg/kg/dose
Synergy (for gram-positive infections): 1 mg/kg/dose

Ophthalmic: Children ≥2 months and Adults: Instill 1-2 drops of solution every 4 hours; apply ointment 2-3 times/day; for severe infections apply ointment every 3-4 hours, or solution 2 drops every 30-60 minutes initially, then reduce to less frequent intervals

Inhalation: Pulmonary infections:
Standard aerosolized tobramycin:
Children: 40-80 mg 2-3 times/day
Adults: 60-80 mg 3 times/day

(Continued)

tobramycin *(Continued)*

High-dose regimen: Children ≥6 years and Adults: 300 mg every 12 hours (do not administer doses less than 6 hours apart); administer in repeated cycles of 28 days on drug followed by 28 days off drug

Dosage Forms [DSC] = Discontinued product

Injection, powder for reconstitution (Nebcin® [DSC]): 1.2 g

Injection, solution, as sulfate: 10 mg/mL (2 mL, 8 mL); 40 mg/mL (2 mL, 30 mL, 50 mL) [may contain sodium metabisulfite]

Nebcin®: 40 mg/mL (2 mL) [contains sodium bisulfite] [DSC]

Ointment, ophthalmic (Tobrex®): 0.3% (3.5 g)

Solution for nebulization [preservative free] (TOBI®): 60 mg/mL (5 mL)

Solution, ophthalmic (AKTob®, Tobrex®): 0.3% (5 mL) [contains benzalkonium chloride]

tobramycin and dexamethasone (toe bra MYE sin & deks a METH a sone)

Sound-Alike/Look-Alike Issues

TobraDex® may be confused with Tobrex®

Synonyms dexamethasone and tobramycin

U.S./Canadian Brand Names TobraDex® [US/Can]

Therapeutic Category Antibiotic/Corticosteroid, Ophthalmic

Use Treatment of external ocular infection caused by susceptible gram-negative bacteria and steroid responsive inflammatory conditions of the palpebral and bulbar conjunctiva, lid, cornea, and anterior segment of the globe

Usual Dosage Children and Adults: Ophthalmic: Instill 1-2 drops of solution every 4 hours; apply ointment 2-3 times/day; for severe infections apply ointment every 3-4 hours, or solution 2 drops every 30-60 minutes initially, then reduce to less frequent intervals

Dosage Forms

Ointment, ophthalmic: Tobramycin 0.3% and dexamethasone 0.1% (3.5 g)

Suspension, ophthalmic: Tobramycin 0.3% and dexamethasone 0.1% (2.5 mL, 5 mL, 10 mL) [contains benzalkonium chloride]

tobramycin sulfate *see* tobramycin *on page 866*

Tobrex® [US/Can] *see* tobramycin *on page 866*

tocophersolan *(Discontinued)* *see page 1042*

Tofranil® [US/Can] *see* imipramine *on page 467*

Tofranil-PM® [US] *see* imipramine *on page 467*

tolazamide (tole AZ a mide)

Sound-Alike/Look-Alike Issues

tolazamide may be confused with tolazoline, tolbutamide

Tolinase® may be confused with Orinase®

Tall-Man TOLAZamide

U.S./Canadian Brand Names Tolinase® [US/Can]

Therapeutic Category Antidiabetic Agent, Oral

Use Adjunct to diet for the management of mild to moderately severe, stable, type 2 diabetes mellitus (noninsulin dependent, NIDDM)

Usual Dosage Oral (doses >1000 mg/day normally do not improve diabetic control):

Adults:

Initial: 100-250 mg/day with breakfast or the first main meal of the day

Fasting blood sugar <200 mg/dL: 100 mg/day

Fasting blood sugar >200 mg/dL: 250 mg/day

Patient is malnourished, underweight, elderly, or not eating properly: 100 mg/day

Adjust dose in increments of 100-250 mg/day at weekly intervals to response. If >500 mg/day is required, give in divided doses twice daily; maximum daily dose: 1 g (doses >1 g/day are not likely to improve control)

Conversion from insulin → tolazamide
10 units day = 100 mg/day
20-40 units/day = 250 mg/day
>40 units/day = 250 mg/day and 50% of insulin dose
Doses >500 mg/day should be given in 2 divided doses
Dosage Forms Tablet: 100 mg, 250 mg, 500 mg
Tolinase®: 100 mg, 250 mg

tolbutamide (tole BYOO ta mide)

Sound-Alike/Look-Alike Issues
tolbutamide may be confused with terbutaline, tolazamide
Synonyms tolbutamide sodium
Tall-Man TOLBUTamide
U.S./Canadian Brand Names Apo-Tolbutamide® [Can]; Tol-Tab® [US]
Therapeutic Category Antidiabetic Agent, Oral
Use Adjunct to diet for the management of mild to moderately severe, stable, type 2 diabetes mellitus (noninsulin dependent, NIDDM)
Usual Dosage Divided doses may improve gastrointestinal tolerance
Adults:
Oral: Initial: 1-2 g/day as a single dose in the morning or in divided doses throughout the day. Total doses may be taken in the morning; however, divided doses may allow increased gastrointestinal tolerance. Maintenance dose: 0.25-3 g/day; however, a maintenance dose >2 g/day is seldom required.
I.V. bolus: 1 g over 2-3 minutes
Dosage Forms [DSC] = Discontinued product
Injection, powder for reconstitution, as sodium (Orinase Diagnostic® [DSC]): 1 g
Tablet (Tol-Tab®): 500 mg

tolbutamide sodium *see* tolbutamide *on this page*

tolcapone (TOLE ka pone)

U.S./Canadian Brand Names Tasmar® [US]
Therapeutic Category Anti-Parkinson Agent
Use Adjunct to levodopa and carbidopa for the treatment of signs and symptoms of idiopathic Parkinson disease
Usual Dosage Adults: Oral: Initial: 100-200 mg 3 times/day; levodopa therapy may need to be decreased upon initiation of tolcapone
Dosage Forms Tablet: 100 mg, 200 mg

Tolectin® [US/Can] *see* tolmetin *on this page*

Tolectin® DS [US] *see* tolmetin *on this page*

Tolinase® [US/Can] *see* tolazamide *on previous page*

tolmetin (TOLE met in)

Synonyms tolmetin sodium
U.S./Canadian Brand Names Tolectin® DS [US]; Tolectin® [US/Can]
Therapeutic Category Analgesic, Nonnarcotic; Nonsteroidal Antiinflammatory Drug (NSAID)
Use Treatment of rheumatoid arthritis and osteoarthritis, juvenile rheumatoid arthritis
Usual Dosage Oral:
Children ≥2 years:
Antiinflammatory: Initial: 20 mg/kg/day in 3 divided doses, then 15-30 mg/kg/day in 3 divided doses
Analgesic: 5-7 mg/kg/dose every 6-8 hours
Adults: 400 mg 3 times/day; usual dose: 600 mg to 1.8 g/day; maximum: 2 g/day
Dosage Forms
Capsule, as sodium (Tolectin® DS): 400 mg
Tablet, as sodium: 200 mg, 600 mg
Tolectin®: 600 mg

tolmetin sodium *see* tolmetin *on previous page*

tolnaftate (tole NAF tate)

Sound-Alike/Look-Alike Issues
tolnaftate may be confused with Tornalate®
Tinactin® may be confused with Talacen®

U.S./Canadian Brand Names Absorbine Jr.® Antifungal [US-OTC]; Aftate® Antifungal [US-OTC]; Blis-To-Sol® [US-OTC]; Dermasept Antifungal [US-OTC]; Fungi-Guard [US-OTC]; Gold Bond® Antifungal [US-OTC]; Pitrex [Can]; Tinactin® Antifungal Jock Itch [US-OTC]; Tinactin® Antifungal [US-OTC]; Tinaderm [US-OTC]; Ting® [US-OTC]; Tip Tap Toe [US-OTC]

Therapeutic Category Antifungal Agent

Use Treatment of tinea pedis, tinea cruris, tinea corporis

Usual Dosage Children ≥2 years and Adults: Topical: Wash and dry affected area; spray aerosol or apply 1-3 drops of solution or a small amount of cream, gel, or powder and rub into the affected areas 2 times/day

Note: May use for up to 4 weeks for tinea pedis or tinea corporis, and up to 2 weeks for tinea cruris

Dosage Forms
Aerosol, liquid, topical:
Aftate®: 1% (120 mL) [contains alcohol]
Tinactin® Antifungal: 1% (120 mL) [contains alcohol]
Ting®: 1% (90 mL)
Aerosol, powder, topical:
Aftate®: 1% (105 g) [contains alcohol]
Tinactin® Antifungal: 1% (45 g, 90 g, 100 g, 150 g) [contains alcohol]
Tinactin® Antifungal Jock Itch: 1% (100 g) [contains alcohol]
Ting®: 1% (90 g)
Cream, topical: 1% (15 g, 30 g)
Fungi-Guard: 1% (15 g)
Tinactin® Antifungal: 1% (15 g, 30 g)
Tinactin® Antifungal Jock Itch: 1% (15 g)
Gel, topical (Absorbine Jr.® Antifungal): 1% (21 g)
Liquid, topical:
Blis-To-Sol®: 1% (30 mL, 55 mL)
Dermasept Antifungal: 1% (30 mL) [contains benzyl alcohol and benzoic acid]
Powder, topical: 1% (45 g)
Solution, topical: 1% (10 mL)
Absorbine Jr.® Antifungal: 1% (60 mL)
Tinaderm: 1% (10 mL)
Swab, topical [liquid-filled swabstick]: 1% (36s)
Gold Bond® Antifungal: 1% (24s)
Tip Tap Toe: 1% (72s)

Tol-Tab® [US] *see* tolbutamide *on previous page*

tolterodine (tole TER oh dine)

Sound-Alike/Look-Alike Issues
Detrol® may be confused with Demerol®, Ditropan®

Synonyms tolterodine tartrate

U.S./Canadian Brand Names Detrol® [US/Can]; Detrol® LA [US]; Unidet® [Can]

Therapeutic Category Anticholinergic Agent

Use Treatment of patients with an overactive bladder with symptoms of urinary frequency, urgency, or urge incontinence

Usual Dosage

Children: Safety and efficacy in pediatric patients have not been established

Adults: Treatment of overactive bladder: Oral:

Immediate release tablet: 2 mg twice daily; the dose may be lowered to 1 mg twice daily based on individual response and tolerability

Dosing adjustment in patients concurrently taking CYP3A4 inhibitors: 1 mg twice daily

Extended release capsule: 4 mg once a day; dose may be lowered to 2 mg daily based on individual response and tolerability

Dosing adjustment in patients concurrently taking CYP3A4 inhibitors: 2 mg daily

Dosage Forms

Capsule, extended release, as tartrate (Detrol® LA): 2 mg, 4 mg

Tablet, as tartrate (Detrol®): 1 mg, 2 mg

tolterodine tartrate *see* tolterodine *on previous page*

Tolu-Sed® DM [US-OTC] *see* guaifenesin and dextromethorphan *on page 416*

Tomocat® [US] *see* radiological/contrast media (ionic) *on page 759*

tomoxetine *see* atomoxetine *on page 86*

Tomudex® [Can] *see* raltitrexed *(Canada only) on page 762*

Tomycine® ***(Discontinued)*** *see page 1042*

Tomycine™ [Can] *see* tobramycin *on page 866*

Tonocard® ***(Discontinued)*** *see page 1042*

Tonopaque® [US] *see* radiological/contrast media (ionic) *on page 759*

Topamax® [US/Can] *see* topiramate *on this page*

Topicaine® [US-OTC] *see* lidocaine *on page 518*

Topicort® [US/Can] *see* desoximetasone *on page 253*

Topicort®-LP [US] *see* desoximetasone *on page 253*

Topicycline® Topical ***(Discontinued)*** *see page 1042*

topiramate (toe PYE ra mate)

U.S./Canadian Brand Names Topamax® [US/Can]

Therapeutic Category Anticonvulsant

Use In adults and pediatric patients, adjunctive therapy for partial onset seizures and adjunctive therapy of primary generalized tonic-clonic seizures; treatment of seizures associated with Lennox-Gastaut syndrome; prophylaxis of migraine headache

Usual Dosage Oral:

Children 2-16 years: Partial seizures (adjunctive therapy), primary generalized tonic-clonic seizures (adjunctive therapy), or seizure associated with Lennox-Gastaut syndrome: Initial dose titration should begin at 25 mg (or less, based on a range of 1-3 mg/kg/day) nightly for the first week; dosage may be increased in increments of 1-3 mg/kg/day (administered in 2 divided doses) at 1- or 2-week intervals to a total daily dose of 5-9 mg/kg/day.

Adults:

Partial onset seizures (adjunctive therapy), primary generalized tonic-clonic seizures (adjunctive therapy): Initial: 25-50 mg/day; titrate in increments of 25-50 mg per week until an effective daily dose is reached; the daily dose may be increased by 25 mg at weekly intervals for the first 4 weeks; thereafter, the daily dose may be increased by 25-50 mg weekly to an effective daily dose (usually at least 400 mg); usual maximum dose: 1600 mg/day

Note: A more rapid titration schedule has been previously recommended (ie, 50 mg/week), and may be attempted in some clinical situations; however, this may reduce the patient's ability to tolerate topiramate.

Migraine: Initial: 25 mg/day, titrated at weekly intervals in 25 mg increments, up to the recommended total daily dose of 100 mg/day given in 2 divided doses

(Continued)

topiramate *(Continued)*

Dosage Forms

Capsule, sprinkle: 15 mg, 25 mg

Tablet: 25 mg, 50 mg, 100 mg, 200 mg

Topisone® [Can] *see* betamethasone (topical) *on page 116*

TOPO *see* topotecan *on this page*

Toposar® [US] *see* etoposide *on page 351*

topotecan (toe poe TEE kan)

Sound-Alike/Look-Alike Issues

Hycamtin® may be confused with Hycomine®

Synonyms hycamptamine; NSC-609699; SK and F 104864; SKF 104864; SKF 104864-A; TOPO; topotecan hydrochloride; TPT

U.S./Canadian Brand Names Hycamtin® [US/Can]

Therapeutic Category Antineoplastic Agent

Use Treatment of ovarian cancer, small cell lung cancer

Usual Dosage Adults (refer to individual protocols): Metastatic ovarian cancer and small cell lung cancer:

IVPB: 1.5 mg/m^2/day for 5 days; repeated every 21 days (neutrophil count should be >1500/mm^3 and platelet count should be >100,000/mm^3)

I.V. continuous infusion: 0.2-0.7 mg/m^2/day for 7-21 days

Dosage adjustment for hematological effects: If neutrophil count <1500/mm^3, reduce dose by 0.25 mg/m^2/day for 5 days for next cycle

Dosage Forms Injection, powder for reconstitution, as hydrochloride: 4 mg [base]

topotecan hydrochloride *see* topotecan *on this page*

Toprol-XL® [US/Can] *see* metoprolol *on page 575*

Topsyn® [Can] *see* fluocinonide *on page 375*

Toradol® [US/Can] *see* ketorolac *on page 496*

Toradol® IM [Can] *see* ketorolac *on page 496*

Torecan® (all products) ***(Discontinued)*** *see page 1042*

toremifene (TORE em i feen)

Synonyms FC1157a; toremifene citrate

U.S./Canadian Brand Names Fareston® [US/Can]

Therapeutic Category Antineoplastic Agent

Use Treatment of advanced breast cancer; management of desmoid tumors and endometrial carcinoma

Usual Dosage Refer to individual protocols.

Adults: Oral: 60 mg once daily, generally continued until disease progression is observed

Dosage Forms Tablet, as citrate: 60 mg

toremifene citrate *see* toremifene *on this page*

Tornalate® ***(Discontinued)*** *see page 1042*

torsemide (TOR se mide)

Sound-Alike/Look-Alike Issues

torsemide may be confused with furosemide

Demadex® may be confused with Denorex®

U.S./Canadian Brand Names Demadex® [US]

Therapeutic Category Diuretic, Loop

Use Management of edema associated with congestive heart failure and hepatic or renal disease; used alone or in combination with antihypertensives in treatment of hypertension; I.V. form is indicated when rapid onset is desired

Usual Dosage Adults: Oral, I.V.:

Congestive heart failure: 10-20 mg once daily; may increase gradually for chronic treatment by doubling dose until the diuretic response is apparent (for acute treatment, I.V. dose may be repeated every 2 hours with double the dose as needed)

Chronic renal failure: 20 mg once daily; increase as described above

Hepatic cirrhosis: 5-10 mg once daily with an aldosterone antagonist or a potassium-sparing diuretic; increase as described above

Hypertension: 2.5-5 mg once daily; increase to 10 mg after 4-6 weeks if an adequate hypotensive response is not apparent; if still not effective, an additional antihypertensive agent may be added

Dosage Forms

Injection, solution: 10 mg/mL (2 mL, 5 mL)

Tablet: 5 mg, 10 mg, 20 mg, 100 mg

tositumomab and iodine I 131 tositumomab

(toe si TYOO mo mab & EYE oh dyne eye one THUR tee one toe si TYOO mo mab)

Synonyms anti-CD20-murine monoclonal antibody I-131; B1; B1 antibody; 131 I anti-B1 antibody; 131 I-anti-B1 monoclonal antibody; iodine I 131 tositumomab and tositumomab; tositumomab I-131

U.S./Canadian Brand Names Bexxar® [US]

Therapeutic Category Antineoplastic Agent, Monoclonal Antibody; Radiopharmaceutical

Use Treatment of relapsed or refractory CD20 positive, follicular, non-Hodgkin lymphoma

Usual Dosage I.V.: Adults: Dosing consists of four components administered in 2 steps. Thyroid protective agents (SSKI, Lugol's solution or potassium iodide), acetaminophen and diphenhydramine should be given with treatment.

Step 1: Dosimetric step (Day 0):

Tositumomab 450 mg in NS 50 mL administered over 60 minutes

Iodine I 131 tositumomab (containing I-131 5.0 mCi and tositumomab 35mg) in NS 30 mL administered over 20 minutes

Note: Whole body dosimetry and biodistribution should be determined on Day 0; days 2, 3, or 4; and day 6 or 7 prior to administration of Step 2. If biodistribution is not acceptable, do not administer the therapeutic step. On day 6 or 7, calculate the patient specific activity of iodine I 131 tositumomab to deliver 75 cGy TBD or 65 cGy TBD (in mCi).

Step 2: Therapeutic step (Day 7):

Tositumomab 450 mg in NS 50 mL administered over 60 minutes

Iodine I 131 tositumomab:

Platelets ≥150,000/mm^3: Iodine I 131 calculated to deliver 75 cGy total body irradiation and tositumomab 35 mg over 20 minutes

Platelets ≥100,000/mm^3 and <150,000/mm^3: Iodine I 131 calculated to deliver 65 cGy total body irradiation and tositumomab 35 mg over 20 minutes

Dosage Forms Note: Not all components are shipped from the same facility. When ordering, ensure that all will arrive on the same day.

Kit [dosimetric package] (Bexxar®): Tositumomab 225 mg/16.1 mL [2 vials], tositumomab 35 mg/2.5 mL [1 vial], and iodine I 131 tositumomab 0.1 mg/mL and 0.61mCi/mL (20 mL) [1 vial]

Kit [therapeutic package] (Bexxar®): Tositumomab 225 mg/16.1 mL [2 vials], tositumomab 35 mg/2.5 mL [1 vial], and iodine I 131 tositumomab 1.1 mg/mL and 5.6 mCi/mL (20 mL) [1 or 2 vials]

tositumomab I-131 *see* tositumomab and iodine I 131 tositumomab *on this page*

Totacillin® ***(Discontinued)*** *see page 1042*

Totacillin-N® ***(Discontinued)*** *see page 1042*

Touro™ Allergy [US] *see* brompheniramine and pseudoephedrine *on page 129*

Touro™ CC [US] *see* guaifenesin, pseudoephedrine, and dextromethorphan *on page 422*

Touro® DM [US] *see* guaifenesin and dextromethorphan *on page 416*

Touro Ex® *(Discontinued)* *see* *page 1042*

Touro LA® [US] *see* guaifenesin and pseudoephedrine *on page 419*

tPA *see* alteplase *on page 36*

T-Phyl® [US] *see* theophylline *on page 854*

TPT *see* topotecan *on page 872*

trace metals (trase MET als)

Synonyms chromium; copper; iodine; manganese; molybdenum; neonatal trace metals; selenium; zinc

U.S./Canadian Brand Names Iodopen® [US]; Molypen® [US]; M.T.E.-4® [US]; M.T.E.-5® [US]; M.T.E.-6® [US]; M.T.E.-7® [US]; Multitrace™-4 [US]; Multitrace™-4 Neonatal [US]; Multitrace™-4 Pediatric [US]; Multitrace™-5 [US]; Neotrace-4® [US]; Pedtrace-4® [US]; P.T.E.-4® [US]; P.T.E.-5® [US]; Selepen® [US]

Therapeutic Category Trace Element

Use Prevention and correction of trace metal deficiencies

Usual Dosage To be added to total parenteral solutions

Dosage Forms

Injection, solution [combination products]:

M.T.E.-4®: Chromium 4 mcg, copper 0.4 mg, manganese 0.1 mg, and zinc 1 mg per mL (3 mL, 10 mL, 30 mL) [30 mL contains benzyl alcohol]

M.T.E.-4® Concentrate: Chromium 10 mcg, copper 1 mg, manganese 0.5 mg, and zinc 5 mg per mL (1 mL, 10 mL) [10 mL contains benzyl alcohol]

M.T.E.-5® [preservative free]: Chromium 4 mcg, copper 0.4 mg, manganese 0.1 mg, selenium 20 mcg, and zinc 1 mg per mL (10 mL)

M.T.E.-5® Concentrate: Chromium 10 mcg, copper 1 mg, manganese 0.5 mg, selenium 60 mcg, and zinc 5 mg per mL (1 mL, 10 mL) [10 mL contains benzyl alcohol]

M.T.E.-6® [preservative free]: Chromium 4 mcg, copper 0.4 mg, iodide 25 mcg, manganese 0.1 mg, selenium 20 mcg, and zinc 1 mg per mL (10 mL)

M.T.E.-6® Concentrate: Chromium 10 mcg, copper 1 mg, iodide 75 mcg, manganese 0.5 mg, selenium 60 mcg, and zinc 5 mg per mL (10 mL) [contains benzyl alcohol]

M.T.E.-7® [preservative free]: Chromium 4 mcg, copper 0.4 mg, iodide 25 mcg, manganese 0.1 mg, molybdenum 25 mcg, selenium 20 mcg, and zinc 1 mg per mL (10 mL)

Multitrace™-4: Chromium 4 mcg, copper 0.4 mg, manganese 0.1 mg, and zinc 1 mg per mL (10 mL) [contains benzyl alcohol]

Multitrace™-4 Neonatal: Chromium 0.85 mcg, copper 0.1 mg, manganese 0.025 mg, and zinc 1.5 mg per mL (2 mL)

Multitrace™-4 Pediatric: Chromium 1 mcg, copper 0.1 mg, manganese 0.025 mg, and zinc 1 mg per mL (3 mL)

Multitrace™-4 Concentrate: Chromium 10 mcg, copper 1 mg, manganese 0.5 mg, and zinc 5 mg per mL (1 mL, 10 mL) [10 mL contains benzyl alcohol]

Multitrace™-5: Chromium 4 mcg, copper 0.4 mg, manganese 0.1 mg, selenium 20 mcg, and zinc 1 mg per mL (10 mL) [contains benzyl alcohol]

Multitrace™-5 Concentrate: Chromium 10 mcg, copper 1 mg, manganese 0.5 mg, selenium 60 mcg, and zinc 5 mg per mL (1 mL, 10 mL) [10 mL contains benzyl alcohol]

Neotrace-4® [preservative free]: Chromium 0.85 mcg, copper 0.1 mg, manganese 0.025 mg, and zinc 1.5 mg per mL (2 mL)

Pedtrace-4® [preservative free]: Chromium 0.85 mcg, copper 0.1 mg, manganese 0.025mg, and zinc 0.5 mg per mL (3 mL, 10 mL)

P.T.E.-4® [preservative free]: Chromium 1 mcg, copper 0.1 mg, manganese 0.025 mg, and zinc 1 mg per mL (3 mL)

P.T.E.-5® [preservative free]: Chromium 1 mcg, copper 0.1 mg, manganese 0.025 mg, selenium 15 mcg, and zinc 1 mg per mL (3 mL)
Trace elements pediatric: Chromium 1 mcg, copper 0.1 mg, manganese 0.03 mg, and zinc 0.5 mg per mL (10 mL) [contains benzyl alcohol]
Injection, solution [elemental equivalence]:
Chromium, as chromic chloride (hexahydrate) [preservative free]: 0.0205 mg/mL [0.004 mg/mL] (10 mL)
Copper, as cupric chloride: 1.07 mg/mL [0.4 mg/mL] (10 mL)
Iodine, as iodine sodium (Iodopen®): 0.118 mg/mL [0.1 mg/mL] (10 mL)
Manganese:
As chloride: 0.36 mg/mL [0.1 mg/mL] (10 mL)
As sulfate [preservative free]: 0.31 mg/mL [0.1 mg/mL] (10 mL)
Molybdenum, as ammonium molybdate (tetrahydrate) (Molypen®): 46 mcg/mL [25 mcg/mL] (10 mL)
Selenium, as selenious acid: 0.0654 mg/mL [0.04 mg/mL] (10 mL)
Selepen®: 0.0654 mg/mL [0.04 mg/mL] (10 mL, 30 mL) [30 mL contains benzyl alcohol]
Zinc:
As chloride: 2.09 mg/mL [1 mg/mL] (10 mL, 50 mL)
As sulfate, anhydrous [preservative free]: 2.46 mg/mL [1 mg/mL] (10 mL)
As sulfate, anhydrous, concentrate [preservative free]: 12.32 mg/mL [5 mg/mL] (5 mL)

Tracleer® [US/Can] *see* bosentan *on page 124*

Tracrium® [US] *see* atracurium *on page 87*

Tral® ***(Discontinued)*** *see page 1042*

tramadol (TRA ma dole)

Sound-Alike/Look-Alike Issues
tramadol may be confused with Toradol®, Trandate®, Voltaren®
Ultram® may be confused with Ultane®, Voltaren®

Synonyms tramadol hydrochloride

U.S./Canadian Brand Names Ultram® [US/Can]

Therapeutic Category Analgesic, Nonnarcotic

Use Relief of moderate to moderately-severe pain

Usual Dosage Oral: Adults: Moderate to severe chronic pain: 50-100 mg every 4-6 hours, not to exceed 400 mg/day
For patients not requiring rapid onset of effect, tolerability may be improved by starting dose at 25 mg/day and titrating dose by 25 mg every 3 days, until reaching 25 mg 4 times/day. Dose may then be increased by 50 mg every 3 days as tolerated, to reach dose of 50 mg 4 times/day.

Dosage Forms Tablet, as hydrochloride: 50 mg

tramadol hydrochloride *see* tramadol *on this page*

tramadol hydrochloride and acetaminophen *see* acetaminophen and tramadol *on page 10*

Trandate® [US/Can] *see* labetalol *on page 499*

trandolapril (tran DOE la pril)

U.S./Canadian Brand Names Mavik® [US/Can]

Therapeutic Category Angiotensin-Converting Enzyme (ACE) Inhibitor

Use Management of hypertension alone or in combination with other antihypertensive agents; treatment of left ventricular dysfunction after myocardial infarction

Usual Dosage Adults: Oral:
Hypertension: Initial dose in patients not receiving a diuretic: 1 mg/day (2 mg/day in black patients). Adjust dosage according to the blood pressure response. Make dosage adjustments at intervals of ≥1 week. Most patients have required dosages of 2-4 mg/day. There is a little experience with doses >8 mg/day. Patients inadequately
(Continued)

trandolapril *(Continued)*

treated with once daily dosing at 4 mg may be treated with twice daily dosing. If blood pressure is not adequately controlled with trandolapril monotherapy, a diuretic may be added.

Usual dose range (JNC 7): 1-4 mg once daily

Heart failure postmyocardial infarction or left ventricular dysfunction postmyocardial infarction: Initial: 1 mg/day; titrate patients (as tolerated) towards the target dose of 4 mg/day. If a 4 mg dose is not tolerated, patients can continue therapy with the greatest tolerated dose.

Dosage Forms Tablet: 1 mg, 2 mg, 4 mg

trandolapril and verapamil (tran DOE la pril & ver AP a mil)

Synonyms verapamil and trandolapril

U.S./Canadian Brand Names Tarka® [US/Can]

Therapeutic Category Antihypertensive Agent, Combination

Use Combination drug for the treatment of hypertension, however, not indicated for initial treatment of hypertension; replacement therapy in patients receiving separate dosage forms (for patient convenience); when monotherapy with one component fails to achieve desired antihypertensive effect, or when dose-limiting adverse effects limit upward titration of monotherapy

Usual Dosage Dose is individualized

Dosage Forms Tablet, combination [trandolapril component is immediate release, verapamil component is sustained release]:

Trandolapril 1 mg and verapamil hydrochloride 240 mg
Trandolapril 2 mg and verapamil hydrochloride 180 mg
Trandolapril 2 mg and verapamil hydrochloride 240 mg
Trandolapril 4 mg and verapamil hydrochloride 240 mg

tranexamic acid (tran eks AM ik AS id)

Sound-Alike/Look-Alike Issues

Cyklokapron® may be confused with cyclosporine

U.S./Canadian Brand Names Cyklokapron® [US/Can]

Therapeutic Category Antihemophilic Agent

Use Short-term use (2-8 days) in hemophilia patients during and following tooth extraction to reduce or prevent hemorrhage

Usual Dosage Children and Adults: I.V.: 10 mg/kg immediately before surgery, then 25 mg/kg/dose orally 3-4 times/day for 2-8 days

Alternatively:

Oral: 25 mg/kg 3-4 times/day beginning 1 day prior to surgery

I.V.: 10 mg/kg 3-4 times/day in patients who are unable to take oral

Dosage Forms

Injection, solution: 100 mg/mL (10 mL)

Tablet: 500 mg [Not marketed in U.S.; available from manufacturer for select cases]

transamine sulphate *see* tranylcypromine *on next page*

Transdermal-NTG® Patch *(Discontinued)* *see page 1042*

Transderm-Nitro® [Can] *see* nitroglycerin *on page 623*

Transderm Scōp® [US] *see* scopolamine *on page 796*

Transderm-V® [Can] *see* scopolamine *on page 796*

Trans-Plantar® [Can] *see* salicylic acid *on page 789*

Trans-Plantar® Transdermal Patch *(Discontinued)* *see page 1042*

***trans*-retinoic acid** *see* tretinoin (topical) *on page 879*

Trans-Ver-Sal® [US-OTC/Can] *see* salicylic acid *on page 789*

Tranxene® [US] *see* clorazepate *on page 217*

Tranxene® SD™ [US] *see* clorazepate *on page 217*

Tranxene® SD™-Half Strength [US] *see* clorazepate *on page 217*

tranxene T-Tab® *see* clorazepate *on page 217*

tranylcypromine (tran il SIP roe meen)

Synonyms transamine sulphate; tranylcypromine sulfate

U.S./Canadian Brand Names Parnate® [US/Can]

Therapeutic Category Antidepressant, Monoamine Oxidase Inhibitor

Use Treatment of major depressive episode without melancholia

Usual Dosage Adults: Oral: 10 mg twice daily, increase by 10 mg increments at 1- to 3-week intervals; maximum: 60 mg/day

Dosage Forms Tablet, as sulfate: 10 mg

tranylcypromine sulfate *see* tranylcypromine *on this page*

Trasicor® [Can] *see* oxprenolol *(Canada only) on page 654*

trastuzumab (tras TU zoo mab)

U.S./Canadian Brand Names Herceptin® [US/Can]

Therapeutic Category Antineoplastic Agent

Use

Single agent for the treatment of patients with metastatic breast cancer whose tumors overexpress the HER-2/*neu* protein and who have received one or more chemotherapy regimens for their metastatic disease

Combination therapy with paclitaxel for the treatment of patients with metastatic breast cancer whose tumors overexpress the HER-2/*neu* protein and who have not received chemotherapy for their metastatic disease

Usual Dosage I.V. infusion: Adults:

Initial loading dose: 4 mg/kg intravenous infusion over 90 minutes

Maintenance dose: 2 mg/kg intravenous infusion over 90 minutes (can be administered over 30 minutes if prior infusions are well tolerated) weekly until disease progression

Dosage Forms Injection, powder for reconstitution: 440 mg [packaged with bacteriostatic water for injection; diluent contains benzyl alcohol]

Trasylol® [US/Can] *see* aprotinin *on page 74*

Travase® ***(Discontinued)*** *see page 1042*

Travatan® [US/Can] *see* travoprost *on this page*

travoprost (TRA voe prost)

Sound-Alike/Look-Alike Issues

Travatan® may be confused with Xalatan®

U.S./Canadian Brand Names Travatan® [US/Can]

Therapeutic Category Prostaglandin, Ophthalmic

Use Reduction of elevated intraocular pressure in patients with open-angle glaucoma or ocular hypertension who are intolerant of the other IOP-lowering medications or insufficiently responsive (failed to achieve target IOP determined after multiple measurements over time) to another IOP-lowering medication

Usual Dosage Ophthalmic: Adults: Glaucoma (open angle) or ocular hypertension: Instill 1 drop into affected eye(s) once daily in the evening; do not exceed once-daily dosing (may decrease IOP-lowering effect). If used with other topical ophthalmic agents, separate administration by at least 5 minutes.

Dosage Forms Solution, ophthalmic: 0.004% (2.5 mL, 5 mL) [contains benzalkonium chloride]

trazodone (TRAZ oh done)

Sound-Alike/Look-Alike Issues

Desyrel® may be confused with Demerol®, Delsym®, Zestril®

(Continued)

trazodone *(Continued)*

Synonyms trazodone hydrochloride

U.S./Canadian Brand Names Alti-Trazodone [Can]; Apo-Trazodone® [Can]; Apo-Trazodone D®; Desyrel® [US/Can]; Gen-Trazodone [Can]; Novo-Trazodone [Can]; Nu-Trazodone [Can]; PMS-Trazodone [Can]

Therapeutic Category Antidepressant, Triazolopyridine

Use Treatment of depression

Usual Dosage Oral: Therapeutic effects may take up to 6 weeks to occur; therapy is normally maintained for 6-12 months after optimum response is reached to prevent recurrence of depression

Children 6-12 years: Depression: Initial: 1.5-2 mg/kg/day in divided doses; increase gradually every 3-4 days as needed; maximum: 6 mg/kg/day in 3 divided doses

Adolescents: Depression: Initial: 25-50 mg/day; increase to 100-150 mg/day in divided doses

Adults: Depression: Initial: 150 mg/day in 3 divided doses (may increase by 50 mg/day every 3-7 days); maximum: 600 mg/day

Dosage Forms Tablet, as hydrochloride: 50 mg, 100 mg, 150 mg, 300 mg

trazodone hydrochloride *see* trazodone *on previous page*

Trecator®-SC [US/Can] *see* ethionamide *on page 348*

Trelstar™ Depot [US/Can] *see* triptorelin *on page 890*

Trelstar™ LA [US] *see* triptorelin *on page 890*

Trendar® *(Discontinued)* *see page 1042*

Trental® [US/Can] *see* pentoxifylline *on page 680*

treprostinil (tre PROST in il)

Synonyms treprostinil sodium

U.S./Canadian Brand Names Remodulin™ [US]

Therapeutic Category Vasodilator

Use Treatment of pulmonary arterial hypertension (PAH) in patients with NYHA Class II-IV symptoms to decrease exercise-associated symptoms

Usual Dosage SubQ infusion: Adults: PAH: Initial: 1.25 ng/kg/minute continuous; if dose cannot be tolerated, reduce to 0.625 ng/kg/minute. Increase at rate not >1.25 ng/kg/minute per week for first 4 weeks, and not >2.5 ng/kg/minute per week for remainder of therapy. Limited experience with doses >40 ng/kg/minute.

Note: Dose must be carefully and individually titrated (symptom improvement with minimal adverse effects).

Dosage Forms Injection, solution; 1 mg/mL (20 mL); 2.5 mg/mL (20 mL); 5 mg/mL (20 mL); 10 mg/mL (20 mL)

treprostinil sodium *see* treprostinil *on this page*

tretinoin and mequinol *see* mequinol and tretinoin *on page 555*

tretinoin, fluocinolone acetonide, and hydroquinone *see* fluocinolone, hydroquinone, and tretinoin *on page 375*

tretinoin (oral) (TRET i noyn oral)

Sound-Alike/Look-Alike Issues

tretinoin may be confused with trientine

U.S./Canadian Brand Names Vesanoid® [US/Can]

Therapeutic Category Antineoplastic Agent

Use Induction of remission in patients with acute promyelocytic leukemia (APL), French American British (FAB) classification M3 (including the M3 variant)

Usual Dosage Oral: Children and Adults:

Remission induction: 45 mg/m^2/day in 2-3 divided doses for up to 30 days after complete remission (maximum duration of treatment: 90 days)

Remission maintenance: 45-200 mg/m²/day in 2-3 divided doses for up to 12 months. **Note:** Optimal consolidation or maintenance regimens have not been determined. All patients should therefore receive a standard consolidation or maintenance chemotherapy regimen for APL after induction therapy with tretinoin unless otherwise contraindicated.

Dosage Forms Capsule: 10 mg

tretinoin (topical) (TRET i noyn TOP i kal)

Sound-Alike/Look-Alike Issues

tretinoin may be confused with trientine

Synonyms retinoic acid; *trans*-retinoic acid; vitamin A acid

U.S./Canadian Brand Names Altinac™ [US]; Avita® [US]; Rejuva-A® [Can]; Renova® [US]; Retin-A® [US/Can]; Retin-A® Micro [US/Can]; Retinova® [Can]

Therapeutic Category Retinoic Acid Derivative

Use Treatment of acne vulgaris; photodamaged skin; palliation of fine wrinkles, mottled hyperpigmentation, and tactile roughness of facial skin as part of a comprehensive skin care and sun avoidance program

Usual Dosage Topical:

Children >12 years and Adults: Acne vulgaris: Begin therapy with a weaker formulation of tretinoin (0.025% cream, 0.04% microsphere gel, or 0.01% gel) and increase the concentration as tolerated; apply once daily to acne lesions before retiring or on alternate days; if stinging or irritation develop, decrease frequency of application

Adults ≥18: Palliation of fine wrinkles, mottled hyperpigmentation, and tactile roughness of facial skin: Pea-sized amount of the 0.02% or 0.05% cream applied to entire face once daily in the evening

Dosage Forms

Cream, topical: 0.025% (20 g, 45 g); 0.05% (20 g, 45 g); 0.1% (20 g, 45 g)
- Altinac™: 0.025% (20 g, 45 g); 0.05% (20 g, 45 g); 0.1% (20 g, 45 g)
- Avita®: 0.025% (20 g, 45 g)
- Renova®: 0.02% (40 g); 0.05% (40 g, 60 g)
- Retin-A®: 0.025% (20 g, 45 g); 0.05% (20 g, 45 g); 0.1% (20 g, 45 g)

Gel, topical: 0.025% (15 g, 45 g)
- Avita®: 0.025% (15 g, 45 g)
- Retin-A®: 0.01% (15 g, 45 g); 0.025% (15 g, 45 g)
- Retin-A® Micro [microsphere gel]: 0.04% (20 g, 45 g); 0.1% (20 g, 45 g)

Liquid, topical (Retin-A®): 0.05% (28 mL)

Trexall™ [US] *see* methotrexate *on page 565*

TRH *see* protirelin *on page 744*

triacetin (trye a SEE tin)

Sound-Alike/Look-Alike Issues

triacetin may be confused with Triacin®

Synonyms glycerol triacetate

U.S./Canadian Brand Names Myco-Nail [US-OTC]

Therapeutic Category Antifungal Agent

Use Fungistat for athlete's foot and other superficial fungal infections

Usual Dosage Apply twice daily, cleanse areas with dilute alcohol or mild soap and water before application; continue treatment for 7 days after symptoms have disappeared

Dosage Forms Liquid, topical: 25% (30 mL)

Triacet™ Topical [US] *see* triamcinolone (topical) *on page 882*

triacetyloleandomycin *see* troleandomycin *on page 891*

Triacin-C® ***(Discontinued)*** *see page 1042*

triaconazole *see* terconazole *on page 846*

Triaderm [Can] *see* triamcinolone (topical) *on page 882*

Triafed® ***(Discontinued)*** *see page 1042*

triamcinolone acetonide, aerosol *see* triamcinolone (systemic) *on next page*

triamcinolone acetonide, aerosol *see* triamcinolone (topical) *on page 882*

triamcinolone acetonide, parenteral *see* triamcinolone (systemic) *on next page*

triamcinolone and nystatin *see* nystatin and triamcinolone *on page 638*

triamcinolone diacetate, oral *see* triamcinolone (systemic) *on next page*

triamcinolone diacetate, parenteral *see* triamcinolone (systemic) *on next page*

triamcinolone hexacetonide *see* triamcinolone (systemic) *on next page*

triamcinolone (inhalation, nasal)

(trye am SIN oh lone in hil LA shun, NAY sal)

Sound-Alike/Look-Alike Issues

Nasacort® may be confused with Nasalcrom®

U.S./Canadian Brand Names Nasacort® [HFA] [US]; Nasacort® AQ [US/Can]; Trinasal® [Can]

Therapeutic Category Corticosteroid, Topical

Use

Nasal inhalation: Management of seasonal and perennial allergic rhinitis in patients ≥6 years of age

Oral inhalation: Control of bronchial asthma and related bronchospastic conditions

Oral topical: Adjunctive treatment and temporary relief of symptoms associated with oral inflammatory lesions and ulcerative lesions resulting from trauma

Systemic: Adrenocortical insufficiency, rheumatic disorders, allergic states, respiratory diseases, systemic lupus erythematosus (SLE), and other diseases requiring antiinflammatory or immunosuppressive effects

Topical: Inflammatory dermatoses responsive to steroids

Usual Dosage Children >12 years and Adults: Intranasal: 2 sprays in each nostril once daily; may increase after 4-7 days up to 4 sprays once daily or 1 spray 4 times/day in each nostril

Dosage Forms

Aerosol for nasal inhalation, as acetonide [CFC free] (Nasacort® [HFA]): 55 mcg/inhalation (9.3 g) [100 doses]

Aerosol for nasal inhalation, as acetonide [spray]:

Nasacort® AQ: 55 mcg/inhalation (16.5 g) [120 doses]

Tri-Nasal®: 50 mcg/inhalation (15 mL) [120 doses]

triamcinolone (inhalation, oral) (trye am SIN oh lone in hil LA shun, OR al)

U.S./Canadian Brand Names Azmacort® [US]

Therapeutic Category Adrenal Corticosteroid

Use

Nasal inhalation: Management of seasonal and perennial allergic rhinitis in patients ≥6 years of age

Oral inhalation: Control of bronchial asthma and related bronchospastic conditions

Oral topical: Adjunctive treatment and temporary relief of symptoms associated with oral inflammatory lesions and ulcerative lesions resulting from trauma

Systemic: Adrenocortical insufficiency, rheumatic disorders, allergic states, respiratory diseases, systemic lupus erythematosus (SLE), and other diseases requiring antiinflammatory or immunosuppressive effects

Topical: Inflammatory dermatoses responsive to steroids

Usual Dosage Oral inhalation: Asthma:

Children 6-12 years: 100-200 mcg 3-4 times/day **or** 200-400 mcg twice daily; maximum dose: 1200 mg/day

Children >12 years and Adults: 200 mcg 3-4 times/day **or** 400 mcg twice daily; maximum dose: 1600 mcg/day

Dosage Forms

Aerosol for oral inhalation, as acetonide (Azmacort®): 100 mcg per actuation (20 g) [240 actuations]

triamcinolone, oral *see* triamcinolone (systemic) *on this page*

triamcinolone (systemic) (trye am SIN oh lone sis TEM ik)

Sound-Alike/Look-Alike Issues

Kenalog® may be confused with Ketalar®

Synonyms triamcinolone acetonide, aerosol; triamcinolone acetonide, parenteral; triamcinolone diacetate, oral; triamcinolone diacetate, parenteral; triamcinolone hexacetonide; triamcinolone, oral

U.S./Canadian Brand Names Aristocort® Forte Injection [US]; Aristocort® Intralesional Injection [US]; Aristocort® Tablet [US/Can]; Aristospan® Intraarticular Injection [US/Can]; Aristospan® Intralesional Injection [US/Can]; Kenalog® Injection [US/Can]

Therapeutic Category Adrenal Corticosteroid

Use

Nasal inhalation: Management of seasonal and perennial allergic rhinitis in patients ≥6 years of age

Oral inhalation: Control of bronchial asthma and related bronchospastic conditions

Oral topical: Adjunctive treatment and temporary relief of symptoms associated with oral inflammatory lesions and ulcerative lesions resulting from trauma

Systemic: Adrenocortical insufficiency, rheumatic disorders, allergic states, respiratory diseases, systemic lupus erythematosus (SLE), and other diseases requiring antiinflammatory or immunosuppressive effects

Topical: Inflammatory dermatoses responsive to steroids

Usual Dosage In general, single I.M. dose of 4-7 times oral dose will control patient from 4-7 days up to 3-4 weeks

Children 6-12 years: I.M.: Acetonide or hexacetonide: 0.03-0.2 mg/kg at 1- to 7-day intervals

Children >12 years and Adults:

Oral: 4-100 mg/day

I.M.: Acetonide or hexacetonide: 60 mg (of 40 mg/mL), additional 20-100 mg doses (usual: 40-80 mg) may be administered when signs and symptoms recur, best at 6-week intervals to minimize HPA suppression

Intra-articularly, intrasynovially, intralesionally: 2.5-40 mg as diacetate salt or acetonide salt, dose may be repeated when signs and symptoms recur

Intra-articularly: Hexacetonide: 2-20 mg every 3-4 weeks as hexacetonide salt

Intralesional (use 10 mg/mL): Diacetate or acetonide: 1 mg/injection site, may be repeated one or more times/week depending upon patients response; maximum; 30 mg at any one time; may use multiple injections if they are more than 1 cm apart

Intra-articular, intrasynovial, and soft-tissue injection (use 10 mg/mL or 40 mg/mL): Diacetate or acetonide: 2.5-40 mg depending upon location, size of joints, and degree of inflammation; repeat when signs and symptoms recur

Sublesionally (as acetonide): Up to 1 mg per injection site and may be repeated one or more times weekly; multiple sites may be injected if they are 1 cm or more apart, not to exceed 30 mg

Dosage Forms

Injection, suspension, as acetonide:

Kenalog-10®: 10 mg/mL (5 mL) [contains benzyl alcohol; not for I.V. or I.M. use]

Kenalog-40®: 40 mg/mL (1 mL, 5 mL, 10 mL) [contains benzyl alcohol; not for I.V. or intradermal use]

Injection, suspension, as diacetate:

Aristocort®: 25 mg/mL (5 mL) [contains benzyl alcohol; not for I.V. use]

Aristocort® Forte: 40 mg/mL (1 mL, 5mL) [contains benzyl alcohol; not for I.V. use]

Injection, suspension, as hexacetonide (Aristospan®): 5 mg/mL (5 mL); 20 mg/mL (1 mL, 5 mL) [contains benzyl alcohol; not for I.V. use]

Tablet (Aristocort®): 4 mg [contains lactose and sodium benzoate]

triamcinolone (topical) (trye am SIN oh lone TOP i kal)

Synonyms triamcinolone acetonide, aerosol

U.S./Canadian Brand Names Aristocort® A Topical [US]; Aristocort® Topical [US]; Kenalog® in Orabase® [US/Can]; Kenalog® Topical [US/Can]; Oracort [Can]; Triacet™ Topical [US]; Triaderm [Can]; Triderm® [US]

Therapeutic Category Corticosteroid, Topical

Use

Nasal inhalation: Management of seasonal and perennial allergic rhinitis in patients ≥6 years of age

Oral inhalation: Control of bronchial asthma and related bronchospastic conditions

Oral topical: Adjunctive treatment and temporary relief of symptoms associated with oral inflammatory lesions and ulcerative lesions resulting from trauma

Systemic: Adrenocortical insufficiency, rheumatic disorders, allergic states, respiratory diseases, systemic lupus erythematosus (SLE), and other diseases requiring antiinflammatory or immunosuppressive effects

Topical: Inflammatory dermatoses responsive to steroids

Usual Dosage Topical:

Cream, Ointment: Apply thin film to affected areas 2-4 times/day

Spray: Apply to affected area 3-4 times/day

Dosage Forms

Aerosol, topical, as acetonide (Kenalog®): 0.2 mg/2-second spray (63 g)

Cream, as acetonide: 0.025% (15 g, 80 g); 0.1% (15 g, 80 g, 454 g, 2270 g); 0.5% (15 g)

Aristocort® A: 0.025% (15 g, 60 g); 0.1% (15 g, 60 g); 0.5% (15 g) [contains benzyl alcohol]

Kenalog®: 0.1% (15 g, 60 g, 80 g); 0.5% (20 g)

Triderm®: 0.1% (30 g, 85 g)

Lotion, as acetonide (Kenalog®): 0.025% (60 mL); 0.1% (60 mL)

Ointment, topical, as acetonide: 0.025% (80 g); 0.1% (15 g, 80 g, 454 g)

Aristocort® A, Kenalog®: 0.1% (15 g, 60 g)

Paste, oral, topical, as acetonide (Kenalog® in Orabase®): 0.1% (5 g)

Tablet (Aristocort®): 4 mg [contains lactose and sodium benzoate]

Triaminic® Allergy Congestion [US-OTC/Can] *see* pseudoephedrine *on page 745*

Triaminic® Allergy Tablet *(Discontinued)* *see page 1042*

Triaminic® Cold and Allergy [US-OTC/Can] *see* chlorpheniramine and pseudoephedrine *on page 189*

Triaminic® Cold Tablet *(Discontinued)* *see page 1042*

Triaminic® Cough and Sore Throat [US-OTC] *see* acetaminophen, dextromethorphan, and pseudoephedrine *on page 12*

Triaminic® Expectorant *(Discontinued)* *see page 1042*

Triaminicol® Multi-Symptom Cold Syrup *(Discontinued)* *see page 1042*

Triaminic® Oral Infant, Drops *(Discontinued)* *see page 1042*

Triaminic® Syrup *(Discontinued)* *see page 1042*

Triamonide® Injection *(Discontinued)* *see page 1042*

triamterene (trye AM ter een)

Sound-Alike/Look-Alike Issues

triamterene may be confused with trimipramine

Dyrenium® may be confused with Pyridium®

U.S./Canadian Brand Names Dyrenium® [US]

Therapeutic Category Diuretic, Potassium Sparing

Use Alone or in combination with other diuretics in treatment of edema and hypertension; decreases potassium excretion caused by kaliuretic diuretics

Usual Dosage Adults: Oral: 100-300 mg/day in 1-2 divided doses; maximum dose: 300 mg/day; usual dosage range (JNC 7): 50-100 mg/day
Dosage Forms Capsule: 50 mg, 100 mg [contains benzyl alcohol]

triamterene and hydrochlorothiazide *see* hydrochlorothiazide and triamterene *on page 443*

Triapin® *(Discontinued)* *see page 1042*

Triatec-8 [Can] *see* acetaminophen and codeine *on page 6*

Triatec-8-Strong [Can] *see* acetaminophen and codeine *on page 6*

Triatec-30 [Can] *see* acetaminophen and codeine *on page 6*

Triavil® [US/Can] *see* amitriptyline and perphenazine *on page 48*

Triavil® 4-50 *(Discontinued)* *see page 1042*

Triaz® [US] *see* benzoyl peroxide *on page 109*

Triaz® Cleanser [US] *see* benzoyl peroxide *on page 109*

triazolam (trye AY zoe lam)

Sound-Alike/Look-Alike Issues
triazolam may be confused with alprazolam
Halcion® may be confused with halcinonide, Haldol®
U.S./Canadian Brand Names Apo-Triazo® [Can]; Gen-Triazolam [Can]; Halcion® [US/Can]
Therapeutic Category Benzodiazepine
Controlled Substance C-IV
Use Short-term treatment of insomnia
Usual Dosage Oral (onset of action is rapid, patient should be in bed when taking medication):
Children <18 years: Dosage not established
Adults:
Hypnotic: 0.125-0.25 mg at bedtime (maximum dose: 0.5 mg/day)
Preprocedure sedation (dental): 0.25 mg taken the evening before oral surgery; or 0.25 mg 1 hour before procedure
Dosage Forms Tablet: 0.125 mg, 0.25 mg [contains sodium benzoate]

tribavirin *see* ribavirin *on page 774*

tricalcium phosphate *see* calcium phosphate (tribasic) *on page 150*

Tricardio B [Can] *see* folic acid, cyanocobalamin, and pyridoxine *on page 386*

Tri-Chlor® [US] *see* trichloroacetic acid *on this page*

Trichlorex® [Can] *see* trichlormethiazide *on this page*

trichlormethiazide (trye klor meth EYE a zide)

U.S./Canadian Brand Names Metahydrin® [Can]; Metatensin® [Can]; Naqua® [US/Can]; Trichlorex® [Can]
Therapeutic Category Diuretic, Thiazide
Use Management of mild to moderate hypertension; treatment of edema in congestive heart failure and nephrotic syndrome
Usual Dosage Adults: Oral: 1-4 mg/day; initially doses may be given twice daily.
Dosage Forms Tablet: 4 mg

trichloroacetaldehyde monohydrate *see* chloral hydrate *on page 181*

trichloroacetic acid (trye klor oh a SEE tik AS id)

U.S./Canadian Brand Names Tri-Chlor® [US]
Therapeutic Category Keratolytic Agent
Use Debride callous tissue
(Continued)

trichloroacetic acid *(Continued)*

Usual Dosage Topical: Apply to verruca, cover with bandage for 5-6 days, remove verruca, reapply as needed

Dosage Forms Liquid: 80% (15 mL)

trichloromonofluoromethane and dichlorodifluoromethane *see* dichlorodifluoromethane and trichloromonofluoromethane *on page 265*

Trichophyton skin test (trye koe FYE ton skin test)

Therapeutic Category Diagnostic Agent

Use Assess cell-mediated immunity

Usual Dosage 0.1 mL intradermally, examine reaction site in 24-48 hours; induration of ≥5 mm in diameter is a positive reaction

Dosage Forms Injection, solution: 1:500 (1 mL)

Tri-Clear® Expectorant *(Discontinued)* *see page 1042*

TriCor® [US/Can] *see* fenofibrate *on page 360*

tricosal *see* choline magnesium trisalicylate *on page 197*

Tri-Cyclen® [Can] *see* ethinyl estradiol and norgestimate *on page 346*

Triderm® [US] *see* triamcinolone (topical) *on page 882*

Tridesilon® [US] *see* desonide *on page 253*

Tridil® Injection *(Discontinued)* *see page 1042*

Tridione® *(Discontinued)* *see page 1042*

trientine (TRYE en teen)

Sound-Alike/Look-Alike Issues

trientine may be confused with Trental®, tretinoin

Synonyms trientine hydrochloride

U.S./Canadian Brand Names Syprine® [US/Can]

Therapeutic Category Chelating Agent

Use Treatment of Wilson's disease in patients intolerant to penicillamine

Usual Dosage Oral (administer on an empty stomach):

Children <12 years: 500-750 mg/day in divided doses 2-4 times/day; maximum: 1.5 g/day

Adults: 750-1250 mg/day in divided doses 2-4 times/day; maximum dose: 2 g/day

Dosage Forms Capsule, as hydrochloride: 250 mg

trientine hydrochloride *see* trientine *on this page*

triethanolamine polypeptide oleate-condensate

(trye eth a NOLE a meen pol i PEP tide OH lee ate-KON den sate)

U.S./Canadian Brand Names Cerumenex® [US/Can]

Therapeutic Category Otic Agent, Ceruminolytic

Use Removal of ear wax (cerumen)

Usual Dosage Children and Adults: Otic: Fill ear canal, insert cotton plug; allow to remain 15-30 minutes; flush ear with lukewarm water as a single treatment; if a second application is needed for unusually hard impactions, repeat the procedure

Dosage Forms Solution, otic: 10% (6 mL, 12 mL)

triethanolamine salicylate (trye eth a NOLE a meen sa LIS i late)

Sound-Alike/Look-Alike Issues

Myoflex® may be confused with Mycelex®

U.S./Canadian Brand Names Antiphlogistine Rub A-535 No Odour [Can]; Mobisyl® [US-OTC]; Myoflex® [US-OTC/Can]; Sportscreme® [US-OTC]

Therapeutic Category Analgesic, Topical

Use Relief of pain of muscular aches, rheumatism, neuralgia, sprains, arthritis on intact skin

Usual Dosage Topical: Apply to area as needed

Dosage Forms Cream, topical: 10% (90 g)

Mobisyl®: 10% (35 g, 100 g, 227 g) [odorless]

Myoflex®: 10% (60 g, 120 g, 240 g, 480 g) [odorless]

Sportscreme®: 10% (40 g, 90 g) [odorless fresh scent]

triethylenethiophosphoramide *see* thiotepa *on page 858*

Trifed-C® *(Discontinued)* *see page 1042*

trifluoperazine (trye floo oh PER a zeen)

Sound-Alike/Look-Alike Issues

trifluoperazine may be confused with triflupromazine, trihexyphenidyl

Stelazine® may be confused with selegiline

Synonyms trifluoperazine hydrochloride

U.S./Canadian Brand Names Apo-Trifluoperazine® [Can]; Novo-Trifluzine [Can]; PMS-Trifluoperazine [Can]; Terfluzine [Can]

Therapeutic Category Phenothiazine Derivative

Use Treatment of schizophrenia

Usual Dosage

Children 6-12 years: Schizophrenia/psychoses:

Oral: Hospitalized or well-supervised patients: Initial: 1 mg 1-2 times/day, gradually increase until symptoms are controlled or adverse effects become troublesome; maximum: 15 mg/day

I.M.: 1 mg twice daily

Adults:

Schizophrenia/psychoses:

Outpatients: Oral: 1-2 mg twice daily

Hospitalized or well-supervised patients: Initial: 2-5 mg twice daily with optimum response in the 15-20 mg/day range; do not exceed 40 mg/day

I.M.: 1-2 mg every 4-6 hours as needed up to 10 mg/24 hours maximum

Nonpsychotic anxiety: Oral: 1-2 mg twice daily; maximum: 6 mg/day; therapy for anxiety should not exceed 12 weeks; do not exceed 6 mg/day for longer than 12 weeks when treating anxiety; agitation, jitteriness, or insomnia may be confused with original neurotic or psychotic symptoms

Dosage Forms [DSC] = Discontinued product

Injection, solution, as hydrochloride (Stelazine®): 2 mg/mL (10 mL) [contains benzyl alcohol] [DSC]

Tablet, as hydrochloride: 1 mg, 2 mg, 5 mg, 10 mg

Stelazine®: 5 mg [DSC]

trifluoperazine hydrochloride *see* trifluoperazine *on this page*

trifluorothymidine *see* trifluridine *on this page*

trifluridine (trye FLURE i deen)

Sound-Alike/Look-Alike Issues

Viroptic® may be confused with Timoptic®

Synonyms F_3T; trifluorothymidine

U.S./Canadian Brand Names Viroptic® [US/Can]

Therapeutic Category Antiviral Agent

Use Treatment of primary keratoconjunctivitis and recurrent epithelial keratitis caused by herpes simplex virus types I and II

Usual Dosage Adults: Instill 1 drop into affected eye every 2 hours while awake, to a maximum of 9 drops/day, until re-epithelialization of corneal ulcer occurs; then use 1 drop every 4 hours for another 7 days; do **not** exceed 21 days of treatment; if improvement has not taken place in 7-14 days, consider another form of therapy

Dosage Forms Solution, ophthalmic: 1% (7.5 mL)

triglycerides, medium chain *see* medium chain triglycerides *on page 547*

trihexyphenidyl (trye heks ee FEN i dil)

Sound-Alike/Look-Alike Issues
trihexyphenidyl may be confused with trifluoperazine

Synonyms benzhexol hydrochloride; trihexyphenidyl hydrochloride

U.S./Canadian Brand Names Apo-Trihex® [Can]

Therapeutic Category Anticholinergic Agent; Anti-Parkinson Agent

Use Adjunctive treatment of Parkinson disease; treatment of drug-induced extrapyramidal symptoms

Usual Dosage Adults: Oral: Initial: 1-2 mg/day, increase by 2 mg increments at intervals of 3-5 days; usual dose: 5-15 mg/day in 3-4 divided doses

Dosage Forms
Elixir, as hydrochloride: 2 mg/5 mL (480 mL)
Tablet, as hydrochloride: 2 mg, 5 mg

trihexyphenidyl hydrochloride *see* trihexyphenidyl *on this page*

TriHIBit® [US] *see* diphtheria, tetanus toxoids, and acellular pertussis vaccine and *Haemophilus* b conjugate vaccine *on page 281*

Tri-Immunol® *(Discontinued)* *see page 1042*

Tri-K® [US] *see* potassium acetate, potassium bicarbonate, and potassium citrate *on page 711*

Trikacide® [Can] *see* metronidazole *on page 576*

TRIKOF-D® *(Discontinued)* *see page 1042*

Tri-Kort® Injection *(Discontinued)* *see page 1042*

Trilafon® *(Discontinued)* *see page 1042*

Trilafon® [Can] *see* perphenazine *on page 683*

Trileptal® [US/Can] *see* oxcarbazepine *on page 653*

Tri-Levlen® [US] *see* ethinyl estradiol and levonorgestrel *on page 339*

Trilisate® *(Discontinued)* *see page 1042*

Trilog® Injection *(Discontinued)* *see page 1042*

Trilone® Injection *(Discontinued)* *see page 1042*

Tri-Luma™ [US] *see* fluocinolone, hydroquinone, and tretinoin *on page 375*

TriLyte™ [US] *see* polyethylene glycol-electrolyte solution *on page 706*

Trimazide® *(Discontinued)* *see page 1042*

trimebutine *(Canada only)* (trye me BYOO teen)

Synonyms trimebutine maleate

U.S./Canadian Brand Names Apo-Trimebutine® [Can]; Modulon® [Can]

Therapeutic Category Antispasmodic Agent, Gastrointestinal

Use Treatment and relief of symptoms associated with irritable bowel syndrome (IBS) (spastic colon). In postoperative paralytic ileus in order to accelerate the resumption of the intestinal transit following abdominal surgery.

Usual Dosage Children ≥12 years and Adults: Oral: 200 mg 3 times/day before meals

Dosage Forms Tablet, as maleate: 100 mg, 200 mg

trimebutine maleate *see* trimebutine *(Canada only)* *on this page*

trimeprazine *(Canada only)* (trye MEP re zeen)

Therapeutic Category Antihistamine

Use Perennial and seasonal allergic rhinitis and other allergic symptoms including urticaria

Usual Dosage Oral:
Children:
6 months to 3 years: 1.25 mg at bedtime or 3 times/day if needed
>3 years: 2.5 mg at bedtime or 3 times/day if needed
>6 years: 5 mg/day
Adults: 2.5 mg 4 times/day
Dosage Forms Tablet, as tartrate: 2.5 mg, 5 mg

trimethobenzamide (trye meth oh BEN za mide)

Sound-Alike/Look-Alike Issues
Tigan® may be confused with Tiazac®, Ticar®
Synonyms trimethobenzamide hydrochloride
U.S./Canadian Brand Names Tigan® [US/Can]
Therapeutic Category Anticholinergic Agent; Antiemetic
Use Treatment of nausea and vomiting
Usual Dosage Rectal use is contraindicated in neonates and premature infants
Children:
<14 kg: Oral, rectal: 100 mg 3-4 times/day
14-40 kg: Oral, rectal: 100-200 mg 3-4 times/day
Adults:
Oral: 250-300 mg 3-4 times/day
I.M., rectal: 200 mg 3-4 times/day
Dosage Forms [DSC] = Discontinued product
Capsule, as hydrochloride: 250 mg [DSC]
Tigan®: 300 mg
Injection, solution, as hydrochloride: 100 mg/mL (2 mL)
Tigan®: 100 mg/mL (2 mL, 20 mL)
Suppository, rectal, as hydrochloride (Tigan®): 100 mg, 200 mg [contains benzocaine]

trimethobenzamide hydrochloride *see* trimethobenzamide *on this page*

trimethoprim (trye METH oh prim)

Sound-Alike/Look-Alike Issues
trimethoprim may be confused with trimethaphan
Proloprim® may be confused with Prolixin®, Protropin®
Synonyms TMP
U.S./Canadian Brand Names Apo-Trimethoprim® [Can]; Primsol® [US]; Proloprim® [US/Can]
Therapeutic Category Antibiotic, Miscellaneous
Use Treatment of urinary tract infections due to susceptible strains of *E. coli*, *P. mirabilis*, *K. pneumoniae*, *Enterobacter* sp and coagulase-negative *Staphylococcus* including *S. saprophyticus*; acute otitis media in children; acute exacerbations of chronic bronchitis in adults; in combination with other agents for treatment of toxoplasmosis, *Pneumocystis carinii*; treatment of superficial ocular infections involving the conjunctiva and cornea
Usual Dosage Oral:
Children: 4 mg/kg/day in divided doses every 12 hours
Adults: 100 mg every 12 hours or 200 mg every 24 hours for 10 days; longer treatment periods may be necessary for prostatitis (ie, 4-16 weeks); in the treatment of *Pneumocystis carinii* pneumonia; dose may be as high as 15-20 mg/kg/day in 3-4 divided doses
Dosage Forms
Solution, oral (Primsol®): 50 mg (base)/5 mL (480 mL) [contains sodium benzoate; bubblegum flavor]
Tablet: 100 mg
Proloprim®: 100 mg, 200 mg

trimethoprim and polymyxin B (trye METH oh prim & pol i MIKS in bee)

Synonyms polymyxin B and trimethoprim

U.S./Canadian Brand Names PMS-Polytrimethoprim [Can]; Polytrim® [US/Can]

Therapeutic Category Antibiotic, Ophthalmic

Use Treatment of surface ocular bacterial conjunctivitis and blepharoconjunctivitis

Usual Dosage Instill 1-2 drops in eye(s) every 4-6 hours

Dosage Forms Solution, ophthalmic: Trimethoprim sulfate 1 mg and polymyxin B sulfate 10,000 units per mL (10 mL) [contains benzalkonium chloride]

trimethoprim and sulfamethoxazole *see* sulfamethoxazole and trimethoprim *on page 831*

trimetrexate glucuronate (tri me TREKS ate gloo KYOOR oh nate)

Synonyms NSC-352122

U.S./Canadian Brand Names NeuTrexin® [US]

Therapeutic Category Antibiotic, Miscellaneous

Use Alternative therapy for the treatment of moderate-to-severe *Pneumocystis carinii* pneumonia (PCP) in immunocompromised patients, including patients with acquired immunodeficiency syndrome (AIDS), who are intolerant of, or are refractory to, co-trimoxazole therapy or for whom co-trimoxazole and pentamidine are contraindicated. **Concurrent folinic acid (leucovorin) must always be administered.**

Usual Dosage Note: Concurrent leucovorin 20 mg/m^2 every 6 hours must be administered daily (oral or I.V.) during treatment and for 72 hours past the last dose of trimetrexate glucuronate.

Adults: I.V.: *Pneumocystis carinii*: 45 mg/m^2 once daily for 21 days; **alternative dosing based on weight:**

<50 kg:Trimetrexate glucuronate 1.5 mg/kg/day; leucovorin 0.6 mg/kg 4 times/day
50-80 kg:Trimetrexate glucuronate 1.2 mg/kg/day; leucovorin 0.5 mg/kg/4 times/day
>80 kg: Trimetrexate glucuronate 1 mg/kg/day; leucovorin 0.5 mg/kg/4 times/day

Note: Oral doses of leucovorin should be rounded up to the next higher 25 mg increment.

Dosage Forms Injection, powder for reconstitution: 25 mg, 200 mg

trimipramine (trye MI pra meen)

Sound-Alike/Look-Alike Issues

trimipramine may be confused with triamterene, trimeprazine

Synonyms trimipramine maleate

U.S./Canadian Brand Names Apo-Trimip® [Can]; Novo-Tripramine [Can]; Nu-Trimipramine [Can]; Rhotrimine® [Can]; Surmontil® [US/Can]

Therapeutic Category Antidepressant, Tricyclic (Tertiary Amine)

Use Treatment of depression

Usual Dosage Oral: Adults: 50-150 mg/day as a single bedtime dose up to a maximum of 200 mg/day outpatient and 300 mg/day inpatient

Dosage Forms Capsule, as maleate: 25 mg, 50 mg, 100 mg

trimipramine maleate *see* trimipramine *on this page*

Trimox® [US] *see* amoxicillin *on page 51*

Trimox® 500 mg *(Discontinued)* *see page 1042*

Trimpex® *(Discontinued)* *see page 1042*

Trinasal® [Can] *see* triamcinolone (inhalation, nasal) *on page 880*

Trinate [US] *see* vitamins (multiple/prenatal) *on page 927*

Tri-Nefrin® Extra Strength Tablet *(Discontinued)* *see page 1042*

TriNessa™ [US] *see* ethinyl estradiol and norgestimate *on page 346*

Tri-Norinyl® [US] *see* ethinyl estradiol and norethindrone *on page 342*

Trinsicon® [US] *see* vitamin B complex combinations *on page 915*

Triofed® Syrup *(Discontinued)* *see page 1042*

Triostat® [US] *see* liothyronine *on page 523*

Tripedia® [US] *see* diphtheria, tetanus toxoids, and acellular pertussis vaccine *on page 280*

Triphasil® [US/Can] *see* ethinyl estradiol and levonorgestrel *on page 339*

Tri-Phen-Chlor® *(Discontinued)* *see page 1042*

Triphenyl® Expectorant *(Discontinued)* *see page 1042*

Triphenyl® Syrup *(Discontinued)* *see page 1042*

triple antibiotic *see* bacitracin, neomycin, and polymyxin B *on page 97*

Triple Care® Antifungal [OTC] *see* miconazole *on page 578*

triple sulfa *see* sulfabenzamide, sulfacetamide, and sulfathiazole *on page 829*

Tri-P® Oral Infant Drops *(Discontinued)* *see page 1042*

Triposed® Syrup *(Discontinued)* *see page 1042*

Tri-Previfem™ [US] *see* ethinyl estradiol and norgestimate *on page 346*

triprolidine and pseudoephedrine

(trye PROE li deen & soo doe e FED rin)

Sound-Alike/Look-Alike Issues

Aprodine® may be confused with Aphrodyne®

Synonyms pseudoephedrine and triprolidine

U.S./Canadian Brand Names Actifed® [Can]; Actifed® Cold and Allergy [US-OTC]; Allerfrim® [US-OTC]; Allerphed® [US-OTC]; Aphedrid™ [US-OTC]; Aprodine® [US-OTC]; Genac® [US-OTC]; Silafed® [US-OTC]; Tri-Sudo® [US-OTC]; Uni-Fed® [US-OTC]

Therapeutic Category Antihistamine/Decongestant Combination

Use Temporary relief of nasal congestion, decongest sinus openings, running nose, sneezing, itching of nose or throat and itchy, watery eyes due to common cold, hay fever, or other upper respiratory allergies

Usual Dosage Oral:

Children:

Syrup:

4 months to 2 years: 1.25 mL 3-4 times/day

2-4 years: 2.5 mL 3-4 times/day

4-6 years: 3.75 mL 3-4 times/day

6-12 years: 5 mL every 4-6 hours; do not exceed 4 doses in 24 hours

Tablet: $^{1}/_{2}$ every 4-6 hours; do not exceed 4 doses in 24 hours

Children >12 years and Adults:

Syrup: 10 mL every 4-6 hours; do not exceed 4 doses in 24 hours

Tablet: 1 every 4-6 hours; do not exceed 4 doses in 24 hours

Dosage Forms

Syrup: Triprolidine hydrochloride 1.25 mg and pseudoephedrine hydrochloride 30 mg per 5 mL (120 mL)

Allerfrim®: Triprolidine hydrochloride 1.25 mg and pseudoephedrine hydrochloride 30 mg per 5 mL (120 mL, 480 mL)

Allerphed®, Aprodine®: Triprolidine hydrochloride 1.25 mg and pseudoephedrine hydrochloride 30 mg per 5 mL (120 mL)

Silafed®: Triprolidine hydrochloride 1.25 mg and pseudoephedrine hydrochloride 30 mg per 5 mL (120 mL, 240 mL)

Tablet (Actifed® Cold and Allergy, Allerfrim®, Aphedrid™, Aprodine®, Genac®, Tri-Sudo®, Uni-Fed®): Triprolidine hydrochloride 2.5 mg and pseudoephedrine hydrochloride 60 mg

triprolidine, codeine, and pseudoephedrine *see* triprolidine, pseudoephedrine, and codeine *on next page*

triprolidine, pseudoephedrine, and codeine

(trye PROE li deen, soo doe e FED rin, & KOE deen)

Synonyms codeine, pseudoephedrine, and triprolidine; pseudoephedrine, triprolidine, and codeine pseudoephedrine, codeine, and triprolidine; triprolidine, codeine, and pseudoephedrine; triprolidine, pseudoephedrine, and codeine, triprolidine, and pseudoephedrine

U.S./Canadian Brand Names CoActifed® [Can]; Covan® [Can]; ratio-Cotridin [Can]

Therapeutic Category Antihistamine/Decongestant/Antitussive

Controlled Substance C-V

Use Symptomatic relief of upper respiratory symptoms and cough

Usual Dosage Oral:

Children:

2-6 years: 2.5 mL 4 times/day

7-12 years: 5 mL 4 times/day **or** 1/2 tablet 4 times/day

Children >12 years and Adults: 10 mL 4 times/day **or** 1 tablet 4 times/day

Dosage Forms

Syrup:

Triprolidine hydrochloride 1.25 mg, pseudoephedrine hydrochloride 30 mg, and codeine phosphate 10 mg per 5 mL [contains alcohol 4.3%]

CoActifed®, CoVan®, ratio-Cotridin: Triprolidine hydrochloride 2 mg, pseudoephedrine hydrochloride 30 mg, and codeine phosphate 10 mg per 5 mL [available in Canada; not available in U.S.]

Tablet (CoActifed®): Triprolidine hydrochloride 4 mg, pseudoephedrine hydrochloride 60 mg, and codeine phosphate 20 mg (50s) [available in Canada; not available in U.S.]

triprolidine, pseudoephedrine, and codeine, triprolidine, and pseudoephedrine *see* triprolidine, pseudoephedrine, and codeine *on this page*

Tri-Pseudo® *(Discontinued)* *see page 1042*

TripTone® [US-OTC] *see* dimenhydrinate *on page 274*

triptoraline *see* triptorelin *on this page*

triptorelin (trip toe REL in)

Synonyms AY-25650; CL-118,532; D-Trp(6)-LHRH; triptoraline; triptorelin pamoate; tryptoreline

U.S./Canadian Brand Names Trelstar™ Depot [US/Can]; Trelstar™ LA [US]

Therapeutic Category Luteinizing Hormone-Releasing Hormone Analog

Use Palliative treatment of advanced prostate cancer as an alternative to orchiectomy or estrogen administration

Usual Dosage I.M.: Adults: Prostate cancer:

Trelstar™ Depot: 3.75 mg once every 28 days

Trelstar™ LA: 11.25 mg once every 84 days

Dosage Forms Injection, powder for reconstitution, as pamoate [also available packaged with Debioclip™ (prefilled syringe containing sterile water)]:

Trelstar™ Depot: 3.75 mg

Trelstar™ LA: 11.25 mg

triptorelin pamoate *see* triptorelin *on this page*

Triquilar® [Can] *see* ethinyl estradiol and levonorgestrel *on page 339*

tris buffer *see* tromethamine *on next page*

Trisenox™ [US] *see* arsenic trioxide *on page 78*

tris(hydroxymethyl)aminomethane *see* tromethamine *on next page*

Trisoject® Injection *(Discontinued)* *see page 1042*

Trisoralen® *(Discontinued)* *see page 1042*

Tri-Sprintec™ [US] *see* ethinyl estradiol and norgestimate *on page 346*

Tri-Statin® II Topical ***(Discontinued)*** *see page 1042*

Trisudex® ***(Discontinued)*** *see page 1042*

Tri-Sudo® [US-OTC] *see* triprolidine and pseudoephedrine *on page 889*

Tri-Tannate Plus® ***(Discontinued)*** *see page 1042*

Tritec® ***(Discontinued)*** *see page 1042*

Trivagizole-3® [Can] *see* clotrimazole *on page 218*

Trivagizole-3® ***(Discontinued)*** *see page 1042*

Tri-Vent™ DM [US] *see* guaifenesin, pseudoephedrine, and dextromethorphan *on page 422*

Tri-Vent™ DPC [US] *see* chlorpheniramine, phenylephrine, and dextromethorphan *on page 191*

Tri-Vi-Flor® [US] *see* vitamins (multiple/pediatric) *on page 927*

Tri-Vi-Flor® with Iron [US] *see* vitamins (multiple/pediatric) *on page 927*

Tri-Vi-Sol® [US-OTC] *see* vitamins (multiple/pediatric) *on page 927*

Tri-Vi-Sol® with Iron [US-OTC] *see* vitamins (multiple/pediatric) *on page 927*

Trivora® [US] *see* ethinyl estradiol and levonorgestrel *on page 339*

Trizivir® [US] *see* abacavir, lamivudine, and zidovudine *on page 2*

Trobicin® [US] *see* spectinomycin *on page 820*

Trocaine® [US-OTC] *see* benzocaine *on page 107*

Trocal® ***(Discontinued)*** *see page 1042*

Trofan® ***(Discontinued)*** *see page 1042*

Trofan DS® ***(Discontinued)*** *see page 1042*

troleandomycin (troe lee an doe MYE sin)

Synonyms triacetyloleandomycin

U.S./Canadian Brand Names Tao® [US]

Therapeutic Category Macrolide (Antibiotic)

Use Antibiotic with spectrum of activity similar to erythromycin

Usual Dosage Oral:

Children 7-13 years: 25-40 mg/kg/day divided every 6 hours (125-250 mg every 6 hours)

Adults: 250-500 mg 4 times/day (around-the-clock every 6 hours)

Dosage Forms Capsule: 250 mg

tromethamine (troe METH a meen)

Synonyms tris buffer; tris(hydroxymethyl)aminomethane

U.S./Canadian Brand Names THAM® [US]

Therapeutic Category Alkalinizing Agent

Use Correction of metabolic acidosis associated with cardiac bypass surgery or cardiac arrest; to correct excess acidity of stored blood that is preserved with acid citrate dextrose; to prime the pump-oxygenator during cardiac bypass surgery; indicated in infants needing alkalinization after receiving maximum sodium bicarbonate (8-10 mEq/kg/24 hours); (advantage of THAM® is that it alkalinizes without increasing pCO_2 and sodium)

Usual Dosage

Neonates and Infants: Metabolic acidosis associated with RDS: Initial: Approximately 1 mL/kg for each pH unit below 7.4; additional doses determined by changes in PaO_2, pH, and pCO_2; **Note:** Although THAM® solution does not raise pCO_2 when treating metabolic acidosis with concurrent respiratory acidosis, bicarbonate may be preferred because the osmotic effects of THAM® are greater.

(Continued)

tromethamine *(Continued)*

Adults: Dose depends on buffer base deficit; when deficit is known: tromethamine (mL of 0.3 M solution) = body weight (kg) x base deficit (mEq/L); when base deficit is not known: 3-6 mL/kg/dose I.V. (1-2 mEq/kg/dose)

Metabolic acidosis with cardiac arrest:

I.V.: 3.5-6 mL/kg (1-2 mEq/kg/dose) into large peripheral vein; 500-1000 mL if needed in adults

I.V. continuous drip: Infuse slowly by syringe pump over 3-6 hours

Acidosis associated with cardiac bypass surgery: Average dose: 9 mL/kg (2.7 mEq/kg); 500 mL is adequate for most adults; maximum dose: 500 mg/kg in ≤1 hour

Excess acidity of acid citrate dextrose priming blood: 14-70 mL of 0.3 molar solution added to each 500 mL of blood

Dosage Forms Injection, solution (THAM®): 18 g [0.3 molar] (500 mL)

Tronolane® [US-OTC] *see* pramoxine *on page 720*

Tropicacyl® [US] *see* tropicamide *on this page*

tropicamide (troe PIK a mide)

Synonyms bistropamide

U.S./Canadian Brand Names Diotrope® [Can]; Mydriacyl® [US/Can]; Opticyl® [US]; Tropicacyl® [US]

Therapeutic Category Anticholinergic Agent

Use Short-acting mydriatic used in diagnostic procedures; as well as preoperatively and postoperatively; treatment of some cases of acute iritis, iridocyclitis, and keratitis

Usual Dosage Ophthalmic: Children and Adults (individuals with heavily pigmented eyes may require larger doses):

Cycloplegia: Instill 1-2 drops (1%); may repeat in 5 minutes

Exam must be performed within 30 minutes after the repeat dose; if the patient is not examined within 20-30 minutes, instill an additional drop

Mydriasis: Instill 1-2 drops (0.5%) 15-20 minutes before exam; may repeat every 30 minutes as needed

Dosage Forms Solution, ophthalmic: 0.5% (15 mL); 1% (2 mL, 3 mL, 15 mL) [contains benzalkonium chloride]

Mydriacyl®: 0.5% (15 mL); 1% (3 mL, 15 mL) [contains benzalkonium chloride]

Opticyl®, Tropicacyl®: 0.5% (15 mL); 1% (15 mL) [contains benzalkonium chloride]

trospium (TROSE pee um)

Synonyms trospium chloride

U.S./Canadian Brand Names Sanctura™ [US]

Therapeutic Category Anticholinergic Agent

Use Treatment of overactive bladder with symptoms of urgency, incontinence, and urinary frequency

Usual Dosage Oral: Adults: 20 mg twice daily

Dosage Forms Tablet, as chloride: 20 mg

trospium chloride *see* trospium *on this page*

Trovan® *(Discontinued)* *see page 1042*

Truphylline® *(Discontinued)* *see page 1042*

Trusopt® [US/Can] *see* dorzolamide *on page 290*

Truvada™ [US] *see* emtricitabine and tenofovir *on page 307*

trypsin, balsam peru, and castor oil

(TRIP sin, BAL sam pe RUE, & KAS tor oyl)

Sound-Alike/Look-Alike Issues

Granulex® may be confused with Regranex®

Synonyms balsam peru, trypsin, and castor oil; castor oil, trypsin, and balsam peru

U.S./Canadian Brand Names Granulex® [US]

Therapeutic Category Protectant, Topical

Use Treatment of decubitus ulcers, varicose ulcers, debridement of eschar, dehiscent wounds and sunburn

Usual Dosage Topical: Apply a minimum of twice daily or as often as necessary

Dosage Forms Aerosol, topical: Trypsin 0.12 mg, balsam Peru 87 mg, and castor oil 788 mg per gram (60 g, 120 g)

Tryptacin® ***(Discontinued)*** *see page 1042*

tryptoreline *see* triptorelin *on page 890*

Trysul® ***(Discontinued)*** *see page 1042*

TSH *see* thyrotropin alpha *on page 860*

TSPA *see* thiotepa *on page 858*

TST *see* tuberculin tests *on this page*

T-Stat® ***(Discontinued)*** *see page 1042*

T-Tab® [US] *see* clorazepate *on page 217*

tuberculin purified protein derivative *see* tuberculin tests *on this page*

tuberculin skin test *see* tuberculin tests *on this page*

tuberculin tests (too BER kyoo lin tests)

Sound-Alike/Look-Alike Issues

Aplisol® may be confused with Anusol®, A.P.L.®, Aplitest®, Atropisol®

Synonyms Mantoux; PPD; tine test; TST; tuberculin purified protein derivative; tuberculin skin test

U.S./Canadian Brand Names Aplisol® [US]; Tubersol® [US]

Therapeutic Category Diagnostic Agent

Use Skin test in diagnosis of tuberculosis, cell-mediated immunodeficiencies

Usual Dosage Children and Adults: Intradermal: 0.1 mL about 4" below elbow; use 1/4" to 1/2" or 26- or 27-gauge needle; significant reactions are ≥5 mm in diameter

Interpretation of induration of tuberculin skin test injections: Positive: ≥10 mm; inconclusive: 5-9 mm; negative: <5 mm

Interpretation of induration of Tine test injections: Positive: >2 mm and vesiculation present; inconclusive: <2 mm (give patient Mantoux test of 5 TU/0.1 mL - base decisions on results of Mantoux test); negative: <2 mm or erythema of any size (no need for retesting unless person is a contact of a patient with tuberculosis or there is clinical evidence suggestive of the disease)

Dosage Forms Injection, solution: 5 TU/0.1 mL (1 mL, 5 mL)

Tubersol® [US] *see* tuberculin tests *on this page*

tubocurarine ***(Discontinued)*** *see page 1042*

Tucks® Cream ***(Discontinued)*** *see page 1042*

Tucks® [US-OTC] *see* witch hazel *on page 934*

Tuinal® ***(Discontinued)*** *see page 1042*

Tums® 500 [US-OTC] *see* calcium carbonate *on page 144*

Tums® E-X [US-OTC] *see* calcium carbonate *on page 144*

Tums® Smooth Dissolve [US-OTC] *see* calcium carbonate *on page 144*

Tums® Ultra [US-OTC] *see* calcium carbonate *on page 144*

Tums® [US-OTC] *see* calcium carbonate *on page 144*

Tusal® ***(Discontinued)*** *see page 1042*

Tusibron® ***(Discontinued)*** *see page 1042*

Tusibron-DM® ***(Discontinued)*** *see page 1042*

Tussafed® [US] *see* carbinoxamine, pseudoephedrine, and dextromethorphan *on page 159*

Tussafin® Expectorant *(Discontinued)* *see page 1042*

Tuss-Allergine® Modified T.D. Capsule *(Discontinued)* *see page 1042*

Tussend® Expectorant [US] *see* hydrocodone, pseudoephedrine, and guaifenesin *on page 447*

Tussi-12® [US] *see* carbetapentane and chlorpheniramine *on page 156*

Tussi-12 S™ [US] *see* carbetapentane and chlorpheniramine *on page 156*

Tussigon® [US] *see* hydrocodone and homatropine *on page 446*

Tussin [US-OTC] *see* guaifenesin *on page 415*

Tussionex® [US] *see* hydrocodone and chlorpheniramine *on page 445*

Tussi-Organidin® *(Discontinued)* *see page 1042*

Tussi-Organidin® DM *(Discontinued)* *see page 1042*

Tussi-Organidin® DM NR [US] *see* guaifenesin and dextromethorphan *on page 416*

Tussi-Organidin® NR [US] *see* guaifenesin and codeine *on page 416*

Tussi-Organidin® S-NR [US] *see* guaifenesin and codeine *on page 416*

Tussizone-12 RF™ [US] *see* carbetapentane and chlorpheniramine *on page 156*

Tuss-LA® *(Discontinued)* *see page 1042*

Tusso-DM® *(Discontinued)* *see page 1042*

Tussogest® Extended Release Capsule *(Discontinued)* *see page 1042*

Tuss-Ornade® *(Discontinued)* *see page 1042*

Tusstat® [US] *see* diphenhydramine *on page 277*

Twelve Resin-K® [US] *see* cyanocobalamin *on page 232*

Twice-A-Day® [US-OTC] *see* oxymetazoline *on page 658*

Twilite® [US-OTC] *see* diphenhydramine *on page 277*

Twin-K® *(Discontinued)* *see page 1042*

Twinrix® *(Discontinued)* *see page 1042*

Two-Dyne® *(Discontinued)* *see page 1042*

Tylenol® 8 Hour [US-OTC] *see* acetaminophen *on page 5*

Tylenol® Allergy Sinus [US-OTC/Can] *see* acetaminophen, chlorpheniramine, and pseudoephedrine *on page 11*

Tylenol® Arthritis Pain [US-OTC] *see* acetaminophen *on page 5*

Tylenol® Children's [US-OTC] *see* acetaminophen *on page 5*

Tylenol® Cold Day Non-Drowsy [US-OTC] *see* acetaminophen, dextromethorphan, and pseudoephedrine *on page 12*

Tylenol® Cold Daytime [Can] *see* acetaminophen, dextromethorphan, and pseudoephedrine *on page 12*

Tylenol® Cold Effervescent Medication Tablet *(Discontinued)* *see page 1042*

Tylenol® Cold, Infants [US-OTC] *see* acetaminophen and pseudoephedrine *on page 9*

Tylenol® Decongestant [Can] *see* acetaminophen and pseudoephedrine *on page 9*

Tylenol® Elixir with Codeine [Can] *see* acetaminophen and codeine *on page 6*

Tylenol® Extra Strength [US-OTC] *see* acetaminophen *on page 5*

Tylenol® Flu Non-Drowsy Maximum Strength [US-OTC] *see* acetaminophen, dextromethorphan, and pseudoephedrine *on page 12*

Tylenol® Infants [US-OTC] *see* acetaminophen *on page 5*

Tylenol® Junior Strength [US-OTC] *see* acetaminophen *on page 5*

Tylenol® No. 1 [Can] *see* acetaminophen and codeine *on page 6*

Tylenol® No. 1 Forte [Can] *see* acetaminophen and codeine *on page 6*

Tylenol® No. 2 with Codeine [Can] *see* acetaminophen and codeine *on page 6*

Tylenol® No. 3 with Codeine [Can] *see* acetaminophen and codeine *on page 6*

Tylenol® No. 4 with Codeine [Can] *see* acetaminophen and codeine *on page 6*

Tylenol® PM Extra Strength [US-OTC] *see* acetaminophen and diphenhydramine *on page 7*

Tylenol® Severe Allergy [US-OTC] *see* acetaminophen and diphenhydramine *on page 7*

Tylenol® Sinus [Can] *see* acetaminophen and pseudoephedrine *on page 9*

Tylenol® Sinus, Children's [US-OTC] *see* acetaminophen and pseudoephedrine *on page 9*

Tylenol® Sinus Day Non-Drowsy [US-OTC] *see* acetaminophen and pseudoephedrine *on page 9*

Tylenol® Sore Throat [US-OTC] *see* acetaminophen *on page 5*

Tylenol® [US-OTC/Can] *see* acetaminophen *on page 5*

Tylenol® with Codeine [US/Can] *see* acetaminophen and codeine *on page 6*

Tylenol® with Codeine (Elixir) ***(Discontinued)*** *see page 1042*

Tylox® [US] *see* oxycodone and acetaminophen *on page 656*

Typhim Vi® [US] *see* typhoid vaccine *on this page*

typhoid vaccine (TYE foid vak SEEN)

Synonyms typhoid vaccine live oral Ty21a

U.S./Canadian Brand Names Typhim Vi® [US]; Vivotif Berna® [US/Can]

Therapeutic Category Vaccine, Inactivated Bacteria

Use Typhoid vaccine: Live, attenuated Ty21a typhoid vaccine should not be administered to immunocompromised persons, including those known to be infected with HIV. Parenteral inactivated vaccine is a theoretically safer alternative for this group.

Parenteral: Promotes active immunity to typhoid fever for patients intimately exposed to a typhoid carrier or foreign travel to a typhoid fever endemic area

Oral: For immunization of children >6 years of age and adults who expect intimate exposure of or household contact with typhoid fever, travelers to areas of world with risk of exposure to typhoid fever, and workers in microbiology laboratories with expected frequent contact with *S. typhi*

Usual Dosage Immunization:

Oral: Children ≥6 years and Adults:

Primary immunization: One capsule on alternate days (day 1, 3, 5, and 7) for a total of 4 doses; all doses should be complete at least 1 week prior to potential exposure

Booster immunization: Repeat full course of primary immunization every 5 years

I.M. (Typhim Vi®): Children ≥2 years and Adults: 0.5 mL given at least 2 weeks prior to expected exposure

Re-immunization: 0.5 mL; optimal schedule has not been established; a single dose every 2 years is currently recommended for repeated or continued exposure

(Continued)

typhoid vaccine *(Continued)*

Dosage Forms

Capsule, enteric coated (Vivotif Berna®): Viable *S. typhi* Ty21a colony-forming units 2-6 x 10^9 and nonviable *S. typhi* Ty21a colony-forming units 50 x 10^9 [also contains sucrose, ascorbic acid, amino acid mixture, lactose, and magnesium stearate]

Injection, solution (Typhim Vi®): Purified Vi capsular polysaccharide 25 mcg/0.5 mL (0.5 mL)

typhoid vaccine live oral Ty21a *see* typhoid vaccine *on previous page*

Tyrodone® Liquid *(Discontinued)* *see page 1042*

tyropanoate sodium *see* radiological/contrast media (ionic) *on page 759*

Tyzine® [US] *see* tetrahydrozoline *on page 852*

Tyzine® Pediatric [US] *see* tetrahydrozoline *on page 852*

U-90152S *see* delavirdine *on page 248*

UAD Otic® *(Discontinued)* *see page 1042*

UCB-P071 *see* cetirizine *on page 178*

Ucephan® [US] *see* sodium phenylacetate and sodium benzoate *on page 814*

UK *see* urokinase *on page 899*

UK-68-798 *see* dofetilide *on page 286*

UK92480 *see* sildenafil *on page 803*

UK109496 *see* voriconazole *on page 932*

Ulcerease® [US-OTC] *see* phenol *on page 687*

ULR-LA® *(Discontinued)* *see page 1042*

Ultane® [US] *see* sevoflurane *on page 803*

Ultiva™ [US/Can] *see* remifentanil *on page 767*

Ultracet™ [US] *see* acetaminophen and tramadol *on page 10*

Ultralente® U *(Discontinued)* *see page 1042*

Ultram® [US/Can] *see* tramadol *on page 875*

UltraMide 25™ [Can] *see* urea *on next page*

Ultra Mide® [US-OTC] *see* urea *on next page*

Ultramop™ [Can] *see* methoxsalen *on page 567*

Ultra NatalCare® [US] *see* vitamins (multiple/prenatal) *on page 927*

Ultraprin [US-OTC] *see* ibuprofen *on page 462*

Ultraquin™ [Can] *see* hydroquinone *on page 454*

Ultrase® MT [US/Can] *see* pancrelipase *on page 663*

Ultrase® MT24 *(Discontinued)* *see page 1042*

Ultra Tears® [US-OTC] *see* artificial tears *on page 78*

Ultravate® [US/Can] *see* halobetasol *on page 428*

Unasyn® [US/Can] *see* ampicillin and sulbactam *on page 57*

undecylenic acid and derivatives (un de sil EN ik AS id & dah RIV ah tivs)

Synonyms zinc undecylenate

U.S./Canadian Brand Names Fungi-Nail® [US-OTC]

Therapeutic Category Antifungal Agent

Use Treatment of athlete's foot (tinea pedis); ringworm (except nails and scalp)

Usual Dosage Children and Adults: Topical: Apply twice daily to affected area for 4 weeks; apply to clean, dry area

Dosage Forms Solution, topical: Undecylenic acid 25% (29.57 mL)

Unguentine® *(Discontinued)* *see page 1042*

Uni-Bent® Cough Syrup *(Discontinued)* *see page 1042*

Uni-Decon® *(Discontinued)* *see page 1042*

Unidet® [Can] *see* tolterodine *on page 870*

Uni-Dur® *(Discontinued)* *see page 1042*

Uni-Fed® [US-OTC] *see* triprolidine and pseudoephedrine *on page 889*

Unipen® *(Discontinued)* *see page 1042*

Unipen® [Can] *see* nafcillin *on page 600*

Uniphyl® [US] *see* theophylline *on page 854*

Uniphyl® SRT [Can] *see* theophylline *on page 854*

Unipres® *(Discontinued)* *see page 1042*

Uni-Pro® *(Discontinued)* *see page 1042*

Uniretic® [US/Can] *see* moexipril and hydrochlorothiazide *on page 588*

Unisom® Maximum Strength SleepGels® [US-OTC] *see* diphenhydramine *on page 277*

Unithroid® [US] *see* levothyroxine *on page 516*

Unitrol® *(Discontinued)* *see page 1042*

Uni-tussin® *(Discontinued)* *see page 1042*

Uni-tussin® DM *(Discontinued)* *see page 1042*

Univasc® [US] *see* moexipril *on page 588*

Univol® [Can] *see* aluminum hydroxide and magnesium hydroxide *on page 40*

unna's boot *see* zinc gelatin *on page 940*

unna's paste *see* zinc gelatin *on page 940*

unoprostone (yoo noe PROS tone)

Synonyms unoprostone isopropyl

U.S./Canadian Brand Names Rescula® [US]

Therapeutic Category Ophthalmic Agent, Miscellaneous

Use To lower intraocular pressure (IOP) in patients with open-angle glaucoma or ocular hypertension; should be used in patients who are not tolerant of, or failed treatment with other IOP-lowering medications

Usual Dosage Ophthalmic: Adults: Instill 1 drop into affected eye(s) twice daily

Dosage Forms Solution, ophthalmic: 0.15% (5 mL) [contains benzalkonium chloride]

unoprostone isopropyl *see* unoprostone *on this page*

Urabeth® *(Discontinued)* *see page 1042*

Uracel® *(Discontinued)* *see page 1042*

Urasal® [Can] *see* methenamine *on page 563*

urea (yoor EE a)

Synonyms carbamide

U.S./Canadian Brand Names Amino-Cerv™ [US]; Aquacare® [US-OTC]; Aquaphilic® With Carbamide [US-OTC]; Carmol® 10 [US-OTC]; Carmol® 20 [US-OTC]; Carmol® 40 [US]; Carmol® Deep Cleaning [US]; DPM™ [US-OTC]; Gormel® [US-OTC]; Kerlac® [US]; Lanaphilic® [US-OTC]; Nutraplus® [US-OTC]; Rea-Lo® [US-OTC]; UltraMide 25™ [Can]; Ultra Mide® [US-OTC]; Ureacin® [US-OTC]; Uremol® [Can]; Urisec® [Can]; Vanamide™ [US]

Therapeutic Category Diuretic, Osmotic; Topical Skin Product

Use

Topical: Keratolytic agent to soften nails or skin; OTC: Moisturizer for dry, rough skin

(Continued)

urea *(Continued)*

Vaginal: Treatment of cervicitis

Usual Dosage Adults:

Hyperkeratotic conditions, dry skin: Topical: Apply 1-3 times/day

Cervicitis: Vaginal: Insert 1 applicatorful in vagina at bedtime for 2-4 weeks

Dosage Forms

Cream: 40% (30 g, 85 g, 199 g)
- Aquacare®: 10% (75 g)
- Carmol® 20: 20% (90 g)
- Carmol® 40: 40% (30 g, 90 g, 210 g)
- DPM™: 20% (118 g) [contains menthol and peppermint oil]
- Gormel®: 20% (75 g, 120 g, 454 g, 2270 g)
- Nutraplus®: 10% (90 g, 454 g)
- Rea-Lo®: 30% (60 g, 240 g)
- Ureacin®-20: 20% (120 g)
- Vanamide™: 40% (85 g, 199 g)

Cream, vaginal (Amino-Cerv™): 8.34% [83.4 mg/g] (82.5 g)

Gel:
- Carmol® 40: 40% (15 mL)
- Kerlac®: 50% (18 mL) [contains lactic acid and zinc]

Lotion: 40% (240 mL)
- Aquacare®: 10% (240 mL)
- Carmol® 10: 10% (180 mL)
- Carmol® 40: 40% (240 mL)
- Kerlac®: 35% (207 mL, 325 mL) [contains lactic acid, vitamin E, and zinc]
- Nutraplus®: 10% (240 mL, 480 mL)
- Ultra Mide®: 25% (120 mL, 240 mL)
- Ureacin®-10: 10% (240 mL)

Ointment:
- Aquaphilic® with Carbamide: 10% (180 g, 480 g); 20% (480 g)
- Lanaphilic®: 10% (454 g); 20% (454 g)

Shampoo: Carmol® Deep Cleaning: 10% (240 mL)

urea and hydrocortisone (yoor EE a & hye droe KOR ti sone)

Synonyms hydrocortisone and urea

U.S./Canadian Brand Names Carmol-HC® [US]; Ti-U-Lac® H [Can]; Uremol® HC [Can]

Therapeutic Category Corticosteroid, Topical

Use Inflammation of corticosteroid-responsive dermatoses

Usual Dosage Apply thin film and rub in well 1-4 times/day. Therapy should be discontinued when control is achieved; if no improvement is seen, reassessment of diagnosis may be necessary.

Dosage Forms Cream: Urea 10% and hydrocortisone acetate 1% (30 g) [in water soluble vanishing cream base]

Ureacin®-40 Topical *(Discontinued)* *see page 1042*

Ureacin® [US-OTC] *see* urea *on previous page*

urea peroxide *see* carbamide peroxide *on page 155*

Urecholine® [US] *see* bethanechol *on page 117*

Uremol® [Can] *see* urea *on previous page*

Uremol® HC [Can] *see* urea and hydrocortisone *on this page*

Urex® [US/Can] *see* methenamine *on page 563*

Urisec® [Can] *see* urea *on previous page*

Urispas® [US/Can] *see* flavoxate *on page 369*

Uristat® [US-OTC] *see* phenazopyridine *on page 685*

Uri-Tet® *(Discontinued)* *see page 1042*

Urobak® ***(Discontinued)*** *see page 1042*

Urobiotic-25® ***(Discontinued)*** *see page 1042*

Urocit®-K [US] *see* potassium citrate *on page 714*

Urodine® ***(Discontinued)*** *see page 1042*

urofollitropin (yoor oh fol li TROE pin)

Therapeutic Category Ovulation Stimulator

Use Induction of ovulation in patients with polycystic ovarian disease and to stimulate the development of multiple oocytes

Usual Dosage Adults: Female: S.C.: 75 units/day for 7-12 days, used with hCG may repeat course of treatment 2 more times

Dosage Forms Injection: 0.83 mg [75 units FSH activity] (2 mL)

urokinase (yoor oh KIN ase)

Synonyms UK

U.S./Canadian Brand Names Abbokinase® [US]

Therapeutic Category Fibrinolytic Agent

Use Thrombolytic agent for the lysis of acute massive pulmonary emboli or pulmonary emboli with unstable hemodynamics

Usual Dosage Adults: I.V.: Acute pulmonary embolism: Loading: 4400 int. units/kg over 10 minutes; maintenance: 4400 int. units/kg/hour for 12 hours. Following infusion, anticoagulation treatment is recommended to prevent recurrent thrombosis. Do not start anticoagulation until aPTT has decreased to less than twice the normal control value. If heparin is used, do not administer loading dose. Treatment should be followed with oral anticoagulants.

Dosage Forms Injection, powder for reconstitution: 250,000 int. units [contains human albumin 250 mg and mannitol 25 mg]

Uro-KP-Neutral® [US] *see* potassium phosphate and sodium phosphate *on page 717*

Urolene Blue® [US] *see* methylene blue *on page 570*

Uro-Mag® [US-OTC] *see* magnesium oxide *on page 539*

Uromitexan™ [Can] *see* mesna *on page 557*

Uroplus® DS ***(Discontinued)*** *see page 1042*

Uroplus® SS ***(Discontinued)*** *see page 1042*

Urovist Cysto® [US] *see* radiological/contrast media (ionic) *on page 759*

Urovist® Meglumine [US] *see* radiological/contrast media (ionic) *on page 759*

Urovist® Sodium 300 [US] *see* radiological/contrast media (ionic) *on page 759*

Uroxatral™ [US] *see* alfuzosin *on page 31*

Urso® [US/Can] *see* ursodiol *on this page*

ursodeoxycholic acid *see* ursodiol *on this page*

ursodiol (ER soe dye ole)

Synonyms ursodeoxycholic acid

U.S./Canadian Brand Names Actigall® [US]; Urso® [US/Can]

Therapeutic Category Gallstone Dissolution Agent

Use Actigall®: Gallbladder stone dissolution; prevention of gallstones in obese patients experiencing rapid weight loss; Urso®: Primary biliary cirrhosis

Usual Dosage Adults: Oral:

Gallstone dissolution: 8-10 mg/kg/day in 2-3 divided doses; use beyond 24 months is not established; obtain ultrasound images at 6-month intervals for the first year of therapy; 30% of patients have stone recurrence after dissolution

Gallstone prevention: 300 mg twice daily

(Continued)

ursodiol *(Continued)*

Primary biliary cirrhosis: 13-15 mg/kg/day in 2-4 divided doses (with food)

Dosage Forms

Capsule (Actigall®): 300 mg

Tablet [film coated] (Urso®): 250 mg, 500 mg

Uticort® ***(Discontinued)*** *see page 1042*

UTI Relief® [US-OTC] *see* phenazopyridine *on page 685*

Utradol™ [Can] *see* etodolac *on page 350*

Uvadex® [US/Can] *see* methoxsalen *on page 567*

vaccinia vaccine *see* smallpox vaccine *on page 808*

Vagifem® [US/Can] *see* estradiol *on page 324*

Vagi-Gard® [US-OTC] *see* povidone-iodine *on page 718*

Vagistat®-1 [US-OTC] *see* tioconazole *on page 865*

Vagitrol® ***(Discontinued)*** *see page 1042*

valacyclovir (val ay SYE kloe veer)

Synonyms valacyclovir hydrochloride

U.S./Canadian Brand Names Valtrex® [US/Can]

Therapeutic Category Antiviral Agent

Use Treatment of herpes zoster (shingles) in immunocompetent patients; treatment of first-episode genital herpes; episodic treatment of recurrent genital herpes; suppression of recurrent genital herpes and reduction of heterosexual transmission of genital herpes in immunocompetent patients; suppression of genital herpes in HIV-infected individuals; treatment of herpes labialis (cold sores)

Usual Dosage Oral:

Adolescents and Adults: Herpes labialis (cold sores): 2 g twice daily for 1 day (separate doses by ~12 hours)

Adults:

Herpes zoster (shingles): 1 g 3 times/day for 7 days

Genital herpes:

Initial episode: 1 g twice daily for 10 days

Recurrent episode: 500 mg twice daily for 3 days

Reduction of transmission: 500 mg once daily (source partner)

Suppressive therapy: Immunocompetent patients: 1000 mg once daily (500 mg once daily in patients with <9 recurrences per year) HIV-infected patients (CD4 ≥100 cells/mm^3): 500 mg twice daily

Dosage Forms Caplet, as hydrochloride: 500 mg, 1000 mg

valacyclovir hydrochloride *see* valacyclovir *on this page*

Valadol® ***(Discontinued)*** *see page 1042*

Valcyte™ [US/Can] *see* valganciclovir *on next page*

valdecoxib (val de KOX ib)

U.S./Canadian Brand Names Bextra® [US/Can]

Therapeutic Category Nonsteroidal Antiinflammatory Drug (NSAID), COX-2 Selective

Use Relief of signs and symptoms of osteoarthritis and adult rheumatoid arthritis; treatment of primary dysmenorrhea

Usual Dosage Oral: Adults:

Osteoarthritis and rheumatoid arthritis: 10 mg once daily; **Note:** No additional benefits seen with 20 mg/day

Primary dysmenorrhea: 20 mg twice daily as needed

Dosage Forms Tablet: 10 mg, 20 mg

23-valent pneumococcal polysaccharide vaccine *see* pneumococcal polysaccharide vaccine (polyvalent) *on page 704*

Valergen® Injection *(Discontinued)* *see page 1042*

Valertest No. 1® *(Discontinued)* *see page 1042*

valganciclovir (val gan SYE kloh veer)

Sound-Alike/Look-Alike Issues

Valcyte™ may be confused with Valium®

Synonyms valganciclovir hydrochloride

U.S./Canadian Brand Names Valcyte™ [US/Can]

Therapeutic Category Antiviral Agent

Use Treatment of cytomegalovirus (CMV) retinitis in patients with acquired immunodeficiency syndrome (AIDS); prevention of CMV disease in high-risk patients (donor CMV positive/recipient CMV negative) undergoing kidney, heart, or kidney/pancreas transplantation

Usual Dosage Oral: Adults:

CMV retinitis:

Induction: 900 mg twice daily for 21 days (with food)

Maintenance: Following induction treatment, or for patients with inactive CMV retinitis who require maintenance therapy: Recommended dose: 900 mg once daily (with food)

Prevention of CMV disease following transplantation: 900 mg once daily (with food) beginning within 10 days of transplantation; continue therapy until 100 days post-transplantation

Dosage Forms Tablet, as hydrochloride: 450 mg [valganciclovir hydrochloride 496.3 mg equivalent to valganciclovir 450 mg]

valganciclovir hydrochloride *see* valganciclovir *on this page*

Valisone® Scalp Lotion [Can] *see* betamethasone (topical) *on page 116*

Valisone® Topical *(Discontinued)* *see page 1042*

Valium® [US/Can] *see* diazepam *on page 263*

Valmid® Capsule *(Discontinued)* *see page 1042*

Valorin Extra [US-OTC] *see* acetaminophen *on page 5*

Valorin [US-OTC] *see* acetaminophen *on page 5*

Valpin® 50 *(Discontinued)* *see page 1042*

valproate semisodium *see* valproic acid and derivatives *on this page*

valproate sodium *see* valproic acid and derivatives *on this page*

valproic acid *see* valproic acid and derivatives *on this page*

valproic acid and derivatives (val PROE ik AS id & dah RIV ah tives)

Sound-Alike/Look-Alike Issues

Depakene® may be confused with Depakote®

Depakote® may be confused with Depakene®, Senokot®

Synonyms dipropylacetic acid; divalproex sodium; DPA; 2-propylpentanoic acid; 2-propylvaleric acid; valproate semisodium; valproate sodium; valproic acid

U.S./Canadian Brand Names Alti-Divalproex [Can]; Apo-Divalproex® [Can]; Depacon® [US]; Depakene® [US/Can]; Depakote® Delayed Release [US]; Depakote® ER [US]; Depakote® Sprinkle® [US]; Epival® ER [Can]; Epival® I.V. [Can]; Gen-Divalproex [Can]; Novo-Divalproex [Can]; Nu-Divalproex [Can]; PMS-Valproic Acid [Can]; PMS-Valproic Acid E.C. [Can]; Rhoxal-valproic [Can]

Therapeutic Category Anticonvulsant

Use Monotherapy and adjunctive therapy in the treatment of patients with complex partial seizures; monotherapy and adjunctive therapy of simple and complex absence

(Continued)

valproic acid and derivatives *(Continued)*

seizures; adjunctive therapy patients with multiple seizure types that include absence seizures

Mania associated with bipolar disorder (Depakote®)

Migraine prophylaxis (Depakote®, Depakote® ER)

Usual Dosage

Seizures: Children >10 years and Adults:

Oral: Initial: 10-15 mg/kg/day in 1-3 divided doses; increase by 5-10 mg/kg/day at weekly intervals until therapeutic levels are achieved; maintenance: 30-60 mg/kg/day. Adult usual dose: 1000-2500 mg/day. **Note:** Regular release and delayed release formulations are usually given in 2-4 divided doses/day, extended release formulation (Depakote® ER) is usually given once daily. Conversion to Depakote® ER from a stable dose of Depakote® may require an increase in the total daily dose between 8% and 20% to maintain similar serum concentrations. Children receiving more than one anticonvulsant (ie, polytherapy) may require doses up to 100 mg/kg/day in 3-4 divided doses

I.V.: Administer as a 60-minute infusion (≤20 mg/minute) with the same frequency as oral products; switch patient to oral products as soon as possible. Alternatively, rapid infusions have been given: ≤15 mg/kg over 5-10 minutes (1.5-3 mg/kg/minute).

Mania: Adults: Oral: 750-1500 mg/day in divided doses; dose should be adjusted as rapidly as possible to desired clinical effect; a loading dose of 20 mg/kg may be used; maximum recommended dosage: 60 mg/kg/day

Migraine prophylaxis: Adults: Oral:

Extended release tablets: 500 mg once daily for 7 days, then increase to 1000 mg once daily; adjust dose based on patient response; usual dosage range 500-1000 mg/day

Delayed release tablets: 250 mg twice daily; adjust dose based on patient response, up to 1000 mg/day

Dosage Forms

Capsule, as valproic acid (Depakene®): 250 mg

Capsule, sprinkles, as divalproex sodium (Depakote® Sprinkle®): 125 mg

Injection, solution, as valproate sodium (Depacon®): 100 mg/mL (5 mL)

Syrup, as valproic acid: 250 mg/5 mL (5 mL, 480 mL)

Depakene®: 250 mg/5 mL (480 mL)

Tablet, delayed release, as divalproex sodium (Depakote®): 125 mg, 250 mg, 500 mg

Tablet, extended release, as divalproex sodium (Depakote® ER): 250 mg, 500 mg

Valrelease® ***(Discontinued)*** *see page 1042*

valrubicin (val ru BYE cin)

Sound-Alike/Look-Alike Issues

Valstar® may be confused with valsartan

Synonyms AD3L; *N*-trifluoroacetyladriamycin-14-valerate

U.S./Canadian Brand Names Valstar® [Can]; Valtaxin® [Can]

Therapeutic Category Antineoplastic Agent, Anthracycline

Use Intravesical therapy of BCG-refractory carcinoma *in situ* of the urinary bladder

Usual Dosage Adults: Intravesical: 800 mg once weekly for 6 weeks

Dosage Forms [DSC] = Discontinued product

Injection, solution [DSC]: 40 mg/mL (5 mL) [contains Cremophor® EL 50% (polyoxyethyleneglycol triricinoleate) and dehydrated alcohol 50%]

valsartan (val SAR tan)

Sound-Alike/Look-Alike Issues

valsartan may be confused with losartan, Valstar™

Diovan® may be confused with Darvon®, Dioval®, Zyban™

U.S./Canadian Brand Names Diovan® [US/Can]

Therapeutic Category Angiotensin II Receptor Antagonist

Use Alone or in combination with other antihypertensive agents in treating essential hypertension; treatment of heart failure (NYHA Class II-IV) in patients intolerant to angiotensin converting enzyme (ACE) inhibitors

Usual Dosage Adults: Oral:

Hypertension: Initial: 80 mg or 160 mg once daily (in patients who are not volume depleted); majority of effect within 2 weeks, maximal effects in 4-6 weeks; dose may be increased to achieve desired effect; maximum recommended dose: 320 mg/day

Heart failure: Initial: 40 mg twice daily; titrate dose to 80-160 mg twice daily, as tolerated; maximum daily dose: 320 mg. **Note:** Do not use with ACE inhibitors and beta blockers.

Dosage Forms [DSC] = Discontinued product

Capsule [DSC]: 80 mg, 160 mg, 320 mg

Tablet: 40 mg, 80 mg, 160 mg, 320 mg

valsartan and hydrochlorothiazide

(val SAR tan & hye droe klor oh THYE a zide)

Sound-Alike/Look-Alike Issues

Diovan® may be confused with Darvon®, Dioval®, Zyban™

Synonyms hydrochlorothiazide and valsartan

U.S./Canadian Brand Names Diovan HCT® [US/Can]

Therapeutic Category Antihypertensive Agent, Combination

Use Treatment of hypertension (not indicated for initial therapy)

Usual Dosage Oral: Adults: Dose is individualized (combination substituted for individual components); dose may be titrated after 3-4 weeks of therapy.

Usual recommended starting dose of valsartan: 80 mg or 160 mg once daily when used as monotherapy in patients who are not volume depleted

Dosage Forms Tablet:

80 mg/12.5 mg: Valsartan 80 mg and hydrochlorothiazide 12.5 mg

160 mg/12.5 mg: Valsartan 160 mg and hydrochlorothiazide 12.5 mg

160 mg/25 mg: Valsartan 160 mg and hydrochlorothiazide 25 mg

Valstar® *(Discontinued)* *see page 1042*

Valstar® [Can] *see* valrubicin *on previous page*

Valtaxin® [Can] *see* valrubicin *on previous page*

Valtrex® [US/Can] *see* valacyclovir *on page 900*

Vamate® Oral *(Discontinued)* *see page 1042*

Vanamide™ [US] *see* urea *on page 897*

Vanatrip® *(Discontinued)* *see page 1042*

Vancenase® AQ 84 mcg *(Discontinued)* *see page 1042*

Vancenase® Pockethaler® *(Discontinued)* *see page 1042*

Vanceril® *(Discontinued)* *see page 1042*

Vanceril® AEM [Can] *see* beclomethasone *on page 102*

Vancocin® [US/Can] *see* vancomycin *on this page*

vancomycin (van koe MYE sin)

Sound-Alike/Look-Alike Issues

vancomycin may be confused with vecuronium

Synonyms vancomycin hydrochloride

U.S./Canadian Brand Names Vancocin® [US/Can]

Therapeutic Category Antibiotic, Miscellaneous

Use Treatment of patients with infections caused by staphylococcal species and streptococcal species; used orally for staphylococcal enterocolitis or for antibiotic-associated pseudomembranous colitis produced by *C. difficile*

(Continued)

vancomycin *(Continued)*

Usual Dosage Initial dosage recommendation:

Neonates: I.V.:

Postnatal age ≤7 days:

<1200 g: 15 mg/kg/dose every 24 hours

1200-2000 g: 10 mg/kg/dose every 12 hours

>2000 g: 15 mg/kg/dose every 12 hours

Postnatal age >7 days:

<1200 g: 15 mg/kg/dose every 24 hours

≥1200 g: 10 mg/kg/dose divided every 8 hours

Infants >1 month and Children: I.V.:

40 mg/kg/day in divided doses every 6 hours

Prophylaxis for bacterial endocarditis:

Dental, oral, or upper respiratory tract surgery: 20 mg/kg 1 hour prior to the procedure

GI/GU procedure: 20 mg/kg plus gentamicin 2 mg/kg 1 hour prior to surgery

Infants >1 month and Children with staphylococcal central nervous system infection: I.V.: 60 mg/kg/day in divided doses every 6 hours

Adults: I.V.:

With normal renal function: 1 g **or** 10-15 mg/kg/dose every 12 hours

Prophylaxis for bacterial endocarditis:

Dental, oral, or upper respiratory tract surgery: 1 g 1 hour before surgery

GI/GU procedure: 1 g plus 1.5 mg/kg gentamicin 1 hour prior to surgery

Antibiotic lock technique (for catheter infections): 2 mg/mL in SWI/NS or D_5W; instill 3-5 mL into catheter port as a flush solution instead of heparin lock (**Note:** Do not mix with any other solutions)

Intrathecal: Vancomycin is available as a powder for injection and may be diluted to 1-5 mg/mL concentration in preservative-free 0.9% sodium chloride for administration into the CSF

Neonates: 5-10 mg/day

Children: 5-20 mg/day

Adults: Up to 20 mg/day

Oral: Pseudomembranous colitis produced by *C. difficile*:

Neonates: 10 mg/kg/day in divided doses

Children: 40 mg/kg/day in divided doses, added to fluids

Adults: 125 mg 4 times/day for 10 days

Dosage Forms [DSC] = Discontinued product

Capsule, as hydrochloride (Vancocin®): 125 mg, 250 mg

Infusion [premixed in iso-osmotic dextrose]: 500 mg (100 mL); 1 g (200 mL)

Injection, powder for reconstitution, as hydrochloride: 500 mg, 1 g, 5 g, 10 g

Vancocin® [DSC]: 500 mg, 1 g, 10 g

vancomycin hydrochloride *see* vancomycin *on previous page*

Vanex Forte™-D *(Discontinued)* *see page 1042*

Vanex-LA® *(Discontinued)* *see page 1042*

Vaniqa™ [US] *see* eflornithine *on page 305*

Vanoxide® *(Discontinued)* *see page 1042*

Vanoxide-HC® [US/Can] *see* benzoyl peroxide and hydrocortisone *on page 111*

Vanquish® Extra Strength Pain Reliever [US-OTC] *see* acetaminophen, aspirin, and caffeine *on page 10*

Vanseb-T® Shampoo *(Discontinued)* *see page 1042*

Vansil™ *(Discontinued)* *see page 1042*

Vantin® [US/Can] *see* cefpodoxime *on page 170*

Vaponefrin® *(Discontinued)* *see page 1042*

Vaponefrin® [Can] *see* epinephrine *on page 311*

VAQTA® [US/Can] *see* hepatitis A vaccine *on page 432*

vardenafil (var DEN a fil)

Sound-Alike/Look-Alike Issues

Levitra® may be confused with Lexiva™

Synonyms vardenafil hydrochloride

U.S./Canadian Brand Names Levitra® [US]

Therapeutic Category Phosphodiesterase (Type 5) Enzyme Inhibitor

Use Treatment of erectile dysfunction

Usual Dosage Oral: Adults: Erectile dysfunction: 10 mg 60 minutes prior to sexual activity; dosing range: 5-20 mg; to be given as one single dose and not given more than once daily

Dosing adjustment with concomitant medications:

Erythromycin: Maximum vardenafil dose: 5 mg/24 hours

Indinavir: Maximum vardenafil dose: 2.5 mg/24 hours

Itraconazole:

200 mg/day: Maximum vardenafil dose: 5 mg/24 hours

400 mg/day: Maximum vardenafil dose: 2.5 mg/24 hours

Ketoconazole:

200 mg/day: Maximum vardenafil dose: 5 mg/24 hours

400 mg/day: Maximum vardenafil dose: 2.5 mg/24 hours

Ritonavir: Maximum vardenafil dose: 2.5 mg/72 hours

Dosage Forms Tablet, as hydrochloride [film-coated]: 2.5 mg, 5 mg, 10 mg, 20 mg

vardenafil hydrochloride *see* vardenafil *on this page*

varicella virus vaccine (var i SEL a VYE rus vak SEEN)

Synonyms chicken pox vaccine; varicella-zoster virus (VZV) vaccine

U.S./Canadian Brand Names Varilrix® [Can]; Varivax® [US/Can]

Therapeutic Category Vaccine, Live Virus

Use Immunization against varicella in children ≥12 months of age and adults. The American Association of Pediatrics recommends that the chickenpox vaccine should be given to all healthy children between 12 months and 18 years; children between 12 months and 13 years who have not been immunized or who have not had chickenpox should receive 1 vaccination while children 13-18 years of age require 2 vaccinations 4-8 weeks apart; the vaccine has been added to the childhood immunization schedule for infants 12-28 months of age and children 11-12 years of age who have not been vaccinated previously or who have not had the disease; it is recommended to be given with the measles, mumps, and rubella (MMR) vaccine

Usual Dosage SubQ:

Children 12 months to 12 years: 0.5 mL

Children 12 years to Adults: 2 doses of 0.5 mL separated by 4-8 weeks

Dosage Forms Injection, powder for reconstitution [preservative free; single-dose vial]: 1350 plaque-forming units (PFU) [contains gelatin and trace amounts of neomycin]

varicella-zoster immune globulin (human)

(var i SEL a-ZOS ter i MYUN GLOB yoo lin HYU man)

Synonyms VZIG

Therapeutic Category Immune Globulin

Use Passive immunization of susceptible immunodeficient patients after exposure to varicella; most effective if begun within 96 hours of exposure; there is no evidence VZIG modifies established varicella-zoster infections.

Restrict administration to those patients meeting the following criteria:

Neoplastic disease (eg, leukemia or lymphoma)

Congenital or acquired immunodeficiency

Immunosuppressive therapy with steroids, antimetabolites or other immunosuppressive treatment regimens

Newborn of mother who had onset of chickenpox within 5 days before delivery or within 48 hours after delivery

(Continued)

varicella-zoster immune globulin (human) *(Continued)*

Premature (≥28 weeks gestation) whose mother has no history of chickenpox
Premature (<28 weeks gestation or ≤1000 g VZIG) regardless of maternal history

One of the following types of exposure to chickenpox or zoster patient(s) may warrant administration:

Continuous household contact
Playmate contact (>1 hour play indoors)
Hospital contact (in same 2-4 bedroom or adjacent beds in a large ward or prolonged face-to-face contact with an infectious staff member or patient)
Susceptible to varicella-zoster
Age <15 years; administer to immunocompromised adolescents and adults and to other older patients on an individual basis

An acceptable alternative to VZIG prophylaxis is to treat varicella, if it occurs, with high-dose I.V. acyclovir

Age is the most important risk factor for reactivation of varicella zoster; persons <50 years of age have incidence of 2.5 cases per 1000, whereas those 60-79 have 6.5 cases per 1000 and those >80 years have 10 cases per 1000

Usual Dosage High-risk susceptible patients who are exposed again more than 3 weeks after a prior dose of VZIG should receive another full dose; there is no evidence VZIG modifies established varicella-zoster infections.

I.M.: Administer by deep injection in the gluteal muscle or in another large muscle mass. Inject 125 units/10 kg (22 lb); maximum dose: 625 units (5 vials); minimum dose: 125 units; do not administer fractional doses. Do not inject I.V.

Dosage Forms Injection, solution [single-dose vial]: 125 units (1.25 mL); 625 units (6.25 mL)

varicella-zoster virus (VZV) vaccine *see* varicella virus vaccine *on previous page*

Varilrix® [Can] *see* varicella virus vaccine *on previous page*

Varivax® [US/Can] *see* varicella virus vaccine *on previous page*

Vascor® [Can] *see* bepridil *on page 112*

Vascor® *(Discontinued)* *see page 1042*

Vascoray® [US] *see* radiological/contrast media (ionic) *on page 759*

Vaseretic® [US/Can] *see* enalapril and hydrochlorothiazide *on page 308*

Vasocidin® [US/Can] *see* sulfacetamide and prednisolone *on page 829*

VasoClear® [US-OTC] *see* naphazoline *on page 604*

Vasocon® [Can] *see* naphazoline *on page 604*

Vasocon-A® [US-OTC/Can] *see* naphazoline and antazoline *on page 604*

Vasocon Regular® Ophthalmic *(Discontinued)* *see page 1042*

Vasodilan® *(Discontinued)* *see page 1042*

vasopressin (vay soe PRES in)

Sound-Alike/Look-Alike Issues

Pitressin® may be confused with Pitocin®

Synonyms ADH; antidiuretic hormone; 8-arginine vasopressin; vasopressin tannate

U.S./Canadian Brand Names Pitressin® [US]; Pressyn® [Can]; Pressyn® AR [Can]

Therapeutic Category Hormone, Posterior Pituitary

Use Treatment of diabetes insipidus; prevention and treatment of postoperative abdominal distention; differential diagnosis of diabetes insipidus

Usual Dosage

Diabetes insipidus (highly variable dosage; titrated based on serum and urine sodium and osmolality in addition to fluid balance and urine output):

I.M., SubQ:

Children: 2.5-10 units 2-4 times/day as needed
Adults: 5-10 units 2-4 times/day as needed (dosage range 5-60 units/day)

Continuous I.V. infusion: Children and Adults: 0.5 milliunit/kg/hour (0.0005 unit/kg/hour); double dosage as needed every 30 minutes to a maximum of 0.01 unit/kg/hour
Intranasal: Administer on cotton pledget, as nasal spray, or by dropper
Abdominal distention: Adults: I.M.: 5 units stat, 10 units every 3-4 hours
Pulseless VT/VF (ACLS protocol): I.V.: 40 units (as a single dose only); if no I.V. access, administer 40 units diluted with NS (to a total volume of 10 mL) endotracheally
Dosage Forms Injection, solution, aqueous: 20 pressor units/mL (0.5 mL, 1 mL, 10 mL)
Pitressin®: 20 pressor units/mL (1 mL)

vasopressin tannate *see* vasopressin *on previous page*

Vasosulf® Ophthalmic *(Discontinued)* *see page 1042*

Vasotec® [US/Can] *see* enalapril *on page 307*

Vasoxyl® *(Discontinued)* *see page 1042*

Vaxigrip® [Can] *see* influenza virus vaccine *on page 473*

VCF™ [US-OTC] *see* nonoxynol 9 *on page 626*

V-Cillin K® *(Discontinued)* *see page 1042*

VCR *see* vincristine *on page 912*

Vectrin® *(Discontinued)* *see page 1042*

vecuronium (ve KYOO roe nee um)

Sound-Alike/Look-Alike Issues
vecuronium may be confused with vancomycin
Norcuron® may be confused with Narcan®

Synonyms ORG NC 45

U.S./Canadian Brand Names Norcuron® [Can]

Therapeutic Category Skeletal Muscle Relaxant

Use Adjunct to general anesthesia to facilitate endotracheal intubation and to relax skeletal muscles during surgery; to facilitate mechanical ventilation in ICU patients; does not relieve pain or produce sedation

Usual Dosage Administer I.V.; dose to effect; doses will vary due to interpatient variability; use ideal body weight for obese patients
Surgery:
Neonates: 0.1 mg/kg/dose; maintenance: 0.03-0.15 mg/kg every 1-2 hours as needed
Infants >7 weeks to 1 year: Initial: 0.08-0.1 mg/kg/dose; maintenance: 0.05-0.1 mg/kg every 60 minutes as needed
Children >1 year and Adults: Initial: 0.08-0.1 mg/kg or 0.04-0.06 mg/kg after initial dose of succinylcholine for intubation; maintenance: 0.01-0.015 mg/kg 25-40 minutes after initial dose, then 0.01-0.015 mg/kg every 12-15 minutes (higher doses will allow less frequent maintenance doses); may be administered as a continuous infusion at 0.8-2 mcg/kg/minute
Pretreatment/priming: Adults: 10% of intubating dose given 3-5 minutes before initial dose
ICU: Adults: 0.05-0.1 mg/kg bolus followed by 0.8-1.7 mcg/kg/minute once initial recovery from bolus observed or 0.1-0.2 mg/kg/dose every 1 hour

Note: Children (1-10 years) may require slightly higher initial doses and slightly more frequent supplementation; infants >7 weeks to 1 year may be more sensitive to vecuronium and have a longer recovery time

Dosage Forms Injection, powder for reconstitution, as bromide: 10 mg, 20 mg [may be supplied with diluent containing benzyl alcohol]

Veetids® [US] *see* penicillin V potassium *on page 677*

Velban® *(Discontinued)* *see page 1042*

Velban® [Can] *see* vinblastine *on page 911*

Velcade™ [US] *see* bortezomib *on page 124*

Velivet™ [US] *see* ethinyl estradiol and desogestrel *on page 335*

Velosef® [US] *see* cephradine *on page 177*

Velosulin® BR (Buffered) *(Discontinued)* *see page 1042*

Velsar® Injection *(Discontinued)* *see page 1042*

venlafaxine (VEN la faks een)

U.S./Canadian Brand Names Effexor® [US/Can]; Effexor® XR [US/Can]

Therapeutic Category Antidepressant, Phenethylamine

Use Treatment of major depressive disorder; generalized anxiety disorder (GAD), social anxiety disorder (social phobia)

Usual Dosage Oral: Adults:

Depression: Immediate-release tablets: 75 mg/day, administered in 2 or 3 divided doses, taken with food; dose may be increased in 75 mg/day increments at intervals of at least 4 days, up to 225-375 mg/day

Depression, GAD, social anxiety disorder: Extended-release capsules: 75 mg once daily taken with food; for some new patients, it may be desirable to start at 37.5 mg/day for 4-7 days before increasing to 75 mg once daily; dose may be increased by up to 75 mg/day increments every 4 days as tolerated, up to a maximum of 225 mg/day

Dosage Forms

Capsule, extended release, as hydrochloride (Effexor® XR): 37.5 mg, 75 mg, 150 mg

Tablet, as hydrochloride (Effexor®): 25 mg, 37.5 mg, 50 mg, 75 mg, 100 mg

Venofer® [US/Can] *see* iron sucrose *on page 485*

Venoglobulin®-I *(Discontinued)* *see page 1042*

Venoglobulin®-S [US] *see* immune globulin (intravenous) *on page 468*

Ventolin® [Can] *see* albuterol *on page 25*

Ventolin® *(Discontinued)* *see page 1042*

Ventolin® Diskus [Can] *see* albuterol *on page 25*

Ventolin® HFA [US] *see* albuterol *on page 25*

Ventolin® Inhaler Aerosol *(Discontinued)* *see page 1042*

Ventrodisk [Can] *see* albuterol *on page 25*

VePesid® [US/Can] *see* etoposide *on page 351*

Veracolate [US-OTC] *see* bisacodyl *on page 120*

verapamil (ver AP a mil)

Sound-Alike/Look-Alike Issues

verapamil may be confused with Verelan®

Calan® may be confused with Colace®

Covera-HS® may be confused with Provera®

Isoptin® may be confused with Isopto® Tears

Verelan® may be confused with verapamil, Virilon®, Voltaren®

Synonyms iproveratril hydrochloride; verapamil hydrochloride

U.S./Canadian Brand Names Alti-Verapamil [Can]; Apo-Verap® [Can]; Calan® [US/Can]; Calan® SR [US]; Chronovera® [Can]; Covera® [Can]; Covera-HS® [US]; Gen-Verapamil [Can]; Gen-Verapamil SR [Can]; Isoptin® [Can]; Isoptin® I.V. [Can]; Isoptin® SR [US/Can]; Novo-Veramil [Can]; Novo-Veramil SR [Can]; Verelan® [US]; Verelan® PM [US]

Therapeutic Category Antiarrhythmic Agent, Class IV; Calcium Channel Blocker

Use Orally for treatment of angina pectoris (vasospastic, chronic stable, unstable) and hypertension; I.V. for supraventricular tachyarrhythmias (PSVT, atrial fibrillation, atrial flutter)

Usual Dosage

Children: SVT:

I.V.:

<1 year: 0.1-0.2 mg/kg over 2 minutes; repeat every 30 minutes as needed

1-15 years: 0.1-0.3 mg/kg over 2 minutes; maximum: 5 mg/dose, may repeat dose in 15 minutes if adequate response not achieved; maximum for second dose: 10 mg/dose

Oral (dose not well established):

1-5 years: 4-8 mg/kg/day in 3 divided doses **or** 40-80 mg every 8 hours

>5 years: 80 mg every 6-8 hours

Adults:

SVT: I.V.: 2.5-5 mg (over 2 minutes); second dose of 5-10 mg (~0.15 mg/kg) may be given 15-30 minutes after the initial dose if patient tolerates, but does not respond to initial dose; maximum total dose: 20 mg

Angina: Oral: Initial dose: 80-120 mg 3 times/day (elderly or small stature: 40 mg 3 times/day); range: 240-480 mg/day in 3-4 divided doses

Hypertension: Oral:

Immediate release: 80 mg 3 times/day; usual dose range (JNC 7): 80-320 mg/day in 2 divided doses

Sustained release: 240 mg/day; usual dose range (JNC 7): 120-360 mg/day in 1-2 divided doses; 120 mg/day in the elderly or small patients (no evidence of additional benefit in doses >360 mg/day).

Extended release: Covera-HS®: Usual dose range (JNC 7): 120-360 mg once daily (once-daily dosing is recommended at bedtime) Verelan® PM: Usual dose range: 200-400 mg once daily at bedtime

Dosage Forms

Caplet, sustained release (Calan® SR): 120 mg, 180 mg, 240 mg

Capsule, extended release: 120 mg, 180 mg, 240 mg

Verelan® PM: 100 mg, 200 mg, 300 mg

Capsule, sustained release, as hydrochloride (Verelan®): 120 mg, 180 mg, 240 mg, 360 mg

Injection, solution, as hydrochloride: 2.5 mg/mL (2 mL, 4 mL)

Tablet, as hydrochloride (Calan®): 40 mg, 80 mg, 120 mg

Tablet, extended release: 120 mg, 180 mg, 240 mg

Covera HS®: 180 mg, 240 mg

Tablet, sustained release, as hydrochloride (Isoptin® SR): 120 mg, 180 mg, 240 mg

verapamil and trandolapril *see* trandolapril and verapamil *on page 876*

verapamil hydrochloride *see* verapamil *on previous page*

Verazinc® Oral *(Discontinued)* *see page 1042*

Vercyte® *(Discontinued)* *see page 1042*

Verelan® [US] *see* verapamil *on previous page*

Verelan® PM [US] *see* verapamil *on previous page*

Vergogel® Gel *(Discontinued)* *see page 1042*

Vergon® *(Discontinued)* *see page 1042*

Vermizine® *(Discontinued)* *see page 1042*

Vermox® [US/Can] *see* mebendazole *on page 545*

Verr-Canth™ *(Discontinued)* *see page 1042*

Verrex-C&M® *(Discontinued)* *see page 1042*

Verrusol® *(Discontinued)* *see page 1042*

Versed® *(Discontinued)* *see page 1042*

Versel® [Can] *see* selenium sulfide *on page 799*

Versiclear™ [US] *see* sodium thiosulfate *on page 817*

verteporfin (ver te POR fin)

U.S./Canadian Brand Names Visudyne® [US/Can]

Therapeutic Category Ophthalmic Agent

(Continued)

verteporfin *(Continued)*

Use Treatment of predominantly classic subfoveal choroidal neovascularization due to macular degeneration, presumed ocular histoplasmosis, or pathologic myopia

Usual Dosage Therapy is a two-step process; first the infusion of verteporfin, then the activation of verteporfin with a nonthermal diode laser

Adults: I.V.: 6 mg/m^2 body surface area

Dosage Forms Injection, powder for reconstitution: 15 mg

Verukan® Solution *(Discontinued)* *see page 1042*

Vesanoid® [US/Can] *see* tretinoin (oral) *on page 878*

Vesprin® *(Discontinued)* *see page 1042*

Vexol® [US/Can] *see* rimexolone *on page 778*

VFEND® [US] *see* voriconazole *on page 932*

V-Gan® Injection *(Discontinued)* *see page 1042*

Viadur® [US/Can] *see* leuprolide acetate *on page 509*

Viagra® [US/Can] *see* sildenafil *on page 803*

Vibazine® *(Discontinued)* *see page 1042*

Vibramycin® [US] *see* doxycycline *on page 294*

Vibramycin® I.V. *(Discontinued)* *see page 1042*

Vibra-Tabs® [US/Can] *see* doxycycline *on page 294*

Vicks® 44® Cough Relief [US-OTC] *see* dextromethorphan *on page 261*

Vicks® 44D Cough & Head Congestion [US-OTC] *see* pseudoephedrine and dextromethorphan *on page 746*

Vicks® 44E [US-OTC] *see* guaifenesin and dextromethorphan *on page 416*

Vicks® 44® Non-Drowsy Cold & Cough Liqui-Caps *(Discontinued)* *see page 1042*

Vicks® Children's Chloraseptic® *(Discontinued)* *see page 1042*

Vicks® Chloraseptic® Sore Throat *(Discontinued)* *see page 1042*

Vicks® DayQuil® Allergy Relief 4 Hour Tablet *(Discontinued)* *see page 1042*

Vicks® DayQuil® Multi-Symptom Cold and Flu [US-OTC] *see* acetaminophen, dextromethorphan, and pseudoephedrine *on page 12*

Vicks® DayQuil® Sinus Pressure & Congestion Relief *(Discontinued)* *see page 1042*

Vicks® Formula 44® *(Discontinued)* *see page 1042*

Vicks® Formula 44® Pediatric Formula *(Discontinued)* *see page 1042*

Vicks® Pediatric Formula 44E [US-OTC] *see* guaifenesin and dextromethorphan *on page 416*

Vicks® Sinex® 12 Hour Ultrafine Mist [US-OTC] *see* oxymetazoline *on page 658*

Vicks® Sinex® Nasal [US-OTC] *see* phenylephrine *on page 689*

Vicks® Sinex® UltraFine Mist [US-OTC] *see* phenylephrine *on page 689*

Vicks® Vatronol® *(Discontinued)* *see page 1042*

Vicodin® [US] *see* hydrocodone and acetaminophen *on page 443*

Vicodin® ES [US] *see* hydrocodone and acetaminophen *on page 443*

Vicodin® HP [US] *see* hydrocodone and acetaminophen *on page 443*

Vicodin Tuss® [US] *see* hydrocodone and guaifenesin *on page 445*

Vicon Forte® [US] *see* vitamins (multiple/oral) *on page 927*

Vicon Plus® [US-OTC] *see* vitamins (multiple/oral) *on page 927*

Vicoprofen® [US/Can] *see* hydrocodone and ibuprofen *on page 446*

Vi-Daylin® ADC + Iron [US-OTC] *see* vitamins (multiple/pediatric) *on page 927*

Vi-Daylin® ADC [US-OTC] *see* vitamins (multiple/pediatric) *on page 927*

Vi-Daylin® Drops [US-OTC] *see* vitamins (multiple/pediatric) *on page 927*

Vi-Daylin®/F [US] *see* vitamins (multiple/pediatric) *on page 927*

Vi-Daylin®/F ADC [US] *see* vitamins (multiple/pediatric) *on page 927*

Vi-Daylin®/F ADC + Iron [US] *see* vitamins (multiple/pediatric) *on page 927*

Vi-Daylin®/F + Iron [US] *see* vitamins (multiple/pediatric) *on page 927*

Vi-Daylin® + Iron Drops [US-OTC] *see* vitamins (multiple/pediatric) *on page 927*

Vi-Daylin® + Iron Liquid [US-OTC] *see* vitamins (multiple/oral) *on page 927*

Vi-Daylin® Liquid [US-OTC] *see* vitamins (multiple/oral) *on page 927*

Vidaza™ [US] *see* azacitidine *on page 92*

Videx® [US/Can] *see* didanosine *on page 268*

Videx® EC [US/Can] *see* didanosine *on page 268*

vigabatrin *(Canada only)* (vye GA ba trin)

Synonyms GVG; MDL-71754

U.S./Canadian Brand Names Sabril® [Can]

Therapeutic Category Anticonvulsant

Use Active management of partial or secondary generalized seizures not controlled by usual treatments; treatment of infantile spasms

Usual Dosage Oral:

Children: **Note:** Administer daily dose in 2 divided doses, especially in the higher dosage ranges:

Adjunctive treatment of seizures: Initial: 40 mg/kg/day; maintenance dosages based on patient weight:

10-15 kg: 0.5-1 g/day
16-30 kg: 1-1.5 g/day
31-50 kg: 1.5-3 g/day
>50 kg: 2-3 g/day

Infantile spasms: 50-100 mg/kg/day, depending on severity of symptoms; higher doses (up to 150 mg/kg/day) have been used in some cases.

Adults: Adjunctive treatment of seizures: Initial: 1 g/day (severe manifestations may require 2 g/day); dose may be given as a single daily dose or divided into 2 equal doses. Increase daily dose by 0.5 g based on response and tolerability. Optimal dose range: 2-3 g/day (maximum dose: 3 g/day)

Dosage Forms

Powder for oral suspension [sachets]: 0.5 g [contains povidone]

Tablet: 500 mg

Vigamox™ [US] *see* moxifloxacin *on page 593*

vinblastine (vin BLAS teen)

Sound-Alike/Look-Alike Issues

vinblastine may be confused with vincristine, vinorelbine

Synonyms NSC-49842; vinblastine sulfate; VLB

Tall-Man vin**BLAS**tine

U.S./Canadian Brand Names Velban® [Can]

Therapeutic Category Antineoplastic Agent

Use Treatment of Hodgkin and non-Hodgkin lymphoma, testicular, lung, head and neck, breast, and renal carcinomas, Mycosis fungoides, Kaposi sarcoma, histiocytosis, choriocarcinoma, and idiopathic thrombocytopenic purpura

(Continued)

vinblastine *(Continued)*

Usual Dosage Refer to individual protocols.

Children and Adults: I.V.: 4-20 mg/m² (0.1-0.5 mg/kg) every 7-10 days **or** 5-day continuous infusion of 1.5-2 mg/m²/day **or** 0.1-0.5 mg/kg/week

Dosage Forms

Injection, powder for reconstitution, as sulfate: 10 mg

Injection, solution, as sulfate: 1 mg/mL (10 mL) [contains benzyl alcohol]

vinblastine sulfate *see* vinblastine *on previous page*

Vincasar® PFS® [US/Can] *see* vincristine *on this page*

vincristine (vin KRIS teen)

Sound-Alike/Look-Alike Issues

vincristine may be confused with vinblastine

Oncovin® may be confused with Ancobon®

Synonyms LCR; leurocristine sulfate; NSC-67574; VCR; vincristine sulfate

Tall-Man vin**CRIS**tine

U.S./Canadian Brand Names Oncovin® [Can]; Vincasar® PFS® [US/Can]

Therapeutic Category Antineoplastic Agent

Use Treatment of leukemias, Hodgkin disease, non-Hodgkin lymphomas, Wilms tumor, neuroblastoma, rhabdomyosarcoma

Usual Dosage **Note:** Doses are often capped at 2 mg; however, this may reduce the efficacy of the therapy and may not be advisable. Refer to individual protocols; orders for single doses >2.5 mg or >5 mg/treatment cycle should be verified with the specific treatment regimen and/or an experienced oncologist prior to dispensing. I.V.:

Children ≤10 kg or BSA <1 m²: Initial therapy: 0.05 mg/kg once weekly then titrate dose; maximum single dose: 2 mg

Children >10 kg or BSA ≥1 m²: 1-2 mg/m², may repeat once weekly for 3-6 weeks; maximum single dose: 2 mg

Neuroblastoma: I.V. continuous infusion with doxorubicin: 1 mg/m²/day for 72 hours

Adults: 0.4-1.4 mg/m², may repeat every week **or**

0.4-0.5 mg/day continuous infusion for 4 days every 4 weeks **or**

0.25-0.5 mg/m²/day for 5 days every 4 weeks

Dosage Forms Injection, solution, as sulfate: 1 mg/mL (1 mL, 2 mL)

vincristine sulfate *see* vincristine *on this page*

vindesine (VIN de seen)

Synonyms DAVA; deacetyl vinblastine carboxamide; desacetyl vinblastine amide sulfate; DVA; eldisine lilly 99094; Lilly CT-3231; NSC-245467; vindesine sulfate

Therapeutic Category Antineoplastic Agent, Vinca Alkaloid

Use Management of acute lymphocytic leukemia, chronic myelogenous leukemia; breast, head, neck, and lung cancers; lymphomas (Hodgkin and non-Hodgkin)

Usual Dosage Refer to individual protocols. I.V.: Adults:

3-4 mg/m² /week **or**

1-2 mg/m² days 1 and 2 every 2 weeks **or**

1-2 mg/m² days 1-5 (continuous infusion) every 2-4 weeks **or**

1-2 mg/m² days 1-5 every 3-4 weeks

Dosage Forms Injection, powder for reconstitution: 5 mg

vindesine sulfate *see* vindesine *on this page*

vinorelbine (vi NOR el been)

Sound-Alike/Look-Alike Issues

vinorelbine may be confused with vinblastine

Synonyms dihydroxydeoxynorvinkaleukoblastine; NVB; vinorelbine tartrate

U.S./Canadian Brand Names Navelbine® [US/Can]

Therapeutic Category Antineoplastic Agent
Use Treatment of nonsmall-cell lung cancer
Usual Dosage Refer to individual protocols.
Adults: I.V.:
Single-agent therapy: 30 mg/m^2 every 7 days
Combination therapy with cisplatin: 25 mg/m^2 every 7 days (with cisplatin 100 mg/m^2 every 4 weeks); **Alternatively:** 30 mg/m^2 in combination with cisplatin 120 mg/m^2 on days 1 and 29, then every 6 weeks
For patients who, during treatment, have experienced fever and/or sepsis while granulocytopenic or had 2 consecutive weekly doses held due to granulocytopenia, subsequent doses of vinorelbine should be:
75% of starting dose for granulocytes ≥1500 cells/mm^3
37.5% of starting dose for granulocytes 1000-1499 cells/mm^3
Dosage Forms Injection, solution, as tartrate [preservative free]: 10 mg/mL (1 mL, 5 mL)

vinorelbine tartrate *see* vinorelbine *on previous page*
Vioform® *(Discontinued)* *see page 1042*
Vioform®-Hydrocortisone Topical *(Discontinued)* *see page 1042*
Viokase® [US/Can] *see* pancrelipase *on page 663*
viosterol *see* ergocalciferol *on page 317*
Vioxx® *(Discontinued)* *see page 1042*
Vira-A® *(Discontinued)* *see page 1042*
Viracept® [US/Can] *see* nelfinavir *on page 608*
Viramune® [US/Can] *see* nevirapine *on page 615*
Virazole® [US/Can] *see* ribavirin *on page 774*
Viread™ [US] *see* tenofovir *on page 845*
Virilon® [US] *see* methyltestosterone *on page 573*
Viroptic® [US/Can] *see* trifluridine *on page 885*
Viscoat® [US] *see* chondroitin sulfate and sodium hyaluronate *on page 197*
Visicol™ [US] *see* sodium phosphates *on page 815*
Visine® Advanced Relief [US-OTC] *see* tetrahydrozoline *on page 852*
Visine-A™ [US-OTC] *see* naphazoline and pheniramine *on page 604*
Visine® L.R. [US-OTC] *see* oxymetazoline *on page 658*
Visine® Original [US-OTC] *see* tetrahydrozoline *on page 852*
Visken® *(Discontinued)* *see page 1042*
Visken® [Can] *see* pindolol *on page 696*
Vistacon-50® Injection *(Discontinued)* *see page 1042*
Vistaject-25® *(Discontinued)* *see page 1042*
Vistaject-50® *(Discontinued)* *see page 1042*
Vistaquel® Injection *(Discontinued)* *see page 1042*
Vistaril® [US/Can] *see* hydroxyzine *on page 458*
Vistazine® Injection *(Discontinued)* *see page 1042*
Vistide® [US] *see* cidofovir *on page 199*
Visudyne® [US/Can] *see* verteporfin *on page 909*
Vitaball® [US-OTC] *see* vitamins (multiple/pediatric) *on page 927*
VitaCarn® Oral *(Discontinued)* *see page 1042*
Vitacon Forte [US] *see* vitamins (multiple/oral) *on page 927*
Vita-C® [US-OTC] *see* ascorbic acid *on page 79*

vitamin A (VYE ta min aye)

Sound-Alike/Look-Alike Issues

Aquasol A® may be confused with Anusol®

Synonyms oleovitamin A

U.S./Canadian Brand Names Aquasol A® [US]; Palmitate-A® [US-OTC]

Therapeutic Category Vitamin, Fat Soluble

Use Treatment and prevention of vitamin A deficiency; parenteral (I.M.) route is indicated when oral administration is not feasible or when absorption is insufficient (malabsorption syndrome)

Usual Dosage

RDA:

<1 year: 375 mcg
1-3 years: 400 mcg
4-6 years: 500 mcg*
7-10 years: 700 mcg*
>10 years: 800-1000 mcg*
Male: 1000 mcg
Female: 800 mcg
* mcg retinol equivalent (0.3 mcg retinol = 1 unit vitamin A)

Vitamin A supplementation in measles (recommendation of the World Health Organization): Children: Oral: Administer as a single dose; repeat the next day and at 4 weeks for children with ophthalmologic evidence of vitamin A deficiency:

6 months to 1 year: 100,000 units
>1 year: 200,000 units

Note: Use of vitamin A in measles is recommended only for patients 6 months to 2 years of age hospitalized with measles and its complications **or** patients >6 months of age who have any of the following risk factors and who are not already receiving vitamin A: immunodeficiency, ophthalmologic evidence of vitamin A deficiency including night blindness, Bitot spots or evidence of xerophthalmia, impaired intestinal absorption, moderate to severe malnutrition including that associated with eating disorders, or recent immigration from areas where high mortality rates from measles have been observed

Note: Monitor patients closely; dosages >25,000 units/kg have been associated with toxicity

Severe deficiency with xerophthalmia: Oral:

Children 1-8 years: 5000-10,000 units/kg/day for 5 days or until recovery occurs
Children >8 years and Adults: 500,000 units/day for 3 days, then 50,000 units/day for 14 days, then 10,000-20,000 units/day for 2 months

Deficiency (without corneal changes): Oral:

Infants <1 year: 100,000 units every 4-6 months
Children 1-8 years: 200,000 units every 4-6 months
Children >8 years and Adults: 100,000 units/day for 3 days then 50,000 units/day for 14 days

Deficiency: I.M.: **Note:** I.M. route is indicated when oral administration is not feasible or when absorption is insufficient (malabsorption syndrome):

Infants: 7500-15,000 units/day for 10 days
Children 1-8 years: 17,500-35,000 units/day for 10 days
Children >8 years and Adults: 100,000 units/day for 3 days, followed by 50,000 units/day for 2 weeks

Note: Follow-up therapy with an oral therapeutic multivitamin (containing additional vitamin A) is recommended:

Low Birth Weight Infants: Additional vitamin A is recommended, however, no dosage amount has been established
Children ≤8 years: 5000-10,000 units/day
Children >8 years and Adults: 10,000-20,000 units/day

Malabsorption syndrome (prophylaxis): Children >8 years and Adults: Oral: 10,000-50,000 units/day of water miscible product

Dietary supplement: Oral:
Infants up to 6 months: 1500 units/day
Children:
6 months to 3 years: 1500-2000 units/day
4-6 years: 2500 units/day
7-10 years: 3300-3500 units/day
Children >10 years and Adults: 4000-5000 units/day

Dosage Forms
Capsule [softgel]: 10,000 units; 25,000 units
Injection, solution (Aquasol A®): 50,000 units/mL (2 mL) [contains polysorbate 80]
Tablet (Palmitate-A®): 5000 units, 15,000 units

vitamin A acid *see* tretinoin (topical) *on page 879*

vitamin A and vitamin D (VYE ta min aye & VYE ta min dee)

Synonyms cod liver oil
U.S./Canadian Brand Names A and D® Ointment [US-OTC]; Baza® Clear [US-OTC]; Clocream® [US-OTC]; Sween Cream® [US-OTC]
Therapeutic Category Protectant, Topical
Use Temporary relief of discomfort due to chapped skin, diaper rash, minor burns, abrasions, as well as irritations associated with ostomy skin care
Usual Dosage Topical: Apply locally with gentle massage as needed
Dosage Forms
Capsule: Vitamin A 1250 int. units and vitamin D 135 int. units; Vitamin A 5000 int. units and vitamin D 400 int. units; Vitamin A 10,000 int. units and vitamin D 400 int. units; Vitamin A 25,000 int. units and vitamin D 400 int. units
Cream:
Sween Cream® [original]: 14 g, 57 g, 142 g, 255 g
Sween Cream®: 14 g, 57 g, 142 g [fresh scent]
Sween Cream®: 57 g [fragrance free]
Ointment: 5 g, 60 g, 120 g, 454 g [in lanolin-petrolatum base]
A and D® Ointment: 45 g, 120 g, 454 g
Baza® Clear: 15 g, 50 g, 150 g, 240 g
Clocream®: 30 g

vitamin B_1 *see* thiamine *on page 856*

vitamin B_2 *see* riboflavin *on page 775*

vitamin B_3 *see* niacin *on page 616*

vitamin B_3 *see* niacinamide *on page 616*

vitamin B_5 *see* pantothenic acid *on page 666*

vitamin B_6 *see* pyridoxine *on page 752*

vitamin B_{12} *see* cyanocobalamin *on page 232*

vitamin B complex combinations

(VYE ta min bee KOM pleks kom bi NAY shuns)

Sound-Alike/Look-Alike Issues
Nephrocaps® may be confused with Nephro-Calci®
Surbex® may be confused with Sebex®, Suprax®, Surfak®
Synonyms B complex combinations; B vitamin combinations
U.S./Canadian Brand Names Allbee® C-800 + Iron [US-OTC]; Allbee® C-800 [US-OTC]; Allbee® with C [US-OTC]; Apatate® [US-OTC]; Diatx™ [US]; DiatxFe™ [US]; Gevrabon® [US-OTC]; NephPlex® Rx [US]; Nephrocaps® [US]; Nephron FA® [US]; Nephro-Vite® [US]; Nephro-Vite® Rx [US]; Stresstabs® B-Complex + Iron [US-OTC]; Stresstabs® B-Complex [US-OTC]; Stresstabs® B-Complex + Zinc [US-OTC]; Surbex-T® [US-OTC]; Trinsicon® [US]; Z-Bec® [US-OTC]
Therapeutic Category Vitamin, Water Soluble
(Continued)

Vitamin B Complex Combinations

Product	B_1 (mg)	B_2 (mg)	B_6 (mg)	B_{12} (mcg)	C (mg)	E (int. units)	Additional Information
Caplet							
Allbee® with C [OTC]	15	10.2	5		300		Niacinamide 50 mg, pantothenic acid 10 mg
Allbee® C-800 [OTC]	15	17	25	12	800	45	Niacinamide 100 mg, pantothenic acid 25 mg
Allbee® C-800 + Iron [OTC]	15	17	25	12	800	45	Fe 27 mg, folic acid 0.4 mcg, niacinamide 100 mg, pantothenic acid 25 mg
Capsule							
Trinsicon®				15			C 75 mg, Fe 110 mg, folic acid 0.5 mg, liver-stomach concentrate (containing intrinsic factor and other vitamin B complex factors) 240 mg
Liquid							
Apatate® [OTC] (per 5 mL) [OTC]	15		0.5	25			Cherry flavor (120 mL)
Gevrabon® [OTC] (per 30 mL) [OTC]	5	2.5	1	1			Choline 10 mg, Fe 15 mg, iodine 100 mcg, Mg 2 mg, Mn 2 mg, niacinamide 60 mg, pantothenic acid 10 mg, Zn 2 mg; alcohol, benzoic acid; sherry wine flavor (480 mL)
Softgel							
Nephrocaps®	1.5	1.7	10	6	100		Biotin 150 mcg, folic acid 1 mcg, niacinamide 20 mg, pantothenic acid 5 mg
Tablet							
Diatx™	1.5	1.5	50		60		Biotin 300 mcg, cobalamin 1 mg, folacin 5 mg, niacinamide 20 mg, pantothenic acid 10 mg [dye free, lactose free, sugar free]
DiatxFe™	1.5	1.5	50		60		Biotin 300 mcg, cobalamin 1 mg, ferrous fumarate 304 mg, folacin 5 mg, niacinamide 20 mg, pantothenic acid 10 mg [dye free, lactose free, sugar free]
NephPlex® Rx	1.5	1.7	10	6	60		Biotin 300 mcg, folic acid 1 mg, niacinamide 20 mg, pantothenic acid 10 mg, zinc 12.5 mg
Nephro-Vite®	1.5	1.7	10	6	60		Biotin 300 mcg, folic acid 0.8 mcg, niacinamide 20 mg, pantothenic acid 10 mg
Nephro-Vite® Rx	1.5	1.7	10	6	60		Biotin 300 mcg, folic acid 1 mcg, niacinamide 20 mg, pantothenic acid 10 mg
Nephron FA®	1.5	1.7	10	6	40		Biotin 300 mcg, docusate sodium 75 mg, ferrous fumarate 200 mg, folic acid 1 mg, pantothenic acid 10 mg

Vitamin B Complex Combinations *(continued)*

Product	B_1 (mg)	B_2 (mg)	B_6 (mg)	B_{12} (mcg)	C (mg)	E (int. units)	Additional Information
Olay® Vitamins Essential Folic Acid w/ B_{12} Complex [OTC]		25	25	200		200	Folic acid 600 mcg, Se 50 mcg
Olay® Vitamins Super B-Stress Defense [OTC]	10	10	5	12	500	30	Biotin 100 mcg, folic acid 400 mcg, niacin 100 mg, pantothenic acid 20 mg
Stresstabs® B-Complex [OTC]	10	10	5	12	500	30	Biotin 45 mcg, folic acid 0.4 mcg, niacinamide 100 mg, pantothenic acid 20 mg
Stresstabs® B-Complex + Iron [OTC]	10	10	5	12	500	30	Biotin 45 mcg, Fe 18 mg, folic acid 0.4 mcg, niacinamide 100 mg, pantothenic acid 20 mg
Stresstabs® B-Complex + Zinc [OTC]	10	10	5	12	500	30	Biotin 45 mcg, Cu 3 mg, folic acid 0.4 mcg, niacinamide 100 mg, pantothenic acid 20 mg, Zn 23.9 mg
Surbex-T® [OTC]	15	10	5	10	500		Ca 20 mg, niacinamide 100 mg
Z-Bec® [OTC]	15	10.2	10	6	600	45	Niacinamide 100 mg, pantothenic acid 25 mg, Zn 22.5 mg
Tablet, Chewable							
Apatate® [OTC]	15		0.5	25			Cherry flavor

Ca = calcium, Cu = copper, Fe = iron, Mg = magnesium, Mn = manganese, Se = selenium, Zn = zinc.

vitamin B complex combinations *(Continued)*

Use Supplement for use in the wasting syndrome in chronic renal failure, uremia, impaired metabolic functions of the kidney, dialysis; labeled for OTC use as a dietary supplement

Usual Dosage Oral: Adults:

Dietary supplement: One tablet daily

Aptate® liquid: One teaspoonful daily, 1 hour prior to mid-day meal

Gevabron® liquid: Two tablespoonsful (30 mL) once daily; shake well before use

Renal patients: One tablet or capsule daily between meals; take after treatment if on dialysis

Nephron FA®: Two tablets once daily, between meals

Dosage Forms Content varies depending on product used. For more detailed information on ingredients see table on page 916.

vitamin B complex with vitamin C

(VYE ta min bee KOM pleks with VYE ta min see)

Therapeutic Category Vitamin, Water Soluble

Use Supportive nutritional supplementation in conditions in which water-soluble vitamins are required like GI disorders, chronic alcoholism, pregnancy, severe burns, and recovery from surgery

Usual Dosage Adults: Oral: 1 tablet/capsule daily

Dosage Forms Content varies depending on product used. For more detailed information on ingredients see table on page 916.

vitamin B complex with vitamin C and folic acid

(VYE ta min bee KOM pleks with VYE ta min see & FOE lik AS id)

Therapeutic Category Vitamin, Water Soluble

Use Supportive nutritional supplementation in conditions in which water-soluble vitamins are required like GI disorders, chronic alcoholism, pregnancy, severe burns, and recovery from surgery

Usual Dosage Adults: Oral: 1 capsule/day

Dosage Forms Content varies depending on product used. For more detailed information on ingredients see table on page 916.

vitamin C *see* ascorbic acid *on page 79*

vitamin D_2 *see* ergocalciferol *on page 317*

vitamin E (VYE ta min ee)

Sound-Alike/Look-Alike Issues

Aquasol E® may be confused with Anusol®

Synonyms *d*-alpha tocopherol; *dl*-alpha tocopherol

U.S./Canadian Brand Names Aqua Gem E® [US-OTC]; Aquasol E® [US-OTC]; E-Gems® [US-OTC]; Key-E® Kaps [US-OTC]; Key-E® [US-OTC]

Therapeutic Category Vitamin, Fat Soluble; Vitamin, Topical

Use Prevention and treatment hemolytic anemia secondary to vitamin E deficiency, dietary supplement

Usual Dosage One unit of vitamin E = 1 mg *dl*-alpha-tocopherol acetate. Oral:

Recommended daily allowance (RDA):

Premature infants ≤3 months: 17 mg (25 units)

Infants:

≤6 months: 3 mg (4.5 units)

7-12 months: 4 mg (6 units)

Children:

1-3 years: 6 mg (9 units); upper limit of intake should not exceed 200 mg/day

4-8 years: 7 mg (10.5 units); upper limit of intake should not exceed 300 mg/day

9-13 years: 11 mg (16.5 units); upper limit of intake should not exceed 600 mg/day

14-18 years: 15 mg (22.5 units); upper limit of intake should not exceed 800 mg/day

Adults: 15 mg (22.5 units); upper limit of intake should not exceed 1000 mg/day
Pregnant female:
≤18 years: 15 mg (22.5 units); upper level of intake should not exceed 800 mg/day
19-50 years: 15 mg (22.5 units); upper level of intake should not exceed 1000 mg/day
Lactating female:
≤18 years: 19 mg (28.5 units); upper level of intake should not exceed 800 mg/day
19-50 years: 19 mg (28.5 units); upper level of intake should not exceed 1000 mg/day
Vitamin E deficiency:
Children (with malabsorption syndrome): 1 unit/kg/day of water miscible vitamin E (to raise plasma tocopherol concentrations to the normal range within 2 months and to maintain normal plasma concentrations)
Adults: 60-75 units/day
Prevention of vitamin E deficiency: Adults: 30 units/day
Prevention of retinopathy of prematurity or BPD secondary to O_2 therapy (AAP considers this use investigational and routine use is not recommended):
Retinopathy prophylaxis: 15-30 units/kg/day to maintain plasma levels between 1.5-2 mcg/mL (may need as high as 100 units/kg/day)
Cystic fibrosis, beta-thalassemia, sickle cell anemia may require higher daily maintenance doses:
Children:
Cystic fibrosis: 100-400 units/day
Beta-thalassemia: 750 units/day
Adults:
Sickle cell: 450 units/day
Alzheimer's disease: 1000 units twice daily
Tardive dyskinesia: 1600 units/day

Dosage Forms
Capsule: 100 units, 200 units, 400 units, 500 units, 600 units, 1000 units
Aqua Gem E®: 200 units, 400 units
E-Gems®: 30 units, 100 units, 600 units, 800 units, 1000 units, 1200 units
Key-E Kaps®: 200 units, 400 units
Cream: 100 units/g (60 g)
Key-E®: 30 units/g (60 g, 120 g, 480 g)
Oil: 100 units/0.25 mL (60 mL); 1150 units/0.25 mL (30 mL, 60 mL, 120 mL)
E-Gem®: 100 units/10 drops (15 mL, 60 mL)
Ointment, topical (Key-E®): 30 units/g (60 g, 120 g, 480 g)
Powder (Key-E®): 700 units/dose (15 g, 75 g, 1000 g)
Solution, oral drops (Aquasol E®): 15 units/0.3 mL (12 mL, 30 mL)
Spray (Key-E®): 30 units/3 seconds (105 g)
Suppository (Key-E®): 30 units (12s, 24s)
Tablet: 100 units, 200 units, 400 units, 500 units, 800 units
Key-E®: 100 units, 200 units, 400 units

vitamin G *see* riboflavin *on page 775*
vitamin K_1 *see* phytonadione *on page 693*

vitamins (multiple/injectable) (VYE ta mins MUL ti pul/in JEC ta bul)

U.S./Canadian Brand Names Infuvite® Adult [US]; Infuvite® Pediatric [US]; M.V.I.®-12 [US]; M.V.I.-Adult® [US]; M.V.I.-Pediatric® [US]
Therapeutic Category Vitamin
Use Nutritional supplement in patients receiving parenteral r nous administration
Usual Dosage I.V.: Not for direct infusion
Children: ≥3 kg to 11 years: Pediatric formulation: 5 mL/da of appropriate solution
Children >11 years and Adults: Adult formulation: 10 mL/da of appropriate solution
Dosage Forms Content varies depending on product used. tion on ingredients see table on next page.

Injectable Formulations

Product	A (int. units)	B_1 (mg)	B_2 (mg)	B_6 (mg)	B_{12} (mcg)	C (mg)	D (int. units)	E (int. units)	K (mcg)	Additional Information
Solution										
Infuvite® Adult (per 10 mL)	3300	6	3.6	6	5	200	200	10	150	Supplied as two 5mL vials. Biotin 60 mcg, folic acid 600 mcg, niacinamide 40mg, dexpanthenol 15mg
Infuvite® Pediatric (per 5 mL)	2300	1.6	1.4	1	1	80	400	7	200	Supplied as one 4 mL vial and one 1 mL vial. Biotin 20 mcg, folic acid 140 mcg, niacinamide 17mg, dexpanthenol 5mg
M.V.I.®-12 (per 10 mL)	3300	3	3.6	4	12.5	100	200	10	–	Supplied as two 5 mL vials or a single 2-chambered 10mL vial. Biotin 60 mcg, folic acid 400 mcg, niacinamide 40mg, dexpanthenol 15mg
M.V.I. Adult™ (per 10 mL)	3300	6	3.6	6	5	200	200	10	150	Supplied as two 5 mL vials or a single 2-chambered 10mL vial. Biotin 60 mcg, folic acid 600 mcg, niacinamide 40mg, dexpanthenol 15mg
Powder for Reconstitution										
M.V.I.® Pediatric	2300	1.2	1.4	1	1	80	400	7	200	Biotin 20 mcg, folic acid 140 mcg, niacinamide 17mg, dexpanthenol 5mg, aluminum, polysorbate80

Adult Formulations

Product	A (int. units)	B_1 (mg)	B_2 (mg)	B_6 (mg)	B_{12} (mcg)	C (mg)	D (int. units)	E (int. units)	Additional Information
Liquid									
Centrum® [OTC] (per 15 mL)	2500	1.5	1.7	2	6	60	400	30	Biotin 300 mcg, Cr 25 mcg, Fe 9 mg, iodine 150 mcg, Mn 2 mg, Mo 25 mg, niacin 20 mg, pantothenic acid 10 mg, Zn 3 mg; alcohol 5.4%, sodium benzoate (240 mL)
Geritol® Tonic [OTC] (per 15 mL)		2.5	2.5	0.5					Chlorine bitartrate 50 mg, Fe 18 mg, methionine 25 mg, niacin 50 mg, pantothenic acid 2 mg; sugars 7 g, alcohol 12%, benzoic acid (120 mL, 360 mL)
Iberet® [OTC] (per 5 mL)		1.2	1.35	0.925	5.63	33.8			Fe 23.6 mg, niacin 6.8 mg, pantothenic acid 2.4 mg; alcohol (240 mL)
Iberet®-500 [OTC] (per 5 mL)		1.2	1.35	0.925	5.63	125			Fe 23.6 mg, niacin 6.8 mg, pantothenic acid 2.4 mg; alcohol (240 mL)
Vi-Daylin® [OTC] (per 5 mL)	2500	1.05	1.2	1.05	4.5	60	400	15	Niacin 13.5 mg; alcohol <0.5%, benzoic acid; lemon/orange flavor (240 mL, 480 mL)
Vi-Daylin® + Iron [OTC] (per 5 mL)	2500	1.05	1.2	1.05	4.5	60	400	15	Fe 10 mg, niacin 13.5 mg; alcohol <0.5%, benzoic acid; lemon/orange flavor (240 mL, 480mL)
Caplet									
Theragran® Heart Right™ [OTC]	5000	3	3.4	16	30	120	400	400	Alpha-carotene, beta-carotene, biotin 30 mcg, Ca 55 mg, Cr 50 mcg, cryptoxanthin, Cu 1.5 mg, Fe 4 mg, folic acid as folate 0.6 mg, iodine 150 mcg, lutein, lycopene, Mg 150 mg, Mn 2 mg, Mo 75 mcg, niacin 20 mg, pantothenic acid 10 mg, Se 70 mcg, vit K 14 mcg, zeaxanthin, Zn 15 mg
Theragran-M® Advanced Formula [OTC]	5000	3	3.4	6	12	90	400	60	Biotin 30 mcg, boron 150 mcg, Ca 40 mg, chloride 7.5 mg, Cr 50 mcg, Cu 2 mg, Fe 9 mg, folic acid 0.4 mg, iodine 150 mcg, Mg 100 mg, Mn 2 mg, Mo 75 mcg, niacin 20 mg, nickel 5 mcg, pantothenic acid 10 mg, phosphorus 31 mg, potassium 7.5 mg, Se 70 mcg, silicon 2 mg, tin 10 mcg, vanadium 10 mcg, vit K 28 mcg, Zn 15 mg
Capsule									
Vicon Forte®	8000	10	5	2	10	150		50	Folic acid 1 mg, Mg 70 mg, Mn 4 mg, niacinamide 25 mg, Zn 80 mg
Vicon Plus® [OTC]	3400	9.3	4.6	1.5		140		45	Mg 5 mg, Mn 1 mg, niacin 24 mg, pantothenic acid 11 mg, Zn 10 mg
Vitacon Forte	8000	10	5	2	10	150		50	Folic acid 1 mg, Mg 70 mg, Mn 4 mg, niacinamide 25 mg, Zn 80 mg

Adult Formulations *(continued)*

Product	A (int. units)	B_1 (mg)	B_2 (mg)	B_6 (mg)	B_{12} (mcg)	C (mg)	D (int. units)	E (int. units)	Additional Information
Tablet									
Centrum® [OTC]	5000	1.5	1.7	2	6	60	400	30	Biotin 30 mcg, boron 150 mcg, Ca 162 mg, chloride 72 mg, Cr 120 mcg, Cu 2 mg, Fe 18 mg, folic acid 0.4 mg, iodine 150 mcg, lutein 250 mcg, Mg 100 mg, Mn 2 mg, Mo 75 mcg, niacin 20 mg, nickel 5 mcg, pantothenic acid 10 mg, phosphorus 109 mg, potassium 80 mg, Se 20 mcg, silicon 2 mg, tin 10 mcg, vanadium 10 mcg, vit K 25 mcg, Zn 15 mg
Centrum® Performance™ [OTC]	5000	4.5	5.1	6	18	120	400	60	Biotin 40 mcg, boron 60 mcg, chloride 72 mg, folic acid 0.4 mg, Ca 100 mg, Cr 120 mcg, Cu 2 mg, Fe 18 mg, ginkgo biloba leaf 60 mg, ginseng root 50 mg, iodine 150 mcg, Mg 40 mg, Mn 4 mg, Mo 75 mcg, niacin 40 mg, nickel 5 mcg, pantothenic acid 10 mg, phosphorus 48 mg, potassium 80 mg, Se 70 mcg, silicon 4 mg, tin 10 mcg, vanadium 10 mcg, vit K 25 mcg, Zn 15 mg
Centrum® Silver® [OTC]	5000	1.5	1.7	3	25	60	400	45	Biotin 30 mcg, boron 150 mcg, Ca 200 mg, chloride 72 mg, Cr 150 mcg, Cu 2 mg, folic acid 0.4 mg, iodine 150 mcg, lutein 250 mcg, Mg 100 mg, Mn 2 mg, Mo 75 mcg, niacin 20 mg, nickel 5 mcg, pantothenic acid 10 mg, phosphorus 48 mg, potassium 80 mg, Se 20 mcg, silicon 2 mg, vanadium 10 mcg, vit K 10 mcg, Zn 15 mg
Iberet®-500 [OTC]		4.96	5.4	3.7	22.5	500			Fe 95 mg (controlled release), niacin 27.2 mg, pantothenic acid 8.28 mg, sodium 65 mg
Iberet-Folic-500® [OTC]		6	6	5	25	500			Fe 105 mg (controlled release), folic acid 0.8 mg, niacinamde 30 mg, pantothenic acid 10 mg
Olay® Vitamins Complete Women's [OTC]	5000	1.5	1.7	2	6	120	400	50	Biotin 30 mcg, boron 150 mcg, Ca 250 mg, chloride 36 mg, coenzyme Q_{10}2 mg, Cr 120 mcg, Cu 5 mg, Fe 18 mg, folic acid 0.4 mg, iodine 150 mcg, lutein 250 mg, Mg 100 mg, Mn 2 mg, Mo 25 mcg, niacin 20 mg, nickel 5 mcg, pantothenic acid 10 mg, phosphorus 77 mg, potassium 40 mg, Se 25 mcg, silicon 2 mg, vanadium 10 mcg, Zn 15 mg
Olay® Vitamins Complete Women's 50+ [OTC]	5000	3	3.4	4	25	120	400	60	Biotin 30 mcg, boron 150 mcg, Ca 250 mg, chloride 72 mg, coenzyme Q_{10}2 mg, Cr 120 mcg, Cu 5 mg, folic acid 0.4 mg, iodine 150 mcg, lutein 250 mg, Mg 120 mg, Mn 2 mg, Mo 25 mcg, niacin 20 mg, nickel 5 mcg, pantothenic acid 10 mg, phosphorus 48 mg, potassium 80 mg, Se 50 mcg, silicon 2 mg, vanadium 10 mcg, Zn 22 mg

Adult Formulations *(continued)*

Product	A (int. units)	B_1 (mg)	B_2 (mg)	B_6 (mg)	B_{12} (mcg)	C (mg)	D (int. units)	E (int. units)	Additional Information
One-A-Day® 50 Plus Formula [OTC]	5000	4.5	3.4	6	30	120	400	60	Biotin 30 mcg, Ca 120 mg, chloride 34 mg, Cr 180 mcg, Cu 2 mg, folic acid 0.4 mg, iodine 150 mcg, Mg 100 mg, Mn 4 mg, Mo 93.75 mcg, niacin 20 mg, pantothenic acid 15 mg, potassium 37.5 mg, Se 150 mcg, vit K 20 mcg, Zn 22.5 mg
One-A-Day® Active Formula [OTC]	5000	4.5	5.1	6	18	120	400	60	American ginseng 55 mg, biotin 40 mcg, boron 150 mcg, Ca 110 mg, chloride 180 mg, Cr 100 mcg, Cu 2 mg, Fe 9 mg, folic acid 0.4 mg, iodine 150 mcg, Mg 40 mg, Mn 2 mg, Mo 25 mcg, niacin 40 mg, nickel 5 mcg, pantothenic acid 10 mg, phosphorus 48 mg, potassium 200 mg, Se 45 mcg, silicon 6 mg, tin 10 mcg, vanadium 10 mcg, vit K 25 mcg, Zn 15 mg
One-A-Day® Essential Formula [OTC]	5000	1.5	1.7	2	6	60	400	30	Folic acid 0.4 mg, niacin 20 mg, pantothenic acid 10 mg
One-A-Day® Maximum Formula [OTC]	5000	1.5	1.7	2	6	60	400	30	Biotin 30 mcg, boron 150 mcg, Ca 162 mg, chloride 72 mg, Cr 65 mcg, Cu 2 mg, Fe 18 mg, folic acid 0.4 mg, iodine 150 mcg, Mg 100 mg, Mn 3.5 mg, Mo 160 mcg, niacin 20 mg, nickel 5 mcg, pantothenic acid 10 mg, phosphorus 109 mg, potassium 80 mg, Se 20 mcg, silicon 2 mg, tin 10 mcg, vanadium 10 mcg, vit K 25 mcg, Zn 15 mg
One-A-Day® Men's Formula [OTC]	5000	2.25	2.55	3	9	90	400	45	Chloride 34 mg, Cr 150 mcg, Cu 2 mg, folic acid 0.4 mg, iodine 150 mcg, Mg 100 mg, Mn 3.5 mg, Mo 42 mcg, niacin 20 mg, pantothenic acid 10 mg, potassium 37.5 mg, Se 87.5 mcg, Zn 15 mg
One-A-Day® Today [OTC]	3000	1.1	1.7	3	18	75	400	33	Biotin 30 mcg, Ca 240 mg, Cr 120 mcg, Cu 2 mg, folic acid 0.4 mg, Mg 120 mg, Mn 2 mg, niacin 14 mg, pantothenic acid 5 mg, potassium 100 mg, Se 70 mcg, soy extract 10 mg, vit K 20 mcg, Zn 15 mg
One-A-Day® Women's Formula [OTC]	2500	1.5	1.7	2	6	60	400	30	Ca 450 mg, Fe 18 mg, folic acid 0.4 mg, Mg 50 mg, niacin 10mg, pantothenic acid 5 mg, Zn 15 mg
Tablet, Chewable									
Centrum® [OTC]	5000	1.5	1.7	2	6	60	400	30	Biotin 45 mcg, Ca 108 mg, Cr 20 mcg, Cu 2 mg, Fe 18 mg, folic acid 0.4 mg, iodine 150 mcg, Mg 40 mg, Mn 1 mg, Mo 20 mcg, niacin 20 mg, pantothenic acid 10 mg, Zn 15 mg

Ca = calcium, Cr = chromium, Cu = copper, Fe = iron, Mg = magnesium, Mn = manganese, Mo = molybdenum, Se = selenium, Zn = zinc.

Pediatric Formulations

Product	A (int. units)	B_1 (mg)	B_2 (mg)	B_6 (mg)	B_{12} (mcg)	C (mg)	D (int. units)	E (int. units)	Additional Information
Drops									
ADEKs [OTC] (per mL)	1500	0.5	0.6	0.6	4	45	400	40	Beta carotene 1 mg, biotin 15 mcg, niacin 6 mg, vit K 0.1 mg, Zn 5 mg; alcohol free, dye free (60mL)
Poly-Vi-Flor® 0.25 mg (per mL)	1500	0.5	0.6	0.4	2	35	400	5	**Fluoride 0.25 mg**, niacin 8 mg; fruit flavor (50mL)
Poly-Vi-Flor® 0.5 mg (per mL)	1500	0.5	0.6	0.4	2	35	400	5	**Fluoride 0.5 mg**, niacin 8 mg; fruit flavor (50mL)
Poly-Vi-Flor® With Iron 0.25 mg (per mL)	1500	0.5	0.6	0.4		35	400	5	**Fluoride 0.25 mg**, iron 10 mg, niacin 8 mg; fruit flavor (50mL)
Poly-Vi-Sol® [OTC] (per mL)	1500	0.5	0.6	0.4	2	35	400	5	Niacin 8 mg (50mL)
Poly-Vi-Sol® With Iron [OTC] (per mL)	1500	0.5	0.6	0.4		35	400	5	Iron 10 mg, niacin 8 mg (50mL)
Soluvite-F® (per 0.6 mL)	1500					35	400		**Fluoride 0.25 mg**; alcohol free, dye free, orange flavor (57 mL)
Tri-Vi-Flor® 0.25 mg (per mL)	1500					35	400		**Fluoride 0.25 mg**; fruit flavor (50mL)
Tri-Vi-Flor® With Iron 0.25 mg (per mL)	1500					35	400		**Fluoride 0.25 mg**, iron 10 mg; fruit flavor (50mL)
Tri-Vi-Sol® [OTC] (per mL)	1500					35	400		Fruit flavor (50mL)
Tri-Vi-Sol® With Iron [OTC] (per mL)	1500					35	400		Iron 10 mg; fruit flavor (50mL)
Vi-Daylin® [OTC] (per mL)	1500	0.5	0.6	0.4	1.5	35	400	5	Niacin 8 mg; alcohol <0.5%, sugar free, fruit flavor (50mL)
Vi-Daylin® + Iron [OTC] (per mL)	1500	0.5	0.6	0.4		35	400	5	Iron 10 mg, niacin 8 mg; alcohol <0.5%, sugar free, fruit flavor (50 mL)
Vi-Daylin® ADC [OTC] (per mL)	1500					35	400		Alcohol <0.5%, sugar free, fruit flavor (50mL)
Vi-Daylin® ADC + Iron [OTC] (per mL)	1500					35	400		Iron 10 mg; benzoic acid, sugar free, fruit flavor (50mL)
Vi-Daylin®/F (per mL)	1500	0.5	0.6	0.4		35	400	5	**Fluoride 0.25 mg**, niacin 8 mg; alcohol <0.1%, benzoic acid, sugar free, fruit flavor (50mL)
Vi-Daylin®/F + Iron (per mL)	1500	0.5	0.6	0.4		35	400	5	**Fluoride 0.25 mg**, iron 10 mg, niacin 8 mg; alcohol <0.1%, benzoic acid, sugar free, fruit flavor (50mL)
Vi-Daylin®/F ADC (per mL)	1500					35	400		**Fluoride 0.25 mg**; sugar free, fruit flavor (50mL)
Vi-Daylin®/F ADC + Iron (permL)	1500					35	400		**Fluoride 0.25 mg**, iron 10 mg; sugar free, fruit flavor (50mL)

Pediatric Formulations *(continued)*

Product	A (int. units)	B_1 (mg)	B_2 (mg)	B_6 (mg)	B_{12} (mcg)	C (mg)	D (int. units)	E (int. units)	Additional Information
Gum									
Vitaball®	5000	1.5	1.7	2	6	60	400	30	Biotin 45 mcg, folic acid 400 mcg, niacinamide 20 mg, pantothenic acid 10 mg; bubble gum, cherry, grape, and watermelon flavors
Tablet, Chewable									
ADEKs® [OTC]	4000	1.2	1.3	1.5	12	60	400	150	Beta carotene 3 mg, biotin 50 mcg, folic acid 0.2 mg, niacin 10 mg, pantothenic acid 10 mg, vit K 150 mcg, Zn 7.5 mg; dye free
Centrum® Kids Rugrats™ Complete [OTC]	5000	1.5	1.7	2	6	60	400	30	Biotin 45 mcg, Ca 108 mg, Cr 20 mcg, Cu 2 mg, Fe 18 mg, folic acid 0.4 mg, iodine 150 mcg, Mg 40 mg, Mn 1 mg, Mo 20 mcg, niacin 20 mg, pantothenic acid 10 mg, phosphorus 50 mg, vit K 10 mg, Zn 15 mg; cherry, fruit punch, and orange flavors
Centrum® Kids Rugrats™ ExtraC [OTC]	5000	1.5	1.7	1	5	250	400	15	Ca 108 mg, Cu 0.5 mg, folic acid 0.3 mg, niacin 13.5 mg, phosphorus 50 mg, sodium 15 mg, Zn 4 mg; cherry, fruit punch, and orange flavors
Centrum® Kids Rugrats™ Extra Calcium [OTC]	5000	1.5	1.7	1	5	60	400	15	Ca 200 mg, Cu 0.5 mg, folic acid 0.3 mg, niacin 13.5 mg, phosphorus 50 mg, Zn 4 mg; cherry, fruit punch, and orange flavors
Flintstones® Complete [OTC]	5000	1.5	1.7	2	6	60	400	30	Biotin 40 mcg, Ca 100 mg, Cu 2 mg, Fe 18 mg, folic acid 0.4 mg, iodine 150 mcg, Mg 20 mg, niacin 20 mg, pantothenic acid 10 mg, phosphorus 100 mg, Zn 15 mg; **phenylalanine 4.56 mg**; cherry, grape, and orange flavors
Flintstones® Original [OTC]	2500	1.05	1.2	1.05	4.5	60	400	15	Folic acid 0.3 mg, niacin 13.5 mg
Flintstones® Plus Calcium [OTC]	2500	1.05	1.2	1.05	4.5	60	400	15	Ca 200 mg, folic acid 0.3 mg, niacin 13.5 mg; **phenylalanine <4 mg**; cherry, grape, and orange flavors
Flintstones® Plus Extra C [OTC]	2500	1.05	1.2	1.05	4.5	250	400	15	Folic acid 0.3 mg, niacin 13.5 mg; grape, orange, peach-apricot, raspberry, and strawberry flavors
Flintstones® Plus Iron [OTC]	2500	1.05	1.2	1.05	4.5	60	400	15	Fe 15 mg, folic acid 0.3 mg, niacin 13.5 mg; grape, orange, peach-apricot, raspberry, and strawberry flavors
My First Flintstones® [OTC]	2500	1.05	1.2	1.05	4.5	60	400	15	Folic acid 0.3 mg, niacin 13.5 mg; cherry, grape, and orange flavors

Pediatric Formulations *(continued)*

Product	A (int. units)	B_1 (mg)	B_2 (mg)	B_6 (mg)	B_{12} (mcg)	C (mg)	D (int. units)	E (int. units)	Additional Information
One-A-Day® Kids Bugs Bunny and Friends Complete [OTC]	5000	1.5	1.7	2	6	60	400	30	Biotin 40 mcg, Ca 100 mg, Cu 2 mg, Fe 18 mg, folic acid 0.4 mg, iodine 150 mcg, Mg 20 mg, niacin 20 mg, pantothenic acid 10 mg, phosphorus 100 mg, Zn 15 mg; sugar free, fruity flavors
One-A-Day® Kids Bugs Bunny and Friends Plus Extra C [OTC]	2500	1.05	1.2	1.05	4.5	250	400	15	Folic acid 0.3 mg, niacin 13.5 mg, **phenylalanine**; sugar free, fruity flavors
One-A-Day® Kids Extreme Sports [OTC]	5000	1.5	1.2	2	6	60	400	30	Biotin 40 mcg, Ca 100 mg, Cu 2 mg, Fe 18 mg, folic acid 0.4 mg, iodine 150 mcg, Mg 20 mg, niacin 20 mg, pantothenic acid 10 mg, phosphorus 100 mg, Zn 15 mg
One-A-Day® Kids Scooby-Doo! Complete [OTC]	5000	1.5	1.7	2	6	60	400	30	Biotin 40 mcg, Ca 100 mg, Cu 2 mg, Fe 18 mg, folic acid 0.4 mg, iodine 150 mcg, Mg 20 mg, niacin 20 mg, pantothenic acid 10 mg, phosphorus 100 mg, Zn 15 mg; fruity flavors
One-A-Day® Kids Scooby-Doo! Plus Calcium [OTC]	2500	1.05	1.2	1.05	4.5	60	400	15	Ca 200 mg, folic acid 0.3 mg, niacin 13.5 mg; fruity flavors

Ca = calcium, Cr = chromium, Cu = copper, Fe = iron, Mg = magnesium, Mn = manganese, Mo = molybdenum, Zn = zinc.

vitamins (multiple/oral) (VYE ta mins MUL ti pul/OR al)

Sound-Alike/Look-Alike Issues

Theragran® may be confused with Phenergan®

Synonyms multiple vitamins; therapeutic multivitamins; vitamins, multiple (oral); vitamins, multiple (therapeutic); vitamins, multiple with iron

U.S./Canadian Brand Names Centrum® Performance™ [US-OTC]; Centrum® Silver® [US-OTC]; Centrum® [US-OTC]; Geritol® Tonic [US-OTC]; Iberet®-500 [US-OTC]; Iberet-Folic-500® [US]; Iberet® [US-OTC]; One-A-Day® 50 Plus Formula [US-OTC]; One-A-Day® Active Formula [US-OTC]; One-A -Day® Essential Formula [US-OTC]; One-A-Day® Maximum Formula [US-OTC]; One-A-Day® Men's Formula [US-OTC]; One-A-Day® Today [US-OTC]; One-A-Day® Women's Formula [US-OTC]; Theragran® Heart Right™ [US-OTC]; Theragran-M® Advanced Formula [US-OTC]; Vicon Forte® [US]; Vicon Plus® [US-OTC]; Vi-Daylin® + Iron Liquid [US-OTC]; Vi-Daylin® Liquid [US-OTC]; Vitacon Forte [US]

Therapeutic Category Vitamin

Use Prevention/treatment of vitamin and mineral deficiencies; labeled for OTC use as a dietary supplement

Usual Dosage Oral: Adults: Daily dose of adult preparations varies by product. Generally, 1 tablet or capsule or 5-15 mL of liquid per day. Consult package labeling. Prescription doses may be higher for burn or cystic fibrosis patients.

Dosage Forms Content varies depending on product used. For more detailed information on ingredients see table on page 921.

vitamins, multiple (oral) *see* vitamins (multiple/oral) *on this page*

vitamins (multiple/pediatric) (VYE ta mins MUL ti pul/pee dee AT rik)

Synonyms children's vitamins; multivitamins/fluoride

U.S./Canadian Brand Names ADEKs [US-OTC]; Centrum® Kids Rugrats™ Complete [US-OTC]; Centrum® Kids Rugrats™ Extra Calcium [US-OTC]; Centrum® Kids Rugrats™ Extra C [US-OTC]; Flintstones® Complete [US-OTC]; Flintstones® Original [US-OTC]; Flintstones® Plus Calcium [US-OTC]; Flintstones® Plus Extra C [US-OTC]; Flintstones® Plus Iron [US-OTC]; My First Flintstones® [US-OTC]; One-A-Day® Kids Bugs Bunny and Friends Complete [US-OTC]; One-A-Day® Kids Bugs Bunny and Friends Plus Extra C [US-OTC]; One-A-Day® Kids Extreme Sports [US-OTC]; One-A-Day® Kids Scooby-Doo! Complete [US-OTC]; One-A-Day® Kids Scooby Doo! Plus Calcium [US-OTC]; Poly-Vi-Flor® [US]; Poly-Vi-Flor® With Iron [US]; Poly-Vi-Sol® [US-OTC]; Poly-Vi-Sol® with Iron [US-OTC]; Soluvite-F [US]; Tri-Vi-Flor® [US]; Tri-Vi-Flor® with Iron [US]; Tri-Vi-Sol® [US-OTC]; Tri-Vi-Sol® with Iron [US-OTC]; Vi-Daylin® ADC + Iron [US-OTC]; Vi-Daylin® ADC [US-OTC]; Vi-Daylin® Drops [US-OTC]; Vi-Daylin®/F [US]; Vi-Daylin®/F ADC [US]; Vi-Daylin®/F ADC + Iron [US]; Vi-Daylin®/F + Iron [US]; Vi-Daylin® + Iron Drops [US-OTC]; Vitaball® [US-OTC]

Therapeutic Category Vitamin

Use Prevention/treatment of vitamin deficiency; products containing fluoride are used to prevent dental caries; labeled for OTC use as a dietary supplement

Usual Dosage Daily dose varies by product; refer to package insert for specific product labeling

Dosage Forms Content varies depending on product used. For more detailed information on ingredients see table on page 924.

vitamins (multiple/prenatal) (VYE ta mins MUL ti pul/pre NAY tal)

Sound-Alike/Look-Alike Issues

Niferex® may be confused with Nephrox®

PreCare® may be confused with Precose®

Prenatal Formulations

Product	A (int. units)	B_1 (mg)	B_2 (mg)	B_6 (mg)	B_{12} (mcg)	C (mg)	D (int. units)	E (int. units)	Additional Information
Caplet									
PreCare® Prenatal		3	3.4	50	12	50	6 mcg	3.5 mg	Ca 250 mg, Cu 2 mg, Fe 40 mg, folic acid 1 mg, Mg 50 mg, Zn 15 mg; dye free
StrongStart™	1000	3	3	20	12	100	400	30	Ca 200 mg, Fe 29 mg, folic acid 1mg, niacinamide 15 mg, pantothenic acid 7 mg, Zn 20 mg; docusate sodium 25 mg
Capsule									
Anemagen™ OB		1.6	1.8	20	12	60	400	30	Ca 200 mg, Fe 28 mg, folic acid 1mg; docusate calcium 25 mg
Chromagen OB®		1.6	1.8	20	12	60	400	30	Ca 200 mg, Cu 2 mg, Fe 28 mg, folic acid 1mg, Mn 2 mg, niacinamide 5 mg, Zn 25 mg; docusate calcium 25 mg
Prenatal H		10	6	5	15	200			Cu 0.8 mg, Fe 106 mg, folic acid 1 mg, Mg 6.9 mg, Mn 1.3 mg, niacinamide 30 mg, pantothenic acid 10 mg, Zn 18.2 mg
Prenatal U		10	6	5	15	200			Cu 0.8 mg, Fe 106.5 mg, folic acid 1 mg, Mn 1.3 mg, niacinamide 30 mg, pantothenic acid 10 mg
Powder									
Obegyn® (per 4 level tsp/8.25 g)	2500 (as palmatate) 2500 (as beta-carotene)	1.7	2	10	12	120	400	60	Biotin 300 mcg, Ca 455 mg, Cu 2 mg, Fe 18 mg, folic acid 1mg, iodine 150 mcg, Mg 150 mg, niacin 20 mg, pantothenic acid 10 mg, Zn 25 mg; **phenylalanine 84 mg/8.25 g**; orange flavor (495 g/60 doses)
Tablet									
A-Free Prenatal		2	2	1	2	33.3	133.3	10	Calcium 333.3 mg, biotin 10 mcg, Cu 0.1 mg, Fe 9 mg, folic acid 266.6 mcg, Mg 33.3 mg, Mn 0.1 mg, niacinamide 10 mg, pantothenic acid 5 mg, Zn 7.5 mg
Advanced NatalCare®	2700	3	3.4	20	12	120	400	30	Ca 200 mg, Cu 2 mg, Fe 90 mg, folic acid 1mg, Mg 30 mg, niacinamide 20 mg, Zn 25 mg; docusate sodium 50 mg
Aminate Fe-90	4000	3	3.4	20	12	120	400	30	Ca 250 mg, Cu 2 mg, Fe 90 mg, folic acid 1 mg, iodine 150 mcg, niacinamide 20 mg, Zn 25 mg; docusate sodium 50 mg
Cal-Nate™	2700	3	3.4	20		120	400	30	Ca 125 mg, Cu 2 mg, Fe 27 mg, folic acid 1 mg, iodine 150 mcg, niacinamide 20 mg, Zn 25 mg; docusate calcium 50 mg

Prenatal Formulations *(continued)*

Product	A (int. units)	B_1 (mg)	B_2 (mg)	B_6 (mg)	B_{12} (mcg)	C (mg)	D (int. units)	E (int. units)	Additional Information
Citracal® Prenatal Rx	2700	3	3.4	20		120	400	30	Ca 125 mg, Cu 2 mg, Fe 27 mg, folic acid 1mg, iodine 150 mcg, niacinamide 20 mg, Zn 25 mg; docusate sodium 50 mg
Duet®	3000	1.8	4	25	12	120	400	30	Ca 200 mg, Cu 2 mg, Fe 29 mg, folic acid 1mg, Mg 25 mg, niacinamide 20 mg, Zn 25 mg
KPN Prenatal	2666.6	2	2	1	2	33.3	133.3	10	Ca 333.3 mg, biotin 10 mcg, Cu 0.1 mg, Fe 9 mg, folic acid 266.6 mcg, Mg 33.3 mg, Mn 0.1 mg, niacinamide 10 mg, pantothenic acid 5 mg, Zn 7.5 mg
NatalCare® CFe 60 [DSC]	1000	2	3	10	12	120	400	11	Fe 60 mg, folic acid 1 mg, niacinamide 20 mg
NatalCare® GlossTabs™	2700	3	3.4	20	12	120	400	10	Biotin 30 mcg, Ca 200 mg, Cu 2 mg, Fe 90 mg, folic acid 1mg, Mg 30 mg, niacinamide 20 mg, pantothenic acid 6 mg, Zn 15 mg; docusate sodium 50 mg
NatalCare® PIC	4000	2.43	3	1.64	3	50	400		Ca 125 mg, folic acid 1 mg, niacinamide 10 mg, polysaccharide-iron complex 60 mg, Zn 18 mg
NatalCare® PIC Forte	5000	3	3.4	4	12	80	400	30	Ca 250 mg, Cu 2 mg, folic acid 1mg, iodine 200 mcg, Mg 10 mg, niacinamide 20 mg, polysaccharide-iron complex 60 mg, Zn 25 mg
NatalCare® Plus	4000	1.84	3	10	12	120	400	22	Ca 200 mg, Cu 2 mg, Fe 27 mg, folic acid 1mg, niacinamide 20 mg, Zn 25 mg
NatalCare® Rx	2000	0.75	0.8	2	1.25	40	200	7.5	Biotin 15 mcg, Ca 100 mg, Cu 1.5 mg, folate 0.5mg, Fe 27 mg, Mg 50 mg, niacin 8.5 mg, pantothenic acid 3.75 mg, Zn 12.5 mg
NatalCare® Three	3000	1.8	4	25	12	120	400	22	Ca 200 mg, Cu 2 mg, Fe 28 mg, folic acid 1mg, Mg 25 mg, niacinamide 20 mg, Zn 25 mg
NataFort®	1000	2	3	10	12	120	400	11	Fe 60 mg, folic acid 1 mg, niacinamide 20 mg
NataTab™ CFe	4000	3	3	3	8	120	400	30	Ca 200 mg, Fe 50 mg, folic acid 1mg, iodine 150 mcg, niacin 20 mg, Zn 15 mg
NataTab™ FA	4000	3	3	6	8	120	400	30	Ca 200 mg, Fe 29 mg, folic acid 1mg, iodine 150 mcg, niacin 20 mg, Zn 15 mg
NataTab™ Rx	4000	3	3	3	8	120	400	30	Biotin 30 mcg, Ca 200 mg, Cu 3 mg, Fe 29 mg, folic acid 1mg, iodine 150 mcg, Mg 100 mg, niacin 20 mg, pantothenic acid 7 mg, Zn 15 mg
Nestabs® CBF	4000	3	3	3	8	120	400	30	Ca 200 mg, Fe 50 mg, folic acid 1 mg, iodine 150 mcg, niacin 20 mg, Zn 15 mg
Nestabs® FA	4000	3	3	3	8	120	400	30	Ca 200 mg, Fe 29 mg, folic acid 1 mg, iodine 150 mcg, niacin 20 mg, Zn 15 mg

Prenatal Formulations *(continued)*

Product	A (int. units)	B_1 (mg)	B_2 (mg)	B_6 (mg)	B_{12} (mcg)	C (mg)	D (int. units)	E (int. units)	Additional Information
Nestabs® RX	4000	3	3	3	8	120	400	30	Biotin 30 mcg, Ca 200 mg, Cu 3 mg, Fe 29 mg, folic acid 1mg, iodine 150 mcg, Mg 100 mg, niacin 20 mg, pantothenic acid 7 mg, Zn 15 mg
Niferex®-PN	4000	2.43	3	1.64	3	50	400		Ca 125 mg, folic acid 1 mg, niacinamide 10 mg, polysaccharide-iron complex 60 mg, Zn 18 mg
Niferex®-PN Forte	5000	3	3.4	4	12	80	400	30	Ca 250 mg, Cu 2 mg, folic acid 1 mg, iodine 200 mcg, Mg 10 mg, niacinamide 20 mg, polysaccharide-iron complex 60 mg, Zn 25 mg
OB-20	2000	43	0.5	2.5	2	30	100	15	Biotin 37.5 mcg, Ca 125 mg, Cr 6.25 mcg, Fe 12.5 mg, folic acid 2.5 mg, Mg 37.5 mg, Mn 1.25 mg, niacinamide 5 mg, pantothenic acid 2.5 mg, Se 6.25 mcg, Zn 6.2 mg
PreCare® Conceive™		3	3.4	50	12	60		30	Ca 200 mg, Cu 2 mg, Fe 30 mg, folic acid 1mg, Mg 100 mg, niacinamide 20 mg, Zn 15 mg
Prenatal 1-A-Day	4000	2	3	3	10	100	400	15	Biotin 100 mcg, Ca 200 mg, Cu 2 mg, Fe 27 mg, folic acid 800 mcg, Mg 60 mg, Mn 2 mg, niacinamide 20 mg, pantothenic acid 10 mg, Zn 15 mg
Prenatal AD	2700	3	3.4	12	120	120	400	30	Ca 200 mg, Cu 2 mg, Fe 90 mg, folic acid 1 mg, Mg 30 mg, niacinamide 20 mg, Zn 25 mg; docusate sodium 50 mg
Prenatal MR 90 Fe™	4000	3	3.4	20	12	120	400	30	Ca 250 mg, Cu 2 mg, Fe 90 mg, folic acid 1mg, iodine 150 mcg, niacinamide 20 mg, Zn 25 mg; docusate sodium 50 mg
Prenatal MRT with Selenium	5000	3	3.4	10	12	120	400	30	Biotin 30 mcg, Ca 200 mg, Cr 25 mcg, Cu 2 mg, Fe 27 mg, folic acid 1mg, iodine 150 mcg, Mg 25 mg, Mn 5 mg, Mo 25 mcg, niacinamide 20 mg, pantothenic acid 10 mg, Se 20 mcg, Zn 25 mg
Prenatal Plus	4000	1.8	3	10	12	120	400	22	Ca 200 mg, Cu 2 mg, Fe 27 mg, folic acid 1mg, niacinamide 20 mg, Zn 25 mg
Prenatal Rx 1	4000	1.5	1.6	4	2.5	80	400	15	Biotin 30 mcg, Ca 200 mg, Cu 3 mg, Fe 60 mg, folic acid 1mg, Mg 100 mg, niacinamide 17 mg, pantothenic acid 7 mg, Zn 25 mg
Prenatal Z	3000	1.5	1.6	2.2	2.2	70	400	10	Ca 200 mg, Fe 65 mg, folic acid 1 mg, iodine 175 mcg, Mg 100 mg, niacin 17 mg, Zn 15 mg
Prenate Elite™		3	3.4	20	12	120	400	10	Biotin 300 mcg, Ca 200 mg, Cu 2 mg, Fe 90 mg, folate 1mg, Mg 30 mg, niacinamide 20 mg, pantothenic acid 6 mg, Zn 15 mg; docusate sodium 50 mg
Prenate GT™	2700	3	3.4	20	12	120	400	10	Biotin 30 mcg, Ca 200 mg, Cu 2 mg, Fe 90 mg, folic acid 1mg, Mg 30 mg, niacinamide 20 mg, pantothenic acid 6 mg, Zn 15 mg; docusate sodium 50 mg

Prenatal Formulations *(continued)*

Product	A (int. units)	B_1 (mg)	B_2 (mg)	B_6 (mg)	B_{12} (mcg)	C (mg)	D (int. units)	E (int. units)	Additional Information
Stuartnatal® Plus 3™	3000	1.8	4	25	12	120	400	22	Ca 200 mg, Cu 2 mg, Fe 28 mg, folic acid 1mg, Mg 25 mg, niacinamide 20 mg, Zn 25 mg
Stuart Prenatal®	4000	1.8	1.7	2.6	8	120	400	30	Ca 200 mg, Fe 28 mg, folic acid 0.8 mg, niacin 20 mg, Zn 25 mg
Trinate	3000	1.8	4	25	12	120	400	22	Ca 200 mg, Cu 2 mg, Fe 28 mg, folic acid 1 mg, Mg 25 mg, niacin 20 mg, Zn 25 mg
Ultra NatalCare®	2700	3	3.4	20	12	120	400	30	Ca 200 mg, Cu 2 mg, Fe 90 mg, folic acid 1mg, iodine 150 mcg, niacinamide 20 mg, Zn 25 mg; docusate sodium 50 mg
Tablet, Chewable									
Duet®	3000	1.8	4	25	12	120	400	30	Ca 100 mg, Cu 2 mg, Fe 29 mg, folic acid 1mg, Mg 25 mg, niacinamide 20 mg, Zn 25 mg; **phenylalanine 15 mg/tablet**
NataChew™	1000	2	3	10	12	120	400	11	Fe 29 mg, folic acid 1 mg, niacinamide 20 mg; peanut extract, wild berry flavor
NutriNate®	1000	2	3	10	12	120	400	11	Fe 29 mg, folic acid 1 mg, niacinamide 20 mg; wild berry flavor
PreCare®				2		50	6 mcg	3.5 mg	Ca 250 mg, Cu 2 mg, Fe 40 mg, folic acid 1 mg, Mg 50 mg, Zn 15 mg
StrongStart™	1000	1	3	20	15	100	400	30	Ca 200 mg, Fe 29 mg, folic acid 1mg, niacinamide 15 mg, pantothenic acid 7 mg, Zn 20 mg; **phenylalanine 6 mg/tablet**
Combination Package									
CareNate™ 600	3500	2	3	3	12	60	400	30	Tablet: Cu 2 mg, Fe 60 mg, folic acid 1 mg, Mg 25 mg, Zn 20 mg; dioctylsulfosuccinate sodium 50 mg Chewable tablet: Ca 600 mg; wild berry flavor
Duet™ DHA	3000	1.8	4	25	12	120	400	30	Tablet: Ca 200 mg, Cu 2 mg, Fe 29 mg, folic acid 1 mg, Mg 25 mg, niacinamide 20 mg, Zn 25 mg Capsule: Omega-3 fatty acids ≥ DHA 200 mg

Cr = chromium, Cu = copper, Fe = iron, Mg = magnesium, Mn = manganese, Mo = molybdenum, Se = selenium, Zn = zinc.

vitamins (multiple/prenatal) *(Continued)*

Synonyms prenatal vitamins

U.S./Canadian Brand Names Advanced NatalCare® [US]; A-Free Prenatal [US]; Aminate Fe-90 [US]; Anemagen™ OB [US]; Cal-Nate™ [US]; CareNate™ 600 [US]; Chromagen® OB [US]; Citracal® Prenatal Rx [US]; Duet® [US]; Duet® DHA [US]; KPN Prenatal [US]; NataChew™ [US]; NataFort® [US]; NatalCare® CFe 60 [US]; NatalCare® GlossTabs™ [US]; NatalCare® PIC [US]; NatalCare® PIC Forte [US]; NatalCare® Plus [US]; NatalCare® Rx [US]; NatalCare® Three [US]; NataTab™ CFe [US]; NataTab™ FA [US]; NataTab™ Rx [US]; Nestabs® CBF [US]; Nestabs® FA [US]; Nestabs® RX [US]; Niferex®-PN [US]; Niferex®-PN Forte [US]; NutriNate® [US]; OB-20 [US]; Obegyn™ [US]; PreCare® [US]; Prenatal 1-A-Day [US]; Prenatal AD [US]; Prenatal H [US]; Prenatal MR 90 Fe™ [US]; Prenatal MTR with Selenium [US]; Prenatal Plus [US]; Prenatal Rx 1 [US]; Prenatal U [US]; Prenatal Z [US]; Prenate Elite™ [US]; Prenate GT™ [US]; StrongStart™ [US]; Stuartnatal® Plus 3™ [US-OTC]; Stuart Prenatal® [US-OTC]; Trinate [US]; Ultra NatalCare® [US]

Therapeutic Category Vitamin

Use Nutritional supplement for use prior to conception, during pregnancy, and postnatal (in lactating and nonlactating women)

Usual Dosage Oral: Adults:

Capsule, tablet: One daily

Powder: 4 teaspoonfuls/day; given once daily or in divided doses; mix 1 teaspoonful in 1 ounce of water

Dosage Forms Content varies depending on product used. For more detailed information on ingredients see table on page 928.

vitamins, multiple (therapeutic) *see* vitamins (multiple/oral) *on page 927*

vitamins, multiple with iron *see* vitamins (multiple/oral) *on page 927*

Vitelle™ Irospan® ***(Discontinued)*** *see page 1042*

Vitrasert® [US/Can] *see* ganciclovir *on page 396*

Vitravene™ ***(Discontinued)*** *see page 1042*

Vitravene™ [Can] *see* fomivirsen *(Canada only) on page 387*

Vitussin [US] *see* hydrocodone and guaifenesin *on page 445*

Vivactil® [US] *see* protriptyline *on page 744*

Viva-Drops® [US-OTC] *see* artificial tears *on page 78*

Vivelle® [US/Can] *see* estradiol *on page 324*

Vivelle-Dot® [US] *see* estradiol *on page 324*

Vivotif Berna® [US/Can] *see* typhoid vaccine *on page 895*

VLB *see* vinblastine *on page 911*

VM-26 *see* teniposide *on page 844*

Volmax® [US] *see* albuterol *on page 25*

Voltaren® [US/Can] *see* diclofenac *on page 266*

Voltaren Ophthalmic® [US] *see* diclofenac *on page 266*

Voltaren Rapide® [Can] *see* diclofenac *on page 266*

Voltaren®-XR [US] *see* diclofenac *on page 266*

Voltare Ophtha® [Can] *see* diclofenac *on page 266*

Vontrol® ***(Discontinued)*** *see page 1042*

voriconazole (vor i KOE na zole)

Synonyms UK109496

U.S./Canadian Brand Names VFEND® [US]

Therapeutic Category Antifungal Agent

Use Treatment of invasive aspergillosis; treatment of esophageal candidiasis; treatment of serious fungal infections caused by *Scedosporium apiospermum* and *Fusarium* spp (including *Fusarium solani*) in patients intolerant of, or refractory to, other therapy

Usual Dosage

Children <12 years: No data available

Children ≥12 years and Adults:

Invasive aspergillosis and other serious fungal infections: I.V.: Initial: Loading dose: 6 mg/kg every 12 hours for 2 doses; followed by maintenance dose of 4 mg/kg every 12 hours

Conversion to oral dosing:

Patients <40 kg: 100 mg every 12 hours; increase to 150 mg every 12 hours in patients who fail to respond adequately

Patients ≥40 kg: 200 mg every 12 hours; increase to 300 mg every 12 hours in patients who fail to respond adequately

Esophageal candidiasis: Oral:

Patients <40 kg: 100 mg every 12 hours

Patients ≥40 kg: 200 mg every 12 hours

Note: Treatment should continue for a minimum of 14 days, and for at least 7 days following resolution of symptoms.

Dosage Forms

Injection, powder for reconstitution: 200 mg [contains SBECD 3200 mg]

Powder for oral suspension: 200 mg/5 mL (70 mL) [contains sodium benzoate and sucrose; orange flavor]

Tablet: 50 mg, 200 mg [contains lactose]

VōSol® [US] *see* acetic acid *on page 15*

VōSol® HC [US/Can] *see* acetic acid, propylene glycol diacetate, and hydrocortisone *on page 15*

VoSpire ER™ [US] *see* albuterol *on page 25*

VP-16 *see* etoposide *on page 351*

VP-16-213 *see* etoposide *on page 351*

Vumon® [US/Can] *see* teniposide *on page 844*

V.V.S.® [US] *see* sulfabenzamide, sulfacetamide, and sulfathiazole *on page 829*

Vytone® [US] *see* iodoquinol and hydrocortisone *on page 481*

Vytorin™ [US] *see* ezetimibe and simvastatin *on page 354*

VZIG *see* varicella-zoster immune globulin (human) *on page 905*

warfarin (WAR far in)

Sound-Alike/Look-Alike Issues

Coumadin® may be confused with Avandia®, Cardura®, Compazine®, Kemadrin®

Synonyms warfarin sodium

U.S./Canadian Brand Names Apo-Warfarin® [Can]; Coumadin® [US/Can]; Gen-Warfarin [Can]; Taro-Warfarin [Can]

Therapeutic Category Anticoagulant (Other)

Use Prophylaxis and treatment of venous thrombosis, pulmonary embolism and thromboembolic disorders; atrial fibrillation with risk of embolism and as an adjunct in the prophylaxis of systemic embolism after myocardial infarction

Usual Dosage

Oral:

Infants and Children: 0.05-0.34 mg/kg/day; infants <12 months of age may require doses at or near the high end of this range; consistent anticoagulation may be difficult to maintain in children <5 years of age

Adults: Initial dosing must be individualized. Consider the patient (hepatic function, cardiac function, age, nutritional status, concurrent therapy, risk of bleeding) in addition to prior dose response (if available) and the clinical situation. Start 5-10 mg daily for 2 days. Adjust dose according to INR results; usual maintenance dose ranges from

(Continued)

warfarin *(Continued)*

2-10 mg daily (individual patients may require loading and maintenance doses outside these general guidelines).

Note: Lower starting doses may be required for patients with hepatic impairment, poor nutrition, CHF, elderly, or a high risk of bleeding. Higher initial doses may be reasonable in selected patients (ie, receiving enzyme-inducing agents and with low risk of bleeding).

I.V. (administer as a slow bolus injection): 2-5 mg/day

Dosage Forms

Injection, powder for reconstitution, as sodium (Coumadin®): 5 mg

Tablet, as sodium (Coumadin®, Jantoven™): 1 mg, 2 mg, 2.5 mg, 3 mg, 4 mg, 5 mg, 6 mg, 7.5 mg, 10 mg

warfarin sodium *see* warfarin *on previous page*

Wartec® [Can] *see* podofilox *on page 704*

Wart-Off® Maximum Strength [US-OTC] *see* salicylic acid *on page 789*

4-Way® Long Acting [US-OTC] *see* oxymetazoline *on page 658*

Wehamine® Injection *(Discontinued)* *see page 1042*

Wehdryl® *(Discontinued)* *see page 1042*

WelChol® [US/Can] *see* colesevelam *on page 224*

Wellbutrin® [US/Can] *see* bupropion *on page 135*

Wellbutrin SR® [US] *see* bupropion *on page 135*

Wellbutrin XL™ [US] *see* bupropion *on page 135*

Wellcovorin® *(Discontinued)* *see page 1042*

Wesmycin® [US] *see* tetracycline *on page 851*

Wesprin® Buffered *(Discontinued)* *see page 1042*

Westcort® [US/Can] *see* hydrocortisone (topical) *on page 451*

Westhroid® [US] *see* thyroid *on page 860*

40 Winks® *(Discontinued)* *see page 1042*

Winpred™ [Can] *see* prednisone *on page 725*

WinRho SD® *(Discontinued)* *see page 1042*

WinRho SDF® [US] *see* Rh_o(D) immune globulin *on page 771*

Winstrol® [US] *see* stanozolol *on page 822*

witch hazel (witch HAY zel)

Synonyms hamamelis water

U.S./Canadian Brand Names Preparation H® Cleansing Pads [Can]; Tucks® [US-OTC]

Therapeutic Category Astringent

Use After-stool wipe to remove most causes of local irritation; temporary management of vulvitis, pruritus ani and vulva; help relieve the discomfort of simple hemorrhoids, anorectal surgical wounds, and episiotomies

Usual Dosage Apply to anorectal area as needed

Dosage Forms

Liquid, topical: 100% (60 mL, 120 mL, 240 mL, 480 mL)

Pads: 50% (20s, 50s)

Tucks®: 50% (12s, 40s, 100s)

Wolfina® *(Discontinued)* *see page 1042*

wood sugar *see* d-xylose *on page 300*

Wound Wash Saline™ [US-OTC] *see* sodium chloride *on page 810*

WR2721 *see* amifostine *on page 43*

WR-139007 *see* dacarbazine *on page 241*

WR-139013 *see* chlorambucil *on page 182*

WR-139021 *see* carmustine *on page 162*

Wyamine® *(Discontinued)* *see page 1042*

Wyamycin S® *(Discontinued)* *see page 1042*

Wycillin® [Can] *see* penicillin G procaine *on page 676*

Wydase® *(Discontinued)* *see page 1042*

Wygesic® *(Discontinued)* *see page 1042*

Wymox® *(Discontinued)* *see page 1042*

Wytensin® *(Discontinued)* *see page 1042*

Wytensin® [Can] *see* guanabenz *on page 425*

Xalatan® [US/Can] *see* latanoprost *on page 507*

Xanax® [US/Can] *see* alprazolam *on page 35*

Xanax TS™ [Can] *see* alprazolam *on page 35*

Xanax XR® [US] *see* alprazolam *on page 35*

Xeloda® [US/Can] *see* capecitabine *on page 152*

Xenical® [US/Can] *see* orlistat *on page 649*

Xerac AC™ [US] *see* aluminum chloride hexahydrate *on page 39*

Xifaxan™ [US] *see* rifaximin *on page 777*

Xigris™ [US/Can] *see* drotrecogin alfa *on page 297*

Xolair® [US] *see* omalizumab *on page 643*

Xopenex® [US/Can] *see* levalbuterol *on page 510*

X-Prep® [US-OTC] *see* senna *on page 799*

X-Seb™ T [US-OTC] *see* coal tar and salicylic acid *on page 220*

Xylocaine® [US/Can] *see* lidocaine *on page 518*

Xylocaine® MPF [US] *see* lidocaine *on page 518*

Xylocaine® MPF With Epinephrine [US] *see* lidocaine and epinephrine *on page 520*

Xylocaine® Viscous [US] *see* lidocaine *on page 518*

Xylocaine® With Epinephrine [Can] *see* lidocaine and epinephrine *on page 520*

Xylocard® [Can] *see* lidocaine *on page 518*

xylometazoline (zye loe met AZ oh leen)

Sound-Alike/Look-Alike Issues

Otrivin® may be confused with Lotrimin®

Synonyms xylometazoline hydrochloride

U.S./Canadian Brand Names Balminil® [Can]; Decongest [Can]

Therapeutic Category Adrenergic Agonist Agent

Use Symptomatic relief of nasal and nasopharyngeal mucosal congestion

Usual Dosage

Children 2-12 years: Instill 2-3 drops (0.05%) in each nostril every 8-10 hours

Children >12 years and Adults: Instill 2-3 drops or sprays (0.1%) in each nostril every 8-10 hours

Dosage Forms [DSC] = Discontinued product

Solution, intranasal drops, as hydrochloride:

Otrivin® [DSC]: 0.1% (25 mL)

Otrivin® Pediatric [DSC]: 0.05% (25 mL)

Solution, intranasal spray, as hydrochloride (Otrivin® [DSC]): 0.1% (20 mL)

xylometazoline hydrochloride *see* xylometazoline *on previous page*

Xyrem® [US] *see* sodium oxybate *on page 813*

Y-90 zevalin *see* ibritumomab *on page 461*

Yasmin® [US] *see* ethinyl estradiol and drospirenone *on page 337*

yellow fever vaccine (YEL oh FEE ver vak SEEN)

U.S./Canadian Brand Names YF-VAX® [US/Can]

Therapeutic Category Vaccine, Live Virus

Use Induction of active immunity against yellow fever virus, primarily among persons traveling or living in areas where yellow fever infection exists

Usual Dosage Children ≥9 months and Adults: SubQ: One dose (0.5 mL) ≥10 days before travel; Booster: Every 10 years

Dosage Forms Injection, powder for reconstitution: ≥5.04 Log_{10} plaque-forming units (PFU) [single-dose vial; produced in chicken embryos; packaged with diluent; vial stopper contains latex]; ≥25.2 Log_{10} plaque-forming units (PFU) [5-dose vial; produced in chicken embryos; packaged with diluent; vial stopper contains latex]

yellow mercuric oxide *see* mercuric oxide *on page 555*

YF-VAX® [US/Can] *see* yellow fever vaccine *on this page*

YM-08310 *see* amifostine *on page 43*

Yocon® [US/Can] *see* yohimbine *on this page*

Yodoxin® [US] *see* iodoquinol *on page 481*

yohimbine (yo HIM bine)

Sound-Alike/Look-Alike Issues

Aphrodyne® may be confused with Aprodine®

Yocon® may be confused with Zocor®

Synonyms yohimbine hydrochloride

U.S./Canadian Brand Names Aphrodyne® [US]; PMS-Yohimbine [Can]; Yocon® [US/Can]

Therapeutic Category Miscellaneous Product

Use No FDA sanctioned indications

Usual Dosage Adults: Oral:

Male erectile impotence: 5.4 mg tablet 3 times/day have been used. If side effects occur, reduce to ½ tablet (2.7 mg) 3 times/day followed by gradual increases to 1 tablet 3 times/day. Results of therapy >10 weeks are not known.

Orthostatic hypotension: Doses of 12.5 mg/day have been utilized; however, more research is necessary

Dosage Forms Tablet, as hydrochloride: 5.4 mg

yohimbine hydrochloride *see* yohimbine *on this page*

Yohimex™ *(Discontinued)* *see page 1042*

Yutopar® *(Discontinued)* *see page 1042*

Z4942 *see* ifosfamide *on page 464*

Zaditen® [Can] *see* ketotifen *on page 497*

Zaditor™ [US/Can] *see* ketotifen *on page 497*

zafirlukast (za FIR loo kast)

Sound-Alike/Look-Alike Issues

Accolate® may be confused with Accupril®, Accutane®, Aclovate®

Synonyms ICI 204, 219

U.S./Canadian Brand Names Accolate® [US/Can]

Therapeutic Category Leukotriene Receptor Antagonist

Use Prophylaxis and chronic treatment of asthma in adults and children ≥5 years of age

Usual Dosage Oral:
Children <5 years: Safety and effectiveness have not been established
Children 5-11 years: 10 mg twice daily
Children ≥12 years and Adults: 20 mg twice daily
Dosage Forms Tablet: 10 mg, 20 mg

Zagam® [US] *see* sparfloxacin *on page 820*

zalcitabine (zal SITE a been)

Synonyms ddC; dideoxycytidine
U.S./Canadian Brand Names Hivid® [US/Can]
Therapeutic Category Antiviral Agent
Use In combination with at least two other antiretrovirals in the treatment of patients with HIV infection; it is not recommended that zalcitabine be given in combination with didanosine, stavudine, or lamivudine due to overlapping toxicities, virologic interactions, or lack of clinical data
Usual Dosage Oral:
Neonates: Dose unknown
Infants and Children <13 years: Safety and efficacy have not been established; suggested usual dose: 0.01 mg/kg every 8 hours; range: 0.005-0.01 mg/kg every 8 hours
Adolescents and Adults: 0.75 mg 3 times/day
Dosage Forms Tablet: 0.375 mg, 0.75 mg

zaleplon (ZAL e plon)

U.S./Canadian Brand Names Sonata® [US/Can]; Starnoc® [Can]
Therapeutic Category Hypnotic, Nonbenzodiazepine (Pyrazolopyrimidine)
Use Short-term (7-10 days) treatment of insomnia (has been demonstrated to be effective for up to 5 weeks in controlled trial)
Usual Dosage Oral: Adults: 10 mg at bedtime (range: 5-20 mg); has been used for up to 5 weeks of treatment in controlled trial setting
Dosage Forms Capsule: 5 mg, 10 mg [contains tartrazine]

Zanaflex® [US/Can] *see* tizanidine *on page 866*

zanamivir (za NA mi veer)

U.S./Canadian Brand Names Relenza® [US/Can]
Therapeutic Category Antiviral Agent, Inhalation Therapy
Use Treatment of uncomplicated acute illness due to influenza virus in adults and children ≥7 years of age; should not be used in patients with underlying airway disease. Treatment should only be initiated in patients who have been symptomatic for no more than 2 days.
Usual Dosage Children ≥7 years and Adults: 2 inhalations (10 mg total) twice daily for 5 days. Two doses should be taken on the first day of dosing, regardless of interval, while doses should be spaced by approximately 12 hours on subsequent days.
Prophylaxis (investigational use): 2 inhalations (10 mg) once daily for duration of exposure period (6 weeks has been used in clinical trial)
Dosage Forms Powder for oral inhalation: 5 mg/blister (20s) [4 blisters per Rotadisk®, 5 Rotadisk® per package; contains lactose]

Zanosar® [US/Can] *see* streptozocin *on page 825*

Zantac® [US/Can] *see* ranitidine hydrochloride *on page 763*

Zantac® 75 [US-OTC/Can] *see* ranitidine hydrochloride *on page 763*

Zantac® EFFERdose® *(Discontinued)* *see page 1042*

Zantryl® *(Discontinued)* *see page 1042*

Zapzyt® Acne Wash [US-OTC] *see* salicylic acid *on page 789*

zidovudine (zye DOE vyoo deen)

Sound-Alike/Look-Alike Issues

Retrovir® may be confused with ritonavir

azidothymidine may be confused with azathioprine

Synonyms azidothymidine; AZT; compound S; ZDV

U.S./Canadian Brand Names Apo-Zidovudine® [Can]; AZT™ [Can]; Novo-AZT [Can]; Retrovir® [US/Can]

Therapeutic Category Antiviral Agent

Use Management of patients with HIV infections in combination with at least two other antiretroviral agents; for prevention of maternal/fetal HIV transmission as monotherapy

Usual Dosage

Prevention of maternal-fetal HIV transmission:

Neonatal: **Note:** Dosing should begin 6-12 hours after birth and continue for the first 6 weeks of life.

Oral:

Full-term infants: 2 mg/kg/dose every 6 hours

Infants ≥30 weeks and <35 weeks gestation at birth: 2 mg/kg/dose every 12 hours; at 2 weeks of age, advance to 2 mg/kg/dose every 8 hours

Infants <30 weeks gestation at birth: 2 mg/kg/dose every 12 hours; at 4 weeks of age, advance to 2 mg/kg/dose every 8 hours

I.V.: Infants unable to receive oral dosing:

Full term: 1.5 mg/kg/dose every 6 hours

Infants ≥30 weeks and <35 weeks gestation at birth: 1.5 mg/kg/dose every 12 hours; at 2 weeks of age, advance to 1.5 mg/kg/dose every 8 hours

Infants <30 weeks gestation at birth: 1.5 mg/kg/dose every 12 hours; at 4 weeks of age, advance to 1.5 mg/kg/dose every 8 hours

Maternal (may delay treatment until after 10-12 weeks gestation): Oral (per AIDSinfo 2003 guidelines): 200 mg 3 times/day or 300 mg twice daily until start of labor

During labor and delivery, administer zidovudine I.V. at 2 mg/kg over 1 hour followed by a continuous I.V. infusion of 1 mg/kg/hour until the umbilical cord is clamped

Children 3 months to 12 years for HIV infection:

Oral: 160 mg/m^2/dose every 8 hours; dosage range: 90 mg/m^2/dose to 180 mg/m^2/dose every 6-8 hours; some Working Group members use a dose of 180 mg/m^2 every 12 hours when using in drug combinations with other antiretroviral compounds, but data on this dosing in children is limited

I.V. continuous infusion: 20 mg/m^2/hour

I.V. intermittent infusion: 120 mg/m^2/dose every 6 hours

Adults:

Oral: 300 mg twice daily or 200 mg 3 times/day

I.V.: 1-2 mg/kg/dose (infused over 1 hour) administered every 4 hours around-the-clock (6 doses/day)

Dosage Forms

Capsule: 100 mg

Injection, solution: 10 mg/mL (20 mL)

Syrup: 50 mg/5 mL (240 mL) [contains sodium benzoate; strawberry flavor]

Tablet: 300 mg

zidovudine, abacavir, and lamivudine *see* abacavir, lamivudine, and zidovudine *on page 2*

zidovudine and lamivudine (zye DOE vyoo deen & la MI vyoo deen)

Sound-Alike/Look-Alike Issues

Combivir® may be confused with Combivent®, Epivir®

Synonyms AZT + 3TC; lamivudine and zidovudine

U.S./Canadian Brand Names Combivir® [US/Can]

Therapeutic Category Antiviral Agent

Use Treatment of HIV infection when therapy is warranted based on clinical and/or immunological evidence of disease progression. Combivir® given twice daily, provides

(Continued)

zidovudine and lamivudine *(Continued)*

an alternative regimen to lamivudine 150 mg twice daily plus zidovudine 600 mg/day in divided doses; this drug form reduces capsule/tablet intake for these two drugs to 2 per day instead of up to 8.

Usual Dosage Children >12 years and Adults: Oral: One tablet twice daily

Dosage Forms Tablet: Zidovudine 300 mg and lamivudine 150 mg

Zilactin® [Can] *see* lidocaine *on page 518*

Zilactin® Baby [US-OTC/Can] *see* benzocaine *on page 107*

Zilactin®-B [US-OTC/Can] *see* benzocaine *on page 107*

Zilactin-L® [US-OTC] *see* lidocaine *on page 518*

Zinacef® [US/Can] *see* cefuroxime *on page 173*

zinc *see* trace metals *on page 874*

Zincate® [US] *see* zinc sulfate *on next page*

zinc chloride (zingk KLOR ide)

Therapeutic Category Trace Element

Use Cofactor for replacement therapy to different enzymes helps maintain normal growth rates, normal skin hydration and senses of taste and smell

Usual Dosage Clinical response may not occur for up to 6-8 weeks

Supplemental to I.V. solutions:

Premature Infants <1500 g, up to 3 kg: 300 mcg/kg/day

Full-term Infants and Children ≤5 years: 100 mcg/kg/day

Adults:

Stable with fluid loss from small bowel: 12.2 mg zinc/liter TPN or 17.1 mg zinc/kg (added to 1000 mL I.V. fluids) of stool or ileostomy output

Metabolically stable: 2.5-4 mg/day, add 2 mg/day for acute catabolic states

Dosage Forms Injection, solution: 1 mg/mL (10 mL, 50 mL)

Zincfrin® [US-OTC/Can] *see* phenylephrine and zinc sulfate *on page 691*

zinc gelatin (zingk JEL ah tin)

Synonyms dome paste bandage; unna's boot; unna's paste; zinc gelatin boot

U.S./Canadian Brand Names Gelucast® [US]

Therapeutic Category Protectant, Topical

Use As a protectant and to support varicosities and similar lesions of the lower limbs

Usual Dosage Apply externally as an occlusive boot

Dosage Forms Bandage: 3" x 10 yards; 4" x 10 yards

zinc gelatin boot *see* zinc gelatin *on this page*

Zincofax® [Can] *see* zinc oxide *on this page*

Zincon® [US-OTC] *see* pyrithione zinc *on page 754*

zinc oxide (zingk OKS ide)

Synonyms base ointment; Lassar's zinc paste

U.S./Canadian Brand Names Ammens® Medicated Deodorant [US-OTC]; Balmex® [US-OTC]; Boudreaux's® Butt Paste [US-OTC]; Critic-Aid Skin Care® [US-OTC]; Desitin® Creamy [US-OTC]; Desitin® [US-OTC]; Zincofax® [Can]

Therapeutic Category Topical Skin Product

Use Protective coating for mild skin irritations and abrasions, soothing and protective ointment to promote healing of chapped skin, diaper rash

Usual Dosage Infants, Children, and Adults: Topical: Apply as required for affected areas several times daily

Dosage Forms

Ointment, topical: 20% (30 g, 60 g, 480 g)

Balmex®: 11.3% (60 g, 120 g, 480 g)
Desitin®: 40% (30 g, 60 g, 90 g, 120 g, 270 g, 480 g) [contains cod liver oil and lanolin]
Desitin® Creamy: 10% (60 g, 120 g)
Paste, topical:
Boudreaux's® Butt Paste: 16% (30 g, 60 g, 120 g, 480 g) [contains castor oil, boric acid, mineral oil, and Peruvian balsam]
Critic-Aid Skin Care®: 20% (71 g, 170 g)
Powder, topical (Ammens® Medicated Deodorant): 9.1% (187.5 g, 330 g) [original and shower fresh scent]

zinc oxide, cod liver oil, and talc (zingk OKS ide, kod LIV er oyl, & talk)

Therapeutic Category Protectant, Topical

Use Relief of diaper rash, superficial wounds and burns, and other minor skin irritations

Usual Dosage Topical: Apply thin layer as needed

Dosage Forms Ointment, topical: Zinc oxide, cod liver oil and talc in a petrolatum and lanolin base (30 g, 60 g, 120 g, 240 g, 270 g)

zinc sulfate (zingk SUL fate)

U.S./Canadian Brand Names Anuzinc [Can]; Orazinc® [US-OTC]; Rivasol [Can]; Zincate® [US]

Therapeutic Category Electrolyte Supplement, Oral

Use Zinc supplement (oral and parenteral); may improve wound healing in those who are deficient

Usual Dosage

RDA: Oral:
Birth to 6 months: 3 mg elemental zinc/day
6-12 months: 5 mg elemental zinc/day
1-10 years: 10 mg elemental zinc/day
≥11 years: 15 mg elemental zinc/day

Zinc deficiency: Oral:
Infants and Children: 0.5-1 mg elemental zinc/kg/day divided 1-3 times/day; somewhat larger quantities may be needed if there is impaired intestinal absorption or an excessive loss of zinc
Adults: 110-220 mg zinc sulfate (25-50 mg elemental zinc)/dose 3 times/day
Parenteral TPN: I.V.:
Infants (premature, birth weight <1500 g up to 3 kg): 300 mcg/kg/day
Infants (full-term) and Children ≤5 years: 100 mcg/kg/day
Adults:
Acute metabolic states: 4.5-6 mg/day
Metabolically stable: 2.5-4 mg/day
Stable with fluid loss from the small bowel: 12.2 mg zinc/L of TPN solution, or an additional 17.1 mg zinc (added to 1000 mL I.V. fluids) per kg of stool or ileostomy output

Dosage Forms

Capsule (Orazinc®, Zincate®): 220 mg [elemental zinc 50 mg]
Injection, solution [preservative free]: 1 mg elemental zinc/mL (10 mL); 5 mg elemental zinc/mL (5 mL)
Tablet (Orazinc®): 110 mg [elemental zinc 25 mg]

zinc sulfate and phenylephrine *see* phenylephrine and zinc sulfate *on page 691*

zinc undecylenate *see* undecylenic acid and derivatives *on page 896*

Zinecard® [US/Can] *see* dexrazoxane *on page 257*

ziprasidone (zi PRAY si done)

Synonyms zeldox; ziprasidone hydrochloride; ziprasidone mesylate

U.S./Canadian Brand Names Geodon® [US]

(Continued)

ziprasidone *(Continued)*

Therapeutic Category Antipsychotic Agent

Use Treatment of schizophrenia; treatment of acute manic or mixed episodes associated with bipolar disorder with or without psychosis; acute agitation in patients with schizophrenia

Usual Dosage Adults:

Bipolar mania: Oral: Initial: 40 mg twice daily (with food)

Adjustment: May increase to 60 or 80 mg twice daily on second day of treatment; average dose 40-80 mg twice daily

Schizophrenia: Oral: Initial: 20 mg twice daily (with food)

Adjustment: Increases (if indicated) should be made no more frequently than every 2 days; ordinarily patients should be observed for improvement over several weeks before adjusting the dose

Maintenance: Range 20-100 mg twice daily; however, dosages >80 mg twice daily are generally not recommended

Acute agitation (schizophrenia): I.M.: 10 mg every 2 hours **or** 20 mg every 4 hours; maximum: 40 mg/day; oral therapy should replace I.M. administration as soon as possible

Dosage Forms

Capsule, as hydrochloride: 20 mg, 40 mg, 60 mg, 80 mg

Injection, powder for reconstitution, as mesylate: 20 mg

ziprasidone hydrochloride *see* ziprasidone *on previous page*

ziprasidone mesylate *see* ziprasidone *on previous page*

Zithromax® [US/Can] *see* azithromycin *on page 94*

Zithromax® TRI-PAK™ *see* azithromycin *on page 94*

Zithromax® Z-PAK® *see* azithromycin *on page 94*

ZM-182,780 *see* fulvestrant *on page 393*

ZNP® Bar [US-OTC] *see* pyrithione zinc *on page 754*

Zocor® [US/Can] *see* simvastatin *on page 805*

Zofran® [US/Can] *see* ondansetron *on page 645*

Zofran® ODT [US/Can] *see* ondansetron *on page 645*

Zoladex® [US/Can] *see* goserelin *on page 413*

Zoladex® LA [Can] *see* goserelin *on page 413*

zoledronate *see* zoledronic acid *on this page*

zoledronic acid (ZOE le dron ik AS id)

Synonyms CGP-42446; zoledronate

U.S./Canadian Brand Names Zometa® [US/Can]

Therapeutic Category Bisphosphonate Derivative

Use Treatment of hypercalcemia and bone metastases of solid tumors

Usual Dosage I.V.: Adults:

Hypercalcemia of malignancy (albumin-corrected serum calcium ≥12 mg/dL): 4 mg (maximum) given as a single dose infused over **no less than 15 minutes**; patients should be adequately hydrated prior to treatment (restoring urine output to ~2 L/day). Monitor serum calcium and wait at least 7 days before considering retreatment. Dosage adjustment may be needed in patients with decreased renal function following treatment.

Multiple myeloma or metastatic bone lesions from solid tumors: 4 mg given over 15 minutes every 3-4 weeks

Note: Patients should receive a daily calcium supplement and multivitamin containing vitamin D

Dosage Forms

Injection, powder for reconstitution: 4 mg [as monohydrate 4.264 mg]

Injection, solution: 4 mg/5 mL (5 mL) [as monohydrate 4.264 mg]

Zolicef® *(Discontinued)* *see page 1042*

zolmitriptan (zohl mi TRIP tan)

Sound-Alike/Look-Alike Issues

zolmitriptan may be confused with sumatriptan

Synonyms 311C90

U.S./Canadian Brand Names Zomig® [US/Can]; Zomig® Rapimelt [Can]; Zomig-ZMT™ [US]

Therapeutic Category Antimigraine Agent; Serotonin Agonist

Use Acute treatment of migraine with or without aura

Usual Dosage Oral:

Children: Safety and efficacy have not been established

Adults: Migraine:

Tablet: Initial: ≤2.5 mg at the onset of migraine headache; may break 2.5 mg tablet in half

Orally-disintegrating tablet: Initial: 2.5 mg at the onset of migraine headache

Nasal spray: Initial: 1 spray (5 mg) at the onset of migraine headache

Note: Use the lowest possible dose to minimize adverse events. If the headache returns, the dose may be repeated after 2 hours; do not exceed 10 mg within a 24-hour period. Controlled trials have not established the effectiveness of a second dose if the initial one was ineffective

Dosage Forms

Solution, nasal spray [single dose] (Zomig®): 5 mg/0.1 mL (0.1 mL)

Tablet (Zomig®): 2.5 mg, 5 mg

Tablet, orally-disintegrating (Zomig-ZMT™): 2.5 mg [contains phenylalanine 2.81 mg/tablet; orange flavor]; 5 mg [contains phenylalanine 5.62 mg/tablet; orange flavor]

Zoloft® [US/Can] *see* sertraline *on page 801*

zolpidem (zole PI dem)

Synonyms zolpidem tartrate

U.S./Canadian Brand Names Ambien® [US/Can]

Therapeutic Category Hypnotic, Nonbarbiturate

Use Short-term treatment of insomnia

Usual Dosage Duration of therapy should be limited to 7-10 days

Adults: Oral: 10 mg immediately before bedtime; maximum dose: 10 mg

Dosage Forms

Tablet, as tartrate: 5 mg, 10 mg

Ambien® PAK™ [dose pack]: 5 mg (30s), 10 mg (30s)

zolpidem tartrate *see* zolpidem *on this page*

Zolyse® *(Discontinued)* *see page 1042*

Zometa® [US/Can] *see* zoledronic acid *on previous page*

Zomig® [US/Can] *see* zolmitriptan *on this page*

Zomig® Rapimelt [Can] *see* zolmitriptan *on this page*

Zomig-ZMT™ [US] *see* zolmitriptan *on this page*

Zonalon® [US/Can] *see* doxepin *on page 292*

Zone-A® [US] *see* pramoxine and hydrocortisone *on page 720*

Zone-A Forte® [US] *see* pramoxine and hydrocortisone *on page 720*

Zonegran™ [US/Can] *see* zonisamide *on next page*

zonisamide (zoe NIS a mide)

U.S./Canadian Brand Names Zonegran™ [US/Can]

Therapeutic Category Anticonvulsant, Sulfonamide

Use Adjunct treatment of partial seizures in children >16 years of age and adults with epilepsy

Usual Dosage Oral: Children >16 years and Adults: Adjunctive treatment of partial seizures: Initial: 100 mg/day; dose may be increased to 200 mg/day after 2 weeks. Further dosage increases to 300 mg/day and 400 mg/day can then be made with a minimum of 2 weeks between adjustments, in order to reach steady state at each dosage level. Doses of up to 600 mg/day have been studied, however, there is no evidence of increased response with doses above 400 mg/day.

Dosage Forms Capsule: 25 mg, 50 mg, 100 mg

zopiclone *(Canada only)* (ZOE pi clone)

U.S./Canadian Brand Names Alti-Zopiclone [Can]; Apo-Zopiclone® [Can]; Gen-Zopiclone [Can]; Imovane® [Can]; Nu-Zopiclone [Can]; Rhovane® [Can]

Therapeutic Category Hypnotic

Use Symptomatic relief of transient and short-term insomnia

Usual Dosage Administer just before bedtime: Oral:

Adults: 5-7.5 mg

Patients with chronic respiratory insufficiency: 3.75 mg; may increase up to 7.5 mg with caution in appropriate cases

Dosage Forms Tablet: 5 mg, 7.5 mg

Zorbtive™ [US] *see* human growth hormone *on page 437*

ZORprin® [US] *see* aspirin *on page 80*

Zostrix®-HP [US-OTC/Can] *see* capsaicin *on page 153*

Zostrix® [US-OTC/Can] *see* capsaicin *on page 153*

Zosyn® [US] *see* piperacillin and tazobactam sodium *on page 697*

Zovia™ [US] *see* ethinyl estradiol and ethynodiol diacetate *on page 338*

Zovirax® [US/Can] *see* acyclovir *on page 19*

zuclopenthixol acetate *see* zuclopenthixol *(Canada only) on this page*

zuclopenthixol *(Canada only)* (zoo kloe pen THIX ol)

Synonyms Z-chlopenthixol; zuclopenthixol acetate; zuclopenthixol decanoate; zuclopenthixol dihydrochloride

U.S./Canadian Brand Names Clopixol-Acuphase® [Can]; Clopixol® [Can]; Clopixol® Depot [Can]

Therapeutic Category Antipsychotic Agent

Use Management of schizophrenia; acetate injection is intended for short-term acute treatment; decanoate injection is for long-term management; dihydrochloride tablets may be used in either phase

Usual Dosage Adults:

Oral: Zuclopenthixol dihydrochloride: Initial: 20-30 mg/day in 2-3 divided doses; usual maintenance dose: 20-40 mg/day; maximum daily dose: 100 mg

I.M.:

Zuclopenthixol acetate: 50-150 mg; may be repeated in 2-3 days; no more than 4 injections should be given in the course of treatment; maximum dose during course of treatment: 400 mg (maximum treatment period: 2 weeks)

Transfer of patients from I.M. acetate (Acuphase®) to oral (tablets): 50 mg = 20 mg daily 100 mg = 40 mg daily 150 mg = 60 mg daily

Zuclopenthixol decanoate: 100 mg by deep I.M. injection; additional I.M. doses of 100-200 mg may be given over the following 1-4 weeks; maximum weekly dose: 600 mg; usual maintenance dose: 150-300 mg every 2 weeks

Transfer of patients from oral (tablets) to I.M. decanoate (depot): ≤20 mg daily = 100 mg every 2 weeks 25-40 mg daily = 200 mg every 2 weeks 50-75 mg daily = 300 mg every 2 weeks >75 mg/day = 400 mg every 2 weeks

Transfer of patients from I.M. acetate (Acuphase®) to I.M. decanoate (depot): 50 mg every 2-3 days = 100 mg every 2 weeks 100 mg every 2-3 days = 200 mg every 2 weeks 150 mg every 2-3 days = 300 mg every 2 weeks

Dosage Forms

Injection:

Clopixol Acuphase®, as acetate: 50 mg/mL [zuclopenthixol 42.5 mg/mL] (1 mL, 2 mL)

Clopixol® Depot, as decanoate: 200 mg/mL [zuclopenthixol 144.4 mg/mL] (10 mL)

Tablet, as dihydrochloride (Clopixol®): 10 mg, 25 mg, 40 mg

zuclopenthixol decanoate *see* zuclopenthixol *(Canada only)* *on previous page*

zuclopenthixol dihydrochloride *see* zuclopenthixol *(Canada only)* *on previous page*

Zyban® [US/Can] *see* bupropion *on page 135*

Zyban™ 100 mg *(Discontinued)* *see page 1042*

Zydone® [US] *see* hydrocodone and acetaminophen *on page 443*

Zyflo™ *(Discontinued)* *see page 1042*

Zyloprim® [US/Can] *see* allopurinol *on page 33*

Zymar™ [US] *see* gatifloxacin *on page 397*

Zymase® *(Discontinued)* *see page 1042*

Zyprexa® [US/Can] *see* olanzapine *on page 641*

Zyprexa® Zydis® [US/Can] *see* olanzapine *on page 641*

Zyrtec® [US] *see* cetirizine *on page 178*

Zyrtec-D 12 Hour™ [US] *see* cetirizine and pseudoephedrine *on page 178*

Zyvox™ [US] *see* linezolid *on page 522*

Zyvoxam® [Can] *see* linezolid *on page 522*

APPENDIX

ABBREVIATIONS & SYMBOLS COMMONLY USED IN MEDICAL ORDERS

Abbreviation	From	Meaning
<		less than
>		greater than
≤		less than or equal to
≥		greater than or equal to
$\overline{aa}$, aa	ana	of each
AA		Alcoholics Anonymous
ABG		arterial blood gas
ac	ante cibum	before meals or food
ACA		Adult Children of Alcoholics
ACLS		advanced cardiac life support
ad	ad	to, up to
a.d.	aurio dextra	right ear
ADHD		attention-deficit/hyperactivity disorder
ADLs		activities of daily living
ad lib	ad libitum	at pleasure
AIDS		acquired immune deficiency syndrome
AIMS		Abnormal Involuntary Movement Scale
a.l.	aurio laeva	left ear
ALS		amyotrophic lateral sclerosis
AM	ante meridiem	morning
AMA		against medical advice
amp		ampul
amt		amount
aq	aqua	water
aq. dest.	aqua destillata	distilled water
ARC		AIDS-related complex
ARDS		adult respiratory distress syndrome
ARF		acute renal failure
a.s.	aurio sinister	left ear
ASAP		as soon as possible
a.u.	aures utrae	each ear
AUC		area under the curve
BDI		Beck Depression Inventory
bid	bis in die	twice daily
BLS		basic life support
bm		bowel movement
BMI		body mass index
bp		blood pressure
BPH		benign prostatic hypertrophy
BPRS		Brief Psychiatric Rating Scale
BSA		body surface area
c	cong	a gallon
$\bar{c}$	cum	with
CA		cancer
CABG		coronary artery bypass graft
CAD		coronary artery disease
cal		calorie
cap	capsula	capsule
CBT		cognitive behavioral therapy
cc		cubic centimeter
CCL		creatinine clearance
CF		cystic fibrosis
CGI		Clinical Global Impression
CIE		chemotherapy-induced emesis
CIV		continuous I.V. infusion
cm		centimeter
CNS		central nervous system
comp	compositus	compound
cont		continue

(continued)

Abbreviation	From	Meaning
COPD		chronic obstructive pulmonary disease
CRF		chronic renal failure
CT		computed tomography
d	dies	day
DBP		diastolic blood pressure
d/c		discontinue
dil	dilue	dilute
disp	dispensa	dispense
div	divide	divide
DOE		dyspnea on exertion
DSM-IV		Diagnostic and Statistical Manual
DTs		delirium tremens
dtd	dentur tales doses	give of such a dose
DVT		deep vein thrombosis
Dx		diagnosis
ECG		electrocardiogram
ECT		electroconvulsive therapy
EEG		electroencephalogram
elix, el	elixir	elixir
emp		as directed
EPS		extrapyramidal side effects
ESRD		end stage renal disease
et	et	and
EtOH		alcohol
ex aq		in water
f, ft	fac, fiat, fiant	make, let be made
FDA		Food and Drug Administration
FMS		fibromyalgia syndrome
g	gramma	gram
GA		Gamblers Anonymous
GABA		gamma-aminobutyric acid
GAD		generalized anxiety disorder
GAF		Global Assessment of Functioning Scale
GERD		gastroesophageal reflux disease
GFR		glomerular filtration rate
GITS		gastrointestinal therapeutic system
gr	granum	grain
gtt	gutta	a drop
GVHD		graft versus host disease
h	hora	hour
HAM-A		Hamilton Anxiety Scale
HAM-D		Hamilton Depression Scale
hs	hora somni	at bedtime
HSV		herpes simplex virus
HTN		hypertension
IBD		inflammatory bowel disease
IBS		irritable bowel syndrome
ICH		intracranial hemorrhage
IHSS		idiopathic hypertrophic subaortic stenosis
I.M.		intramuscular
IOP		intraocular pressure
IU		international unit
I.V.		intravenous
kcal		kilocalorie
kg		kilogram
KIU		kallikrein inhibitor unit
L		liter
LAMM		L-α-acetyl methadol
liq	liquor	a liquor, solution
LVH		left ventricular hypertrophy
M	misce	mix; Molar

(continued)

Abbreviation	From	Meaning
MADRS		Montgomery Asbery Depression Rating Scale
MAOIs		monoamine oxidase inhibitors
mcg		microgram
MDEA		3.4-methylene-dioxy amphetamine
m. dict	more dictor	as directed
MDMA		3,4-methylene-dioxy methamphetamine
mEq		milliequivalent
mg		milligram
mixt	mixtura	a mixture
mL		milliliter
mm		millimeter
mM		millimolar
MMSE		Mini-Mental State Examination
MPPP		l-methyl-4-proprionoxy-4-phenyl pyridine
MR		mental retardation
MRI		magnetic resonance image
MS		multiple sclerosis
NF		National Formulary
NKA		no known allergies
NMS		neuroleptic malignant syndrome
no.	numerus	number
noc	nocturnal	in the night
non rep	non repetatur	do not repeat, no refills
NPO		nothing by mouth
NSAID		nonsteroidal antiinflammatory drug
NV		nausea and vomiting
O, Oct	octarius	a pint
OA		osteoarthritis
OCD		obsessive-compulsive disorder
o.d.	oculus dexter	right eye
o.l.	oculus laevus	left eye
o.s.	oculus sinister	left eye
o.u.	oculo uterque	each eye
PANSS		Positive and Negative Symptom Scale
PAT		paroxysmal artrial tachycardia
pc, post cib	post cibos	after meals
PCP		phencyclidine
PD		Parkinson disease
PE		pulmonary embolus
per		through or by
PID		pelvic inflammatory disease
PM	post meridiem	afternoon or evening
P.O.	per os	by mouth
PONV		postoperative nausea and vomiting
P.R.	per rectum	rectally
prn	pro re nata	as needed
PSVT		paroxysmal supraventricular tachycardia
PTA		prior to admission
PTSD		post-traumatic stress disorder
PUD		peptic ulcer disease
pulv	pulvis	a powder
PVD		peripheral vascular disease
q		every
qad	quoque alternis die	every other day
qd		every day, daily
qh	quiaque hora	every hour
qid	quater in die	four times a day
qod		every other day
qs	quantum sufficiat	a sufficient quantity
qs ad		a sufficient quantity to make
qty		quantity

(continued)

Abbreviation	From	Meaning
qv	quam volueris	as much as you wish
RA		rheumatoid arthritis
REM		rapid eye movement
Rx	recipe	take, a recipe
rep	repetatur	let it be repeated
$\bar{s}$	sine	without
sa	secundum artem	according to art
SAH		subarachnoid hemorrhage
sat	sataratus	saturated
SBE		subacute bacterial endocarditis
SBP		systolic blood pressure
SIADH		syndrome of inappropriate antidiuretic hormone secretion
sig	signa	label, or let it be printed
SL		sublingual
SLE		systemic lupus erythematosus
SOB		shortness of breath
sol	solutio	solution
solv		dissolve
$\overline{ss}$, ss	semis	one-half
sos	si opus sit	if there is need
SSKI		saturated solution of potassium iodide
SSRIs		selective serotonin reuptake inhibitors
stat	statim	at once, immediately
STD		sexually transmitted disease
SubQ		subcutaneous
supp	suppositorium	suppository
SVT		supraventricular tachycardia
Sx		symptom
syr	syrupus	syrup
tab	tabella	tablet
tal		such
TCA		tricyclic antidepressant
TD		tardive dyskinesia
tid	ter in die	three times a day
TKO		to keep open
TPN		total parenteral nutrition
tr, tinct	tincture	tincture
trit		triturate
tsp		teaspoonful
Tx		treatment
u.d., ut dict		as directed
ULN		upper limits of normal
ung	unguentum	ointment
URI		upper respiratory infection
USAN		United States Adopted Names
USP		United States Pharmacopeia
UTI		urinary tract infection
v.o.		verbal order
VTE		venous thromboembolism
VZV		varicella zoster virus
w.a.		while awake
x3		3 times
x4		4 times
YBOC		Yale Brown Obsessive-Compulsive Scale
YMRS		Young Mania Rating Scale

NORMAL LABORATORY VALUES FOR ADULTS

Automated Chemistry (CHEMISTRY A)

Test	Values	Remarks
SERUM PLASMA		
Acetone	Negative	
Albumin	3.2-5 g/dL	
Alcohol, ethyl	Negative	
Aldolase	1.2-7.6 IU/L	
Ammonia	20-70 mcg/dL	Specimen to be placed on ice as soon as collected
Amylase	30-110 units/L	
Bilirubin, direct	0-0.3 mg/dL	
Bilirubin, total	0.1-1.2 mg/dL	
Calcium	8.6-10.3 mg/dL	
Calcium, ionized	2.24-2.46 mEq/L	
Chloride	95-108 mEq/L	
Cholesterol, total	≤200 mg/dL	Fasted blood required --- normal value affected by dietary habits This reference range is for a general adult population
HDL cholesterol	40-60 mg/dL	Fasted blood required --- normal value affected by dietary habits
LDL cholesterol	<160 mg/dL	If triglyceride is >400 mg/dL, LDL cannot be calculated accurately (Friedewald equation). Target LDL-C depends on patient's risk factors.
CO_2	23-30 mEq/L	
Creatine kinase (CK) isoenzymes		
CK-BB	0%	
CK-MB (cardiac)	0%-3.9%	
CK-MM (muscle)	96%-100%	

CK-MB levels must be both ≥4% and 10 IU/L to meet diagnostic criteria for CK-MB positive result consistent with myocardial injury.

Test	Values	Remarks
Creatine phosphokinase (CPK)	8-150 IU/L	
Creatinine	0.5-1.4 mg/dL	
Ferritin	13-300 ng/mL	
Folate	3.6-20 ng/dL	
GGT (gamma-glutamyltranspeptidase)		
male	11-63 IU/L	
female	8-35 IU/L	
GLDH	To be determined	
Glucose (preprandial)	<115 mg/dL	Goals different for diabetics
Glucose, fasting	60-110 mg/dL	Goals different for diabetics
Glucose, nonfasting (2-h postprandial)	<120 mg/dL	Goals different for diabetics
Hemoglobin A_{1c}	<8	
Hemoglobin, plasma free	<2.5 mg/100 mL	
Hemoglobin, total glycosolated (Hb A_1)	4%-8%	
Iron	65-150 mcg/dL	
Iron binding capacity, total (TIBC)	250-420 mcg/dL	
Lactic acid	0.7-2.1 mEq/L	Specimen to be kept on ice and sent to lab as soon as possible
Lactate dehydrogenase (LDH)	56-194 IU/L	
Lactate dehydrogenase (LDH) isoenzymes		
LD_1	20%-34%	
LD_2	29%-41%	
LD_3	15%-25%	
LD_4	1%-12%	
LD_5	1%-15%	

Test	Values	Remarks
Flipped LD_1/LD_2 ratios (>1 may be consistent with myocardial injury) particularly when considered in combination with a recent CK-MB positive result		
Lipase	23-208 units/L	
Magnesium	1.6-2.5 mg/dL	Increased by slight hemolysis
Osmolality	289-308 mOsm/kg	
Phosphatase, alkaline		
adults 25-60 y	33-131 IU/L	
adults 61 y or older	51-153 IU/L	
infancy-adolescence	Values range up to 3-5 times higher than adults	
Phosphate, inorganic	2.8-4.2 mg/dL	
Potassium	3.5-5.2 mEq/L	Increased by slight hemolysis
Prealbumin	>15 mg/dL	
Protein, total	6.5-7.9 g/dL	
SGOT (AST)	<35 IU/L (20-48)	
SGPT (ALT) (10-35)	<35 IU/L	
Sodium	134-149 mEq/L	
Transferrin	>200 mg/dL	
Triglycerides	45-155 mg/dL	Fasted blood required
Troponin I	<1.5 ng/mL	
Urea nitrogen (BUN)	7-20 mg/dL	
Uric acid		
male	2-8 mg/dL	
female	2-7.5 mg/dL	

Test	Values	Remarks
CEREBROSPINAL FLUID		
Glucose	50-70 mg/dL	
Protein		
adults and children	15-45 mg/dL	CSF obtained by lumbar puncture
newborn infants	60-90 mg/dL	

On CSF obtained by cisternal puncture: About 25 mg/dL

On CSF obtained by ventricular puncture: About 10 mg/dL

Note: Bloody specimen gives erroneously high value due to contamination with blood proteins

Test	Values	Remarks
URINE		
(24-hour specimen is required for all these tests unless specified)		
Amylase	32-641 units/L	The value is in units/L and **not** calculated for total volume
Amylase, fluid (random samples)		Interpretation of value left for physician, depends on the nature of fluid
Calcium	Depends upon dietary intake	
Creatine		
male	150 mg/24 h	Higher value on children and during pregnancy
female	250 mg/24 h	
Creatinine	1000-2000 mg/24 h	
Creatinine clearance (endogenous)		
male	85-125 mL/min	A blood sample must accompany urine specimen
female	75-115 mL/min	
Glucose	1 g/24 h	
5-hydroxyindoleacetic acid	2-8 mg/24 h	
Iron	0.15 mg/24 h	Acid washed container required
Magnesium	146-209 mg/24 h	
Osmolality	500-800 mOsm/kg	With normal fluid intake
Oxalate	10-40 mg/24 h	
Phosphate	400-1300 mg/24 h	
Potassium	25-120 mEq/24 h	Varies with diet; the interpretation of urine electrolytes and osmolality should be left for the physician
Sodium	40-220 mEq/24 h	
Porphobilinogen, qualitative	Negative	
Porphyrins, qualitative	Negative	
Proteins	0.05-0.1 g/24 h	
Salicylate	Negative	
Urea clearance	60-95 mL/min	A blood sample must accompany specimen
Urea N	10-40 g/24 h	Dependent on protein intake
Uric acid	250-750 mg/24 h	Dependent on diet and therapy
Urobilinogen	0.5-3.5 mg/24 h	For qualitative determination on random urine, send sample to urinalysis section in Hematology Lab
Xylose absorption test		
children	16%-33% of ingested xylose	
FECES		
Fat, 3-day collection	<5 g/d	Value depends on fat intake of 100 g/d for 3 days preceding and during collection
GASTRIC ACIDITY		
Acidity, total, 12 h	10-60 mEq/L	Titrated at pH 7

BLOOD GASES

	Arterial	Capillary	Venous
pH	7.35-7.45	7.35-7.45	7.32-7.42
pCO_2 (mm Hg)	35-45	35-45	38-52
pO_2 (mm Hg)	70-100	60-80	24-48
HCO_3 (mEq/L)	19-25	19-25	19-25
TCO_2 (mEq/L)	19-29	19-29	23-33
O_2 saturation (%)	90-95	90-95	40-70
Base excess (mEq/L)	-5 to +5	-5 to +5	-5 to +5

HEMATOLOGY

Complete Blood Count

Age	Hgb (g/dL)	Hct (%)	MCV (fL)	MCH (pg)	MCHC (%)	RBC (mill/mm^3)	RDW	PLTS (x $10^3/mm^3$)
0-3 d	15.0-20.0	45-61	95-115	31-37	29-37	4.0-5.9	<18.0	250-450
1-2 wk	12.5-18.5	39-57	86-110	28-36	28-38	3.6-5.5	<17.0	250-450
1-6 mo	10.0-13.0	29-42	74-96	25-35	30-36	3.1-4.3	<16.5	300-700
7 mo - 2 y	10.5-13.0	33-38	70-84	23-30	31-37	3.7-4.9	<16.0	250-600
2-5 y	11.5-13.0	34-39	75-87	24-30	31-37	3.9-5.0	<15.0	250-550
5-8 y	11.5-14.5	35-42	77-95	25-33	31-37	4.0-4.9	<15.0	250-550
13-18 y	12.0-15.2	36-47	78-96	25-35	31-37	4.5-5.1	<14.5	150-450
Adult male	13.5-16.5	41-50	80-100	26-34	31-37	4.5-5.5	<14.5	150-450
Adult female	12.0-15.0	36-44	80-100	26-34	31-37	4.0-4.9	<14.5	150-450

WBC and Diff

Age	WBC (x 10^3/mm^3)	Segs	Bands	Eos	Basos	Lymphs	Atypical Lymphs	Monos	# of NRBCs
0-3 d	9.0-35.0	32-62	10-18	0-2	0-1	19-29	0-8	5-7	0-2
1-2 wk	5.0-20.0	14-34	6-14	0-2	0-1	36-45	0-8	6-10	0
1-6 mo	6.0-17.5	13-33	4-12	0-3	0-1	41-71	0-8	4-7	0
7 mo - 2 y	6.0-17.0	15-35	5-11	0-3	0-1	45-76	0-8	3-6	0
2-5 y	5.5-15.5	23-45	5-11	0-3	0-1	35-65	0-8	3-6	0
5-8 y	5.0-14.5	32-54	5-11	0-3	0-1	28-48	0-8	3-6	0
13-18 y	4.5-13.0	34-64	5-11	0-3	0-1	25-45	0-8	3-6	0
Adults	4.5-11.0	35-66	5-11	0-3	0-1	24-44	0-8	3-6	0

Erythrocyte Sedimentation Rates and Reticulocyte Counts

Sedimentation rate, Westergren

Children	0-20 mm/hour
Adult male	0-15 mm/hour
Adult female	0-20 mm/hour

Sedimentation rate, Wintrobe

Children	0-13 mm/hour
Adult male	0-10 mm/hour
Adult female	0-15 mm/hour

Reticulocyte count

Newborns	2%-6%
1-6 mo	0%-2.8%
Adults	0.5%-1.5%

NORMAL LABORATORY VALUES FOR CHILDREN

CHEMISTRY		Normal Values
Albumin	0-1 y	2.0-4.0 g/dL
	1 y - adult	3.5-5.5 g/dL
Ammonia	Newborns	90-150 mcg/dL
	Children	40-120 mcg/dL
	Adults	18-54 mcg/dL
Amylase	Newborns	0-60 units/L
	Adults	30-110 units/L
Bilirubin, conjugated, direct	Newborns	<1.5 mg/dL
	1 mo - adult	0-0.5 mg/dL
Bilirubin, total	0-3 d	2.0-10.0 mg/dL
	1 mo - adult	0-1.5 mg/dL
Bilirubin, unconjugated, indirect		0.6-10.5 mg/dL
Calcium	Newborns	7.0-12.0 mg/dL
	0-2 y	8.8-11.2 mg/dL
	2 y - adult	9.0-11.0 mg/dL
Calcium, ionized, whole blood		4.4-5.4 mg/dL
Carbon dioxide, total		23-33 mEq/L
Chloride		95-105 mEq/L
Cholesterol	Newborns	45-170 mg/dL
	0-1 y	65-175 mg/dL
	1-20 y	120-230 mg/dL
Creatinine	0-1 y	≤0.6 mg/dL
	1 y - adult	0.5-1.5 mg/dL
Glucose	Newborns	30-90 mg/dL
	0-2 y	60-105 mg/dL
	Children to Adults	70-110 mg/dL
Iron	Newborns	110-270 mcg/dL
	Infants	30-70 mcg/dL
	Children	55-120 mcg/dL
	Adults	70-180 mcg/dL
Iron binding	Newborns	59-175 mcg/dL
	Infants	100-400 mcg/dL
	Adults	250-400 mcg/dL
Lactic acid, lactate		2-20 mg/dL
Lead, whole blood		<10 mcg/dL
Lipase	Children	20-140 units/L
	Adults	0-190 units/L
Magnesium		1.5-2.5 mEq/L
Osmolality, serum		275-296 mOsm/kg

CHEMISTRY		Normal Values
Osmolality, urine		50-1400 mOsm/kg
Phosphorus	Newborns	4.2-9.0 mg/dL
	6 wk to 19 mo	3.8-6.7 mg/dL
	19 mo to 3 y	2.9-5.9 mg/dL
	3-15 y	3.6-5.6 mg/dL
	>15 y	2.5-5.0 mg/dL
Potassium, plasma	Newborns	4.5-7.2 mEq/L
	2 d - 3 mo	4.0-6.2 mEq/L
	3 mo - 1 y	3.7-5.6 mEq/L
	1-16 y	3.5-5.0 mEq/L
Protein, total	0-2 y	4.2-7.4 g/dL
	>2 y	6.0-8.0 g/dL
Sodium		136-145 mEq/L
Triglycerides	Infants	0-171 mg/dL
	Children	20-130 mg/dL
	Adults	30-200 mg/dL
Urea nitrogen, blood	0-2 y	4-15 mg/dL
	2 y - adult	5-20 mg/dL
Uric acid	Male	3.0-7.0 mg/dL
	Female	2.0-6.0 mg/dL

ENZYMES

Alanine aminotransferase (ALT) (SGPT)	0-2 mo	8-78 units/L
	>2 mo	8-36 units/L
Alkaline phosphatase (ALKP)	Newborns	60-130 units/L
	0-16 y	85-400 units/L
	>16 y	30-115 units/L
Aspartate aminotransferase (AST) (SGOT)	Infants	18-74 units/L
	Children	15-46 units/L
	Adults	5-35 units/L
Creatine kinase (CK)	Infants	20-200 units/L
	Children	10-90 units/L
	Adult Male	0-206 units/L
	Adult Female	0-175 units/L
Lactate dehydrogenase (LDH)	Newborns	290-501 units/L
	1 mo - 2 y	110-144 units/L
	>16 y	60-170 units/L

THYROID FUNCTION TESTS

Test	Age	Value
T_4 (thyroxine)	1-7 d	10.1-20.9 mcg/dL
	8-14 d	9.8-16.6 mcg/dL
	1 mo - 1 y	5.5-16.0 mcg/dL
	>1 y	4.0-12.0 mcg/dL
FTI	1-3 d	9.3-26.6
	1-4 wk	7.6-20.8
	1-4 mo	7.4-17.9
	4-12 mo	5.1-14.5
	1-6 y	5.7-13.3
	>6 y	4.8-14.0
T_3 by RIA	Newborns	100-470 ng/dL
	1-5 y	100-260 ng/dL
	5-10 y	90-240 ng/dL
	10 y - adult	70-210 ng/dL
T_3 uptake		35%-45%
TSH	Cord	3-22 μIU/mL
	1-3 d	<40 μIU/mL
	3-7 d	<25 μIU/mL
	>7 d	0-10 μIU/mL

APOTHECARY/METRIC CONVERSIONS

Approximate Liquid Measures

Basic equivalent: 1 fluid ounce = 30 mL

Examples:

1 gallon	3800 mL	4 fluid oz	120 mL
1 quart	960 mL	15 minims	1 mL
1 pint	480 mL	10 minims	0.6 mL
8 fluid oz	240 mL		

1 gallon	128 fluid ounces
1 quart	32 fluid ounces
1 pint	16 fluid ounces

Approximate Household Equivalents

1 teaspoonful	5 mL	1 tablespoonful	15 mL

Weights

Basic equivalents:

1 oz = 30 g　　　15 gr = 1 g

Examples:

4 oz	120 g	1 gr	60 mg
2 oz	60 g	$^{1}/_{100}$ gr	600 mcg
10 gr	600 mg	$^{1}/_{150}$ gr	400 mcg
7 $^{1}/_{2}$ gr	500 mg	$^{1}/_{200}$ gr	300 mcg
16 oz	1 pound		

Metric Conversions

Basic equivalents:

1 g	1000 mg	1 mg	1000 mcg

Examples:

5 g	5000 mg	5 mg	5000 mcg
0.5 g	500 mg	0.5 mg	500 mcg
0.05 g	50 mg	0.05 mg	50 mcg

Exact Equivalents

1 g = 15.43 grains	0.1 mg = $^{1}/_{600}$ gr
1 milliliter (mL) = 16.23 minims	0.12 mg = $^{1}/_{500}$ gr
1 minim = 0.06 milliliter	0.15 mg = $^{1}/_{400}$ gr
1 gr = 64.8 milligrams	0.2 mg = $^{1}/_{300}$ gr
1 pint (pt) = 473.2 milliliters	0.3 mg = $^{1}/_{200}$ gr
1 oz = 28.35 grams	0.4 mg = $^{1}/_{150}$ gr
1 lb = 453.6 grams	0.5 mg = $^{1}/_{120}$ gr
1 kg = 2.2 pounds	0.6 mg = $^{1}/_{100}$ gr
1 qt = 946.4 milliliters	0.8 mg = $^{1}/_{80}$ gr
	1 mg = $^{1}/_{65}$ gr

Solids*

¼ grain = 15 mg
½ grain = 30 mg
1 grain = 60 mg
1½ grains = 90 mg
5 grains = 300 mg
10 grains = 600 mg

*Use exact equivalents for compounding and calculations requiring a high degree of accuracy.

POUNDS/KILOGRAMS CONVERSION

1 pound = 0.45359 kilograms
1 kilogram = 2.2 pounds

lb	= kg	lb	= kg	lb	= kg
1	0.45	70	31.75	140	63.50
5	2.27	75	34.02	145	65.77
10	4.54	80	36.29	150	68.04
15	6.80	85	38.56	155	70.31
20	9.07	90	40.82	160	72.58
25	11.34	95	43.09	165	74.84
30	13.61	100	45.36	170	77.11
35	15.88	105	47.63	175	79.38
40	18.14	110	49.90	180	81.65
45	20.41	115	52.16	185	83.92
50	22.68	120	54.43	190	86.18
55	24.95	125	56.70	195	88.45
60	27.22	130	58.91	200	90.72
65	29.48	135	61.24		

TEMPERATURE CONVERSION

Centigrade to Fahrenheit = (°C x 9/5) + 32 = °F
Fahrenheit to Centigrade = (°F - 32) x 5/9 = °C

°C	= °F	°C	= °F	°C	= °F
100.0	212.0	39.0	102.2	36.8	98.2
50.0	122.0	38.8	101.8	36.6	97.9
41.0	105.8	38.6	101.5	36.4	97.5
40.8	105.4	38.4	101.1	36.2	97.2
40.6	105.1	38.2	100.8	36.0	96.8
40.4	104.7	38.0	100.4	35.8	96.4
40.2	104.4	37.8	100.1	35.6	96.1
40.0	104.0	37.6	99.7	35.4	95.7
39.8	103.6	37.4	99.3	35.2	95.4
39.6	103.3	37.2	99.0	35.0	95.0
39.4	102.9	37.0	98.6	0	32.0
39.2	102.6				

ACQUIRED IMMUNODEFICIENCY SYNDROME (AIDS) — LAB TESTS AND APPROVED DRUGS FOR HIV INFECTION AND AIDS-RELATED CONDITIONS

This list of tests is not intended in any way to suggest patterns of physician's orders, nor is it complete. These tests may support possible clinical diagnoses or rule out other diagnostic possibilities. Each laboratory test relevant to AIDS is listed and weighted. Two symbols (**) indicate that the test is diagnostic, that is, documents the diagnosis if the expected is found. A single symbol (*) indicates a test frequently used in the diagnosis or management of the disease. The other listed tests are useful on a selective basis with consideration of clinical factors and specific aspects of the case.

Acid-Fast Stain
Acid-Fast Stain, Modified, *Nocardia* Species
Antimicrobial Susceptibility Testing, Fungi
Antimicrobial Susceptibility Testing, Mycobacteria
Arthropod Identification
Babesiosis Serological Test
Bacteremia Detection, Buffy Coat Micromethod
Bacterial Culture, Blood
Bacterial Culture, Bronchoscopy Specimen
Bacterial Culture, Sputum
Bacterial Culture, Stool
Bacterial Culture, Throat
Bacterial Culture, Urine, Clean Catch
Beta$_2$-Microglobulin
Blood and Fluid Precautions, Specimen Collection
Bronchial Washings Cytology
Bronchoalveolar Lavage Cytology
Brushings Cytology
Candida Antigen
Candidiasis Serologic Test
Cat Scratch Disease Serology
CD4/CD8 Enumeration
Cerebrospinal Fluid Cytology
Cryptococcal Antigen Titer
Cryptosporidium Diagnostic Procedures
Cytomegalic Inclusion Disease Cytology
Cytomegalovirus Antibody
Cytomegalovirus Antigen Detection
Cytomegalovirus Culture
Cytomegalovirus DNA Detection
Darkfield Examination, Syphilis
Electron Microscopy
Folic Acid, Serum
Fungal Culture, Biopsy or Body Fluid
Fungal Culture, Blood
Fungal Culture, Cerebrospinal Fluid
Fungal Culture, Sputum
Fungal Culture, Stool
Fungal Culture, Urine
Hemoglobin A_2
Hepatitis B Surface Antigen
Herpes Cytology
Herpes Simplex Virus Antigen Detection
Herpes Simplex Virus Culture
Histopathology
Histoplasmosis Antibody

Histoplasmosis Antigen
**HIV-1/HIV-2 Serology
HTLV-I/II Antibody
*Human Immunodeficiency Virus Culture
*Human Immunodeficiency Virus DNA Amplification
India Ink Preparation
Inhibitor, Lupus, Phospholipid Type
KOH Preparation
Leishmaniasis Serological Test
Leukocyte Immunophenotyping
Lymphocyte Transformation Test
Microsporidia Diagnostic Procedures
Mycobacteria by DNA Probe
Mycobacterial Culture, Biopsy or Body Fluid
Mycobacterial Culture, Cerebrospinal Fluid
Mycobacterial Culture, Cutaneous and Subcutaneous Tissue
Mycobacterial Culture, Sputum
Mycobacterial Culture, Stool
Neisseria gonorrhoeae Culture and Smear
Nocardia Culture
Ova and Parasites, Stool
*p24 Antigen
Platelet Count
Pneumocystis carinii Preparation
Pneumocystis Immunofluorescence
Polymerase Chain Reaction
Red Blood Cell Indices
Risks of Transfusion
Skin Biopsy
Sputum Cytology
Toxoplasmosis Serology
VDRL, Serum
Viral Culture
Viral Culture, Blood
Viral Culture, Body Fluid
Viral Culture, Central Nervous System Symptoms
Viral Culture, Dermatological Symptoms
Viral Culture, Tissue
Virus, Direct Detection by Fluorescent Antibody
White Blood Count

CURRENTLY APPROVED ANTIRETROVIRAL DRUGS

Fusion Protein Inhibitors

enfuvirtide (Fuzeon™)

Non-Nucleoside Reverse Transcriptase Inhibitors (NNRTIs)

lopinavir and ritonavir (Kaletra™)
efavirenz (Sustiva®)

Nucleoside/Nucleotide Reverse Transcriptase Inhibitors (NRTIs)

abacavir (Ziagen®)
abacavir and lamivudine (Epzicom™)
abacavir, lamivudine, and zidovudine (Trizivir®)
delavirdine (Rescriptor®)
didanosine (Videx®, Videx® EC)
emtricitabine (Emtriva™)
emtricitabine and tenofovir (Truvada™)
lamivudine (Epivir®, Epivir-HBV®)
nevirapine (Viramune®)
tenofovir (Viread™)
stavudine (Zerit®)
zalcitabine (Hivid®)
zidovudine (Retrovir®)
zidovudine + lamivudine (Combivir®)

Protease Inhibitors (PIs)

amprenavir (Agenerase®)
atazanavir (Reyataz™)
fosamprenavir (Lexiva™)
indinavir (Crixivan®)
nelfinavir (Viracept®)
ritonavir (Norvir®, Norvir® SEC)
saquinavir (Fortovase®, Invirase®)

DRUGS USED TO TREAT COMPLICATIONS OF HIV / AIDS

Generic Name (Synonym)	Brand Name	Use
alitretinoin gel 0.1%	Panretin® Gel	AIDS-related Kaposi sarcoma
amphotericin B, lipid complex (ABLC)	Abelcet®, AmBisome®	Antifungal for aspergillosis
atovaquone	Mepron®	Antiprotozoal antibiotic used to treat and prevent *Pneumocystis carinii* pneumonia
azithromycin	Zithromax®	Antibiotic used to treat *Mycobacterium avium*
cidofovir	Vistide®	Antiviral used to treat cytomegalovirus (CMV)
clarithromycin (Cla)	Biaxin®	Antibiotic used to treat and prevent *Mycobacterium avium*
daunorubicin citrate (liposomal)	DaunoXome®	Chemotherapy for Kaposi sarcoma
doxorubicin (liposomal)	Doxil®	Chemotherapy for Kaposi sarcoma
dronabinol	Marinol®	Treat loss of appetite
epoetin alfa (erythropoietin, EPO)	Procrit®, Epogen®	Treat anemia related to AZT therapy
famciclovir	Famvir®	Antiviral used to treat herpes
fluconazole	Diflucan®	Antifungal used to treat candidiasis and cryptococcal meningitis
fomivirsen sodium injection	Vitravene™ intravitreal injection	Antiviral used to treat CMV retinitis
foscarnet	Foscavir®	Antiviral used to treat herpes and CMV retinitis
ganciclovir insert	Vitrasert® Implant	Antiviral used to treat CMV retinitis
ganciclovir (DHPG)	Cytovene®	Antiviral used to treat CMV retinitis
immune globulin, intravenous (IVIG)	Gamimune® N	Immune booster used to prevent bacterial infections in children
interferon alfa-2a (IFLrA, rIFN-A)	Roferon-A®	Treat Kaposi sarcoma and hepatitis C
interferon alfa-2b (INF-alpha 2)	Intron®-A	Treat Kaposi sarcoma and hepatitis C
itraconazole	Sporanox®	Antifungal used to treat blastomycosis, histoplasmosis, aspergillosis, and candidiasis
megestrol acetate	Megace®	Treat loss of appetite and weight
paclitaxel	Taxol®	Kaposi sarcoma
pentamidine	NebuPent®	Antiprotozoal antibiotic used to prevent *Pneumocystis carinii* pneumonia
rifabutin (ansamycin)	Mycobutin®	Antimycobacterial used to prevent *Mycobacterium avium*
human growth hormone (somatrem, somatropin)	Serostim®	Treat weight loss
sulfamethoxazole and trimethoprim (co-trimoxazole)	Bactrim™, Septra®	Antiprotozoal antibiotic used to treat and prevent *Pneumocystis carinii* pneumonia
trimetrexate glucuronate	Neutrexin®	Antiprotozoal antibiotic used to treat *Pneumocystis carinii* pneumonia
valganciclovir	Valcyte™	Antiviral used to treat CMV retinitis

CHEMOTHERAPY REGIMENS

5 + 2

Use: Leukemia, acute myeloid (induction)

Regimen:

Cytarabine: I.V.: 100-200 mg/m^2/day continuous infusion days 1-5
with
Daunorubicin: I.V.: 45 mg/m^2 days 1 and 2
or
Mitoxantrone: I.V.: 12 mg/m^2 days 1 and 2

7 + 3 (Daunorubicin)

Use: Leukemia, acute myeloid (induction)

Regimen:

Cytarabine: I.V.: 100-200 mg/m^2 continuous infusion days 1-7
Daunorubicin: I.V.: 45 mg/m^2 days 1-3
Administer one cycle only

7 + 3 (Idarubicin)

Use: Leukemia, acute myeloid (induction)

Regimen:

Cytarabine: I.V.: 100-200 mg/m^2/day continuous infusion days 1-7
Idarubicin: I.V.: 12 mg/m^2 days 1-3
Administer one cycle only

7 + 3 (Mitoxantrone)

Use: Leukemia, acute myeloid (induction)

Regimen:

Cytarabine: I.V.: 100-200 mg/m^2 continuous infusion days 1-7
Mitoxantrone: I.V.: 12 mg/m^2 days 1-3
Administer one cycle only

7 + 3 + 7

Use: Leukemia, acute myeloid

Regimen:

Cytarabine: I.V.: 100 mg/m^2 continuous infusion days 1-7
Daunorubicin: I.V.: 50 mg/m^2 days 1-3
Etoposide: I.V.: 75 mg/m^2 days 1-7
Repeat cycle every 21 days; up to 3 cycles may be given based on individual response

8 in 1 (Brain Tumors)

Use: Brain tumors

Regimen:

Variation 1:

Methylprednisolone: I.V.: 300 mg/m^2 every 6 hours day 1 (3 doses)
Vincristine: I.V.: 1.5 mg/m^2 (maximum 2 mg) day 1
Lomustine: Oral: 75 mg/m^2 day 1
Procarbazine: Oral: 75 mg/m^2 day 1; 1 hour after methylprednisolone and vincristine
Hydroxyurea: Oral: 3000 mg/m^2 day 1; 2 hours after methylprednisolone and vincristine
Cisplatin: I.V.: 90 mg/m^2 day 1; 3 hours after methylprednisolone and vincristine
Cytarabine: I.V.: 300 mg/m^2 day 1; 9 hours after methylprednisolone and vincristine
Dacarbazine: I.V.: 150 mg/m^2 day 1; 12 hours after methylprednisolone and vincristine
Repeat cycle every 14 days

Variation 2:

Methylprednisolone: I.V.: 300 mg/m^2 every 6 hours day 1 (3 doses)
Vincristine: I.V.: 1.5 mg/m^2 (maximum 2 mg) day 1
Lomustine: Oral: 75 mg/m^2 day 1
Procarbazine: Oral: 75 mg/m^2 day 1; 1 hour after methylprednisolone and vincristine
Hydroxyurea: Oral: 3000 mg/m^2 day 1; 2 hours after methylprednisolone and vincristine
Cisplatin: I.V.: 60 mg/m^2 day 1; 3 hours after methylprednisolone and vincristine
Cytarabine: I.V.: 300 mg/m^2 day 1; 9 hours after methylprednisolone and vincristine
Cyclophosphamide: I.V.: 300 mg/m^2 day 1; 12 hours after methylprednisolone and vincristine
Repeat cycle every 14 days

8 in 1 (Retinoblastoma)

Use: Retinoblastoma

Regimen:

Vincristine: I.V.: 1.5 mg/m^2 day 1
Methylprednisolone: I.V.: 300 mg/m^2 day 1
Lomustine: Oral: 75 mg/m^2 day 1
Procarbazine: Oral: 75 mg/m^2 day 1
Hydroxyurea: Oral: 1500 mg/m^2 day 1
Cisplatin: I.V.: 60 mg/m^2 day 1
Cytarabine: I.V.: 300 mg/m^2 day 1
Repeat cycle every 28 days

AAV (DD)

Use: Wilms Tumor

Regimen:

Dactinomycin: I.V.: 15 mcg/kg days 1-5 of weeks 0, 13, 26, 39, 52, 65
Doxorubicin: I.V.: 20 mg/m^2 days 1-3 of weeks 6, 19, 32, 45, 58
Vincristine: I.V.: 1.5 mg/m^2 day 1 of weeks 0-10, 13, 14, 26, 27, 39, 40, 52, 53, 65, 66

ABVD

Use: Lymphoma, Hodgkin disease

Regimen:

Variation 1:

Doxorubicin: I.V.: 25 mg/m^2 days 1 and 15
Bleomycin: I.V.: 10 units/m^2 days 1 and 15
Vinblastine: I.V.: 6 mg/m^2 days 1 and 15
Dacarbazine: I.V.: 375 mg/m^2 days 1 and 15
Repeat cycle every 28 days for 6-8 cycles

Variation 2:

Doxorubicin: I.V.: 25 mg/m^2 days 1 and 14
Bleomycin: I.V.: 10 units/m^2 days 1 and 14
Vinblastine: I.V.: 6 mg/m^2 days 1 and 14
Dacarbazine: I.V.: 150 mg/m^2 days 1-5
Repeat cycle every 28 days for 6 cycles

AC

Use: Breast cancer

Regimen:

Variation 1:

Doxorubicin: I.V.: 60 mg/m^2 day 1

Cyclophosphamide: I.V.: 600 mg/m^2 day 1

Repeat cycle every 21 days

Variation 2 (dose dense):

Doxorubicin: I.V.: 60 mg/m^2 day 1

Cyclophosphamide: I.V.: 600 mg/m^2 day 1

Filgrastim: SubQ: 5 mcg/kg for 7-10 days, beginning day 3

Repeat cycle every 14 days

ACAV (J)

Use: Wilms tumor

Regimen:

Dactinomycin: I.V.: 15 mcg/kg days 1-5 of weeks 0, 13, 26, 39, 52, 65

Cyclophosphamide: I.V.: 10 mg/kg days 1-3 of weeks 0, 6, 13, 19, 26, 32, 39, 45, 52, 58, 65

Doxorubicin: I.V.: 20 mg/m^2 days 1-3 of weeks 6, 19, 32, 45, 58

Vincristine: I.V.: 1.5 mg/m^2 day 1 of weeks 0-10, 13, 14, 19, 20, 26, 27, 32, 33, 39, 40, 45, 52, 53, 56, 57, 65, 66

AC/Paclitaxel, Sequential

Use: Breast cancer

Regimen:

Doxorubicin: I.V.: 60 mg/m^2 day 1

Cyclophosphamide: I.V.: 600 mg/m^2 day 1

Repeat cycle every 21 days for 4 cycles

followed by:

Paclitaxel: I.V.: 175 mg/m^2 day 1

Repeat cycle every 21 days for 4 cycles

AP

Use: Endometrial Cancer

Regimen:

Doxorubicin: I.V.: 60 mg/m^2 day 1

Cisplatin: I.V.: 60 mg/m^2 day 1

Repeat cycle every 21 days

AV (EE)

Use: Wilms Tumor

Regimen:

Dactinomycin: I.V.: 15 mcg/kg days 1-5 of weeks 0, 5, 13, 26

Vincristine: I.V.: 1.5 mg/m^2/dose day 1 of weeks 0-10, 13, 14, 16, 17

AV (K)

Use: Wilms tumor

Regimen:

Dactinomycin: I.V.: 15 mcg/kg days 1-5 of weeks 0, 5, 13, 22, 31, 40, 49, 58

Vincristine: I.V.: 1.5 mg/m^2/dose day 1 of weeks 0-10, 15-20, 24-29, 33-38, 42-47, 51-56, 60-65

AV (L)

Use: Wilms tumor

Regimen:

Dactinomycin: I.V.: 15 mcg/kg days 1-5 of weeks 0 and 5

Vincristine: I.V.: 1.5 mg/m^2 day 1 of weeks 0-10

AV (Wilms tumor)

Use: Wilms tumor

Regimen:

Dactinomycin: I.V.: 15 mcg/kg days 1-5 of weeks 0, 13, 26, 39, 52, 65

Vincristine: I.V.: 1.5 mg/m^2/dose day 1 of weeks 0-8, 13, 14, 26, 27, 39, 40, 52, 53, 65, 66

AVD

Use: Wilms tumor

Regimen:

Dactinomycin: I.V.: 15 mcg/kg days 1-5 of weeks 0, 13, 26, 39, 52, 65

Doxorubicin: I.V.: 20 mg/m^2 days 1-3 of weeks 6, 19, 32, 45, 58

Vincristine: I.V.: 1.5 mg/m^2 day 1 of weeks 0-8, 13, 14, 26, 27, 39, 40, 52, 53, 65, 66

AVDP

Use: Leukemia, acute lymphocytic (relapse)

Regimen:

Asparaginase: I.V.: 15,000 units/m^2 days 1-5, 8-12, 15-19, 22-26

Vincristine: I.V.: 2 mg/m^2 (maximum 2 mg) days 8, 15, 22

Daunorubicin: I.V.: 30-60 mg/m^2 days 8, 15, 22

Prednisone: Oral: 40 mg/m^2 days 8-12, 15-19, 22-26

BACOP

Use: Lymphoma, non-Hodgkin

Regimen:

Bleomycin: I.V.: 5 units/m^2 days 15 and 22

Doxorubicin: I.V.: 25 mg/m^2 days 1 and 8

Cyclophosphamide: I.V.: 650 mg/m^2 days 1 and 8

Vincristine: I.V.: 1.4 mg/m^2 (maximum 2 mg) days 1 and 8

Prednisone: Oral: 60 mg/m^2 days 15-28

Repeat cycle every 28 days

BEACOPP

Use: Lymphoma, Hodgkin disease

Regimen:

Bleomycin: I.V.: 10 units/m^2 day 8

Etoposide: I.V.: 100 mg/m^2 days 1-3

Doxorubicin: I.V.: 25 mg/m^2 day 1

Cyclophosphamide: I.V.: 650 mg/m^2 day 1

Vincristine: I.V.: 1.4 mg/m^2 (maximum 2 mg) day 1

Procarbazine: Oral: 100 mg/m^2 days 1-7

Prednisone: Oral: 40 mg/m^2 days 1-14

Filgrastim: SubQ: 300-480 mcg daily from day 8 until leukocytes >2000 cells/mm^3 for 3 days

Repeat cycle every 21 days

BEP (Ovarian, Testicular)

Use: Ovarian cancer; Testicular cancer

Regimen:

Bleomycin: I.V.: 30 units days 2, 9, 15
Etoposide: I.V.: 100 mg/m^2 days 1-5 **or** 120 mg/m^2 days 1-3
Cisplatin: I.V.: 20 mg/m^2 days 1-5
Repeat cycle every 21 days

BEP (Testicular)

Use: Testicular cancer

Regimen:

Variation 1:
Bleomycin: I.V.: 30 units days 2, 9, 15
Etoposide: I.V.: 100 mg/m^2 days 1-5
Cisplatin: I.V.: 20 mg/m^2 days 1-5
Repeat cycle every 21 days

Variation 2:
Bleomycin: I.V.: 30 units once weekly
Etoposide: I.V.: 120 mg/m^2 days 1, 3, 5
Cisplatin: I.V.: 20 mg/m^2 days 1-5
Repeat cycle every 21 days

Variation 3:
Bleomycin: I.V.: 30 units days 1, 8, 15
Etoposide: I.V.: 165 mg/m^2 days 1-3
Cisplatin: I.V.: 50 mg/m^2 days 1, 2
Repeat cycle every 21 days

Bicalutamide + LHRH-A

Use: Prostate Cancer

Regimen:

Bicalutamide: Oral: 50 mg/day **with**
Goserelin acetate: SubQ: 3.6 mg day 1 **or**
Leuprolide depot: I.M.: 7.5 mg day 1
Repeat cycle every 28 days

BOLD

Use: Melanoma

Regimen:

Dacarbazine: I.V.: 200 mg/m^2 days 1-5
Vincristine: I.V.: 1 mg/m^2 days 1 and 4
Bleomycin: I.V.: 15 units days 2 and 5
Lomustine: Oral: 80 mg day 1
Repeat cycle every 4 weeks

CA

Use: Leukemia, acute myeloid

Regimen: Induction:

Cytarabine: I.V.: 3000 mg/m^2 every 12 hours days 1 and 2 (4 doses)
Asparaginase: I.M.: 6000 units/m^2 at hour 42
Repeat cycle every 7 days for 2 or 3 cycles

CABO

Use: Head and neck cancer

Regimen:

Cisplatin: I.V.: 50 mg/m^2 day 4
Methotrexate: I.V.: 40 mg/m^2 days 1 and 15
Bleomycin: I.V.: 10 units days 1, 8, and 15
Vincristine: I.V.: 2 mg days 1, 8, and 15
Repeat cycle every 21 days

CAD/MOPP/ABV

Use: Lymphoma, Hodgkin disease

Regimen:

CAD:
Lomustine: Oral: 100 mg/m^2 day 1
Melphalan: Oral: 6 mg/m^2 days 1-4
Vindesine: I.V.: 3 mg/m^2 days 1 and 8
MOPP:
Mechlorethamine: I.V.: 6 mg/m^2 days 1 and 8
Vincristine: I.V.: 1.4 mg/m^2 days 1 and 8
Procarbazine: Oral: 100 mg/m^2 days 1-14
Prednisone: Oral: 40 mg/m^2 days 1-14
ABV:
Doxorubicin: I.V.: 25 mg/m^2 days 1 and 14
Bleomycin: SubQ: 6 units/m^2 days 1 and 14
Vinblastine: I.V.: 2 mg/m^2 continuous infusion days 4-12 and 18-26
CAD is administered first, then MOPP begins on day 29 or day 37 following CAD. ABV is administered on day 29 following MOPP; CAD recycles on day 29 following ABV.

CAF

Use: Breast cancer

Regimen:

Variation 1:
Cyclophosphamide: Oral: 100 mg/m^2 days 1-14
Doxorubicin: I.V.: 30 mg/m^2 days 1 and 8
Fluorouracil: I.V.: 500 mg/m^2 days 1 and 8
Repeat cycle every 28 days
Variation 2:
Cyclophosphamide: Oral: 100 mg/m^2 days 1-14
Doxorubicin: I.V.: 25 mg/m^2 days 1 and 8
Fluorouracil: I.V.: 500 mg/m^2 days 1 and 8
Repeat cycle every 28 days

CAP

Use: Bladder Cancer

Regimen:

Cyclophosphamide: I.V.: 400 mg/m^2 day 1
Doxorubicin: I.V.: 40 mg/m^2 day 1
Cisplatin: I.V.: 60 mg/m^2 day 1
Repeat cycle every 21 days

Carbo-Tax (Adenocarcinoma)

Use: Adenocarcinoma, unknown primary

Regimen:

Paclitaxel: I.V.: 135 mg/m^2 infused over 24 hours day 1
followed by:
Carboplatin: I.V.: Target AUC 7.5
Repeat cycle every 21 days

Carbo-Tax (Nonsmall Cell Lung Cancer)

Use: Nonsmall Cell lung cancer

Regimen:

Paclitaxel: I.V.: 135-215 mg/m^2 infused over 24 hours day 1 **or** 175 mg/m^2 infused over 3 hours day 1 **followed by:**

Carboplatin: I.V.: Target AUC 7.5

Repeat cycle every 21 days

Carbo-Tax (Ovarian Cancer)

Use: Ovarian cancer

Regimen:

Variation 1:

Paclitaxel: I.V.: 135 mg/m^2 infused over 24 hours day 1 **or** 175 mg/m^2 over 3 hours day 1, **followed by:**

Carboplatin: I.V.: Target AUC 5

Repeat cycle every 21 days

Variation 2:

Paclitaxel: I.V.: 175 mg/m^2 day 1

Carboplatin: I.V.: AUC 7.5 day 1

Repeat cycle every 21 days

Variation 3:

Paclitaxel: I.V.: 185 mg/m^2 day 1

Carboplatin: I.V.: AUC 6 day 1

Repeat cycle every 21 days

CaT (Nonsmall Cell Lung Cancer)

Use: Nonsmall cell lung cancer

Regimen:

Variation 1:

Paclitaxel: I.V.: 175 mg/m^2 day 1 **or** 135 mg/m^2 continuous infusion day 1

Carboplatin: I.V.: AUC 7.5 day 1 or 2

Repeat cycle every 21 days

Variation 2:

Paclitaxel: I.V.: 225 mg/m^2 day 1

Carboplatin: I.V.: AUC 6 day 1

Repeat cycle every 21 days

CaT (Ovarian Cancer)

Use: Ovarian cancer

Regimen:

Paclitaxel: I.V.: 175 mg/m^2 day 1 **or** 135 mg/m^2 continuous infusion day 1

Carboplatin: I.V.: AUC 7.5 day 1 or 2

Repeat cycle every 21 days

CAVE

Use: Small cell lung cancer

Regimen:

Cyclophosphamide: I.V.: 750 mg/m^2 day 1

Doxorubicin: I.V.: 50 mg/m^2 day 1

Vincristine: I.V.: 1.4 mg/m^2 (maximum 2 mg) day 1

Etoposide: I.V.: 60-100 mg/m^2 days 1-3

Repeat cycle every 21 days

CAV-P/VP

Use: Neuroblastomas

Regimen:

Course 1, 2, 4, 6:
Cyclophosphamide: I.V.: 70 mg/kg days 1 and 2
Doxorubicin: I.V.: 25 mg/m^2 continuous infusion days 1-3
Vincristine: I.V.: 0.033 mg/kg continuous infusion days 1-3
Vincristine: I.V.: 1.5 mg/m^2 day 9
Course 3, 5, 7
Etoposide: I.V.: 200 mg/m^2 days 1-3
Cisplatin: I.V.: 50 mg/m^2 days 1-4

CC

Use: Ovarian cancer

Regimen:

Carboplatin: I.V.: Target AUC 5-7.5 day 1
Cyclophosphamide: I.V.: 600 mg/m^2 day 1
Repeat cycle every 28 days

CCCDE (Retinoblastoma)

Use: Retinoblastoma

Regimen:

Cyclophosphamide: I.V.: 150 mg/m^2 days 1-7
Cyclophosphamide: Oral: 150 mg/m^2 days 22-28, 43-49
Doxorubicin: I.V.: 35 mg/m^2 days 10 and 52
Cisplatin: I.V.: 90 mg/m^2 days 8, 50, 71
Etoposide: I.V.: 150 mg/m^2 continuous infusion days 29-31, 73-75

CCDDT (Neuroblastomas)

Use: Neuroblastomas

Regimen:

Cyclophosphamide: I.V.: 40 mg/kg days 1 and 2
Cisplatin: I.V.: 20 mg/m^2 days 1-5
Teniposide: I.V.: 100 mg/m^2 day 7
Doxorubicin: I.V.: 60 mg/m^2 day 1
Dacarbazine: I.V.: 250 mg/m^2 days 1-5
Repeat cycle every 21-28 days

CCDLMV (Burkitt Lymphoma)

Use: Lymphoma, non-Hodgkin (Burkitt)

Regimen:

Methotrexate: I.T.: 10 mg/m^2 at hour 0
Cytarabine: I.T.: 50 mg/m^2 at hour 0
Cyclophosphamide: I.V.: 300 mg/m^2 every 12 hours (for 6 doses) at hours 0, 12, 24, 36, 48, 60
Vincristine: I.V.: 1.5 mg/m^2 at hour 72
Doxorubicin: I.V.: 50 mg/m^2 at hour 72
Followed after hematopoietic recovery by
Methotrexate: I.T.: 12 mg/m^2 at hour 0
Methotrexate: I.V. push: 200 mg/m^2, then 800 mg/m^2 as a 24-hour infusion from hours 0-24
Cytarabine: I.T.: 50 mg/m^2 at hour 24
Cytarabine: I.V.: 400 mg/m^2 over 48 hours from hours 24-72, with escalating doses in succeeding courses
Leucovorin: I.V.: 30 mg/m^2 at hours 36 and 42, then 3 mg/m^2 at hours 54, 66, 78

CCDT (Melanoma)

Use: Melanoma

Regimen:

Dacarbazine: I.V.: 220 mg/m^2 days 1-3, every 21-28 days
Carmustine: I.V.: 150 mg/m^2 day 1, every 42-56 days
Cisplatin: I.V.: 25 mg/m^2 days 1-3, every 21-28 days
Tamoxifen: Oral: 20 mg/day (use of tamoxifen is optional)

CCT (Neuroblastomas)

Use: Neuroblastomas

Regimen:

Cyclophosphamide: I.V.: 40 mg/kg days 1 and 2
Cisplatin: I.V.: 20 mg/m^2 days 22-26
Teniposide: I.V.: 100 mg/m^2 day 28
Repeat every 42 days for 3 cycles

CD (Rhabdomyosarcoma)

Use: Rhabdomyosarcoma

Regimen:

Doxorubicin: I.V.: 35-60 mg/m^2 day 1
Cyclophosphamide: I.V.: 500-1500 mg/m^2 day 1
Repeat cycle every 21-28 days

CDDP/VP-16

Use: Brain tumors

Regimen:

Variation 1:
Cisplatin: I.V.: 90 mg/m^2 day 1
Etoposide: I.V.: 150 mg/m^2 days 3 and 4
Repeat cycle every 21 days

Variation 2:
Cisplatin: I.V.: 40 mg/m^2 days 1-5
Etoposide: I.V.: 100 mg/m^2 days 1-5
Repeat cycle every 28 days

CDLPV (Leukemia)

Use: Leukemia, acute lymphocytic (induction)

Regimen:

Cyclophosphamide: I.V.: 1200 mg/m^2 day 1
Daunorubicin: I.V.: 45 mg/m^2 days 1-3
Prednisone: Oral: 60 mg/m^2 days 1-21
Vincristine: I.V.: 2 mg/m^2/week
Asparaginase: I.V.: 6000 units/m^2 3 times/week
or
Pegaspargase: I.M., I.V.: 2500 units/m^2 every 14 days if patient develops hypersensitivity to native L-asparaginase

CE (Neuroblastomas)

Use: Neuroblastomas

Regimen:

Carboplatin: I.V.: 500 mg/m^2 days 1 and 2
Etoposide: I.V.: 100 mg/m^2 days 1-3
Repeat cycle every 21-28 days

CE (Retinoblastoma)

Use: Retinoblastoma
Regimen:

Etoposide: I.V.: 100 mg/m^2 days 1-5
Carboplatin: I.V.: 160 mg/m^2 days 1-5
Repeat cycle every 21 days

CE (Wilms Tumor)

Use: Wilms Tumor
Regimen:

Etoposide: I.V.: 100 mg/m^2 days 1-5
Carboplatin: I.V.: 160 mg/m^2 days 1-5

CE-CAdO

Use: Neuroblastomas
Regimen:

Carboplatin: I.V.: 160 mg/m^2 days 1-5
Etoposide: I.V.: 100 mg/m^2 days 1-5
or
Carboplatin: I.V.: 200 mg/m^2 days 1-3
Etoposide: I.V.: 150 mg/m^2 days 1-3
and
Cyclophosphamide: I.V.: 300 mg/m^2 days 1-5
Doxorubicin: I.V.: 60 mg/m^2 day 5
Vincristine: I.V.: 1.5 mg/m^2 days 1 and 5
Repeat cycle every 21 days

CEF

Use: Breast cancer
Regimen:

Cyclophosphamide: Oral: 75 mg/m^2 days 1-14
Epirubicin: I.V.: 60 mg/m^2 days 1 and 8
Fluorouracil: I.V.: 500 mg/m^2 days 1 and 8
Repeat cycle every 28 days

CEV

Use: Rhabdomyosarcoma
Regimen:

Carboplatin: I.V.: 500 mg/m^2 day 1
Epirubicin: I.V.: 150 mg/m^2 day 1
Vincristine: I.V.: 1.5 mg/m^2 days 1 and 7
Repeat cycle every 21 days

CF

Use: Head and neck cancer
Regimen:

Variation 1:
Cisplatin: I.V.: 100 mg/m^2 day 1
Fluorouracil: I.V.: 1000 mg/m^2 continuous infusion days 1-4 or days 1-5
Repeat cycle every 21-28 days
Variation 2:
Carboplatin: I.V.: 400 mg/m^2 day 1
Fluorouracil: I.V.: 1000 mg/m^2 continuous infusion days 1-4 or days 1-5
Repeat cycle every 21-28 days

CHAMOCA

Use: Gestational trophoblastic tumor
Regimen:

Hydroxyurea: Oral: 500 mg every 6 hours for 4 doses, day 1 (start at 6 AM)
Dactinomycin: I.V.: 0.2 mg days 1-3 (give at 7 PM) **followed by** 0.5 mg days 4 and 5 (give at 7 PM)
Cyclophosphamide: I.V.: 500 mg/m^2 days 3 and 8 (give at 7 PM)
Vincristine: I.V.: 1 mg/m^2 (maximum 2 mg) day 2 (give at 7 AM)
Methotrexate: I.V. push: 100 mg/m^2 day 2 (give at 7 PM) **followed by** 200 mg/m^2 over 12 hours day 2
Leucovorin: I.M.: 14 mg every 6 hours for 6 doses days 3-5 (begin at 7 PM on day 3)
Doxorubicin: I.V.: 30 mg/m^2 day 8 (give at 7 PM)
Repeat cycle every 18 days or as toxicity permits

ChlVPP

Use: Lymphoma, Hodgkin disease
Regimen:

Chlorambucil: Oral: 6 mg/m^2 (maximum 10 mg) days 1-14
Vinblastine: I.V.: 6 mg/m^2 (maximum 10 mg) days 1 and 8
Procarbazine: Oral: 100 mg/m^2 (maximum 150 mg) days 1-14
Prednisone: Oral: 40-50 mg/m^2 days 1-14
Repeat cycle every 28 days

CHL + PRED

Use: Leukemia, chronic lymphocytic
Regimen:

Chlorambucil: Oral: 0.4 mg/kg/day for 1 day every other week; increase initial dose of 0.4 mg/kg by 0.1 mg/kg every 2 weeks until toxicity or disease control is achieved
Prednisone: Oral: 100 mg/day for 2 days every other week

CHOP

Use: Lymphoma, non-Hodgkin
Regimen:

Cyclophosphamide: I.V.: 750 mg/m^2 day 1
Doxorubicin: I.V.: 50 mg/m^2 day 1
Vincristine: I.V.: 1.4 mg/m^2 (maximum 2 mg) day 1
Prednisone: Oral: 100 mg days 1-5 **or** 50-57 mg/m^2 days 1-5
Repeat cycle every 21 days

CHOP-Bleo

Use: Lymphoma, non-Hodgkin
Regimen:

Cyclophosphamide: I.V.: 750 mg/m^2 day 1
Doxorubicin: I.V.: 50 mg/m^2 day 1
Vincristine: I.V.: 2 mg days 1 and 5
Prednisone: Oral: 100 mg days 1-5
Bleomycin: I.V.: 15 units days 1 and 5
Repeat cycle every 21-28 days

CI (Neuroblastomas)

Use: Neuroblastomas
Regimen:

Ifosfamide: I.V.: 1500 mg/m^2 days 1-3
Carboplatin: I.V.: 400 mg/m^2 day 4
Repeat cycle every 21-28 days

CISCA

Use: Bladder cancer

Regimen:

Cyclophosphamide: I.V.: 650 mg/m^2 day 1
Doxorubicin: I.V.: 50 mg/m^2 day 1
Cisplatin: I.V.: 100 mg/m^2 day 2
Repeat cycle every 21-28 days

Cisplatin-Docetaxel

Use: Bladder cancer

Regimen:

Cisplatin: I.V.: 30 mg/m^2 day 1
Docetaxel: I.V.: 40 mg/m^2 day 4
Repeat cycle weekly for 8 weeks

Cisplatin-Fluorouracil

Use: Cervical cancer

Regimen:

Variation 1:
Cisplatin: I.V.: 75 mg/m^2 day 1
Fluorouracil: I.V.: 1000 mg/m^2 continuous infusion days 1-4 (96 hours)
Repeat cycle every 21 days
Variation 2:
Cisplatin: I.V.: 50 mg/m^2 day 1 starting 4 hours before radiotherapy
Fluorouracil: I.V.: 1000 mg/m^2 continuous infusion days 2-5 (96 hours)
Repeat cycle every 28 days

Cisplatin-Vinorelbine

Use: Cervical cancer

Regimen:

Cisplatin: I.V.: 80 mg/m^2 day 1
Vinorelbine: I.V.: 25 mg/m^2 days 1 and 8
Repeat cycle every 21 days

CMF

Use: Breast cancer

Regimen:

Variation 1:
Methotrexate: I.V.: 40 mg/m^2 days 1 and 8
Fluorouracil: I.V.: 600 mg/m^2 days 1 and 8
Cyclophosphamide: Oral: 100 mg/m^2 days 1-14
Repeat cycle every 28 days
Variation 2 (older than 60 years):
Methotrexate: I.V.: 30 mg/m^2 days 1 and 8
Fluorouracil: I.V.: 400 mg/m^2 days 1 and 8
Cyclophosphamide: Oral: 100 mg/m^2 days 1-14
Repeat cycle every 28 days

CMF-IV

Use: Breast cancer

Regimen:

Cyclophosphamide: I.V.: 600 mg/m^2 day 1
Methotrexate: I.V.: 40 mg/m^2 day 1
Fluorouracil: I.V.: 600 mg/m^2 day 1
Repeat cycle every 21 or 28 days

CMV

Use: Bladder cancer

Regimen:

Cisplatin: I.V.: 100 mg/m^2 infused over 4 hours (start 12 hours after methotrexate) day 2

Methotrexate: I.V.: 30 mg/m^2 days 1 and 8

Vinblastine: I.V.: 4 mg/m^2 days 1 and 8

Repeat cycle every 21 days

CNF

Use: Breast cancer

Regimen:

Variation 1:

Cyclophosphamide: I.V: 500 mg/m^2 day 1

Mitoxantrone: I.V.: 10 mg/m^2 day 1

Fluorouracil: I.V.: 500 mg/m^2 day 1

Repeat cycle every 21 days

Variation 2:

Cyclophosphamide: I.V.: 500-600 mg/m^2 day 1

Fluorouracil: I.V.: 500-600 mg/m^2 day 1

Mitoxantrone: I.V.: 10-12 mg/m^2 day 1

Repeat cycle every 21 days

CNOP

Use: Lymphoma, non-Hodgkin

Regimen:

Cyclophosphamide: I.V.: 750 mg/m^2 day 1

Mitoxantrone: I.V.: 10 mg/m^2 day 1

Vincristine: I.V.: 1.4 mg/m^2 day 1

Prednisone: Oral: 50 mg/m^2 days 1-5

Repeat cycle every 21 days

CO

Use: Retinoblastoma

Regimen:

Cyclophosphamide: I.V.: 10 mg/kg days 1-3

Vincristine: I.V.: 1.5 mg/m^2 day 1

Repeat cycle every 21 days

COMLA

Use: Lymphoma, non-Hodgkin

Regimen:

Cyclophosphamide: I.V.: 1500 mg/m^2 day 1

Vincristine: I.V.: 1.4 mg/m^2 (maximum 2.5 mg) days 1, 8, 15

Methotrexate: I.V.: 120 mg/m^2 days 22, 29, 36, 43, 50, 57, 64, 71

Leucovorin calcium rescue: Oral: 25 mg/m^2 every 6 hours for 4 doses (beginning 24 hours after each methotrexate dose)

Cytarabine: I.V.: 300 mg/m^2 days 22, 29, 36, 43, 50, 57, 64, 71

Repeat cycle every 21 days

COMP

Use: Lymphoma, Hodgkin disease

Regimen:

Cyclophosphamide: I.V.: 1200 mg/m^2 day 1, cycle 1 **followed by** 1000 mg/m^2 day 1 on subsequent cycles

Vincristine: I.V.: 2 mg/m^2 (maximum 2 mg) days 3, 10, 17, 24, cycle 1 **followed by** 1.5 mg/m^2 days 1 and 4, on subsequent cycles

Methotrexate: I.V.: 300 mg/m^2 day 12

Prednisone: Oral: 60 mg/m^2 (maximum 60 mg) days 3-30 then taper for 7 days, cycle 1 **followed by** 60 mg/m^2 (maximum 60 mg) days 1-5, on subsequent cycles

Maintenance cycles repeat every 28 days

COP

Use: Lymphoma, non-Hodgkin

Regimen:

Cyclophosphamide: I.V.: 800 mg/m^2 day 1

Vincristine: I.V.: 1.4 mg/m^2 (maximum 2 mg) day 1

Prednisone: Oral: 60 mg/m^2 days 1-5

Repeat cycle every 21 days

COP-BLAM

Use: Lymphoma, non-Hodgkin

Regimen:

Cyclophosphamide: I.V.: 400 mg/m^2 day 1

Vincristine: I.V.: 1 mg/m^2 day 1

Prednisone: Oral: 40 mg/m^2 days 1-10

Bleomycin: I.V.: 15 mg day 14

Doxorubicin: I.V.: 40 mg/m^2 day 1

Procarbazine: Oral: 100 mg/m^2 days 1-10

COPE or Baby Brain I

Use: Brain cancer

Regimen:

Cycle A:

Vincristine: I.V.: 0.065 mg/kg (max: 1.5 mg) days 1, 8

Cyclophosphamide: I.V.: 65 mg/kg day 1

Cycle B:

Cisplatin: I.V.: 4 mg/m^2 day 1

Etoposide: I.V.: 6.5 mg/kg days 3, 4

Repeat cycle every 28 days in the following sequence: AABAAB

COPP (C MOPP)

Use: Lymphoma, non-Hodgkin

Regimen:

Cyclophosphamide: I.V.: 400-650 mg/m^2 days 1 and 8

Vincristine: I.V.: 1.4-2 mg/m^2 (maximum 2 mg) days 1 and 8

Procarbazine: Oral: 100 mg/m^2 days 1-14

Prednisone: Oral: 40 mg/m^2 days 1-14

Repeat cycle every 28 days

CP (Leukemia)

Use: Leukemia, chronic lymphocytic

Regimen:

Chlorambucil: Oral: 30 mg/m^2 day 1
Prednisone: Oral: 80 mg days 1-5
Repeat cycle every 14 days

CP (Ovarian Cancer)

Use: Ovarian cancer

Regimen:

Cyclophosphamide: I.V.: 750 mg/m^2 day 1
Cisplatin: I.V.: 75 mg/m^2 day 1
Repeat cycle every 21 days

CT

Use: Ovarian cancer

Regimen:

Paclitaxel: I.V.: 135 mg/m^2 continuous infusion day 1
Cisplatin: I.V.: 75 mg/m^2 day 2
Repeat cycle every 21 days

CV

Use: Retinoblastoma

Regimen:

Cyclophosphamide: I.V.: 300 mg/m^2
Vincristine: I.V.: 1.5 mg/m^2
Repeat weekly for 6 weeks
followed by:
Cyclophosphamide: I.V.: 200 mg/m^2
Vincristine: I.V.: 1.5 mg/m^2
Repeat weekly for 42 weeks

CVD

Use: Melanoma

Regimen:

Vinblastine: I.V.: 1.6 mg/m^2 days 1-5
Dacarbazine: I.V.: 800 mg/m^2 day 1
Cisplatin: I.V.: 20 mg/m^2 days 2-5
Repeat cycle every 21 days

CVP (Leukemia)

Use: Leukemia, chronic lymphocytic

Regimen:

Variation 1:
Cyclophosphamide: Oral: 400 or 300 mg/m^2 days 1-5
Vincristine: I.V.: 1.4 mg/m^2 (maximum 2 mg) day 1
Prednisone: Oral: 100 mg/m^2 days 1-5
Repeat cycle every 21 days
Variation 2:
Cyclophosphamide: I.V.: 800 mg/m^2 day 1
Vincristine: I.V.: 1.4 mg/m^2 (maximum 2 mg) day 1
Prednisone: Oral: 100 mg/m^2 days 1-5
Repeat cycle every 21 days

CVP (Lymphoma, non-Hodgkin)

Use: Lymphoma, non-Hodgkin

Regimen:

Cyclophosphamide: Oral: 400 mg/m^2 days 1-5
Vincristine: I.V.: 1.4 mg/m^2 day 1
Prednisone: Oral: 100 mg/m^2 days 1-5
Repeat cycle every 21 days

Cyclophosphamide + Doxorubicin

Use: Prostate cancer

Regimen:

Doxorubicin: I.V.: 40 mg/m^2 day 1
Cyclophosphamide: I.V.: 800-2000 mg/m^2 day 1
Filgrastim: SubQ: 5 mcg/kg days 2-10 (or until ANC >10,000 cells/µL
Repeat cycle every 21 days

Cyclophosphamide + Estramustine

Use: Prostate cancer

Regimen:

Cyclophosphamide: Oral: 2 mg/kg days 1-14
Estramustine: Oral: 10 mg/kg days 1-14
Repeat cycle every 28 days

Cyclophosphamide + Etoposide

Use: Prostate cancer

Regimen:

Cyclophosphamide: Oral: 100 mg days 1-14
Etoposide: Oral: 50 mg days 1-14
Repeat cycle every 28 days

Cyclophosphamide + Vincristine + Dexamethasone

Use: Prostate cancer

Regimen:

Cyclophosphamide: Oral: 250 mg days 1-14
Vincristine: I.V.: 1 mg days 1, 8, and 15
Dexamethasone: Oral: 0.75 mg twice daily days 1-14
Repeat cycle every 28 days

CYVADIC

Use: Sarcoma

Regimen:

Cyclophosphamide: I.V.: 500 mg/m^2 day 1
Vincristine: I.V.: 1.4 mg/m^2 days 1 and 5
Doxorubicin: I.V.: 50 mg/m^2 day 1
Dacarbazine: I.V.: 250 mg/m^2 days 1-5
Repeat cycle every 21 days

DA

Use: Leukemia, acute myeloid (induction)

Regimen: Induction:

Daunorubicin: I.V.: 45 mg/m^2 days 1-3
Cytarabine: I.V.: 100 mg/m^2 continuous infusion days 1-7

Dacarbazine/Tamoxifen

Use: Melanoma
Regimen:

Dacarbazine: I.V.: 250 mg/m^2 days 1-5, every 21 days
Tamoxifen: Oral: 20 mg/day (use of tamoxifen is optional)

Dartmouth Regimen

Use: Melanoma
Regimen:

Tamoxifen: Oral: 10 mg twice daily starting 1 week prior to chemotherapy and continuing indefinitely
Carmustine: I.V.: 150 mg/m^2 day 1 (every other cycle)
Cisplatin: I.V.: 25 mg/m^2 days 1-3
Dacarbazine: I.V.: 220 mg/m^2 days 1-3
Repeat cycle every 21 days

DAT

Use: Leukemia, acute myeloid (induction)
Regimen: Induction:

Daunorubicin: I.V. bolus: 45 mg/m^2 days 1-3
Cytarabine: I.V. bolus: 200 mg/m^2
Thioguanine: Oral: 100 mg/m^2 days 1-7

DAV

Use: Leukemia, acute myeloid
Regimen: Induction:

Daunorubicin: I.V.: 60 mg/m^2 days 3-5
Cytarabine: I.V.: 100 mg/m^2 continuous infusion days 1-2 **followed by** 100 mg/m^2 every 12 hours days 3-8 (12 doses)
Etoposide: I.V.: 150 mg/m^2 days 6-8
Administer one cycle only

DDV

Use: Wilms tumor
Regimen:

Vincristine: I.V.: 1.5 mg/m^2/dose (maximum 2 mg/dose) every 7 days for 10 weeks
Dactinomycin: I.V.: 0.45 mg/m^2 every 21 days
alternating with:
Vincristine: I.V.: 1.5 mg/m^2/dose (maximum 2 mg/dose) every 7 days for 10 weeks
Doxorubicin: I.V.: 30 mg/m^2 every 21 days

DHAP

Use: Lymphoma, non-Hodgkin

Regimen:

Variation 1:

Dexamethasone: I.V.: 10 mg every 6 hours days 1-4

Cytarabine: I.V.: 2 g/m^2 every 12 hours for 2 doses day 2

Cisplatin: I.V.: 100 mg/m^2 continuous infusion day 1

Repeat cycle every 21-28 days

Variation 2:

Dexamethasone: I.V. or Oral: 40 mg days 1-4

Cisplatin: I.V.: 100 mg/m^2 day 1

Cytarabine: I.V.: 2000 mg/m^2 every 12 hours for 2 doses day 2 (begins at the end of the cisplatin infusion)

Repeat cycle every 3-4 weeks for 6-10 cycles (salvage therapy) or 1-2 cycles (mobilization prior to high-dose therapy with peripheral hematopoietic progenitor cell support)

Variation 3:

Dexamethasone: I.V. or Oral: 40 mg days 1-4

Oxaliplatin: I.V.: 130 mg/m^2 day 1

Cytarabine: I.V.: 2000 mg/m^2 every 12 hours for 2 doses day 2

Repeat cycle every 3 weeks

DMC

Use: Gestational trophoblastic tumor

Regimen:

Dactinomycin: I.V.: 0.37 mg/m^2 days 1-5

Methotrexate: I.V.: 11 mg/m^2 days 1-5

Cyclophosphamide: I.V.: 110 mg/m^2 days 1-5

Repeat cycle every 21 days

Docetaxel-Cisplatin

Use: Nonsmall cell lung cancer

Regimen:

Docetaxel: I.V.: 75 mg/m^2 day 1

Cisplatin: I.V.: 75 mg/m^2 day 1

Repeat cycle every 21 days

Doxorubicin + Ketoconazole

Use: Prostate cancer

Regimen:

Doxorubicin: I.V.: 20 mg/m^2 continuous infusion day 1

Ketoconazole: Oral: 400 mg 3 times/day days 1-7

Repeat cycle every 7 days

Doxorubicin + Ketoconazole/Estramustine + Vinblastine

Use: Prostate cancer

Regimen:

Doxorubicin: I.V.: 20 mg/m^2 days 1, 15, and 29

Ketoconazole: Oral: 400 mg 3 times/day days 1-7, 15-21, and 29-35

Estramustine: Oral: 140 mg 3 times/day days 8-14, 22-28, and 36-42

Vinblastine: I.V.: 5 mg/m^2 days 8, 22, and 36

Repeat cycle every 8 weeks

DVP

Use: Leukemia, acute lymphocytic
Regimen: Induction:

Daunorubicin: I.V.: 25 mg/m^2 days 1, 8, and 15
Vincristine: I.V.: 1.5 mg/m^2 (maximum 2 mg) days 1, 8, 15, and 22
Prednisone: Oral: 60 mg/m^2 days 1-28 then taper over next 14 days
Administer single cycle; used in conjunction with intrathecal chemotherapy

EAP

Use: Gastric cancer
Regimen:

Etoposide: I.V.: 120 mg/m^2 days 4, 5, 6
Doxorubicin: I.V.: 20 mg/m^2 days 1 and 7
Cisplatin: I.V.: 40 mg/m^2 days 2 and 8
Repeat cycle every 28 days

EC (Nonsmall Cell Lung Cancer)

Use: Nonsmall cell lung cancer
Regimen:

Etoposide: I.V.: 120 mg/m^2 days 1-3
Carboplatin: I.V.: AUC 6 day 1
Repeat cycle every 21-28 days

EC (Small Cell Lung Cancer)

Use: Small cell lung cancer
Regimen:

Variation 1:
Etoposide: I.V.: 100-120 mg/m^2 days 1-3
Carboplatin: I.V.: 325-400 mg/m^2 day 1
Repeat cycle every 28 days
Variation 2:
Etoposide: I.V.: 120 mg/m^2 days 1-3
Carboplatin: I.V.: AUC 6 day 1
Repeat cycle every 21-28 days

EDAP

Use: Multiple myeloma
Regimen:

Etoposide: I.V.: 100-200 mg/m^2 days 1-4
Dexamethasone: Oral, I.V.: 40 mg/m^2 days 1-5
Cytarabine: I.V.: 1000 mg day 5
Cisplatin: I.V.: 20 mg continuous infusion days 1-4

EE

Use: Wilms tumor
Regimen:

Dactinomycin: I.V.: 15 mcg/kg days 1-5 of weeks 0, 5, 13, 24
Vincristine: I.V.: 1.5 mg/m^2 day 1 of weeks 1-10, 13, 14, 24, 25

EE-4A

Use: Wilms tumor
Regimen:

Dactinomycin: I.V.: 45 mcg/kg day 1 of weeks 0, 3, 6, 9, 12, 15, 18
Vincristine: I.V.: 2 mg/m^2 day 1 of weeks 1-10, 12, 15, 18

ELF

Use: Gastric cancer

Regimen:

Leucovorin calcium: I.V.: 300 mg/m^2 days 1-3, **followed by:**

Etoposide: I.V.: 120 mg/m^2 days 1-3, **followed by:**

Fluorouracil: I.V.: 500 mg/m^2 days 1-3

Repeat cycle every 21-28 days

EMA 86

Use: Leukemia, acute myeloid

Regimen: Induction:

Mitoxantrone: I.V.: 12 mg/m^2 days 1-3

Etoposide: I.V.: 200 mg/m^2 continuous infusion days 8-10

Cytarabine: I.V.: 500 mg/m^2 continuous infusion days 1-3 and 8-10

Administer one cycle only

EMA/CO

Use: Gestational trophoblastic tumor

Regimen:

Etoposide: I.V.: 100 mg/m^2 days 1 and 2

Methotrexate: I.V.: 300 mg/m^2 infused over 12 hours day 1

Dactinomycin: I.V. push: 0.5 mg days 1 and 2

Leucovorin: Oral, I.M.: 15 mg twice daily for 2 days (start 24 hours after the start of methotrexate) days 2, 3

Alternate weekly with:

Cyclophosphamide: I.V.: 600 mg/m^2 infused over 30 minutes day 1

Vincristine: I.V. push: 0.8 mg/m^2 (maximum 2 mg) day 1

EP (Adenocarcinoma)

Use: Adenocarcinoma, unknown primary

Regimen:

Cisplatin: I.V.: 60-100 mg/m^2 day 1

Etoposide: I.V.: 80-100 mg/m^2 days 1-3

Repeat cycle every 21 days

EP (Nonsmall Cell Lung Cancer)

Use: Nonsmall cell lung cancer

Regimen:

Etoposide: I.V.: 80-120 mg/m^2 days 1-3

Cisplatin: I.V.: 80-100 mg/m^2 day 1

Repeat cycle every 21-28 days

EP (Small Cell Lung Cancer)

Use: Small cell lung cancer

Regimen:

Variation 1:
Etoposide: I.V.: 100 mg/m^2 days 1-3
Cisplatin: I.V.: 25 mg/m^2 days 1-3
Repeat cycle every 21 days for 4-6 cycles

Variation 2:
Etoposide: I.V.: 100 mg/m^2 days 1-3
Cisplatin: I.V.: 100 mg/m^2 day 1
Repeat cycle every 21 days

Variation 3:
Etoposide: I.V.: 80 mg/m^2 days 1-3
Cisplatin: I.V.: 80 mg/m^2 day 1
Repeat cycle every 21-28 days

EP (Testicular Cancer)

Use: Testicular cancer

Regimen:

Variation 1:
Etoposide: I.V.: 100 mg/m^2 days 1-5
Cisplatin: I.V.: 20 mg/m^2 days 1-5
Repeat cycle every 21 days

Variation 2:
Etoposide: I.V.: 120 mg/m^2 days 1-3
Cisplatin: I.V.: 20 mg/m^2 days 1-5
Repeat cycle every 3 or 4 weeks

Variation 3:
Etoposide: I.V.: 120 mg/m^2 days 1, 3, and 5
Cisplatin: I.V.: 20 mg/m^2 days 1-5
Repeat cycle every 3 or 4 weeks

EP/EMA

Use: Gestational trophoblastic tumor

Regimen:

Etoposide: I.V.: 150 mg/m^2 day 1
Cisplatin: I.V.: 25 mg/m^2 infused over 4 hours for 3 consecutive doses, day 1 (total: 75 mg/m^2)

Alternate weekly with:
Etoposide: I.V.: 100 mg/m^2 day 1
Methotrexate: I.V.: 300 mg/m^2 infused over 12 hours day 1
Dactinomycin: I.V. push: 0.5 mg day 1
Leucovorin: Oral, I.M.: 15 mg twice daily for 2 days (start 24 hours after the start of methotrexate) days 2, 3

EPOCH

Use: Lymphoma, non-Hodgkin

Regimen:

Etoposide: I.V.: 50 mg/m^2 continuous infusion days 1-4
Vincristine: I.V.: 0.4 mg/m^2 continuous infusion days 1-4
Doxorubicin: I.V.: 10 mg/m^2 continuous infusion days 1-4
Cyclophosphamide: I.V.: 750 mg/m^2 day 6
Prednisone: Oral: 60 mg/m^2 days 1-6
Repeat cycle every 21 days

EP/PE

Use: Nonsmall cell lung cancer

Regimen:

Etoposide: I.V.: 120 mg/m^2 days 1-3
Cisplatin: I.V.: 60-120 mg/m^2 day 1
Repeat cycle every 21-28 days

ESHAP

Use: Lymphoma, non-Hodgkin

Regimen:

Variation 1:
Etoposide: I.V.: 40 mg/m^2 days 1-4
Methylprednisolone: I.V.: 500 mg days 1-5
Cytarabine: I.V.: 2 g/m^2 day 1
Cisplatin: I.V.: 25 mg/m^2 continuous infusion days 1-4
Repeat cycle every 21-28 days

Variation 2:
Etoposide: I.V.: 40 mg/m^2 days 1-4
Methylprednisolone: I.V.: 500 mg days 1-5
Cytarabine: I.V.: 2 g/m^2 day 5
Cisplatin: I.V.: 25 mg/m^2 continuous infusion days 1-4
Repeat cycle every 21-28 days

Variation 3:
Etoposide: I.V.: 60 mg/m^2 days 1-4
Methylprednisolone: I.V.: 500 mg days 1-4
Cytarabine: I.V.: 2 g/m^2 day 5
Cisplatin: I.V.: 25 mg/m^2 continuous infusion days 1-4
Repeat cycle every 21 days

Estramustine + Docetaxel

Use: Prostate cancer

Regimen:

Variation 1:
Docetaxel: I.V.: 20-80 mg/m^2 day 2
Estramustine: Oral: 280 mg 3 times/day days 1-5
Repeat cycle every 21 days

Variation 2:
Docetaxel: I.V.: 20-80 mg/m^2 day 2
Estramustine: Oral: 14 mg/kg days 1-21
Repeat cycle every 21 days

Variation 3:
Docetaxel: I.V.: 35 mg/m^2 days 2 and 9
Estramustine: Oral: 420 mg 3 times/day for 4 doses, then 280 mg 3 times/day for 5 doses days 1, 2, 3, 8, 9, and 10
Repeat cycle every 21 days

Estramustine + Docetaxel + Carboplatin

Use: Prostate cancer

Regimen:

Docetaxel: I.V.: 70 mg/m^2 day 2
Estramustine: Oral: 280 mg 3 times/day days 1-5
Carboplatin: I.V.: Target AUC 5 day 2
Repeat cycle every 3 weeks

Estramustine + Docetaxel + Hydrocortisone

Use: Prostate cancer

Regimen:

Docetaxel: I.V.: 70 mg/m^2 day 2
Estramustine: Oral: 10 mg/kg days 1-5
Hydrocortisone: Oral: 40 mg daily
Repeat cycle every 3 weeks

Estramustine + Etoposide

Use: Prostate cancer

Regimen:

Variation 1:
Estramustine: Oral: 15 mg/kg days 1-21
Etoposide: Oral: 50 mg/m^2 days 1-21
Repeat cycle every 4 weeks

Variation 2:
Estramustine: Oral: 10 mg/kg/day days 1-21
Etoposide: Oral: 50 mg/m^2 days 1-21
Repeat cycle every 4 weeks

Variation 3:
Estramustine: Oral: 140 mg 3 times/day days 1-21
Etoposide: Oral: 50 mg/m^2 days 1-21
Repeat cycle every 4 weeks

Estramustine + Vinorelbine

Use: Prostate cancer

Regimen:

Variation 1:
Estramustine: Oral: 140 mg 3 times/day days 1-14
Vinorelbine: I.V.: 25 mg/m^2 days 1 and 8
Repeat cycle every 21 days

Variation 2:
Estramustine: Oral: 280 mg 3 times/day days 1-3
Vinorelbine: I.V.: 15 or 20 mg/m^2 day 2
Give weekly for 8 weeks, then every other week

EV

Use: Prostate cancer

Regimen:

Variation 1:
Estramustine: Oral: 10 mg/kg days 1-42
Vinblastine: I.V.: 4 mg/m^2 days 1, 8, 15, 22, 29, and 36
Repeat cycle every 8 weeks

Variation 2:
Estramustine: Oral: 600 mg/m^2 days 1-42
Vinblastine: I.V.: 4 mg/m^2 days 1, 8, 15, 22, 29, and 36
Repeat cycle every 8 weeks

EVA

Use: Lymphoma, Hodgkin disease

Regimen:

Etoposide: I.V.: 100 mg/m^2 days 1-3
Vinblastine: I.V.: 6 mg/m^2 day 1
Doxorubicin: I.V.: 50 mg/m^2 day 1
Repeat cycle every 28 days

FAC

Use: Breast cancer

Regimen:

Variation 1:

Fluorouracil: I.V.: 500 mg/m^2 days 1 and 8 **or** 500 mg/m^2 day 1
Doxorubicin: I.V.: 50 mg/m^2 day 1
Cyclophosphamide: I.V.: 500 mg/m^2 day 1
Repeat cycle every 21-28 days

Variation 2:

Fluorouracil: I.V.: 200 mg/m^2 days 1-3
Doxorubicin: I.V.: 40 mg/m^2 day 1
Cyclophosphamide: I.V.: 400 mg/m^2 day 1
Repeat cycle every 28 days

Variation 3:

Fluorouracil: I.V.: 400 mg/m^2 days 1 and 8
Doxorubicin: I.V.: 40 mg/m^2 day 1
Cyclophosphamide: I.V.: 400 mg/m^2 day 1
Repeat cycle every 28 days

Variation 4:

Fluorouracil: I.V.: 600 mg/m^2 days 1 and 8
Doxorubicin: I.V.: 60 mg/m^2 day 1
Cyclophosphamide: I.V.: 600 mg/m^2 day 1
Repeat cycle every 28 days

Variation 5:

Fluorouracil: I.V.: 300 mg/m^2 days 1 and 8
Doxorubicin: I.V.: 30 mg/m^2 day 1
Cyclophosphamide: I.V.: 300 mg/m^2 day 1
Repeat cycle every 28 days

FAM

Use: Gastric cancer; Pancreatic cancer

Regimen:

Fluorouracil: I.V.: 600 mg/m^2 days 1, 8, 29, 36
Doxorubicin: I.V.: 30 mg/m^2 days 1 and 29
Mitomycin C: I.V.: 10 mg/m^2 day 1
Repeat cycle every 8 weeks

FAMTX

Use: Gastric cancer

Regimen:

Variation 1:

Methotrexate: I.V.: 1500 mg/m^2 day 1
Fluorouracil: I.V.: 1500 mg/m^2 (1 hour after methotrexate) day 1
Leucovorin: Oral: 15 mg/m^2 every 6 hours for 48 hours (start 24 hours after methotrexate) day 2
Doxorubicin: I.V.: 30 mg/m^2 day 15
Repeat cycle every 28 days

Variation 2:

Methotrexate: I.V.: 1500 mg/m^2 day 1
Fluorouracil: I.V.: 1500 mg/m^2 day 1
Leucovorin: Oral: 15 mg/m^2 every 6 hours for 8 doses, 30 mg/m^2 every 6 hours for 8 more doses if 24-hour methotrexate level ≥2.5 mol/L (start 24 hours after methotrexate)
Doxorubicin: I.V.: 30 mg/m^2 day 15
Repeat cycle every 28 days

F-CL

Use: Colorectal cancer

Regimen:

Variation 1 (Mayo Regimen):
Fluorouracil: I.V.: 425 mg/m^2 days 1-5
Leucovorin: I.V.: 20 mg/m^2 days 1-5
Repeat cycle every 28 days

Variation 2:
Fluorouracil: I.V.: 400 mg/m^2 days 1-5
Leucovorin: I.V.: 20 mg/m^2 days 1-5
Repeat cycle every 28 days

Variation 3:
Fluorouracil: I.V.: 500 mg/m^2 day 1
Leucovorin: I.V.: 20 mg/m^2 (2-hour infusion) day 1
or 500 mg/m^2 (2-hour infusion) day 1
Repeat cycle weekly

Variation 4:
Fluorouracil: I.V.: 600 mg/m^2 weekly for 6 weeks
Leucovorin: I.V.: 500 mg/m^2 (3-hour infusion) weekly for 6 weeks
Repeat cycle every 8 weeks

Variation 5:
Fluorouracil: I.V.: 600 mg/m^2 weekly for 6 weeks
Leucovorin: I.V.: 500 mg/m^2 weekly for 6 weeks
Repeat cycle every 8 weeks

Variation 6:
Fluorouracil: I.V.: 600 mg/m^2 weekly
Leucovorin: I.V.: 500 mg/m^2 (2-hour infusion) weekly
Repeat cycle weekly

Variation 7:
Fluorouracil: I.V.: 2600 mg/m^2 continuous infusion day 1
Leucovorin: I.V.: 500 mg/m^2 continuous infusion day 1
Repeat cycle weekly

Variation 8:
Fluorouracil: I.V.: 2600 mg/m^2 continuous infusion day 1
Leucovorin: I.V.: 300 mg/m^2 (maximum 500 mg) continuous infusion day 1
Repeat cycle weekly

Variation 9:
Fluorouracil: I.V.: 2600 mg/m^2 continuous infusion once weekly for 6 weeks
Leucovorin: I.V.: 500 mg/m^2 weekly for 6 weeks
Repeat cycle every 8 weeks

Variation 10:
Fluorouracil: I.V.: 2300 mg/m^2 continuous infusion day 1
Leucovorin: I.V.: 50 mg/m^2 continuous infusion day 1
Repeat cycle weekly

Variation 11:
Fluorouracil: I.V.: 200 mg/m^2 continuous infusion days 1-14
Leucovorin: I.V.: 5 mg/m^2 days 1-14
Repeat cycle every 28 days

Variation 12:
Fluorouracil: I.V.: 200 mg/m^2 continuous infusion daily for 4 weeks
followed by (starting week 5): 200 mg/m^2 continuous infusion days 1-21
Leucovorin: I.V.: 20 mg/m^2 days 1, 8, and 15
Repeat cycle every 4 weeks

FEC

Use: Breast cancer

Regimen:

Fluorouracil: I.V.: 500 mg/m^2 day 1
Cyclophosphamide: I.V.: 500 mg/m^2 day 1
Epirubicin: I.V.: 100 mg/m^2 day 1
Repeat cycle every 21 days

FIS-HAM

Use: Leukemia, acute lymphocytic; Leukemia, acute myeloid

Regimen:

Fludarabine: I.V.: 15 mg/m^2 every 12 hours days 1, 2, 8, and 9
Cytarabine: I.V.: 750 mg/m^2 every 3 hours days 1, 2, 8, and 9
Mitoxantrone: I.V.: 10 mg/m^2 days 3, 4, 10, and 11

FL

Use: Prostate cancer

Regimen:

Variation 1:
Flutamide: Oral: 250 mg every 8 hours
Leuprolide acetate: SubQ: 1 mg daily
Variation 2:
Flutamide: Oral: 250 mg every 8 hours
Leuprolide acetate depot: I.M.: 22.5 mg day 1
Repeat cycle every 3 months

FLAG

Use: Leukemia, acute myeloid

Regimen:

Fludarabine: I.V.: 30 mg/m^2 days 1-5
Cytarabine: I.V.: 2 g/m^2 days 1-5 (3.5 hours after end of fludarabine infusion)
Filgrastim: SubQ: 5 mcg/kg day 1
followed by 300 mcg daily until ANC >500-1000 cells/mcL postnadir
Repeat cycle every 3-4 weeks

FLe

Use: Colorectal cancer

Regimen:

Fluorouracil: I.V.: 450 mg/m^2 for 5 days, then after a pause of 4 weeks, 450 mg/m^2/week for 48 weeks
Levamisole: Oral: 50 mg 3 times/day for 3 days, repeated every 2 weeks for 1 year

Fludarabine-Rituximab

Use: Leukemia, chronic lymphocytic

Regimen:

Rituximab: I.V.: 375 mg/m^2 days 1 and 4 (cycle 1); day 1 (cycles 2-6)
Fludarabine: I.V.: 25 mg/m^2 days 1-5
Repeat cycle every 4 weeks

FOIL

Use: Colorectal cancer

Regimen:

Irinotecan: I.V.: 175 mg/m^2 day 1
Oxaliplatin: I.V.: 100 mg/m^2 day 1
Leucovorin: I.V.: 200 mg/m^2 day 1
Fluorouracil: I.V.: 3800 mg/m^2 continuous infusion days 1 and 2
Repeat cycle every 14 days

FOLFOX 2

Use: Colorectal cancer

Regimen:

Oxaliplatin: I.V.: 100 mg/m^2 day 1
Leucovorin: I.V.: 500 mg/m^2 (2-hour infusion) days 1 and 2
Fluorouracil: I.V.: 1.5-2 g/m^2 (24-hour infusion) days 1 and 2
Repeat cycle every 2 weeks

FOLFOX 3

Use: Colorectal cancer

Regimen:

Oxaliplatin: I.V.: 85 mg/m^2 day 1
Leucovorin: I.V.: 500 mg/m^2 (2-hour infusion) days 1 and 2
Fluorouracil: I.V.: 1500 mg/m^2 (22-hour infusion) days 1 and 2
Repeat cycle every 2 weeks

FOLFOX 4

Use: Colorectal cancer

Regimen:

Oxaliplatin: I.V.: 85 mg/m^2 day 1
Leucovorin: I.V.: 200 mg/m^2 (2-hour infusion) days 1 and 2
Fluorouracil: I.V. bolus: 400 mg/m^2 days 1 and 2
 followed by 600 mg/m^2 (22-hour infusion) days 1 and 2
Repeat cycle every 2 weeks

FOLFOX 7

Use: Colorectal cancer

Regimen:

Oxaliplatin: I.V.: 130 mg/m^2 day 1
Leucovorin: I.V.: 400 mg/m^2 (2-hour infusion) day 1
Fluorouracil: I.V.: 400 mg/m^2 day 1
 followed by 1200 mg/m^2 continuous infusion days 1 and 2
Repeat cycle every 2 weeks

FU HURT

Use: Head and neck cancer

Regimen:

Hydroxyurea: Oral: 1000 mg every 12 hours for 11 doses days 0-5
Fluorouracil: I.V.: 800 mg/m^2/day continuous infusion (start AM after admission) days 1-5
Paclitaxel: I.V.: 5-25 mg/m^2/day continuous infusion days 1-5
Filgrastim: SubQ: 5 mcg/kg/day days 6-12 (start ≥12 hours after completion of fluorouracil infusion)
5-7 cycles may be administered

FU/LV/CPT-11

Use: Colorectal cancer

Regimen:

Irinotecan: I.V.: 350 mg/m^2 day 1
Leucovorin: I.V.: 20 mg/m^2 days 22-26
Fluorouracil: I.V.: 425 mg/m^2 days 22-26
Repeat cycle every 6 weeks

FU/LV/CPT-11 (Saltz Regimen)

Use: Colorectal cancer

Regimen:

Fluorouracil: I.V.: 500 mg/m^2 days 1, 8, 15, and 22
Leucovorin: I.V.: 20 mg/m^2 days 1, 8, 15, and 22
Irinotecan: I.V.: 125 mg/m^2 days 1, 8, 15, and 22
Repeat cycle every 42 days

FUP

Use: Gastric cancer

Regimen:

Fluorouracil: I.V.: 1000 mg/m^2 continuous infusion days 1-5
Cisplatin: I.V.: 100 mg/m^2 day 2
Repeat cycle every 28 days

FZ

Use: Prostate cancer

Regimen:

Variation 1:
Flutamide: Oral: 250 mg every 8 hours
Goserelin acetate: SubQ: 3.6 mg day 1
Repeat cycle every 28 days

Variation 2:
Flutamide: Oral: 250 mg every 8 hours
Goserelin acetate: SubQ: 10.8 mg day 1
Repeat cycle every 3 months

GC

Use: Nonsmall cell lung cancer

Regimen:

Gemcitabine: I.V.: 1000 mg/m^2 days 1, 8, 15
Cisplatin: I.V.: 100 mg/m^2 day 1 **or** 2 **or** 15
Repeat cycle every 28 days for 2-6 cycles

Gemcitabine/Capecitabine

Use: Pancreatic cancer

Regimen:

Gemcitabine: I.V.: 1000 mg/m^2 days 1 and 8
Capecitabine: Oral: 650 mg/m^2 twice daily days 1-14
Repeat cycle every 21 days

Gemcitabine-Carboplatin

Use: Nonsmall cell lung cancer

Regimen:

Gemcitabine: I.V.: 1000 or 1100 mg/m^2 days 1 and 8
Carboplatin: I.V.: AUC 5 day 8
Repeat cycle every 28 days

Gemcitabine-Cis

Use: Nonsmall cell lung cancer
Regimen:

Variation 1:
Gemcitabine: I.V.: 1000 mg/m^2 days 1, 8, and 15
Cisplatin: I.V.: 100 mg/m^2 day 2 **or** 15
Repeat cycle every 28 days

Variation 2:
Gemcitabine: I.V.: 1000-1200 mg/m^2 days 1, 8, and 15
Cisplatin: I.V.: 100 mg/m^2 day 1 **or** 2 **or** 15
Repeat cycle every 28 days

Gemcitabine-Cisplatin

Use: Bladder cancer
Regimen:

Gemcitabine: I.V.: 1000 mg/m^2 days 1, 8, and 15
Cisplatin: I.V.: 70 mg/m^2 day 2
Repeat cycle every 28 days for 6 cycles

Gemcitabine/Irinotecan

Use: Pancreatic cancer
Regimen:

Gemcitabine: I.V.: 1000 mg/m^2 days 1 and 8
Irinotecan: I.V.: 100 mg/m^2 days 1 and 8
Repeat cycle every 21 days

Gemcitabine-Vinorelbine

Use: Nonsmall cell lung cancer
Regimen:

Variation 1:
Gemcitabine: I.V.: 1200 mg/m^2 days 1 and 8
Vinorelbine: I.V.: 30 mg/m^2 days 1 and 8
Repeat cycle every 21 days for 6 cycles

Variation 2:
Gemcitabine: I.V.: 1000 mg/m^2 days 1, 8, and 15
Vinorelbine: I.V.: 20 mg/m^2 days 1, 8, and 15
Repeat cycle every 28 days for 6 cycles

HDMTX (Osteosarcoma)

Use: Osteosarcoma
Regimen:

Methotrexate: I.V.: 12 g/m^2/week for 2-12 weeks
Leucovorin calcium rescue: Oral, I.V.: 15 mg/m^2 every 6 hours (beginning 30 hours after the beginning of the 4-hour methotrexate infusion) for 10 doses; **serum methotrexate levels must be monitored**

HDMTX (Sarcoma)

Use: Sarcoma
Regimen:

Methotrexate: I.V.: 8-12 g/m^2
Leucovorin calcium: Oral, I.V.: 15-25 mg every 6 hours (beginning 24 hours after methotrexate dose) for at least 10 doses
Courses repeated weekly for 2-4 weeks, alternating with various cancer chemotherapy combination regimens

HI-CDAZE

Use: Leukemia, acute myeloid (induction)

Regimen:

Daunorubicin: I.V.: 30 mg/m^2 days 1-3
Cytarabine: I.V.: 3 g/m^2 every 12 hours days 1-4
Etoposide: I.V.: 200 mg/m^2 days 1-3, 6-8
Azacitidine: I.V.: 150 mg/m^2 days 3-5, 8-10

HIPE-IVAD

Use: Neuroblastomas

Regimen:

Cisplatin: I.V.: 40 mg/m^2 days 1-5
Etoposide: I.V.: 100 mg/m^2 days 1-5
Ifosfamide: I.V.: 3 g/m^2 days 21-23
Mesna: I.V.: 3 g/m^2 continuous infusion days 21-23
Vincristine: I.V.: 1.5 mg/m^2 day 21
Doxorubicin: I.V.: 60 mg/m^2 day 23
Repeat cycle every 28 days

Hyper-CVAD

Use: Leukemia, acute myeloid

Regimen:

Course 1, 3, 5, and 7:
Cyclophosphamide: I.V.: 300 mg/m^2 every 12 hours days 1-3
Mesna: I.V.: 3600 mg/m^2 continuous infusion days 1-3
Methotrexate: I.T.: 12 mg day 2
Vincristine: I.V.: 2 mg days 4 and 11
Doxorubicin: I.V.: 50 mg/m^2 day 4
Cytarabine: I.T.: 100 mg day 8
Dexamethasone: Oral or I.V.: 40 mg days 1-4 and 11-14
Course 2, 4, 6, and 8:
Methotrexate: I.V.: 200 mg/m^2 day 1
  followed by 800 mg/m^2 continuous infusion day 1
Cytarabine: I.V.: 3 g/m^2 every 12 hours days 2 and 3
Methotrexate: I.T.: 12 mg day 2
Leucovorin: I.V.: 15 mg every 6 hours days 3 and 4
Methylprednisolone: I.V.: 50 mg twice daily days 1-3
Cytarabine: I.T.: 100 mg day 8
Cycles are given when WBC is ≥3, Plt ≥60

ICE (Sarcoma)

Use: Osteosarcoma; Soft tissue sarcoma

Regimen:

Ifosfamide: I.V.: 1500 mg/m^2 days 1-3 (with mesna uroprotection)
Carboplatin: I.V.: 635 mg/m^2 day 3
Etopside: I.V.: 100 mg/m^2 days 1-3

Idarubicin, Cytarabine, Etoposide (ICE Protocol)

Use: Leukemia, acute myeloid

Regimen:

Idarubicin: I.V.: 6 mg/m^2 days 1-5
Cytarabine: I.V.: 600 mg/m^2 days 1-5
Etoposide: I.V.: 150 mg/m^2 days 1-3
Administer one cycle only

Idarubicin, Cytarabine, Etoposide (IDA-Based BF12)

Use: Leukemia, acute myeloid

Regimen:

Idarubicin: I.V.: 5 mg/m^2 days 1-5

Cytarabine: I.V.: 2000 mg/m^2 every 12 hours for 10 doses days 1-5

Etoposide: I.V.: 100 mg/m^2 days 1-5

Second cycle may be given based on individual respone; time between cycles not specified

IDMTX/6-MP

Use: Leukemia, acute lymphocytic

Regimen:

Week 1:

Methotrexate: I.V.: 200 mg/m^2
followed by 800 mg/m^2 continuous infusion day 1

Mercaptopurine: I.V.: 200 mg/m^2
followed by 800 mg/m^2 over 8 hours day 1

Leucovorin: Oral or I.V.: 5 mg/m^2 every 6 hours for 5-13 doses beginning 24 hours after end of methotrexate infusion

Week 2:

Methotrexate: I.M.: 20 mg/m^2 day 8

Mercaptopurine: Oral: 50 mg/m^2 days 8-14

Repeat cycle every 2 weeks up to 12 cycles

IE

Use: Soft tissue sarcoma

Regimen:

Etoposide: I.V.: 100 mg/m^2 days 1-3

Ifosfamide: I.V.: 2500 mg/m^2 days 1-3

Mesna: I.V.: 20% of ifosfamide dose prior to and at 4-, 8-, and 12 hours after ifosfamide administration

Repeat cycle every 28 days

IL-2 + IFN

Use: Melanoma

Regimen:

Cisplatin: I.V.: 20 mg/m^2 days 1-4

Vinblastine: I.V.: 1.6 mg/m^2 days 1-4

Dacarbazine: I.V.: 800 mg/m^2 day 1

Aldesleukin: I.V.: 9 million units/m^2 continuous infusion days 1-4

Interferon alfa-2b: SubQ: 5 million units/m^2 days 1-5, 7, 9, 11, 13

Repeat cycle every 21 days

IMVP-16

Use: Lymphoma, non-Hodgkin

Regimen:

Ifosfamide: I.V.: 4 g/m^2 continuous infusion over 24 hours day 1

Mesna: I.V.: 800 mg/m^2 bolus prior to ifosfamide, then 4 g/m^2 continuous infusion over 12 hours concurrent with ifosfamide; then 2.4 g/m^2 continuous infusion over 12 hours after ifosfamide infusion day 1

Methotrexate: I.V.: 30 mg/m^2 days 3 and 10

Etoposide: I.V.: 100 mg/m^2 days 1-3

Repeat cycle every 21-28 days

Interleukin 2-Interferon Alfa 2

Use: Renal cell cancer

Regimen:

Weeks 1 and 4:

Aldesleukin: SubQ: 20 million units/m^2 3 times weekly

Interferon alfa: SubQ: 6 million units/m^2 once weekly

Weeks 2, 3, 5, and 6:

Aldesleukin: SubQ: 5 million units/m^2 3 times weekly

Interferon alfa: SubQ: 6 million units/m^2 3 times weekly

Repeat cycle every 56 days

Interleukin 2-Interferon Alfa 2-Fluorouracil

Use: Renal cell cancer

Regimen:

Weeks 1 and 4:

Aldesleukin: SubQ: 20 million units/m^2 3 times weekly

Interferon alfa: SubQ: 6 million units/m^2 once weekly

Weeks 2 and 3:

Aldesleukin: SubQ: 5 million units/m^2 3 times weekly

Weeks 5-8:

Interferon alfa: SubQ: 9 million units/m^2 3 times weekly

Fluorouracil: I.V.: 750 mg/m^2 once weekly

Repeat cycle every 56 days

IPA

Use: Hepatoblastoma

Regimen:

Ifosfamide: I.V.: 500 mg/m^2 day 1 **followed by**

1000 mg/m^2 continuous infusion days 1-3

Cisplatin: I.V.: 20 mg/m^2 days 4-8

Doxorubicin: I.V.: 30 mg/m^2 continuous infusion days 9 and 10

Repeat cycle every 21 days

Larson Regimen

Use: Leukemia, acute lymphocytic

Regimen:

Cyclophosphamide: I.V.: 1200 mg/m^2 day 1

Daunorubicin: I.V.: 45 mg/m^2 days 1-3

Vincristine: I.V.: 2 mg days 1, 8, 15, and 22

Prednisone: Oral or I.V.: 60 mg/m^2 days 1-21

Asparaginase: SubQ: 6000 units/m^2 days 5, 8, 11, 15, 18, and 22

Administer one cycle only

Linker Protocol

Use: Leukemia, acute lymphocytic

Regimen:

Remission induction:

Daunorubicin: I.V.: 50 mg/m^2 days 1-3

Vincristine: I.V.: 2 mg days 1, 8, 15, and 22

Prednisone: Oral: 60 mg/m^2 days 1-28

Asparaginase: I.M.: 6000 units/m^2 days 17-28

If residual leukemia in bone marrow on day 14:

Daunorubicin: I.V.: 50 mg/m^2 day 15

If residual leukemia in bone marrow on day 28:

Daunorubicin: I.V.: 50 mg/m^2 days 29 and 30

Vincristine: I.V.: 2 mg days 29 and 36

Prednisone: Oral: 60 mg/m^2 days 29-42

Asparaginase: I.M.: 6000 units/m^2 days 29-35

Consolidation therapy:

Treatment A (cycles 1, 3, 5, and 7)

Daunorubicin: I.V.: 50 mg/m^2 days 1 and 2

Vincristine: I.V.: 2 mg days 1 and 8

Prednisone: Oral: 60 mg/m^2 days 1-14

Asparaginase: I.M.: 12,000 units/m^2 days 2, 4, 7, 9, 11, and 14

Treatment B (cycles 2, 4, 6, and 8)

Teniposide: I.V.: 165 mg/m^2 days 1, 4, 8, and 11

Cytarabine: I.V.: 300 mg/m^2 days 1, 4, 8, and 11

Treatment C (cycle 9)

Methotrexate: I.V.: 690 mg/m^2 continuous infusion day 1 (over 42 hours)

Leucovorin: I.V.: 15 mg/m^2 every 6 hours for 12 doses (start at end of methotrexate infusion)

Administer remission induction regimen for one cycle only. Repeat consolidation cycle every 28 days

LOPP

Use: Lymphoma, Hodgkin disease

Regimen:

Chlorambucil: Oral: 10 mg days 1-10

Vincristine: I.V.: 1.4 mg/m^2 (maximum 2 mg) days 1 and 8

Procarbazine: Oral: 100 mg/m^2 days 1-10

Prednisone: Oral: 25 mg/m^2 (maximum 60 mg) days 1-14

or

Prednisolone: Oral: 25 mg/m^2 (maximum 60 mg) days 1-14

Repeat cycle every 28 days

M-2

Use: Multiple myeloma

Regimen:

Vincristine: I.V.: 0.03 mg/kg (maximum 2 mg) day 1

Carmustine: I.V.: 0.5-1 mg/kg day 1

Cyclophosphamide: I.V.: 10 mg/kg day 1

Melphalan: Oral: 0.25 mg/kg days 1-4 **or** 0.1 mg/kg days 1-7 **or** 1-10

Prednisone: Oral: 1 mg/kg days 1-7

Repeat cycle every 35-42 days

MACOP-B

Use: Lymphoma, non-Hodgkin

Regimen:

Methotrexate: I.V.: 400 mg/m^2 weeks 2, 6, 10
Doxorubicin: I.V.: 50 mg/m^2 weeks 1, 3, 5, 7, 9, 11
Cyclophosphamide: I.V.: 350 mg/m^2 weeks 1, 3, 5, 7, 9, 11
Vincristine: I.V.: 1.4 mg/m^2 (maximum 2 mg) weeks 2, 4, 8, 10, 12
Bleomycin: I.V.: 10 units/m^2 weeks 4, 8, 12
Prednisone: Oral: 75 mg/day for 12 weeks, then taper over 2 weeks
Leucovorin calcium: Oral: 15 mg/m^2 every 6 hours for 6 doses (beginning 24 hours after methotrexate) weeks 2, 6, 10
Sulfamethoxazole/trimethoprim (800 mg/160 mg): Oral: Tablet twice daily for 12 weeks
Ketoconazole: Oral: 200 mg/day
Administer one cycle

MAID

Use: Soft tissue sarcoma

Regimen:

Mesna: I.V.: 2500 mg/m^2 continuous infusion days 1-4
Doxorubicin: I.V.: 20 mg/m^2 continuous infusion days 1-3
Ifosfamide: I.V.: 2500 mg/m^2 continuous infusion days 1-3
Dacarbazine: I.V.: 300 mg/m^2 continuous infusion days 1-3
Repeat cycle every 21-28 days

m-BACOD

Use: Lymphoma, non-Hodgkin

Regimen:

Methotrexate: I.V.: 200 mg/m^2 days 8 and 15
Leucovorin calcium: Oral: 10 mg/m^2 every 6 hours for 8 doses (beginning 24 hours after each methotrexate dose) days 9 and 16
Bleomycin: I.V.: 4 units/m^2 day 1
Doxorubicin: I.V.: 45 mg/m^2 day 1
Cyclophosphamide: I.V.: 600 mg/m^2 day 1
Vincristine: I.V.: 1 mg/m^2 day 1
Dexamethasone: Oral: 6 mg/m^2 days 1-5
Repeat cycle every 21 days

MINE

Use: Lymphoma, non-Hodgkin

Regimen:

Mesna: I.V.: 1.33 g/m^2/day concurrent with ifosfamide dose, then 500 mg orally (4 hours after each ifosfamide infusion) days 1-3
Ifosfamide: I.V.: 1.33 g/m^2 days 1-3
Mitoxantrone: I.V.: 8 mg/m^2 day 1
Etoposide: I.V.: 65 mg/m^2 days 1-3
Repeat cycle every 28 days

MINE-ESHAP

Use: Lymphoma, non-Hodgkin

Regimen:

Mesna: I.V.: 1.33 g/m^2 concurrent with ifosfamide dose, then 500 mg orally (4 hours after ifosfamide) days 1-3
Ifosfamide: I.V.: 1.33 g/m^2 days 1-3
Mitoxantrone: I.V.: 8 mg/m^2 day 1
Etoposide: I.V.: 65 mg/m^2 days 1-3
Repeat cycle every 21 days for 6 cycles, followed by 3-6 cycles of ESHAP

mini-BEAM

Use: Lymphoma, Hodgkin disease

Regimen:

Carmustine: I.V.: 60 mg/m^2 day 1

Etoposide: I.V.: 75 mg/m^2 days 2-5

Cytarabine: I.V.: 100 mg/m^2 every 12 hours for 8 doses days 2-5

Melphalan: I.V.: 30 mg/m^2 day 6

Repeat cycle every 4-6 weeks

Mitoxantrone + Hydrocortisone

Use: Prostate cancer

Regimen:

Mitoxantrone: I.V.: 14 mg/m^2 day 1

Hydrocortisone: Oral: 40 mg daily

Repeat cycle every 3 weeks

MM

Use: Leukemia, acute lymphocytic (maintenance)

Regimen:

Mercaptopurine: Oral: 50-75 mg/m^2 days 1-7

Methotrexate: Oral, I.V.: 20 mg/m^2 day 1

Repeat cycle every 7 days

MOP

Use: Brain tumors

Regimen:

Mechlorethamine: I.V.: 6 mg/m^2 days 1 and 8

Vincristine: I.V.: 1.5 mg/m^2 (maximum 2 mg) days 1 and 8

Procarbazine: Oral: 100 mg/m^2 days 1-14

Repeat cycle every 28 days

MOPP (Lymphoma, Hodgkin Disease)

Use: Lymphoma, Hodgkin disease

Regimen:

Variation 1:

Mechlorethamine: I.V.: 6 mg/m^2 days 1 and 8

Vincristine: I.V.: 1.4 mg/m^2 days 1 and 8

Procarbazine: Oral: 100 mg/m^2 days 1-14

Prednisone: Oral: 40 mg/m^2 days 1-14 (cycles 1 and 4)

Repeat cycle every 28 days for 6-8 cycles

MOPP (Lymphoma, Hodgkin Disease) *(continued)*

Variation 2:

Mechlorethamine: I.V.: 6 mg/m^2 (maximum 15 mg) days 1 and 8
Vincristine: I.V.: 1.4 mg/m^2 (maximum 2 mg) days 1 and 8
Procarbazine: Oral: 100 mg/m^2 days 1-10
Prednisone: Oral: 25 mg/m^2 (maximum 60 mg) days 1-14

or

Prednisolone: Oral: 25 mg/m^2 (maximum 60 mg) days 1-14
Repeat cycle every 28 days

Variation 3:

Mechlorethamine: I.V.: 6 mg/m^2 days 1 and 8
Vincristine: I.V.: 1.4 mg/m^2 days 1 and 8
Procarbazine: Oral: 50 mg day 1, 100 mg day 2, 100 mg/m^2 days 3-14
Prednisone: Oral: 40 mg/m^2 days 1-14
Repeat cycle every 28 days

Variation 4:

Mechlorethamine: I.V.: 6 mg/m^2 days 1 and 8
Vincristine: I.V.: 1.4 mg/m^2 days 1 and 8
Procarbazine: Oral: 50 mg day 1, 100 mg day 2, 100 mg/m^2 days 3-10
Prednisone: Oral: 40 mg/m^2 days 1-14
Repeat cycle every 28 days

Variation 5:

Mechlorethamine: I.V.: 6 mg/m^2 days 1 and 8
Vincristine: I.V.: 1.4 mg/m^2 days 1 and 8
Procarbazine: Oral: 50 mg/m^2 day 1, then 100 mg/m^2 days 2-14
Prednisone: Oral: 40 mg/m^2 days 1-14
Repeat cycle every 28 days

MOPP (Medulloblastoma)

Use: Brain cancer

Regimen:

Mechlorethamine: I.V.: 3 mg/m^2, days 1 and 8
Vincristine: I.V.: 1.4 mg/m^2 (maximum 2 mg) days 1 and 8
Prednisone: Oral: 40 mg/m^2 days 1-10
Procarbazine: Oral: 50 mg day 1 **followed by**
100 mg day 2 **followed by**
100 mg/m^2 days 3-10
Repeat cycle every 28 days

MOPP/ABVD

Use: Lymphoma, Hodgkin disease

Regimen:

Variation 1:

Mechlorethamine: I.V.: 6 mg/m^2 days 1 and 8
Vincristine: I.V.: 1.4 mg/m^2 (maximum 2 mg) days 1 and 8
Procarbazine: I.V.: 100 mg/m^2 days 1-14
Prednisone: Oral: 40 mg/m^2 days 1-14 (during cycles 1, 4, 7, and 10 only)
Doxorubicin: Oral: 25 mg/m^2 days 29 and 43
Bleomycin: I.V.: 10 units/m^2 day 29 and 43
Vinblastine: I.V.: 6 mg/m^2 days 29 and 43
Dacarbazine: I.V.: 375 mg/m^2 days 29 and 43
Repeat cycle every 56 days

Variation 2:

Mechlorethamine: I.V.: 6 mg/m^2 days 1 and 8
Vincristine: I.V.: 1.4 mg/m^2 (maximum 2 mg) days 1 and 8
Procarbazine: I.V.: 100 mg/m^2 days 1-14
Prednisone: Oral: 40 mg/m^2 days 1-14 (during cycles 1 and 7 only)
Doxorubicin: Oral: 25 mg/m^2 days 29 and 43
Bleomycin: I.V.: 10 units/m^2 days 29 and 43
Vinblastine: I.V.: 6 mg/m^2 days 29 and 43
Dacarbazine: I.V.: 375 mg/m^2 days 29 and 43
Repeat cycle every 56 days

Variation 3:

Mechlorethamine: I.V.: 6 mg/m^2 days 1 and 8
Vincristine: I.V.: 1.4 mg/m^2 (maximum 2 mg) days 1 and 8
Procarbazine: I.V.: 100 mg/m^2 days 1-14
Prednisone: Oral: 40 mg/m^2 days 1-14 (every cycle)
Doxorubicin: Oral: 25 mg/m^2 days 29 and 43
Bleomycin: I.V.: 10 units/m^2 days 29 and 43
Vinblastine: I.V.: 6 mg/m^2 days 29 and 43
Dacarbazine: I.V.: 375 mg/m^2 days 29 and 43
Repeat cycle every 56 days

Variation 4:

MOPP Regimen:

Mechlorethamine: I.V.: 6 mg/m^2 days 1 and 8
Vincristine: I.V.: 1.4 mg/m^2 (maximum 2 mg) days 1 and 8
Procarbazine: I.V.: 100 mg/m^2 days 1-14
Prednisone: Oral: 25 mg/m^2 days 1-14

ABVD Regimen:

Doxorubicin: Oral: 25 mg/m^2 days 1 and 15
Bleomycin: I.V.: 6 units/m^2 days 1 and 15
Vinblastine: I.V.: 6 mg/m^2 days 1 and 15
Dacarbazine: I.V.: 250 mg/m^2 days 1 and 15
Each regimen cycle is 28 days. Administer regimens in alternating fashion as follows: 2 cycles of MOPP alternating with 2 cycles of ABVD for a total of 8 cycles

Variation 5 (pediatrics):

Mechlorethamine: I.V.: 6 mg/m^2 days 1 and 8
Vincristine: I.V.: 1.4 mg/m^2 days 1 and 8
Procarbazine: Oral: 100 mg/m^2 days 1-14
Prednisone: Oral: 40 mg/m^2 days 1-14
Doxorubicin: Oral: 25 mg/m^2 days 29 and 42
Bleomycin: I.V.: 10 units/m^2 days 29 and 42
Vinblastine: I.V.: 6 mg/m^2 days 29 and 42
Dacarbazine: I.V.: 150 mg/m^2 days 29-33
Repeat cycle evey 56 days for 4 cycles

Variation 6 (pediatrics):

Mechlorethamine: I.V.: 6 mg/m^2 days 1 and 8
Vincristine: I.V.: 1.4 mg/m^2 days 1 and 8
Procarbazine: Oral: 100 mg/m^2 days 1-14
Prednisone: Oral: 40 mg/m^2 days 1-14
Doxorubicin: Oral: 25 mg/m^2 days 29 and 42
Bleomycin: I.V.: 10 units/m^2 days 29 and 42
Vinblastine: I.V.: 6 mg/m^2 days 29 and 42
Dacarbazine: I.V.: 375 mg/m^2 days 29 and 43
Repeat cycle evey 56 days for 4 cycles

MOPP/ABV Hybrid

Use: Lymphoma, Hodgkin disease

Regimen:

Mechlorethamine: I.V.: 6 mg/m^2 day 1
Vincristine: I.V.: 1.4 mg/m^2 day 1
Procarbazine: Oral: 100 mg/m^2 days 1-7
Prednisone: Oral: 40 mg/m^2 days 1-14
Doxorubicin: I.V.: 35 mg/m^2 day 8
Bleomycin: I.V.: 10 units/m^2 day 8
Vinblastine: I.V.: 6 mg/m^2 day 8
Repeat cycle every 28 days

MP (Multiple Myeloma)

Use: Multiple myeloma

Regimen:

Melphalan: Oral: 8-10 mg/m^2 days 1-4
Prednisone: Oral: 40-60 mg/m^2 days 1-4
Repeat cycle every 28-42 days

MP (Prostate Cancer)

Use: Prostate cancer

Regimen:

Mitoxantrone: I.V.: 12 mg/m^2 day 1
Prednisone: Oral: 5 mg twice daily
Repeat cycle every 21 days

MTX/6-MP/VP (Maintenance)

Use: Leukemia, acute lymphocytic

Regimen:

Methotrexate: Oral: 20 mg/m^2 weekly
Mercaptopurine: Oral: 75 mg/m^2 daily
Vincristine: I.V.: 1.5 mg/m^2 day 1
Prednisone: Oral: 40 mg/m^2 days 1-5
Repeat monthly for 2-3 years

MTX-CDDPAdr

Use: Osteosarcoma

Regimen:

Cisplatin: I.V.: 75 mg/m^2 day 1 of cycles 1-7, then 120 mg/m^2 for cycles 8-10
Doxorubicin: I.V.: 25 mg/m^2 days 1-3 of cycles 1-7
Methotrexate: I.V.: 12 g/m^2 days 21 and 28
Leucovorin calcium rescue: I.V.: 20 mg/m^2 every 3 hours (beginning 16 hours after completion of methotrexate) for 8 doses, then orally every 6 hours for 8 doses

MV

Use: Leukemia, acute myeloid

Regimen:

Mitoxantrone: I.V.: 10 mg/m^2 days 1-5
Etoposide: I.V.: 100 mg/m^2 days 1-5
Second cycle may be given based on individual respone; time between cycles not specified

M-VAC

Use: Bladder cancer

Regimen:

Methotrexate: I.V.: 30 mg/m^2 days 1, 15, 22

Vinblastine: I.V.: 3 mg/m^2 days 2, 15, 22

Doxorubicin: I.V.: 30 mg/m^2 day 2

Cisplatin: I.V.: 70 mg/m^2 day 2

Repeat cycle every 28 days

MVPP

Use: Lymphoma, Hodgkin disease

Regimen:

Variation 1:

Mechlorethamine: I.V.: 6 mg/m^2 days 1 and 8

Vinblastine: I.V.: 6 mg/m^2 days 1 and 8

Procarbazine: Oral: 100 mg/m^2 days 1-14

Prednisone: Oral: 40 mg/m^2 days 1-14

Repeat cycle every 42 days

Variation 2:

Mechlorethamine: I.V.: 6 mg/m^2 days 1 and 8

Vinblastine: I.V.: 4 mg/m^2 days 1 and 8

Procarbazine: Oral: 100 mg/m^2 days 1-14

Prednisone: Oral: 40 mg/m^2 days 1-14

Repeat cycle every 4-6 weeks

N4SE Protocol

Use: Neuroblastomas

Regimen:

Vincristine: I.V.: 0.05 mg/kg days 1 and 2

Doxorubicin: I.V.: 15 mg/m^2 days 1 and 2

Cyclophosphamide: I.V.: 30 mg/kg days 1 and 2

Fluorouracil: I.V.: 1 mg/kg days 3, 8, and 9

Cytarabine: I.V.: 3 mg/kg days 3, 8, and 9

Hydroxyurea: Oral: 40 mg/kg days 3, 8, and 9

Repeat cycle every 21-28 days

N6 Protocol

Use: Neuroblastomas

Regimen:

Course 1, 2, 4, 6

Cyclophosphamide: I.V.: 70 mg/kg days 1 and 2

Doxorubicin: I.V.: 25 mg/m^2 continuous infusion days 1-3

Vincristine: I.V.: 0.033 mg/kg continuous infusion days 1-3

Vincristine: I.V.: 1.5 mg/m^2 day 9

Course 3, 5, 7

Etoposide: I.V.: 200 mg/m^2 days 1-3

Cisplatin: I.V.: 50 mg/m^2 days 1-4

NFL

Use: Breast cancer

Regimen:

Variation 1:

Mitoxantrone: I.V.: 12 mg/m^2 day 1

Fluorouracil: I.V.: 350 mg/m^2 days 1-3

Leucovorin: I.V.: 300 mg/m^2 days 1-3

Variation 2:

Mitoxantrone: I.V.: 10 mg/m^2 day 1

Fluorouracil: I.V.: 1000 mg/m^2 continuous infusion days 1-3

Leucovorin: I.V.: 100 mg/m^2 days 1-3

Repeat cycle every 21 days

OPA

Use: Lymphoma, Hodgkin disease

Regimen:

Vincristine: I.V.: 1.5 mg/m^2 (maximum 2 mg) days 1, 8, and 15

Prednisone: Oral: 60 mg/m^2 days 1-15 in 3 divided doses

Doxorubicin: I.V.: 40 mg/m^2 days 1 and 15

Second cycle may be given based on individual response; time between cycles not specified

OPEC

Use: Neuroblastomas

Regimen:

Vincristine: I.V.: 1.5 mg/m^2 day 1

Cyclophosphamide: I.V.: 600 mg/m^2 day 1

Cisplatin: I.V.: 100 mg/m^2 day 2

Teniposide: I.V.: 150 mg/m^2 day 4

Repeat cycle every 21 days

OPEC-D

Use: Neuroblastomas

Regimen:

Vincristine: I.V.: 1.5 mg/m^2 day 1

Cyclophosphamide: I.V.: 600 mg/m^2 day 1

Doxorubicin: I.V.: 40 mg/m^2 day 1

Cisplatin: I.V.: 100 mg/m^2 day 2

Teniposide: I.V.: 150 mg/m^2 day 4

Repeat cycle every 21 days

OPPA

Use: Lymphoma, Hodgkin disease

Regimen:

Vincristine: I.V.: 1.5 mg/m^2 (maximum 2 mg) days 1, 8, and 15

Prednisone: Oral: 60 mg/m^2 days 1-15 in 3 divided doses

Doxorubicin: I.V.: 40 mg/m^2 days 1 and 15

Procarbazine: Oral: 100 mg/m^2 days 1-15 in 2 or 3 divided doses

Second cycle may be given based on individual response; time between cycles not specified

PAC (CAP)

Use: Ovarian cancer

Regimen:

Cisplatin: I.V.: 50 mg/m^2 day 1
Doxorubicin: I.V.: 50 mg/m^2 day 1
Cyclophosphamide: I.V.: 1000 mg/m^2 day 1
Repeat cycle every 21 days for 8 cycles

PA-CI

Use: Hepatoblastoma

Regimen:

Variation 1:
Cisplatin: I.V.: 90 mg/m^2 day 1
Doxorubicin: I.V.: 20 mg/m^2 continuous infusion days 2-5
Repeat cycle every 21 days

Variation 2:
Cisplatin: I.V.: 20 mg/m^2 days 1-4
Doxorubicin: I.V.: 100 mg/m^2 continuous infusion day 1
Repeat cycle every 21-28 days

Paclitaxel, Carboplatin, Etoposide

Use: Adenocarcinoma, unknown primary

Regimen:

Paclitaxel: I.V.: 200 mg/m^2 infused over 1 hour day 1 **followed by:**
Carboplatin: I.V.: Target AUC 6
Etoposide: Oral: 50 mg, alternate with 100 mg, days 1-10
Repeat cycle every 21 days

Paclitaxel + Estramustine + Carboplatin

Use: Prostate cancer

Regimen:

Paclitaxel: I.V.: 100 mg/m^2 day 3 each week
Estramustine: Oral: 10 mg/kg daily days 1-5 each week
Carboplatin: I.V.: Target AUC 6 day 3
Repeat cycle every 28 days

Paclitaxel + Estramustine + Etoposide

Use: Prostate cancer

Regimen:

Paclitaxel: I.V.: 135 mg/m^2 day 2
Estramustine: Oral: 280 mg 3 times/day days 1-14
Etoposide: Oral: 100 mg days 1-14
Repeat cycle every 21 days

Paclitaxel-Vinorelbine

Use: Breast cancer

Regimen:

Paclitaxel: I.V.: 135 mg/m^2 day 1
Vinorelbine: I.V.: 30 mg/m^2 days 1 and 8
Repeat cycle every 28 days

PC (Bladder Cancer)

Use: Bladder cancer

Regimen:

Paclitaxel: I.V.: 200 mg/m^2 or 225 mg/m^2 day 1
Carboplatin: I.V.: AUC 5-6 day 1
Repeat cycle every 21 days

PC (Nonsmall Cell Lung Cancer)

Use: Nonsmall cell lung cancer

Regimen:

Variation 1:
Paclitaxel: I.V.: 175-225 mg/m^2 day 1
Carboplatin: I.V.: Target AUC 5-7 day 1
Repeat cycle every 21 days for 2-8 cycles

Variation 2:
Paclitaxel: I.V.: 175 mg/m^2 day 1
Cisplatin: I.V.: 80 mg/m^2 day 1
Repeat cycle every 21 days

Variation 3:
Paclitaxel: I.V.: 135 mg/m^2 continuous infusion day 1
Carboplatin: I.V.: AUC 7.5 day 2
Repeat cycle every 21 days

Variation 4:
Paclitaxel: I.V.: 135 mg/m^2 continuous infusion day 1
Cisplatin: I.V.: 75 mg/m^2 day 2
Repeat cycle every 21 days

PCV

Use: Brain tumors

Regimen:

Lomustine: Oral: 110 mg/m^2 day 1
Procarbazine: Oral: 60 mg/m^2 days 8-21
Vincristine: I.V.: 1.4 mg/m^2 (maximum 2 mg) days 8 and 29
Repeat cycle every 6-8 weeks

PE

Use: Prostate cancer

Regimen:

Variation 1:
Paclitaxel: I.V.: 30-35 mg/m^2/day continuous infusion days 1-4 or 2-5
Estramustine: Oral: 600 mg/m^2 days 1-21
Repeat cycle every 21 days

Variation 2:
Paclitaxel: I.V. 60-107 mg/m^2 infused over 3 hours weekly
Estramustine: Oral: 280 mg twice daily 3 days/week

Variation 3:
Paclitaxel: I.V. 150 mg/m^2 weekly
Estramustine: Oral: 280 mg 3 times/day 3 days/week

Variation 4:
Paclitaxel: I.V.: 100 mg/m^2 days 1, 8, and 15
Estramustine: Oral: 280 mg 3 times/day days 1, 2, and 3 every week
Repeat cycle every 4 weeks

Variation 5:
Paclitaxel: I.V.: 90 mg/m^2 over 1 hour weekly for 6 weeks
Estramustine: Oral: 280 mg twice daily 3 days/week for 6 weeks (the day before, day of, and day after paclitaxel)
Repeat cycle every 8 weeks

PE-CAdO

Use: Neuroblastomas

Regimen:

Cisplatin: I.V.: 100 mg/m^2 day 1

Teniposide: I.V.: 160 mg/m^2 day 3

alternating with

Cyclophosphamide: I.V.: 300 mg/m^2 days 1-5

Doxorubicin: I.V.: 60 mg/m^2 day 5

Vincristine: I.V.: 1.5 mg/m^2 days 1 and 5

Repeat cycle every 21 days

PFL (Colorectal Cancer)

Use: Colorectal cancer

Regimen:

Cisplatin: I.V.: 25 mg/m^2 continuous infusion days 1-5

Fluorouracil: I.V.: 800 mg/m^2 continuous infusion days 2-5

Leucovorin calcium: I.V.: 500 mg/m^2 continuous infusion days 1-5

Repeat cycle every 28 days

PFL (Head and Neck Cancer)

Use: Head and neck cancer

Regimen:

Variation 1:

Cisplatin: I.V.: 25 mg/m^2 continuous infusion days 1-5

Fluorouracil: I.V.: 800 mg/m^2 continuous infusion days 2-6

Leucovorin: I.V.: 500 mg/m^2 continuous infusion days 1-6

Repeat cycle every 28 days

Variation 2:

Cisplatin: I.V.: 100 mg/m^2 day 1

Fluorouracil: I.V.: 600-1000 mg/m^2 continuous infusion days 1-5

Leucovorin: Oral: 50 mg/m^2 every 4-6 hours days 1-6

Repeat cycle every 21 days

PFL + IFN

Use: Head and neck cancer

Regimen:

Cisplatin: I.V.: 100 mg/m^2 day 1

Fluorouracil: I.V.: 640 mg/m^2/day continuous infusion days 1-5

Leucovorin calcium: Oral: 100 mg every 4 hours days 1-5

Interferon alfa-2b: SubQ: 2 x 10^6 units/m^2 days 1-6

POC

Use: Brain tumors

Regimen:

Prednisone: Oral: 40 mg/m^2 days 1-14

Lomustine: Oral: 100 mg/m^2 day 1

Vincristine: I.V.: 1.5 mg/m^2 (maximum 2 mg) days 1, 8, and 15

Repeat cycle every 6 weeks

POMP

Use: Leukemia, acute myeloid

Regimen: Maintenance:

Mercaptopurine: Oral: 50 mg 3 times a day
Methotrexate: Oral: 20 mg/m^2 once weekly
Vincristine: I.V.: 2 mg day 1
Prednisone: Oral: 200 mg days 1-5
Repeat cycle monthly for 2 years

Pro-MACE

Use: Lymphoma, non-Hodgkin

Regimen:

Prednisone: Oral: 60 mg/m^2 days 1-14
Methotrexate: I.V.: 1.5 g/m^2 day 14
Leucovorin calcium: I.V.: 50 mg/m^2 every 6 hours for 5 doses (beginning 24 hours after methotrexate dose) day 14
Doxorubicin: I.V.: 25 mg/m^2 days 1 and 8
Cyclophosphamide: I.V.: 650 mg/m^2 days 1 and 8
Etoposide: I.V.: 120 mg/m^2 days 1 and 8
Repeat cycle every 28 days

Pro-MACE-CytaBOM

Use: Lymphoma, non-Hodgkin

Regimen:

Prednisone: Oral: 60 mg/m^2 days 1-14
Doxorubicin: I.V.: 25 mg/m^2 day 1
Cyclophosphamide: I.V.: 650 mg/m^2 day 1
Etoposide: I.V.: 120 mg/m^2 day 1
Cytarabine: I.V.: 300 mg/m^2 day 8
Bleomycin: I.V.: 5 units/m^2 day 8
Vincristine: I.V.: 1.4 mg/m^2 (maximum 2 mg) day 8
Methotrexate: I.V.: 120 mg/m^2 day 8
Leucovorin calcium: Oral: 25 mg/m^2 every 6 hours for 4 doses day 9
Concomitant sulfamethoxazole/trimethoprim (800 mg/160 mg); Oral: Tablet twice daily
Repeat cycle every 21-28 days

Pt-FU

Use: Head and neck cancer

Regimen:

Cisplatin: I.V.: 100 mg/m^2 day 1
Fluorouracil: I.V.: 1000 mg/m^2 continuous infusion days 1-5
Repeat cycle every 21 days for 2 cycles

PV

Use: Breast cancer

Regimen:

Variation 1:
Paclitaxel: I.V.: 135 mg/m^2 day 1
Vinorelbine: I.V.: 30 mg/m^2 day 1
Repeat cycle every 21 days

Variation 2:
Paclitaxel: I.V.: 150 mg/m^2 day 1
Vinorelbine: I.V.: 25 mg/m^2 day 1
Repeat cycle every 21 days

PVA (POG 8602)

Use: Leukemia, acute lymphocytic

Regimen:

Induction:

Prednisone: Oral: 40 mg/m^2 (maximum 60 mg) days 0-28 (given in 3 divided doses)

Vincristine: I.V.: 1.5 mg/m^2 (maximum 2 mg) days 0, 7, 14, and 21

Asparaginase: I.M.: 6000 units/m^2 3 times per week for 2 weeks

Intrathecal therapy: Days 0 and 22

Administer one cycle only

CNS consolidation:

Mercaptopurine: Oral: 75 mg/m^2 days 29-42

Intrathecal therapy: Days 29 and 36

Administer one cycle only

Intensification:

Regimen A:

Methotrexate: I.V.: 1000 mg/m^2 continuous infusion day 1

Cytarabine: I.V.: 1000 mg/m^2 continuous infusion day 1 (start 12 hours after methotrexate)

Leucovorin: I.M., I.V., or Oral: 30 mg/m^2 24 and 36 hours after the **start** of methotrexate **followed by** 3 mg/m^2 48, 60, and 72 hours after the **start** of methotrexate

Intrathecal therapy: Weeks 9, 12, 15, and 18

Repeat cycle every 3 weeks for 6 cycles

or

Regimen B:

Methotrexate: I.V.: 1000 mg/m^2 continuous infusion day 1

Cytarabine: I.V.: 1000 mg/m^2 continuous infusion day 1 (start 12 hours after methotrexate)

Leucovorin: I.M., I.V., or Oral: 30 mg/m^2 24 and 36 hours after the **start** of methotrexate **followed by** 3 mg/m^2 48, 60, and 72 hours after the **start** of methotrexate

Intrathecal therapy: Weeks 9, 12, 15, and 18

Repeat cycle every 12 weeks for 6 cycles

Maintenance:

Regimen A:

Methotrexate: I.M.: 20 mg/m^2 weekly

Mercaptopurine: Oral: 75 mg/m^2 daily

Intrathecal therapy: Day 1 every 8 weeks for 10 doses beginning at week 25

Prednisone: Oral: 40 mg/m^2 (maximum 60 mg) days 1-7 (given in 3 divided doses)

Vincristine: I.V.: 1.5 mg/m^2 (maximum 2 mg) days 1 and 8

Repeat 8-day cycle beginning weeks 8, 17, 25, 41, 57, 73, 89, 105

or

Regimen B:

Methotrexate: I.M.: 20 mg/m^2 weekly for 7 weeks

Mercaptopurine: Oral: 75 mg/m^2 daily for 7 weeks

Repeat cycle every 12 weeks for 4 cycles (begins weeks 22, 34, 46, 58, 70)

followed by

Methotrexate: I.M.: 20 mg/m^2 weekly

Mercaptopurine: Oral: 75 mg/m^2 daily

Repeat cycle weekly during weeks 70-156

Intrathecal therapy: Day 1 every 8 weeks for 10 doses beginning at week 25

Prednisone: Oral: 40 mg/m^2 days 1-7 (given in 3 divided doses)

Vincristine: I.V.: 1.5 mg/m^2 (maximum 2 mg) days 1 and 8

Repeat 8-day cycle beginning weeks 8, 17, 25, 41, 57, 73, 89, and 105

PVA (POG 9005)

Use: Leukemia, acute lymphocytic

Regimen:

Induction:

Prednisone: Oral: 40 mg/m^2 (maximum 60 mg) days 1-28 (given in 3 divided doses)

Vincristine: I.V.: 1.5 mg/ m^2 (maximum 2 mg) days 1, 8, 15, and 22

Asparaginase: I.M.: 6000 units/m^2 days 2, 5, 8, 12, 15, 19

Intrathecal therapy: Day 1

Administer one cycle only

Intensification:

Regimen A:

Methotrexate: I.V: 1000 mg/m^2 continuous infusion day 1

Mercaptopurine: I.V.: 1000 mg/m^2 day 2

Leucovorin: I.M., I.V., or Oral: 5 mg/m^2 every 6 hours for 5 doses day 3 (start 48 hours after the start of methotrexate)

Repeat cycle every 2 weeks for 12 cycles

or

Regimen B:

Methotrexate: Oral: 30 mg/m^2 every 6 hours for 6 doses day 1

Mercaptopurine: I.V.: 1000 mg/m^2 day 2 (start after last methotrexate dose)

Leucovorin: I.M., I.V., or Oral: 5 mg/m^2 every 6 hours for 5 doses day 3 (start 48 hours after the start of methotrexate)

Repeat cycle every 2 weeks for 12 cycles

Maintenance:

Methotrexate: I.M.: 20 mg/m^2 weekly

Mercaptopurine: Oral: 50 mg/m^2 daily

Repeat cycle weekly during weeks 25-130

Intrathecal therapy: Day 1 every 12 weeks weeks 25-130

PVB

Use: Testicular cancer

Regimen:

Variation 1:

Cisplatin: I.V.: 20 mg/m^2 days 1-5

Vinblastine: I.V.: 0.2 mg/m^2 days 1 and 2

Bleomycin: I.V.: 30 units days 2, 9, and 16

Repeat cycle every 3 weeks

Variation 2:

Cisplatin: I.V.: 20 mg/m^2 days 1-5

Vinblastine: I.V.: 0.15 mg/m^2 days 1 and 2

Bleomycin: I.V.: 30 units days 2, 9, and 16

Repeat cycle every 3 weeks

Variation 3:

Cisplatin: I.V.: 20 mg/m^2 days 1-5

Vinblastine: I.V.: 6 mg/m^2 days 1 and 2

Bleomycin: I.M.: 30 units days 2, 9, and 16

Repeat cycle every 3 weeks

PVD

Use: Leukemia, acute lymphocytic (induction)

Regimen:

Prednisone: Oral: 40 mg/m^2 for 28 days

Vincristine: I.V.: 1.5 mg/m^2/week for 4 weeks

Asparaginase: I.M.: 5000 int. units/m^2 days 2, 5, 8, 12, 15, 18

PVDA

Use: Leukemia, acute lymphocytic (induction)

Regimen:

Variation 1:

Prednisone: Oral: 40 mg/m^2 days 1-28

Vincristine: I.V.: 1.5 mg/m^2 days 2, 8, 15, and 22

Daunorubicin: I.V.: 25 mg/m^2 days 2, 8, 15, and 22

Asparaginase: I.M.: 5000 units/m^2 3 times weekly for 4 weeks

Variation 2:

Prednisone: Oral: 60 mg/m^2 days 1-28

Vincristine: I.V.: 1.5 mg/m^2 days 1, 8, 15, and 22

Daunorubicin: I.V.: 25 mg/m^2 days 1, 8, 15, and 22

Asparaginase: I.M., SubQ, or I.V.: 5000 units/m^2 days 1-14

Administer one cycle only; used in conjuction with intrathecal chemotherapy

R-CHOP

Use: Lymphoma, non-Hodgkin

Regimen:

Rituximab: I.V.: 375 mg/m^2 day 1

Cyclophosphamide: I.V.: 750 mg/m^2 day 3

Doxorubicin: I.V.: 50 mg/m^2 day 3

Vincristine: I.V.: 1.4 mg/m^2 (maximum 2 mg) day 3

Prednisone: Oral: 100 mg days 3-7

Repeat cycle every 21 days

Regimen A1

Use: Neuroblastomas

Regimen:

Cyclophosphamide: I.V.: 1.2 g/m^2 day 1

Vincristine: I.V.: 1.5 mg/m^2 day 1

Doxorubicin: I.V.: 40 mg/m^2 day 3

Cisplatin: I.V.: 90 mg/m^2 day 5

Repeat cycle every 28 days

Regimen A2

Use: Neuroblastomas

Regimen:

Cyclophosphamide: I.V.: 1.2 g/m^2 day 1

Etoposide: I.V.: 100 mg/m^2 days 1-5

Doxorubicin: I.V.: 40 mg/m^2 day 3

Cisplatin: I.V.: 90 mg/m^2 day 5

Repeat cycle every 28 days

Sequential Dox-CMF

Use: Breast cancer

Regimen:

Doxorubicin: I.V.: 75 mg/m^2 every 21 days for 4 cycles followed by 21- or 28-day CMF for 8 cycles

Stanford V

Use: Lymphoma, Hodgkin disease

Regimen:

Mechlorethamine: I.V.: 6 mg/m^2 day 1

Doxorubicin: I.V.: 25 mg/m^2 days 1 and 15

Vinblastine: I.V.: 6 mg/m^2 days 1 and 15

Vincristine: I.V.: 1.4 mg/m^2 (maximum 2 mg) days 8 and 22

Bleomycin: I.V.: 5 units/m^2 days 8 and 22

Etoposide: I.V.: 60 mg/m^2 days 15 and 16

Prednisone: Oral: 40 mg/m^2 every other day for 10 weeks
followed by tapering of dose by 10 mg every other day for next 14 days

Repeat cycle every 28 days

Note: In patients >50 years of age, vinblastine dose decreased to 4 mg/m^2 and vincristine dose decreased to 1 mg/m^2 on weeks 9-12. Concomitant sulfamethoxazole/trimethoprim (800 mg/160 mg) twice daily orally; acyclovir 200 mg 3 times/day orally; ketoconazole 200 mg/day orally, and stool softeners used.

TAD

Use: Leukemia, acute myeloid

Regimen:

Induction:

Daunorubicin: I.V.: 60 mg/m^2 days 3-5

Cytarabine: I.V.: 100 mg/m^2 continuous infusion days 1 and 2 **followed by** 100 mg/m^2 every 12 hours days 3-8

Thioguanine: Oral: 100 mg/m^2 every 12 hours days 3-9

Administer one cycle only

Tamoxifen-Epirubicin

Use: Breast cancer

Regimen:

Tamoxifen: Oral: 20 mg daily

Epirubicin: I.V.: 50 mg/m^2 days 1 and 8

Repeat epirubicin cycle every 28 days for 6 cycles; continue tamoxifen for 4 years

TCF

Use: Esophageal cancer

Regimen:

Paclitaxel: I.V.: 175 mg/m^2 day 1

Cisplatin: I.V.: 20 mg/m^2 days 1-5

Fluorouracil: I.V.: 750 mg/m^2 continuous infusion days 1-5

Repeat cycle every 28 days

TIP

Use: Esophageal cancer; Head and neck cancer

Regimen:

Paclitaxel: I.V.: 175 mg/m^2 day 1

Ifosfamide: I.V.: 1000 mg/m^2 days 1-3

Mesna: I.V.: 400 mg/m^2 before ifosfamide days 1-3

followed by: 200 mg/m^2 4 hours after ifosfamide days 1-3

Cisplatin: I.V.: 60 mg/m^2 day 1

Repeat cycle every 21-28 days

Trastuzumab-Paclitaxel

Use: Breast cancer

Regimen:

Paclitaxel: I.V.: 175 mg/m^2 day 1

Trastuzumab: I.V.: 4 mg/kg (loading dose) day 1 cycle 1 **followed by** 2 mg/kg days 1, 8, and 15

Repeat cycle every 21 days for at least 6 cycles

TVTG

Use: Leukemia, acute lymphocytic; Leukemia, acute myeloid

Regimen:

Topotecan: I.V.: 1 mg/m^2 continuous infusion days 1-5

Vinorelbine: I.V.: 20 mg/m^2 days 0, 7, 14, and 21

Thiotepa: I.V.: 15 mg/m^2 day 2

Gemcitabine: I.V.: 3600 mg/m^2 day 7

Dexamethasone: Oral or I.V.: 45 mg/m^2 days 7-14 (given in 3 divided doses)

Repeat cycle when ANC >500 cells/mcL and platelet count >75,000 cells/mcL

VAB VI

Use: Testicular cancer

Regimen:

Vinblastine: I.V.: 4 mg/m^2 day 1

Dactinomycin: I.V.: 1 mg/m^2 day 1

Bleomycin: I.V. push: 30 units day 1, then 20 units/m^2 continuous infusion days 1-3

Cisplatin: I.V.: 120 mg/m^2 day 4

Cyclophosphamide: I.V.: 600 mg/m^2 day 1

Repeat cycle every 21 days

VAC (Ovarian Cancer)

Use: Ovarian cancer

Regimen:

Vincristine: I.V.: 1.2-1.5 mg/m^2 (maximum 2 mg) weekly for 10-12 weeks **or** every 2 weeks for 12 doses

Dactinomycin: I.V.: 0.3-0.4 mg/m^2 days 1-5

Cyclophosphamide: I.V.: 150 mg/m^2 days 1-5

Repeat every 28 days

VAC (Retinoblastoma)

Use: Retinoblastoma

Regimen:

Vincristine: I.V.: 1.5 mg/m^2 day 1

Dactinomycin: I.V.: 0.015 mg/kg days 1-5

Cyclophosphamide: I.V.: 200 mg/m^2 days 1-5

VAC (Rhabdomyosarcoma)

Use: Rhabdomyosarcoma

Regimen:

Induction:

Vincristine: I.V. push: 1.5 mg/m^2 (maximum 2 mg) weekly for 12 weeks, then at week 16

Dactinomycin: I.V. push: 0.015 mg/kg (maximum 0.5 mg) days 1-5, repeat every 3 weeks for 3 cycles, then stop for 2 cycles; repeat at week 16

Cyclophosphamide: I.V.: 10 mg/kg days 1-3 (alternately: 2.2 g/m^2 day 1), repeat every 3 weeks for 5 cycles; then at week 16

Continuation:

Vincristine: I.V. push: 1.5 mg/m^2 (maximum 2 mg) weeks 20-25, 29-34, 38-43

Dactinomycin: I.V. push: 0.015 mg/kg (maximum 0.5 mg) weeks 20 and 23, 29 and 32, 38 and 41

Cyclophosphamide: I.V.: 2.2 mg/m^2 weeks 20 and 23, 29 and 32, 38 and 41

VAC Pulse

Use: Rhabdomyosarcoma

Regimen:

Vincristine: I.V.: 2 mg/m^2/dose (maximum 2 mg/dose) every 7 days for 12 weeks

Dactinomycin: I.V.: 0.015 mg/kg/day (maximum 0.5 mg/day) days 1-5, weeks 1 and 13

Cyclophosphamide: Oral, I.V.: 10 mg/kg/day for 7 days, repeat every 6 weeks

VAD

Use: Multiple myeloma

Regimen:

Vincristine: I.V.: 0.4 mg continuous infusion days 1-4

Doxorubicin: I.V.: 9 mg/m^2 continuous infusion days 1-4

Dexamethasone: Oral: 40 mg days 1-4, 9-12, 17-20

Repeat cycle every 28-35 days

VAD/CVAD

Use: Leukemia, acute lymphocytic

Regimen:

Induction:

Vincristine: I.V.: 0.4 mg continuous infusion days 1-4 and 24-27

Doxorubicin: I.V.: 12 mg/m^2 continuous infusion days 1-4 and 24-27

Dexamethasone: Oral: 40 mg days 1-4, 9-12 and 17-20

Cyclophosphamide: I.V.: 1 g/m^2 day 24

Dexamethasone: Oral: 40 mg days 24-27, 32-35 and 40-43

Administer one cycle only

VATH

Use: Breast cancer

Regimen:

Vinblastine: I.V.: 4.5 mg/m^2 day 1

Doxorubicin: I.V.: 45 mg/m^2 day 1

Thiotepa: I.V.: 12 mg/m^2 day 1

Fluoxymesterone: Oral: 10 mg 3 times/day days 1-21

Repeat cycle every 21 days

VBAP

Use: Multiple myeloma

Regimen:

Vincristine: I.V.: 1 mg day 1
Carmustine: I.V.: 30 mg/m^2 day 1
Doxorubicin: I.V.: 30 mg/m^2 day 1
Prednisone: Oral: 100 mg days 1-4
Repeat cycle every 21 days

VBMCP

Use: Multiple myeloma

Regimen:

Vincristine: I.V.: 1.2 mg/m^2 day 1
Carmustine: I.V.: 20 mg/m^2 day 1
Melphalan: Oral: 8 mg/m^2 days 1-4
Cyclophosphamide: I.V.: 400 mg/m^2 day 1
Prednisone: Oral: 40 mg/m^2 days 1-7 (all cycles), then 20 mg/m^2 days 8-14 (first 3 cycles only)
Repeat cycle every 35 days

VBP (PVB)

Use: Testicular cancer

Regimen:

Vinblastine: I.V.: 6 mg/m^2 days 1 and 2
Bleomycin: I.V.: 30 units days 1, 8, 15, (22)
Cisplatin: I.V.: 20 mg/m^2 days 1-5
Repeat cycle every 21-28 days

VC

Use: Nonsmall cell lung cancer

Regimen:

Variation 1:
Vinorelbine: I.V.: 25 mg/m^2 days 1, 8, 15, 22
Cisplatin: I.V.: 100 mg/m^2 day 1
Repeat cycle every 28 days for 2-8 cycles

Variation 2:
Vinorelbine: I.V.: 30 mg/m^2 weekly
Cisplatin: I.V.: 120 mg/m^2 days 1 and 29 (cycle 1); day 1 only on subsequent cycles
Repeat cycle every 6 weeks

VCAP

Use: Multiple myeloma

Regimen:

Vincristine: I.V.: 1 mg day 1
Cyclophosphamide: Oral: 100 mg/m^2 days 1-4
Doxorubicin: I.V.: 25 mg/m^2 day 2
Prednisone: Oral: 60 mg/m^2 days 1-4
Repeat cycle every 28 days

Vinorelbine-Cis

Use: Nonsmall cell lung cancer

Regimen:

Vinorelbine: I.V.: 30 mg/m^2 every 7 days
Cisplatin: I.V.: 120 mg/m^2 day 1 and 29, then every 6 weeks

Vinorelbine/Doxorubicin

Use: Breast cancer

Regimen:

Vinorelbine: I.V.: 25 mg/m^2 days 1 and 8

Doxorubicin: I.V.: 50 mg/m^2 day 1

Repeat cycle every 21 days

Vinorelbine-Gemcitabine

Use: Nonsmall cell lung cancer

Regimen:

Vinorelbine: I.V.: 20 mg/m^2 days 1, 8, and 15

Gemcitabine: I.V.: 800 mg/m^2 days 1, 8, and 15

Repeat cycle every 28 days

VIP (Etoposide) (Testicular Cancer)

Use: Testicular cancer

Regimen:

Variation 1:

Etoposide: I.V.: 75 mg/m^2 days 1-5

Ifosfamide: I.V.: 1200 mg/m^2 days 1-5

Cisplatin: I.V.: 20 mg/m^2 days 1-5

Repeat cycle every 21 days

Variation 2:

Etoposide: I.V.: 100 mg/m^2 days 1-5

Ifosfamide: I.V.: 1200 mg/m^2 days 1-5

Cisplatin: I.V.: 20 mg/m^2 days 1-5

Repeat cycle every 21 days

Variation 3:

Ifosfamide: I.V.: 2500 mg/m^2 days 1 and 2

Mesna: I.V.: 2400 mg/m^2 days 1 and 2

Etoposide: I.V.: 100 mg/m^2 days 3, 4, and 5

Cisplatin: I.V.: 40 mg/m^2 days 3, 4, and 5

Repeat cycle every 21 days

Variation 4:

Etoposide: I.V.: 75 mg/m^2 days 1-5

Ifosfamide: I.V.: 1200 mg/m^2 days 1-5

Cisplatin: I.V.: 20 mg/m^2 days 1-5

Mesna: I.V.: 400 mg/m^2, then 1200 mg/m^2 continuous infusion days 1-5

Repeat cycle every 21 days

VIP (Small Cell Lung Cancer)

Use: Small cell lung cancer

Regimen:

Etoposide: I.V.: 75 mg/m^2 days 1-4 **or**
100 mg/m^2 days 1-4

Ifosfamide: I.V.: 1200 mg/m^2 days 1-4

Cisplatin: I.V.: 20 mg/m^2 days 1-4

Mesna: I.V.: 300 mg/m^2 day 1 **followed by**
1200 mg/m^2 continuous infusion days 1-4

Repeat cycle every 21 days

VIP (Vinblastine) (Testicular Cancer)

Use: Testicular Cancer

Regimen:

Variation 1:

Vinblastine: I.V.: 0.11 mg/kg days 1 and 2

Ifosfamide: I.V.: 1200 mg/m^2 days 1-5

Cisplatin: I.V.: 20 mg/m^2 days 1-5

Repeat cycle every 21 days

Variation 2:

Vinblastine: I.V.: 6 mg/m^2 days 1 and 2

Ifosfamide: I.V.: 1500 mg/m^2 days 1-5

Cisplatin: I.V.: 20 mg/m^2 days 1-5

Repeat cycle every 21 days

VP (Leukemia, Acute Lymphocytic)

Use: Leukemia, acute lymphocytic (induction)

Regimen:

Vincristine: I.V.: 2 mg/m^2/week for 4-6 weeks (maximum 2 mg)

Prednisone: Oral: 60 mg/m^2/day in divided doses for 4 weeks, taper weeks 5-7

VP (Small Cell Lung Cancer)

Use: Small cell lung cancer

Regimen:

Etoposide: I.V.: 100 mg/m^2 days 1-4

Cisplatin: I.V.: 20 mg/m^2 days 1-4

Repeat cycle every 21 days

V-TAD

Use: Leukemia, acute myeloid

Regimen:

Induction:

Etoposide: I.V.: 50 mg/m^2 days 1-3

Thioguanine: Oral: 75 mg/m^2 every 12 hours days 1-5

Daunorubicin: I.V.: 20 mg/m^2 days 1 and 2

Cytarabine: I.V.: 75 mg/m^2 continuous infusion days 1-5

Up to 3 cycles may be given based on individual response; time between cycles not specified

XelOx

Use: Colorectal cancer

Regimen:

Oxaliplatin: I.V.: 130 mg/m^2 day 1

Capecitabine: Oral: 1000 or 1250 mg/m^2 twice daily days 1-14

Repeat cycle every 3 weeks

CHEMOTHERAPY REGIMEN INDEX

Adenocarcinoma, Unknown Primary

Brain

Neuroblastomas

Breast

Eye

Retinoblastoma

Gastrointestinal

Genitourinary

Genitourinary *(continued)*

Prostate Cancer

Renal Cell Cancer

Testicular Cancer

Wilms Tumor

Head and Neck Cancer

Hematologic/Leukemia

Lung

Lung *(continued)*

Small Cell

Lymphoid Tissue (Lymphoma)

Lymphoma, Hodgkin Disease

Lymphoma, Non-Hodgkin

Lymphoma, Non-Hodgkin (Burkitt)

Myeloma

Multiple Myeloma

Sarcoma

Osteosarcoma

Rhabdomyosarcoma

Soft Tissue Sarcoma

Skin

Melanoma

HERBS AND COMMON NATURAL AGENTS

The authors have chosen to include this list of natural products and their reported uses. Due to limited scientific evidence to support these uses, the information provided here is not intended as a cure for any disease, and should not be construed as curative or healing. In addition, the reader is strongly encouraged to seek other references that discuss this information in more detail, and that discuss important issues such as contraindications, warnings, precautions, adverse reactions, and interactions.

PROPOSED CLAIMS

Herb	Reported Uses
Acetyl-L-carnitine (ALC)	Alzheimer disease; depression; diabetic peripheral neuropathy; Parkinson disease
Adrenal extract	Depression; fatigue; stress; fibromylagia
Aloe (*Aloe supp*)	Gingivitis; healing agent for wounds, minor burns, and other minor skin irritations
Alpha-Lipoic acid	Diabetes, diabetic peripheral neuropathy; glaucoma; prevention of cataracts; prevention of neurologic disorders, including stroke; chemotherapy and radiation (adjunct); circulation; multiple sclerosis; hypertension
Androstenedione	Athletic performance (enhancement)
Aortic extract	Circulation structure, function, and integrity (arteries and veins); prevention of vascular disease including atherosclerosis, cerebral and peripheral arterial insufficiency, varicose veins, hemorrhoids, and vascular retinopathies such as macular degeneration
Arabinoxylane	Chemotherapy-induced leukopenia; immune system enhancement (antiviral and anticancer activity); HIV infection
Arginine	Cardiovascular disease; chronic heart failure; hypercholesterolemia; circulation; increases lean body mass; inflammatory bowel disease; immune support; male infertility; sexual vitality and enhancement; wound healing
Artichoke (*Cynara scolymus*)	Eczema and other dermatologic problems; hepatic protection/stimulation; hypercholesterolemia; bile flow; indigestion
Ashwagandha (*Withania somnifera*)	Adaptogen/tonic (promote wellness); chemotherapy and radiation (adjunct); stress, fatigue, nervous exhaustion
Astragalus (*Astragalus membranaceus*) [Milk Vetch]	Adaptogen/tonic (promote wellness); chemotherapy and radiation (adjunct); immune support; multiple sclerosis; otitis media; tissue oxygenation
Bacopa (*Bacopa monniera*)	Alzheimer disease/senility; memory enhancement and improvement of cognitive function
Beta-Carotene	Asthma; cervical dysplasia; coronary heart disease (risk reduction; in combination); immune support; photoprotection (erythropoietic protoporphyria); prevention of lung cancer
Betaine hydrochloride	Digestive aid (hypochlorhydria and achlorhydria); rosacea
Bifidobacterium bifidum (*bifidus*)	Crohn disease; diarrhea; gastrointestinal microflora recolonization (anaerobic); ulcerative colitis
Bilberry (*Vaccinium myrtillus*)	Diarrhea; hemorrhoids; ophthalmologic disorders (antioxidant) including myopia, diminished acuity, glaucoma; dark adaptation, macular degeneration, night blindness, diabetic retinopathy, cataracts; scleroderma; vascular disorders including varicose veins, capillary permeability/stability, phlebitis
Biotin (Vitamin H)	Brittle nails; diabetes; diabetic peripheral neuropathy; seborrheic dermatitis; uncombable hair syndrome
Bismuth	Ulcers

(continued)

Herb	Reported Uses
Bitter melon (*Momordica charantia*)	Antiviral; diabetes, including impaired glucose tolerance (IGT)
Black cohosh (*Cimicifuga racemosa*)	Arthritis; menopause symptoms (including vasomotor); premenstrual syndrome (PMS); mild depression
Bladderwrack (*Fucus vesiculosus*)	Fibrocystic breast disease; hypothyroidism; nutrient (rich source of iodine, potassium, magnesium, calcium, and iron)
Boron	Osteoarthritis; osteoporosis; rheumatoid arthritis
Boswellia (*Boswellia serrata*)	Antiinflammatory; arthritis; ulcerative colitis
Branched-chain amino acids (BCAAs)	Muscle development and lean body mass (increase)
Bromelain (*Anas comosus*)	Arthritis (antiinflammatory; proteolytic); cervical dysplasia; digestive enzyme; sinusitis
Bupleurum (*Bupleurum falcatum*)	Chronic inflammatory disease; fatigue; hepatic protection; systemic lupus erythematosus (SLE)
Calcium	Blood pressure regulation; cancer prevention; hypercholesterolemia; hypertension; kidney stones; poison ivy (topical; lactate form); premenstrual syndrome (PMS); pregnancy; prevention of osteoporosis
Calendula (*Calendula officinalis*)	Antibacterial, antifungal, antiviral, antiprotozoal; vulnerary; wound-healing (immune stimulant)
Caprylic acid	Antifungal/antiyeast; candidiasis; Crohn disease; dysbiosis
Carnitine	Athletic performance (enhancement); congestive heart failure (CHF); hypercholesterolemia; male infertility; weight loss
Cascara (*Rhamnus purshiana*)	Laxative
Cat's claw (*Uncaria tomentosa*)	Antiinflammatory; antimicrobial (antibacterial, antifungal, antiviral); antioxidant; cervical dysplasia; Crohn disease; diverticulitis; endometriosis; fibromyalgia; immune support; multiple sclerosis; rosacea; systemic lupus erythematosus (SLE)
Cayenne (*Capsicum annuum, Capsicum frutescens*)	Antiinflammatory and analgesic (topical); cardiovascular circulatory support; digestive stimulant
Chamomile, German (*Matricaria chamomilla, Matricaria recutita*)	Minor injury (topical antiinflammatory); carminative, antispasmodic; insomnia (mild sedative); anxiolytic; colic; diaper rash; indigestion; nausea/vomiting; oral health (as mouth rinse/gargle); stress/anxiety; teething; uterine tonic
Chasteberry (*Vitex agnus-castus*)	Acne vulgaris; cervical dysplasia; corpus luteum insufficiency; hyperprolactinemia and insufficient lactation; menopause; menorrhagia; menstrual disorders including amenorrhea, endometriosis, premenstrual syndrome (PMS); rosacea
Chitosan	Weight reduction
Chlorophyll	Antiinflammatory, antioxidant, and wound-healing properties; bacteriostatic; odor absorbent/suppressant (breath freshener, toothpaste, mouthwash, and deodorant); protectant
Chondroitin sulfate	Osteoarthritis
Chromium	Atherosclerosis; diabetes, type 1; diabetes, type 2; glaucoma; hypercholesterolemia; hypertriglyceridemia; hypothyroidism; premenstrual syndrome (PMS); weight loss
Clove (*Syzygium aromaticum*)	Antiseptic; analgesic (toothache and teething)

(continued)

Herb	Reported Uses
Coenzyme Q_{10}	Angina; cancer (preventive); chemotherapy (adjunct); chronic fatigue syndrome; congestive heart failure (CHF); fibromyalgia; gingivitis; hypercholesterolemia; hypertension; HMG-CoA reductase inhibitors may cause depletion of this nutraceutical; multiple sclerosis; muscular dystrophy; periodontal disease; weight loss
Coleus (*Coleus forskohlii*)	Asthma and allergies; eczema; hypertension and congestive heart failure (CHF); psoriasis
Collagen (Type II)	Arthritis (rheumatoid and osteo); burns (first- and second-degree); ulcers (pressure, venous stasis, diabetic); surgical and traumatic wounds; wound healing (topical)
Colostrum	Antiviral (mild); athletic performance (enhancement); diarrhea; immune support
Conjugated linoleic acid (CLA)	Muscle development and lean body mass (increase)
Copper	Anemia; osteoporosis; rheumatoid arthritis
Cordyceps (*Cordyceps sinensis*)	Adaptogen/tonic (promote wellness); antioxidant; chemotherapy and radiation (adjunct); endurance and stamina; fibromyalgia; hepatoprotection; lung, liver, and kidney function (general support); sexual vitality (males and females); tissue oxygenation; fatigue; immunomodulator
Cranberry (*Vaccinium macrocarpon*)	Nephrolithiasis (preventive); urinary tract infection, including prevention
Creatine	Enhancement of athletic performance (energy production and protein synthesis for muscle building)
Cyclo-hispro	Diabetes, type 2; hypoglycemia
Dandelion (*Taraxacum officinale*)	Leaf used as a diuretic; root used for disorders of bile secretion (choleretic), appetite stimulation, dyspepsia
Dehydroepiandrosterone (DHEA)	Antiaging; depression; diabetes, type 2; fatigue; lupus
Devil's claw (*Harpagophytum procumbens*)	Antiinflammatory; back pain; osteoarthritis, gout, and other inflammatory conditions
Docosahexaenoic acid (DHA)	Alzheimer disease; attention deficit disorder (ADD) and attention deficit hyperactivity disorder (ADHD); coronary heart disease (risk reduction); Crohn disease; diabetes; eczema; hypertension; hypertriglyceridemia; psoriasis; rheumatoid arthritis; stroke (risk reduction)
Dong quai (*Angelica sinensis*)	Anemia; energy enhancement (particularly in females); hypertension; menopause, dysmenorrhea, premenstrual syndrome (PMS), and amenorrhea; menorrhagia; phytoestrogen
Echinacea (*Echinacea purpurea, Echinacea angustifolia*)	Antibacterial (topical; boils, abscesses, tonsillitis, poison ivy); antiviral; arthritis (*E. augustifolia*); immune support (cold and other upper respiratory infections); otitis media
Elder (*Sambucus nigra, Sambucus canadensis*)	Berry used as an antiviral, antioxidant, and for influenza; flower used as an antiinflammatory, colds and influenza, diaphoretic, diuretic, fever, sinusitis, and sore throat
Ephedra (*Ephedra sinica*)	Allergies, sinusitis, hay fever; asthma; weight loss
Evening primrose (*Oenothera biennis*)	Amenorrhea; attention deficit disorder (ADD); depression; diabetes; diabetic peripheral neuropathy; eczema, dermatitis, and psoriasis; endometriosis; fatigue; fibrocystic breast disease (FBD); hypercholesterolemia; irritable bowel syndrome; menorrhagia; multiple sclerosis; omega-6 fatty acid supplementation; premenstrual syndrome (PMS) and menopause; rheumatoid arthritis; rosacea; scleroderma
Eyebright (*Euphrasia officinalis*)	Eye fatigue; catarrh of the eyes

(continued)

Herb	Reported Uses
Fenugreek (*Trigonella foenum-graecum*)	Diabetes; hypercholesterolemia
Feverfew (*Tanacetum parthenium*)	Antiinflammatory, rheumatoid arthritis; migraine headache (preventive); muscle soreness
Fish oils	Acne vulgaris; asthma; cardiac death (sudden; preventive); cardiac support (general; proposed benefits); circulation; coronary heart disease (preventive); Crohn disease; diabetes; dysmenorrhea; eczema, psoriasis; fatigue; headache; heart disease and heart attack (risk reduction), including women; herpes simplex 2; hypertension; hypertriglyceridemia; memory enhancement; multiple sclerosis; premenstrual syndrome (PMS); rheumatoid arthritis; rosacea; scleroderma; stroke (risk reduction)
Flaxseed oil	Acne vulgaris; arthritis (rheumatoid); asthma; constipation; coronary heart disease (risk reduction); hemorrhoids; hypertension; multiple sclerosis; omega-3 essential fatty acid source (cell wall and cellular membrane structure; cholesterol transport and oxidation); premenstrual syndrome (PMS); prostaglandins production; psoriasis; stroke (risk reduction); systemic lupus erythematosus (SLE)
Folic acid	Alcoholism; anemia; atherosclerosis; cancer prevention (colon and breast); cervical dysplasia; coronary heart disease (risk reduction); coronary restenosis (rate reduction by decreasing plasma homocysteine levels); Crohn disease; dementia and Alzheimer disease (risk reduction); depression; gingivitis; osteoporosis; pregnancy (prevention of birth defects) and lactation; schizophrenia (risk reduction, by decreasing homocysteine levels); ulcer, aphthous
Garcinia (*Garcinia cambogia*)	Pancreatic function (supportive) and glucose regulation; weight loss
Garlic (*Allium sativum*)	Antimicrobial (bacterial and fungal); antioxidant (practitioners should be aware that aged garlic extracts have been reported to improve this benefit); coagulation (mild inhibitor of platelet-activating factor); hyperlipidemia; hypertension; immune support
Ginger (*Zingiber officinale*)	Antiemetic, for nausea and vomiting in pregnancy; motion sickness; antiinflammatory (musculoskeletal); diverticulitis; indigestion/heartburn; osteoarthritis
Ginkgo (*Ginkgo biloba*)	Alzheimer disease, dementia; asthma; depression; epilepsy; headaches; intermittent claudication; macular degeneration; memory enhancement; Parkinson disease; peripheral blood flow (cerebral vascular disease, peripheral vascular insufficiency, impotence, tinnitus, and depression); seizures; sexual dysfunction (antidepressant-induced)
Ginseng, Panax (*Panax ginseng*)	Adrenal tonic; diabetes; physical and mental performance, [energy enhancement], chemotherapy and radiation (adjunct); immune support
Ginseng, Siberian (*Eleutherococcus senticosus*)	Adaptogen/tonic (promote wellness); athletic performance (enhancement); stress (decreased fatigue); immune support
Glucosamine	Osteoarthritis and joint structure support; rheumatoid arthritis and other inflammatory conditions
Glutamine	Alcoholism; athletic performance (enhancement); cancer (adjunct); catabolic wasting; chemotherapy (prevention of adverse effects); fibromyalgia; HIV infection (adjunct); immune support; peptic ulcer disease; postsurgical healing; ulcerative colitis and other inflammatory bowel diseases
Glutathione	Hepatoprotection (alcohol-induced liver damage); immune support; peptic ulcer disease
Goldenseal (*Hydrastis canadensis*)	Fever; gallbladder; mucous membrane tonifying (used in inflammation of mucosal membranes); gastritis; antimicrobial (antibacterial/antifungal); bronchitis, cystitis, and infectious diarrhea; sinusitis; sore throat; urinary tract infection (UTI)

(continued)

Herb	Reported Uses
Gotu kola (*Centella asiatica*)	Connective tissue (support); hemorrhoids (topical); macular degeneration; memory enhancement; psoriasis; venous insufficiency; wound healing (topical)
Grapefruit seed (*Citrus paradisi*)	Antifungal, antibacterial, antiparasitic; diarrhea; diverticulitis; eczema; endometriosis; irritable bowel syndrome (IBS); rosacea; sinusitis; sore throat; ulcerative colitis; urinary tract infection (UTI)
Grape seed (*Vitis vinifera*)	Allergies, antiinflammatory, asthma; antioxidant; circulation, platelet aggregation inhibitor, capillary fragility, arterial/venous insufficiency (intermittent claudification, varicose veins); gingivitis; glaucoma; macular degeneration; multiple sclerosis; Parkinson disease; scleroderma
Green tea (*Camellia sinensis*)	Antioxidant; cancer and cardiovascular disease (preventive); chemotherapy and radiation (adjunct); diarrhea; gingivitis; hypercholesterolemia; macular degeneration; platelet-aggregation inhibitor
Ground ivy (*Hedera helix*)	Croup; mucolytic; upper respiratory congestion and cough
Guggul (*Commiphora mukul*)	Hypercholesterolemia; hypothyroidism; osteoarthritis; weight loss
Gymnema (*Gymnema sylvestre*)	Diabetes, blood sugar regulation
Hawthorn (*Crataegus oxyacantha*)	Angina, hypotension, hypertension, peripheral vascular disease, tachycardia; cardiotonic; congestive heart failure
Hops (*Humulus lupulus*)	Sedative/hypnotic (mild)
Horse chestnut (*Aesculus hippocastanum*)	Scleroderma; venous insufficiency (varicose veins, hemorrhoids, deep venous thrombosis, lower extremity edema [oral and topical])
Horsetail (*Equisetum arvense*)	Diuretic; high mineral content (including silicic acid); bone and connective tissue strengthening, including osteoporosis
Huperzine A (*Huperzia serrata*)	Senile dementia and Alzheimer disease
Hydroxymethyl butyrate (HMB)	Athletic performance (enhancement)
5-Hydroxytryptophan (5-HTP)	Anxiety; depression; fibromyalgia; headache; migraine; sleep disorders, insomnia (stimulates the production of melatonin); weight loss
Inositol hexaphosphate (IP-6)	Cancer (preventive)
Iodine	Fibrocystic breast disease; goiter (preventive); hypothyroidism; mucolytic agent
Ipriflavone	Prevention of osteoporosis (men and women)
Iron	Anemia; menorrhagia; pregnancy; restless legs syndrome
Isoflavones (soy)	Benign prostatic hyperplasia (BPH); cancer (preventive); cervical dysplasia; chemotherapy (adjunct); endometriosis; hypercholesterolemia; menopausal symptoms; osteoarthritis; osteoporosis; premenstrual syndrome (PMS)
Kava kava (*Piper methysticum*)	Fibromyalgia; insomnia; anxiety/stress, skeletal muscle relaxation, postischemic episodes; muscle soreness
Lactobacillus acidophilus	Constipation; diarrhea (infantile); eczema (preventive); gastrointestinal microflora recolonization; hypercholesterolemia; immune support; lactose intolerance; vaginal candidiasis
Lavender (*Lavendula officinalis*)	Wound healing including minor burns (topical)

(continued)

Herb	Reported Uses
Lemon balm/Melissa (*Melissa officinalis*)	Antiviral (oral herpes virus); attention deficit hyperactivity disorder (ADHD); sedation (pediatrics); teething (topical)
Licorice (*Glycyrrhiza glabra*)	Adrenal insufficiency (licorice); Crohn disease; croup; expectorant and antitussive (licorice); gastrointestinal ulceration (DGL chewable products)
Liver extract	Liver tonic
Lutein	Cataracts; macular degeneration
Lycopene	Atherosclerosis; cancer (preventive; especially lung and prostate); macular degeneration
Lysine	Angina pectoris; herpes simplex; osteoporosis; ulcer, aphthous
Magnesium	Asthma; attention deficit hyperactivity disorder (ADHD); cardiovascular disease; circulation; colic (magnesium salt); congestive heart failure (CHF); diabetes; dysmenorrhea; epilepsy; fatigue; fibromyalgia (magnesium salt); gallbladder (magnesium salt); heart disease; hypertension; hypoglycemia; insomnia; kidney stones; migraine headache; mitral valve prolapse (MVP); muscle cramps; nervousness; osteoporosis; premenstrual syndrome (PMS); stress/anxiety; multiple sclerosis
Malic acid	Aluminum toxicity; fibromyalgia
Manganese	Diabetes; epilepsy; osteoporosis
Marshmallow (*Althaea officinalis*)	Cough; croup; mucilaginous, demulcent; peptic ulcer disease; sore throat
Mastic (*Pistacia lentiscus*)	*H. pylori* inhibitor; peptic ulcer disease
Melatonin	Insomnia; jet lag; oxidative stress in dialysis patients (preventive)
Methionine	Liver detoxification
Methyl sulfonyl methane (MSM)	Allergies; analgesic; arthritis (osteo and rheumatoid); interstitial cystitis; lupus
Milk thistle (*Silybum marianum*)	Antidote for poisoning by Death Cup mushroom; antioxidant (specifically hepatic cells), liver diseases including acute/chronic hepatitis, jaundice, and stimulation of bile secretion/cholagogue; chemotherapy and radiation (adjunct); constipation; eczema; gallbladder; halitosis; hepatoprotective, including drug toxicities (ie, phenothiazines, butyrophenones, ethanol, and acetaminophen); hyperthyroidism; psoriasis; rosacea
Modified citrus pectin (MCP)	Anticarcinogenic; hypercholesterolemia
Muira puama (*Ptychopetalum olacoides*)	Athletic performance (enhancement); sexual vitality (males)
N-Acetyl cysteine (NAC)	Acetaminophen toxicity; AIDS; asthma (mucolytic, antioxidant); bronchitis; cardioprotection (during chemotherapy); fatigue; glutathione production; heavy metal detoxification; hyperthyroidism; hypothyroidism; macular degeneration; multiple sclerosis; nephropathy (preventive); Parkinson disease; scleroderma; systemic lupus erythematosus (SLE)
Nicotinamide adenine dinucleotide (NADH)	Chronic fatigue; Parkinson disease; stamina and energy
Olive leaf (*Olea europaea*)	Acne vulgaris; antibacterial; antifungal, antiviral; Crohn disease; diabetes; diarrhea; diverticulitis; eczema; endometriosis; hypertension; multiple sclerosis; scleroderma; ulcerative colitis; urinary tract infection (UTI)
Pancreatic extract	Antiinflammatory; cancer (adjunct); celiac disease; digestive disturbances; food allergies; immune complex diseases
Para-Aminobenzoic acid (PABA)	Peyronie disease; scleroderma; vitiligo

(continued)

Herb	Reported Uses
Parsley (*Petroselinum crispum*)	Halitosis; antibacterial, antifungal
Passion flower (*Passiflora spp*)	Hyperthyroidism; insomnia (sedative)
Peppermint (*Mentha piperita*)	Carminative, spasmolytic; colic; indigestion; irritable bowel syndrome; motion sickness
Phenylalanine	Reward deficiency syndrome in addiction; analgesic; depression; vitiligo
Phosphatidyl choline (PC)	Alcohol-induced liver damage; Alzheimer disease; gallstones; hepatitis
Phosphatidyl serine (PS)	Alzheimer disease; depression; memory enhancement
Potassium	Cardiac arrhythmias; congestive heart failure (CHF); hypertension; kidney stones
Pregnenolone	Arthritis; hormone precursor (DHEA, cortisol, progesterone, estrogens, and testosterone); mental performance
Progesterone	Breast cancer (preventive); dysmenorrhea; endometriosis; menopause symptoms; osteoporosis; premenstrual syndromes (PMS)
Psyllium (*Plantago ovata, Plantago isphagula*)	Bulk-forming laxative (containing 10% to 30% mucilage); halitosis
Pygeum (*Pygeum africanum, Prunus africana*)	Benign prostatic hyperplasia (BPH)
Pyruvate	Athletic performance (enhancement); weight loss
Quercetin	Allergies; asthma; atherosclerosis; cataracts; peptic ulcer disease; sinusitis
Red clover (*Trifolium pratense*)	Endometriosis; liver and kidney detoxification (liquid extract); menopause symptoms (proprietary extract contains 4 phytoestrogens); menorrhagia
Red yeast rice (*Monascus purpureus*)	Hypercholesterolemia
Rehmannia (*Rehmannia glutinosa*)	Rheumatoid arthritis; systemic lupus erythematosus (SLE)
Reishi (*Ganoderma lucidum*)	Chemotherapy and radiation (adjunct); hypertension; seizure disorder; immune support; fatigue
SAMe (S-adenosyl methionine)	Cardiovascular disease; depression; fibromyalgia; headache; insomnia; liver disease; osteoarthritis; rheumatoid arthritis
Saw palmetto (*Serenoa repens*)	Benign prostatic hyperplasia (BPH)
Schisandra (*Schizandra chinensis*)	Adaptogen/tonic (to promote wellness); hepatic protection and detoxification; chemotherapy and radiation (adjunct); endurance, stamina, and work performance (enhancement); decreases fatigue
Selenium	Acne vulgaris (with vitamin E); AIDS; atherosclerosis; bronchial asthma; cancer (preventive); cardiomyopathy; cataracts; chemotherapy and radiation (adjunct); circulation; eczema; epilepsy; hemorrhoids; herpes simplex 1 and 2; hypothyroidism; macular degeneration; prostate cancer (preventive); ulcerative colitis
Senna (*Cassia senna*)	Laxative
Shark cartilage	Cancer; osteoarthritis, rheumatoid arthritis
Spleen extract	Chemotherapy and radiation (adjunct); cold/flu; fatigue; spleen function (supportive)
Stinging nettle (*Urtica dioica*)	Leaf used for allergic rhinitis, allergy and hay fever symptoms, uric acid excretion, and sinusitis; root used for benign prostatic hyperplasia (BPH)

(continued)

Herb	Reported Uses
St John's wort (*Hypericum perforatum*)	Antibacterial, antiinflammatory (topical: minor wounds, infections, bruises, muscle soreness, and sprains); mild to moderate depression, melancholia, stress and anxiety
Taurine	Congestive heart failure (CHF); diabetes; gallbladder; hypertension; seizure disorders
Tea tree (*Melaleuca alternifolia*)	**Not for ingestion**; acne vulgaris; antifungal, antibacterial; mouthwash for dental and oral health; burns, cuts, scrapes, insect bites
Thyme (*Thymus vulgaris*)	Antifungal; cough (upper respiratory origin); croup
Thymus extract	Fatigue; immune support; otitis media; sinusitis; systemic lupus erythematosus (SLE)
Thyroid extract	Fatigue; immune support; fibromyalgia
Tocotrienols	Cancer (preventive); heart disease; hypercholesterolemia; skin (supportive, protective)
Tribulus (*Tribulus terrestris*)	Athletic performance (enhancement), sexual vitality
Turmeric (*Curcuma longa*)	Antioxidant; antiinflammatory; antirheumatic; hypercholesterolemia; dysmenorrhea; muscle soreness
Tylophora (*Tylophora asthmatica*)	Allergies; asthma
Tyrosine	Alzheimer disease; depression; hypothyroidism; phenylketonuria (PKU); substance abuse
Uva-Ursi (*Arctostaphylos uva-ursi*)	Urinary tract infections and kidney stone prevention
Valerian (*Valeriana officinalis*)	Hyperthyroidism; insomnia (sedative/hypnotic); premenstrual syndrome (PMS), menopause; restless motor syndromes and muscle spasms
Vanadium	Diabetes, type 1; diabetes, type 2; hypoglycemia
Vinpocetine	Cognitive function; Alzheimer disease and senility
Vitamin A (Retinol)	Acne vulgaris; AIDS; cancer (preventive); cervical dysplasia; circulation; cold/flu; Crohn disease; diverticulitis; eczema; fibrocystic breast disease (FBD); glaucoma; hemorrhoids; measles; menorrhagia; night blindness; otitis media; premenstrual syndrome (PMS); psoriasis; rosacea; sore throat; ulcerative colitis; urinary tract infection (UTI)
Vitamin B_1 (Thiamine)	Alcoholism; Alzheimer disease; anemia (megaloblastic); congestive heart failure (CHF); diabetes; fibromyalgia; insomnia; neurological conditions (Bell palsy, trigeminal neuralgia, sciatica, sensory neuropathies); psychiatric illness
Vitamin B_2	Cataracts; depression; migraine
Vitamin B_3	Acne vulgaris (4% niacinamide topical gel); cataracts; coronary disease (preventive); diabetes, type 1; diabetes, type 2; hyperlipidemia (hypercholesterolemia, hypertriglyceridemia); impaired glucose tolerance; intermittent claudication; myocardial infarction (risk reduction); osteoarthritis; Raynaud syndrome; rheumatoid arthritis; schizophrenia; antioxidant
Vitamin B_5 (Pantothenic acid)	Adrenal support; allergies; arthritis; constipation; hyperlipidemia (pantethine, but not pantothenic acid, lowers cholesterol and triglycerides); rheumatoid arthritis; wound healing
Vitamin B_6 (Pyridoxine)	Arthritis; asthma; autism; cardiovascular disease; carpal tunnel syndrome; coronary heart disease (risk reduction); coronary restenosis (rate reduction by lowering plasma homocysteine levels); dementia and Alzheimer disease (risk reduction); depression (associated with oral contraceptives); diabetic peripheral neuropathy; epilepsy, B_6-dependant; headache; insomnia; kidney stones; monosodium glutamate (MSG) sensitivity; nausea and vomiting (in pregnancy); peptic ulcer disease; PMS

(continued)

Herb	Reported Uses
Vitamin B_{12} (Cobalamin)	AIDS; asthma; atherosclerosis (due to homocysteine elevation); coronary restenosis (rate reduction by lowering plasma homocysteine levels); Crohn disease; dementia and Alzheimer disease (risk reduction); depression; diabetic peripheral neuropathy; male infertility; memory loss; multiple sclerosis; pernicious anemia; sulfite sensitivity
Vitamin B complex-25	See individual B vitamins
Vitamin C	AIDS; allergies; antioxidant; asthma; atherosclerosis; cancer; cataracts; cervical dysplasia; circulation; cold; constipation; coronary heart disease (preventive, in patients laking lipid-lowering agents); Crohn disease; diabetes; diverticulitis; eczema; endometriosis; fatigue; fever; fibrocystic breast disease (FBD); fibromyalgia; gallbladder disease (risk reduction); gingivitis; glaucoma; herpes simplex virus 1 and 2; immune support; irritable bowel syndrome (IBS); multiple sclerosis; myocardial infarction (risk reduction); nitrate tolerance (preventive); osteoporosis; otitis media; Parkinson disease; peptic ulcer disease; psoriasis; reflex sympathetic dystrophy (preventive); sinusitis; sore throat; stress/anxiety; sunburn; ulcerative colitis; urinary tract infection (UTI); wound healing
Vitamin D	Crohn disease; epilepsy (during anticonvulsant therapy); hearing loss; osteoporosis; psoriasis; rickets; scleroderma
Vitamin E	Acne vulgaris (with selenium); Alzheimer disease; atherosclerosis; Benign prostatic hyperplasia (BPH); cancer (preventive); cataracts; cervical dysplasia; circulation; diabetes; dyslipidemias; eczema; endometriosis; epilepsy; fibrocystic breast disease (FBD); gallbladder; hemorrhoids; macular degeneration; multiple sclerosis; myocardial infarction (risk reduction); osteoarthritis; peptic ulcer disease; peripheral circulation; premenstrual syndrome (PMS); psoriasis; rheumatoid arthritis; scleroderma; sunburn; systemic lupus erythematosus; ulcerative colitis
Vitamin K	Osteoporosis; synthesis of blood clotting factors
White oak (*Quercus alba*)	Antiinflammatory (mild: throat and mouth as a soothing agent)
White willow (*Salix alba*)	Antipyretic; antiinflammatory
Wild yam (*Dioscorea villosa*)	Female vitality (conversion to progesterone in the body is poor)
Yohimbe (*Pausinystalia yohimbe*)	Sexual vitality (men and women); male erectile dysfunction
Zinc	Acne vulgaris; aphthous ulcers; benign prostatic hyperplasia (BPH); common cold; Crohn disease; diabetes; diaper rash; diverticulitis; gastric ulcer healing; immune support; macular degeneration; osteoporosis; otitis media; sexual vitality (men); skin conditions, eczema, psoriasis; sore throat; ulcerative colitis; wound healing

TOP 200 PRESCRIBED DRUGS*

Brand Name (if appropriate)	Generic Name	Rank
Accupril®	quinapril	56
----	acetaminophen and codeine	54
Aciphex®	rabeprazole	81
Actonel®	risedronate	96
Actos®	pioglitazone	70
Adderall XR™	dextroamphetamine and amphetamine	106
Advair™ Diskus®	fluticasone and salmeterol	48
----	albuterol (aerosol)	13
----	albuterol (sulfate)	169
Allegra®	fexofenadine	25
Allegra-D®	fexofenadine and pseudoephedrine	91
----	allopurinol	146
Alphagan® P	brimonidine	177
----	alprazolam	11
Altace®	ramipril	58
Amaryl®	glimepiride	101
Ambien®	zolpidem	24
----	amitriptyline	52
----	amoxicillin	6
----	amoxicillin and clavulanate potassium	51
Amoxil®	amoxicillin	95
Apri®	ethinyl estradiol and desogestrel	200
Aricept®	donepezil	156
Atacand®	candesartan	175
----	atenolol	4
Atrovent®	ipratropium	197
Augmentin ES-600®	amoxicillin and clavulanate potassium	138
Avalide®	irbesartan and hydrochlorothiazide	190
Avandia®	rosiglitazone	77
Avapro®	irbesartan	116
Avelox®	moxifloxacin	178
Aviane™	ethinyl estradiol and levonorgestrel	158
Bactroban®	mupirocin	153
Bextra®	valdecoxib	67
Biaxin®	clarithromycin	161
Biaxin® XL	clarithromycin	129
----	carisoprodol	113
Cartia® XT	diltiazem	130
Cefzil®	cefprozil	151
Celebrex®	celecoxib	23
Celexa™	citalopram	39
----	cephalexin	26
Cipro®	ciprofloxacin	83
----	ciprofloxacin	162

*NDC Health, "The Top 200 Prescriptions for 2003 by Number of U.S. Prescriptions Dispensed," Available at: http://www.rxlist.com/top200.htm

(continued)

Brand Name (if appropriate)	Generic Name	Rank
----	clonazepam	38
----	clonidine	92
----	betamethasone and clotrimazole	179
Combivent®	ipratropium and albuterol	105
Concerta™	methylphenidate	102
Coreg®	carvedilol	121
Cotrim®	sulfamethoxazole and trimethoprim	98
Coumadin®	warfarin	75
Cozaar®	losartan	69
----	cyclobenzaprine	63
Depakote®	valproic acid and derivatives	111
Detrol® LA	tolterodine	118
----	diazepam	117
Diflucan®	fluconazole	65
Digitek®	digoxin	82
Dilantin®	phenytoin	147
----	diltiazem	90
Diovan®	valsartan	59
Diovan HCT®	valsartan and hydrochlorothiazide	74
Ditropan® XL	oxybutynin	160
----	doxycycline	141
Duragesic®	fentanyl	152
Effexor® XR	venlafaxine	35
Elidel®	pimecrolimus	166
----	enalapril	122
Endocet®	oxycodone and acetaminophen	125
Evista®	raloxifene	88
Flomax®	tamsulosin	80
Flonase®	fluticasone	49
Flovent®	fluticasone	103
----	fluoxetine	34
----	folic acid	133
Fosamax®	alendronate	28
----	furosemide	7
----	gemfibrozil	126
Glucophage®	metformin	86
Glucotrol® XL	glipizide	64
Glucovance™	glyburide and metformin	104
----	glyburide	72
Humalog®	insulin preparations	150
Humulin® 70/30	insulin preparations	155
Humulin® N	insulin preparations	119
----	hydrochlorothiazide	8
----	hydrocodone and acetaminophen	1
Hyzaar®	losartan and hydrochlorothiazide	94
Imitrex®	sumatriptan	142
Inderal® LA	propranolol	165
----	isosorbide mononitrate	114
Kariva™	ethinyl estradiol and desogestrel	191

(continued)

Brand Name (if appropriate)	Generic Name	Rank
Klor-Con®	potassium chloride	144
Klor-Con® M20	potassium chloride	145
Lanoxin®	digoxin	93
Lantus®	insulin preparations	120
----	ibuprofen	19
Lescol® XL	fluvastatin	181
Levaquin™	levofloxacin	57
Levothroid®	levothyroxine	115
Levoxyl®	levothyroxine	20
Lexapro™	escitalopram	55
Lipitor®	atorvastatin	2
----	lisinopril	10
----	lorazepam	37
Lotensin®	benazepril	87
Lotrel®	amlodipine and benazepril	60
Low-Ogestrel®	ethinyl estradiol and norgestrel	192
Macrobid®	nitrofurantoin	139
----	meclizine	136
----	metformin	50
----	methylprednisolone	171
----	metoprolol	33
Miacalcin®	calcitonin	182
Microgestin™ Fe	ethinyl estradiol and norethindrone	149
MiraLax™	polyethylene glycol-electrolyte solution	157
MOBIC®	meloxicam	173
Monopril®	fosinopril	131
----	naproxen	73
Nasacort® AQ	triamcinolone	137
Nasonex®	mometasone	84
Necon®	ethinyl estradiol and norethindrone	143
Neurontin®	gabapentin	36
Nexium™	esomeprazole	27
Niaspan®	Niacin	163
----	nifedipine	170
NitroQuick®	nitroglycerin	186
Norvasc®	amlodipine	9
----	omeprazole	62
Omnicef®	cefdinir	135
Ortho Evra™	ethinyl estradiol and norelgestromin	76
Ortho Tri-Cyclen®	ethinyl estradiol and norgestimate	31
Ortho-Novum®	ethinyl estradiol and norethindrone	183
----	oxycodone and acetaminophen	85
Oxycontin®	oxycodone	97
Patanol®	olopatadine	154
Paxil®	paroxetine	42
Paxil CR™	paroxetine	78
----	penicillin V potassium	68
Percocet®	oxycodone and acetaminophen	196

(continued)

Brand Name (if appropriate)	Generic Name	Rank
----	phenytoin	176
Plavix®	clopidogrel	44
Plendil®	felodipine	184
----	potassium chloride	46
Pravachol®	pravastatin	43
----	prednisone	32
Premarin®	estrogens (conjugated)	16
Prempro™	estrogens (conjugated/equine) and medroxyprogesterone	112
Prevacid®	lansoprazole	17
Prilosec®	omeprazole	107
----	promethazine	124
----	promethazine and codeine	185
----	propoxyphene and acetaminophen	21
----	propranolol	198
Proscar®	finasteride	189
Protonix®	pantoprazole	47
Pulmicort Respules®	budesonide	167
----	ranitidine hydrochloride	53
Remeron®	mirtazapine	194
Rhinocort® Aqua™	budesonide	134
Risperdal®	risperidone	79
Roxicet™	oxycodone and acetaminophen	195
Seroquel®	quetiapine	108
Singulair®	montelukast	30
Skelaxin®	metaxalone	128
----	sulfamethoxazole and trimethoprim	148
----	spironolactone	187
Strattera™	atomoxetine	164
Synthroid®	levothyroxine	3
----	temazepam	140
----	terazosin	188
----	timolol	174
TobraDex®	tobramycin and dexamethasone	193
Topamax®	topiramate	127
Toprol-XL®	metoprolol	14
----	trazodone	71
----	triamcinolone	180
----	hydrochlorothiazide and triamterene	22
TriCor®	fenofibrate	100
Trimox®	amoxicillin	45
Trivora®-28	ethinyl estradiol and levonorgestrel	168
Tussionex®	hydrocodone and chlorpheniramine	172
Ultracet™	acetaminophen and tramadol	123
Valtrex®	valacyclovir	110
----	verapamil	66
Viagra®	sildenafil	40
Vioxx®	rofecoxib	29
----	warfarin	61

(continued)

Brand Name (if appropriate)	Generic Name	Rank
Wellbutrin® SR	bupropion	41
Xalatan®	latanoprost	99
Yasmin®	ethinyl estradiol and drospirenone	109
Zetia™	ezetimibe	132
Zithromax®	azithromycin	5
Zocor®	simvastatin	15
Zoloft®	sertraline	12
Zyprexa®	olanzapine	89
Zyrtec®	cetirizine	18
Zyrtec-D 12 Hour™	cetirizine and pseudoephedrine	159

NEW DRUGS ADDED SINCE LAST EDITION

Brand Name	Generic Name	Use
Alimta®	pemetrexed	Malignant pleural mesothelioma
Alinia®	nitazoxanide	Diarrhea
Apokyn™	apomorphine	Treatment of hypomobility
Avastin™	bevacizumab	Metastatic colorectal cancer
BabyBIG®	botulism immune globulin (intravenous-human)	Treatment of infant botulism
Betaxon®	levobetaxolol	Glaucoma
Bexxar®	tositumomab and iodine I 131 tositumomab	Lymphoma
Caduet®	amlodipine and atorvastatin	Hypertension, hypercholesterolemia
Campral®	acamprosate	Alcohol dependence
Cialis®	tadalafil	Treatment of erectile dysfunction
Ciprodex®	ciprofloxacin and dexamethasone	Treatment of acute otitis media, externa
ClimaraPro™	estradiol and levonorgestrel	Menopause symptoms
Copaxone®	glatiramer acetate	Multiple sclerosis
Coversyl Plus®, Preterex® (Canada only)	perindopril and indapamide	Hypertension
Cubicin™	daptomycin	Gram-positive infections caused by complicated skin and skin structure infections
Epzicom™	abacavir and lamivudine	HIV infections
Erbitux™	cetuximab	Treatment of epidermal growth factor receptor
Ertaczo™	sertaconazole	Treatment of athlete's foot
Ketek™ (Canada only)	telithromycin	Anti-infective
Lexiva™	fosamprenavir	HIV infections
Namenda™	memantine	Dementia of the Alzheimer type
Norprolac® (Canada only)	quinagolide	Treatment of hyperprolactinemia
Plenaxis™	abarelix	Prostate cancer
Prevacid® NapraPAC™	lansoprazole and naproxen	Reduction of the risk of NSAID-associated gastric ulcers
Raptiva™	efalizumab	Psoriasis
Sanctura™	trospium	Treatment of overactive bladder
Sensipar™	cinacalcet	Treatment of secondary hyperparathyroidism, hypercalcemia
Symbyax™	olanzapine and fluoxetine	Depression, bipolar disorder
Tindamax™	tinidazole	Treatment of trichomoniasis
Truvada™	emtricitabine and tenofovir	HIV infections
Vidaza™	azacitidine	Treatment of myelodysplastic syndrome (MDS)
Vytorin™	ezetimibe and simvastatin	Hypercholesterolemia
Xalacom® (Canada only)	latanoprost and timolol	Glaucoma
Xifaxan™	rifaximin	Treatment of travelers' diarrhea

PENDING DRUGS OR DRUGS IN CLINICAL TRIALS

Proposed Brand Name or Synonym	Generic Name	Use
Ariflo™	cilomast	Chronic obstructive pulmonary disease
Boniva™	ibandronate sodium	Osteoporosis
Certican™	everlimus	Prevention of organ rejection after transplant
Enablex™	darifenacin	Overactive bladder
Entereg™	alvimopan	Postoperative ileus
Estorra™	eszopoclone	Insomnia
Exanta™	ximelagatran	Prevention of venous thromboembolism
Genasense™	oblimersen sodium	Malignant melanoma
LY303366	anidulafungin	Esophageal candidiasis
Macugen™	pegaptanib sodium	Macular degeneration
NN304	insulin determir	Long-acting insulin
Orathecin™	rubitecan	Pancreatic cancer
Prestara™	prasterone	Lupus
Prexige™	lumiracoxib	Nonsteroidal antiinflammatory drug
Prialt™	ziconotide	Chronic pain
Ranexa™	ranolazine	Angina
Raptiva™	efalizumab	Psoriasis
Riquent™	LJP 394	Lupus
Surfaxin™	lucinactant	Respiratory distress syndrome
Symlin™	pramlinitide	Diabetes
Tarceva™	erlotinib	Lung cancer
Vanlev™	omapatrilat	Hypertension

DRUG PRODUCTS NO LONGER AVAILABLE (U.S.)

Brand Name	Generic Name
Absorbine® Antifungal	tolnaftate
Absorbine® Jock Itch	tolnaftate
AccuHist® Pediatric	brompheniramine and pseudoephedrine
Aches-N-Pain®	ibuprofen
Achromycin® Parenteral	tetracycline
Achromycin® V Capsule	tetracycline
Achromycin® V Oral Suspension	tetracycline
Aci-jel®	acetic acid
ACT®	fluoride
Actagen-C®	triprolidine, pseudoephedrine, and codeine
Actagen® Syrup	triprolidine and pseudoephedrine
Actagen® Tablet	triprolidine and pseudoephedrine
Act-A-Med®	triprolidine and pseudoephedrine
ACTH-40®	corticotropin
Actidil®	triprolidine
Actifed® Allergy Tablet (Night)	diphenhydramine and pseudoephedrine
Actifed® Syrup	triprolidine and pseudoephedrine
Actifed® With Codeine	triprolidine, pseudoephedrine, and codeine
Actinex®	masoprocol
Acutrim® 16 Hours	phenylpropanolamine
Acutrim® Late Day	phenylpropanolamine
Acutrim® II, Maximum Strength	phenylpropanolamine
Adalat®	nifedipine
Adipost®	phendimetrazine tartrate
Adlone® Injection	methylprednisolone
Adphen®	phendimetrazine tartrate
Adrin®	nylidrin hydrochloride
Adsorbocarpine® Ophthalmic	pilocarpine
Adsorbonac®	sodium chloride
Adsorbotear® Ophthalmic Solution	artificial tears
Advanced Formula Oxy® Sensitive Gel	benzoyl peroxide
Aeroaid®	thimerosal
Aerodine®	povidone-iodine
Aerolate® Oral Solution	theophylline
Aerosporin® Injection	polymyxin B
Afrin® Children's Nose Drops	oxymetazoline
Afrinol®	pseudoephedrine
Afrin® Saline Mist	sodium chloride
Agoral® Plain	mineral oil
Airet®	albuterol
AKBeta®	levobunolol
Ak-Chlor® Ophthalmic	chloramphenicol
Ak-Homatropine® Ophthalmic	homatropine
AK-Mycin®	erythromycin (systemic)
Akoline® C.B. Tablet	vitamin
AK-Pentolate®	cyclopentolate
AK-Spore® H.C. Ophthalmic	bacitracin, neomycin, polymyxin B, and hydrocortisone
AK-Spore® H.C. Otic	neomycin, polymyxin B, and hydrocortisone
AK-Spore® Ophthalmic Ointment	bacitracin, neomycin, and polymyxin B
AK-Taine®	proparacaine
AK-Tracin®	bacitracin
AK-Zol®	acetazolamide

(continued)

Brand Name	Generic Name
Ala-Cort®	hydrocortisone
Ala-Scalp®	hydrocortisone
Ala-Tet®	tetracycline
Alazide®	hydrochlorothiazide and spironolactone
Albalon-A® Ophthalmic	naphazoline and antazoline
Albumisol®	albumin
Albunex®	albumin
Alconefrin® Nasal Solution	phenylephrine
Aldoclor®	chlorothiazide and methyldopa
Aldomet®	methyldopa
Aldoril® D50	methyldopa and hydrochlorothiazide
Allegra® 60 mg Capsule	fexofenadine
Allercon® Tablet	triprolidine and pseudoephedrine
Allerest® 12 Hour Capsule	chlorpheniramine and phenylpropanolamine
Allerest® 12 Hour Nasal Solution	oxymetazoline
Allerest® Eye Drops	naphazoline
Allerfrin® Syrup	triprolidine and pseudoephedrine
Allerfrin® Tablet	triprolidine and pseudoephedrine
Allerfrin® with Codeine	triprolidine, pseudoephedrine, and codeine
Alor® 5/500	hydrocodone and aspirin
Alphagan®	brimonidine
Alphamul®	castor oil
AL-Rr® Oral	chlorpheniramine
Altocor™	lovastatin
Aludrox®	aluminum hydroxide and magnesium hydroxide
Alupent® Inhalation Solution	metaproterenol
Alu-Tab®	aluminum hydroxide
Amaphen®	butalbital compound and acetaminophen
Ambi 10®	benzoyl peroxide
Ambi® Skin Tone	hydroquinone
Amcort® Injection	triamcinolone (systemic)
Amen®	medroxyprogesterone acetate
Amibid LA	guaifenesin
Amin-Aid®	amino acid
Amipaque®	radiological/contrast media (non-ionic)
Amonidrin® Tablet	guaifenesin
AMO Vitrax®	sodium hyaluronate
Amphojel®	aluminum hydroxide
Amvisc®	sodium hyaluronate
Amvisc® Plus	sodium hyaluronate
Anabolin®	nandrolone
Anacin-3® (all products)	acetaminophen
Anacin® PM Aspirin Free	acetaminophen and diphenhydramine
Anaids® Tablet	alginic acid and sodium bicarbonate
Anamine® Syrup	chlorpheniramine and pseudoephedrine
Anaplex® Liquid	chlorpheniramine and pseudoephedrine
Anatuss®	guaifenesin, phenylpropanolamine, and dextromethorphan
Andro/Fem®	estradiol and testosterone
Andro-L.A.® Injection	testosterone
Androlone®	nandrolone
Androlone®-D	nandrolone
Andropository® Injection	testosterone
Anectine®	succinylcholine
Anergan® 25 Injection	promethazine hydrochloride
Anodynos-DHC®	hydrocodone and acetaminophen
Anoquan®	butalbital compound and acetaminophen

(continued)

Brand Name	Generic Name
Antazoline-V® Ophthalmic	naphazoline and antazoline
Anthra-Derm®	anthralin
Antiben®	antipyrine and benzocaine
Antihist-1®	clemastine
Antihist-D®	clemastine and phenylpropanolamine
Antilirium®	physostigmine
Antiminth®	pyrantel pamoate
Antinea® Cream	benzoic acid and salicylic acid
Antispas® Injection	dicyclomine
Anti-Tuss® Expectorant	guaifenesin
Antivert® Chewable Tablet	meclizine hydrochloride
Antrizine®	meclizine
Antrocol® Capsule & Tablet	atropine and belladonna
Anturane®	sulfinpyrazone
Anxanil® Oral	hydroxyzine
Apacet®	acetaminophen
Apaphen®	acetaminophen and phenyltoloxamine
A.P.L.®	chorionic gonadotropin (human)
Aplitest®	tuberculin tests
Apresazide®	hydralazine and hydrochlorothiazide
Apresoline®	hydralazine
AquaMEPHYTON®	phytonadione
Aquaphyllin®	theophylline
AquaTar®	coal tar
Aquest®	estrone
Aralen® Phosphate With Primaquine Phosphate	chloroquine phosphate and primaquine phosphate
Aramine®	metaraminol
Arcotinic® Tablet	iron and liver combination
Arduan®	pipecuronium
Argyrol® S.S.	silver protein, mild
Arlidin®	nylidrin (all products)
Arm-a-Med® Isoetharine	isoetharine
Arm-a-Med® Isoproterenol	isoproterenol
Arm-a-Med® Metaproterenol	metaproterenol sulfate
A.R.M® Caplet	chlorpheniramine and phenylpropanolamine
Arrestin®	trimethobenzamide
Artane®	trihexyphenidyl
Artha-G®	salsalate
Arthritis Foundation® Ibuprofen	ibuprofen
Arthritis Foundation® Nighttime	acetaminophen and diphenhydramine
Arthritis Foundation® Pain Reliever, Aspirin Free	acetaminophen
Arthropan®	choline salicylate
Articulose-50® Injection	prednisolone
A.S.A.®	aspirin
Asbron-G® Elixir	theophylline and guaifenesin
Asbron-G® Tablet	theophylline and guaifenesin
Ascorbicap®	ascorbic acid
Asendin®	amoxapine
Asmalix®	theophylline
A-Spas®	hyoscyamine
Aspirin Free Anacin®	acetaminophen
Asproject®	sodium thiosalicylate
AsthmaHaler® Mist	epinephrine
AsthmaNefrin®	epinephrine
Atabrine® Tablet	quinacrine hydrochloride
Atapryl®	quinacrine hydrochloride

(continued)

Brand Name	Generic Name
Atolone® Oral	triamcinolone (systemic)
Atozine® Oral	hydroxyzine
Atrohist® Plus	chlorpheniramine, phenylephrine, phenylpropanolamine, and belladonna alkaloids
Atromid-S®	clofibrate
Atropair®	atropine
----	atropine soluble tablet
Atropisol®	atropine
Aureomycin®	chlortetracycline
AVC™	sulfanilamide
Avlosulfon®	dapsone
Axotal®	butalbital compound and aspirin
Azdone®	hydrocodone and aspirin
Azlin® Injection	azlocillin
Azo Gantanol®	sulfamethoxazole and phenazopyridine
Azo Gantrisin®	sulfisoxazole and phenazopyridine
Azulfidine® Suspension	sulfasalazine
B-A-C®	butalbital compound with aspirin
Bactocill®	oxacillin
BactoShield®	chlorhexidine gluconate
Bactrim™ I.V. Infusion	sulfamethoxazole and trimethoprim
Baldex®	dexamethasone (ophthalmic)
Bancap®	butalbital compound with acetaminophen
Banesin®	acetaminophen
Banophen® Decongestant Capsule	diphenhydramine and pseudoephedrine
Banthine®	methantheline
Bantron®	lobeline (all products)
Barbidonna®	hyoscyamine, atropine, scopolamine, and phenobarbital
Barbita®	phenobarbital
Barc™ Liquid	pyrethrins
Basaljel®	aluminum carbonate
Baycol®	cerivastatin
Baypress®	nitrendipine
Beclovent®	beclomethasone
Becomject-100®	vitamin B complex
Beconase®	beclomethasone
Becotin® Pulvules®	vitamins (multiple)
Beepen-VK®	penicillin V potassium
Beesix®	pyridoxine hydrochloride
Belix® Oral	diphenhydramine
Bellafoline®	levorotatory alkaloids of belladonna (all products)
Bellatal®	hyoscyamine, atropine, scopolamine, and phenobarbital
Bellergal-S®	belladonna, phenobarbital, and ergotamine tartrate
Bemote®	dicyclomine
Bena-D®	diphenhydramine
Benadryl® 50 mg Capsule	diphenhydramine hydrochloride
Benadryl® Cold/Flu	acetaminophen, diphenhydramine, and pseudoephedrine
Benahist® Injection	diphenhydramine hydrochloride
Ben-Allergin-50® Injection	diphenhydramine
Ben-Aqua®	benzoyl peroxide
Benemid®	probenecid
Benoject®	diphenhydramine hydrochloride
Bentyl® Injection	dicyclomine
Benylin® Cough Syrup	diphenhydramine
Benylin DM®	dextromethorphan
Benzac® AC Gel	benzoyl peroxide
Benzac® W Gel	benzoyl peroxide

(continued)

Brand Name	Generic Name
Benzocol®	benzocaine
Berocca®	vitamin (multiple)
Berocca® Plus	vitamin (multiple)
Berubigen®	cyanocobalamin
Beta-2®	isoetharine
Betachron®	propranolol
Betalene® Topical	betamethasone (topical)
Betalin® S	thiamine
Betapen®-VK	penicillin V potassium
Beta-Val® Ointment (only)	betamethasone
Betaxon®	levobetaxolol
Betoptic®	betaxolol
Bexophene®	propoxyphene and aspirin
Biamine® Injection	thiamine hydrochloride
Biavax® II	rubella and mumps vaccine, combined
Bilezyme® Tablet	pancrelipase
Bilopaque®	radiological/contrast media (ionic)
Bioclate®	antihemophilic factor (recombinant)
BioCox®	coccidioidin skin test
Biodine®	povidone-iodine
Biomox®	amoxicillin
Biopatch®	chlorhexidine gluconate
Biozyme-C®	collagenase
Biphetamine®	amphetamine and dextroamphetamine
Blanex® Capsule	chlorzoxazone and acetaminophen
BlemErase® Lotion	benzoyl peroxide
Breezee® Mist Antifungal	miconazole
Breonesin®	guaifenesin
Brethaire®	terbutaline
Bretylol®	bretylium
Bricanyl®	terbutaline
Bromaline® Elixir	brompheniramine and phenylpropanolamine
Bromanate® DC	brompheniramine, phenylpropanolamine, and codeine
Bromarest®	brompheniramine
Bromatapp®	brompheniramine and phenylpropanolamine
Brombay®	brompheniramine
Bromfed®	brompheniramine and pseudoephedrine
Bromfed-PD®	brompheniramine and pseudoephedrine
Bromphen®	brompheniramine
Bromphen® DC With Codeine	brompheniramine, phenylpropanolamine, and codeine
Brompheril®	dexbrompheniramine and pseudoephedrine
Bronchial®	theophylline and guaifenesin
Bronchial Mist®	epinephrine
Bronitin® Mist	epinephrine
Bronkephrine®	ethylnorepinephrine hydrochloride
Bronkometer®	isoetharine
Bronkosol®	isoetharine
Brotane®	brompheniramine
Bucladin®-S Softab®	buclizine
Buffered®, Tri-buffered	aspirin
Buf-Puf® Acne Cleansing Bar	salicylic acid
Bumex® Injection	bumetanide
Butace®	butalbital compound
Butalan®	butabarbital sodium
Buticaps®	butabarbital sodium
Byclomine® Injection	dicyclomine
Bydramine® Cough Syrup	diphenhydramine

(continued)

Brand Name	Generic Name
Cafatine-PB®	ergotamine
Cafetrate®	ergotamine
Caladryl® Spray	diphenhydramine and calamine
Calciday-667®	calcium carbonate
Calcimar®	calcitonin
Calciparine® Injection	heparin calcium
----	calcium gluceptate
Calderol®	calcifediol
Calm-X® Oral	dimenhydrinate
Calphron®	calcium acetate
Cal-Plus®	calcium carbonate
Caltrate Jr.®	calcium carbonate
Camalox® Suspension & Tablet	aluminum hydroxide, calcium carbonate, and magnesium hydroxide
Cantharone®	cantharidin
Cantharone Plus®	cantharidin
Capzasin-P®	capsaicin
Carbastat®	carbachol
Carbiset® Tablet	carbinoxamine and pseudoephedrine
Carbiset-TR® Tablet	carbinoxamine and pseudoephedrine
Carbocaine®	mepivacaine
Carbodec® Syrup	carbinoxamine and pseudoephedrine
Carbodec® Tablet	carbinoxamine and pseudoephedrine
Carbodec® TR Tablet	carbinoxamine and pseudoephedrine
Cardem®	celiprolol
Cardilate®	erythrityl tetranitrate
Cardio-Green®	indocyanine green
Cardioquin®	quinidine
Cardizem® Injection	diltiazem
Cardizem® SR	diltiazem
Caroid®	cascara sagrada and phenolphthalein
Carter's Little Pills®	bisacodyl
Cartrol® Ocupress®	carteolol
Catarase® 1:5000	chymotrypsin (all products)
C-Crystals®	ascorbic acid
Cebid®	ascorbic acid
Cedilanid-D® Injection	deslanoside
Ceepryn®	cetylpyridinium
Cefadyl®	cephapirin
Cefanex®	cephalexin
Cefobid®	cefoperazone
Ceftin® Tablet 125 mg	cefuroxime
Celectol®	celiprolol
Cena-K®	potassium chloride
Cenocort® A-40	triamcinolone
Cenocort® Forte	triamcinolone
Centrax® Capsule & Tablet	prazepam
Cephulac®	lactulose
Ceptaz®	ceftazidime
Cerespan®	papaverine hydrochloride
Cesamet®	nabilone
Cetane®	ascorbic acid
Cetapred® Ophthalmic	sulfacetamide and prednisolone
Cevalin®	ascorbic acid
CharcoAid®	charcoal
Chealamide®	edetate disodium
Chenix® Tablet	chenodiol
Chibroxin®	norfloxacin

(continued)

Brand Name	Generic Name
Children's Hold®	dextromethorphan
Children's Kaopectate®	attapulgite
Chirocaine®	levobupivacaine
Chlo-Amine® Oral	chlorpheniramine
Chlorafed® Liquid	chlorpheniramine and pseudoephedrine
Chlorate® Oral	chlorpheniramine
Chlorgest-HD® Elixir	chlorpheniramine, phenylephrine, and hydrocodone
Chlorofon-A® Tablet	chlorzoxazone
Chloromycetin® Cream	chloramphenicol
Chloromycetin® Kapseals®	chloramphenicol
Chloromycetin® Ophthalmic	chloramphenicol
Chloromycetin® Otic	chloramphenicol
Chloromycetin® Palmitate Oral Suspension	chloramphenicol
Chloroptic® Ophthalmic Solution	chloramphenicol
Chloroptic-P® Ophthalmic	chloramphenicol and prednisolone
Chloroptic® SOP	chloramphenicol
Chloroserpine®	reserpine and hydrochlorothiazide
Chlorphed®	brompheniramine
Chlorphed®-LA Nasal Solution	oxymetazoline
Chlor-Pro® Injection	chlorpheniramine
Chlor-Rest® Tablet	chlorpheniramine and phenylpropanolamine
Chlortab®	chlorpheniramine maleate
Chlor-Trimeton® Syrup	chlorpheniramine
Cholan-HMB®	dehydrocholic acid
Choledyl®	oxtriphylline
Choledyl SA®	oxtriphylline
---	cholera vaccine (all products)
Choloxin®	dextrothyroxine
Chorex®	chorionic gonadotropin
Choron®	chorionic gonadotropin (human)
Chronulac®	lactulose
Chymex®	bentiromide (all products)
Cibacalcin®	calcitonin
Cipralan®	cifenline
Cithalith-S® Syrup	lithium citrate
Citro-Nesia™ Solution	magnesium citrate
Clear Away® Disc	salicylic acid
Clear By Design® Gel	benzoyl peroxide
Clearsil® Maximum Strength	benzoyl peroxide
Clear Tussin® 30	guaifenesin and dextromethorphan
Clindex®	clidinium and chlordiazepoxide
---	clioquinol (all products)
Clistin® Tablet	carbinoxamine maleate
Clopra®	metoclopramine
Clorpactin® XCB Powder	oxychlorosene sodium
Cloxapen®	cloxacillin
Clysodrast®	bisacodyl
Cobalasine® Injection	adenosine phosphate
Cobex®	cyanocobalamin
Codamine®	hydrocodone and phenylpropanolamine
Codamine® Pediatric	hydrocodone and phenylpropanolamine
Codehist® DH	chlorpheniramine, pseudoephedrine, and codeine
Codimal-A® Injection	brompheniramine maleate
Codimal® Expectorant	guaifenesin and phenylpropanolamine
ColBenemid®	colchicine and probenecid
Cold & Allergy® Elixir	brompheniramine and phenylpropanolamine

(continued)

Brand Name	Generic Name
Coldlac-LA®	guaifenesin and phenylpropanolamine
Coldloc®	guaifenesin, phenylpropanolamine, and phenylephrine
Coly-Mycin® S Oral	colistin sulfate
Combipres®	clonidine and chlorthalidone
Comfort® Ophthalmic	naphazoline
Comfort® Tears Solution	artificial tears
Compazine®	prochlorperazine
Conex®	guaifenesin and phenylpropanolamine
Congess® Jr	guaifenesin and pseudoephedrine
Congess® Sr	guaifenesin and pseudoephedrine
Congestant D®	chlorpheniramine, phenylpropanolamine, and acetaminophen
Constant-T® Tablet	theophylline
Contac® Cold 12 Hour Relief Non-Drowsy	pseudoephedrine
Contac® Cough Formula Liquid	guaifenesin and dextromethorphan
Control®	phenylpropanolamine
Control-L®	pyrethrins
Contuss®	guaifenesin, phenylpropanolamine, and phenylephrine
Contuss® XT	guaifenesin and phenylpropanolamine
Cophene-B®	brompheniramine
Cophene XP®	hydrocodone, pseudoephedrine, and guaifenesin
Co-Pyronil® 2 Pulvules®	chlorpheniramine and pseudoephedrine
Corgonject®	chorionic gonadotropin
Corliprol®	celiprolol
Cortaid® Ointment	hydrocortisone
Cortatrigen® Otic	neomycin, polymyxin B, and hydrocortisone
Cortef® Suspension	hydrocortisone
Cortenema®	hydrocortisone
Cortisporin® Topical Cream	neomycin, polymyxin B, and hydrocortisone
Cortone®	cortisone acetate
Cortrophin-Zinc®	corticotropin
Cotazym®	pancrelipase
Cotazym-S®	pancrelipase
Cotrim®	co-trimoxazole
Cotrim® DS	co-trimoxazole
Crystamine®	cyanocobalamin
Crysticillin® A.S.	penicillin G procaine
Crysti 1000®	cyanocobalamin
Crystodigin®	digitoxin
Cyanoject®	cyanocobalamin
Cyclospasmol®	cyclandelate (all products)
Cycofed® Pediatric	guaifenesin, pseudoephedrine, and codeine
Cycrin® 10 mg Tablet	medroxyprogesterone acetate
Cyomin®	cyanocobalamin
Dacodyl®	bisacodyl
Dakrina® Ophthalmic Solution	artificial tears
Dalgan®	dezocine
Dallergy-D® Syrup	chlorpheniramine and phenylephrine
D-Amp®	ampicillin
Danex® Shampoo	pyrithione zinc
Dapacin® Cold Capsule	chlorpheniramine, phenylpropanolamine, and acetaminophen
Darbid® Tablet	isopropamide iodide (all products)
Daricon®	oxyphencyclimine (all products)
Darvon® 32 mg Capsule	propoxyphene hydrochloride
Darvon-N® Oral Suspension	propoxyphene napsylate
Datril® Extra Strength	acetaminophen
Dayto Himbin®	yohimbine

(continued)

Brand Name	Generic Name
DC 240® Softgel®	docusate
Debrisan®	dextranomer
Decadron® Elixir	dexamethasone
Decadron® 0.25 mg & 6 mg Tablets	dexamethasone
Decadron® Phosphate	dexamethasone
Decadron® Phosphate Ophthalmic Ointment	dexamethasone
Deca-Durabolin®	nandrolone
Decaspray®	dexamethasone
Decholin®	dehydrocholic acid
Defen-LA®	guaifenesin and pseudoephedrine
Deficol®	bisacodyl
Degest® 2 Ophthalmic	naphazoline
Dehist®	brompheniramine maleate
Deladumone®	estradiol and testosterone
Delatest® Injection	testosterone
Del-Mycin® Topical	erythromycin (ophthalmic/topical)
Delta-Cortef®	prednisolone (systemic)
Deltalin® Capsule	ergocalciferol
Delta-Tritex® Topical	triamcinolone (topical)
Del-Vi-A®	vitamin A
Demazin® Syrup	chlorpheniramine and phenylpropanolamine
depAndrogyn®	estradiol and testosterone
depAndro® Injection	testosterone
depGynogen® Injection	estradiol
depMedalone® Injection	methylprednisolone
Depoject® Injection	methylprednisolone
Deponit® Patch	nitroglycerin
Depo-Provera® 100 mg/mL	medroxyprogesterone
Depo-Testadiol®	estradiol and testosterone
Depotest® Injection	testosterone
Depotestogen®	estradiol and testosterone
Deprol®	meprobamate and benactyzine hydrochloride
Dermaflex® Gel	lidocaine
Dermatophytin-O	candida albicans (monilia)
Dermoxyl® Gel	benzoyl peroxide
Despec® Liquid	guaifenesin, phenylpropanolamine, and phenylephrine
Desquam-X® Wash	benzoyl peroxide
Detussin® Expectorant	hydrocodone, pseudoephedrine, and guaifenesin
Dexacen-4®	dexamethasone
Dexacen® LA-8	dexamethasone
Dexatrim® Pre-Meal	phenylpropanolamine
Dexchlor®	dexchlorpheniramine
Dexedrine® Elixir	dextroamphetamine sulfate
Dey-Dose® Isoproterenol	isoproterenol
Dey-Dose® Metaproterenol	metaproterenol sulfate
Dey-Lute® Isoetharine	isoetharine
DHC®	hydrocodone and acetaminophen
DHC Plus®	dihydrocodeine compound
Dialose® Capsule	docusate sodium
Dialose® Plus Capsule	docusate and casanthranol
Dialose® Tablet	docusate
Dialume®	aluminum hydroxide
Diamine T.D.®	brompheniramine
Diamox® 250 mg Tablet	acetazolamide
Diaparene® Cradol®	methylbenzethonium
Diapid® Nasal Spray	lypressin

(continued)

Brand Name	Generic Name
Diar-aid®	loperamide
Diasorb®	attapulgite
Diazemuls® Injection	diazepam
Dibent® Injection	dicyclomine
Dicarbosil®	calcium carbonate
---	dicumarol (all products)
Digepepsin®	pancreatin
Dihyrex® Injection	diphenhydramine
Dilantin-30® Pediatric Suspension	phenytoin
Dilantin® With Phenobarbital	phenytoin with phenobarbital
Dilaudid® 1 mg & 3 mg Tablet	hydromorphone hydrochloride
Dilaudid® Cough Syrup	hydromorphone
Dilocaine® Injection	lidocaine
Dilomine® Injection	dicyclomine
Dimaphen® Elixir	brompheniramine and phenylpropanolamine
Dimaphen® Tablets	brompheniramine and phenylpropanolamine
Dimetabs® Oral	dimenhydrinate
Dimetane®	brompheniramine maleate
Dimetane®-DC	brompheniramine, phenylpropanolamine, and codeine
Dimetane® Decongestant Elixir	brompheniramine and phenylephrine
Dimetapp® 4-Hour Liqui-Gel Capsule	brompheniramine and phenylpropanolamine
Dimetapp® Elixir	brompheniramine and phenylpropanolamine
Dimetapp® Extentabs®	brompheniramine and phenylpropanolamine
Dimetapp® Sinus Caplets	pseudoephedrine and ibuprofen
Dimetapp® Tablet	brompheniramine and phenylpropanolamine
Dinate® Injection	dimenhydrinate
Diocto C®	docusate and casanthranol
Diocto-K®	docusate
Diocto-K Plus®	docusate
Dioctolose Plus®	docusate and casanthranol
Dioval® Injection	estradiol
Diphenacen 50® Injection	diphenhydramine
Diphenatol®	diphenoxylate and atropine
Diphenylan Sodium®	phenytoin
Diprosone®	betamethasone
Disalcid®	salsalate
Disanthrol®	docusate and casanthranol
Disobrom®	dexbrompheniramine and pseudoephedrine
Disonate®	docusate
Disotate®	edetate disodium
Di-Spaz® Injection	dicyclomine
Di-Spaz® Oral	dicyclomine
Dispos-a-Med® Isoproterenol	isoproterenol
Dital®	phendimetrazine
Diucardin®	hydroflumethiazide
Diupress®	chlorothiazide and reserpine
Diurigen®	chlorothiazide
Dizac® Injectable Emulsion	diazepam
Dizmiss®	meclizine
Dizymes® Tablet	pancreatin
D-Med® Injection	methylprednisolone
Docusoft Plus™	docusate and casanthranol
Doktors® Nasal Solution	phenylephrine
Dolacet® Forte	hydrocodone and acetaminophen
Dolene®	propoxyphene
Dolorac™	capsaicin

(continued)

Brand Name	Generic Name
Dolorex®	capsaicin
Dommanate® Injection	dimenhydrinate
Donnamar®	hyoscyamine
Donnapectolin-PG®	hyoscyamine, atropine, scopolamine, kaolin, pectin, and opium
Donnapine®	hyoscyamine, atropine, scopolamine, and phenobarbital
Donnazyme®	pancreatin
Donphen® Tablet	hyoscyamine, atropine, scopolamine, and phenobarbital
Dopar®	levodopa
Dopastat® Injection	dopamine hydrochloride
Doriden® Tablet	glutethimide
Dormarex® 2 Oral	diphenhydramine
Doxidan®	docusate and casanthranol
Doxinate® Capsule	docusate sodium
D-Pan®	dexpanthenol
Dramamine® Injection	dimenhydrinate
Dramilin® Injection	dimenhydrinate
Dramocen®	dimenhydrinate
Dramoject®	dimenhydramine
Drinex®	acetaminophen, chlorpheniramine, and pseudoephedrine
Dristan® Long Lasting Nasal Solution	oxymetazoline
Dristan® Saline Spray	sodium chloride
Drithocreme® HP 1%	anthralin
Drixoral® Cough & Congestion Liquid Caps	pseudoephedrine and dextromethorphan
Drixoral® Cough Liquid Caps	dextromethorphan
Drixoral® Non-Drowsy	pseudoephedrine
Dry Eye® Therapy Solution	artificial tears
Dryox® Gel	benzoyl peroxide
Dryox® Wash	benzoyl peroxide
DSMC Plus®	docusate and casanthranol
D-S-S Plus®	docusate and casanthranol
Duadacin® Capsule	chlorpheniramine, phenylpropanolamine, and acetaminophen
DuoCet™	hydrocodone and acetaminophen
Duo-Cyp®	estradiol and testosterone
Duo-Medihaler®	isoproterenol and phenylephrine
DuoPlant®	salicylic acid
Duo-Trach® Injection	lidocaine
Duotrate®	pentaerythritol tetranitrate
Duphalac®	lactulose
Duracid®	aluminum hydroxide, magnesium carbonate, and calcium carbonate
Duract®	bromfenac (all products)
Duradyne DHC®	hydrocodone and acetaminophen
Dura-Gest®	guaifenesin, phenylpropanolamine, and phenylephrine
Duralone® Injection	methylprednisolone
Duranest® (plain and with epinephrine)	etidocaine
Duratest® Injection	testosterone
Duratestrin®	estradiol and testosterone
Durathate® Injection	testosterone
Dura-Vent®	guaifenesin and phenylpropanolamine
Dura-Vent®/DA	chlorpheniramine, phenylephrine, and methscopolamine
Duricef® Oral Suspension 125 mg/5 mL	cefadroxil
Durrax® Oral	hydroxyzine
Duvoid®	bethanechol
DV® Vaginal Cream	dienestrol
Dwelle® Ophthalmic Solution	artificial tears

(continued)

Brand Name	Generic Name
Dycill®	dicloxacillin
Dyclone®	dyclonine
Dyflex-400® Tablet	dyphylline
Dymelor®	acetohexamide
Dymenate® Injection	dimenhydrinate
Dynapen®	dicloxacillin
Dyrexan-OD®	phendimetrazine
ED-SPAZ®	hyoscyamine
Effer-Syllium®	psyllium
Eflone®	fluorometholone
Efodine®	povidone-iodine
Elase® (all products)	fibrinolysin and desoxyribonuclease
Elase®-Chloromycetin® Ointment	fibrinolysin and desoxyribonuclease
Elavil®	amitriptyline
Eldepryl® Tablet (only)	selegiline
Eldoquin® Lotion	hydroquinone
Elixomin®	theophylline
Elixophyllin SR®	theophylline
E-Lor® Tablet	propoxyphene and acetaminophen
Emecheck®	phosphorated carbohydrate solution
Emete-Con® Injection	benzquinamide
----	emetine hydrochloride
Emitrip®	amitriptyline
Emulsoil®	castor oil
E-Mycin®	erythromycin (systemic)
E-Mycin-E®	erythromycin (systemic)
Endep® 25 mg, 50 mg, 100 mg	amitriptyline hydrochloride
Endocodone®	oxycodone
Endolor®	butalbital compound and acetaminophen
Enduron® 2.5 mg Tablet	methyclothiazide
Ener-B®	cyanocobalamin
Enisyl®	l-lysine
Enkaid®	encainide
Enomine®	guaifenesin, phenylpropanolamine, and phenylephrine
Enovid®	mestranol and norethynodrel
Enovil®	amitriptyline
E.N.T.®	brompheniramine and phenylpropanolamine
Entozyme®	pancreatin
Entuss-D® Liquid	hydrocodone and pseudoephedrine
Epifrin®	epinephrine
E-Pilo-x® Ophthalmic	pilocarpine and epinephrine
Epinal®	epinephryl borate
E.P. Mycin® Capsule	oxytetracycline
Equanil®	meprobamate
Equilet®	calcium carbonate
Ercaf®	ergotamine
Ergostat®	ergotamine
Ergotamine Tartrate and Caffeine Cafatine®	ergotamine
Ergotrate® Maleate Injection	ergonovine
Eridium®	phenazopyridine hydrochloride
Ery-Sol® Topical Solution	erythromycin, topical
Esidrix®	hydrochlorothiazide
E-Solve-2® Topical	erythromycin (ophthalmic/topical)
Estivin® II Ophthalmic	naphazoline
Estradurin® Injection	polyestradiol phosphate
Estra-L® Injection	estradiol

(continued)

Brand Name	Generic Name
Estratab®	estrogens (esterified)
Estro-Cyp® Injection	estradiol
Estroject-2® Injection	estradiol
Estroject-L.A.® Injection	estradiol
Estronol® Injection	estrone
Estrostep® 21	ethinyl estradiol and norethindrone
Estrovis®	quinestrol
Ethaquin®	ethaverine hydrochloride
Ethatab®	ethaverine hydrochloride
ETS-2% Topical	erythromycin (ophthalmic/topical)
Euthroid® Tablet	liotrix
Eutron®	methyclothiazide and pargyline
Evac-Q-Mag®	magnesium citrate
Evalose®	lactulose
Everone® Injection	testosterone
Excedrin® IB	ibuprofen
Exidine® Scrub	chlorhexidine gluconate
Exna®	benzthiazide
Exosurf Neonatal®	colfosceril palmitate
Exsel®	selenium sulfide
Extra Action Cough Syrup	guaifenesin and dextromethorphan
Eye-Lube-A® Solution	artificial tears
Eye-Sed® Ophthalmic	zinc sulfate
Ezide®	hydrochlorothiazide
Fastin®	phentermine
Fedahist® Expectorant	guaifenesin and pseudoephedrine
Fedahist® Expectorant Pediatric	guaifenesin and pseudoephedrine
Fedahist® Tablet	chlorpheniramine and pseudoephedrine
Feen-A-Mint®	bisacodyl
FemCare®	clotrimazole
Femcet®	butalbital compound and acetaminophen
Femguard®	sulfabenzamide, sulfacetamide, and sulfathiazole
Femstat®	butoconazole nitrate
Fentanyl Oralet®	fentanyl
Feosol® Elixir	ferrous sulfate
Ferancee®	ferrous sulfate and ascorbic acid
Fergon Plus®	iron with vitamin B
Fer-In-Sol® Capsule	ferrous sulfate
Fer-In-Sol® Syrup	ferrous sulfate
Fermalox®	ferrous sulfate, magnesium hydroxide, and docusate
Ferndex®	dextroamphetamine sulfate
Fero-Gradumet®	ferrous sulfate
Ferospace®	ferrous sulfate
Ferralet®	ferrous gluconate
Ferralyn® Lanacaps®	ferrous sulfate
Ferra-TD®	ferrous sulfate
Fiorgen PF®	butalbital compound and aspirin
Fiorital®	butalbital compound and aspirin
Flavorcee®	ascorbic acid
Flaxedil®	gallamine triethiodide
Fleet® Flavored Castor Oil	castor oil
Fleet® Laxative	bisacodyl
Fleet® Sof-Lax® Overnight	docusate and casanthranol
Flexaphen®	chlorzoxazone
Flonase® 9 g	fluticasone
Florone E®	diflorasone

(continued)

Brand Name	Generic Name
Floropryl® Ophthalmic	isoflurophate
Fluonid® Topical	fluocinolone
FluorCare® Neutral	fluoride
Fluoritab®	fluoride
Fluor-Op®	fluorometholone
Fluothane®	halothane
Flura®	fluoride
Flurate® Ophthalmic Solution	fluorescein sodium
Flurosyn® Topical	fluocinolone
FluShield®	influenza virus vaccine
Flutex® Topical	triamcinolone (topical)
Folex® Injection	methotrexate
Folex® PFS™	methotrexate
Follutein®	chorionic gonadotropin
Folvite®	folic acid
Formula Q®	quinine
FS Shampoo® Topical	fluocinolone
Fumasorb®	ferrous fumarate
Fumerin®	ferrous fumarate
Funduscein® Injection	fluorescein sodium
Furacin® Topical	nitrofurazone
Furalan®	nitrofurantoin
Furamide®	diloxanide furoate
Furan®	nitrofurantoin
Furanite®	nitrofurantoin
Furoxone®	furazolidone
G-1®	butalbital compound and acetaminophen
Gamastan®	immune globulin, intramuscular
Gammagard® Injection	immune globulin, intravenous
Gammar®	immune globulin, intramuscular
Gamulin® Rh	Rh_o(D) immune globulin (intramuscular)
Ganite™	gallium nitrate
Gantanol®	sulfamethoxazole
Gantrisin® Ophthalmic	sulfisoxazole
Gantrisin® Tablet	sulfisoxazole
Garamycin®	gentamicin
Gas-Ban DS®	aluminum hydroxide, magnesium hydroxide, and simethicone
Gastrosed™	hyoscyamine
Gee Gee®	guaifenesin
Gel-Tin®	fluoride
Gelusil® Liquid	aluminum hydroxide, magnesium hydroxide, and simethicone
Genabid®	papaverine hydrochloride
Genagesic®	guaifenesin and phenylpropanolamine
Genamin® Cold Syrup	chlorpheniramine and phenylpropanolamine
Genamin® Expectorant	guaifenesin and phenylpropanolamine
Genasoft® Plus	docusate and casanthranol
Genatap® Elixir	brompheniramine and phenylpropanolamine
Genatuss®	guaifenesin
Gencalc® 600	calcium carbonate
Gen-D-phen®	diphenhydramine hydrochloride
Gen-K®	potassium chloride
Genora® 0.5/35	ethinyl estradiol and norethindrone
Genora® 1/35	ethinyl estradiol and norethindrone
Genora® 1/50	mestranol and norethindrone
Gentacidin®	gentamicin
Gentrasul®	gentamicin
Geref®	sermorelin acetate

(continued)

Brand Name	Generic Name
Geridium®	phenazopyridine
GG-Cen®	guaifenesin
Glaucon®	epinephrine
Glukor®	chorionic gonadotropin
Glyate®	guaifenesin
Glycerol-T®	theophylline and guaifenesin
Glycofed®	guaifenesin and pseudoephedrine
Glycotuss®	guaifenesin
Glycotuss-dM®	guaifenesin and dextromethorphan
G-myticin®	gentamicin
Gonic®	chorionic gonadotropin
Goniosol®	hydroxypropyl methylcellulose
Grifulvin® V Tablet 250 mg and 500 mg	griseofulvin
Grisactin®	griseofulvin
Grisactin® Ultra	griseofulvin
Guaifenex®	guaifenesin, phenylpropanolamine, and phenylephrine
Guaifenex® PPA 75	guaifenesin and phenylpropanolamine
Guaipax®	guaifenesin and phenylpropanolamine
Guaitab®	guaifenesin and pseudoephedrine
Guaivent®	guaifenesin and pseudoephedrine
GuiaCough®	guaifenesin and dextromethorphan
GuiaCough® Expectorant	guaifenesin
Guiatex®	guaifenesin, phenylpropanolamine, and phenylephrine
Guaituss CF®	guaifenesin, phenylpropanolamine, and dextromethorphan
G-well®	lindane
Gyne-Sulf®	sulfabenzamide, sulfacetamide, and sulfathiazole
Gynogen® Injection	estradiol
Gynogen L.A.® Injection	estradiol
----	halazone tablet
Haldrone®	paramethasone acetate
Halenol® Tablet	acetaminophen
Halfan®	halofantrine
Halog®-E	halcinonide
Halotex®	haloprogin
Halotussin®	guaifenesin
Halotussin® DM	guaifenesin and dextromethorphan
Halotussin® PE	guaifenesin and pseudoephedrine
Haltran®	ibuprofen
Harmonyl®	deserpidine
H-BIG®	hepatitis B immune globulin
Healon®	sodium hyaluronate
Healon® GV	sodium hyaluronate
Healon® 5	sodium hyaluronate
HemFe®	iron with vitamins
Hep-B-Gammagee®	hepatitis B immune globulin
Heptalac®	lactulose
Herplex®	idoxuridine
Hetrazan®	diethylcarbamazine citrate
Hismanal®	astemizole
Histaject®	brompheniramine maleate
Histalet Forte® Tablet	chlorpheniramine, pyrilamine, phenylephrine, and phenylpropanolamine
Histalet® X	guaifenesin and pseudoephedrine
Hista-Vadrin® Tablet	chlorpheniramine, phenylephrine, and phenylpropanolamine
Histerone® Injection	testosterone
Histinex® D Liquid	hydrocodone and pseudoephedrine
Histolyn-CYL®	histoplasmin

(continued)

Brand Name	Generic Name
Histor-D® Syrup	chlorpheniramine and phenylephrine
Histor-D® Timecelles®	chlorpheniramine, phenylephrine, and methscopolamine
Histrodrix®	dexbrompheniramine and pseudoephedrine
Humalog® Mix 50/50 Insulin	insulin
Humegon™	menotropins
Humibid® LA	guaifenesin
Humibid® Pediatric	guaifenesin
Humibid® Sprinkle	guaifenesin
Humorsol® Ophthalmic	demecarium
HycoClear Tuss®	hydrocodone and guaifenesin
Hycomine®	hydrocodone and phenylpropanolamine
Hycomine® Pediatric	hydrocodone and phenylpropanolamine
Hydeltra-T.B.A.®	prednisolone
Hydergine®	ergoloid mesylates
Hydramyn® Syrup	diphenhydramine hydrochloride
Hydrate®	dimenhydrinate
Hydrobexan® Injection	hydroxocobalamin
Hydrocet®	hydrocodone and acetaminophen
Hydro Cobex®	hydroxocobalamin
Hydrocodone PA® Syrup	hydrocodone and phenylpropanolamine
Hydrocortone® Acetate	hydrocortisone
Hydro-Crysti-12®	hydroxocobalamin
HydroDIURIL®	hydrochlorothiazide
Hydrogesic®	hydrocodone and acetaminophen
Hydromox®	quinethazone
Hydro-Par®	hydrochlorothiazide
Hydrophed®	theophylline, ephedrine, and hydroxyzine
Hydropres®	hydrochlorothiazide and reserpine
Hydrotropine®	hydrocodone and homatropine
Hydroxacen®	hydroxyzine
Hygroton®	chlorthalidone
Hylorel®	guanadrel
----	hyoscyamine, atropine, scopolamine, kaolin, and pectin
Hy-Pam® Oral	hydroxyzine
Hyperab®	rabies immune globulin (human)
Hyper-Tet®	tetanus immune globulin (human)
Hy-Phen®	hydrocodone and acetaminophen
HypRho®-D	$Rh_o(D)$ immune globulin (intramuscular)
HypRho®-D Mini-Dose	$Rh_o(D)$ immune globulin (intramuscular)
Hyprogest® 250	hydroxyprogesterone caproate
Hyzine®	hydroxyzine
Ibuprin®	ibuprofen
Idamycin®	idarubicin
Ilopan-Choline® Oral	dexpanthenol
Ilopan® Injection	dexpanthenol
Ilosone® Pulvules®	erythromycin (systemic)
Ilozyme®	pancrelipase
I-Naphline® Ophthalmic	naphazoline
Innovar®	droperidol and fentanyl
Inocor®	inamrinone (amrinone)
Intal® Inhalation Capsule	cromolyn sodium
Intensol® Solution	metoclopramide
Intercept™	nonoxynol 9
Intropin®	dopamine
Iodex-p®	povidone-iodine
Iodo-Niacin® Tablet	potassium iodide and niacinamide hydroiodide
Iophen®	iodinated glycerol

(continued)

Brand Name	Generic Name
Iophen-C®	iodinated glycerol and codeine
Iophen-DM®	iodinated glycerol and dextromethorphan (all products)
Iophen NR	guaifenesin
Iophylline®	iodinated glycerol and theophylline
Iotuss®	iodinated glycerol and codeine
Iotuss-DM®	iodinated glycerol and dextromethorphan (all products)
I-Pentolate®	cyclopentolate
I-Phrine® Ophthalmic Solution	phenylephrine
I-Picamide®	tropicamide
Ismelin®	guanethidine
Ismotic®	isosorbide
Iso-Bid®	isosorbide dinitrate
Isollyl® Improved	butalbital compound and aspirin
Isoptin®	verapamil
Isopto® Cetapred®	sulfacetamide sodium and prednisolone
Isopto® Eserine	physostigmine
Isopto® Frin Ophthalmic Solution	phenylephrine
Isopto® P-ES	pilocarpine and physostigmine
Isopto® Plain Solution	artificial tears
Isovex®	ethaverine hydrochloride
Isuprel® Glossets®	isoproterenol
I-Tropine®	atropine
Janimine®	imipramine
Jenamicin®	gentamicin
Jenest™-28	ethinyl estradiol and norethindrone
Just Tears® Solution	artificial tears
Kabikinase®	streptokinase
Kalcinate®	calcium gluconate
Kaochlor®	potassium chloride
Kaochlor-Eff®	potassium bicarbonate, potassium chloride, and potassium citrate
Kaochlor® SF	potassium chloride
Kaodene®	kaolin and pectin
Kaopectate® Advanced Formula	attapulgite
Kaopectate® Maximum Strength Caplets	attapulgite
Kaopectate® II	loperamide
Kapectolin PG®	hyoscyamine, atropine, scopolamine, kaolin, pectin, and opium
Karidium®	fluoride
Karigel®	fluoride
Karigel®-N	fluoride
Kasof®	docusate
Kato® Powder	potassium chloride
Kaybovite-1000®	cyanocobalamin
Keflin®	cephalothin sodium
Kefurox® Injection	cefuroxime
Kefzol®	cefazolin
K-Electrolyte® Effervescent	potassium bicarbonate
Kenacort® Oral	triamcinolone (systemic)
Kenaject® Injection	triamcinolone (systemic)
Kenonel® Topical	triamcinolone (topical)
Kestrin® Injection	estrone
Key-Pred®	prednisolone (systemic)
Key-Pred-SP®	prednisolone (systemic)
K-G®	potassium gluconate
K-Gen® Effervescent	potassium bicarbonate
K-Ide®	potassium bicarbonate and potassium citrate, effervescent

(continued)

Brand Name	Generic Name
Kinerase®	hyaluronidase
Kinesed®	hyoscyamine, atropine, scopolamine, and phenobarbital
K-Lease®	potassium chloride
Klerist-D® Tablet	chlorpheniramine and pseudoephedrine
Klorominr® Oral	chlorpheniramine
Klorvess®	potassium chloride
Klorvess® Effervescent	potassium bicarbonate and potassium chloride, effervescent
K-Lyte® Effervescent	potassium bicarbonate
K-Norm®	potassium chloride
Koate®-HP	antihemophilic factor (human)
Koate®-HS Injection	antihemophilic factor (human)
Koate®-HT Injection	antihemophilic factor (human)
Kogenate®	antihemophilic factor (recombinant)
Kolyum® Powder	potassium chloride and potassium gluconate
Konakion® Injection	phytonadione
Kondon's Nasal®	ephedrine
Konyne-HT® Injection	factor IX complex (human)
K-Pek®	attapulgite
Kwell®	lindane
LA-12®	hydroxocobalamin
Lacril® Ophthalmic Solution	artificial tears
Lactulose PSE®	lactulose
Lamprene® 100 mg	clofazimine
Laniazid® Tablet	isoniazid
Lanorinal®	butalbital compound and aspirin
Largon®	propiomazine
Larodopa®	levodopa
Lasan™ HP-1 Topical	anthralin
Lasan™ Topical	anthralin
Ledercillin VK®	penicillin V potassium
Lente® Iletin® II	insulin preparations
Lente® Insulin	insulin preparations
Lente® L	insulin preparations
----	levodopa
Levo-T™	levothyroxine
Libritabs® (all products)	chlordiazepoxide
Lice-Enz® Shampoo	pyrethrins
LidoPen® I.M. Injection Auto-Injector	lidocaine
Lincorex®	lincomycin
Liquaemin®	heparin
Liquibid®	guaifenesin
Liquibid® 1200	guaifenesin
Liqui-Char®	charcoal
Liquid Pred®	prednisone
Liquifilm® Forte Solution	artificial tears
Liquifilm® Tears Solution	artificial tears
Listerex® Scrub	salicylic acid
Listermint® With Fluoride	fluoride
Lithane®	lithium
Lithonate®	lithium
Lithotabs®	lithium
LoCHOLEST®	cholestyramine resin
LoCHOLEST® Light	cholestyramine resin
Logen®	diphenoxylate and atropine
Lomanate®	diphenoxylate and atropine
Lorcet®	hydrocodone and acetaminophen

(continued)

Brand Name	Generic Name
Lorelco®	probucol
Lorsin®	acetaminophen, chlorpheniramine, and pseudoephedrine
Lortab® ASA	hydrocodone and aspirin
Losopan®	magaldrate and simethicone
Lotrimin® AF Cream	clotrimazole
Lotrimin® AF Lotion	clotrimazole
Lotrimin® AF Solution	clotrimazole
Loxitane® I.M.	loxapine
Lozi-Tab®	fluoride
LubriTears® Solution	artificial tears
Ludiomil®	maprotiline
Luride®-SF	fluoride
Luvox®	fluvoxamine
Lycolan® Elixir	l-lysine
LYMErix™	lyme disease
Lyphocin® Injection	vancomycin
3M™ Avagard®	chlorhexidine gluconate
Maalox® Anti-Gas	aluminum hydroxide, magnesium hydroxide, and simethicone
Maalox® Anti-Gas Extra Strength	aluminum hydroxide, magnesium hydroxide, and simethicone
Maalox® Extra Strength	aluminum hydroxide and magnesium hydroxide
Maalox® Plus	aluminum hydroxide, magnesium hydroxide, and simethicone
Maalox® TC (Therapeutic Concentrate)	aluminum hydroxide and magnesium hydroxide
Macrodex®	dextran
Magalox Plus®	aluminum hydroxide, magnesium hydroxide, and simethicone
Magan®	magnesium salicylate
Magsal®	magnesium salicylate
Malatal®	hyoscyamine, atropine, scopolamine, and phenobarbital
Mallisol®	povidone-iodine
Malotuss® Syrup	guaifenesin
Mandol® (all products)	cefamandole
Mantadil® Cream	chlorcyclizine
Maolate®	chlorphenesin
Maox®	magnesium oxide
Marax®	theophylline, ephedrine, and hydroxyzine
Marmine® Injection	dimenhydrinate
Marmine® Oral	dimenhydrinate
Marthritic®	salsalate
Max-Caro®	beta-carotene
Maxidex® Ophthalmic Ointment	dexamethasone
Maxiflor®	diflorasone
Maximum Strength Desenex® Antifungal Cream	miconazole
Maximum Strength Dex-A-Diet®	phenylpropanolamine
Maximum Strength Dexatrim®	phenylpropanolamine
Maxolon®	metoclopramide
Mazanor®	mazindol
Measurin®	aspirin
Meclan® Topical	meclocycline
Meclomen®	meclofenamate sodium
Medidin® Liquid	hydrocodone and guaifenesin
Medihaler-Epi®	epinephrine
Medihaler Ergotamine®	ergotamine
Medihaler-Iso®	isoproterenol
Medipain 5®	hydrocodone and acetaminophen
Medipren®	ibuprofen

(continued)

Brand Name	Generic Name
Medi-Quick® Topical Ointment	bacitracin, neomycin, and polymyxin B
Medispaz®	hyoscyamine
Medi-Tuss®	guaifenesin
Medralone® Injection	methylprednisolone
Medrapred®	prednisolone and atropine
Medrol® Acetate Topical	methylprednisolone
Mellaril® (all products)	thioridazine
Mellaril-S®	thioridazine
Meni-D®	meclizine
Meprospan®	meprobamate
Mesantoin®	mephenytoin
Mestinon® Injection	pyridostigmine
Metahydrin®	trichlormethiazide
Metaprel® Aerosol	metaproterenol sulfate
Metaprel® Inhalation Solution	metaproterenol sulfate
Metaprel® Syrup	metaproterenol sulfate
Metaprel® Tablet	metaproterenol sulfate
Metasep®	parachlorometaxylenol
---	methicillin
Meticorten®	prednisone
Metizol® Tablet	metronidazole
Metra®	phendimetrazine tartrate
Metreton®	prednisolone (ophthalmic)
Metrodin®	urofollitropin
Metro I.V.® Injection	metronidazole
Metubine® Iodide	metocurine iodide
Mezlin®	mezlocillin
Micro-K® LS	potassium chloride
microNefrin®	epinephrine
Midamor®	amiloride
Miflex® Tablet	chlorzoxazone and acetaminophen
Migrapap®	acetaminophen, isometheptene, and dichloralphenazone
Migratine®	acetaminophen, isometheptene, and dichloralphenazone
Milkinol®	mineral oil
Milontin®	phensuximide
Milophene®	clomiphene
Milprem®	meprobamate and conjugated estrogens
Mini-Gamulin® Rh	Rh_0(D) immune globulin (intramuscular)
Minocin® Tablet	minocycline
Minute-Gel®	fluoride
Miochol®	acetylcholine
Mithracin®	plicamycin
Mito-Carn®	levocarnitine
Mitran® Oral	chlordiazepoxide
Mobidin®	magnesium salicylate
Moctanin®	monoctanoin
Modane® Soft	docusate
Moduretic®	amiloride and hydrochlorothiazide
Moisturel® Lotion	dimethicone
Monafed®	guaifenesin
Monafed® DM	guaifenesin and dextromethorphan
Monistat i.v.™ Injection	miconazole
Monocete® Topical Liquid	monochloroacetic acid
Monocid®	cefonicid
Motrin® IB Sinus	pseudoephedrine and ibuprofen
Moxam® Injection	moxalactam
M-Prednisol® Injection	methylprednisolone

(continued)

Brand Name	Generic Name
M-R-VAX® II	measles and rubella vaccines (combined)
MSTA®	mumps skin test antigen
Mucosil™	acetylcysteine
Multitest CMI®	skin test antigens, multiple
Muroptic-5®	sodium chloride
Mus-Lax®	chlorzoxazone
Mycelex®-G	clotrimazole
Mycifradin® Sulfate	neomycin
Mycolog®-II	nystatin and triamcinolone
Myconel® Topical	nystatin and triamcinolone
Mykrox®	metolazone
Mylanta AR®	famotidine
Mylanta®-II	aluminum hydroxide, magnesium hydroxide, and simethicone
Mylaxen® Injection	hexafluorenium bromide
Myminic® Expectorant	guaifenesin and phenylpropanolamine
Myochrysine®	gold sodium thiomalate
Myotonachol™	bethanechol
Myphetane DC®	brompheniramine, phenylpropanolamine, and codeine
Nafazair® Ophthalmic	naphazoline
Nafcil™	nafcillin
Naldecon®	chlorpheniramine, phenyltoloxamine, phenylpropanolamine, and phenylephrine
Naldecon® DX Adult Liquid	guaifenesin, phenylpropanolamine, and dextromethorphan
Naldecon-EX® Children's Syrup	guaifenesin and phenylpropanolamine
Naldelate®	chlorpheniramine, phenyltoloxamine, phenylpropanolamine, and phenylephrine
Nalgest®	chlorpheniramine, phenyltoloxamine, phenylpropanolamine, and phenylephrine
Nallpen®	nafcillin
Nalspan®	chlorpheniramine, phenyltoloxamine, phenylpropanolamine, and phenylephrine
Nandrobolic® Injection	nandrolone phenpropionate
Naphcon Forte® Ophthalmic	naphazoline
Nasacort®	triamcinolone
Nasahist B®	brompheniramine
Natabec®	vitamin (multiple/prenatal)
Natabec® FA	vitamin (multiple/prenatal)
Natabec® Rx	vitamin (multiple/prenatal)
Natalins® Rx	vitamin (multiple/prenatal)
Naturetin®	bendroflumethiazide
Naus-A-Way®	phosphorated carbohydrate solution
N-B-P® Ointment	bacitracin, neomycin, and polymyxin B
Nebcin®	tobramycin
Nelova™ 0.5/35E	ethinyl estradiol and norethindrone
Nelova™ 1/35E	ethinyl estradiol and norethindrone
Nelova™ 1/50M	mestranol and norethindrone
Nelova™ 10/11	ethinyl estradiol and norethindrone
Neo-Calglucon®	calcium glubionate
Neo-Castaderm®	resorcinol, boric acid, acetone
Neo-Cortef®	neomycin and hydrocortisone
NeoDecadron® Topical	neomycin and dexamethasone
Neo-Dexameth® Ophthalmic	neomycin and dexamethasone
Neo-Durabolic®	nandrolone
Neofed®	pseudoephedrine
Neo-Medrol® Acetate Topical	methylprednisolone and neomycin
Neomixin® Topical	bacitracin, neomycin, and polymyxin B
Neoquess® Injection	dicyclomine hydrochloride
Neoquess® Tablet	hyoscyamine sulfate

(continued)

Brand Name	Generic Name
Neo-Synalar® Topical	neomycin and fluocinolone
Neo-Tabs®	neomycin
NeoVadrin®	vitamins (multiple)
Nephrox Suspension	aluminum hydroxide
Neptazane®	methazolamide
Nervocaine® Injection	lidocaine
Nestrex®	pyridoxine
Netromycin®	netilmicin
Neucalm-50® Injection	hydroxyzine
Neuramate®	meprobamate
Neutra-Phos® Capsule	potassium phosphate and sodium phosphate
New Decongestant®	chlorpheniramine, phenyltoloxamine, phenylpropanolamine, and phenylephrine
N.G.A.® Topical	nystatin and triamcinolone
Niac®	niacin
Niacels™	niacin
N'ice®	ascorbic acid
Niclocide®	niclosamide
Nicobid®	niacin
Nicolar®	niacin
Nico-Vert®	meclizine
Nidryl®	diphenhydramine hydrochloride
Niferex Forte®	iron with vitamins
Niloric®	ergoloid mesylates
Nilstat®	nystatin
Nipride® Injection	nitroprusside sodium
Nisaval®	pyrilamine maleate
Nitro-Bid® I.V. Injection	nitroglycerin
Nitro-Bid® Oral	nitroglycerin
Nitrocine® Oral	nitroglycerin
Nitrodisc® Patch	nitroglycerin
Nitrol®	nitroglycerin
Nitrong® Oral Tablet	nitroglycerin
Nitrostat® 0.15 mg Tablet	nitroglycerin
Noctec®	chloral hydrate
Nolamine®	chlorpheniramine, phenindamine, and phenylpropanolamine
Nolex® LA	guaifenesin and phenylpropanolamine
Noludar®	methyprylon
No Pain-HP®	capsaicin
Norcet®	hydrocodone and acetaminophen
Norcuron®	vecuronium
Nordryl® Injection	diphenhydramine
Nordryl® Oral	diphenhydramine
Norethin™ 1/35E	ethinyl estradiol and norethindrone
Norlutate®	norethindrone
Norlutin®	norethindrone
Normiflo®	ardeparin
Norplant® Implant	levonorgestrel
Norzine®	thiethylperazine
Novacet®	sulfur and sulfacetamide
Novafed®	pseudoephedrine
Novafed® A	chlorpheniramine and pseudoephedrine
Novahistine® DMX Liquid	guaifenesin, pseudoephedrine, and dextromethorphan
Novahistine® Elixir	chlorpheniramine and phenylephrine
Novahistine® Expectorant	guaifenesin, pseudoephedrine, and codeine
Novolin® L Insulin	insulin
Novo Nordisk® (all products)	insulin

(continued)

Brand Name	Generic Name
NP-27®	tolnaftate
NPH Iletin® I Insulin	insulin
NTZ® Long Acting Nasal Solution	oxymetazoline
Numzident®	benzocaine
Nuprin®	ibuprofen
Nursoy®	enteral nutritional therapy
Nutropin Depot®	human growth hormone
Nydrazid®	isoniazid
Nystex®	nystatin
OCL®	polyethylene glycol-electrolyte solution
Octamide®	metoclopramide
Octicair® Otic	neomycin, polymyxin B, and hydrocortisone
Octocaine®	lidocaine and epinephrine
OcuClear®	oxymetazoline
Ocupress®	carteolol
Ocusert Pilo-20®	pilocarpine
Ocusert Pilo-40®	pilocarpine
Ocu-Sul®	sulfacetamide
Ocutricin® Topical Ointment	bacitracin, neomycin, and polymyxin B
OmniHIB™	*Haemophilus* B conjugate vaccine
Omnipen®	ampicillin
Omnipen®-N	ampicillin
Oncet®	hydrocodone and homatropine
Ony-Clear	benzalkonium chloride
Opcon® Ophthalmic	naphazoline
Oncovin®	vincristine
Ophthaine®	proparacaine
Ophthalgan® Ophthalmic	glycerin
Ophthifluor®	fluorescein sodium
Ophthochlor® Ophthalmic	chloramphenicol
Ophthocort®	chloramphenicol, polymyxin B, and hydrocortisone
Optimine®	azatadine
Optimoist® Solution	saliva substitute
Orabase®-O	benzocaine
Oradex-C®	dyclonine
Orajel® Brace-Aid Oral Anesthetic	benzocaine
Orasone®	prednisone
Oratect®	benzocaine
Ordrine AT® Extended Release Capsule	caramiphen and phenylpropanolamine
Oreticyl®	deserpidine and hydrochlorothiazide
Oreton® Methyl	methyltestosterone
Organidin®	iodinated glycerol
Orgaran®	danaparoid
Orimune®	poliovirus vaccine (live/trivalent/oral)
Orinase Diagnostic®	tolbutamide
Orinase® Oral	tolbutamide
ORLAAM®	levomethadyl acetate hydrochloride
Ormazine®	chlorpromazine
Ornade® Spansule® Capsules	chlorpheniramine and phenylpropanolamine
Ornidyl® Injection	eflornithine
Or-Tyl® Injection	dicyclomine
Orudis®	ketoprofen
Osteocalcin®	calcitonin
Otic-Care® Otic	neomycin, polymyxin B, and hydrocortisone
Otic Domeboro®	aluminum acetate and acetic acid

(continued)

Brand Name	Generic Name
Otic Tridesilon®	desonide and acetic acid
Otobiotic®	polymyxin B and hydrocortisone
Otocort® Otic	neomycin, polymyxin B, and hydrocortisone
Otosporin® Otic	neomycin, polymyxin B, and hydrocortisone
Otrivin®	xylometazoline
Otrivin® Pediatric	xylometazoline
Ovral®	ethinyl estradiol and norgestrel
O-V Staticin®	nystatin
Oxsoralen® Oral	methoxsalen
Oxy-5®	benzoyl peroxide
----	oxyphenbutazone
Pamprin IB®	ibuprofen
Panadol®	acetaminophen
Panasal® 5/500	hydrocodone and aspirin
Panscol® Lotion	salicylic acid
Panscol® Ointment	salicylic acid
Pantopon®	opium alkaloids
Panwarfarin®	warfarin sodium
Paplex®	salicylic acid
Paradione®	paramethadione
Paraflex®	chlorzoxazone
Para-Hist AT®	promethazine, phenylephrine, and codeine
---	paraldehyde
Par Decon®	chlorpheniramine, phenyltoloxamine, phenylpropanolamine, and phenylephrine
Paredrine®	hydroxyamphetamine
Paremyd® Ophthalmic	hydroxyamphetamine and tropicamide
Parepectolin®	kaolin and pectin with opium
Pargen Fortified®	chlorzoxazone
Par Glycerol®	iodinated glycerol
Parsidol®	ethopropazine (all products)
Partuss® LA	guaifenesin and phenylpropanolamine
Pathilon®	tridihexethyl
Pathocil®	dicloxacillin
Pavabid® (all products)	papaverine hydrochloride
Pavasule®	papaverine hydrochloride
Pavatine®	papaverine hydrochloride
Pavatym®	papaverine hydrochloride
Pavesed®	papaverine hydrochloride
Pavulon®	pancuronium
Paxene®	paclitaxel
Paxipam®	halazepam
PBZ® (all products)	tripelennamine
PediaPatch Transdermal Patch	salicylic acid
Pedia-Profen™	ibuprofen
Pediatric Triban®	trimethobanzamide
Penetrex®	enoxacin
Pentacarinat® Injection	pentamidine
Penthrane®	methoxyflurane
Pentids®	penicillin G potassium, oral (all products)
Pentothal® Sodium Rectal Suspension	thiopental
Pen.Vee® K	penicillin V potassium
Pepcid RPD™	famotidine
Peptavlon®	pentagastrin
Pepto® Diarrhea Control	loperamide
Percodan®-Demi	oxycodone and aspirin
Percolone®	oxycodone

(continued)

Brand Name	Generic Name
Perfectoderm® Gel	benzoyl peroxide
Periactin®	cyproheptadine
Peri-Colace®	docusate and casanthranol
Peritrate®	pentaerythritol tetranitrate
Peritrate® SA	pentaerythritol tetranitrate
Permitil® Oral	fluphenazine
Peroxin A5®	benzoyl peroxide
Peroxin A10®	benzoyl peroxide
Persa-Gel®	benzoyl peroxide
Pertussin® CS	dextromethorphan
Pertussin® ES	dextromethorphan
Pfizerpen-AS®	penicillin G procaine
Phazyme®	simethicone
Phenadex® Senior	guaifenesin and dextromethorphan
Phenahist-TR®	chlorpheniramine, phenylephrine, phenylpropanolamine, and belladonna alkaloids
Phenameth® DM	promethazine and dextromethorphan
Phenaphen®	acetaminophen
Phenaphen®/Codeine #4	acetaminophen and codeine
Phenaseptic®	phenol
Phenazine® Injection	promethazine
Phencen-50®	promethazine
Phenchlor® S.H.A.	chlorpheniramine, phenylephrine, phenylpropanolamine, and belladonna alkaloids
Phendry® Oral	diphenhydramine
Phenerbel-S®	belladonna, phenobarbital, and ergotamine tartrate
Phenergan® VC With Codeine	promethazine, phenylephrine, and codeine
Phenergan® With Dextromethorphan	promethazine and dextromethorphan
Phenetron®	chlorpheniramine
Phenoxine®	phenylpropanolamine
Phenurone®	phenacemide
Phenyldrine®	phenylpropanolamine
Phenylfenesin® L.A.	guaifenesin and phenylpropanolamine
Pherazine® VC With Codeine	promethazine, phenylephrine, and codeine
Pherazine® With Codeine	promethazine and codeine
Pherazine® With DM	promethazine and dextromethorphan
Phos-Ex® 62.5	calcium acetate
Phos-Ex® 125	calcium acetate
Phos-Ex® 167	calcium acetate
Phos-Ex® 250	calcium acetate
pHos-pHaid®	ammonium biphosphate, sodium biphosphate, and sodium acid pyrophosphate
Phosphaljel®	aluminum phosphate
Pilagan® Ophthalmic	pilocarpine
Pilostat® Ophthalmic	pilocarpine
Pindac®	pinacidil
Pin-Rid®	pyrantel pamoate
Pipracil®	piperacillin
Placidyl®	ethchlorvynol
Plaquase®	collagenase
Plasma-Plex®	plasma protein fraction
Plasmatein®	plasma protein fraction
Plegine®	phendimetrazine
Pneumomist®	guaifenesin
Pnu-Imune® 23	pneumococcal polysaccharide vaccine
Pod-Ben-25®	podophyllum resin

(continued)

Brand Name	Generic Name
Podofin®	podophyllum resin
Point-Two®	fluoride
Poladex®	dexchlorpheniramine
Polaramine®	dexchlorpheniramine
Polargen®	dexchlorpheniramine maleate
Poliovax® Injection	poliovirus vaccine, inactivated
Polycillin-N® Injection	ampicillin
Polycillin® Oral	ampicillin
Polycillin-PRB®	ampicillin and probenecid (all products)
Polyflex® Tablet	chlorzoxazone
Polygam® Injection	immune globulin, intravenous
Poly-Histine CS®	brompheniramine, phenylpropanolamine, and codeine
Poly-Histine-D® Capsule	phenyltoloxamine, phenylpropanolamine, pyrilamine, and pheniramine
Polymox®	amoxicillin
Pondimin®	fenfluramine
Porcelana® Sunscreen	hydroquinone
Posicor®	mibefradil (all products)
Potasalan®	potassium chloride
Pramet® FA	vitamin (multiple/prenatal)
Pramilet® FA	vitamin (multiple/prenatal)
Predair®	prednisolone
Predaject-50®	prednisolone
Predalone®	prednisolone
Predcor®	prednisolone
Predcor-TBA®	prednisolone
Predicort-50®	prednisolone
Prednicen-M®	prednisone
Prefrin™	phenylephrine
Preludin®	phenmetrazine hydrochloride
Premarin® With Methyltestosterone	estrogens and methyltestosterone
Prescription Strength Desenex®	miconazole
Priscoline®	tolazoline
Proampacin®	ampicillin and probenecid (all products)
Pro-Banthine®	propantheline
Pro-Bionate®	lactobacillus
Pro-Cal-Sof®	docusate
Procan™ SR	procainamide
Profasi®	chorionic gonadotropin
Profenal®	suprofen
Profen LA®	guaifenesin and phenylpropanolamine
Profilate-HP®	antihemophilic factor (human)
Progestaject® Injection	progesterone
ProHIBiT®	*Haemophilus* B conjugate vaccine
Prokine™ Injection	sargramostim
Prolamine®	phenylpropanolamine
Prolixin®	fluphenazine
Prolixin Enanthate®	fluphenazine
Proloid®	thyroglobulin
Prometa®	metaproterenol sulfate
Prometh®	promethazine
Promethist® With Codeine	promethazine, phenylephrine, and codeine
Prometh® VC Plain Liquid	promethazine and phenylephrine
Prometh® VC With Codeine	promethazine, phenylephrine, and codeine
Pronestyl-SR®	procainamide
Pronestyl®	procainamide

(continued)

Brand Name	Generic Name
Propacet®	propoxyphene and acetaminophen
Propagest®	phenylpropanolamine
Proplex® SX-T Injection	factor IX complex (human)
Propoxacet-N®	propoxyphene and acetaminophen
Pro-Sof®	docusate sodium
Pro-Sof® Plus	docusate and casanthranol
Prostaphlin®	oxacillin
ProStep® Patch	nicotine
Prostin F_2 Alpha®	dinoprost tromethamine
Protenate®	plasma protein fraction
Prothazine-DC®	promethazine and codeine
Protilase®	pancrelipase
Protopam® Tablet	pralidoxime chloride
Protostat® Oral	metronidazole
Protuss®-DM	guaifenesin, pseudoephedrine, and dextromethorphan
Provatene®	beta-carotene
Proventil® Inhaler	albuterol
Proventil® Solution	albuterol
Proventil® Tablet	albuterol
Pseudo-Gest Plus® Tablet	chlorpheniramine and pseudoephedrine
Psorion® Topical	betamethasone (topical)
Pyridium Plus®	phenazopyridine, hyoscyamine, and butabarbital
Queltuss®	guaifenesin and dextromethorphan
Questran® Tablet	cholestyramine resin
Quiess® Injection	hydroxyzine
Quinaglute® Dura-Tabs®	quinidine
----	quinagolide
Quinalan®	quinidine
Quinamm®	quinine sulfate
Quinora®	quinidine
Quiphile®	quinine sulfate
Q-vel®	quinine sulfate
Raplon®	rapacuronium
Raudixin®	*Rauwolfia serpentina*
Rauverid®	*Rauwolfia serpentina*
Raxar®	grepafloxacin
R & C® Lice	permethrin
Rectacort® Suppository	hydrocortisone
Redisol®	cyanocobalamin
Redux®	dexfenfluramine
Regitine®	phentolamine
Reglan® Syrup	metoclopramide
Regonol®	pyridostigmine
Regulace®	docusate and casanthranol
Regular Iletin® I Insulin	insulin
Regulax SS®	docusate
Regutol®	docusate
Relefact® TRH	protirelin
Relief® Ophthalmic Solution	phenylephrine
Renografin-60®	radiological/contrast media (ionic)
Renografin-76®	radiological/contrast media (ionic)
Renoquid®	sulfacytine
Renormax®	spirapril
Renovist®	radiological/contrast media (ionic)
Renovist® II	radiological/contrast media (ionic)
Reposans-10® Oral	chlordiazepoxide
Rep-Pred®	methylprednisolone

(continued)

Brand Name	Generic Name
Resa®	reserpine
Resaid®	chlorpheniramine and phenylpropanolamine
Rescaps-D® S.R. Capsule	caramiphen and phenylpropanolamine
Rescon® Liquid	chlorpheniramine and phenylpropanolamine
Respa-GF®	guaifenesin
Respbid®	theophylline
RespiGam®	respiratory syncytial virus immune globulin (intravenous)
Resporal®	dexbrompheniramine and pseudoephedrine
Restall®	hydroxyzine
Rexigen Forte®	phendimetrazine
Rezulin®	troglitazone
R-Gel®	capsaicin
R-Gen®	iodinated glycerol
Rheaban®	attapulgite
Rheomacrodex®	dextran
Rhesonativ® Injection	Rh_o(D) immune globulin
Rhinatate® Tablet	chlorpheniramine, pyrilamine, and phenylephrine
Rhindecon®	phenylpropanolamine
Rhinocort® Nasal Inhaler	budesonide
Rhinolar®	chlorpheniramine, phenylpropanolamine, and methscopolamine
Rhulicaine®	benzocaine
Rhuli® Cream	benzocaine, calamine, and camphor
RID®	pyrethrins and piperonyl butoxide
Riobin®	riboflavin
Riopan®	magaldrate
Riopan® Plus	magaldrate and simethicone
Riopan® Plus Double Strength	magaldrate and simethicone
Robafen® CF	guaifenesin, phenylpropanolamine, and dextromethorphan
Robaxisal®	methocarbamol and aspirin
Robicillin® Tablet	penicillin V potassium
Robitet®	tetracycline
Robitussin® A-C	guaifenesin and codeine
Robitussin®-DAC	guaifenesin, pseudoephedrine, and codeine
Rolatuss® Plain Liquid	chlorpheniramine and phenylephrine
Rondomycin® Capsule	methacycline hydrochloride (all products)
RotaShield®	rotavirus vaccine
Roxanol SR™ Oral	morphine sulfate
Roxiprin®	oxycodone and aspirin
Rubramin-PC®	cyanocobalamin
Rufen®	ibuprofen
Ru-Tuss® Liquid	chlorpheniramine and phenylephrine
Ru-Tuss® Tablet	chlorpheniramine, phenylephrine, phenylpropanolamine, and belladonna alkaloids
Ru-Vert-M®	meclizine
Rymed®	guaifenesin and pseudoephedrine
Rymed-TR®	guaifenesin and phenylpropanolamine
Ryna®	chlorpheniramine and pseudoephedrine
Ryna-C®	chlorpheniramine, pseudoephedrine, and codeine
Salacid® Ointment	salicylic acid
Saleto-200®	ibuprofen
Saleto-400®	ibuprofen
Salgesic®	salsalate
Salmonine®	calcitonin
Salsitab®	salsalate
Saluron®	hydroflumethiazide
Salutensin®	hydroflumethiazide and reserpine
Salutensin-Demi®	hydroflumethiazide and reserpine

(continued)

Brand Name	Generic Name
SangCya™	cyclosporine
Sanorex®	mazindol
Sansert®	methysergide
Scabene®	lindane
Sclavo Test - PPD®	tuberculin purified protein derivative
Sebizon®	sulfacetamide
Secran®	vitamins (multiple)
Seldane®	terfenadine
Seldane-D®	terfenadine and pseudoephedrine
Selecor®	celiprolol
Selectol®	celiprolol
Selestoject®	betamethasone
Selpak®	selegiline
Selsun Gold® for Women	selenium sulfide
Senolax®	senna
Septa® Topical Ointment	bacitracin, neomycin, and polymyxin B
Septisol®	hexachlorophene
Ser-A-Gen®	hydralazine, hydrochlorothiazide, and reserpine
Ser-Ap-Es®	hydralazine, hydrochlorothiazide, and reserpine
Serentil®	mesoridazine
Serevent®	salmeterol
Serpalan®	reserpine
Serpasil®	reserpine
Serpatabs®	reserpine
Serzone®	nefazodone
Siblin®	psyllium
Silain®	simethicone
Silaminic® Cold Syrup	chlorpheniramine and phenylpropanolamine
Silaminic® Expectorant	guaifenesin and phenylpropanolamine
Sildicon-E®	guaifenesin and phenylpropanolamine
Siltussin-CF®	guaifenesin, phenylpropanolamine, and dextromethorphan
Sine-Aid® IB	pseudoephedrine and ibuprofen
Sinubid®	phenyltoloxamine, phenylpropanolamine, and acetaminophen
Sinufed® Timecelles®	guaifenesin and pseudoephedrine
Sinumed®	acetaminophen, chlorpheniramine, and pseudoephedrine
Sinumist®-SR Capsulets®	guaifenesin
Skelex®	chlorzoxazone
Sleep-eze 3® Oral	diphenhydramine
Sleepwell 2-nite®	diphenhydramine
Slim-Mint®	benzocaine
Slo-bid™	theophylline
Slo-Phyllin® (all products)	theophylline
Slo-Phyllin® GG	theophylline and guaifenesin
Slo-Salt®	salt substitute
Slow-K®	potassium chloride
Snaplets-EX®	guaifenesin and phenylpropanolamine
Sodium P.A.S.®	aminosalicylate sodium
----	sodium tetradecyl
Sofarin®	warfarin sodium
Solatene®	beta-carotene
Solfoton®	phenobarbital
Solganal®	aurothioglucose
Sorbitrate®	isosorbide dinitrate
Sotradecol®	sodium tetradecyl
Soyacal®	fat emulsion
Span-FF®	ferrous fumarate
Sparine®	promazine

(continued)

Brand Name	Generic Name
Spasmoject®	dicyclomine
Spasmolin®	hyoscyamine, atropine, scopolamine, and phenobarbital
Spec-T®	benzocaine
Spectrobid® Tablet	bacampicillin
Spherulin®	coccidioidin skin test
Spironazide®	hydrochlorothiazide and spironolactone
Spirozide®	hydrochlorothiazide and spironolactone
SRC® Expectorant	hydrocodone, pseudoephedrine, and guaifenesin
Stadol® NS	butorphanol
Stahist®	chlorpheniramine, phenylephrine, phenylpropanolamine, and belladonna alkaloids
Staphcillin®	methicillin (all products)
Staticin®	erythromycin (systemic)
Statobex®	phendimetrazine tartrate
Stelazine®	trifluoperazine
Stemex®	paramethasone acetate
Stilphostrol®	diethylstilbestrol
St. Joseph® Cough Suppressant	dextromethorphan
St. Joseph® Measured Dose Nasal Solution	phenylephrine
Sucostrin®	succinylcholine chloride
Sucrets® Cough Calmers	dextromethorphan
Sudafed® Cough	guaifenesin, pseudoephedrine, and dextromethorphan
Sudafed® Plus Liquid	chlorpheniramine and pseudoephedrine
Sudex®	guaifenesin and pseudoephedrine
Sufedrin®	pseudoephedrine
Sulfa-Gyn®	sulfabenzamide, sulfacetamide, and sulfathiazole
Sulfamethoprim®	co-trimoxazole
Sulfa-Trip®	sulfabenzamide, sulfacetamide, and sulfathiazole
Sultrin™	sulfabenzamide, sulfacetamide, and sulfathiazole
Superchar®	charcoal
Superchar® With Sorbitol	charcoal
Supprelin®	histrelin
Suppress®	dextromethorphan
Surital®	thiamylal sodium
Sus-Phrine®	epinephrine
Sustaire®	theophylline
Symadine®	amantadine hydrochloride
Symmetrel® Capsule	amantadine hydrochloride
Synalar-HP® Topical	fluocinolone
Synemol® Topical	fluocinolone
Synkayvite®	menadiol sodium
Syntocinon® Nasal	oxytocin
Sytobex®	cyanocobalamin
Tabron®	vitamins, multiple
Tac™-40 Injection	triamcinolone (systemic)
Tacaryl®	methdilazine hydrochloride (all products)
TACE®	chlorotrianisene
Tagamet® 800 mg	cimetidine
Talwin® Compound	pentazocine and aspirin
Tamine®	brompheniramine and phenylpropanolamine
Tanac®	benzocaine
Tanoral® Tablet	chlorpheniramine, pyrilamine, and phenylephrine
Tarabine® PFS	cytarabine
Taractan®	chlorprothixene
Tavist-D®	clemastine and phenylpropanolamine
T-Caine® Lozenge	benzocaine

(continued)

Brand Name	Generic Name
Tear Drop® Solution	artificial tears
TearGard® Ophthalmic Solution	artificial tears
Tebamide®	trimethobenzamide
Teczem®	enalapril and diltiazem
Tedral®	theophylline, ephedrine, and phenobarbital
Tega-Vert® Oral	dimenhydrinate
Tegison®	etretinate
Tegopen®	cloxacillin
Telachlor® Oral	chlorpheniramine
Teladar® Topical	betamethasone (topical)
Teldrin® Oral	chlorpheniramine
Teline®	tetracycline
Temaril®	trimeprazine tartrate
Temazin® Cold Syrup	chlorpheniramine and phenylpropanolamine
Tempra®	acetaminophen
Ten-K®	potassium chloride
Tepanil®	diethylpropion hydrochloride
Tepanil® TenTabs®	diethylpropion hydrochloride
----	terpin hydrate
----	terpin hydrate and codeine
Terra-Cortril® Ophthalmic Suspension	oxytetracycline and hydrocortisone
Terramycin® Oral	oxytetracycline
Tesamone® Injection	testosterone
Tes-Tape®	diagnostic aids (*in vitro*), urine
Testoderm®	testosterone
Testoderm® TTS	testosterone
Testoderm® With Adhesive	testosterone
Testomar®	yohimbine
Testopel® Pellet	testosterone
Tetracap®	tetracycline
Tetralan®	tetracycline
Tetram®	tetracycline
Tetramune®	diphtheria, tetanus toxoids, whole-cell pertussis, and *Haemophilus* B conjugate
Tetrasine® Extra Ophthalmic	tetrahydrozoline
Tetrasine® Ophthalmic	tetrahydrozoline
T-Gen®	trimethobenzamide
Theelin® Aqueous Injection	estrone
Theobid®	theophylline
Theobid® Jr Duracaps®	theophylline
Theoclear-80®	theophylline
Theoclear®-L.A.	theophylline
Theo-Dur® (all products)	theophylline
Theo-Dur® Sprinkle®	theophylline
Theolair-SR™	theophylline
Theo-Organidin®	iodinated glycerol and theophylline
Theo-Sav®	theophylline
Theospan®-SR	theophylline
Theostat-80®	theophylline
Theovent®	theophylline
Theo-X®	theophylline
Therabid®	vitamins (multiple)
Thera-Flu® Severe Cold Non-Drowsy	acetaminophen, dextromethorphan, and pseudoephedrine
Thera-Flur®	fluoride
Thera-Hist® Syrup	chlorpheniramine and phenylpropanolamine
Theramine® Expectorant	guaifenesin and phenylpropanolamine

(continued)

Brand Name	Generic Name
TheraPatch® Warm	capsaicin
Thiacide®	methenamine and potassium acid phosphate
Thioplex®	thiotepa
Thorazine®	chlorpromazine
Thrombinar®	thrombin (topical)
Thrombostat®	thrombin (topical)
Thypinone®	protirelin
Thyrar®	thyroid
Thyrel® TSH	protirelin
Thyro-Block®	potassium iodide
Thyroid Strong®	thyroid
Thytropar®	thyrotropin
Tiamate®	diltiazem
Ticon®	trimethobenzamide
Tiject-20®	trimethobenzamide
Timecelles®	ascorbic acid
TinBen®	benzoin
Tindal®	acetophenazine maleate
Tinver®	sodium thiosulfate
----	tocophersolan
Tomycine®	tobramycin
Tonocard®	tocainide
Topicycline® Topical	tetracycline
Torecan® (all products)	thiethylperazine
Tornalate®	bitolterol
Totacillin®	ampicillin
Totacillin-N®	ampicillin
Touro Ex®	guaifenesin
Tral®	hexocyclium methylsulfate
Transdermal-NTG® Patch	nitroglycerin
Trans-Plantar® Transdermal Patch	salicylic acid
Travase®	sutilains
Trendar®	ibuprofen
Triacin-C®	triprolidine, pseudoephedrine, and codeine
Triafed®	triprolidine and pseudoephedrine
Triaminic® Allergy Tablet	chlorpheniramine and phenylpropanolamine
Triaminic® Cold Tablet	chlorpheniramine and phenylpropanolamine
Triaminic® Expectorant	guaifenesin and phenylpropanolamine
Triaminicol® Multi-Symptom Cold Syrup	chlorpheniramine, phenylpropanolamine, and dextromethorphan
Triaminic® Oral Infant, Drops	pheniramine, phenylpropanolamine, and pyrilamine
Triaminic® Syrup	chlorpheniramine and phenylpropanolamine
Triamonide® Injection	triamcinolone (systemic)
Triapin®	butalbital compound and acetaminophen
Triavil® 4-50	amitriptyline and perphenazine
Tri-Clear® Expectorant	guaifenesin phenylpropanolamine
Tridil® Injection	nitroglycerin
Tridione®	trimethadione
Trifed-C®	triprolidine, pseudoephedrine, and codeine
Tri-Immunol®	diphtheria, tetanus toxoids, and whole-cell pertussis vaccine
Trilafon®	perphenazine
Trilisate®	choline magnesium trisalicylate
TRIKOF-D®	guaifenesin, phenylpropanolamine, and dextromethorphan
Tri-Kort® Injection	triamcinolone (systemic)
Trilog® Injection	triamcinolone (systemic)
Trilone® Injection	triamcinolone (systemic)
Trimazide®	trimethobenzamide

(continued)

Brand Name	Generic Name
Trimox® 500 mg	amoxicillin
Trimpex®	trimethoprim
Tri-Nefrin® Extra Strength Tablet	chlorpheniramine and phenylpropanolamine
Triofed® Syrup	triprolidine and pseudoephedrine
Tri-Phen-Chlor®	chlorpheniramine, phenyltoloxamine, phenylpropanolamine, and phenylephrine
Triphenyl® Expectorant	guaifenesin and phenylpropanolamine
Triphenyl® Syrup	chlorpheniramine and phenylpropanolamine
Tri-P® Oral Infant Drops	pheniramine, phenylpropanolamine, and pyrilamine
Triposed® Syrup	triprolidine and pseudoephedrine
Tri-Pseudo®	triprolidine and pseudoephedrine
Trisoralen®	trioxsalen
Tristoject® Injection	triamcinolone (systemic)
Tri-Statin® II Topical	nystatin and triamcinolone
Trisudex®	triprolidine and pseudoephedrine
Tri-Tannate Plus®	chlorpheniramine, ephedrine, phenylephrine, and carbetapentane
Tritec®	ranitidine bismuth citrate
Trivagizole-3®	clotrimazole
Trocal®	dextromethorphan
Trofan®	L-tryptophan
Trofan DS®	L-tryptophan
Trovan®	trovafloxacin
Truphylline®	aminophylline
Tryptacin®	L-tryptophan
Trysul®	sulfabenzamide, sulfacetamide, and sulfathiazole
T-Stat®	erythromycin (systemic)
----	tubocurarine
Tucks® Cream	witch hazel
Tuinal®	amobarbital and secobarbital
Tusal®	sodium thiosalicylate
Tusibron®	guaifenesin
Tusibron-DM®	guaifenesin and dextromethorphan
Tussafin® Expectorant	hydrocodone, pseudoephedrine, and guaifenesin
Tuss-Allergine® Modified T.D. Capsule	caramiphen and phenylpropanolamine
Tussi-Organidin®	iodinated glycerol and codeine
Tussi-Organidin® DM	iodinated glycerol and dextromethorphan (all products)
Tuss-LA®	guaifenesin and pseudoephedrine
Tusso-DM®	iodinated glycerol and dextromethorphan (all products)
Tussogest® Extended Release Capsule	caramiphen and phenylpropanolamine
Tuss-Ornade®	caramiphen and phenylpropanolamine
Twin-K®	potassium citrate and potassium gluconate
Twinrix®	hepatitis A inactivated and hepatitis B (recombinant) vaccine
Two-Dyne®	butalbital compound and acetaminophen
Tylenol® Cold Effervescent Medication Tablet	chlorpheniramine, phenylpropanolamine, and acetaminophen
Tylenol® with Codeine (Elixir)	acetaminophen and codeine
Tyrodone® Liquid	hydrocodone and pseudoephedrine
UAD Otic®	neomycin, polymyxin B, and hydrocortisone
ULR-LA®	guaifenesin and phenylpropanolamine
Ultralente® U	insulin zinc suspension, extended
Ultrase® MT24	pancrelipase
Unguentine®	benzocaine
Uni-Bent® Cough Syrup	diphenhydramine
Uni-Decon®	chlorpheniramine, phenyltoloxamine, phenylpropanolamine, and phenylephrine

(continued)

Brand Name	**Generic Name**
Uni-Dur®	theophylline
Unipen®	nafcillin
Unipres®	hydralazine, hydrochlorothiazide, and reserpine
Uni-Pro®	ibuprofen
Unitrol®	phenylpropanolamine
Uni-tussin®	guaifenesin
Uni-tussin® DM	guaifenesin and dextromethorphan
Urabeth®	bethanechol
Uracel®	sodium salicylate
Ureacin®-40 Topical	urea
Uri-Tet®	oxytetracycline
Urobak®	sulfamethoxazole
Urobiotic-25®	oxytetracycline and sulfamethizole
Urodine®	phenazopyridine
Uroplus® DS	co-trimoxazole
Uroplus® SS	co-trimoxazole
Uticort®	betamethasone (all products)
Vagitrol®	sulfanilamide
Valadol®	acetaminophen
Valergen® Injection	estradiol
Valertest No. 1®	estradiol and testosterone
Valisone® Topical	betamethasone (topical)
Valmid® Capsule	ethinamate
Valpin® 50	anisotropine methylbromide
Valrelease®	diazepam
Valstar®	valrubicin
Vamate® Oral	hydroxyzine
Vanatrip®	amitriptyline
Vancenase® AQ 84 mcg	beclomethasone
Vancenase® Pockethaler®	beclomethasone
Vanceril®	beclomethasone
Vanex Forte™-D	chlorpheniramine, phenylephrine, and methscoplamine
Vanex-LA®	guaifenesin and phenylpropanolamine
Vanoxide®	benzoyl peroxide
Vanseb-T® Shampoo	coal tar, sulfur, and salicylic acid
Vansil™	oxamniquine
Vaponefrin®	epinephrine
Vascor®	bepridil
Vasodilan®	isoxsuprine
Vasocon Regular® Ophthalmic	naphazoline
Vasosulf® Ophthalmic	sulfacetamide and phenylephrine
Vasoxyl®	methoxamine
V-Cillin K®	penicillin V potassium
Vectrin®	minocycline
Velban®	vinblastine
Velosulin® BR (Buffered)	insulin
Velsar® Injection	vinblastine sulfate
Venoglobulin®-I	immune globulin (intravenous)
Ventolin®	albuterol
Ventolin® Inhaler Aerosol	albuterol
Verazinc® Oral	zinc sulfate
Vercyte®	pipobroman
Vergogel® Gel	salicylic acid
Vergon®	meclizine
Vermizine®	piperazine
Verr-Canth™	cantharidin
Verrex-C&M®	podophyllin and salicylic acid

(continued)

Brand Name	Generic Name
Verrusol®	salicylic acid, podophyllin, and cantharidin
Versed®	midazolam
Verukan® Solution	salicylic acid
Vesprin®	triflupromazine
V-Gan® Injection	promethazine hydrochloride
Vibazine®	buclizine
Vibramycin® I.V.	doxycycline
Vicks® 44® Non-Drowsy Cold & Cough Liqui-Caps	pseudoephedrine and dextromethorphan
Vicks® Children's Chloraseptic®	benzocaine
Vicks® Chloraseptic® Sore Throat	benzocaine
Vicks® DayQuil® Allergy Relief 4 Hour Tablet	brompheniramine and phenylpropanolamine
Vicks® DayQuil® Sinus Pressure & Congestion Relief	guaifenesin and phenylpropanolamine
Vicks® Formula 44® Pediatric Formula	dextromethorphan
Vicks® Formula 44®	dextromethorphan
Vicks® Vatronol®	ephedrine
Vioform®	clioquinol
Vioform®-Hydrocortisone Topical	clioquinol and hydrocortisone
Vioxx®	rofecoxib
Vira-A®	vidarabine
Visken®	pindolol
Vistacon-50® Injection	hydroxyzine
Vistaject-25®	hydroxyzine
Vistaject-50®	hydroxyzine
Vistaquel® Injection	hydroxyzine
Vistazine® Injection	hydroxyzine
VitaCarn® Oral	levocarnitine
Vitelle™ Irospan®	ferrous sulfate and ascorbic acid
Vitravene™	fomivirsen
Vontrol®	diphenidol
Wehamine® Injection	dimenhydrinate
Wehdryl®	diphenhydramine
Wellcovorin®	leucovorin
Wesprin® Buffered	aspirin
40 Winks®	diphenhydramine
WinRho SD®	Rh_o (D) immune globulin (intravenous-human)
Wolfina®	*Rauwolfia serpentina*
Wyamine®	mephentermine
Wyamycin S®	erythromycin
Wydase®	hyaluronidase
Wygesic®	propoxyphene and acetaminophen
Wymox®	amoxicillin
Wytensin®	guanabenz
Yohimex™	yohimbine
Yutopar®	ritodrine
Zantac® EFFERdose®	ranitidine
Zantryl®	phentermine
Zartan®	cephalexin
Zebrax®	clidinium and chlordiazepoxide
Zefazone®	cefmetazole
Zetran®	diazepam
Zolicef®	cefazolin

(continued)

Brand Name	Generic Name
Zolyse®	chymotrypsin alpha (all products)
Zyban™ 100 mg	bupropion
Zyflo™	zileuton
Zymase®	pancrelipase

PHARMACEUTICAL MANUFACTURERS AND DISTRIBUTORS

AAI Development Services
2320 Scientific Park Drive
Wilmington, NC 28405
(800) 575-4224
www.aaiintl.com

Abbott Laboratories
(Pharmaceutical Products Division)
100 Abbott Park Road
Abbott Park, IL 60064-3500
(847) 937-6100
www.abbott.com

Adams Respiratory Therapeutics
409 Main Street
Chester, NJ 07930
(908) 879-1400
www.adamslaboratories.com

A P Pharma
123 Saginaw Drive
Redwood City, CA 94063
(650) 366-2626
www.advancedpolymer.com

Advanced Vision Research
12 Alfred Street
Suite 200
Woburn, MA 01801
(800) 579-8327
www.theratears.com

Akorn, Inc
2500 Millbrook Drive
Buffalo Grove, IL 60089
(800) 535-7155
www.akorn.com

AkPharma, Inc
6840 Old Egg Harbor Road
Pleasantville, NJ 08232
(800) 994-4711
www.akpharma.com

Alcon Laboratories, Inc
6201 South Freeway
Fort Worth, TX 76134
www.alconlabs.com

Allen & Hanburys
Five Moore Drive
Research Triangle Park, NC 27709
(800) 334-0089

Allerderm Laboratories
PO Box 2070
Petaluma, CA 94954
www.allerderm.com

Allergan, Inc
PO Box 19534
Irvine, CA 92623-9534
(800) 347-4500
www.allergan.com

Alliance Pharmaceutical, Inc
6175 Lusk Boulevard
San Diego, CA 92121
(858) 410-5200
www.allp.com

Allscripts Healthcare Solutions
2401 Commerce Avenue
Libertyville, IL 60048-4464
(800) 654-0889
www.allscripts.com

Almay, Inc
1501 Williamsboro Street
Oxford, NC 27565
(800) 473-8566
www.almay.com

Alpharma, Inc
One Executive Drive
Fort Lee, NJ 07024
(800) 645-4216
www.alpharma.com

Alpharma USPD, Inc
200 Elmora Avenue
Elizabeth, NJ 07207
(800) 432-8534
www.alpharmauspd.com

Alpha Therapeutic (see Grifols)

AltaRex Corp
610 Lincoln Street
Waltham, MA 02451
(888) 801-6665
www.altarex.com

Alza Corp
1900 Charleston Road
PO Box 7210
Mountain View, CA 94039-7210
(650) 564-5000
www.alza.com

Amarin Pharmaceuticals, Inc
(see Valeant Pharmaceuticals)

Ambix Laboratories
55 West End Road
Totowa, NJ 07512
(973) 890-9002
www.ambixlabs.com

Amcon Laboratories
40 North Rock Hill Road
St Louis, MO 63119
(800) 255-6161
www.amcon-labs.com

American Lecithin Company
115 Hurley Road
Unit 2B
Oxford, CT 06478
(800) 364-4416
www.americanlecithin.com

American Medical Industries Health Products
330 East Third Street
Suite 2
Dell Rapids, SD 57022-1918
(605) 428-5501
www.ezhealthcare.com

American Pharmaceutical Partners, Inc (APP)
Woodfield Executive Center
1101 Perimeter Drive
Suite 300
Schaumburg, IL 60173-5837
(888) 391-6300
www.appdrugs.com

American Red Cross
2025 E Street Northwest
Washington, DC 20006
(202) 303-4498
www.redcross.org

American Regent Laboratories
One Luitpold Drive
Shirley, NY 11967
(800) 645-1706
www.americanregent.com

Amgen, Inc
One Amgen Center Drive
Thousand Oaks, CA 91320-1799
(800) 772-6436
www.amgen.com

AMSCO Scientific (see Steris Corp)

Amylin Pharmaceuticals, Inc
9360 Towne Centre Drive
Suite 110
San Diego, California 92121
(858) 552-2200
www.amylin.com

Andrew Jergens Company
2535 Spring Grove Avenue
Cincinnati, OH 45214-1773
(800) 742-8798
www.jergens.com

Andrx Corp
4955 Orange Drive
Davie, FL 33314
(954) 584-0300
www.andrx.com

Angelini Pharmaceuticals
50 Tice Boulevard
Woodcliff Lake, NJ 07677
(201) 476-9000
www.angelinipharmaceuticals.com

Antibodies, Inc
PO Box 1560
Davis, CA 95617
(800) 824-8540
www.antibodiesinc.com

Antigenics, Inc
630 Fifth Avenue
Suite 2100
New York, NY 10111
(212) 994-8200
www.antigenic.com

Apotex Corp
2400 North Commerce Parkway
Suite 400
Weston, FL 33326
(800) 706-5575
www.apotexcorp.com

Apothecary Products, Inc
11750 12th Avenue South
Burnsville, MN 55337-1295
(800) 328-2742
www.apothecaryproducts.com

Apothecon
PO Box 4500
Princeton, NJ 08543-4500
(800) 321-1335

Apothecus Pharmaceutical Corp
220 Townsend Square
Oyster Bay, NY 11771-1532
(800) 227-2393
www.apothecus.com

Applied Genetics, Inc Dermatics
205 Buffalo Avenue
Freeport, NY 11520
(516) 868-9026
www.agiderm.com

AstraZeneca Pharmaceuticals, LP
1800 Concord Pike
PO Box 15437
Wilmington, DE 19850-5437
(800) 236-9933
www.astrazeneca-us.com

Atley Pharmaceuticals, Inc
10511 Old Ridge Road
Ashland, VA 23005
(804) 227-2250
www.atley.com

Aventis Behring
1020 First Avenue
PO Box 61501
King of Prussia, PA 19406-0901
(610) 878-4000
www.aventisbehring.com

Aventis Pasteur
Discovery Drive
Box 187
Swiftwater, PA 18370-0187
(570) 839-7187
www.aventispasteur.com

Aventis Pharmaceuticals, Inc
300 Somerset Corporate Boulevard
Bridgewater, NJ 08807-2854
(800) 981-2491
www.aventispharma-us.com

Axcan, Inc
22 Inverness Center Parkway
Birmingham, AL 35242
(205) 991-8085
www.axcanscandipharm.com

Bajamar Chemical Company, Inc
9609 Dielman Rock Island
St Louis, MO 63132
(888) 242-3414
www.vesselvite.com

Banner
4100 Mendenhall Oaks Parkway
Suite 301
High Point, NC 27265
(336) 812-3442
www.banpharm.com

Barre-National, Inc
7250 Windsor Boulevard
Baltimore, MD 21244
(410) 298-1000

Barr Laboratories, Inc
2 Quaker Road
PO Box 2900
Pomona, NY 10970
(800) 222-0190
www.barrlabs.com

Bausch & Lomb Pharmaceuticals (BD)
8500 Hidden River Parkway
Tampa, FL 33637
(800) 323-0000
www.bausch.com

Bausch & Lomb Surgical, Inc
180 Via Verde
San Dimas, CA 91773
(800) 338-2020
www.bausch.com

Baxa Corp
13760 East Arapahoe Road
Englewood, CO 80112-3903
(800) 567-2292
www.baxa.com

Baxter Healthcare Corp
Corp Headquarters
One Baxter Parkway
Deerfield, IL 60015-4625
(800) 422-9837
www.baxter.com

Baxter Pharmaceutical Solutions
927 South Curry Pike
Bloomington, IN 47403
(800) 353-0887
www.baxterdrugdelivery.com

Bayer Corp
(Pharmaceutical Division)
400 Morgan Lane
West Haven, CT 06516-4175
(203) 812-2000
www.bayerus.com

Bayer Corp
(Consumer Care Division)
36 Columbia Road
PO Box 1910
Morristown, NJ 07962-1910
(800) 331-4536
www.bayercare.com

Bayer Corp
(Diagnostic Division)
511 Benedict Avenue
Tarrytown, NY 10591-5097
(914) 631-8000
www.bayerdiag.com

Bayer, Inc
77 Belfield Road
Etobicoke, Ontario, Canada M9W 1G6
(800) 268-1331
www.bayer.ca

B Braun Medical
1601 Wallace Drive
Suite 150
Carrollton, TX 75006
(800) 854-6851
www.bbraunusa.com

BD Medical Pharmaceutical Systems
One Becton Drive
Franklin Lakes, NJ 07417
(201) 847-4017
www.bd.com

BD Biosciences
2350 Qume Drive
San Jose, CA 95131-1807
(877) 232-8995
www.bdbiosciences.com

Beckman Coulter, Inc
4300 North Harbor Boulevard
PO Box 3100
Fullerton, CA 92834-3100
(714) 871-4848
www.beckman.com

Bedford Laboratories
300 Northfield Road
Bedford, OH 44146
(440) 232-3320
www.bedfordlabs.com

Beiersdorf, Inc
Wilton Corporate Center
187 Danbury Road
Wilton, CT 06897
(203) 563-5800
www.beiersdorf.com

Berlex Laboratories, Inc
340 Changebridge Road
PO Box 1000
Montville, NJ 07045-1000
(973) 487-2000
www.berlex.com

Berna Products Corp
4216 Ponce de Leon Boulevard
Coral Gables, FL 33146
(800) 533-5899
www.bernaproducts.com

Bertek Pharmaceuticals, Inc
781 Chestnut Ridge Road
Morgantown, WV 26505
(304) 285-6420
www.bertek.com

Beta Dermaceuticals, Inc
PO Box 691106
San Antonio, TX 78269-1106
(210) 349-9326
www.beta-derm.com

Beutlich Pharmaceuticals
1541 Shields Drive
Waukegan, IL 60085
(800) 238-8542
www.beutlich.com

B. F. Ascher & Company, Inc
15501 West 109th Street
Lenexa, KS 66219-1308
(913) 888-1880
www.bfascher.com

Biocraft Laboratories, Inc
18-01 River Road
Fair Lawn, NJ 07410
(201) 703-0400

BioCryst Pharmaceuticals, Inc
2190 Parkway Lake Drive
Birmingham, AL 35244
(205) 444-4600
www.biocryst.com

Biogen idec
14 Cambridge Center
Cambridge, MA 02142
(617) 679-2000
www.biogen.com

BioGenex
4600 Norris Canyon Road
San Ramon, CA 94583
(800) 421-4149
www.biogenex.net

Bioglan Pharmaceuticals
7 Great Valley Parkway
Suite 301
Malvern, PA 19355
(888) 246-4526
www.bioglan.com

Biomerica, Inc
1533 Monrovia Avenue
Newport Beach, CA 92663
(949) 645-2111
www.biomerica.com

Biomira USA, Inc
70 South Main Street
Suite B and C
Cranbury, NJ 08512
(877) 234-0444
www.biomira.com

Biopure Corp
11 Hurley Street
Cambridge, MA 02141
(617) 234-6500
www.biopure.com

Biospecifics Technologies Corp
35 Wilbur Street
Lynbrook, NY 11563
(516) 593-7000
www.biospecifics.com

BIO-TECH Pharmacal, Inc
PO Box 1992
Fayetteville, AR 72702
(800) 345-1199
www.bio-tech-pharm.com

Birchwood Laboratories, Inc
7900 Fuller Road
Eden Prairie, MN 55344-2195
(800) 328-6156
www.birchlabs.com

Blaine Pharmaceuticals
1717 Dixie Highway
Suite 700
Fort Wright, KY 41011
(800) 633-9353
www.blainepharma.com

Blairex Laboratories, Inc
1600 Brian Drive
PO Box 2127
Columbus, IN 47202-2127
(800) 252-4739
www.blairex.com

Blansett Pharmacal Company, Inc
PO Box 638
North Little Rock, AR 72115
(800) 816-9695
www.blansett.com

Blistex, Inc
1800 Swift Drive
Oak Brook, IL 60523-1574
(800) 837-1800
www.blistex.com

Block Drug Company, Inc
(see GlaxoSmithKline)

Bluco, Inc
28350 Schoolcraft
Livonia, MI 48150
(800) 832-4464
www.blucoinc.com

Bock Pharmaceutical Company
PO Box 419056
St Louis, MO 63141
(314) 579-0770

Boehringer Ingelheim Pharmaceuticals, Inc
900 Ridgebury Road
PO Box 368
Ridgefield, CT 06877-0368
(203) 791-6194
www.boehringer-ingelheim.com

Boehringer Mannheim (see Roche Pharmaceuticals)

Bone Care International
Bone Care Center
1600 Aspen Commons
Middleton, WI 53562
(888) 389-3300
www.bonecare.com

Boots Pharmaceuticals, Inc
(see Knoll Pharmaceuticals Company)

Bracco Diagnostics, Inc
107 College Road East
Princeton, NJ 08540
(800) 631-5245
www.bracco.com

Braintree Laboratories, Inc
PO Box 850929
Braintree, MA 02185-0929
(800) 874-6756
www.braintreeLabs.com

Bristol-Myers Squibb Company (Pharmaceutical Division)
PO Box 4500
Princeton, NJ 08543-4500
(800) 321-1335
www.bms.com

Bristol-Myers Squibb Company (Oncology)
PO Box 4500
Princeton, NJ 08543-4500
(800) 426-7644
www.bmsoncology.com

Bristol-Myers Squibb OTC
1350 Liberty Avenue
Hillside, NJ 07205
(800) 468-7746
www.bms.com

Bryan Corp
4 Plympton Street
Woburn, MA 01801
(800) 343-7711
www.bryancorporation.com

BTG, Inc
3877 Fairfax Ridge Road
Fairfax, VA 22030
(800) 432-4284
www.btg.com

Burroughs Wellcome Company
(see GlaxoSmithKline)

Calmoseptine, Inc
16602 Burke Lane
Huntington Beach, CA 92647
(800) 800-3405
www.calmoseptineointment.com

Capellon Pharmaceuticals, Inc
7462 Dogwood Drive
Fort Worth, TX 76118
(817) 595-5820
www.capellon.com

Caraco Pharmaceutical Laboratories, LTD
1150 Elijah McCoy Drive
Detroit, MI 48202
(800) 818-4555
www.caraco.com

Cardinal Health, Inc
7000 Cardinal Place
Dublin, OH 43017
(800) 234-8701
www.cardinal.com

Cardinal Health, Inc
Nuclear Pharmacy Services
6464 Canoga Avenue
Woodland Hills, CA 91367
(800) 678-6779
www.cardinal.com/nps

Cardiovascular Research, LTD
1061 Shary Circle
Concord, CA 94518
(510) 827-2636

Carma Laboratories, Inc
5801 West Airways Avenue
Franklin, WI 53132
(414) 421-7707
www.carma-labs.com

Carolina Medical Products Company
PO Box 147
Farmville, NC 27828
(800) 227-6637
www.carolinamedical.com

Carrington Laboratories
2001 Walnut Hill Lane
Irving, TX 73038
(972) 518-1300
www.carringtonlabs.com

C. B. Fleet Company, Inc
4615 Murray Place
PO Box 11349
Lynchburg, VA 24506
(434) 528-4000
www.cbfleet.com

CCA Industries, Inc
200 Murray Hill Parkway
East Rutherford, NJ 07073
(201) 330-1400
www.ccaindustries.com

Celgene Corp
7 Powder Horn Drive
Warren, NJ 07059
(732) 271-1001
www.celgene.com

Cellegy Pharmaceuticals, Inc
349 Oyster Point Boulevard
Suite 200
South San Francisco, CA 94080
(650) 616-2200
www.cellegy.com

Celltech Pharmaceuticals, Inc
755 Jefferson Road
Rochester, NY 14623
(800) 234-5535
www.celltechgroup.com

Centeon (see Aventis Behring)

Centers for Disease Control and Prevention
1600 Clifton Road
Atlanta, GA 30333
(800) 311-3435
www.cdc.gov

Centocor, Inc
200 Great Valley Parkway
Malvern, PA 19355
(610) 240-8251
www.centocor.com

Central Pharmaceuticals, Inc
(see Schwarz Pharma, Inc)

Cephalon, Inc
145 Brandywine Parkway
West Chester, PA 19380
(610) 344-0200
www.cephalon.com

Cerenex Pharmaceuticals
Five Moore Drive
Research Triangle Park, NC 27709
(800) 334-0089

Cetylite Industries, Inc
9051 River Road
Pennsauken, NJ 08110
(800) 257-7740
www.cetylite.com

Chattem Consumer Products
1715 West 38th Street
Chattanooga, TN 37409
(800) 366-6833
www.chattem.com

Chesapeake Biological Laboratories, Inc
1111 South Paca Street
Baltimore, MD 21230
(410) 843-5000
www.cblinc.com

Chiron Corp
4560 Horton Street
Emeryville, CA 94608-2916
(510) 655-8730
www.chiron.com

Chronimed, Inc
10900 Red Circle Drive
Minnetonka, MN 55343
(800) 444-5951
www.chronimed.com

Chugai Pharma USA, LLC
6225 Nancy Ridge Drive
San Diego, CA 92121
(858) 535-5900
www.chugai-pharm.com

Ciba-Geigy Pharmaceuticals
(see Novartis Pharmaceuticals Corp)

CIBA Vision
11460 Johns Creek Parkway
Duluth, GA 30097
(678) 415-3937
www.cibavision.com

Circa Pharmaceuticals, Inc
(see Watson Laboratories, Inc)

Cirrus Healthcare Products, LLC
60 Main Street
PO Box 220
Cold Spring Harbor, NY 11724
(800) 327-6151
www.earplanes.com

CIS-US, Inc
10 DeAngelo Drive
Bedford, MA 01730
(800) 221-7554
www.cisusinc.com

Claragen, Inc
387 Technology Drive
College Park, MD 20742
(301) 405-8593
www.claragen.com

Clay-Park Labs, Inc
1700 Bathgate Avenue
Bronx, NY 10457
(800) 933-5550
www.claypark.com

C & M Pharmacal, Inc
(see Genesis Pharmaceutical, Inc)

CNS, Inc
7615 Smetana Lane
Minneapolis, MN 55344
(952) 229-1500
www.cns.com

Colgate Oral Pharmaceuticals
One Colgate Way
Canton, MA 02021
(800) 226-5428
www.colgate.com

Colgate-Palmolive Company
300 Park Avenue
New York, NY 10022
(800) 221-4607
www.colgate.com

CollaGenex Pharmaceuticals, Inc
41 University Drive
Newtown, PA 18940
(888) 339-5678
www.collagenex.com

Columbia Laboratories, Inc
354 Eisenhower Parkway
Second Floor-Plaza 1
Livingston, NJ 07039
(973) 994-3999
www.columbialabs.com

Combe, Inc
1101 Westchester Avenue
White Plains, NY 10604
(800) 873-7400
www.combe.com

Complimed Medical Research Group
1441 West Smith Road
Ferndale, WA 98248
(888) 977-8008
www.complimed.com

Conair Interplak Division
One Cummings Point Road
Stamford, CT 06904
(203) 351-9000
www.conair.com

Connaught Labs (see Aventis Pasteur)

Connective Therapeutics, Inc
3400 West Bayshore Road
Palo Alto, CA 94303
(415) 843-2800
www.connectics.com

Connetics Corp
3290 West Bayshore Road
Palo Alto, CA 94303
(888) 969-2628
www.connetics.com

Contract Pharmacal Corp
135 Adams Avenue
Hauppauge, NY 11788
(631) 231-4610
www.contractpharmacal.com

ConvaTec
(Bristol-Myers Squibb Company)
PO Box 5254
Princeton, NJ 08543-5254
(800) 422-8811
www.convatec.com

CooperVision
370 Woodcliff Drive
Suite 200
Fairport, NY 14450
(800) 538-7850
www.coopervision.com

Corixa
1124 Columbia Street
Suite 200
Seattle, WA 98104
(206) 754-5711
www.corixa.com

C. R. Bard, Inc
8195 Industrial Boulevard
Covington, GA 30014
(800) 526-4455
www.bardmedical.com

Cumberland Pharmaceuticals
2525 West End Avenue
Suite 950
Nashville, TN 37203
(615) 255-0068
www.cumberlandpharma.com

CVS Procare Direct
3651 Ridge Mill Drive
Columbia, OH 43026
(800) 252-6245

Cyanotech Corp
73-4460 Queen Kaahamanu Highway
Suite 102
Kailua-Kona, HI 96740
(800) 395-1353
www.cyanotech.com

Cygnus, Inc
400 Penobscot Drive
Redwood City, CA 94063-4719
(650) 369-4300
www.cygn.com

CYNACON/OCuSOFT
5311 Avenue North
Rosenburg, TX 77471
(800) 233-5469
www.ocusoft.com

Cypress Pharmaceutical, Inc
135 Industrial Boulevard
Madison, MS 39110
(800) 856-4393
www.cypressrx.com

CYTOGEN Corp
650 College Road East
Suite 3100
Princeton, NJ 08540
(800) 833-3533
www.cytogen.com

CytRx Corp
154 Technology Parkway
Suite 200
Norcross, GA 30092
(770) 368-9500
www.cytrx.com

Daiichi Pharmaceutical Corp
11 Philips Parkway
Montvale, NJ 07645-1810
(877) 324-4244
www.daiichius.com

Dakryon Pharmaceuticals
(see Medco Lab, Inc)

Danco Labs, LLC
PO Box 4816
New York, NY 10185
(877) 432-7596
www.earlyoptionpill.com

Daniels Pharmaceuticals
2517 25th Avenue North
St Petersburg, FL 33713-3918
(800) 237-7427

Dartmouth Pharmaceuticals
38 Church Avenue
Wareham, MA 02571
(508) 295-2200
www.ilovemynails.com

Davol, Inc
100 Sockanossett Crossroad
PO Box 8500
Cranston, RI 02920
(800) 556-6756
www.davol.com

Del Laboratories, Inc
178 EAB Plaza
Uniondale, NY 11556
(800) 952-5080
www.dellabs.com

Delmont Laboratories, Inc
715 Harvard Avenue
PO Box 269
Swarthmore, PA 19081
(800) 562-5541
www.delmont.com

Den-Mat Corp
2727 Skyway Drive
Santa Maria, CA 93455
(800) 445-0345
www.den-mat.com

Derma Science
214 Carnegie Center
Suite 100
Princeton, NJ 08540
(800) 825-4325
www.dermasciences.com

Dermik Laboratories
500 Arcola Road
PO Box 1200
Collegeville, PA 19426
(800) 340-7502
www.dermik.com

DeRoyal Industries, Inc
200 DeBusk Lane
Powell, TN 37849
(800) 337-6925
www.deroyal.com

DexGen Pharmaceuticals, Inc
PO Box 675
Manasquan, NJ 08736
(877) DEXGEN1
www.dexgen.com

Dey LP
2751 Napa Valley Corporate Drive
Napa, CA 94558
(707) 224-3200
www.deyinc.com

DiaPharma Group, Inc
8948 Beckett Road
West Chester, OH 45069
(800) 526-5224
www.diapharma.com

Diatide, Inc
9 Delta Drive
Londonderry, NH 03053
(603) 437-8970
www.diatide.com

Dickinson Brands, Inc
31 East High Street
East Hampton, CT 06424
(888) 860-2279
www.dickinsonbrands.com

Digestive Care, Inc
1120 Win Drive
Bethlehem, PA 18017-7059
(610) 882-5950
www.pancrecarb.com

Discovery Laboratories, Inc
350 South Main Street
Suite 307
Doylestown, PA 18901
(215) 340-4699
www.discoverylabs.com

Discus Dental, Inc
8550 Higuera Street
Culver City, CA 90232
(800) 422-9448
www.discusdental.com

Dista Products Company
(see Eli Lilly & Company)

Doak Dermatologics
383 Route 46 West
Fairfield, NJ 07004-2402
(800) 405-3625
www.bradpharm.com

Dow Hickam, Inc
(see Bertek Pharmaceuticals, Inc)

Dreir Pharmaceuticals, Inc
9602 North 122nd Place
Scottsdale, AZ 85259
(800) 541-4044
www.dreirpharmaceuticals.com

DuPont Pharmaceuticals
Chestnut Run Plaza
974 Centre Road
Wilmington, DE 19805
(800) 474-2762
www.dupontpharma.com

Duramed Pharmaceuticals
5040 Duramed Drive
Cincinnati, OH 45213
(513) 731-9900
www.duramed.com

Dura Pharmaceuticals
(see Elan Pharmaceuticals)

Durex Consumer Products
3585 Engineering Drive
Suite 200
Norcross, GA 30092
(888) 566-3468
www.durex.com

Durham Pharmacal Corp
Route 145
Oak Hill, NY 12460
(888) 438-7426
www.durhampharm.com

DUSA Pharmaceuticals, Inc
25 Upton Drive
Wilmington, MA 01887
(978) 657-7500
www.dusapharma.com

Eagle Vison, Inc
8500 Wolf Lake Drive
Suite 110
PO Box 34877
Memphis, TN 38184
(800) 222-7584
www.eaglevis.com

Eckerd Drug Corp
PO Box 4689
Clearwater, FL 33758
(800) 325-3737
www.eckerd.com

ECR Pharmaceuticals
PO Box 71600
Richmond, VA 23255
(804) 527-1950
www.ecrpharma.com

Effcon Laboratories, Inc
PO Box 7499
Marietta, GA 30065-1499
(800) 722-2428
www.effcon.com

E. Fougera & Company
60 Baylis Road
Melville, NY 11747
(800) 645-9833
www.fougera.com

Eisai, Inc
500 Frank W. Burr Boulevard
Teaneck, NJ 07666
(201) 692-1100
www.eisai.com

Elan Corp
800 Gateway Boulevard
South San Francisco, CA 94080
(650) 877-0900
www.elan.com

Eli Lilly & Company
Lilly Corporate Center
Indianapolis, IN 46285
(800) 545-5979
www.lilly.com

Elkins-Sinn, Inc
2 Esterbrook Lane
Cherry Hill, NJ 08003-4099
(610) 688-4400

EMD Chemicals, Inc
480 South Democrat Road
Gibbstown, NJ 08027
(800) 222-0342
www.emdchemicals.com

Endo Pharmaceuticals, Inc
100 Painters Drive
Chadds Ford, PA 19317
(610) 558-9800
www.endo.com

EnviroDerm Pharmaceuticals, Inc
PO Box 32370
Louisville, KY 40232-2370
(800) 991-3376
www.enviroderm.com

Enzon, Inc
685 Route 202/206
Bridgewater, NJ 08807
(908) 575-9457
www.enzon.com

Eon Labs Manufacturing, Inc
227-15 North Conduit Avenue
Laurelton, NY 11413
(800) 526-0225
www.eonlabs.com

E. R. Squibb & Sons, Inc
(see Bristol-Myers Squibb Company)

Ethex Corp
10888 Metro Court
St Louis, MO 63043-2413
(800) 321-1705
www.ethex.com

Ethicon, Inc
(Johnson & Johnson)
US Route 22 West
PO Box 151
Somerville, NJ 08876-0151
(800) 255-2500
www.ethiconinc.com

Everett Laboratories, Inc
29 Spring Street
West Orange, NJ 07052
(973) 324-0200
www.everettlabs.com

E-Z-EM
717 Main Street
Westbury, NY 11590
(800) 544-4624
www.ezem.com

Female Health Company
515 North State Street
Suite 2225
Chicago, IL 60610
(800) 884-1601
www.femalehealth.com

Ferndale Laboratories, Inc
780 West Eight Mile Road
Ferndale, MI 48220
(800) 621-6003
www.ferndalelabs.com

Ferring Pharmaceuticals, Inc
400 Rella Boulevard
Suffern, NY 10901
(888) 337-7464
www.ferringusa.com

Fidia Pharmaceutical Corp
2000 K Street Northwest
Suite 700
Washington, DC 20006
(202) 371-9898
www.fidiapharma.com

First Horizon Pharmaceutical Corp
6195 Shiloh Road
Alpharetta, GA 30005
(770) 442-9707
www.horizonpharm.com

Fischer Pharmaceuticals, Inc
165 Gibraltar Court
Sunnyvale, CA 94089
(800) 782-0222
www.dr-fischer.com

Fisons Corp (see Aventis Behring)

Fleming & Company
1733 Gilsinn Lane
Fenton, MO 63026
(800) 343-0164
www.flemingcompany.com

Forest Laboratories, Inc
909 Third Avenue
New York, NY 10022
(800) 947-5227
www.frx.com

Freeda Vitamins, Inc
36 East 41st Street
New York, NY 10017
(800) 777-3737
www.freedavitamins.com

Fujisawa Healthcare, Inc
Three Parkway North
Deerfield, IL 60015-2548
(800) 727-7003
www.fujisawa.com

Galderma Laboratories, Inc
14501 North Freeway
Fort Worth, TX 76177
(817) 961-5000
www.galdermausa.com

Gallipot, Inc
2020 Silver Bell Road
St Paul, MN 55122
(800) 423-6967
www.gallipot.com

Gambro Healthcare, Inc
10810 West Collins Avenue
Lakewood, CO 80215-4498
(303) 232-6800
www.gambro.com

Gate Pharmaceuticals
PO Box 1090
North Wales, PA 19454-1090
(800) 292-4283
www.gatepharma.com

Gebauer Company
4444 East 153rd Street
Cleveland, OH 44128
(800) 321-9348
www.gebauerco.com

Geigy Pharmaceuticals
(see Novartis Pharmaceuticals Corp)

Genaissance Pharmaceuticals
Five Science Parkway
New Haven, CT 06511
(203) 773-1450
www.genaissance.com

GenDerm Corp (see Medicis Pharmaceutical Corp)

Gen-King (see Kinray)

Genentech, Inc
One DNA Way
South San Francisco, CA 94080-4990
(650) 225-1000
www.gene.com

General Injectables & Vaccines
US Highway 52 South
PO Box 9
Bastian, VA 24314-0009
(540) 688-4121
www.giv.com

General Nutrition, Inc
300 6th Avenue
Pittsburgh, PA 15222
(888) 462-2548
www.gnc.com

Genesis Nutrition
1816 Wall Street
Florence, SC 29501
(800) 451-7933
www.genesisnutrition.com

Genesis Pharmaceutical, Inc
1721 Maplelane Avenue
Hazel Park, MI 48030
(800) 459-8663
www.genesispharm.com

Geneva Pharmaceuticals, Inc
2655 West Midway Boulevard
PO Box 446
Broomfield, CO 80038-0446
(800) 525-8747

GenPharm International, Inc
(see Medarex)

GensiaSicor Pharmaceuticals
(see SICOR Pharmaceuticals, Inc)

GenVec, Inc
65 West Watkins Mill Road
Gaithersburg. MD 20878
(240) 632-0740
www.genvec.com

Genzyme Pharmaceuticals
500 Kendall Street
Cambridge, MA 02142
(617) 252-7500
www.genzyme.com

Geodesic MediTech, Inc
2921 Sandy Pointe No. 3
Del Mar, CA 92014
(888) 357-9399
www.geodesicmeditech.com

Gerber Products Company
445 State Street
Fremont, MI 49413-0001
(800) 443-7237
www.gerber.com

Geron Corp
230 Constitution Drive
Menlo Park, CA 94025
(650) 473-7700
www.geron.com

Gilead
333 Lakeside Drive
Foster City, CA 94404
(800) 445-3235
www.gilead.com

Glades Pharmaceuticals, LLC
6340 Sugarloaf Parkway
Duluth, GA 30097
(888) 445-2337
www.glades.com

GlaxoSmithKline
Five Moore Drive
PO Box 13398
Research Triangle Park, NC 27709
(888) 825-5249
www.gsk.com

GlaxoSmithKline
One Franklin Plaza
Philadelphia, PA 19102
(888) 825-5249
www.gsk.com

GlaxoSmithKline
Consumer Healthcare
PO Box 1467
Pittsburgh, PA 15230
(412) 928-1000
www.gsk.com

GlaxoWellcome, Inc (see GlaxoSmithKline)

Glenwood, LLC
111 Cedar Lane
Englewood, NJ 07631
(800) 542-0772
www.glenwood-llc.com

Global Pharmaceuticals, Inc
3735 Castor Avenue
Philadelphia, PA 19124
(215) 289-2220
www.globalphar.com

Goldline Laboratories, Inc
(see Zenith Goldline Pharmaceuticals)

Gordon Laboratories
6801 Ludlow Street
Upper Darby, PA 19082-2408
(800) 356-7870
www.gordonlabs.com

GF Health Products, Inc
2935 Northeast Parkway
Atlanta, GA 30360
(800) 347-5678
www.grahamfield.com

Grandpa Brands Company
1820 Airport Exchange Boulevard
Erlanger, KY 41018
(800) 684-1468
www.csdent.com

Green Turtle Bay Vitamin Company
56 High Street
Summit, NJ 07901
(800) 887-8535
www.energywave.com

Greer Laboratories, Inc
639 Nuway Circle
PO Box 800
Lenoir, NC 28645-0800
(800) 438-0088
www.greerlabs.com

Grifols
(Bioscience Division)
2410 Lillyvale Avenue
Los Angeles, CA 90032
(888) 474-3657
www.grifolsusa.com

Guilford Pharmaceuticals, Inc
6611 Tributary Street
Baltimore, MD 21224
(410) 631-6300
www.guilfordpharm.com

G & W Laboratories
111 Coolidge Street
South Plainfield, NJ 07080-3895
(800) 922-1038
www.gwlabs.com

Gynetics
PO Box 8509
Somerville, NJ 08876
(800) 311-7378
www.gynetics.com

Halocarbon Products Corp
PO Box 661
River Edge, NJ 07661
(201) 262-8899
www.halocarbon.com

Hart Health & Safety
PO Box 94044
Seattle, WA 98124
(800) 234-4278
www.harthealth.com

Harvard Drug Group, LCC
31778 Enterprise Drive
Livonia, MI 48150
(800) 875-0123
www.harvarddrugs.com

Hauser Pharmaceutical, Inc
4401 East US Highway 30
Valparaiso, IN 46383
(800) 441-2309
www.hauserpharmaceutical.com

Hawthorn Pharmaceuticals, Inc
PO Box 2248
Madison, MS 39130
(888) 455-5253
www.hawthornrx.com

HDC Corp
628 Gibraltar Court
Milpitas, CA 95035
(800) 227-8162
www.hdccorp.com

HealthAsure, Inc
26635 West Agoura Road
Suite 205
Calabasas, CA 91302
(818) 577-1100
www.breathasure.com

Healthfirst Corp
22316 70th Avenue West
Unit A
Mountlake Terrace, WA 98043-2184
(425) 771-5733

Helix Biopharma Corp
215-7080 River Road
Richmond, BC V6X 1X5
(800) 563-4363
www.helixbiopharma.com

Hemacare Corp
21101 Oxnard Street
Woodland HIlls, CA 91367
(877) 310-0717
www.hemacare.com

Hemagen Diagnostics, Inc
9033 Red Branch Road
Columbia, MD 21045
(800) 495-2180
www.hemagen.com

Hemispherx Biopharma, Inc
One Penn Center
1617 John F. Kennedy Boulevard
6th Floor
Philadelphia, PA 19103
(215) 988-0080
www.hemispherx.com

Henry Schein, Inc
135 Duryea Road
Melville, NY 11747
(631) 843-5500
www.henryschein.com

Hill Dermaceuticals, Inc
2650 South Mellonville Avenue
Sanford, FL 32773-9311
(800) 344-5707
www.hillderm.com

Hi-Tech Pharmacal, Inc
369 Bayview Avenue
Amityville, NY 11701
(631) 789-8228
www.hitechpharm.com

Hoechst-Marion Roussel, Inc (see Aventis)

Hoffmann-LaRoche
(see Roche Pharmaceuticals)

Hogil Pharmaceutical Corp
Two Manhattanville Road
Purchase, NY 10577-2118
(914) 696-7600
www.hogil.com

Hollister-Stier Laboratories, LLC
3525 North Regal Street
Spokane, WA 99207-5788
(800) 992-1120
www.hollister-stier.com

Home Access Health Corp
2401 West Hassell Road
Suite 1510
Hoffman Estates, IL 60195
(847) 781-2500
www.homeaccess.com

Hope Pharmaceuticals
8260 East Gelding Drive
Suite 104
Scottsdale, AZ 85260
(800) 755-9595
www.hopepharm.com

Horizon Diagnostics, Inc
2930 East Houston Street
San Antonio, TX 78202
(210) 222-2108
www.horizondiagnostics.com

Horizon Pharmaceutical Corp
(see First Horizon Pharmaceutical Corp)

Hospira, Inc
275 North Field Drive
Lake Forest, IL 60045
(877) 467-7472
www.hospira.com

Hyland Immuno
(Baxter)
550 North Brand Boulevard
Glendale, CA 91203
(800) 423-2090
http://baxdb1.baxter.com

Hyland Laboratories, Inc
(Standard Homeopathic Company)
210 West 131st Street
Los Angeles, CA 90061
(800) 624-9659
www.hylands.com

ICN Pharmaceuticals, Inc
(see Valeant Pharmaceuticals)

IDEC Pharmaceuticals
(see Bogen idec)

Ilex Oncology, Inc
4545 Horizon Hill Boulevard
San Antonio, TX 78229-2263
(210) 949-8200
www.ilexonc.com

Immune Response Corp
5935 Darwin Court
Carlsbad, CA 92008
(760) 431-7080
www.imnr.com

ImmunoGen, Inc
128 Sidney Street
Cambridge, MA 02139
(617) 995-2500
www.immunogen.com

Immunomedics, Inc
300 American Road
Morris Plains, NJ 07950
(973) 605-8200
www.immunomedics.com

Immuno-US, Inc
(see Baxter Healthcare Corp)

IMPAX Laboratories, Inc
30831 Huntwood Avenue
Hayward, CA 94544
(510) 476-2000
www.impaxlabs.com

Incyte Pharmaceuticals, Inc
Experimental Station
Route 141 & Henry Clay Road
Building E336
Wilmington, DE 19880
(800) 305-0670
www.incyte.com

Indevus Pharmaceuticals, Inc
99 Hayden Avenue
Suite 200
Lexington, MA 02421
(781) 861-8444
www.interneuron.com

InKine Pharmaceutical Company, Inc
1787 Sentry Parkway
West Building 18
Suite 440
Blue Bell, PA 19422
(215) 283-6850
www.inkine.com

INO Therapeutics, Inc
54 Old Highway 22
Clinton, NJ 08809
(908) 238-6600
www.inotherapeutics.com

Inspire Pharmaceuticals, Inc
4222 Emperor Boulevard
Suite 200
Durham, NC 27703
(919) 941-9777
www.inspirepharm.com

Interferon Sciences, Inc
783 Jersey Avenue
New Brunswick, NJ 08901-3660
(888) 728-4372
www.interferonsciences.com

InterMune Pharmaceuticals, Inc
3280 Bayshore Boulevard
Brisbane, CA 94005
(415) 466-2200
www.intermune.com

International Medication Systems, Limited (IMS)
1886 Santa Anita Avenue
South El Monte, CA 91733
(800) 423-4136
www.ims-limited.com

IntraBiotics Pharmaceuticals, Inc
2483 East Bayshore Road
Suite 100
Palo Alto, CA 94303
(650) 526-6800

Introgen Therapeutics, Inc
301 Congress Avenue
Austin, TX 78701
(512) 320-5010
www.introgen.com

Inveresk
11000 Westen Parkway
Cary, NC 27513
(919) 460-9005
www.inveresk.com

Inverness Medical Innovations
51 Sawyer Road
Suite 200
Waltham, MA 02453-3448
(781) 647-3900
www.invernessmedical.com

Inwood Laboratories (Forest)
321 Prospect Street
Inwood, NY 11096
(800) 876-5227

Iomed, Inc
2441 South 3850 West
Suite A
Salt Lake City, UT 84120
(800) 621-3347
www.iomed.com

IOP, Inc
3151 Airway Avenue
Costa Mesa, CA 92626
(800) 535-3545
www.iopinc.com

Isis Pharmaceuticals
2292 Faraday Avenue
Carlsbad, CA 92008
(760) 931-9200
www.isispharm.com

Ivax Pharmaceuticals, Inc
4400 Biscayne Boulevard
Miami, FL 33137
(800) 327-4114
www.ivaxpharmaceuticals.com

IVPCARE
7164 Technology Drive
Suite 100
Frisco, TX 75034
(800) 424-9002
www.ivpcare.com

Janssen Pharmaceutica Products, LP
1125 Trenton-Harbourton Road
PO Box 200
Titusville, NJ 08560-0200
(800) 526-7736
www.us.janssen.com

Jerome Stevens Pharmaceuticals, Inc
60 DaVinci Drive
Bohemia, NY 11716-2613
(631) 567-1113

Johnson & Johnson
One Johnson & Johnson Plaza
New Brunswick, NJ 08933
(732) 524-0400
www.jnj.com

Jones Pharma
(see King Pharmaceuticals, Inc)

J. R. Carlson Laboratories, Inc
15 College Drive
Arlington Heights, IL 60004-1985
(847) 255-1600
www.carlsonlabs.com

J. T. Baker, Inc (see Mallinckrodt Baker, Inc)

Kendall Healthcare Products
15 Hampshire Street
Mansfield, MA 02048
(800) 962-9888
www.kendallhq.com

Key Pharmaceuticals (see Schering-Plough Corp)

Kimberly-Clark/Ballard Medical Products
12050 Lone Peak Parkway
Draper, UT 84020
(800) 528-5591
www.kchealthcare.com

King Pharmaceuticals, Inc
501 Fifth Street
Bristol, TN 37620
(800) 776-3637
www.kingpharm.com

Kingswood Laboratories, Inc
10375 Hague Road
Indianapolis, IN 46256
(800) 968-7772
www.kingswood-labs.com

Kinray
152-35 10th Avenue
Whitestone, NY 11357
(800) 854-6729
www.kinray.com

Kirkman Laboratories, Inc
6400 Southwest Rosewood Street
Lake Oswego, OR 97035
(800) 245-8282
www.kirkmanlabs.com

KLI Corp
1119 Third Avenue Southwest
Carmel, IN 46032
(800) 308-7452
www.entertainers-secret.com

Knoll Pharmaceuticals Company
3000 Continental Drive North
Mt Olive, NJ 07828
(800) 526-0221
www.hhplus.com

Konsyl Pharmaceuticals, Inc
10 Kilmer Road
PO Box 1907
Edison, NJ 08818-1907
(732) 819-4402
www.konsyl.com

Kos Pharmaceuticals, Inc
1001 Brickell Bay Drive
25th Floor
Miami, FL 33131
(305) 577-3464
www.kospharm.com

Kramer Laboratories, Inc
8778 Southwest 8th Street
Miami, FL 33174
(800) 824-4894
www.kramerlabs.com

K. V. Pharmaceutical Company
2503 South Hanley Road
St Louis, MO 63144
(314) 645-6600
www.kvpharma.com

Lacrimedics, Inc
PO Box 1209
Eastsound, WA 98245
(800) 367-8327
www.lacrimedics.com

Lactaid, Inc
7050 Camp Hill Road
Fort Washington, PA 19034
(800) 522-8243
www.lactaid.com

Lannett Company, Inc
9000 State Road
Philadelphia, PA 19136
(800) 325-9994
www.lannett.com

LecTec Corp
10701 Red Circle Drive
Minnetonka, MN 55343
(800) 777-2291
www.lectec.com

Lee Laboratories
1475 Athens Highway
Grayson, GA 30017
(770) 972-4450
www.leelabs.com

Lee Pharmaceuticals
1434 Santa Anita Avenue
South El Monte, CA 91733
(800) 950-5337
www.leepharmaceuticals.com

Leiner Health Products
901 East 233rd Street
Carson, CA 90745
(310) 835-8400
www.leiner.com

LifeScan, Inc
(Johnson & Johnson Company)
1000 Gibraltar Drive
Milpitas, CA 95035
(800) 227-8862
www.lifescan.com

LifeSign LLC
71 Veronica Avenue
PO Box 218
Somerset, NJ 08875-0218
(800) 526-2125
www.lifesignmed.com

Ligand Pharmaceuticals
10275 Science Center Drive
San Diego, CA 92121
(858) 550-7500
www.ligand.com

Lilly & Company (see Eli Lilly & Company)

Lincoln Diagnostics
PO Box 1128
Decatur, IL 62525
(217) 877-2531
www.lincolndiagnostics.com

LSI America Corp
4732 Twin Valley Drive
Austin, TX 78731-3537
(800) 720-5936
www.ondrox.com

Lyne Laboratories
10 Burke Drive
Brockton, MA 02301
(800) 525-0450
www.lyne.com

3M Pharmaceuticals
3M Center
Building 275-3W-01
PO Box 33275
St Paul, MN 55133
(800) 328-0255
3m.com/pharma

Magno-Humphries Laboratories
8800 Southwest Commercial Street
Tigard, OR 97223
(503) 684-5464
www.magno-humphries.com

Mallinckrodt Baker, Inc
222 Red School Lane
Phillipsburg, NJ 08865
(800) 582-2537
www.mallbaker.com

Mallinckrodt, Inc
(Corp Headquarters)
675 McDonnell Boulevard
Hazelwood, MO 63042
(314) 654-2000
www.mallinckrodt.com

Marlyn Nutraceuticals, Inc
14851 North Scottsdale Road
Scottsdale, AZ 85254
(800) 462-7596

Martec Pharmaceutical, Inc
1800 North Topping
Kansas City, MO 64120
(800) 822-6782
www.martec-kc.com

Martek Biosciences Corp
6480 Dobbin Road
Columbia, MD 21045
(800) 338-9959
www.martekbio.com

Mason Vitamins, Inc
5105 Northwest 159th Street
Miami Lakes, FL 33014-6370
(800) 327-6005
www.masonvitamins.com

Mayne Pharma (USA), Inc
650 From Road
(Mack-Cali Centre II)
5th Floor South
Paramus, NJ 07652
(201) 225-5500
www.us.maynepharma.com

McGuff Company, Inc
3524 West Lake Center Drive
Santa Ana, CA 92704
(800) 854-7220
www.mcguffmedical.com

McNeil Consumer Healthcare
Camp Hill Road
Mail Stop 278
Fort Washington, PA 19034-2292
(800) 962-5357
www.ortho-mcneil.com

Mead Johnson Laboratories
(see Bristol-Myers Squibb Company)

Medarex
707 State Road
Princeton, NJ 08540-1437
(609) 430-2880
www.medarex.com

Medco Lab, Inc
716 West 7th Street
Sioux City, IA 51103
(712) 255-8770
www.medcolab.com

Medeva Pharmaceuticals
(see Celltech Pharmaceuticals, Inc)

Medicis Pharmaceutical Corp
8125 North Hayden Road
Scottsdale, AZ 85258-2463
(602) 808-8800
www.medicis.com

Medi-Dose, Inc
70 Industrial Drive
Ivyland, PA 18974
(800) 523-8966
www.medidose.com

MedImmune, Inc
One MedImmune Way
Gaithersburg, MD 20878
(877) 633-4411
www.medimmune.com

Medisca, Inc
661 Route 3, Unit C
Plattsburgh, NY 12901
(800) 932-1039
www.medisca.com

MediSense, Inc
(Abbott Laboratories)
4A Crosby Drive
Bedford, MA 01730
(800) 323-9100

Medix Pharmaceuticals Americas, Inc (MPA)
12505 Starkey Road
Suite M
Largo, FL 33773
(888)242-3463
www.biafine.com

MedPointe Pharmaceuticals
265 Davidson Avenue
Suite 300
PO Box 6833
Somerset, NJ 08873-4120
(732) 564-2200
www.medpointeinc.com

Medtronic, Inc
710 Medtronic Parkway
Minneapolis, MN 55432-5604
(763) 514-4000
www.medtronic.com

Menicon America, Inc
1840 Gateway Drive
Second Floor
San Mateo, CA 94404
(650) 378-1424
www.menicon.com

Mentholatum Company, Inc
(Rohto Pharmaceutical Company)
707 Sterling Drive
Orchard Park, NY 14127
(716) 677-2500
www.mentholatum.com

Merck & Company
(Human Health Division)
PO Box 4
West Point, PA 19486-0004
(800) 672-6372
www.merck.com

Mericon Industries, Inc
8819 North Pioneer Road
Peoria, IL 61615-1561
(800) 242-6464
www.mericon-industries.com

Meridian Medical Technologies
(King Pharmaceuticals, Inc)
10240 Old Columbia Road
Columbia, MD 21046
(800) 638-8093
www.meridianmeds.com

Merit Pharmaceuticals
2611 San Fernando Road
Los Angeles, CA 90065
(800) 421-9657
www.meritpharm.com

Merz Pharmaceuticals
4215 Tudor Lane
Greensboro, NC 27410
(800) 334-0514
www.merzusa.com

Methapharm, Inc
11772 West Sample Road
Suite 101
Coral Springs, FL 33065
(800) 287-7686
www.methapharm.com

MGI Pharma, Inc
5775 West Old Shakopee Road
Suite 100
Bloomington, MN 55437-3174
(800) 562-5580
www.mgipharma.com

Mikart, Inc
1750 Chattahoochee Avenue
Atlanta, GA 30318
(404) 351-4510
www.mikart.com

Miles Allergy (see Bayer Corp)

Miles, Inc (see Bayer Corp)

Milex Products, Inc
4311 North Normandy
Chicago, IL 60634-1403
(800) 621-1278
www.milexproducts.com

Miller Pharmacal Group, Inc
350 Randy Road
Suite 2
Carol Stream, IL 60188-1831
(800) 323-2935
www.millerpharmacal.com

Mission Pharmacal Company
10999 IH-10 West
Suite 1000
San Antonio, TX 78230
(210) 696-8400
www.missionpharmacal.com

Monaghan Medical Corp
5 Latour Avenue
Suite 1600
PO Box 2805
Plattsburgh, NY 12901
(800) 833-9653
www.monaghanmed.com

Monarch Pharmaceuticals
(King Pharmaceuticals, Inc)
355 Beecham Street
Bristol, TN 37620
(800) 776-3637
www.monarchpharm.com

Monticello Drug Company
1604 Stockton Street
Jacksonville, FL 32204
(800) 735-0666
www.monticellocompanies.com

Moore Medical Corp
PO Box 1500
New Britain, CT 06050-1500
(800) 234-1464
www.mooremedical.com

Morton Grove Pharmaceuticals
6451 West Main Street
Morton Grove, IL 60053
(800) 346-6854
www.mgp-online.com

Mutual Pharmaceutical Company, Inc/United Research Laboratories
1100 Orthodox Street
Philadelphia, PA 19124
(800) 523-3684
www.urlmutual.com

Mylan Laboratories, Inc
1500 Corporate Drive
Suite 400
Canonsburg, PA 15317
(724) 514-1800
www.mylan.com

Mylan Pharmaceuticals, Inc
P0 Box 4310
Morgantown, WV 26504
(800) 826-9526
www.mylanpharm.com

Nabi
(Corp Headquarters)
5800 Park of Commerce Boulevard Northwest
Boca Raton, FL 33487
(561) 989-5800
www.nabi.com

Nagase Pharmaceuticals
500 Fifth Avenue
Suite 840
New York, NY 10110
(212) 354-3140
www.nagase.com

Nastech Pharmaceutical Company, Inc
45 Adams Avenue
Hauppauge, NY 11788
(631) 273-0101
www.nastech.com

NATREN, Inc
3105 Willow Lane
Westlake Village, CA 91361
(800) 992-3323
www.natren.com

Natrol, Inc
21411 Prairie Street
Chatsworth, CA 91311
(800) 326-1520
www.natrol.com

Natures Bounty, Inc
(NBTY, Inc)
90 Orville Drive
Bohemia, NY 11716
(888) 465-6757
www.naturesbounty.com

Nature's Sunshine Products, Inc
75 East 1700 South
Provo, UT 84606
(800) 223-8225
www.nsponline.com

NeoPharm, Inc
150 Field Drive
Suite 195
Lake Forest, IL 60045
(847) 295-8678
www.neopharm.com

NeoRx Corp
300 Elliott Avenue West
Suite 500
Seattle, WA 98119-4007
(206) 281-7001
www.neorx.com

Nephron Pharmaceuticals Corp
4121 34th Street
Orlando, FL 32811
(800) 443-4313
www.nephronpharm.com

Nestle Clinical Nutrition
3 Parkway North
Suite 500
Deerfield, IL 60015
(800) 422-2752
www.nestleclinicalnutrition.com

NeuroGenesis/Matrix Tech, Inc
120 Park Avenue
League City, TX 77573
(800) 345-8912
www.neurogenesis.com

Neutrogena Corp
5760 West 96th Street
Los Angeles, CA 90045-5595
(800) 582-4048
www.neutrogena.com

Nexstar Pharmaceuticals, Inc
2860 Wilderness Place
Boulder, CO 80301

Niche Pharmaceuticals, Inc
209 North Oak Street
Roanoke, TX 76262
(800) 677-0355
www.niche-inc.com

Nnodum Pharmaceuticals
(Zikspain)
PO Box 19725
Cincinnati, OH 45219
(513) 861-2329
www.zikspain.com

Nomax, Inc
40 North Rock Hill Road
St Louis, MO 63119
(314) 961-2500
www.nomax.com

Noramco, Inc
(Johnson & Johnson)
1440 Olympic Drive
Athens, GA 30601
(706) 353-4400
www.noramco.com

Norstar Consumer Products Company, Inc
5517 95th Avenue
Kenosha, WI 53144
(262) 652-8505
www.norstarcpc.com

Northern Research Laboratories, Inc
4225 White Bear Parkway
Suite 600
St Paul, MN 55110-3389
(888) 884-4675
www.northernresearch.com

Nova Factor
1620 Century Center Parkway
Suite 109
Memphis, TN 38134
(800) 235-8498
www.accredohealth.net

Novartis Pharmaceuticals Corp
One Health Plaza
East Hanover, NJ 07936-1080
(973) 781-8265
www.pharma.us.novartis.com

Noven Pharmaceuticals, Inc
11960 Southwest 144th Street
Miami, FL 33186
(305) 253-5099
www.noven.com

Novocol
(Septodont, Inc)
PO Box 11926
Wilmington, DE 19850
(800) 872-8305
www.septodontinc.com

Novo Nordisk Pharmaceuticals, Inc
100 College Road West
Princeton, NJ 08540
(800) 727-6500
www.novonordisk-us.com

Novopharm USA, Inc
165 East Commerce Drive
Suite 100
Schaumburg, IL 60173-5326
(800) 635-5067

Numark Laboratories, Inc
164 Northfield Avenue
Edison, NJ 08837
(800) 338-8079
www.numarklabs.com

Nutraceutical Solutions
6704 Ranger Avenue
Corpus Christi, TX 78415
(800) 856-7040
www.eliquidsolutions.com

NutraMax Laboratories, Inc
2208 Lakeside Boulevard
Edgewood, MD 21040
(800) 925-5187
www.nutramaxlabs.com

NutriSoy International, Inc
424 South Kentucky Avenue
Evansville, IN 47714
(888) 769-0769
www.nutrisoy.com

Octamer, Inc
100 Shoreline Highway
Mill Valley, CA 94941
(415) 332-6434
www.octamer.com

Odyssey Pharmaceuticals, Inc
72 Eagle Rock Avenue
East Hanover, NJ 07936
(877) 427-9068
www.odysseypharm.com

Ohmeda Pharmaceuticals
(see Baxter Pharmaceutical Products, Inc)

Omnicell
1201 Charleston Road
Mountain View, CA 94043-1337
(800) 850-6664
www.omnicell.com

Omnii Products
1500 North Florida Mango Road
Suite 1
West Palm Beach, FL 33409
(800) 445-3386
www.omniiproducts.com

ONYX Pharmaceuticals
3031 Research Drive
Richmond, CA 94806
(510) 262-8772
www.onyx-pharm.com

Optics Laboratory, Inc
9480 Telstar Avenue #3
El Monte, CA 91731
(626) 350-1926
www.opticslab.com

Optimox Corp
PO Box 3378
Torrance, CA 90510-3378
(800) 223-1601
www.optimox.com

Organogenesis, Inc
150 Dan Road
Canton, MA 02021
(781) 575-0775
www.organogenesis.com

Organon, Inc
375 Mt Pleasant Avenue
West Orange, NJ 07052
(973) 325-4500
www.organon-usa.com

Orphan Medical, Inc
13911 Ridgedale Drive
Suite 250
Minnetonka, MN 55305
(952) 513-6900
www.orphan.com

Ortho Biotech Products, LP
430 Route 22 East
PO Box 6914
Bridgewater, NJ 08807-0914
(908) 541-4000
www.orthobiotech.com

Ortho-Clinical Diagnostics
100 Indigo Creek Drive
Rochester, NY 14626
(800) 828-6316
www.orthoclinical.com

Ortho-McNeil Pharmaceutical, Inc
1000 U.S. Route 202 South
Raritan, NJ 08869
(800) 682-6532
www.ortho-mcneil.com

Oscient Pharmaceuticals
100 Beaver Street
Waltham, MA 02154-8440
(617) 398-2300

Otsuka America Pharmaceutical, Inc
2440 Research Boulevard
Rockville, MD 20850
(800) 562-3974
www.otsuka.com

Oxford Pharmaceutical Services, Inc
One US Highway 46 West
Totowa, NJ 07512
(877) 284-9120
www.oxfordpharm.com

OXIS International, Inc
6040 North Cutter Circle
Suite 317
Portland, OR 97217
(503) 283-3911
www.oxis.com

Paddock Laboratories, Inc
3940 Quebec Avenue North
Minneapolis, MN 55427
(800) 328-5113
www.paddocklabs.com

Pan American Laboratories, LLC
PO Box 8950
Mandeville, LA 70470-8950
(985) 893-4097
www.panamericanlabs.com

Parke-Davis
Pfizer Pharmaceuticals
201 Tabor Road
Morris Plains, NJ 07950
(800) 223-0432

Parnell Pharmaceuticals
1525 Francisco Boulevard
San Rafael, CA 94901
(800) 457-4276
www.parnellpharm.com

Pasteur Merieux Connaught USA
PO Box 187, Route 611
Swiftwater, PA 18370
(717) 839-7187

Par Pharmaceutical, Inc
One Ram Ridge Road
Spring Valley, NY 10977
(800) 828-9393
www.parpharm.com

PDRx Pharmaceuticals, Inc
727 North Ann Arbor
Oklahoma City, OK 73127
(800) 299-7379
www.pdrx.com

Pediatric Pharmaceuticals, Inc
120 Wood Avenue South
Suite 300
Iselin, NJ 08830
(732) 603-7708
www.pediatricpharm.com

Pedinol Pharmacal, Inc
30 Banfi Plaza North
Farmingdale, NY 11735
(800) 733-4665
www.pedinol.com

Perrigo Company
515 Eastern Avenue
Allegan, MI 49010
(800) 719-9260
www.perrigo.com

Person & Covey, Inc
616 Allen Avenue
Glendale, CA 91201
(818) 240-1030
www.personandcovey.com

Pfizer Pharmaceuticals Group (PPG)
235 East 42nd Street
New York, NY 10017-5755
(800) 438-1985
www.pfizer.com

Pharma 21, Inc
1363 Shinly
Suite 100
Escondido, CA 92026
(760) 743-7441
www.pharma21.net

Pharmaceutical Formulations, Inc
PO Box 1904
Edison, NJ 08818-1904
(732) 985-7100
www.pfiotc.com

Pharmaceutical Specialties, Inc
PO Box 6298
Rochester, MN 55903-6298
(800) 325-8232
www.psico.com

Pharmacia Corp
(see Pfizer Pharmaceuticals Group (PPG))

Pharmacia & Upjohn Company
(Ophthalmics Division)
701 East Milham Road
Kalamazoo, MI 49001
(800) 423-4866

Pharmakon Labs
6050 Jet Port Industrial Boulevard
Tampa, FL 33634
(800) 888-4045
www.pharmakonlabs.com

Pharmanex
75 West Center
Provo, UT 84601
(801) 345-9800
www.pharmanex.com

Pharmatek Laboratories, Inc
5626 Oberlin Drive
San Diego, CA 92121
(858) 587-8783
www.pharmatek.com

Pharmics, Inc
PO Box 27554
Salt Lake City, UT 84127
(801) 966-4138
www.pharmics.com

PhytoPharmica, Inc
825 Challenger Drive
Green Bay, WI 54311
(800) 553-2370
www.phytopharmica.com

Plantex USA, Inc
Two University
Suite 305
Hackensack, NJ 07601
(201) 343-4141
www.plantexusa.com

Playtex Company
74 Commerce Drive
Allendale, NJ 07401-1600
(800) 816-5742
www.playtex.com

PLIVA, Inc
72 Eagle Rock Avenue
East Hanover, NJ 07936
(973) 386-5566
www.plivainc.com

Plough, Inc
(see Schering-Plough Corp)

PolyMedica Corp
11 State Street
Woburn, MA 01801
(781) 933-2020
www.polymedica.com

Procter & Gamble Pharmaceuticals, Inc
Sharon Woods Technical Center
11520 Reed Hartman Highway
Cincinnati, OH 45241
(800) 448-4878
www.pgpharma.com

ProCyte Corp
PO Box 808
Redmond, WA 98073-0808
(425) 869-1239
www.procyte.com

Protein Design Labs, Inc
34801 Campus Drive
Fremont, CA 94555
(510) 574-1400
www.pdl.com

Protein Sciences Corp
1000 Research Parkway
Meriden, CT 06450
(800) 488-7099
www.proteinsciences.com

Protherics, Inc
5214 Maryland Way
Suite 405
Brentwood, TN 37027
(615) 327-1027
www.protherics.com

Psychemedics Corp
1280 Massachusetts Avenue
Cambridge, MA 02138
(800) 628-8073
www.psychemedics.com

Purdue Pharma, LP
(The Purdue Frederick Company)
One Stamford Forum
201 Tresser Boulevard
Stamford, CT 06901-3431
(888) 726-7535
www.purduepharma.com

Purepac Pharmaceuticals Company
14 Commerce Drive
Suite 301
Cranford, NJ 07016
(800) 432-8534
www.purepac.com

Puritan's Pride
1233 Montauk Highway
PO Box 9001
Oakdale, NY 11769-9001
(800) 645-1030
www.puritanspride.com

QLT, Inc
887 Great Northern Way
Vancouver, BC
Canada V5T 4T5
(800) 663-5486
www.qlt-pdt.com

Questcor Pharmaceuticals, Inc
3260 Whipple Road
Union City, CA 94587
(510) 400-0700
www.questcor.com

Quidel Corp
10165 McKellar Court
San Diego, CA 92121
(800) 874-1517
www.quidel.com

Ranbaxy Pharmaceuticals, Inc USA
600 College Road East
Princeton, NJ 08540
(609) 720-9200
www.ranbaxy.com

R & D Laboratories
3925 East Watkins
Suite 200
Phoenix, AZ 85034
(800) 927-1034
www.mdlabs.com

Reese Pharmaceutical Company, Inc
10617 Frank Avenue
Cleveland, OH 44106
(800) 321-7178
www.reesechemical.com

Regeneron Pharmaceuticals, Inc
777 Old Saw Mill River Road
Tarrytown, NY 10591
(914) 345-7400
www.regeneron.com

Remel, Inc
12076 Santa Fe Drive
PO Box 14428
Lenexa, KS 66215
(800) 255-6730
www.remelinc.com

Requa, Inc
540 Barnum Avenue
PO Box 2384
Bridgeport, CT 06608
(800) 321-1085
www.requa.com

Research Triangle Institute
PO Box 12194
Research Triangle Park, NC 27709-2194
(919) 485-2666
www.rti.org

Rexall Sundown, Inc
(Royal Numico, N.V.)
6111 Broken Sound Parkway Northwest
Boca Raton, FL 33487
(800) 327-0908
www.rexallsundown.com

Rhone-Poulenc Rorer Pharmaceuticals, Inc
500 Arcola Road
PO Box 1200
Collegeville, PA 19426-0998
(800) 340-7502

Richardson-Vicks, Inc
(see Procter & Gamble Pharmaceuticals, Inc)

Ricola, Inc
51 Gibraltar Drive
Morris Plains, NJ 07950
(973) 984-6811
www.ricolausa.com

R.I.D., Inc
(Bayer Consumer Care Division)
36 Columbia Road
PO Box 1910
Morristown, NJ 07962-1910
(800) 331-4536
www.licerid.com

Rite Aid Corp
30 Hunter Lane
Camp Hill, PA 17011
(717) 761-2633
www.riteaid.com

Roberts Pharmaceuticals Corp
4 Industrial Way West
Eatontown, NJ 07724
(800) 828-2088

Roche Pharmaceuticals
340 Kingsland Street
Nutley, NJ 07110
(973) 235-5000
www.rocheusa.com

Roerig
235 East 42nd Street
New York, NY 10017
(800) 438-1985

Rorer (see Rhone-Poulenc Rorer Pharmaceuticals, Inc)

Ross Products Division, Abbott Labs
625 Cleveland Avenue
Columbus, OH 43215
(800) 230-7677
www.ross.com

Roxane Laboratories, Inc
PO Box 16532
Columbus, OH 43216
(800) 962-8364
www.roxane.com

R. P. Scherer, Inc
(see Cardinal Health, Inc)

Salix Pharmaceuticals, Inc
8540 Colonnade Center Drive
Suite 501
Raleigh, NC 27615
(919) 862-1000
www.salixltd.com

Sandoz Pharmaceuticals (see Novartis Pharmaceuticals Corp)

SangStat, Inc
6300 Dunbarton Circle
Fremont, CA 94555
(510) 789-4300
www.sangstat.com

Sanofi-Synthelabo, Inc
90 Park Avenue
New York, NY 10016
(212) 551-4000
www.sanofi-synthelabous.com

Santen, Inc
555 Gateway Drive
Napa, CA 94558
(707) 254-1750
www.santen-inc.com

Savage Laboratories
(Altana Inc)
60 Baylis Road
Melville, NY 11747-2006
(800) 231-0206
www.savagelabs.com

Scandinavian Naturals
13 North 7th Street
Perkasie, PA 18944
(800) 288-2844
www.scandinaviannaturals.com

Scandipharm
(see Axcan Pharma, Inc)

Schaffer Laboratories
1058 North Allen Avenue
Pasadena, CA 91104
(800) 231-6725
www.schafferlabs.com

Schein Pharmaceutical, Inc
(see Watson Laboratories, Inc)

Schering-Plough Corp
(World Headquarters)
2000 Galloping Hill Road
Kenilworth, NJ 07033-0530
(908) 298-4000
www.schering-plough.com

Schwarz Pharma, Inc
6140 West Executive Drive
Mequon, WI 53092
(262) 238-5400
www.schwarzusa.com

SciClone Pharmaceuticals, Inc
901 Mariner's Island Boulevard
Suite 205
San Mateo, CA 94404
(650) 358-3456
www.sciclone.com

Scios
(Corp Headquarters)
6500 Paseo Padre Parkway
Freemont, CA 94555
(510) 248-2500
www.sciosinc.com

Sepracor
(Corp Headquarters)
84 Waterford Drive
Marlborough, MA 01752
(877) SEPRACOR
www.sepracor.com

Septodont, Inc
PO Box 11926
Wilmington, DE 19850
(800) 872-8305
www.septodontinc.com

Seres Laboratories, Inc
3331-B Industrial Drive
Santa Rosa, CA 95403
(707) 526-4526
www.sereslabs.com

Serono, Inc
One Technology Place
Rockland, MA 02370
(800) 283-8088
www.seronousa.com

Shaklee Corporation
(Corp Headquarters)
4747 Willow Road
Pleasanton, CA 94588
(925) 924-2000
www.shaklee.com

Sheffield Laboratories
(Faria Ltd LLC)
170 Broad Street
New London, CT 06320
(800) 442-4451
www.sheffield-labs.com

Sherwood Davis & Geck
(see Kendall Healthcare Products)

Sherwood Medical
(see Kendall Healthcare Products)

Shire Laboratories
1550 East Gude Drive
Rockville, MD 20850
(301) 838-2500
www.shirelabs.com

SHS North America
PO Box 117
Gaithersburg, MD 20884-0117
(800) 636-2283
www.SHSNA.com

SICOR Pharmaceuticals, Inc
19 Hughes
Irvine, CA 92618
(800) 729-9991
www.gensiasicor.com

Sigma-Tau Pharmaceuticals, Inc
800 South Frederick Avenue
Suite 300
Gaithersburg, MD 20877
(800) 447-0169
www.sigma-tau.com

Silarx Pharmaceuticals, Inc
19 West Street
Spring Valley, NY 10977
(845) 352-4020
www.silarx.com

Sirna Therapeutics
2950 Wilderness Place
Boulder, CO 80301
(303) 449-6500
www.sirna.com

SkyePharma US, Inc
10 East 63rd Street
New York, NY 10021
(212) 753-5780
www.skyepharma.com

Slim Fast Foods Company
PO Box 3625
West Palm Beach, FL 33402
(877) 375-4632
www.slim-fast.com

Smith & Nephew, Inc
150 Minuteman Road
Andover, MA 01810
(978) 749-1000
www.smithnephew.com

Solvay Pharmaceuticals
901 Sawyer Road
Marietta, GA 30062
(770) 578-9000
www.solvaypharmaceuticals-us.com

Somerset Pharmaceuticals, Inc
2202 Northwest Shore Boulevard
Suite 450
Tampa, FL 33607
(800) 892-8889
www.somersetpharm.com

Sonus Pharmaceuticals
22026 20th Avenue Southeast
Suite 102
Bothell, Washington 98021
(206) 487-9500
www.sonuspharma.com

Spectrum Chemical Manufacturing Corp
14422 South San Pedro Street
Gardena, CA 90248-9985
(800) 813-1514
www.spectrumchemical.com

St Jude Medical, Inc
One Lillehei Plaza
St Paul, MN 55117-9913
(800) 328-9634
www.sjm.com

Star Pharmaceuticals, Inc
1881 West State 84
Suite 101
Fort Lauderdale, FL 33315
(800) 845-7827
www.starpharm.com

Squibb (see Bristol-Myers Squibb Company)

Steris Corp
5960 Heisley Road
Mentor, OH 44060-1834
(440) 354-2600
www.americantable.com

Sterling Health
(see Bayer Corp Consumer Care Division)

Sterling Winthrop
(see Sanofi-Synthelabo, Inc)

Stiefel Laboratories, Inc
255 Alhambra Circle
Coral Gables, FL 33134
(888) 784-3335
www.stiefel.com

Stratus Pharmaceuticals, Inc
14377 Southwest 142nd Street
Miami, FL 33186
(800) 442-7882
www.stratuspharmaceuticals.com

SummaRx Laboratories
2525 Ridgmar Boulevard
Suite 404
Ft Worth, TX 76116
(800) 406-6900
www.summalabs.com

Summers Laboratories, Inc
103 G.P. Clement Drive
Collegeville, PA 19426-2044
(800) 533-7546
www.sumlab.com

Summit Pharmaceuticals
(see Novartis Pharmaceuticals Corp)

SuperGen, Inc
4140 Dublin Boulevard
Suite 200
Dublin, CA 94568
(925) 560-0100
www.supergen.com

Superior Pharmaceutical Company
1385 Kemper Meadow Drive
Cincinnati, OH 45240-1635
(800) 826-5035
www.superiorpharm.com

Swiss-American Products, Inc
4641 Nall Road
Dallas, TX 75244
(800) 633-8872
www.elta.net

Syncor
(see Cardinal Health, Inc)

Syntex Laboratories (see Roche Pharmaceuticals)

Takeda Pharmaceuticals North America, Inc
475 Half Day Road
Lincolnshire, IL 60069
(847) 383-3000
www.tpna.com

Tanox, Inc
10301 Stella Link
Houston, TX 77025-5445
(713) 578-4000
www.tanox.com

TAP Pharmaceutical Products, Inc
675 North Field Drive
Lake Forest, IL 60045
(847) 348-2779
www.tap.com

Targeted Genetics Corp
1100 Olive Way
Suite 100
Seattle, WA 98101
(206) 623-7612
www.targen.com

Taro Pharmaceuticals USA, Inc
5 Skyline Drive
Hawthorne, NY 10532
(914) 345-9001
www.tarousa.com

Tec Laboratories, Inc
7100 Tec Labs Way Southwest
Albany, OR 97321
(800) 482-4464
www.teclabsinc.com

Telluride Pharmaceuticals Corp
300 Valley Road
Hillsborough, NJ 08844-4656
(908) 369-1800
www.tellpharm.com

Teva Pharmaceuticals USA
1090 Horsham Road
PO Box 1090
North Wales, PA 19454-1090
(215) 591-3000
www.tevapharmusa.com

The Medicines Company
One Cambridge Center
Cambridge, MA 02142
(617) 225-9099
www.angiomax.com

Therasense
1360 South Loop Road
Alameda, CA 94502
(510) 748-5400
www.therasense.com

Tishcon Corp
30 New York Avenue
Westbury, NY 11590-5910
(516) 333-0829
www.tishcon.com

Tom's of Maine, Inc
302 LaFayette Center
PO Box 710
Kennebunk, ME 04043
(800) 367-8667
www.tomsofmaine.com

Triton Consumer Products, Inc
561 West Golf Road
Arlington Heights, IL 60005-3904
(800) 942-2009
www.tritonconsumerproducts.com

Tweezerman
55 Sea Cliff Avenue
Glen Cove, NY 11542-3695
(800) 645-3340
www.tweezerman.com

TwinLab Corporation
150 Motor Parkway
Suite 210
Hauppauge, NY 11788
(800) 645-5626
www.twinlab.com

UAD Laboratories, Inc
(see Forest Laboratories, Inc)

UCB Pharmaceuticals, Inc
1950 Lake Park Drive
Smyrna, GA 30080
(770) 970-7500
www.ucb-pharma.com

UDL Laboratories, Inc
1718 Northrock Court
Rockford, IL 61103
(800) 848-0462
www.udllabs.com

Unimed Pharmaceuticals
(see Solvay Pharmaceuticals)

Unipath Diagnostics, Inc
51 Sawyer Road
Suite 200
Waltham, MA 02453
(781) 647-3900
www.unipath.com

United Guardian Laboratories
230 Marcus Boulevard
Hauppauge, NY 11788
(800) 645-5566
www.u-g.com

Upjohn (see Pharmacia & Upjohn Company)

Upsher-Smith Laboratories
6701 Evenstad Drive
Maple Grove, MN 55369
(800) 654-2299
www.upsher-smith.com

UroCor, Inc
800 Research Parkway
Oklahoma City, OK 73104
(800) 634-9330
www.urocor.com

Urologix
14405 21st Avenue North
Minneapolis, MN 55447
(800) 475-1403
www.urologix.com

USA Nutritionals, Inc
513 Commack Road
Deerpark, NY 11729
(631) 643-0600
www.USANutritionals.com

US DenTek
307 Excellence Way
Maryville, TN 37801
(800) 433-6835
www.usdentek.com

US Surgical Corp
150 Glover Avenue
Norwalk, CT 06856
(800) 722-8772
www.ussurg.com

Valeant Pharmaceuticals
Valeant Plaza
3300 Hyland Avenue
Costa Mesa, CA 92626
(800) 548-5100
www.valeant.com

Value in Pharmaceuticals
3000 Alt Boulevard
Grand Island, NY 14072
(800) 724-3784
www.vippharm.com

Vertex Pharmaceuticals, Inc
130 Waverly Street
Cambridge, MA 02139
(617) 444-6100
www.vpharm.com

VHA, Inc
220 East Las Colinas Boulevard
Irving, TX 75039
(972) 830-0000
www.vha.com

Vicks Health Care Products
(see Procter & Gamble Pharmaceuticals, Inc)

Vicks Pharmacy Products
(see Procter & Gamble Pharmaceuticals, Inc)

VISION Pharmaceuticals, Inc
1022 North Main Street
PO Box 400
Mitchell, SD 57301
(800) 325-6789
www.visionpharm.com

VistaPharm
2224 Cahaba Valley Drive
Suite B3
Birmingham, AL 35242
(205) 981-1387
www.vistapharm.com

Vitaline Corp
9775 Southwest Circle C5
Wilsonville, OR 97070
(800) 931-1709
www.vitaline.com

Vitamin Research Products
3579 Highway 50 East
Carson City, NV 89701
(800) 877-2447
www.vrp.com

Vivus, Inc
1172 Castro Street
Mountain View, CA 94040
(650) 934-5200
www.vivus.com

Walgreen Company
200 Wilmont Road
Dearfield, IL 60015
(847) 940-2500
www.walgreens.com

Wallace Pharmaceuticals
265 Davidson Avenue
Suite 300
PO Box 6833
Somerset, NJ 08875-6833
(732) 564-2200

Wal-Mart Stores, Inc
702 Southwest 8th Street
Bentonville, AR 72716
(501) 273-4000
www.wal-mart.com

Wampole Laboratories
2 Research Way
Princeton, NJ 08540
(800) 257-9525
www.wampolelabs.com

Warner Chilcott Laboratories
100 Enterprise Drive
Rockaway, NJ 07866
(973) 442-3200
www.warnerchilcott.com

Watson Laboratories, Inc
311 Bonnie Circle
Corona, CA 92880
(800) 272-5525
www.watsonpharm.com

Westwood-Squibb Pharmaceuticals
(Bristol-Myers Squibb)
100 Forest Avenue
Buffalo, NY 14213
(800) 333-0950

W. F. Young, Inc
PO Box 1990
East Longmeadow, MA 01028-5990
(800) 628-9653
www.absorbine.com

Whitehall-Robins Healthcare
(see Wyeth Pharmaceuticals)

Winthrop Pharmaceuticals
(see Sanofi-Synthelabo, Inc)

Wisconsin Pharmacal Company
(WPC Brands)
1 Pharmacal Way
Jackson, WI 53037
(800) 558-6614
www.pharmacalway.com

Wm. Wrigley Jr Company
410 North Michigan Avenue
Chicago, IL 60611
(312) 644-2121
www.wrigley.com

Women First Healthcare, Inc
5355 Mira Sorrento Place
Suite 700
San Diego, CA 92121
(858) 509-1171
www.womenfirst.com

Woodward Laboratories, Inc
11132 Winners Circle
Los Alamitos, CA 90720
(800) 780-6999
www.woodwardlabs.com

Wyeth Pharmaceuticals
5 Giralda Farms
Madison, NJ 07940
www.wyeth.com

Xoma
2910 7th Street
Berkeley, CA 94710
(800) 246-9662
www.xoma.com

Xttrium Laboratories, Inc
415 West Pershing Road
Chicago, IL 60609
(877) 988-2721
www.adultrashcreme.com

Young Dental Manufacturing
13705 Shoreline Court East
Earth City, MO 63045
(800) 325-1881
www.youngdental.com

Zanfel Laboratories, Inc
Morton, IL 61550
(800) 401-4002
www.zanfel.com

Zeneca Pharmaceuticals
(see AstraZeneca Pharmaceuticals, LP)

Zenith Goldline Pharmaceuticals
4400 Biscayne Boulevard
Miami, FL 33137-3227
(305) 575-6000
www.zenithgoldline.com

Zila Pharmaceuticals, Inc
5227 North 7th Street
Phoenix, AZ 85014-2800
(602) 266-6700
www.zila.com

ZLB Behring
1020 First Avenue
PO Box 61501
King of Prussia, PA 19406
(610) 878-4155
www.zlbbehring.com

Zonagen, Inc
2408 Timberloch Place, B-1
The Woodlands, TX 77380
(281) 719-3400
www.zonagen.com

ZymeTx, Inc
655 Research Parkway
Suite 554
Oklahoma City, OK 73104
(888) 817-1314
www.zymetx.com

ZymoGenetics, Inc
1201 Eastlake Avenue East
Seattle, WA 98102-3702
(206) 442-6600
www.zymogenetics.com

INDICATION / THERAPEUTIC CATEGORY INDEX

ABDOMINAL DISTENTION (POSTOPERATIVE)

Hormone, Posterior Pituitary

ABETALIPOPROTEINEMIA

Vitamin, Fat Soluble

ABORTION

Antiprogestin

Oxytocic Agent

Prostaglandin

ACETAMINOPHEN POISONING

Mucolytic Agent

ACHALASIA

Adrenergic Agonist Agent

Calcium Channel Blocker

Vasodilator

ACHLORHYDRIA

Gastrointestinal Agent, Miscellaneous

ACIDOSIS (METABOLIC)

Alkalinizing Agent

Electrolyte Supplement, Oral

ACNE

Acne Products

Antibiotic, Topical

Antiseborrheic Agent, Topical

Estrogen and Androgen Combination

Keratolytic Agent

Retinoic Acid Derivative

Tetracycline Derivative

ANESTHESIA (GENERAL)

Barbiturate

General Anesthetic

ANESTHESIA (LOCAL)

Local Anesthetic

BERIBERI

Vitamin, Water Soluble

BIPOLAR DEPRESSION DISORDER

Anticonvulsant

Antimanic Agent

Antipsychotic Agent

BIRTH CONTROL

Contraceptive

Contraceptive, Implant (Progestin)

Contraceptive, Oral

Antifungal Agent, Systemic

Antifungal/Corticosteroid

CANKER SORE

Antiinfective Agent, Oral

Antiinflammatory Agent, Locally Applied

Local Anesthetic

Protectant, Topical

CARCINOMA

Androgen

Antiandrogen

Antineoplastic Agent

CONGESTION (NASAL)

Adrenergic Agonist Agent

Antihistamine

Antihistamine/Decongestant/Anticholinergic

Antihistamine/Decongestant/Antitussive

Antihistamine/Decongestant Combination

Antitussive/Decongestant

Antitussive/Decongestant/Expectorant

Cold Preparation

Decongestant/Analgesic

Laxative, Stimulant

Stool Softener

CONTRACEPTION

Contraceptive

Contraceptive, Implant (Progestin)

Contraceptive, Oral

Contraceptive, Progestin Only

Estrogen and Progestin Combination

Spermicide

COPROPORPHYRIA

Beta-Adrenergic Blocker

CORNEAL EDEMA

Lubricant, Ocular

COUGH

Antihistamine

Antihistamine/Antitussive

Antihistamine/Decongestant/Antitussive

Antihistamine/Decongestant Combination

Antitussive

Antitussive/Decongestant

Antitussive/Decongestant/Expectorant

DANDRUFF

Antiseborrheic Agent, Topical

DEBRIDEMENT OF CALLOUS TISSUE

Keratolytic Agent

DEBRIDEMENT OF ESCHAR

Protectant, Topical

DECUBITUS ULCERS

Enzyme

Enzyme, Topical Debridement

Protectant, Topical

Topical Skin Product

DEEP VEIN THROMBOSIS (DVT)

Anticoagulant (Other)

Factor Xa Inhibitor

Low Molecular Weight Heparin

DEMENTIA

Acetylcholinesterase Inhibitor

Antidepressant, Tricyclic (Tertiary Amine)

Benzodiazepine

Ergot Alkaloid and Derivative

DENTAL CARIES (PREVENTION)

Mineral, Oral

DERMATOSIS

Anesthetic/Corticosteroid

Antibiotic, Topical

Corticosteroid, Topical

DRY MOUTH

Gastrointestinal Agent, Miscellaneous

DRY SKIN

Topical Skin Product

Vitamin, Topical

DUCTUS ARTERIOSUS (CLOSURE)

Nonsteroidal Antiinflammatory Drug (NSAID)

DUCTUS ARTERIOSUS (TEMPORARY MAINTENANCE OF PATENCY)

Prostaglandin

DUODENAL ULCER

Antacid

Antibiotic, Macrolide Combination

Antibiotic, Penicillin

Gastric Acid Secretion Inhibitor

Gastrointestinal Agent, Gastric or Duodenal Ulcer Treatment

Gastrointestinal Agent, Miscellaneous

EDEMA

Antihypertensive Agent, Combination

Diuretic, Combination

Diuretic, Loop

Diuretic, Miscellaneous

Contraceptive, Progestin Only

Hormone, Posterior Pituitary

Progestin

ENURESIS

Anticholinergic Agent

Antidepressant, Tricyclic (Tertiary Amine)

Antispasmodic Agent, Urinary

Vasopressin Analog, Synthetic

EPICONDYLITIS

Nonsteroidal Antiinflammatory Drug (NSAID)

EYE IRRITATION

Adrenergic Agonist Agent

Ophthalmic Agent, Miscellaneous

EYELID INFECTION

Antibiotic, Ophthalmic

Pharmaceutical Aid

FABRY DISEASE

Enzyme

FACTOR IX DEFICIENCY

Antihemophilic Agent

FACTOR VIII DEFICIENCY

Blood Product Derivative

Uricosuric Agent

Xanthine Oxidase Inhibitor

GRAFT VS HOST DISEASE

Immunosuppressant Agent

GRAM-NEGATIVE INFECTION

Aminoglycoside (Antibiotic)

Antibiotic, Carbapenem

Antibiotic, Miscellaneous

Antibiotic, Penicillin

Antibiotic, Quinolone

Carbapenem (Antibiotic)

Cephalosporin (First Generation)

Cephalosporin (Second Generation)

Antihistamine/Decongestant Combination

HEADACHE (SINUS)

Analgesic, Nonnarcotic

Antihistamine/Analgesic

Antihistamine/Decongestant/Analgesic

Cold Preparation

Decongestant/Analgesic

HYPERPLASIA, VULVAR SQUAMOUS

Estrogen Derivative

HYPERPROLACTINEMIA

Ergot Alkaloid and Derivative

Ergot-like Derivative

HYPERTENSION

Adrenergic Agonist Agent

Alpha-Adrenergic Agonist

Alpha-Adrenergic Blocking Agent

Alpha-/Beta- Adrenergic Blocker

Angiotensin-Converting Enzyme (ACE) Inhibitor

Angiotensin II Antagonist Combination

Angiotensin II Receptor Antagonist

Antihypertensive Agent

Antihypertensive Agent, Combination

Beta-Adrenergic Blocker

Calcium Channel Blocker

Diuretic, Combination

Diuretic, Loop

Diuretic, Miscellaneous

Diuretic, Potassium Sparing

Diuretic, Thiazide

Ganglionic Blocking Agent

Miscellaneous Product

HYPOMAGNESEMIA

Electrolyte Supplement, Oral

HYPOMOBILITY

Anti-Parkinson Agent (Dopamine Agonist)

HYPONATREMIA

Electrolyte Supplement, Oral

HYPOPARATHYROIDISM

Diagnostic Agent

Vitamin D Analog

HYPOPHOSPHATEMIA

Electrolyte Supplement, Oral

Vitamin D Analog

MYDRIASIS

Adrenergic Agonist Agent

Anticholinergic/Adrenergic Agonist

Anticholinergic Agent

MYELODYSPLASTIC SYNDROME (MDS)

Antineoplastic Agent, Antimetabolite (Pyrimidine)

MYELOMA

Antineoplastic Agent

Proteasome Inhibitor

MYOCARDIAL INFARCTION

Anticoagulant (Other)

Antilipemic Agent, HMG-CoA Reductase Inhibitor

Antiplatelet Agent

Beta-Adrenergic Blocker

Nonsteroidal Antiinflammatory Drug (NSAID), COX-2 Selective

Prostaglandin

OSTEODYSTROPHY

Vitamin D Analog

OSTEOMALACIA

Vitamin D Analog

OSTEOMYELITIS

Antibiotic, Miscellaneous

Antifungal Agent, Systemic

Carbapenem (Antibiotic)

Otic Agent, Analgesic

Otic Agent, Antiinfective

Quinolone

OTITIS MEDIA

Antibiotic, Carbacephem

Antibiotic/Corticosteroid, Otic

Antibiotic, Miscellaneous

Antibiotic, Otic

Antibiotic, Penicillin

Cephalosporin (First Generation)

Cephalosporin (Second Generation)

Cephalosporin (Third Generation)

Macrolide (Antibiotic)

Ovulation Stimulator

PAGET DISEASE OF BONE

Bisphosphonate Derivative

Polypeptide Hormone

PAIN

Analgesic, Miscellaneous

Analgesic, Narcotic

Analgesic, Nonnarcotic

PENICILLIN HYPERSENSITIVITY (DIAGNOSTIC)

Diagnostic Agent

PEPTIC ULCER

Antibiotic, Miscellaneous

Anticholinergic Agent

Antidiarrheal

Gastric Acid Secretion Inhibitor

Gastrointestinal Agent, Gastric or Duodenal Ulcer Treatment

Histamine H_2 Antagonist

Macrolide (Antibiotic)

Penicillin

PERCUTANEOUS TRANSLUMINAL CORONARY ANGIOPLASTY (PTCA)

Anticoagulant (Other)

PERIANAL WART

Immune Response Modifier

PERIPHERAL VASCULAR DISEASE

Vasodilator, Peripheral

PERTUSSIS

Toxoid

Vaccine, Inactivated Bacteria

PHARYNGITIS

Antibiotic, Penicillin

Cephalosporin (First Generation)

Cephalosporin (Second Generation)

Cephalosporin (Third Generation)

Macrolide (Antibiotic)

Penicillin

Tetracycline Derivative

PLAGUE

Antibiotic, Aminoglycoside

Antitubercular Agent

Vaccine, Inactivated Bacteria

PLANTARIS

Keratolytic Agent

PLANTAR WARTS

Keratolytic Agent

Topical Skin Product

PLATELET AGGREGATION (PROPHYLAXIS)

Antiplatelet Agent

PNEUMOCYSTIS CARINII

Antibiotic, Miscellaneous

Antiprotozoal

Sulfonamide

Sulfone

PNEUMONIA

Aminoglycoside (Antibiotic)

Contraceptive, Progestin Only

Estrogen and Progestin Combination

Spermicide

PREMATURE LUTEINIZING HORMONE (LH) SURGES

Antigonadotropic Agent

PREMENSTRUAL DYSPHORIC DISORDER (PMDD)

Antidepressant, Selective Serotonin Reuptake Inhibitor

PREOPERATIVE SEDATION

Analgesic, Narcotic

Antihistamine

Barbiturate

Benzodiazepine

General Anesthetic

PSEUDOHYPOPARATHYROIDISM

Vitamin D Analog

PSORIASIS

Antineoplastic Agent

Antipsoriatic Agent

Corticosteroid, Topical

Immunosuppressant Agent

Keratolytic Agent

Monoclonal Antibody

Psoralen

Retinoid-like Compound

Vitamin D Analog

PSYCHOSES

Antipsychotic Agent

Antipsychotic Agent, Benzisoxazole

Antipsychotic Agent, Butyrophenone

Antipsychotic Agent, Dibenzoxazepine

Antipsychotic Agent, Dihydroindoline

Phenothiazine Derivative

Thioxanthene Derivative

PUBERTY (DELAYED)

Androgen

Diagnostic Agent

PUBERTY (PRECOCIOUS)

Hormone, Posterior Pituitary

Luteinizing Hormone-Releasing Hormone Analog

PULMONARY ARTERY HYPERTENSION (PAH)

Endothelin Antagonist

Vasodilator

PULMONARY EMBOLISM

Anticoagulant (Other)

Fibrinolytic Agent

Low Molecular Weight Heparin

RESPIRATORY DISTRESS SYNDROME (RDS)

Lung Surfactant

RESPIRATORY SYNCYTIAL VIRUS (RSV)

Antiviral Agent

Immune Globulin

Monoclonal Antibody

RESPIRATORY TRACT INFECTION

Aminoglycoside (Antibiotic)

Antibiotic, Carbacephem

Antibiotic, Macrolide

Antibiotic, Miscellaneous

Antibiotic, Penicillin

Antibiotic, Quinolone

Cephalosporin (First Generation)

Cephalosporin (Second Generation)

Cephalosporin (Third Generation)

Cephalosporin (Fourth Generation)

Macrolide (Antibiotic)

RHEUMATIC FEVER

Nonsteroidal Antiinflammatory Drug (NSAID)

Penicillin

RHINITIS

Adrenal Corticosteroid

Adrenergic Agonist Agent

Antihistamine

ROUNDWORMS

Anthelmintic

RUBELLA

Vaccine, Live Virus

SALIVATION (EXCESSIVE)

Anticholinergic Agent

SARCOIDOSIS

Corticosteroid, Topical

SCURVY

Vitamin, Water Soluble

SEBORRHEIC DERMATITIS

Antiseborrheic Agent, Topical

Keratolytic Agent

SERUM THYROGLOBULIN (TG) TESTING

Diagnostic Agent

SHOCK

Adrenal Corticosteroid

Cephalosporin (Third Generation)

Cold Preparation

Decongestant/Analgesic

Expectorant/Decongestant

Macrolide (Antibiotic)

Penicillin

UPPER GASTROINTESTINAL MOTILITY DISORDERS

Dopamine Antagonist

UREA CYCLE DISORDER

Miscellaneous Product

URINARY BLADDER SPASM

Anticholinergic Agent

URINARY RETENTION

Antispasmodic Agent, Urinary

Cholinergic Agent

URINARY TRACT INFECTION

Antibiotic, Carbacephem

Antibiotic, Miscellaneous

Antibiotic, Penicillin

Antibiotic, Quinolone

Antibiotic, Urinary Antiinfective

Cephalosporin (First Generation)

Cephalosporin (Second Generation)

Cephalosporin (Third Generation)

Cephalosporin (Fourth Generation)

Genitourinary Irrigant

Irrigating Solution

Penicillin

Quinolone

Sulfonamide

Urinary Tract Product

URTICARIA

Antihistamine

2005

QUICK LOOK DRUG BOOK

Image Guide to Tablets and Capsules

The Quick Look Drug Book 2005 image insert displays actual color photographs of the most commonly prescribed tablets and capsules.

Drugs are listed alphabetically by generic name, and, where applicable, the trade name is listed. Dosages appear under each individual image.

Use the white scale at the bottom of each image to determine the actual size. The distance between each division on the scale is equivalent to 1/8 inch or 3.175 mm.

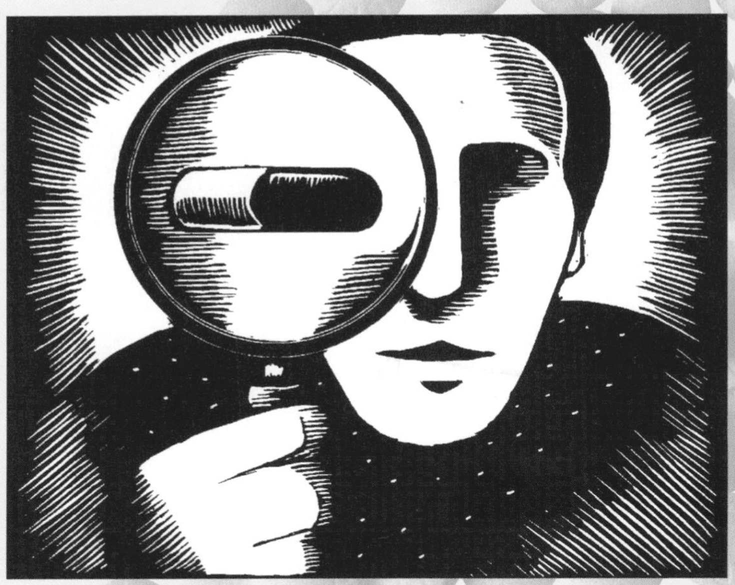

Acetaminophen and Codeine

(generic)

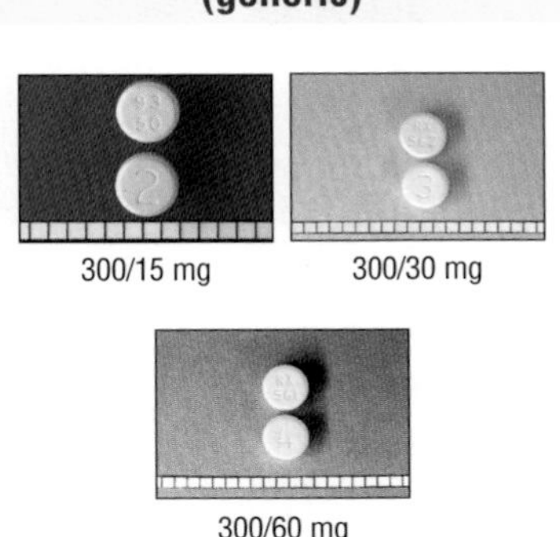

300/15 mg 300/30 mg

300/60 mg

Acetaminophen and Tramadol

Ultracet™

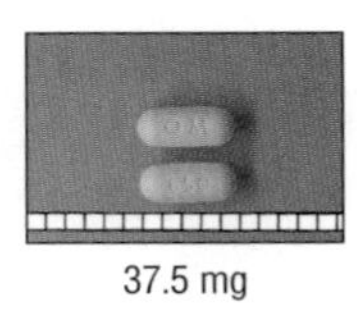

37.5 mg

Alendronate

Fosamax®

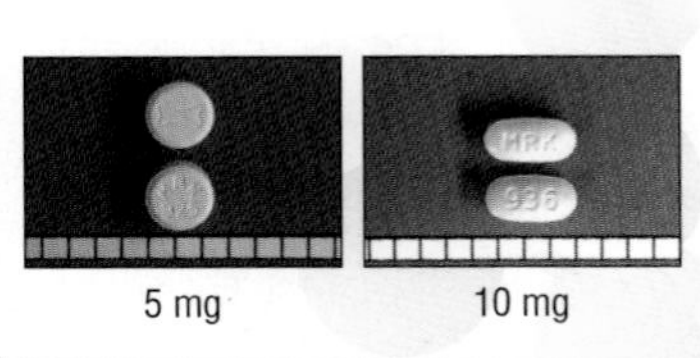

5 mg 10 mg

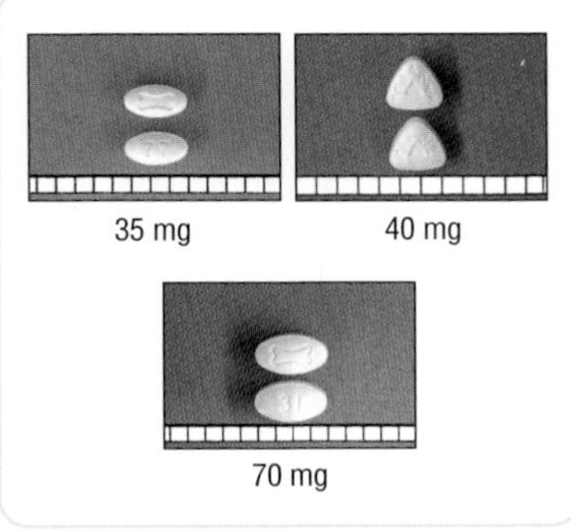

35 mg 40 mg

70 mg

Allopurinol

(generic)

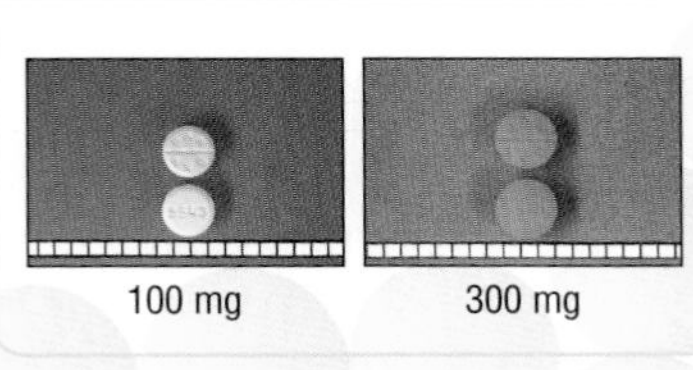

100 mg 300 mg

Alprazolam

(generic)

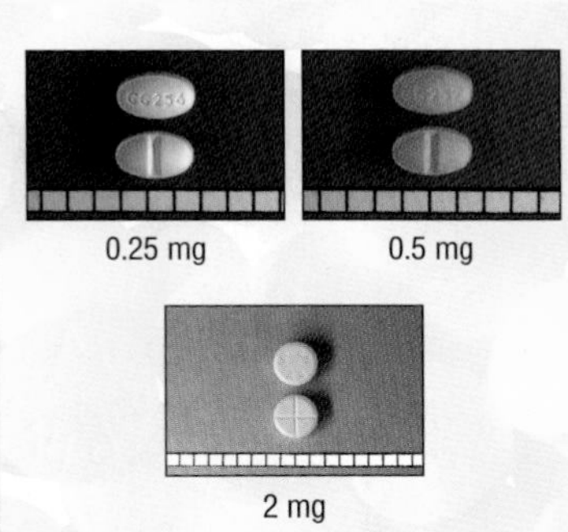

0.25 mg 0.5 mg

2 mg

Xanax®

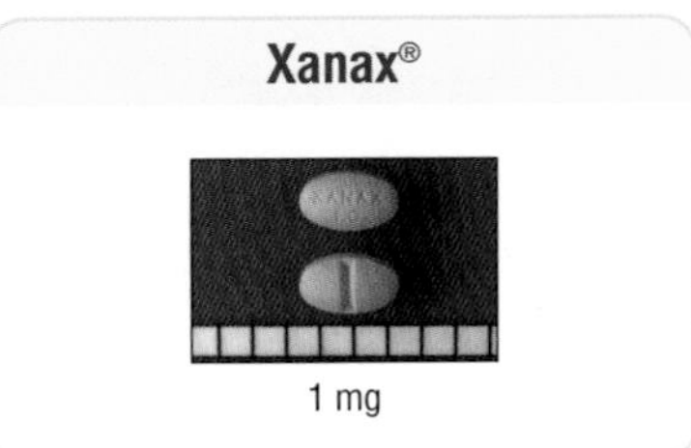

1 mg

Amitriptyline

(generic)

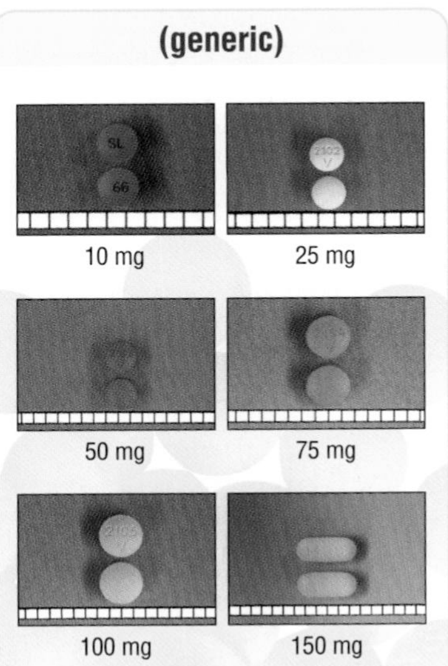

10 mg | 25 mg | 50 mg | 75 mg | 100 mg | 150 mg

Amlodipine

Norvasc®

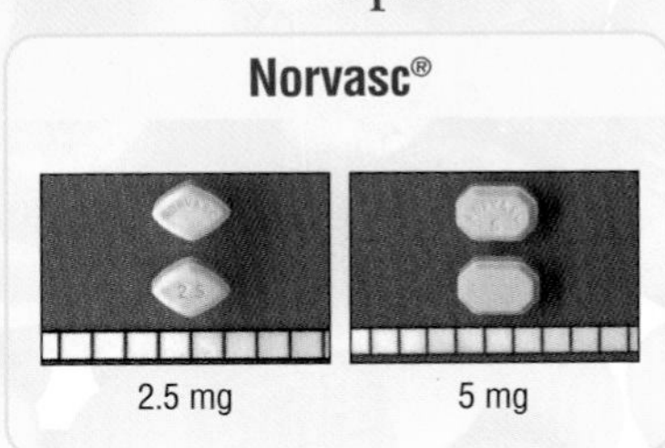

2.5 mg | 5 mg

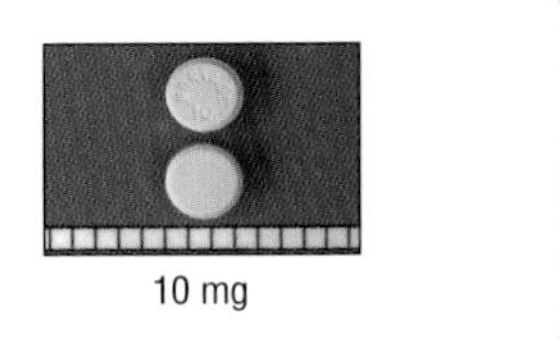

10 mg

Amlodipine and Benzepril

Lotrel®

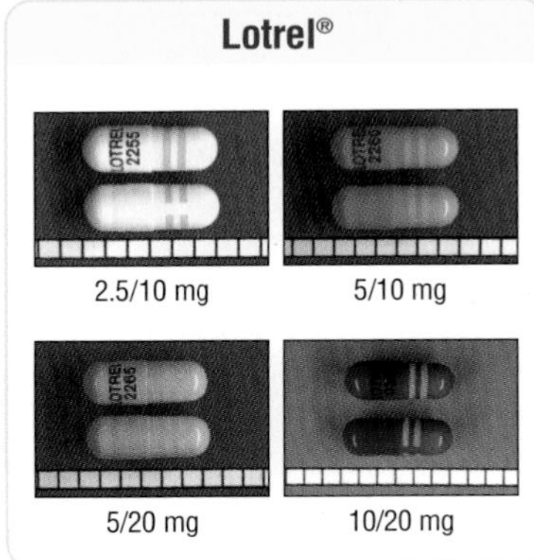

2.5/10 mg | 5/10 mg | 5/20 mg | 10/20 mg

Amoxicillin

(generic)

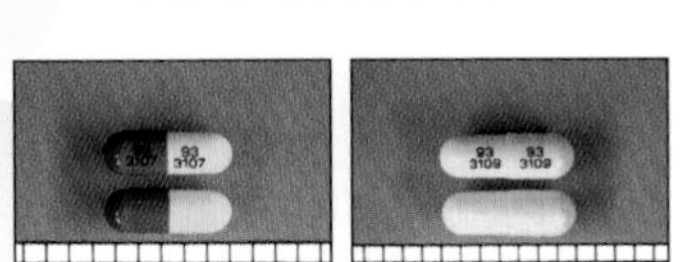

250 mg | 500 mg

Amoxil®

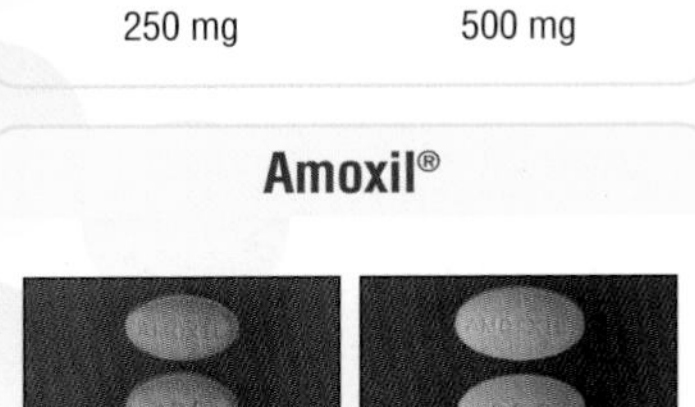

125 mg | 250 mg

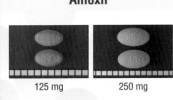

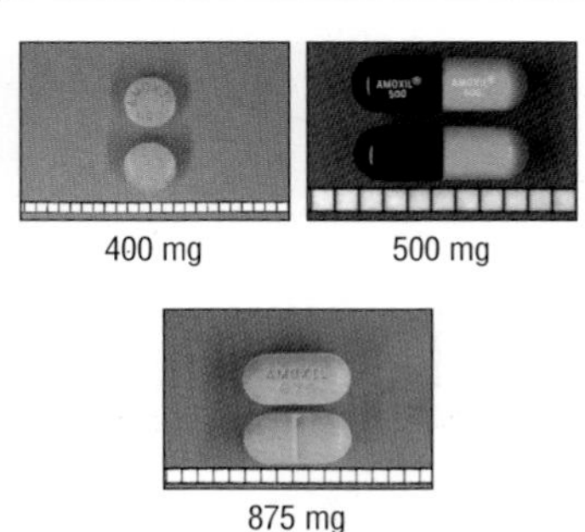

400 mg

500 mg

875 mg

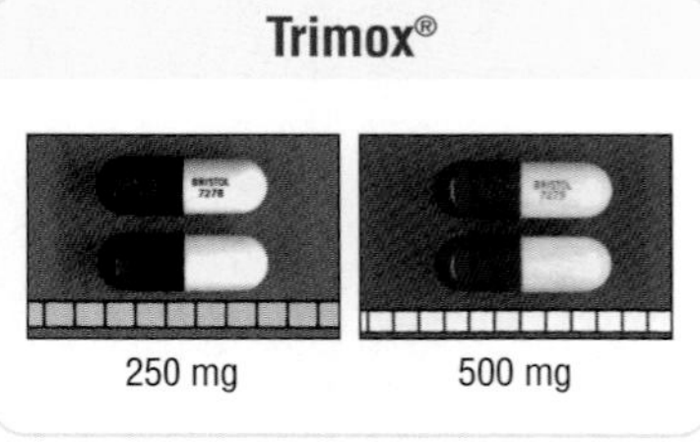

Trimox®

250 mg

500 mg

Amoxicillin and Clavulanate Potassium

(generic)

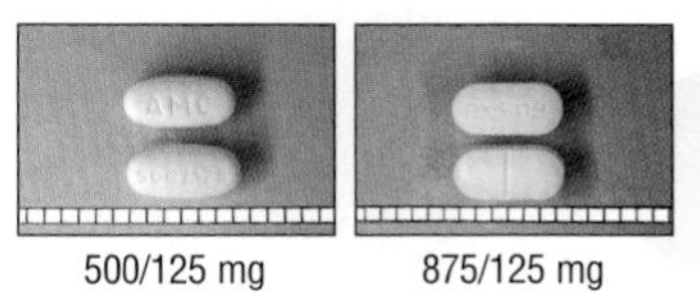

500/125 mg

875/125 mg

Atenolol

(generic)

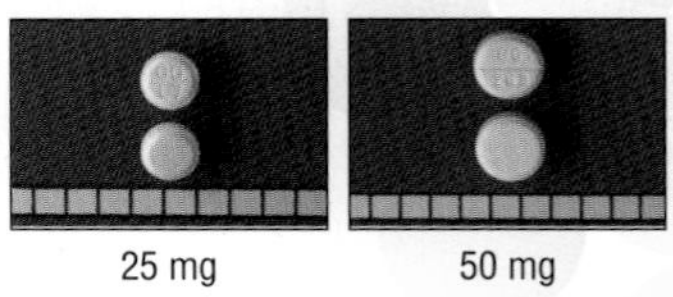

25 mg

50 mg

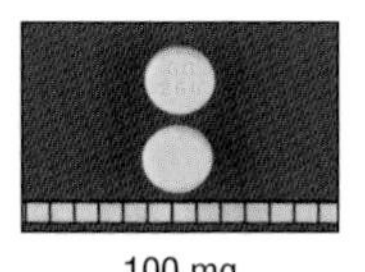

100 mg

Atomoxetine

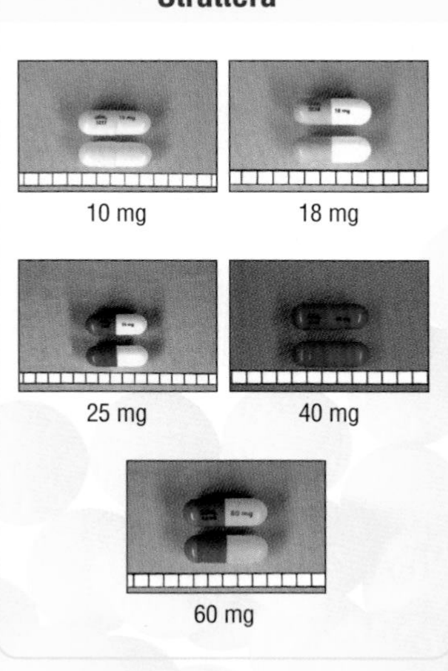

Strattera™

10 mg

18 mg

25 mg

40 mg

60 mg

Atorvastatin

Lipitor®

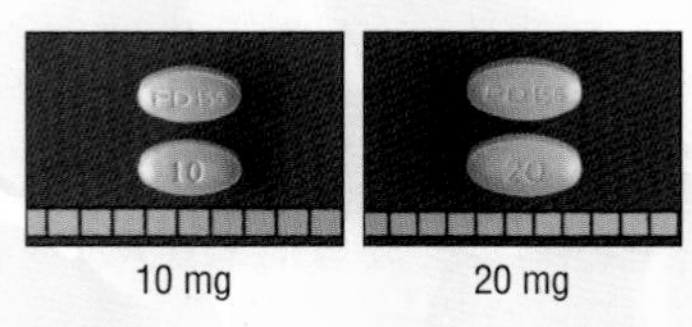

10 mg

20 mg

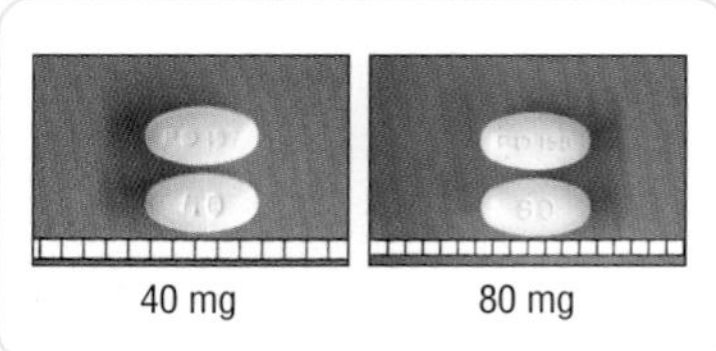

40 mg 80 mg

Azithromycin

Zithromax®

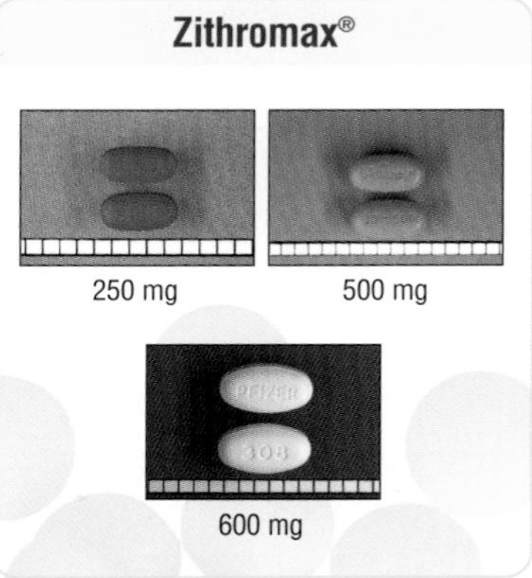

250 mg 500 mg

600 mg

Benazepril

Lotensin®

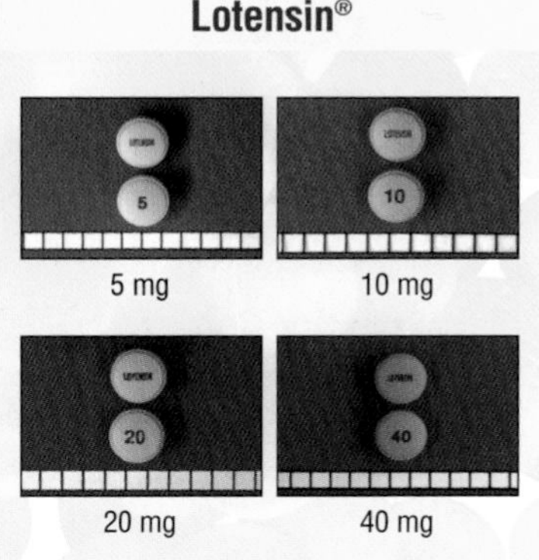

5 mg 10 mg

20 mg 40 mg

Bupropion

Wellbutrin SR®

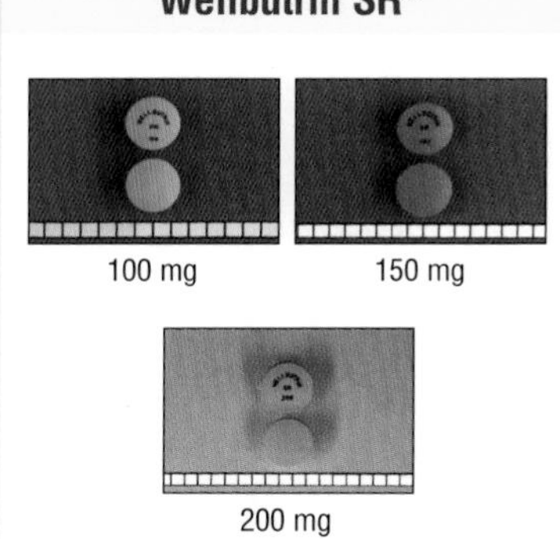

100 mg 150 mg

200 mg

Candesartan

Atacand®

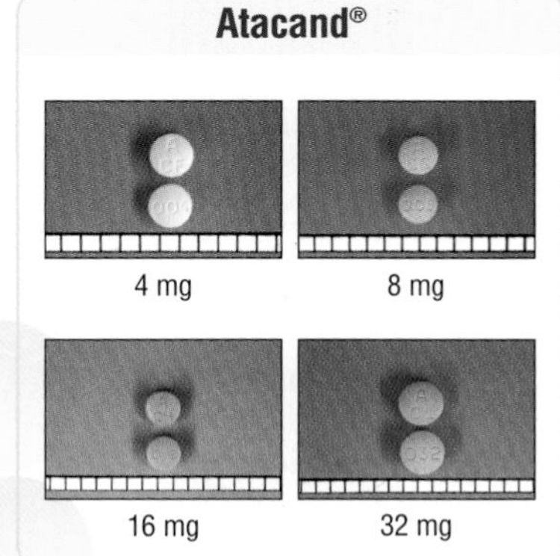

4 mg 8 mg

16 mg 32 mg

Carisoprodol

(generic)

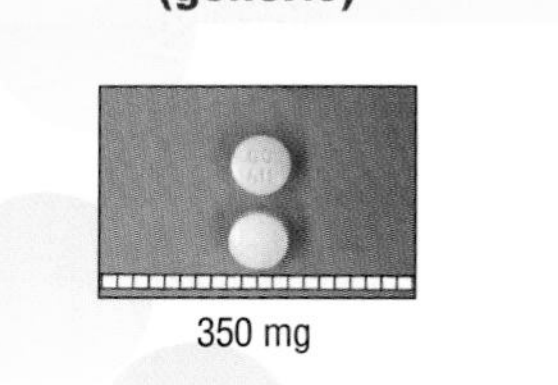

350 mg

Carvedilol

Coreg®

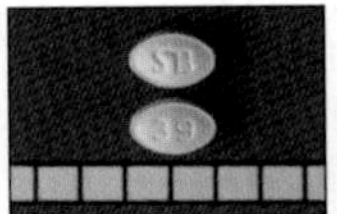

3.125 mg

Coreg Tiltab®

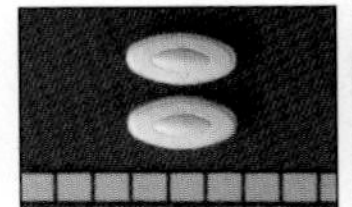

6.25 mg

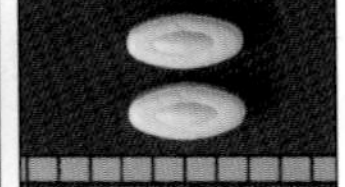

12.5 mg

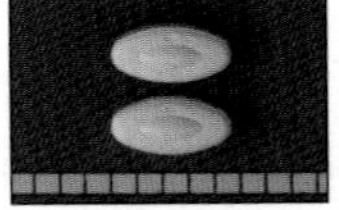

25 mg

Cefdinir

Omnicef®

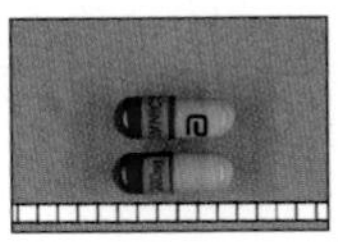

300 mg

Cefprozil

Cefzil®

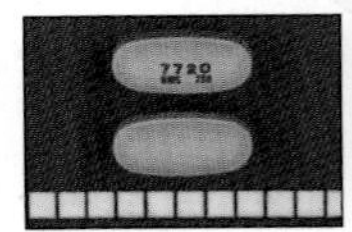

250 mg

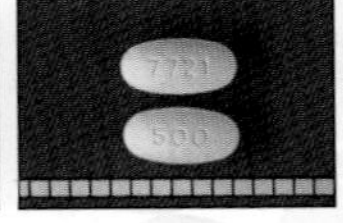

500 mg

Celecoxib

Celebrex™

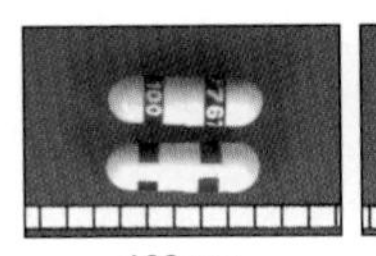

100 mg

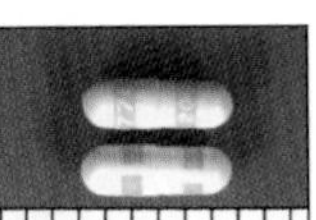

200 mg

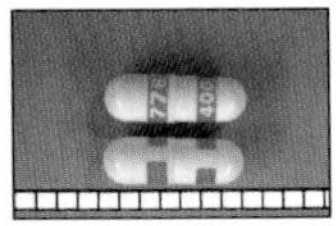

400 mg

Cephalexin

(generic)

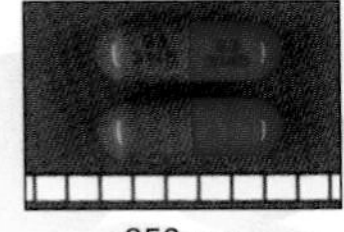

250 mg

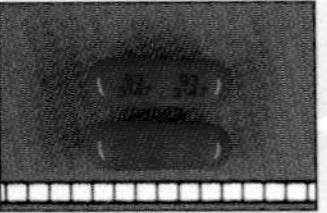

500 mg

Cetirizine

Zyrtec®

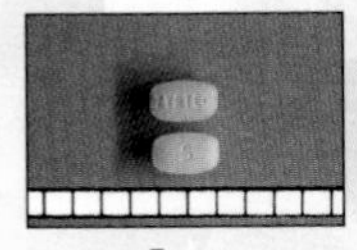

5 mg

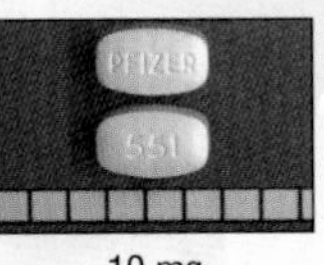

10 mg

Zyrtec–D 12 Hour™

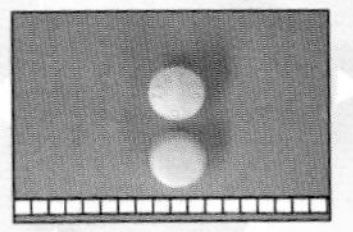

5 mg

Ciprofloxacin

(generic)

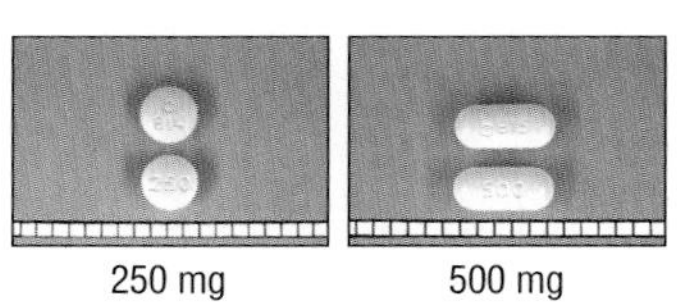
250 mg 500 mg

Cipro®

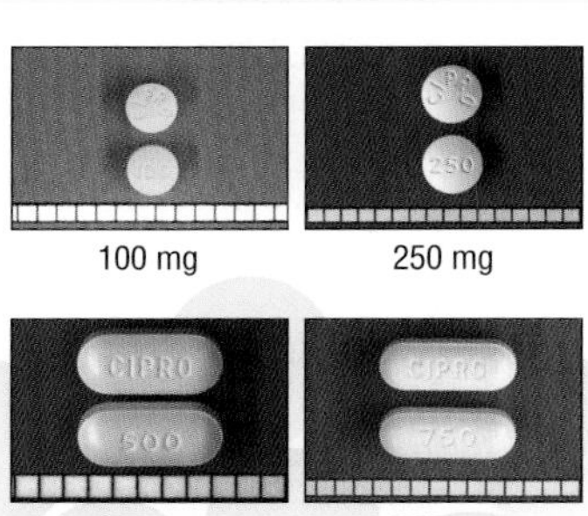
100 mg 250 mg
500 mg 750 mg

Citalopram

Celexa™

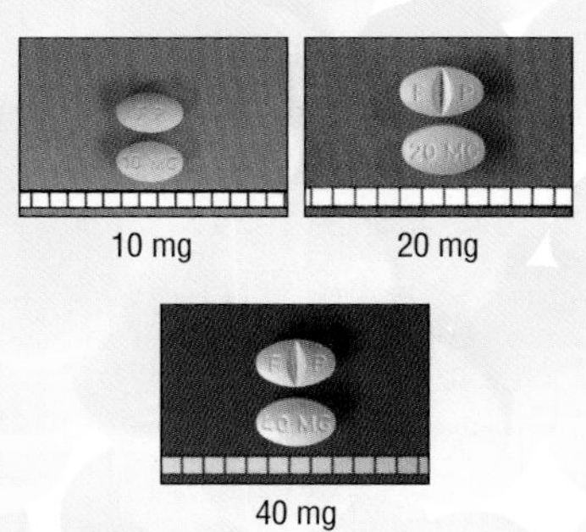
10 mg 20 mg
40 mg

Clarithromycin

Biaxin®

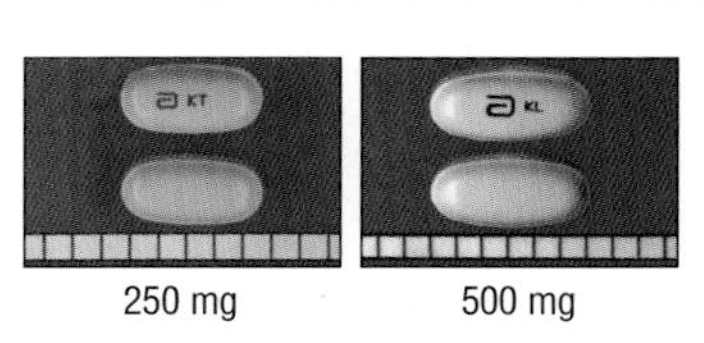
250 mg 500 mg

Biaxin® XL

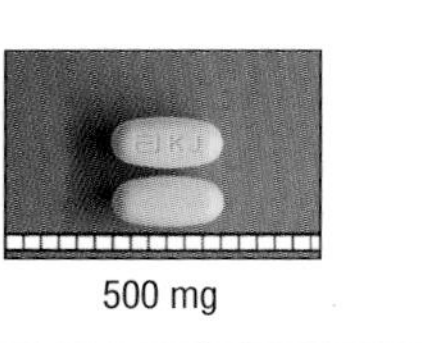
500 mg

Clonazepam

(generic)

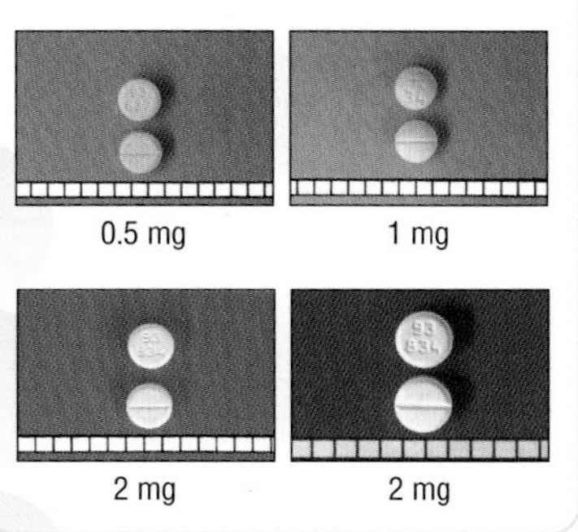
0.5 mg 1 mg
2 mg 2 mg

Clonidine

(generic)

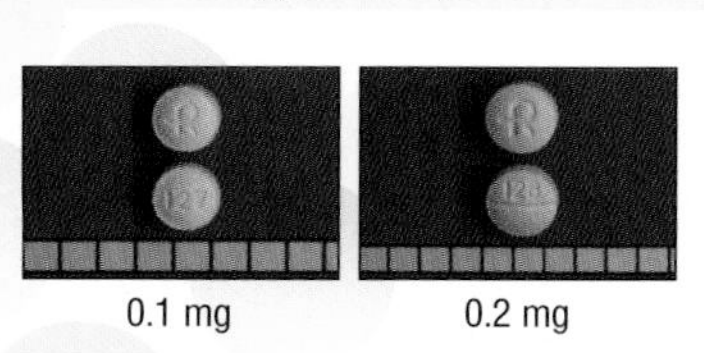
0.1 mg 0.2 mg

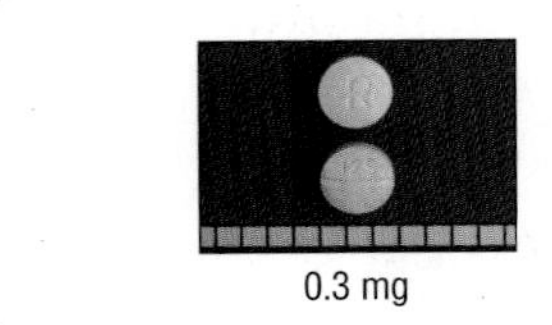

0.3 mg

Clopidogrel

Plavix®

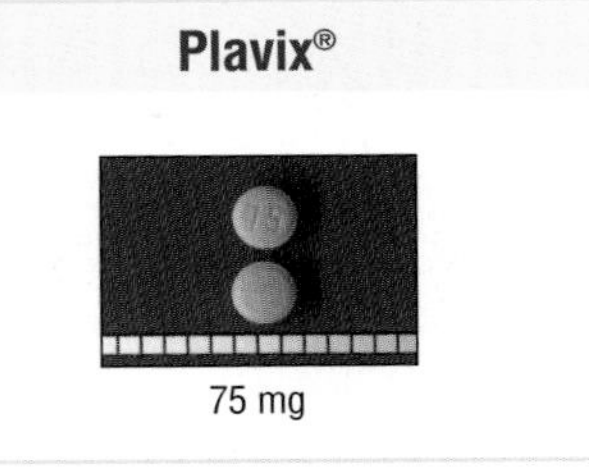

75 mg

Cyclobenzaprine

(generic)

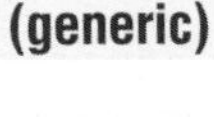

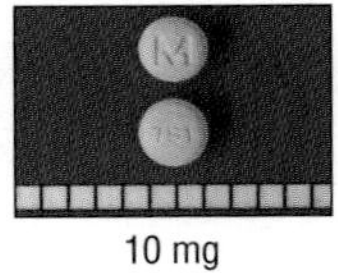

10 mg

Dextroamphetamine and Amphetamine

Adderall XR™

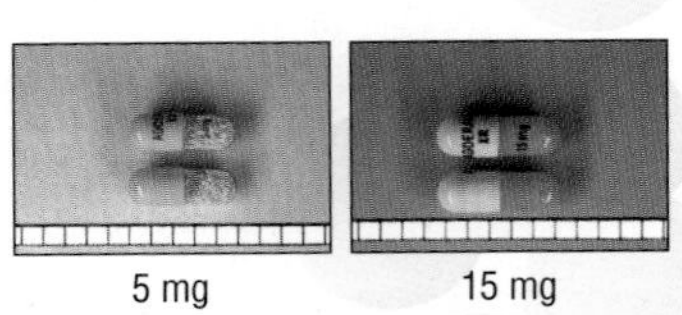

5 mg 15 mg

Diazepam

(generic)

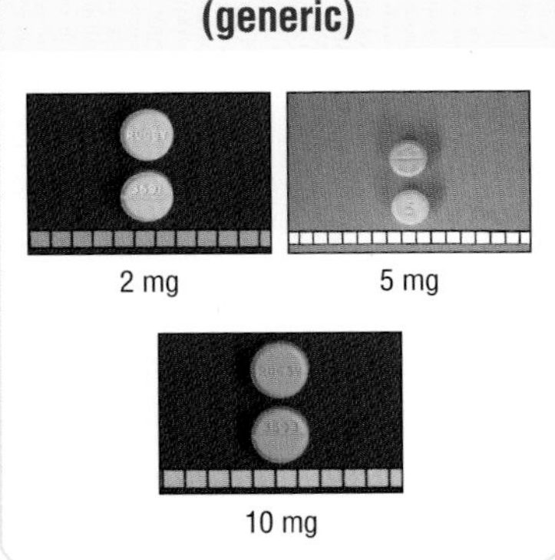

2 mg 5 mg

10 mg

Digoxin

Lanoxin®

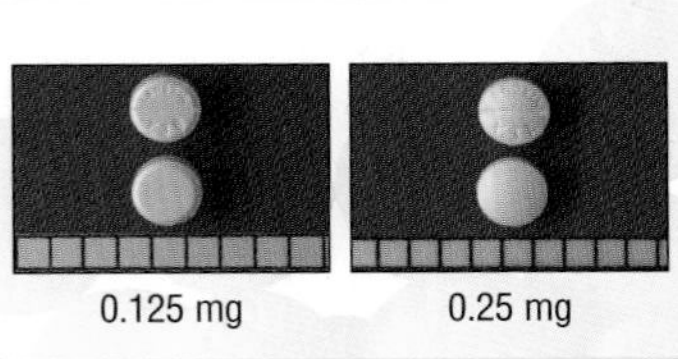

0.125 mg 0.25 mg

Diltiazem

(generic)

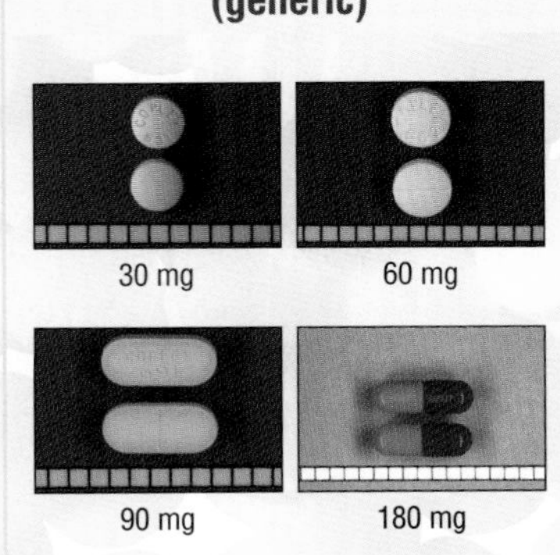

30 mg 60 mg

90 mg 180 mg

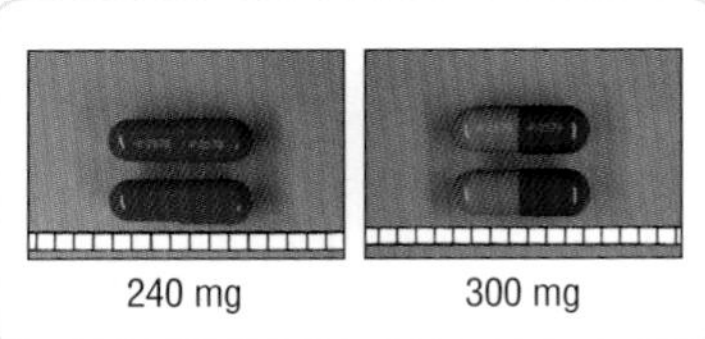

240 mg | 300 mg

Cartia XT™

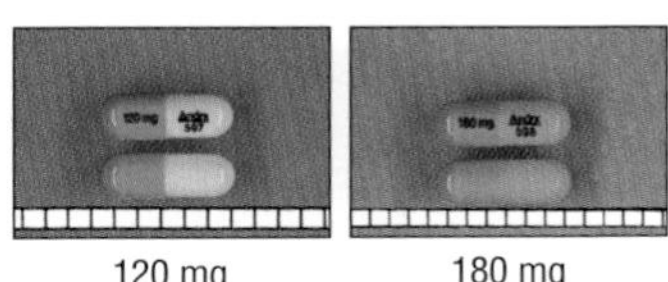

120 mg | 180 mg

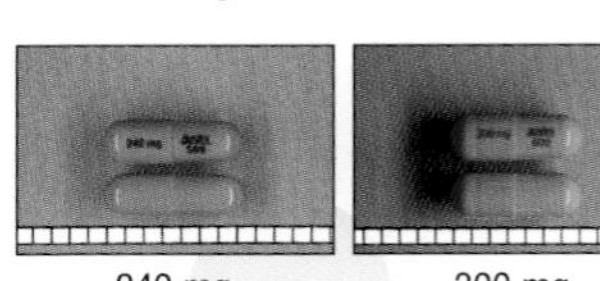

240 mg | 300 mg

Donepezil

Aricept®

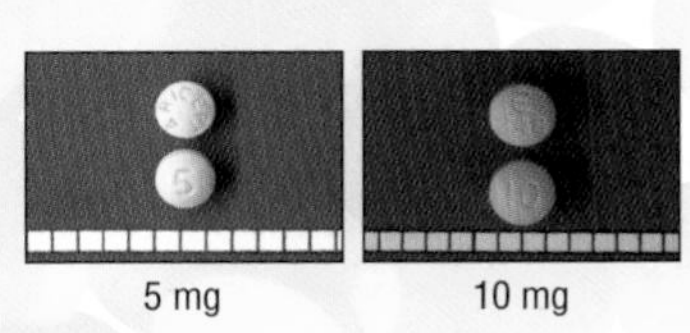

5 mg | 10 mg

Doxycycline

(generic)

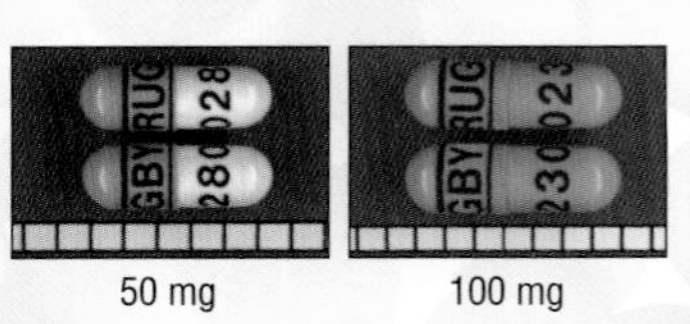

50 mg | 100 mg

Enalapril

(generic)

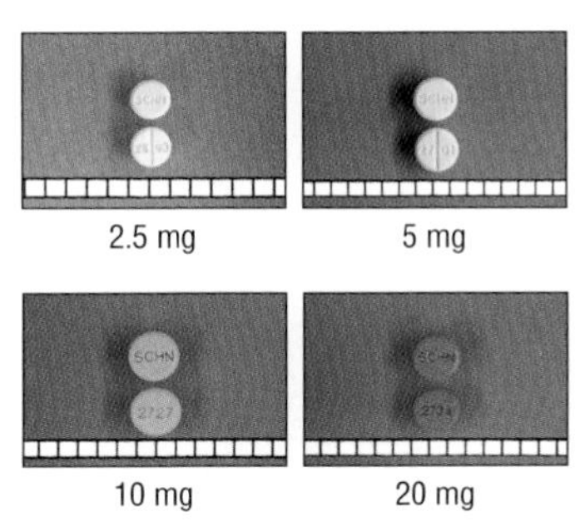

2.5 mg | 5 mg

10 mg | 20 mg

Escitalopram

Lexapro™

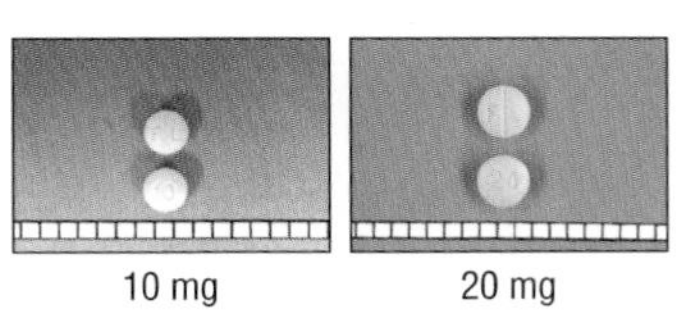

10 mg | 20 mg

Estrogens (Conjugated/Equine)

Premarin®

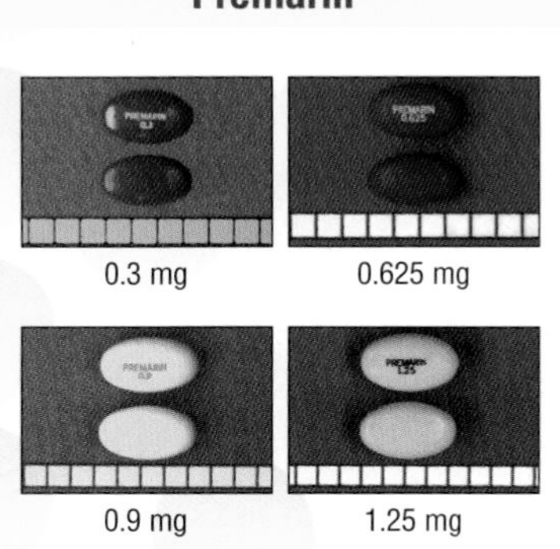

0.3 mg | 0.625 mg

0.9 mg | 1.25 mg

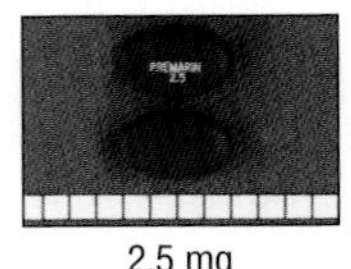

2.5 mg

Estrogens (Conjugated/Equine) and Medroxyprogesterone

Prempro™

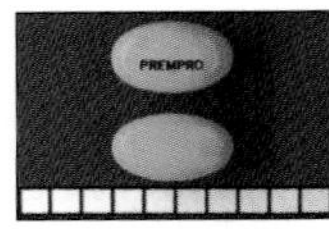

0.625/2.5 mg

Ethinyl Estradiol and Desogestrel

Apri® 28

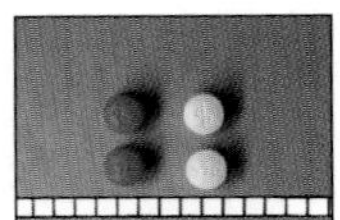
multiple dosages

Kariva™ 28

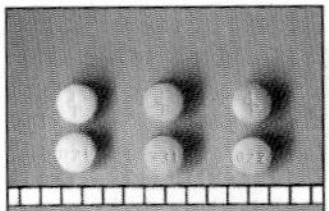
multiple dosages

Ethinyl Estradiol and Drospirenone

Yasmin®

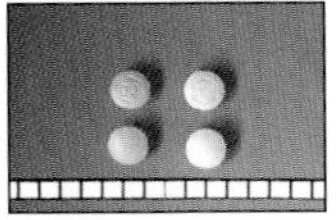
multiple dosages

Ethinyl Estradiol and Norethindrone

Ortho-Novum® 1/35

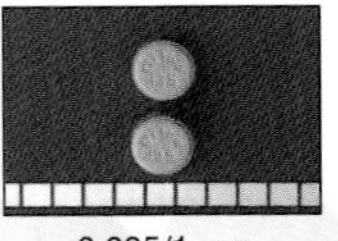
0.035/1 mg

Ortho-Novum® 1/35 28

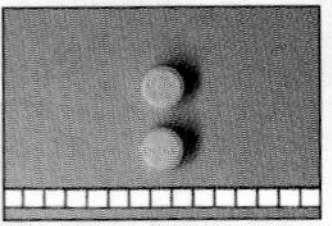
multiple dosages

Ortho-Novum® 7/7/7

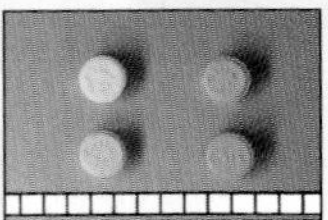
multiple dosages

Ethinyl Estradiol and Norgestimate

Ortho Tri-Cyclen® LO

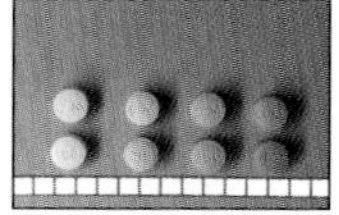

multiple dosages

Ezetimibe

Zetia™

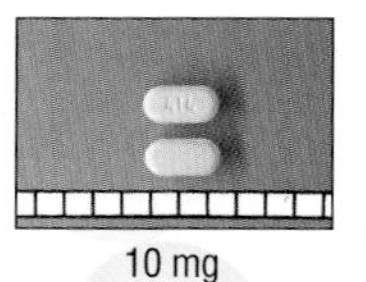

10 mg

Felodipine

Plendil®

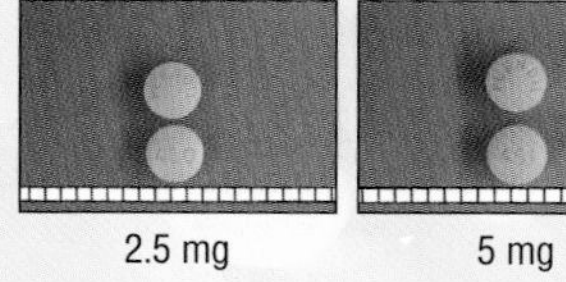

2.5 mg 5 mg

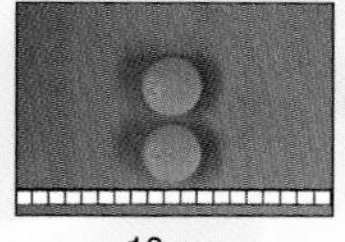

10 mg

Fenofibrate

Tricor®

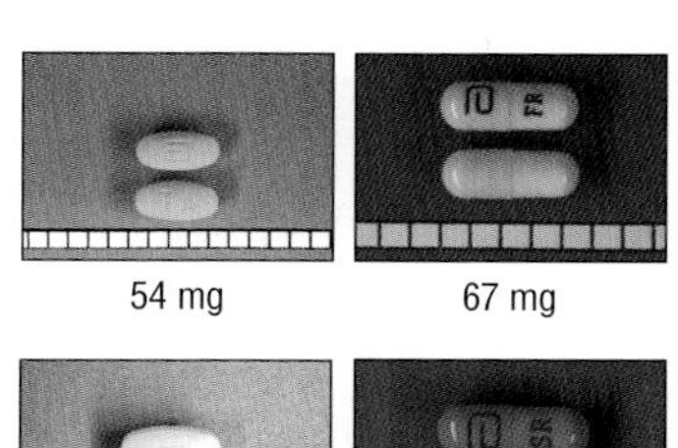

54 mg 67 mg

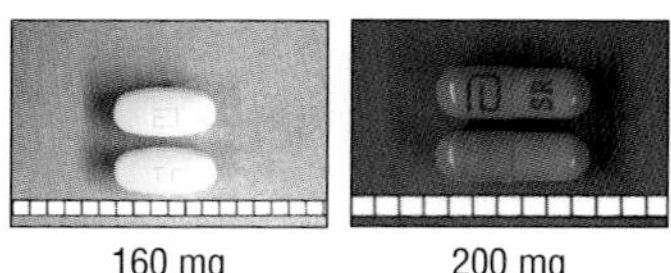

160 mg 200 mg

Fexofenadine

Allegra®

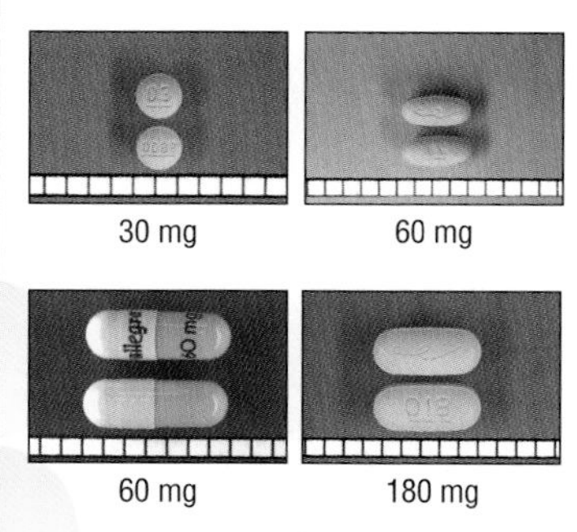

30 mg 60 mg

60 mg 180 mg

Fexofenadine and Pseudoephedrine

Allegra-D®

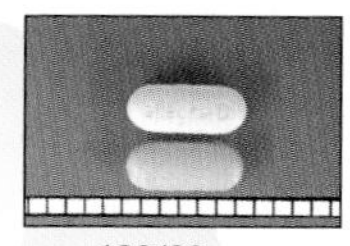

120/60 mg

Finasteride

Proscar®

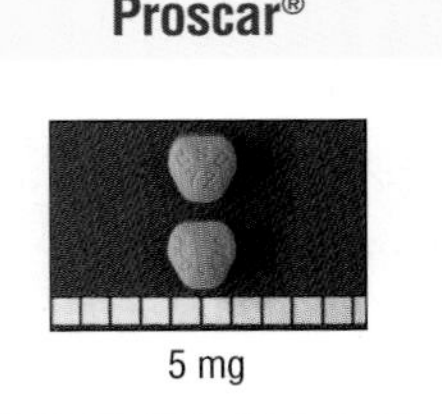

5 mg

Fluconazole

Diflucan®

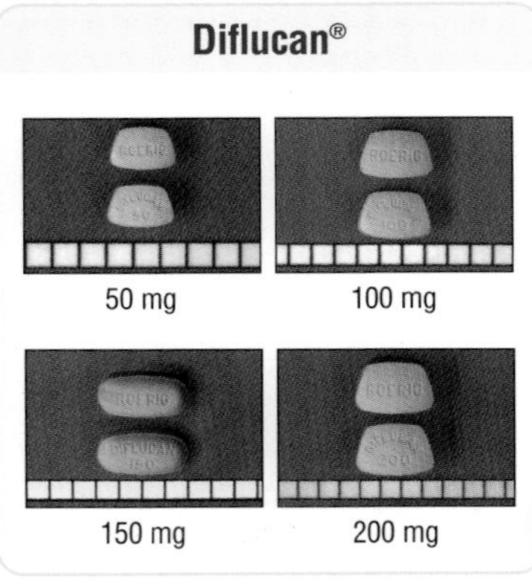

50 mg 100 mg

150 mg 200 mg

Fluoxetine

(generic)

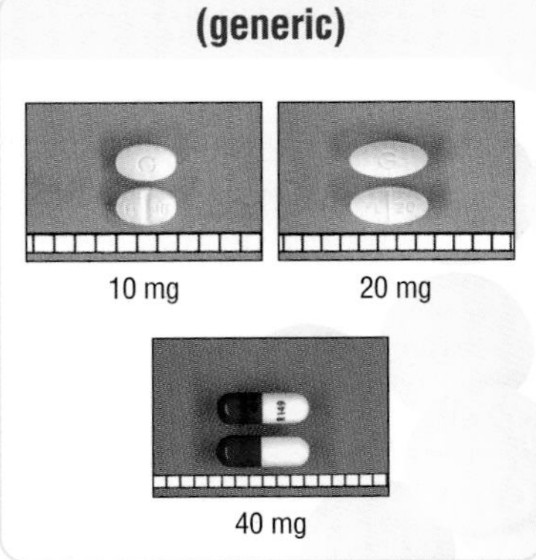

10 mg 20 mg

40 mg

Fluvastatin

Lescol® XL

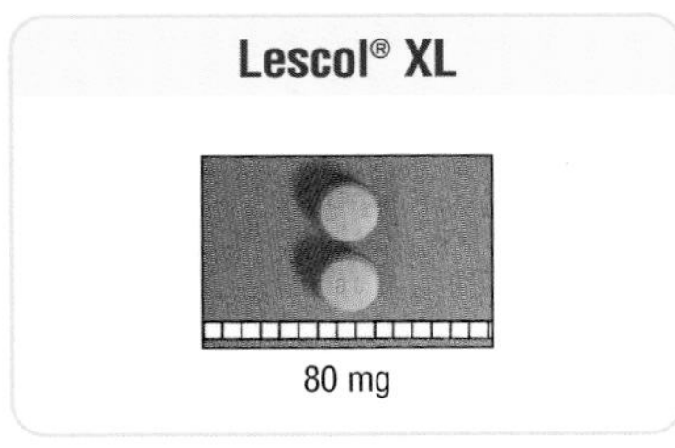

80 mg

Folic Acid

(generic)

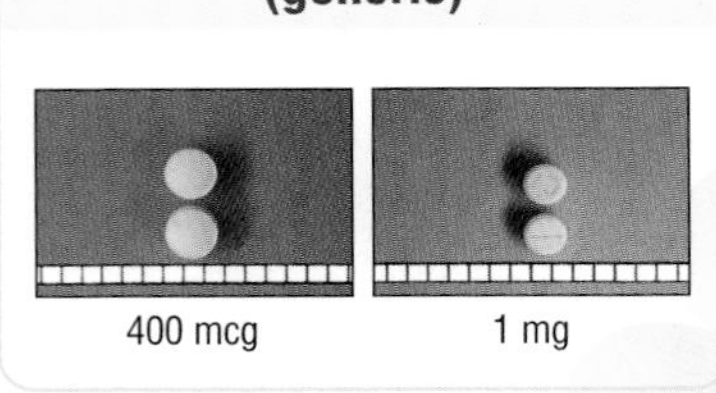

400 mcg 1 mg

Fosinopril

Monopril®

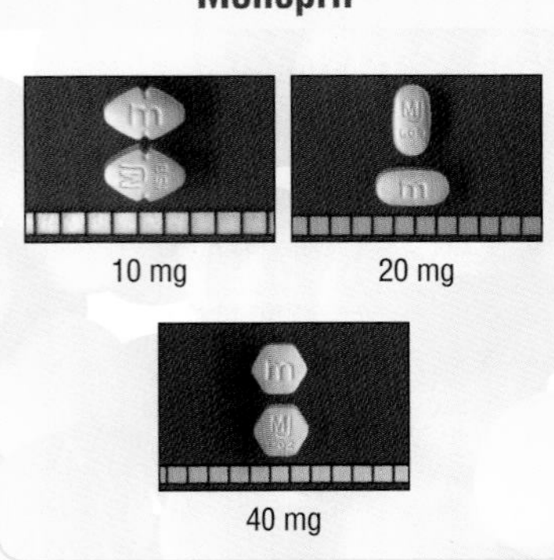

10 mg 20 mg

40 mg

Furosemide

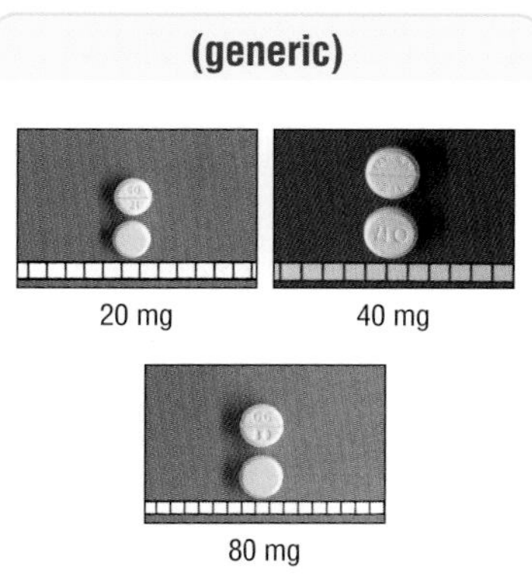

(generic)

20 mg

40 mg

80 mg

Gabapentin

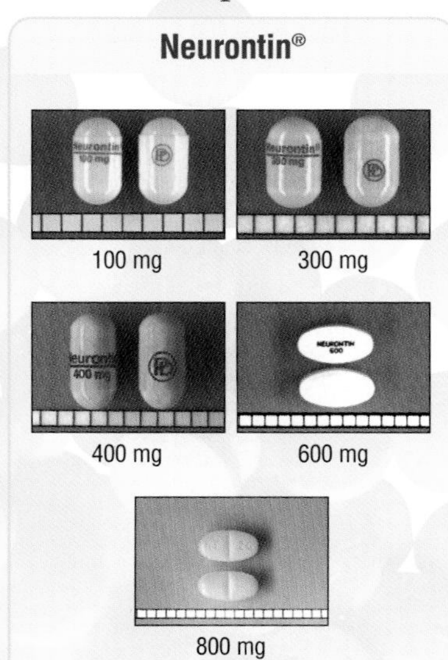

Neurontin®

100 mg

300 mg

400 mg

600 mg

800 mg

Gemfibrozil

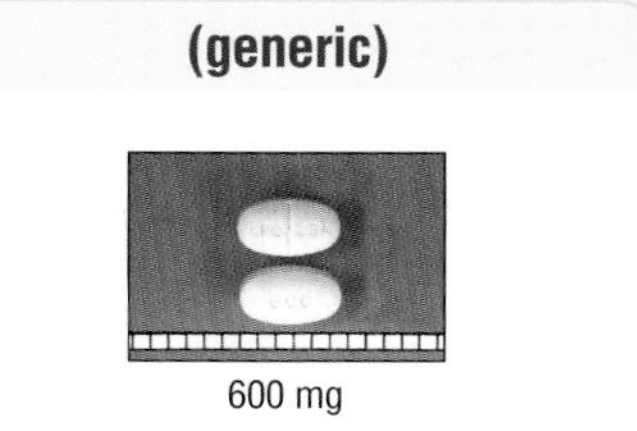

(generic)

600 mg

Glimepiride

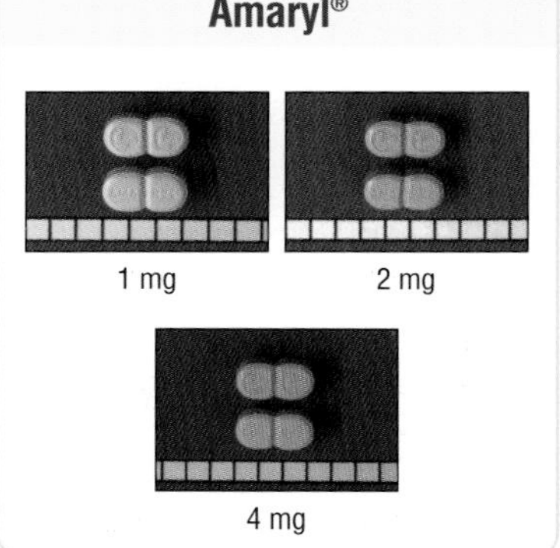

Amaryl®

1 mg

2 mg

4 mg

Glipizide

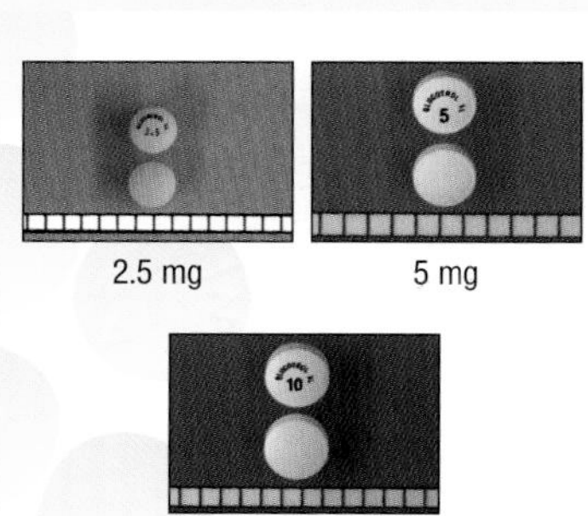

Glucotrol® XL

2.5 mg

5 mg

10 mg

Glyburide

(generic)

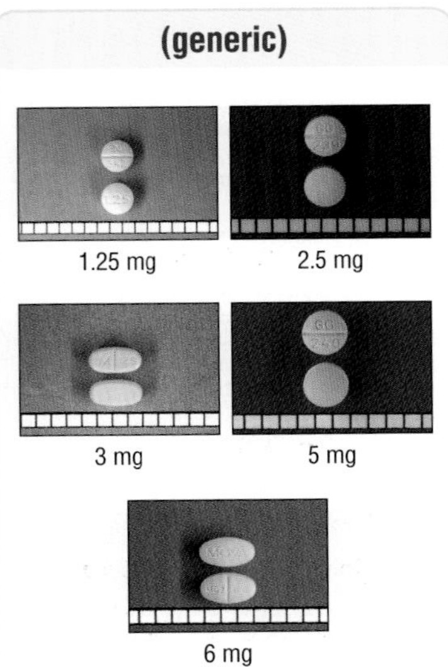

1.25 mg | 2.5 mg | 3 mg | 5 mg | 6 mg

Glyburide and Metformin

Glucovance™

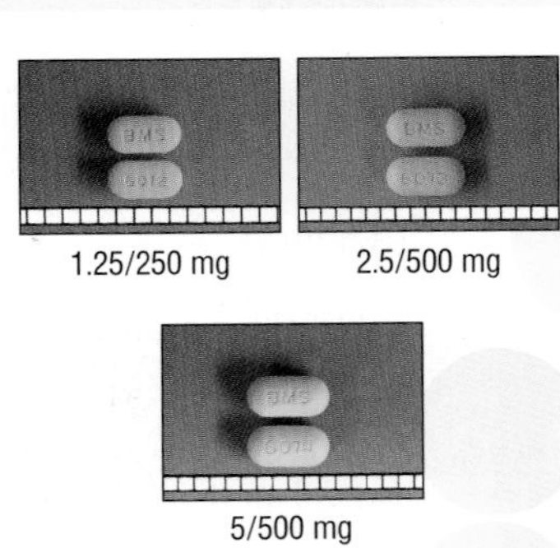

1.25/250 mg | 2.5/500 mg | 5/500 mg

Hydrochlorothiazide

(generic)

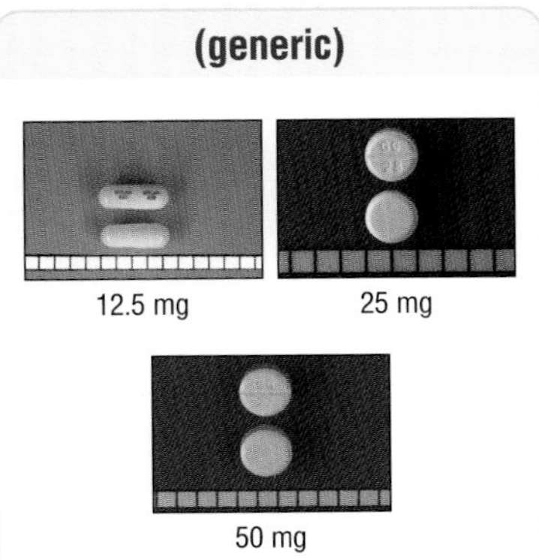

12.5 mg | 25 mg | 50 mg

Hydrochlorothiazide and Triamterine

(generic)

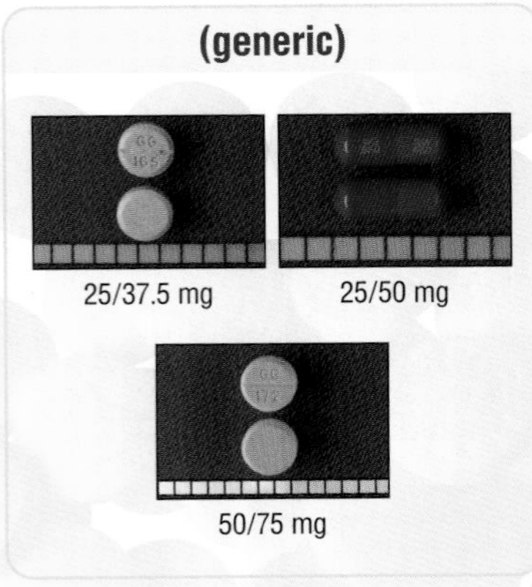

25/37.5 mg | 25/50 mg | 50/75 mg

Hydrocodone and Acetaminophen

(generic)

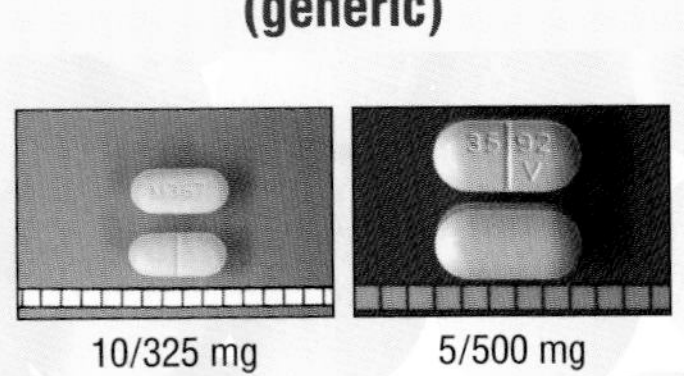

10/325 mg | 5/500 mg

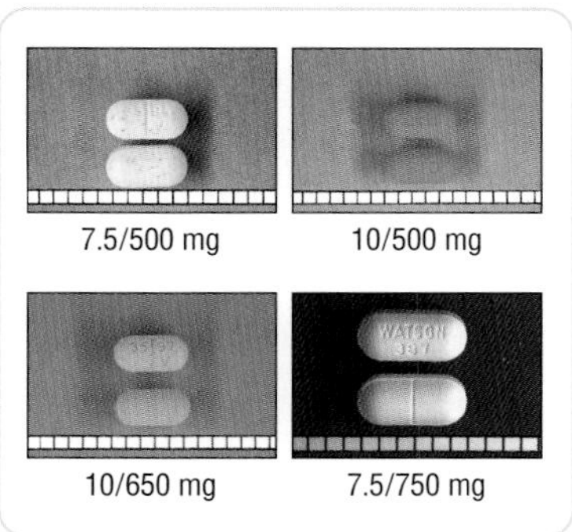

7.5/500 mg 10/500 mg

10/650 mg 7.5/750 mg

Lortab®

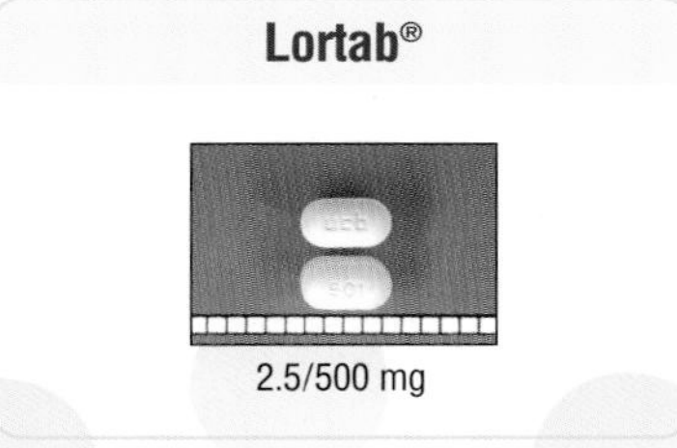

2.5/500 mg

Ibuprofen

(generic)

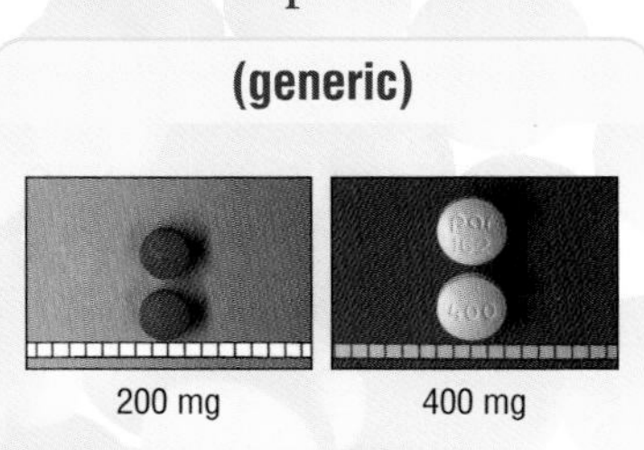

200 mg 400 mg

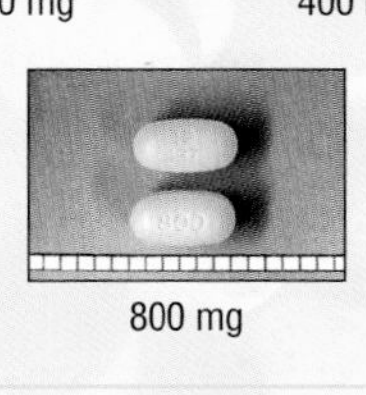

800 mg

Irbesartan

Avalide®

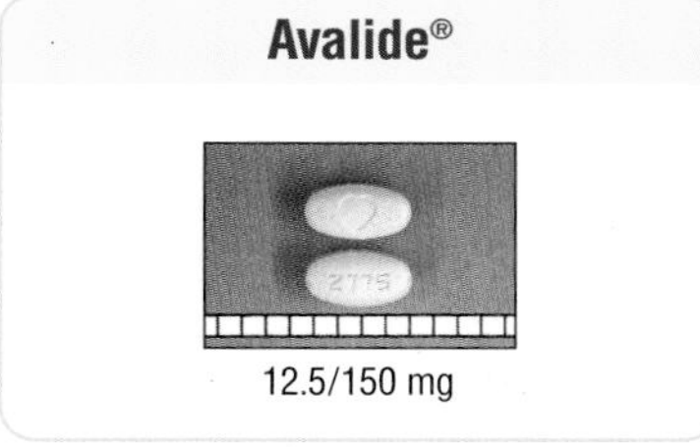

12.5/150 mg

Avapro®

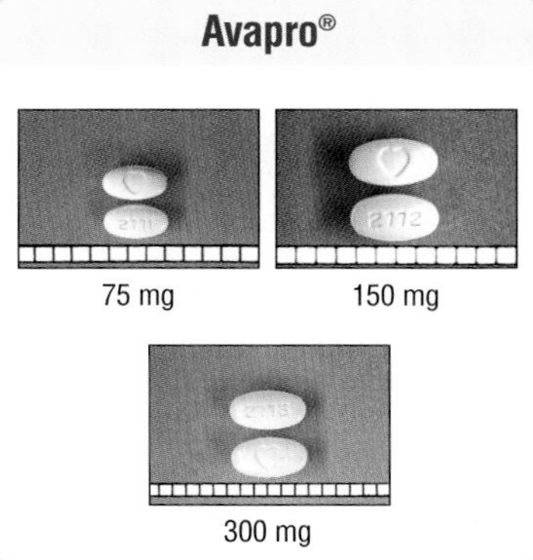

75 mg 150 mg

300 mg

Isosorbide Mononitrate

(generic)

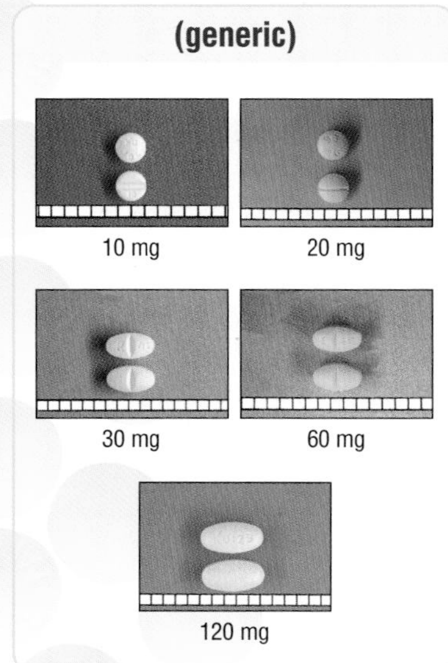

10 mg 20 mg

30 mg 60 mg

120 mg

Lansoprazole

Prevacid®

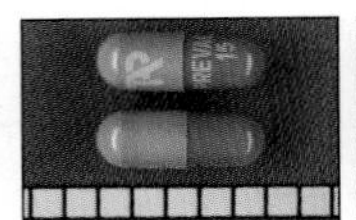
15 mg

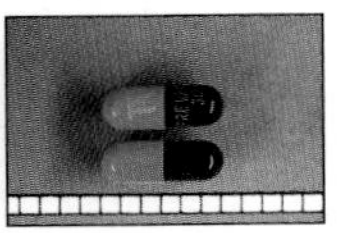
30 mg

Levofloxacin

Levaquin®

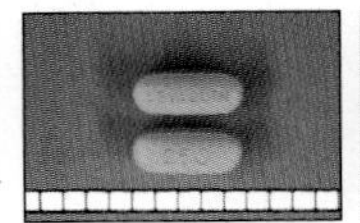
250 mg

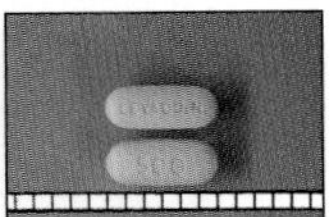
500 mg

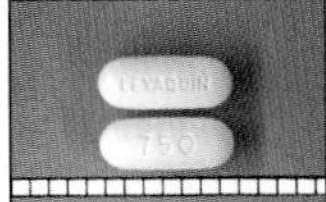
750 mg

Levothyroxine

Levothroid®

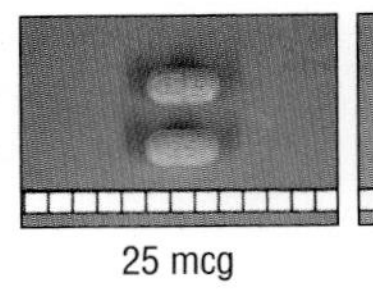
25 mcg

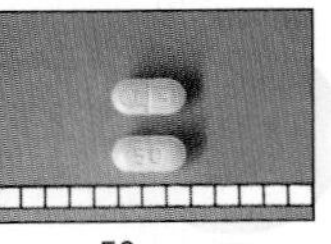
50 mcg

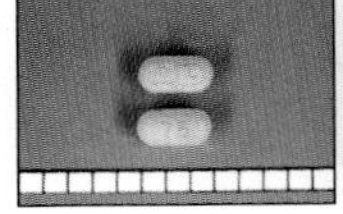
75 mcg

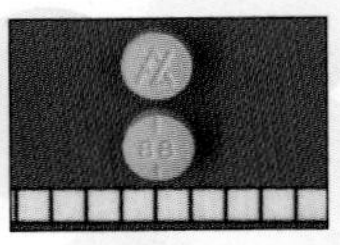
88 mcg

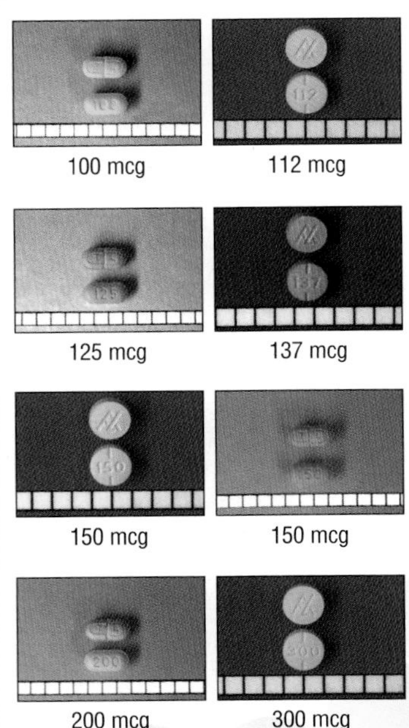
100 mcg

112 mcg

125 mcg

137 mcg

150 mcg

150 mcg

200 mcg

300 mcg

Levoxyl®

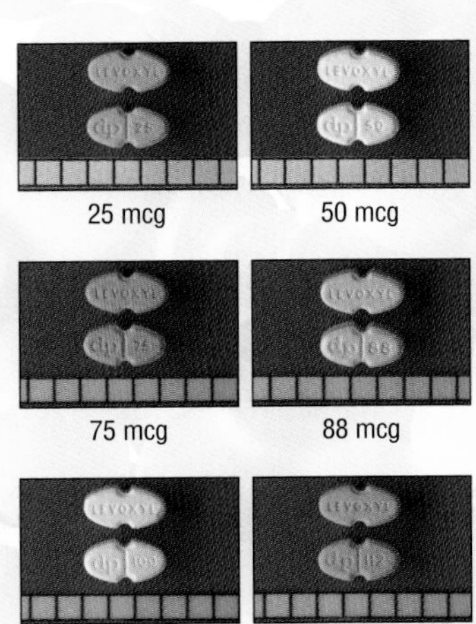
25 mcg

50 mcg

75 mcg

88 mcg

100 mcg

112 mcg

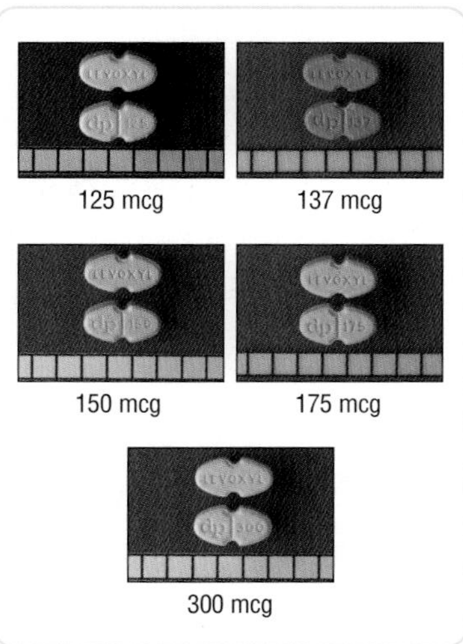

125 mcg 137 mcg

150 mcg 175 mcg

300 mcg

Synthroid®

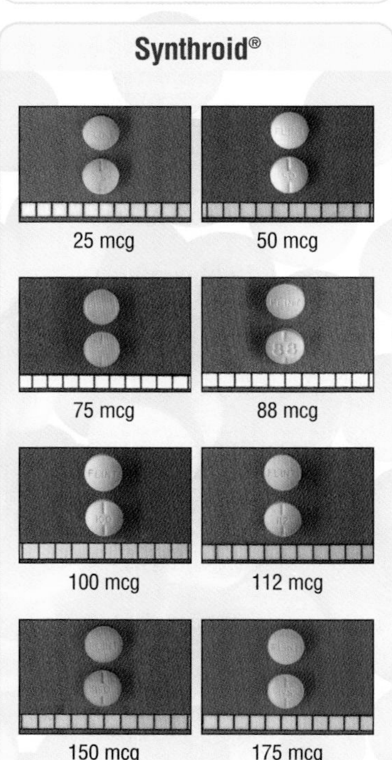

25 mcg 50 mcg

75 mcg 88 mcg

100 mcg 112 mcg

150 mcg 175 mcg

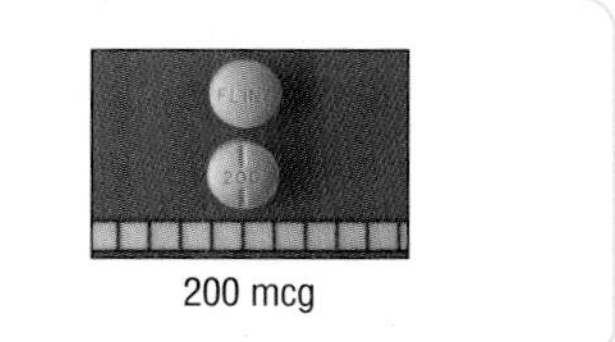

200 mcg

Lisinopril

(generic)

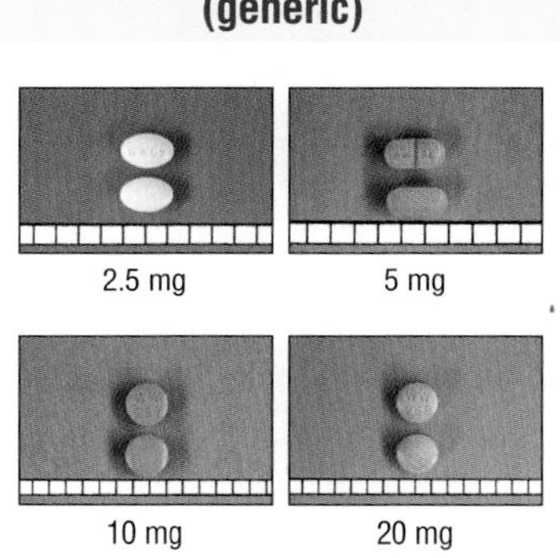

2.5 mg 5 mg

10 mg 20 mg

Lorazepam

(generic)

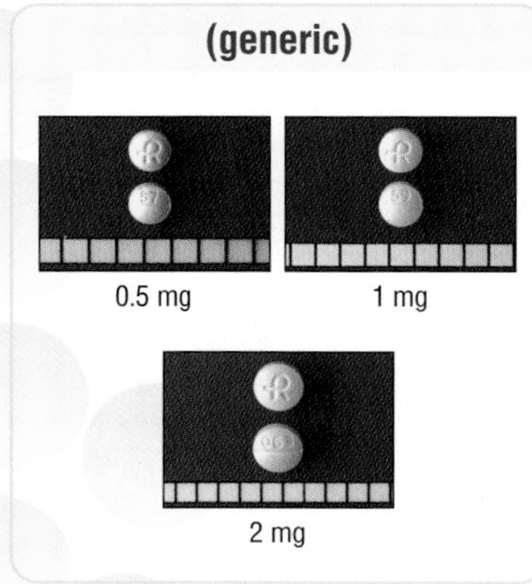

0.5 mg 1 mg

2 mg

Losartan

Cozaar®

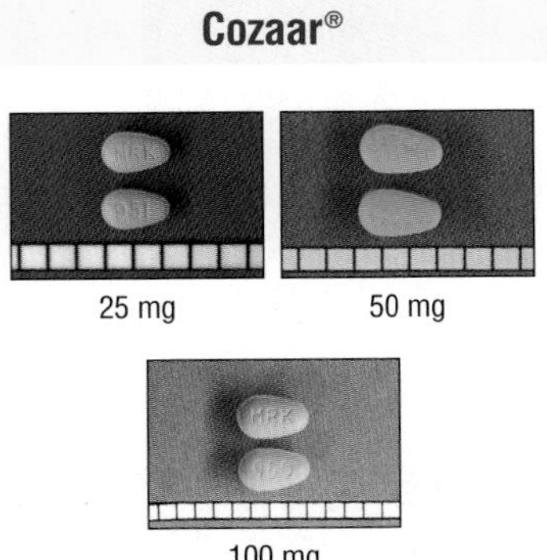

25 mg | 50 mg

100 mg

Losartan and Hydrochlorothiazide

Hyzaar®

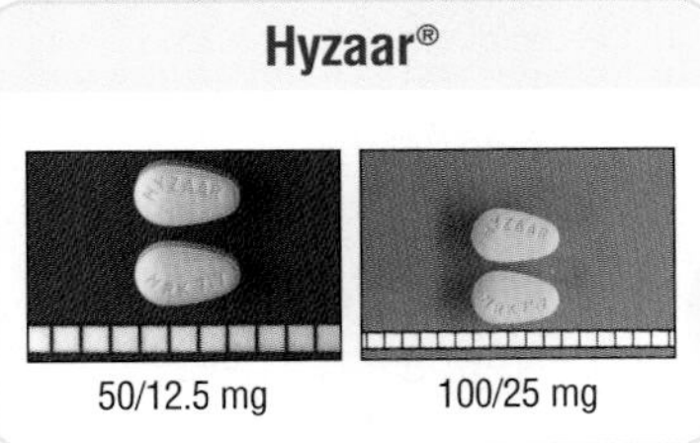

50/12.5 mg | 100/25 mg

Meclizine

(generic)

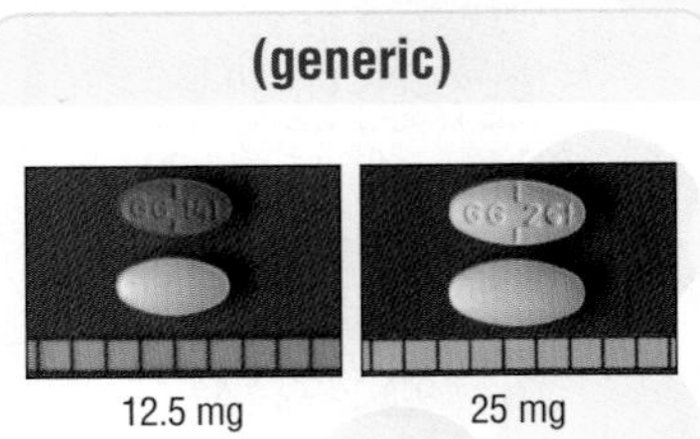

12.5 mg | 25 mg

Meloxicam

Mobic®

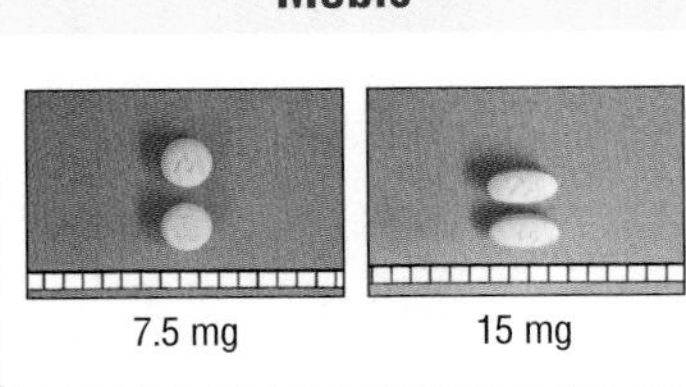

7.5 mg | 15 mg

Mestranol and Norethindrone

Ortho-Novum® 1/50 28

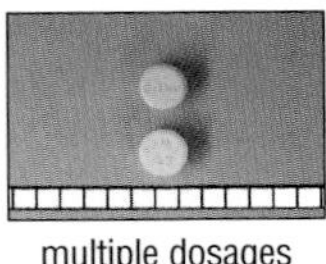

multiple dosages

Metaxalone

Skelaxin®

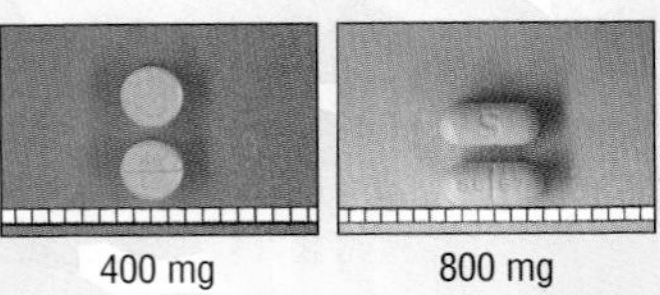

400 mg | 800 mg

Metformin

(generic)

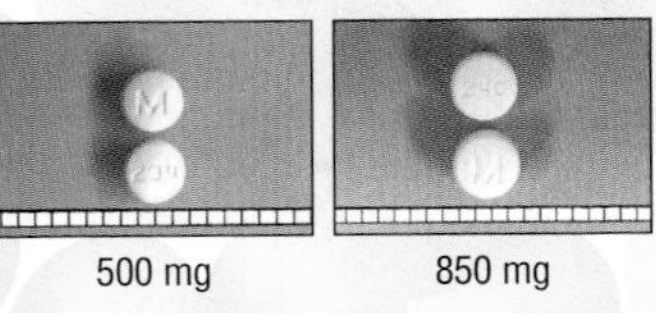

500 mg | 850 mg

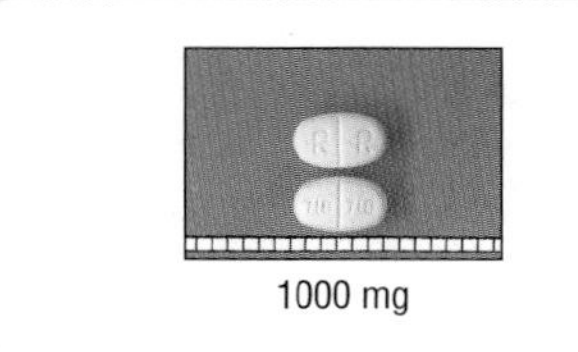
1000 mg

Glucophage® XR

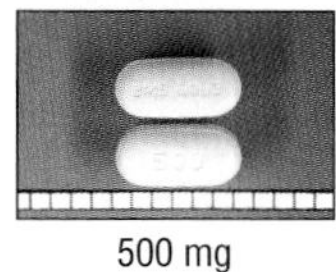
500 mg

Methylphenidate

Concerta™

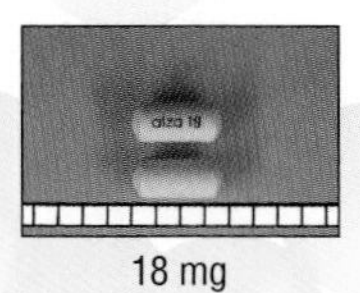

18 mg

Concerta®

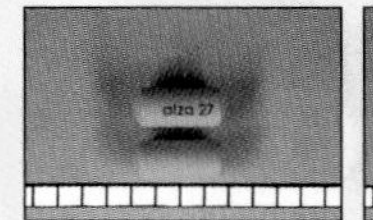

27 mg

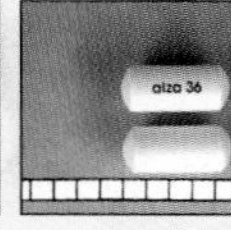

36 mg

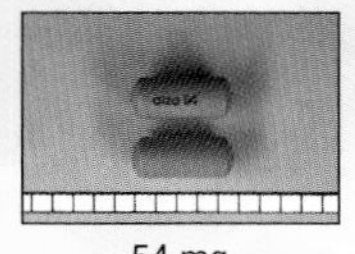
54 mg

Methylprednisolone

(generic)

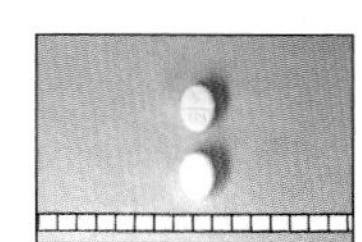
4 mg

Metoprolol

(generic)

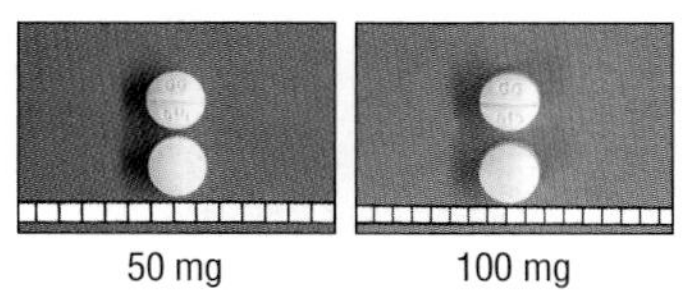
50 mg 100 mg

Toprol XL®

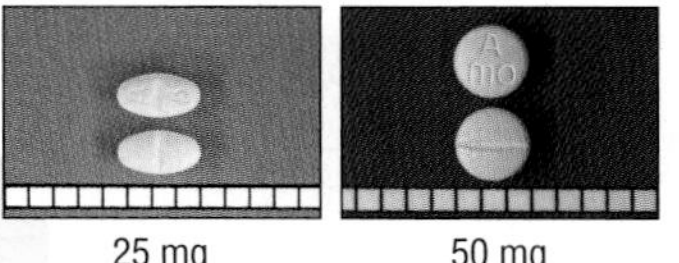

25 mg 50 mg

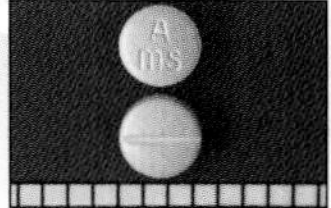

100 mg

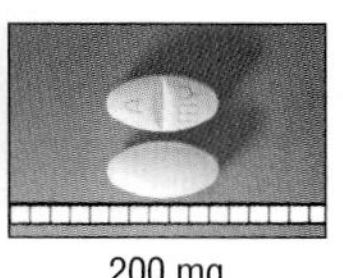
200 mg

Mirtazapine

Remeron®

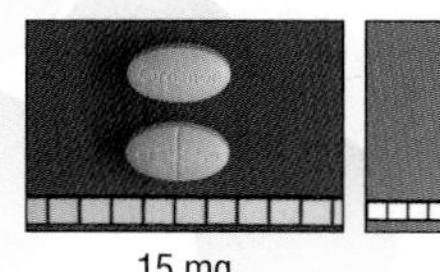
15 mg

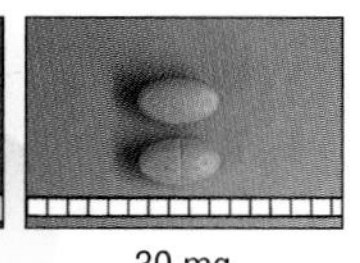
30 mg

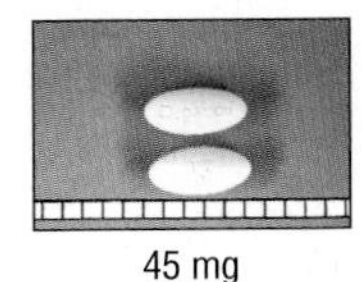

45 mg

Montelukast

Singulair®

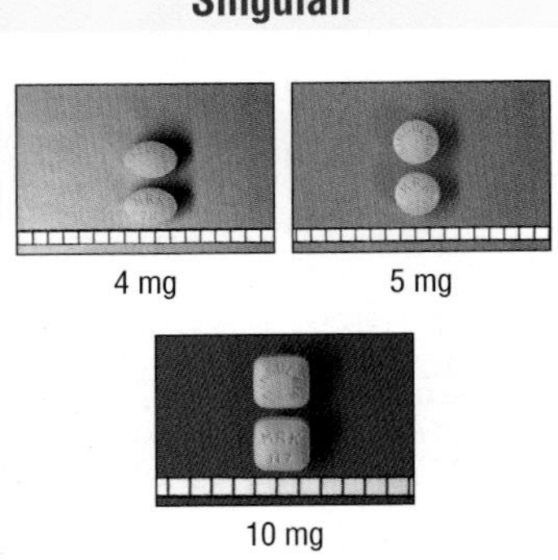

4 mg

5 mg

10 mg

Moxifloxacin

Avelox®

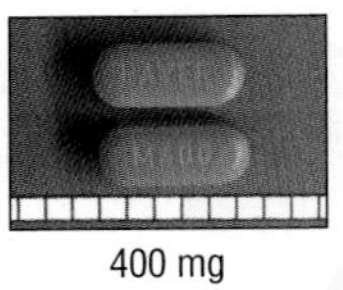

400 mg

Naproxen

(generic)

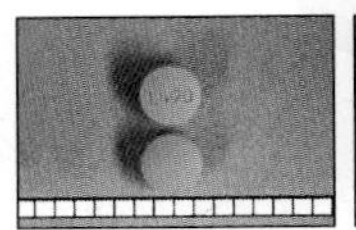

220 mg

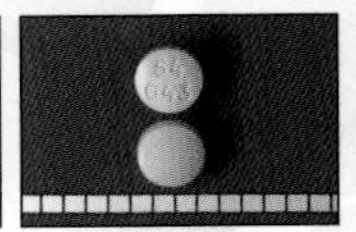

250 mg

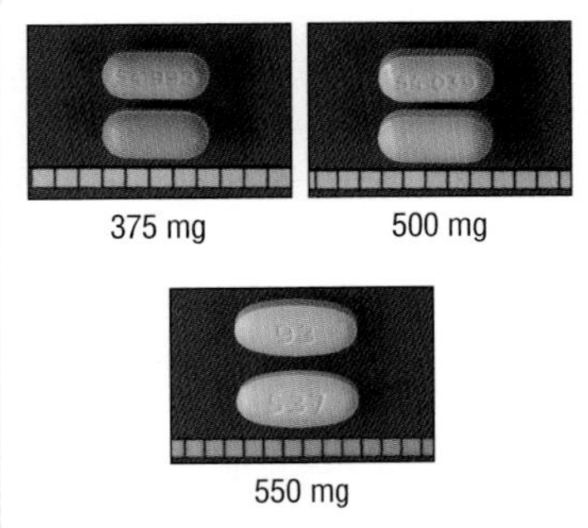

375 mg

500 mg

550 mg

Niacin

Niaspan®

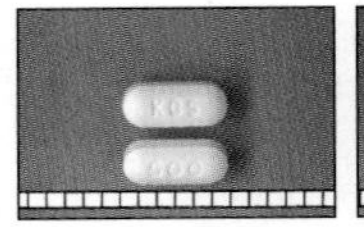

500 mg

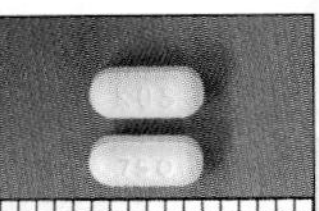

750 mg

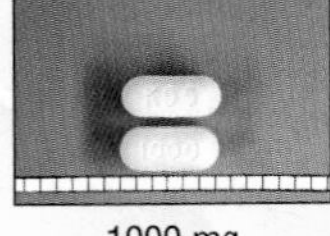

1000 mg

Nifedipine

Nifediac™ CC

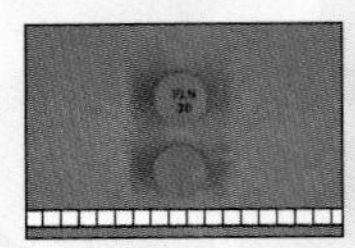

30 mg

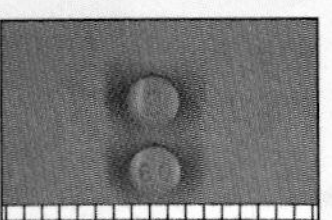

60 mg

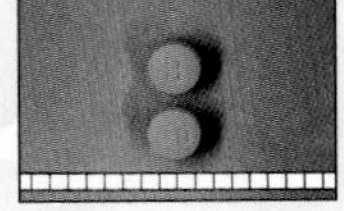

90 mg

Nitrofurantoin

Macrobid®

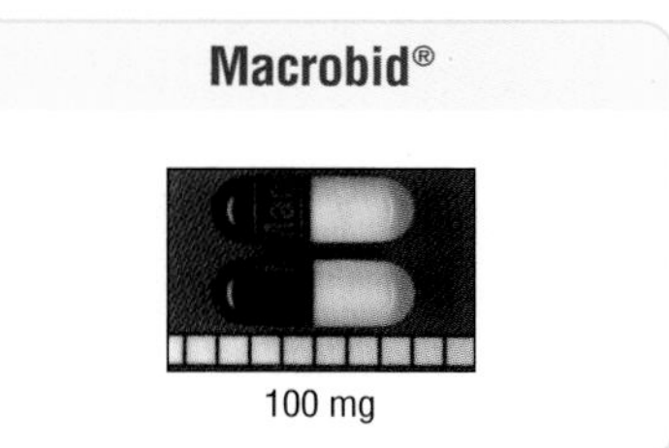

100 mg

Olanzapine

Zyprexa®

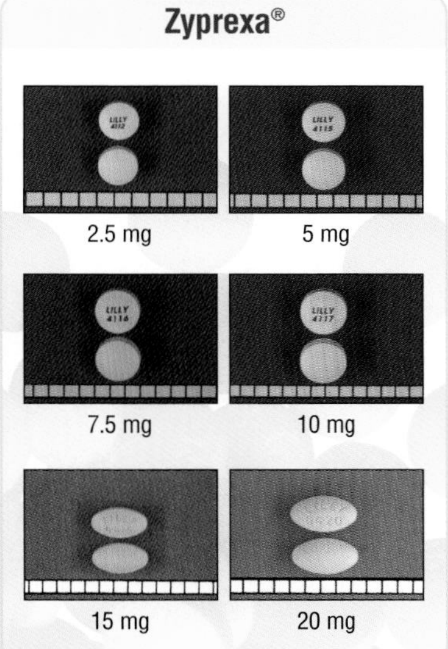

2.5 mg | 5 mg

7.5 mg | 10 mg

15 mg | 20 mg

Omeprazole

(generic)

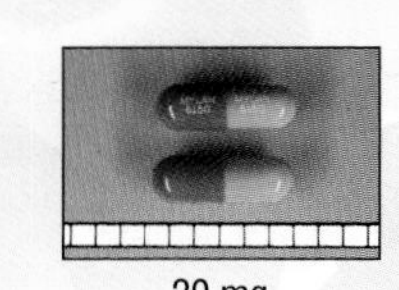

20 mg

Prilosec®

10 mg | 20 mg

40 mg

Oxybutynin

Ditropan® XL

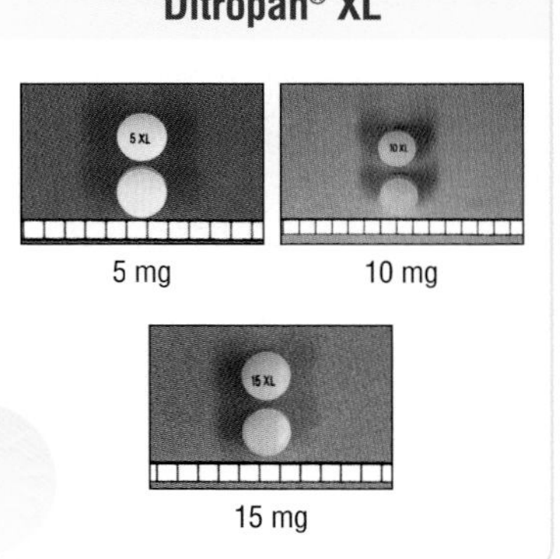

5 mg | 10 mg

15 mg

Oxycodone

Oxycontin®

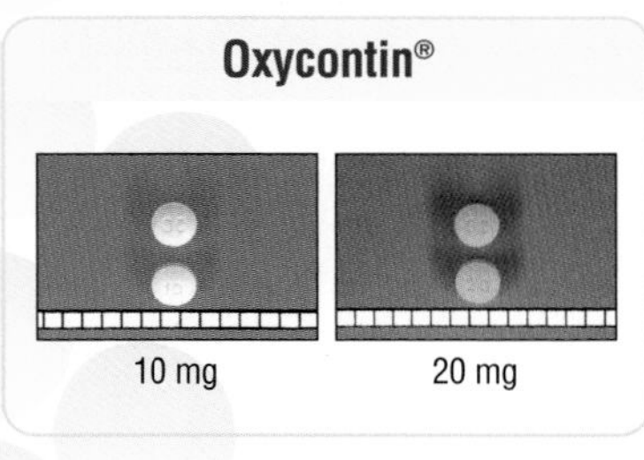

10 mg | 20 mg

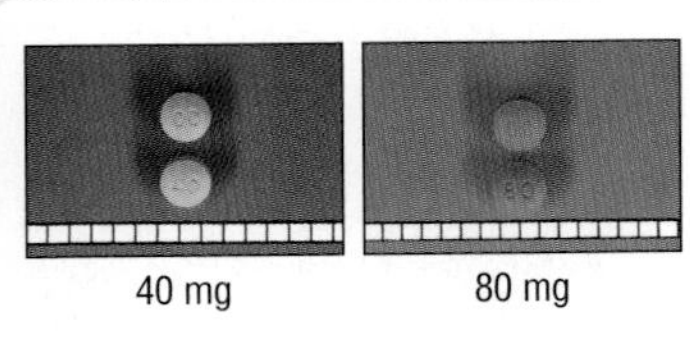

40 mg 80 mg

Oxycodone and Acetaminophen

(generic)

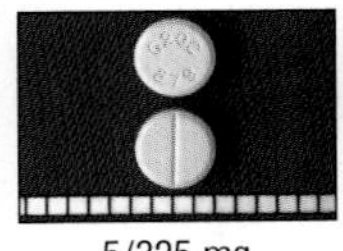

5/325 mg

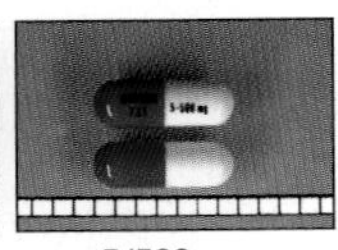

5/500 mg

Endocet®

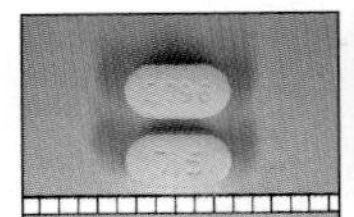

7.5/500 mg

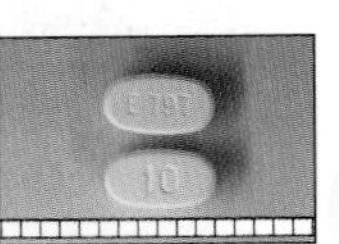

10/650 mg

Percocet®

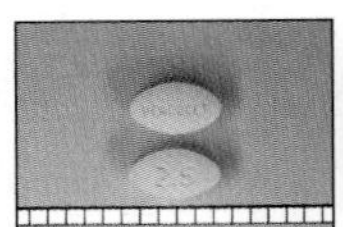

2.5/325 mg

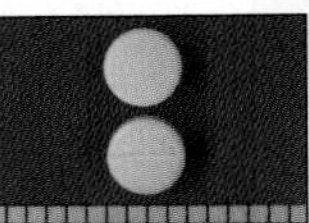

5/325 mg

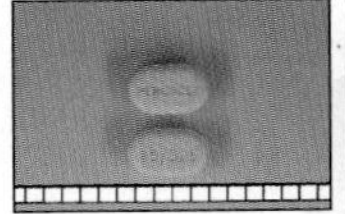

7.5/325 mg

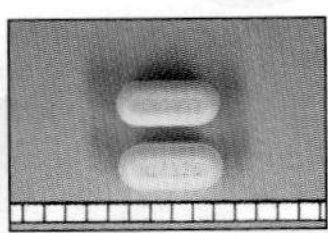

10/325 mg

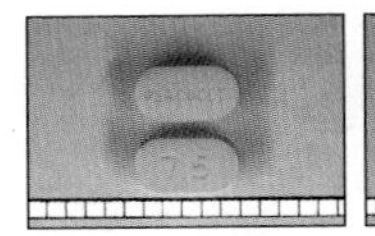

7.5/500 mg

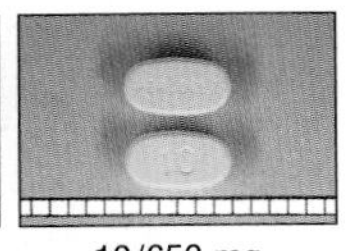

10/650 mg

Roxicet®

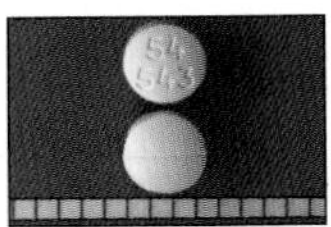

5/325 mg

Pantoprazole

Protonix®

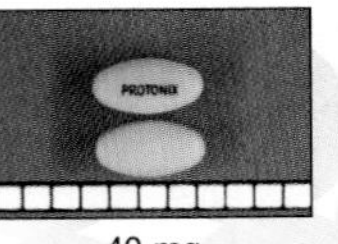

40 mg

Paroxetine

Paxil®

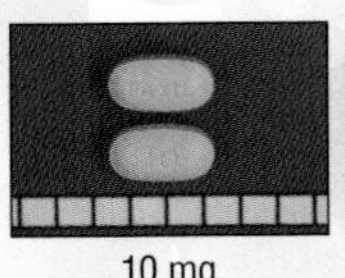

10 mg

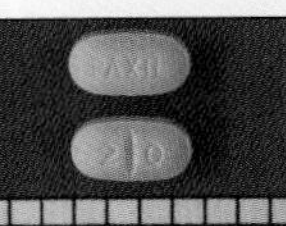

20 mg

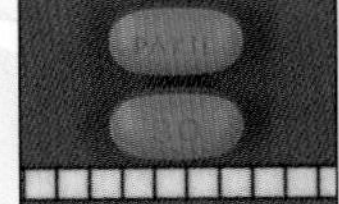

30 mg

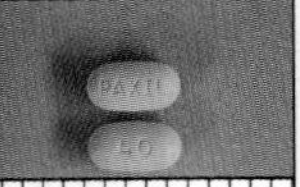

40 mg

Paxil® CR

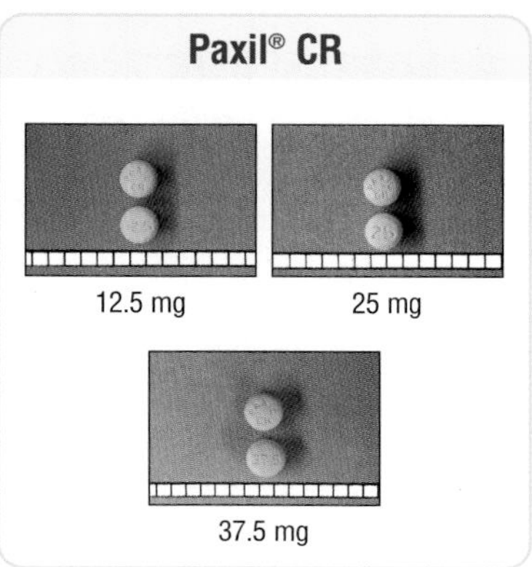

12.5 mg

25 mg

37.5 mg

Penicillin V Potassium

(generic)

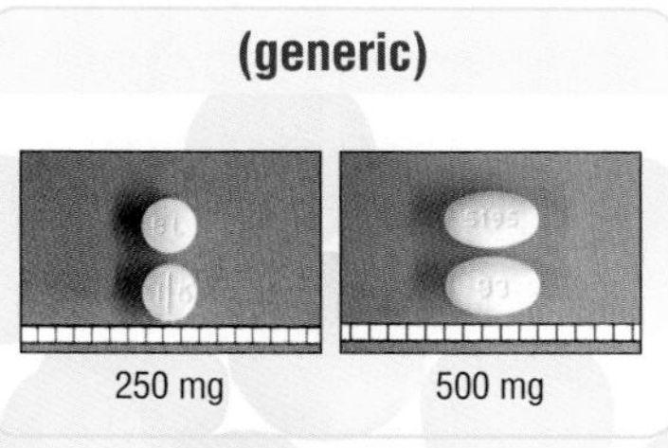

250 mg

500 mg

Phenytoin

(generic)

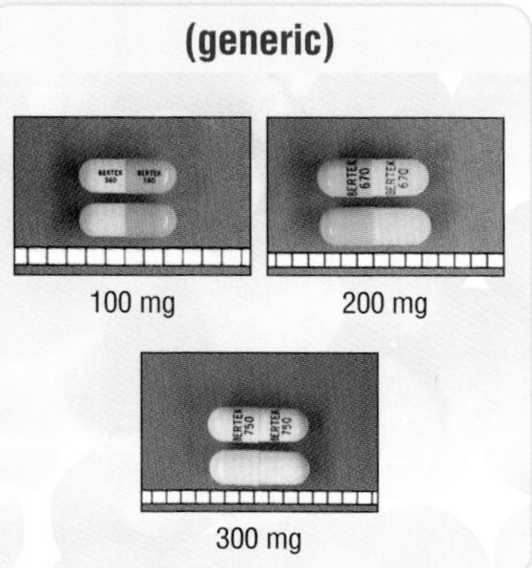

100 mg

200 mg

300 mg

Dilantin® Kapseals®

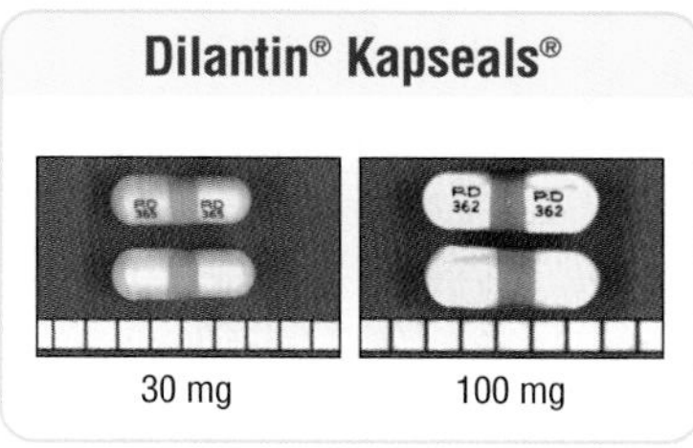

30 mg

100 mg

Pioglitazone

Actos™

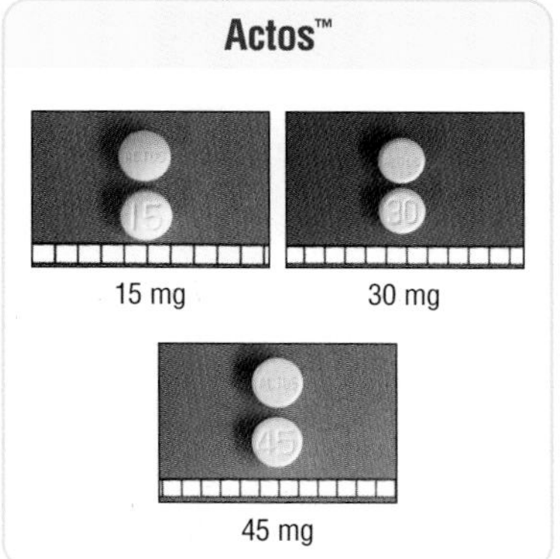

15 mg

30 mg

45 mg

Potassium Chloride

(generic)

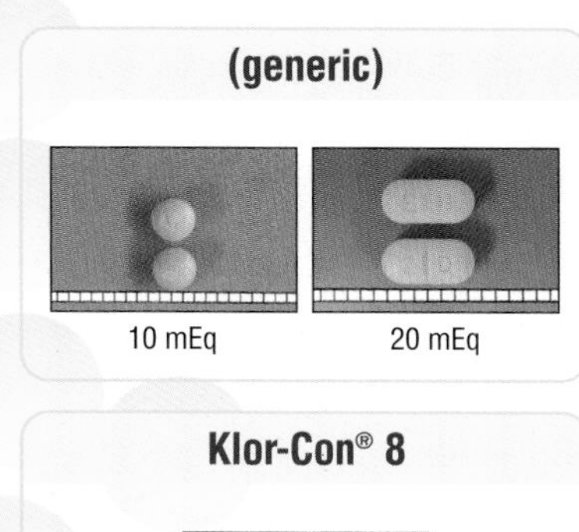

10 mEq

20 mEq

Klor-Con® 8

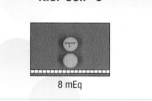

8 mEq

Klor-Con® 10

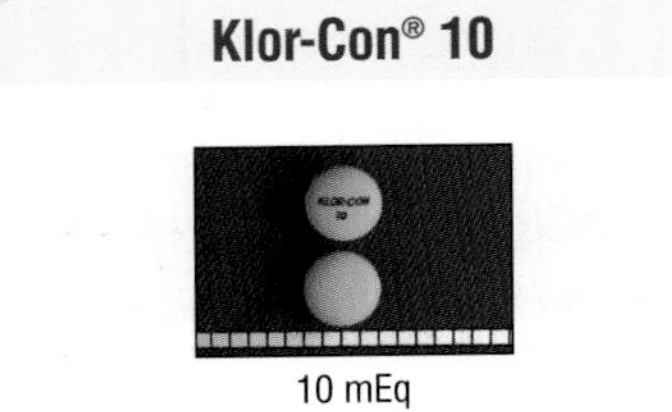

10 mEq

Klor-Con® M20

20 mEq

Pravastatin

Pravachol®

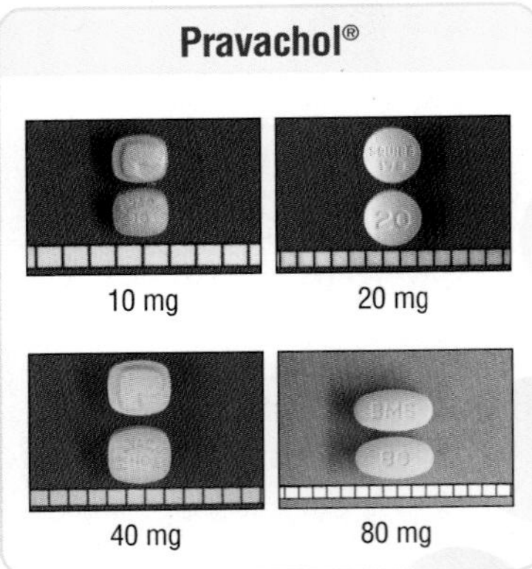

10 mg | 20 mg | 40 mg | 80 mg

Prednisone

(generic)

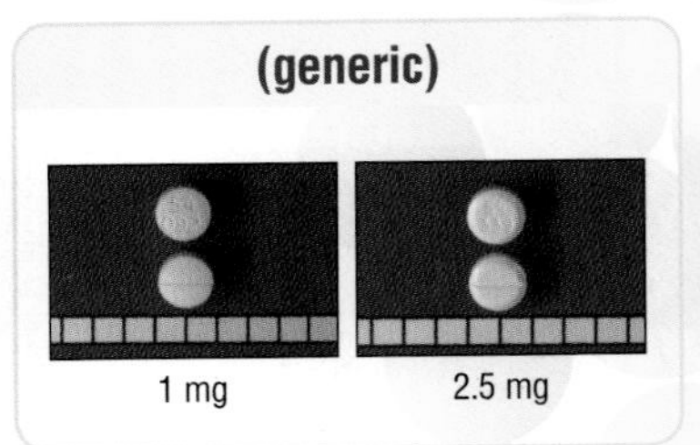

1 mg | 2.5 mg

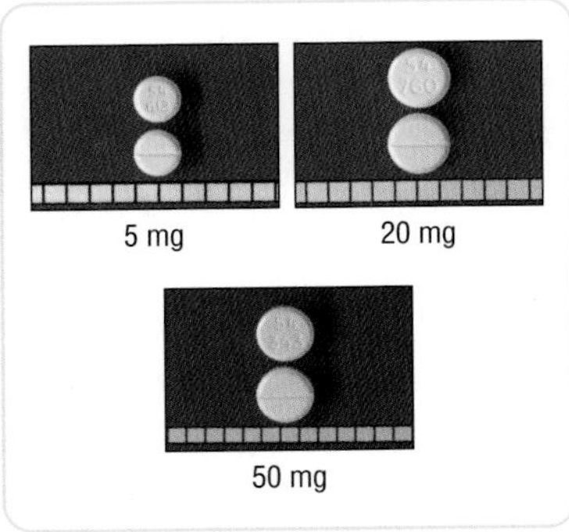

5 mg | 20 mg | 50 mg

Promethazine

(generic)

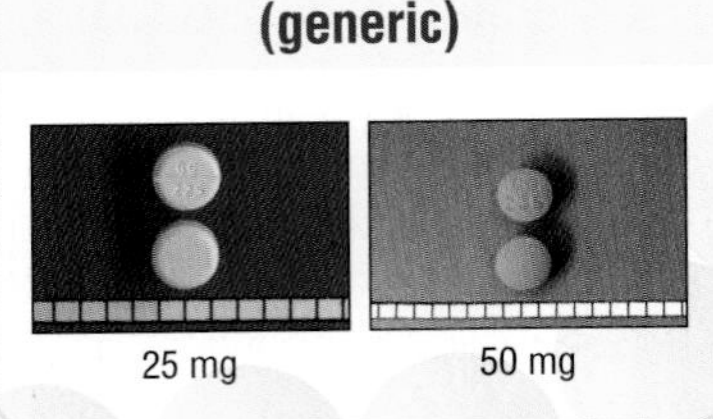

25 mg | 50 mg

Propoxyphene and Acetaminophen

(generic)

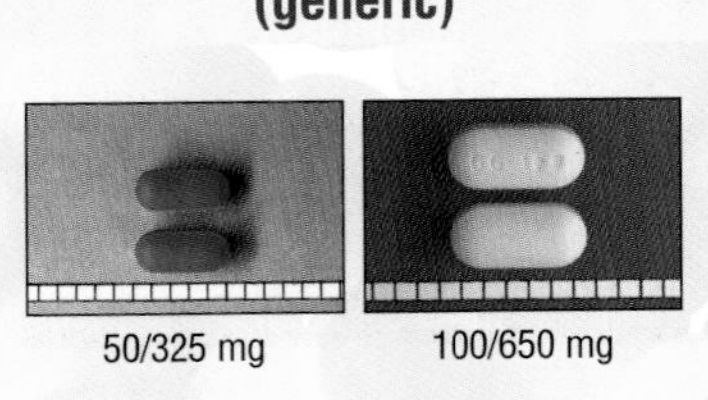

50/325 mg | 100/650 mg

Propranolol

(generic)

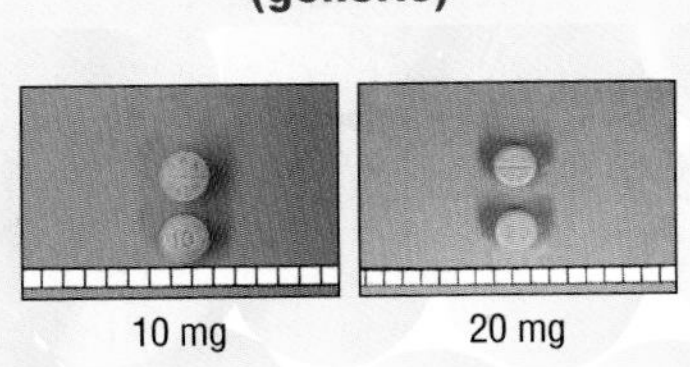

10 mg | 20 mg

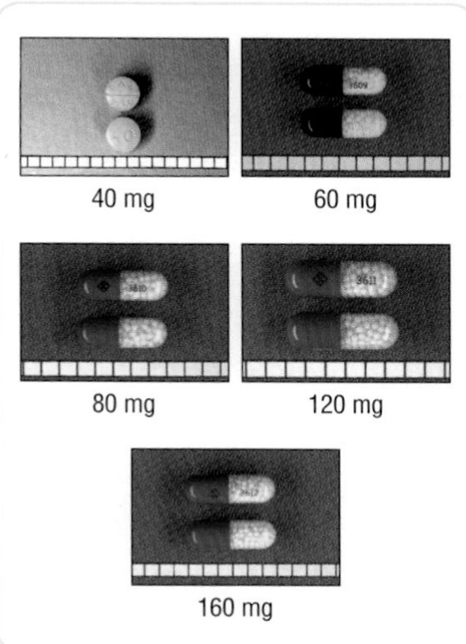

40 mg 60 mg

80 mg 120 mg

160 mg

Inderal® LA

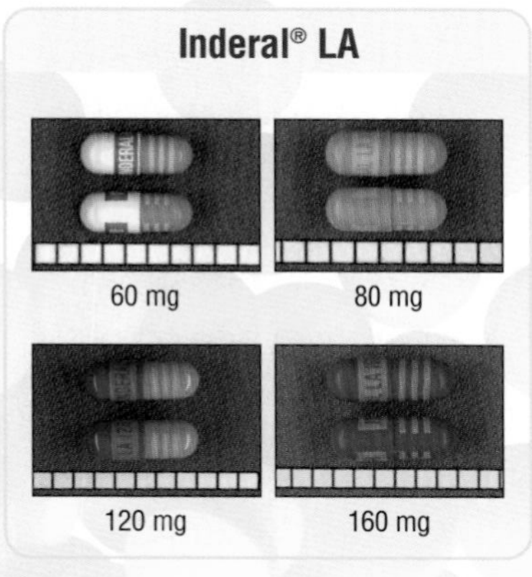

60 mg 80 mg

120 mg 160 mg

Quetiapine

Seroquel®

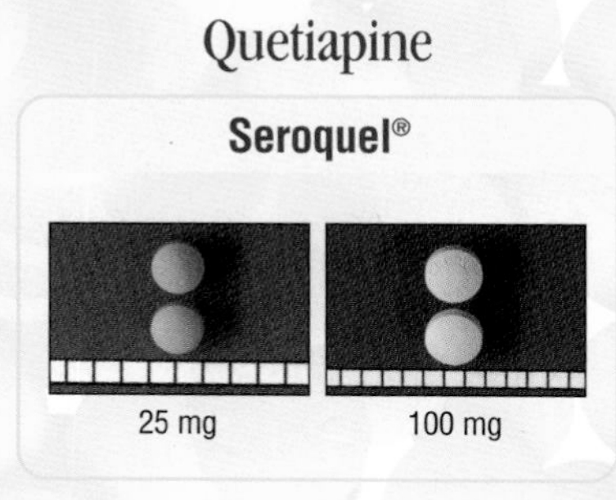

25 mg 100 mg

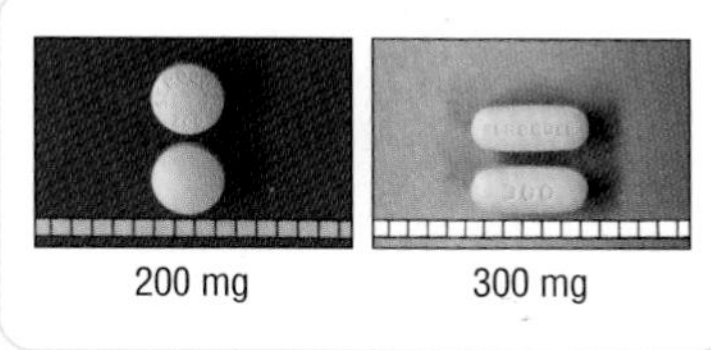

200 mg 300 mg

Quinapril

Accupril®

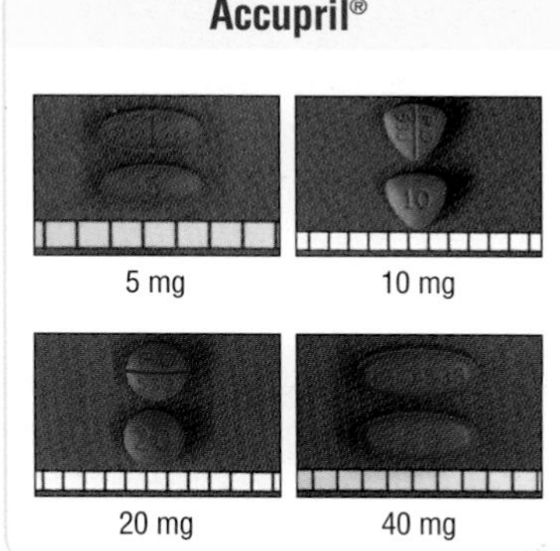

5 mg 10 mg

20 mg 40 mg

Rabeprazole

Aciphex®

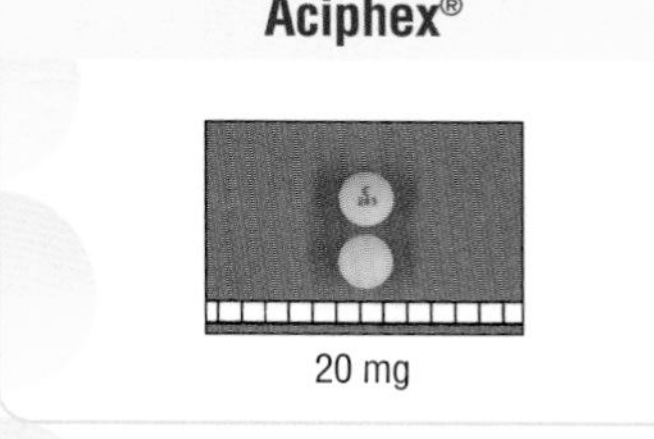

20 mg

Raloxifene

Evista®

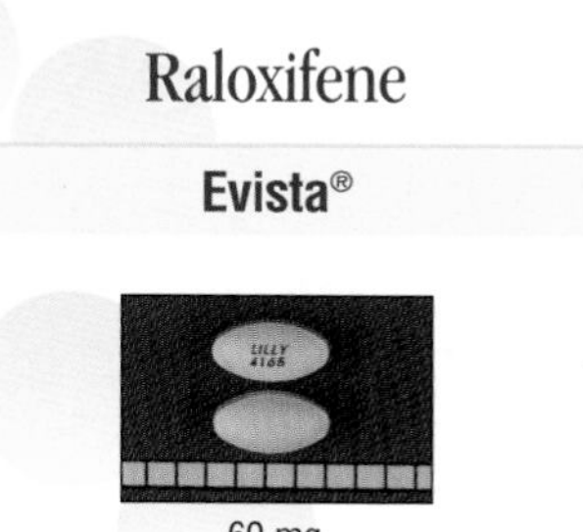

60 mg

Ramipril

Altace™

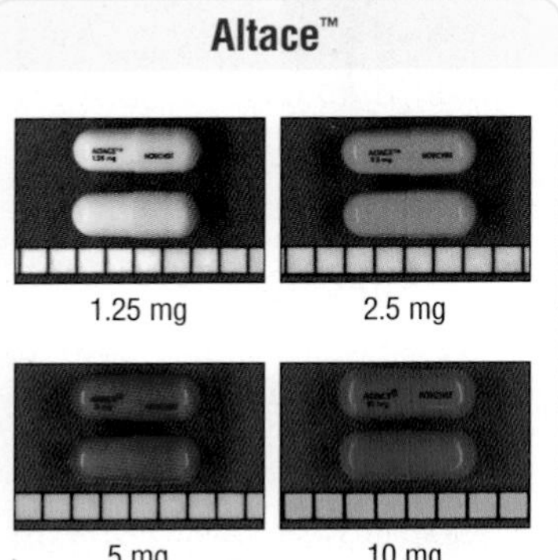

1.25 mg | 2.5 mg | 5 mg | 10 mg

Ranitidine

(generic)

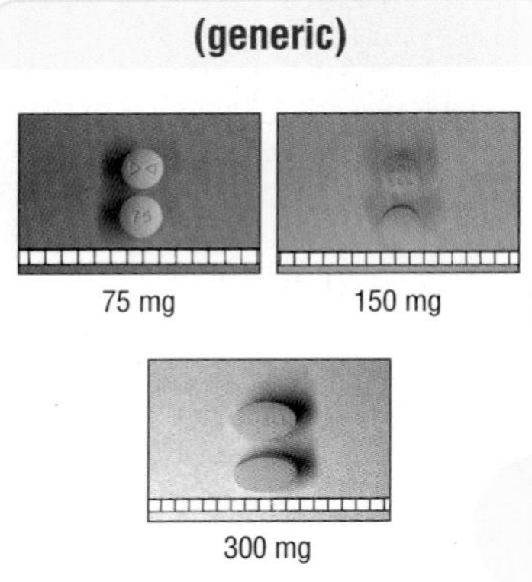

75 mg | 150 mg | 300 mg

Risedronate

Actonel®

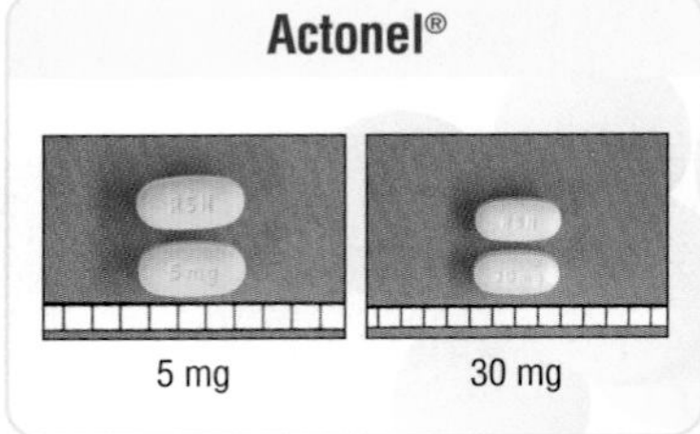

5 mg | 30 mg

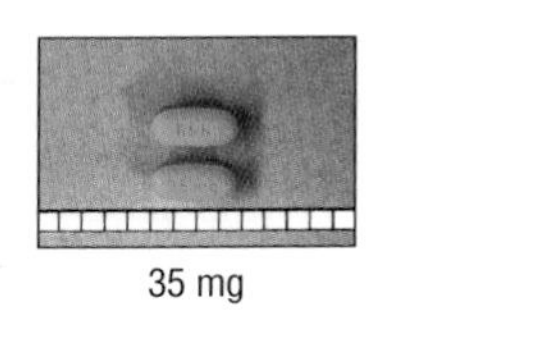

35 mg

Risperidone

Risperdal®

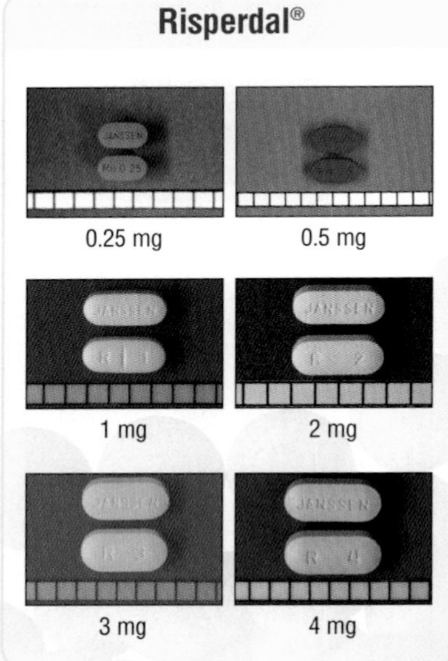

0.25 mg | 0.5 mg | 1 mg | 2 mg | 3 mg | 4 mg

Rosiglitazone

Avandia®

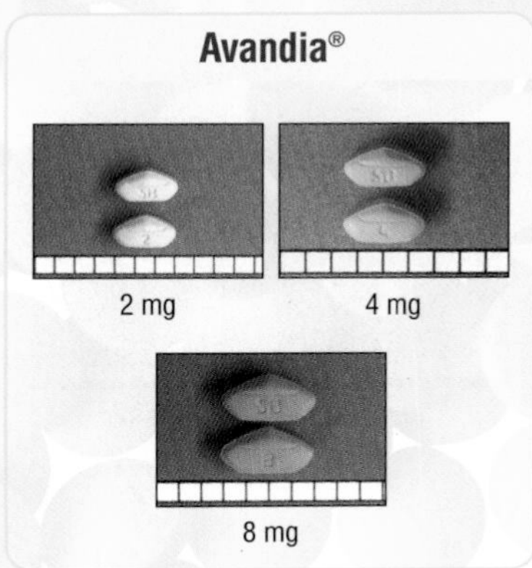

2 mg | 4 mg | 8 mg

Sertraline

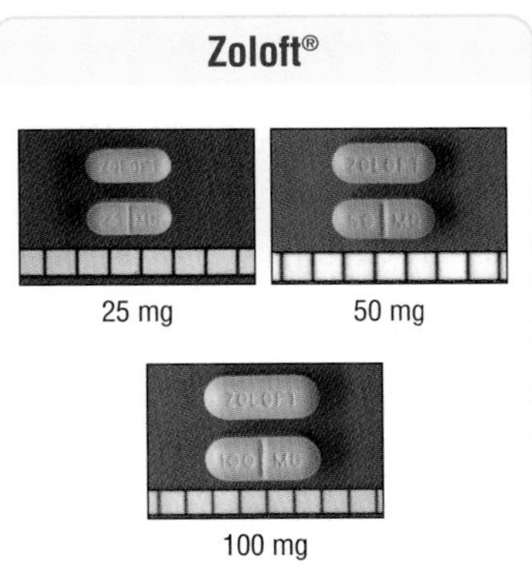

Zoloft®

25 mg 50 mg

100 mg

Sildenafil

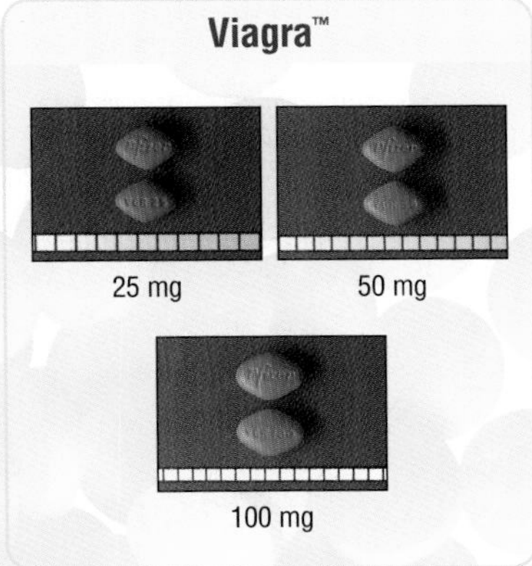

Viagra™

25 mg 50 mg

100 mg

Simvastatin

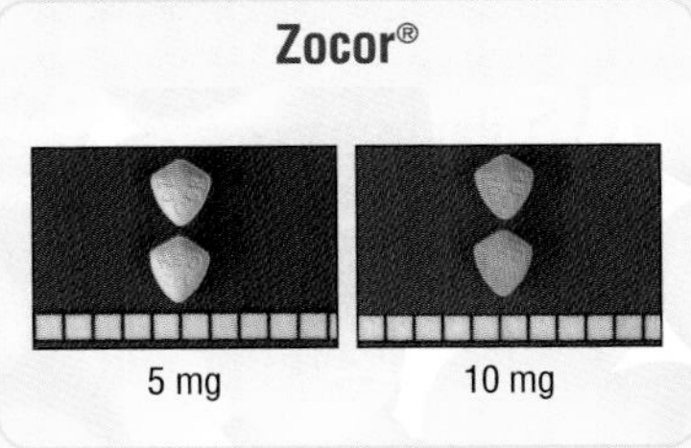

Zocor®

5 mg 10 mg

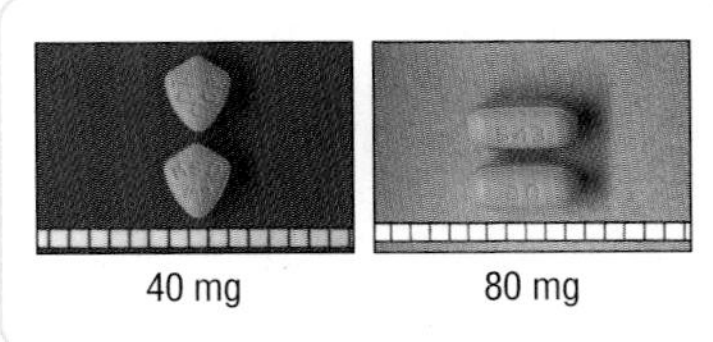

40 mg 80 mg

Spironolactone

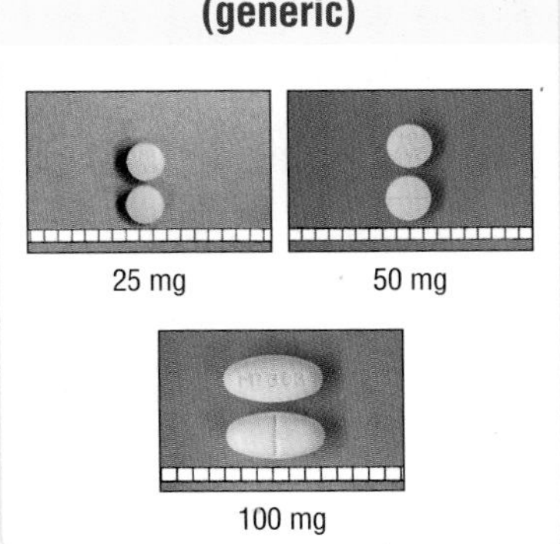

(generic)

25 mg 50 mg

100 mg

Sulfamethoxazole and Trimethoprim

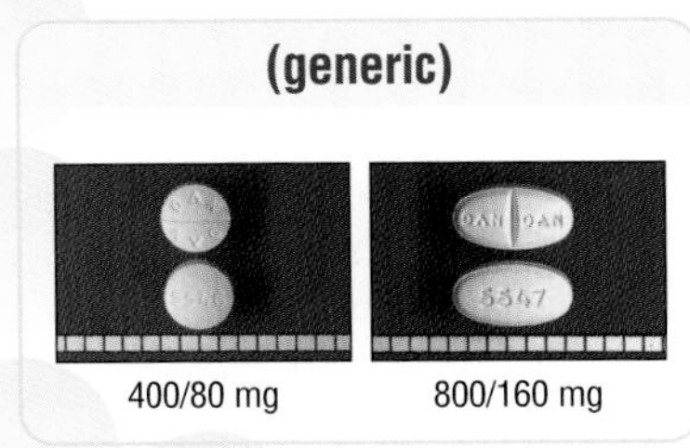

(generic)

400/80 mg 800/160 mg

Tamsulosin

Flomax®

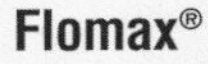

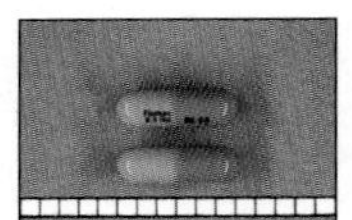

0.4 mg

Temazepam

(generic)

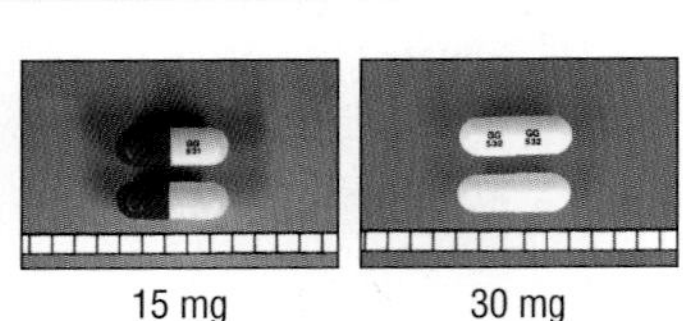

15 mg 30 mg

Terazosin

(generic)

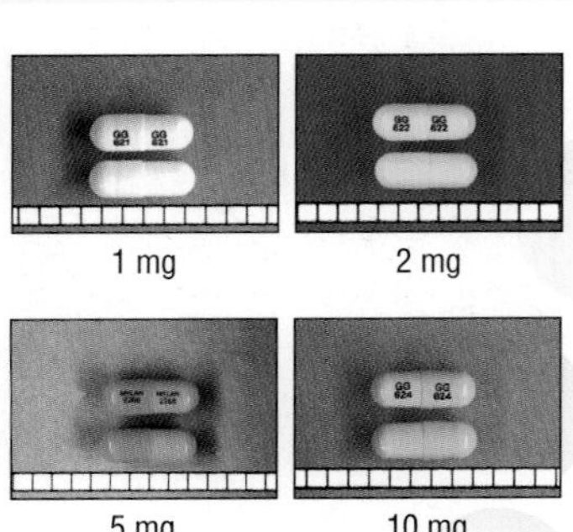

1 mg 2 mg

5 mg 10 mg

Tolterodine

Detrol® LA

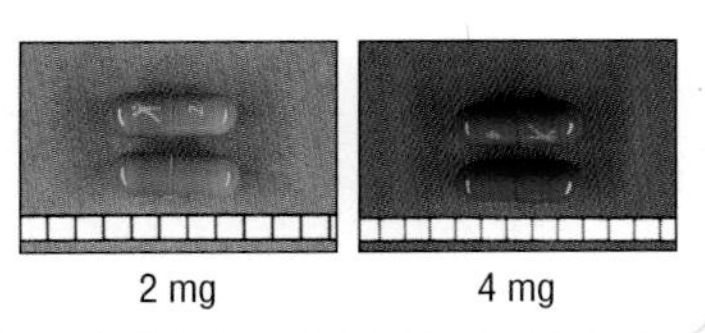

2 mg 4 mg

Topiramate

Topamax®

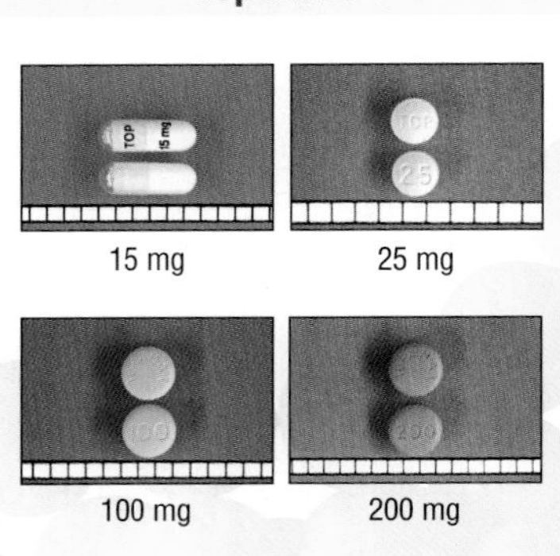

15 mg 25 mg

100 mg 200 mg

Trazodone

(generic)

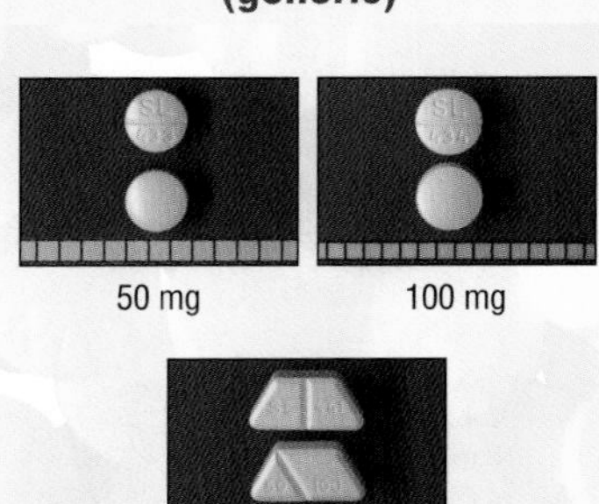

50 mg 100 mg

150 mg

Valacyclovir

Valtrex®

500 mg

1000 mg

Valdecoxib

Bextra™

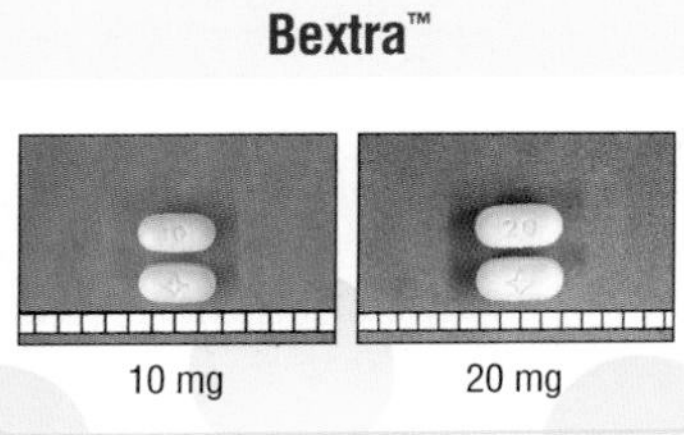

10 mg

20 mg

Valproic Acid and Derivatives

Depakote®

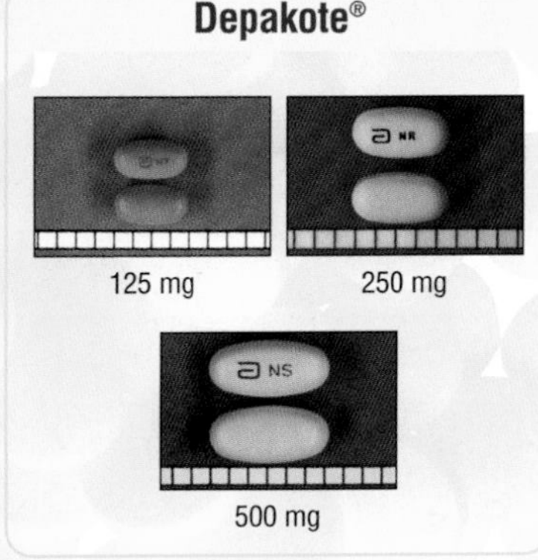

125 mg

250 mg

500 mg

Valsartan

Diovan™

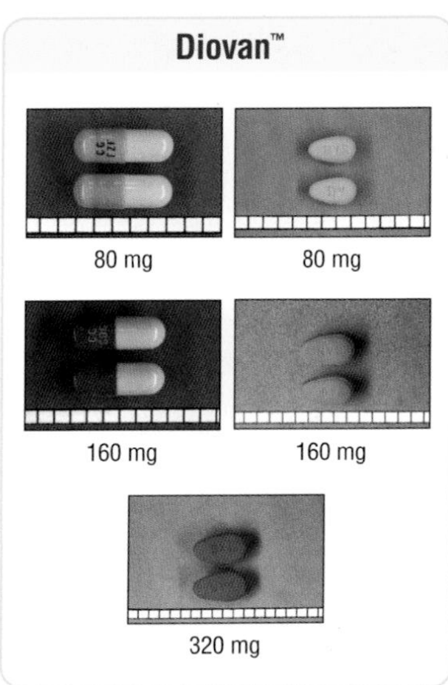

80 mg

80 mg

160 mg

160 mg

320 mg

Valsartan and Hydrochlorothiazide

Diovan HCT®

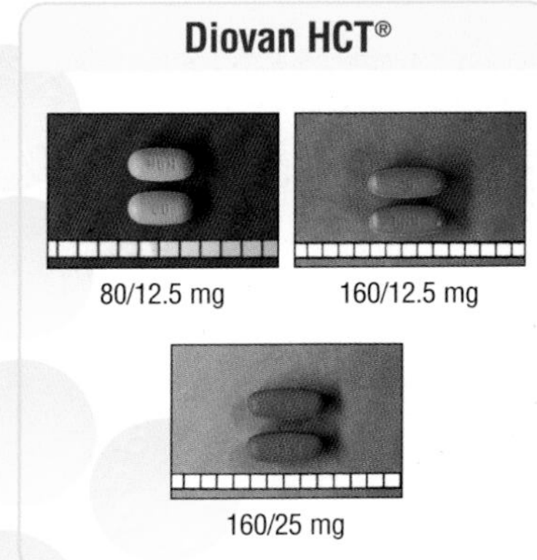

80/12.5 mg

160/12.5 mg

160/25 mg

Venlafaxine

Effexor XR®

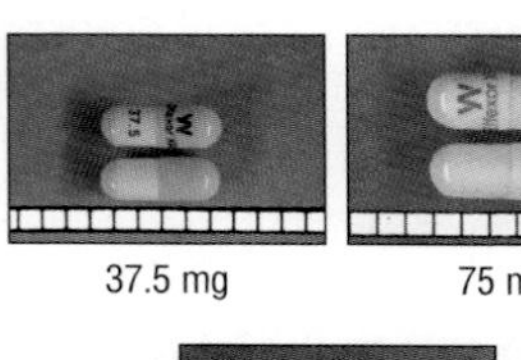

37.5 mg

75 mg

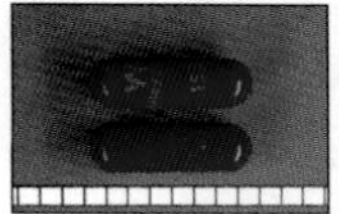

150 mg

Verapamil

(generic)

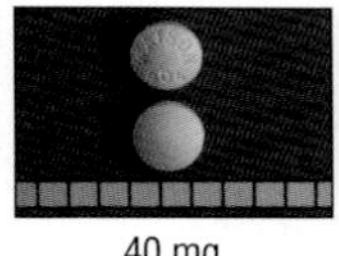

40 mg

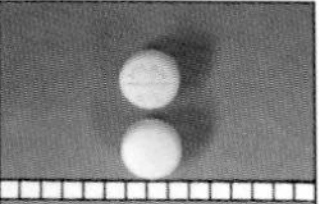

80 mg

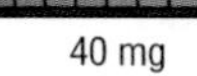

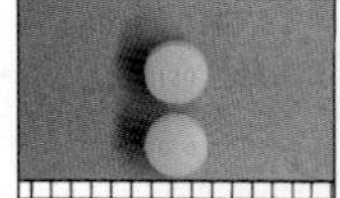

120 mg

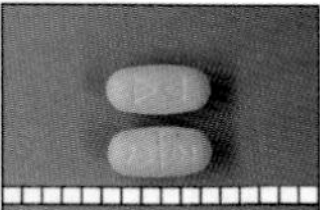

180 mg

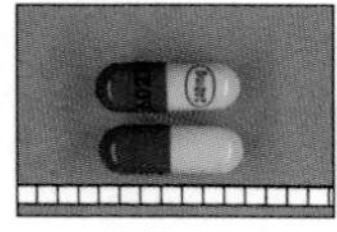

240 mg

Warfarin

(generic)

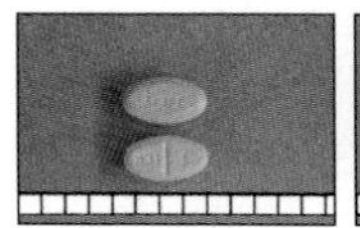

1 mg

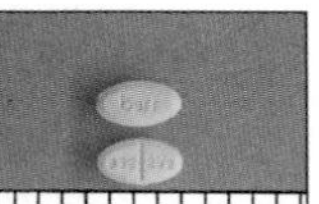

2.5 mg

3 mg

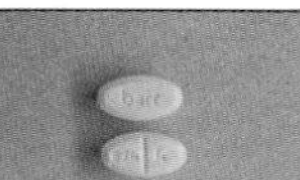

4 mg

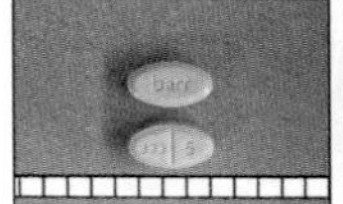

5 mg

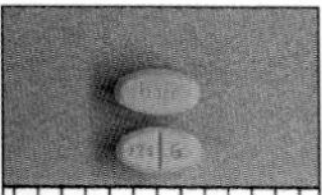

6 mg

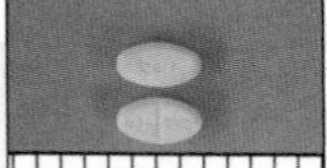

7.5 mg

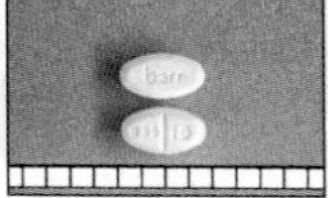

10 mg

Coumadin®

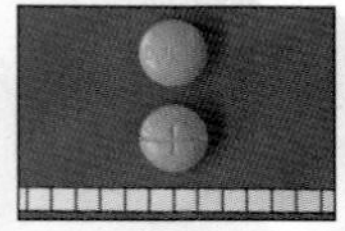

1 mg

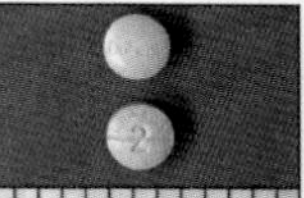

2 mg

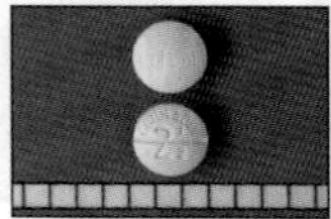

2.5 mg

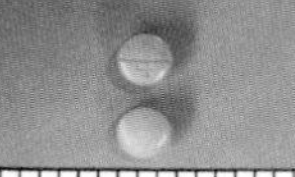

4 mg

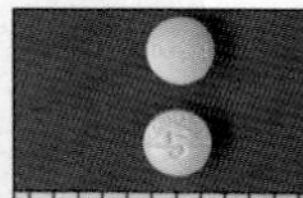

5 mg

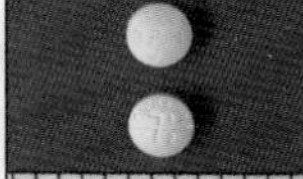

7.5 mg